ACSM's
Foundations of
Strength Training
and Conditioning

Second Edition

ACSM's Foundations of Strength Training and Conditioning

Second Edition

NICHOLAS RATAMESS JR, PHD, CSCS*D, FNSCA
Department of Health Exercise Science
The College of New Jersey
Ewing, New Jersey

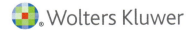

Philadelphia • Baltimore • New York • London
Buenos Aires • Hong Kong • Sydney • Tokyo

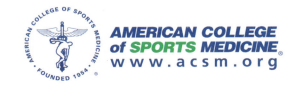

Acquisitions Editor: Lindsey Porambo
Development Editor: Amy Millholen
Editorial Coordinator: Lindsay Ries
Marketing Manager: Phyllis Hitner
Production Project Manager: Barton Dudlick
Design Coordinator: Stephen Druding
Manufacturing Coordinator: Margie Orzech
Prepress Vendor: SPi Global

ACSM Committee on Certification and Registry Boards Chair: Christie Ward-Ritacco, PhD, ACSM-EP, EIM2
ACSM Publications Committee Chair: Jeffrey Potteiger, PhD, FACSM
ACSM Certification-Related Content Advisory Committee Chair: Dierdra Bycura, EdD, ACSM-PT, ACSM-EP
ACSM Chief Operating Officer: Katie Feltman
ACSM Development Editor: Angie Chastain

Second Edition

Copyright © 2022 American College of Sports Medicine

1ˢᵗ edition Copyright © 2010 Wolters Kluwer Health/Lippincott Williams & Wilkins. All rights reserved. This book is protected by copyright. No part of this book may be reproduced or transmitted in any form or by any means, including as photocopies or scanned-in or other electronic copies, or utilized by any information storage and retrieval system without written permission from the copyright owner, except for brief quotations embodied in critical articles and reviews. Materials appearing in this book prepared by individuals as part of their official duties as U.S. government employees are not covered by the above-mentioned copyright. To request permission, please contact Wolters Kluwer at Two Commerce Square, 2001 Market Street, Philadelphia, PA 19103, via email at permissions@lww.com, or via our website at shop.lww.com (products and services).

9 8 7 6 5 4 3 2 1

Printed in China

Cataloging-in-Publication Data available on request from the Publisher

ISBN: 978-1-9751-1875-4

This work is provided "as is," and the publisher disclaims any and all warranties, express or implied, including any warranties as to accuracy, comprehensiveness, or currency of the content of this work.

This work is no substitute for individual patient assessment based upon healthcare professionals' examination of each patient and consideration of, among other things, age, weight, gender, current or prior medical conditions, medication history, laboratory data and other factors unique to the patient. The publisher does not provide medical advice or guidance and this work is merely a reference tool. Healthcare professionals, and not the publisher, are solely responsible for the use of this work including all medical judgments and for any resulting diagnosis and treatments.

Given continuous, rapid advances in medical science and health information, independent professional verification of medical diagnoses, indications, appropriate pharmaceutical selections and dosages, and treatment options should be made and healthcare professionals should consult a variety of sources. When prescribing medication, healthcare professionals are advised to consult the product information sheet (the manufacturer's package insert) accompanying each drug to verify, among other things, conditions of use, warnings and side effects and identify any changes in dosage schedule or contraindications, particularly if the medication to be administered is new, infrequently used or has a narrow therapeutic range. To the maximum extent permitted under applicable law, no responsibility is assumed by the publisher for any injury and/or damage to persons or property, as a matter of products liability, negligence law or otherwise, or from any reference to or use by any person of this work.

Disclaimer

Care has been taken to confirm the accuracy of the information present and to describe generally accepted practices. However, the authors, editors, and publisher are not responsible for errors or omissions or for any consequences from application of the information in this publication and make no warranty, expressed or implied, with respect to the currency, completeness, or accuracy of the contents of the publication. Application of this information in a particular situation remains the professional responsibility of the practitioner; the clinical treatments described and recommended may not be considered absolute and universal recommendations.

The authors, editors, and publisher have exerted every effort to ensure that drug selection and dosage set forth in this text are in accordance with the current recommendations and practice at the time of publication. However, in view of ongoing research, changes in government regulations, and the constant flow of information relating to drug therapy and drug reactions, the reader is urged to check the package insert for each drug for any change in indications and dosage and for added warnings and precautions. This is particularly important when the recommended agent is a new or infrequently employed drug.

Some drugs and medical devices presented in this publication have Food and Drug Administration (FDA) clearance for limited use in restricted research settings. It is the responsibility of the health care provider to ascertain the FDA status of each drug or device planned for use in their clinical practice.

shop.lww.com

This book is dedicated to my wife, Alison; my children, Jessica, Vinnie, and Nicole; and my parents, Nick and Veronica, for their love and support.

PREFACE

Optimizing sports performance through improved athleticism has long been a primary goal among athletes, coaches, and practitioners. Although athleticism is improved substantially by participating in sports via regular practice and competition, most recognize that maximizing athletic performance can only be attained by combining sport participation with an effective strength training and conditioning program. The field of strength training and conditioning has grown immensely over the past 30 years. As a result, the number of practitioners, educators, and students in strength and conditioning–related careers and academic programs has dramatically increased. Greater scientific study, practical recommendations, and dissemination of knowledge to practitioners are needed to meet the needs of a growing field. *ACSM's Foundations of Strength Training and Conditioning* provides a review of scientific and practical information and presents the information in a logical manner. It bridges the gap between scientific study and professional practice and is aimed at coaches, athletes, personal trainers, fitness instructors, and students preparing for a career in a strength training and conditioning–related field.

Organization

The primary objectives of *ACSM's Foundations of Strength Training and Conditioning* are to provide the most pertinent and up-to-date information regarding the training and testing of athletes and a foundation in basic physiology and kinesiology. The book is organized into four basic sections: (1) historical and strength and conditioning field–related foundations; (2) basic biomechanics, nutrition, and physiology; (3) flexibility, sprint, plyometric, balance, agility, aerobic, and resistance training program design and exercise prescription; and (4) testing and evaluation. Chapter 1 provides some historical and field-related information. It is important for strength and conditioning students and professionals to have a basic understanding of its history. Chapters 2 through 9 provide the reader with basic information in human biomechanics and physiology. New to this edition, Chapter 3 covers the basics of nutrition. A foundation in human movement and physiology is paramount for the strength and conditioning professional to understand proper movement and the acute responses and subsequent adaptations that affect human performance. Chapter 10 discusses key strength and conditioning principles that form the basic template of any training program prescribed to athletes. Chapters 11 through 17 provide up-to-date information for improving athletic performance. Training recommendations and several exercise prescription examples are provided to help guide the reader through the program design process. Chapter 18 discusses the importance of training periodization when designing long-term training programs for athletes. Chapter 19 provides current information regarding the testing and evaluation of human performance. In addition, norms are provided for key fitness components and test results.

Features

Various learning tools have been incorporated into each chapter to help facilitate learning and comprehension. **Interpreting Research** boxes draw attention to important research findings and explain their application to strength and conditioning practice. **Myths & Misconceptions** debunk common myths and clarify widespread misconceptions. **Case Studies** throughout the chapters present real-world scenarios. Using the skills and knowledge gained from the text, these case studies require the reader to evaluate the issues and devise effective solutions. **Sidebars** amplify important concepts presented within the chapters. Finally, **Review Questions** at the end of each chapter assess the reader's grasp of key concepts.

Additional Resources

ACSM's Foundations of Strength Training and Conditioning includes additional resources for both instructors and students that are available on the book's companion Web site at http://thepoint.lww.com/ratamess2e.

Instructors

- Image Bank
- PowerPoint Lecture Outlines
- Test Bank

Students

- Videos
- Online-only appendix of exercise variation images
- Animations

Nick Ratamess

USER'S GUIDE

ACSM's Foundations of Strength Training and Conditioning was created and developed to provide a review of scientific and practical information, bridging the gap between scientific study and professional practice. Written for coaches, athletes, personal trainers, fitness instructors, and students preparing for a career in a strength training and conditioning-related field, this text helps link greater scientific study, practical recommendations, and dissemination of knowledge to meet the needs of this growing field. Please take a few moments to look through this User's Guide, which will introduce you to the tools and features that will enhance your learning experience.

Chapter Objectives highlight the main points of the chapter and what important information readers should focus on as they move through the content presented.

OBJECTIVES

After completing this chapter, you will be able to:

- Demonstrate proper breathing during resistance exercise
- Describe the proper performance of several barbell, dumbbell, and machine resistance exercises for lower body, upper body, and core musculature
- Describe how exercises can be combined into a single exercise to increase complexity
- Describe methods of grip strength training
- Describe the proper performance of the Olympic lifts and their variations
- Describe the performance of exercises with different modalities including medicine balls, stability balls, BOSU balls, sand bags, kettlebells, ropes, and other implements

Sidebar: Strength and Conditioning Professional Proficiencies

Sidebars present brief topic points to highlight important material.

- Anatomy and physiology
- Kinesiology
- Sports endocrinology
- Bioenergetics and metabolism
- Neuromuscular physiology
- Connective tissue physiology
- Biomechanics and motor learning
- Cardiorespiratory physiology
- Environmental physiology
- Immune function
- Sport psychology
- Sports nutrition
- Supplements and ergogenic aids
- Overtraining and detraining
- Periodization
- Recovery
- Weight loss/body fat reduction
- CPR administration and first aid
- Special populations (children, older adults, clinical)
- Warm-ups/cooldowns
- Corrective exercise
- Weight training and Olympic lifting
- Plyometric training
- Aerobic endurance training
- Speed, agility, quickness, and mobility training
- Balance and functional training
- Power and ballistic training
- Strength training
- Bodyweight training
- Metabolic/high-intensity interval training
- Flexibility and myofascial release
- Muscle endurance and hypertrophy training
- Implement training
- Sport-specific demands and conditioning
- Advanced program design
- Exercise technique and spotting
- Performance/postural assessment
- Injury prevention
- Facility design and management
- Equipment use and maintenance
- Organization and administration
- Risk management and liability

Case Study 14.1

Steve is a recent college graduate with a degree in Health and Exercise Science and a concentration in Strength and Conditioning. He was hired by a Division III college and was put in charge of strength and conditioning for the school's football team. As part of his lifting program, Steve required all athletes to perform the power clean because of its utility for power and performance enhancement. However, several incoming freshmen have no experience with Olympic lifting. As a student (and athlete), Steve was properly instructed to teach the power clean in stages (using variations) rather than the complete lift. Thus, Steve grouped these athletes together and began instructional sessions to teach proper technique.

Question for Consideration: If you were Steve, what progressions would you use in order to teach this exercise to this group of athletes?

Case Studies throughout the chapters present real-world scenarios. Using the skills and knowledge gained from the text, these case studies require the reader to evaluate the issues and devise effective solutions.

Myths & Misconceptions
An Athlete Should Never Hold His or Her Breath When Lifting

Proper breathing is critical to RT. Breathing patterns may vary depending on the complexity and intensity of exercise. Under many circumstances, it is recommended that the athlete exhale during the more difficult part (the concentric [CON] or positive phase) and inhale during the easier segment (the eccentric [ECC] or negative phase) for several exercises. Breathing patterns for complex lifts may vary corresponding to the difficulty of the phase. However, there are exceptions to this general rule. During the lifting of heavy loads for exercises that require high levels of intra-abdominal pressure (IAP) and lumbar spine support (deadlift, squat, bent-over row, Olympic lifts), many athletes temporarily hold their breath during the most difficult part. During a heavy squat, an athlete may inhale during the decent, temporarily hold his or her breath at the bottom position and during the initial ascent (until the sticking region is surpassed), and then exhale during the upper segment of the ascent. Breath holding helps increase torso rigidity and enables better exercise performance. Valsalva maneuvers are unavoidable during intense resistance exercise (>80% of 1 RM) or when sets approach muscular failure (1). An incremental rise in IAP is seen as intensity and effort increase (1). The greater postural stability enables better strength and power performance from the individual. Valsalva maneuvers are avoided under many circumstances, but there are occasions where holding one's breath is advantageous.

Myths & Misconceptions boxes debunk popular myths and clarify widespread misconceptions about strength and conditioning.

Interpreting Research boxes draw attention to important research findings and explain their application to strength and conditioning practice.

Interpreting Research
Comparison of Various Balance Devices

Wahl MJ, Behm DG. Not all instability training devices enhance muscle activation in highly resistance-trained individuals. *J Strength Cond Res.* 2008;22:1360–1370.

A study by Wahl and Behm (67) examined muscle activation to standing and squatting on Dyna Discs, BOSU ball, wobble board, an SB, and the floor. The results showed:

- During standing, soleus muscle activity was highest on the wobble board compared to other modalities, and lower abdominal muscle activity was highest using the wobble board, and second on an SB.
- During standing, the SB increased rectus femoris muscle activity the most, the wobble board increased biceps femoris activity the highest, and the SB and wobble board increased erector spinae muscle activity the most.
- During squatting, soleus activity was highest on the wobble board, and lower abdominal activity was highest on the wobble board and SB.
- Dyna Discs and BOSU balls provided a minimal muscle stimulus in resistance-trained subjects.

The authors concluded that modalities that provided greater instability (SB and wobble board) were more effective for increasing muscle activation than those that provide mild instability (Dyna Discs, BOSU).

User's Guide ix

Exercises

Lower-Body Plyometric Exercises

Two-Foot Ankle Hop ("Pogo")
Intensity: Low

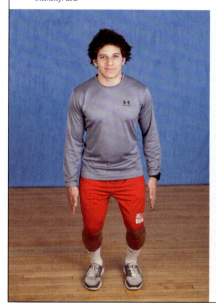
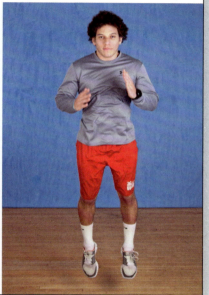

Exercise boxes provide step-by-step instruction for various exercises, along with photos of the proper positioning and movement. With these exercise boxes can be found **Caution! boxes**, which provide warning and reminders about important things to remember while doing the specific exercise. **Variations** of the exercise described are also provided.

At the end of each chapter, an extensive list of **Review Questions** provide students with a chance to apply what they've learned and assess their knowledge through multiple choice and true/false questions.

REVIEW QUESTIONS

1. The maximal amount of force one can generate during a specific movement pattern at a specified velocity of contraction is
   a. Muscle endurance
   b. Muscle power
   c. Muscle strength
   d. Body composition

2. A competitive sport where lifters place based on the amount of weight they lift in the snatch and clean and jerk is
   a. Bodybuilding
   b. Weightlifting
   c. Powerlifting

User's Guide

SUMMARY POINTS

- Strength training is an essential component to improving health and maximizing performance. Virtually all health- and skill-related components of fitness are enhanced when specifically targeted through proper program design.
- Scoring highly on various measures of physical fitness can separate athletes of different caliber.
- Examination of the history of S&C is important for the practitioner as it magnifies the accomplishments of many pioneering individuals in the field and perhaps may provide insight into future S&C trends.
- The key ingredient to RT responses and subsequent training adaptations is proper design of the training program.
- Competitive forms of RT include weightlifting, bodybuilding, powerlifting, strength competitions, and strength/fitness competitions, *e.g.*, CrossFit.
- Education in S&C is gained through scholarly study, personal experience, and professional practice.

Summary Points provide a checklist of the important concepts discussed in each chapter for a quick review.

High-quality, four-color illustrations and photos throughout the text help to draw attention to important concepts in a visually stimulating and intriguing manner. They help to clarify the text and are particularly helpful for visual learners.

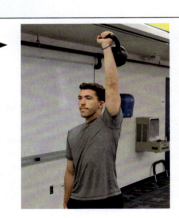

FIGURE 10.2 Overhead single kettlebell walk.

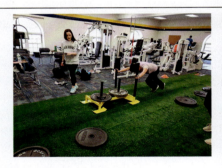

FIGURE 10.3 The sled push exercise.

Overweight/Underweight Implements
A common training tool among athletes is to perform sport-specific exercises against a resistance, *e.g.*, overweight implements. Overweight implements allow the athlete to overload

Student Resources

Inside the front cover of your textbook, you'll find your personal access code. Use it to log on to http://thePoint.lww.com/ratamess2e—the companion Web site for this textbook. On the Web site, you can access various supplemental materials available to help enhance and further your learning. These assets include an interactive quiz bank, animations, and videos. Adopting instructors have access to an image bank and test bank.

REVIEWERS

James R. Bagley, PhD
San Francisco State University
San Francisco, California

Lee E. Brown, EdD, FACSM, CSCS*D
California State University, Fullerton
Fullerton, California

Jared W. Coburn, PhD, FACSM, CSCS*D
California State University, Fullerton
Fullerton, California

Joshua A. Cotter, PhD, FACSM, EIM2, CSCS
California State University, Long Beach
Long Beach, California

Kurt A. Escobar, PhD
California State University, Long Beach
Long Beach, California

Steven J. Fleck, PhD, FACSM
FlecksRx LLC
Ridgway, Colorado

William J. Kraemer, PhD, FACSM
The Ohio State University
Columbus, Ohio

Jonathan Mike, PhD, CSCS
Grand Canyon University
Phoenix, Arizona

Michael T. Nelson, PhD, CSCS
Carrick Institute
Cape Canaveral, Florida

Stacey Privett, MS
Hampton University
Hampton, Virginia

Cory M. Scheadler, PhD, ACSM-CEP, CSCS
Northern Kentucky University
Highland Heights, Kentucky

Allison N. Schroeder, MD
Mayo Clinic Square
Minneapolis, Minnesota

Kevin Valenzuela, PhD, CSCS
California State University Long Beach
Long Beach, California

ACKNOWLEDGMENTS

I would like to thank the American College of Sports Medicine (ACSM) for giving me the opportunity and support to write this new edition of the book. Special thanks go out to the staff at Wolters Kluwer for their support and assistance with this book, especially Acquisitions Editor Lindsey Porambo, Editorial Coordinator Lindsay Ries, and Development Editor Amy Millholen for their project insight and direction. I would like to thank ACSM Development Editor Angie Chastain for all of her guidance and editorial assistance, and Mark Flanders and Chris Merillo for their outstanding work during the photo shoot. I want to thank my colleagues Drs. William Kraemer, Jay Hoffman, Avery Faigenbaum, Jie Kang, Jill Bush, and Tamara Rial Rebullido for their valuable feedback on the book. Lastly, I want to thank Jaclyn Levowsky, Christina Rzeszutko, Jaishon Scott, Nicholas Gambino, Dr. Ryan Ross, Dr. John Farrell, Cameron Richardson, Joseph Rosenberg, Kavan Latham, Brian Fardman, Stephanie Hohn, Cathy Phan, Rebecca Keller, Dr. Tamara Rial Rebullido, Terrence Wilkerson, Idalis Vasquez, Avery Epstein, Tyler Andriopoulos, Joanne Smith-Tavener, Emily Hirsch, Julia Melao, Maria Grill, Christian Mendez, Matthew Pollock, Connor Jarvie, Daniel Kilroy, Jeremy Whaley, Andrew Duff, Anthony Rua, Vincent Ratamess, Jessica Ratamess, Nicole Ratamess, Kayla Kolaritsch, and Eamonn O'Connell for their assistance in demonstrating several exercises portrayed in this book.

CONTENTS

Preface vi

User's Guide vii

Reviewers xi

Acknowledgments xii

PART ONE Foundations 1

1 Introduction to Strength Training and Conditioning 3

2 Biomechanics of Force Production and Performance 22

3 Basic Nutrition 47

PART TWO Physiological Responses and Adaptations 73

4 Neural Adaptations to Training 75

5 Muscular Adaptations to Training 96

6 Connective Tissue Adaptations to Training 126

7 Endocrine System Responses and Adaptations 145

8 Metabolic Responses and Adaptations to Training 178

9 Responses and Adaptations of the Cardiorespiratory System 210

10 Principles of Strength Training and Conditioning 237

PART THREE Strength Training and Conditioning Program Design 249

11 Warm-Up, Flexibility, and Myofascial Release 251

12 Resistance Training Program Design 287

13 Resistance Training Equipment and Safety 336

14 Resistance Training Exercises 367

15 Plyometric Training 447

16 Sprint and Agility Training 500

17 Aerobic Training 535

18 Training Periodization and Tapering 570

PART FOUR Assessment 591

19 Assessment and Evaluation 593

Index 647

PART I

Foundations

CHAPTER 1
Introduction to Strength Training and Conditioning

OBJECTIVES

After completing this chapter, you will be able to:

- Define basic strength and conditioning terms
- Understand a brief history of strength training and conditioning from its early origins to modern times
- Describe common goals associated with resistance training
- Describe the benefits of strength training and conditioning
- Describe health- and skill-related components of fitness
- Describe competitive forms of resistance training
- Discuss the strength and conditioning profession in terms of preparation, proficiencies, and duties/responsibilities

What is Strength Training and Conditioning?

Strength training and conditioning (S&C) is a term that has been adapted to include several modalities of exercise. **Strength training** (*e.g.*, the use of training to target increases in muscular strength) via **resistance training** (RT; *e.g.*, training using any form of resistance including bodyweight to enhance health- and skill-related fitness components) serves as the core, and other modalities of exercises are included depending on the needs of the athlete. For example, an S&C program for strength and power athletes would include RT but also plyometrics, speed/agility/mobility training, flexibility exercises, and aerobic training (in addition to the rigors of practice and competition). For an individual exercising for general fitness, RT would be included in addition to flexibility and cardiovascular training. Multiple modalities of training enhance several health- and skill-related components of muscular fitness. Thus, integration of multiple training modalities is critical to optimizing total conditioning.

The importance of a high-quality S&C program cannot be overemphasized. From an athletic standpoint, improving and establishing good motor skill technique is critical but can only take an athlete to a certain level of achievement. Often, it is the health- and skill-related components of fitness that separate athletic talent. Elite athletes possess greater strength, power, speed, and jumping ability compared to athletes of lesser rank (1). For example, an analysis of National Football League (NFL) drafted players versus undrafted players showed that the drafted players had better 40-yd dash times, vertical jump height, pro-agility shuttle times, and 3-cone drill times compared to undrafted players eligible for the draft (2). Garstecki et al. (3) compared Division I and Division II National Collegiate Athletic Association (NCAA) football players and showed that Division I athletes had greater one-repetition maximum (1 RM) bench press, squat, power clean, vertical jump height, fat-free mass, lower percent body, and faster 40-yd dash times than Division II athletes. Fleisig et al. (4) compared high school, collegiate, and professional baseball pitchers and showed that the professional pitchers had greater muscle strength, shoulder, and elbow throwing velocities compared to lesser-skilled pitchers. Thus, there is a relationship between an athlete's status and several components of physical conditioning.

Brief History of Strength Training and Conditioning

A brief examination of the history of S&C is important for any practitioner (5–8). Knowledge of prominent individuals, eras, events, and training practices is critical to understanding the field. In fact, some important training concepts currently popular are not new; rather, they were used in the past, fell out of popularity, and have resurfaced. One may state that study of the past may be important in preparation of future S&C trends. Nevertheless, it is certainly fascinating to examine this facet of our history.

Early Origins

Feats of muscular strength and evidence of some type of RT date back several thousands of years to ancient times. Ancient artwork depicted strength contests of various types. Weight-throwing contests were held and training for a strong military was desirable because warfare was common.

Perhaps more familiar were the accolades of the ancient Greeks circa sixth century B.C. The ancient Greeks were well known for their pursuit of excellence in physical education and sport. Although the city of Athens valued the aesthetic sides of physical education, Sparta's main objective was to have a strong, powerful army. Men and women were required to be in shape. Boys were sent to military school ~6–7 years of age and were trained rigorously in gymnastics, running, jumping, javelin and discus throwing, swimming, and hunting. Women were not required to leave home but were trained rigorously as well. In addition, sports were popular as the Olympic Games (consisting of events such as foot races, discus and javelin throwing, long jump [with weights], wrestling, boxing, pankration, equestrian, and pentathlon) initiated circa 776 B.C., and many individuals trained at gymnasiums to enhance physical performance. Perhaps the best-known Greek strongman was *Milo of Crotona*. Milo was a 5-time wrestling champion and a 22-time strength champion. He has been credited with the first use of progressive overload during RT. In addition, the ancient Greeks were well known for lifting heavy stones. In fact, one of the earliest bodybuilding events was thought to occur in Sparta. Spartan men were judged on their physiques and punished if found to be lacking adequate development. Strength training for military purposes was continued by the armies of the Roman Empire. After the fall of the Roman Empire, religious opposition to training predominated for the next 1,000 years and not much progress was made during this time.

Connections with Science and Medicine

Throughout early times, a relationship existed between the medical/scientific communities and fascination with muscular strength and development. The famous physician *Galen* (129–199 A.D.) was thought to be the first sports medicine specialist to recommend RT. He promoted the use of handheld weights as he worked extensively with gladiators at the time. Large strides from the scientific community in the development of strength training came during the Renaissance. It was suggested that the famous French writer *Michel de Montaigne* described the benefits of strength training with reference to his father. German educator *Joachim Camerarius* (circa 1544) wrote about weight training and how it could lead to improved health and performance.

Appreciation for the human body (and adaptations to RT) was gained by advances in human anatomy. The landmark text of *Andreas Vesalius* (1514–1564) *De Humani Corporis Fabrica* and several works of *Bernard Siegfried Albinus* (1697–1770) emphasizing the musculoskeletal system vastly increased the understanding of human anatomy and, to some degree, awareness of changes associated with physical exercise. A few publications in the 1700s began to discuss benefits of training with dumbbells, *e.g., Hieronymus Mercurialis' De Arte Gymnastica* and *The Spectator* by Joseph Addison. *Ben Franklin* was also a well-known proponent of dumbbell training during the late 1700s.

Nineteenth-Century Advances

The 1800s were a time in our history where S&C gained increased popularity. Strides in physical education were made. Nationalistic influences were seen where prominent physical educators (from Germany and Sweden) trained several students who brought their ideas and philosophies to the Unites States circa 1825. These philosophies were adopted and modified by several American educators. Some programs were rigorous and comprised mostly of gymnastics exercises, and others were modified and included other modalities such as manual resistance exercise, calisthenics, flexibility exercises, games/sports, and dance. Interestingly, the use of resistance equipment such as ropes, medicine balls (whose variations have been used since the times of the ancient Greeks), dumbbells, clubs, and other implements could be seen in the curricula. The first commercial gym was opened in New York by *William Wood* in 1835. A very influential individual at the time was *Dudley Sargent* (1849–1924), a Harvard-trained medical doctor (Fig. 1.1). He invented several

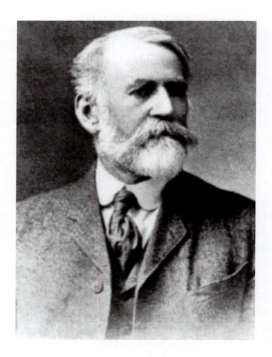

FIGURE 1.1 Dudley Sargent.

exercise machines and developed methods to assess muscular strength and performance (Sargent vertical jump test).

Perhaps one of the most early influential time periods during the mid-1800s to the early 1900s was known as the Era of the Strongmen. This was a time where great feats of strength performance led to the realization of the potential for improving strength and appearance. In Europe and North America, various individuals promoted their muscular strength for entertainment and commercial purposes. Interestingly, many of these strongmen brought to light extraordinary strength performances. However, some were responsible to some extent for some RT myths that perpetuated (5,8). Although a discussion of many of these strength legends is beyond the scope of this chapter, several pioneering strength athletes need to be recognized. *George Barker Windship*, a Harvard-trained medical doctor, toured North America performing feats of strength including what he termed the *Health Lift* (a partial range of motion [ROM] dead lift) and whose motto was "Strength is Health." Canadian strongman *Louis Cyr* (1863–1912) (Fig. 1.2) was a large (~300 lb) individual who possessed phenomenal strength including a 4,337-lb back lift and a famous horse pull demonstration. However, members of the anti-weight training community pointed to Cyr stating that weight training could lead to excessive bulk, slowness, and make an individual "muscle bound." *Louis Uni* (1862–1928), The Great Apollon, was a French circus strongman who performed amazing feats of strength (one-arm snatch with 80–90 kg, juggling with 20-kg weights) and was known to train with what today would be akin to thick bars. *Ludwig Durlacher* (1844–1924), also known as Professor Attila, was a German strongman with incredible core strength who had claimed to invent, adapt, or modify several pieces of training

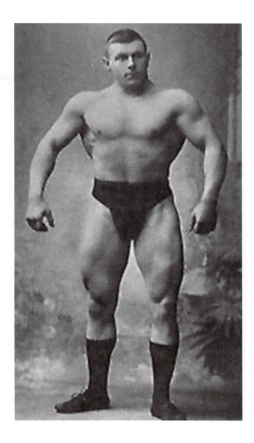

FIGURE 1.3 George Hackenschmidt.

equipment including the Roman Chair. Perhaps his greatest attribute was his ability to train other strongmen. *George Hackenschmidt* (1877–1968), also known as The Russian Lion (Fig. 1.3), was a wrestling champion and strongman who later laid claim to inventing the Hack Squat. *Henry "Milo" Steinborn* (1894–1989) was a renowned wrestler and strongman who set the prototype for the modern-day Olympic-style barbell with revolving ends. *Sigmund Klein* (1902–1987), a strongman from Germany who immigrated to the United States, was known for amazing strength, an excellent physique, and for writing articles on weight training. *Thomas Inch* (1881–1963), known as "Britain's Strongest Youth," was most renowned for being the only man at that time capable of lifting a 3+-in. thick grip, 173-lb dumbbell overhead from the ground with one arm, which today is commonly known as the Thomas Inch Replica Dumbbell and is used by several strength competitors in training. Lastly, *Eugen Sandow* (1867–1925) (Fig. 1.4) was a German strongman who moved to England and performed incredible feats of strength. However, he was renowned for his fabulous physique and is immortalized on the trophy awarded to the winner of the Mr. Olympia bodybuilding contest each year.

Twentieth-Century Advances

The early to mid-1900s were times marked by change. Myths and misconceptions associated with RT began to escalate,

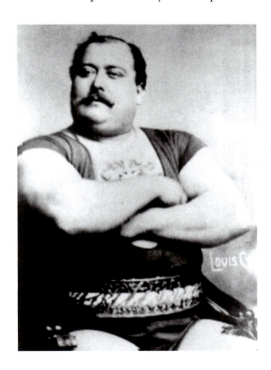

FIGURE 1.2 Louis Cyr.

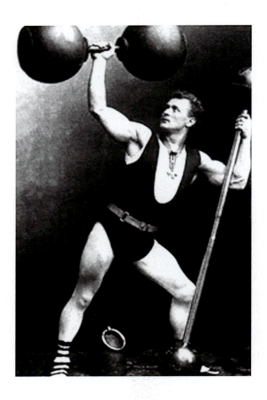

FIGURE 1.4 Eugen Sandow.

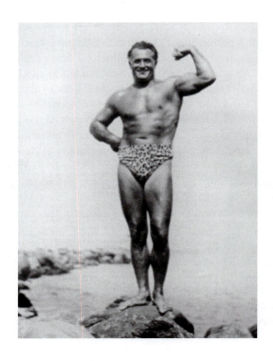

FIGURE 1.5 Charles Atlas.

and despite the fact that strongmen were touring, a number of individuals known for their strength accomplishments became market driven. Although they had all attained their strength and size through weight training methods, they began to market other forms of RT equipment as alternatives that claimed to increase strength without becoming muscle bound. Although many individuals contributed to alternative forms of RT (cable devices, isometrics, etc.), the most popular was Angelo Siciliano. *Angelo Siciliano* (1892–1972), better known as Charles Atlas (Fig. 1.5), became known as the "world's most perfectly developed man who began as a 97-lb weakling."

His landmark advertisements were well known where if one followed his course then he or she could transcend into a strong, well-developed individual.

His training philosophy was known as *Dynamic Tension* and consisted of 12 lessons of resistance exercises (bodyweight, isometrics) that could be performed anywhere for 15 minutes a day. Several million people have read his material to this day and/or incorporated some facet of his training advice, evidence of his marketing genius in the 1920s.

It was around this time when some early weight training magazines, books, and courses were published predominantly by well-known strongmen or lifting practitioners as well as the establishment of the Milo Barbell Company in Philadelphia, PA

Myths & Misconceptions
Resistance Training Will Make One "Muscle Bound," Slower, and Reduce Performance

Throughout the history of S&C, several myths and misconceptions developed and several remain in existence today despite scientific evidence pointing to the contrary. It remains a mystery why certain myths continue to perpetuate; however, it is clear that the S&C professionals need to do their best to dispel these myths whenever possible. One myth is the creation of the muscle-bound individual via RT. This muscle-bound phenomenon is thought to reduce movement mobility, speed, and performance. This myth dates back more than 100 years to the Strongman Era. The reality is that RT enhances virtually all components of fitness and increases athletic performance (9–13). An exception exists in that if one always trains with slow velocities and gains a large amount of mass, it is theoretically possible to become slower. However, specificity of RT tells us that moderate-to-fast lifting velocities can increase speed and performance. The majority of strength/power athletes currently resistance train and few have shown signs of slowing down. Thus, proper program design is critical to increasing speed and performance, and RT will enhance performance when performed properly.

in 1902. In 1899, the first issue of the landmark magazine *Physical Culture* (which was a common term to describe the promotion of muscular growth, strength, and health through exercise at the turn of the century) was published by Bernarr McFadden. Around this time, another magazine called *Health and Strength* was published by Hopton Hadley (an English cycling enthusiast). In 1914, a magazine called *Strength* was published by Alan Calvert (which later became the popular *Strength and Health* magazine published by Bob Hoffman in the 1930s). The longtime running magazine *Iron Man* began circulation in 1936 by Peary and Mabel Rader. Several popular weight training books/courses were published at the time including *Sandow's System of Physical Training* (1894) and *Strength and How to Obtain It* (1897) by Eugen Sandow; *The Way to Live in Health and Physical Fitness* (1908) by George Hackenschmidt; *Milo Barbell Courses* (1902) by Alan Calvert; *The Development of Muscle Power* (1906) and *The Textbook of Weight-Lifting* (1910) by Arthur Saxon; *Muscle Building* (1924) and *Secrets of Strength* (1925) by Earle Liederman; *Muscle Building and Physical Culture* (1927) by George Jowett; *Physical Training Simplified—The Complete Science of Muscular Development* (1930) by Mark Berry; and *The Rader Master Bodybuilding and Weight Gaining System* (1946) by Peary Rader. Therefore, RT literature became popular during this time and continued to rise in popularity until present day.

Competitive Lifting Sports

Competitive lifting sports began in the late 1800s with Olympic weightlifting rising to the forefront. The first USA weightlifting contest was held in 1861 in Chicago, the first weightlifting championship was held in 1891, and weightlifting first entered the Olympic Games in 1896. At first, the lifts contested were the one- and two-hand overhead lifts, with no weight classes. Weightlifting returned to the Olympic Games in 1904 after a brief hiatus. By 1920, the snatch, clean and press, and clean and jerk were the competitive lifts; eventually the clean and press was discontinued in 1972 due to difficulty in judging the lift. The sport of Olympic weightlifting (or just weightlifting) was largely popularized in the United States by legendary strength pioneer Bob Hoffman (Fig. 1.6). *Bob Hoffman* (1898–1985) was known as the "Father of American Weightlifting." He formed the world famous York Lifting Club (as Hoffman had purchased Milo Barbell Co. in 1932 and formed the York Barbell Company). Hoffman's accolades were enormous as he published magazines, wrote several books, manufactured nutrition supplements, and helped make the United States a weightlifting powerhouse through the mid-1950s. Although weightlifting was his passion, Hoffman showed some interest in other lifting sports and was instrumental in encouraging athletes to incorporate weight training in their conditioning programs. After the 1950s, other countries such as the Soviet Union, Turkey, Greece, and China emerged in the sport of weightlifting. Some notable legendary weightlifters during this period include Tommy Kono, Vasily Alexeev, Imre Foldi, Norbert Schemansky, Ken Patera, Naim Suleymanoglu ("Pocket Hercules"; Fig. 1.7), Paul Anderson, and Andrei Chermerkin to name a few.

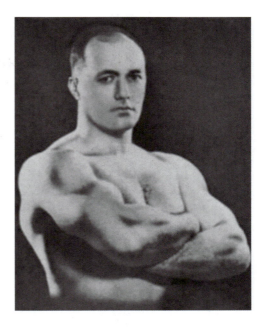

FIGURE 1.6 Bob Hoffman.

The next major lifting sport to develop from weightlifting was bodybuilding. Although interest in physique training was seen throughout history, bodybuilding competition, as we know it, can be traced back to the early 1900s. The first organized competition dates back to Britain in 1901 and was facilitated by Eugen Sandow. In 1903, the first bodybuilding ("Physical Culture") competition was held in Madison Square Garden, NY. However, bodybuilding did not stand alone in competition. That is, athletes who competed in bodybuilding had to compete in weightlifting first. Bodybuilding grew in popularity during the 1930s and 1940s as some notable athletes brought some recognition by successfully competing in Mr. America

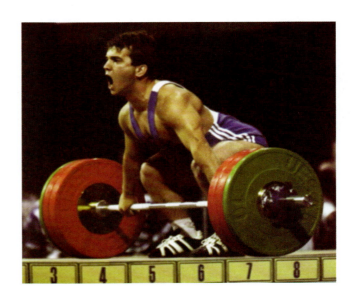

FIGURE 1.7 Naim Suleymanoglu.

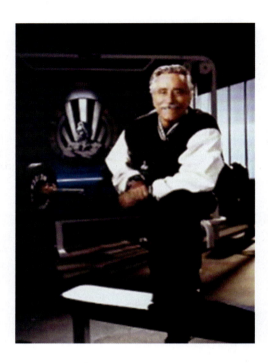

FIGURE 1.8 Joe Weider.

competitions, *e.g.*, John Grimek, Clancy Ross, Steve Reeves, etc. However, the 1940s marked a historical time period due to a large extent of the work of Joe and Ben Weider. The Weiders sought more respect for bodybuilders and subsequently formed the International Federation of Body Builders (to rival the Amateur Athletic Union, which dominated lifting sports). Joe Weider's (Fig. 1.8) status in bodybuilding was truly legendary and is a major reason why bodybuilding is so popular in the United States today. His accolades were enormous. He was well known for his feud with Bob Hoffman, books and publications (*Your Physique*, *Muscle Power*, later *Muscle and Fitness* and *Flex*), coining of training terms and principles, promotion of bodybuilding training and events (the Mr. and Ms. Olympia), and equipment and nutrition supplement manufacturing. Although *Muscle Beach*, Santa Monica, CA, was a popular sport, recreational, and bodybuilding venue from 1934 to 1958, the mecca for bodybuilding later became Venice Beach, CA. Many notable and prominent bodybuilders were seen from the 1950s on but some very influential individuals included Joe Gold, Jack LaLanne, Reg Park, Bill Pearl, Larry Scott, Sergio Oliva, Frank Zane, Arnold Schwarzenegger, Lou Ferrigno, Franco Colombu, Lee Haney, Rachel McLish, Cori Everson, Dorian Yates, Lenda Murray, Ronnie Coleman, Jay Cutler, and Phil Heath.

Powerlifting evolved during the late 1950s. It was initially referred to as the *odd lift* competition because it did not include the Olympic lifts but was composed of the squat, bench press, and deadlift exercises. Although critics of powerlifting claimed that it lacked image, the sport began to increase in popularity during the early 1960s. During its first ~15 years, more than 68 powerlifting records were set. The first US championships were held in 1964 in York, PA, the first world championships were held in 1971, the first US women's championship was held in 1978, and the first women's world championship was contested in 1980. In 1972, the International Powerlifting Federation was formed (with Bob Crist president and Bob Hoffman treasurer) and thereafter other organizations were formed. In the 1980s, the major magazine *Powerlifting USA* began publication and powerlifters became noted for using specialized apparel that substantially enhanced lifting performance, *e.g.*, bench press shirts, squat suits and briefs, and so on. Through the years, the United States has dominated international powerlifting competitions. Some notable powerlifters include Larry Pacifico, Vince Anello, Don Reinhoudt, Ed Coan, Lamar Gant, Dr. Fred Hatfield, Drs. Janice and Terry Todd, Louie Simmons, Anthony Clark, Ted Arcidi, Tamara Grimwood-Rainwater, Scot Mendelson, Ryan Kennelly, Laura Phelps-Sweatt, Becca Swanson, and Tiny Meeker.

The evolution of modern-day strength competitions (*i.e.*, consisting of ~6–8 events) began in 1977 with the World's Strongest Man competition held in Universal Studios in California. This annual competition is very popular and since then many other strength competitions have evolved. Strength competitions initially began with athletes of different backgrounds. For example, Olympic weightlifters, bodybuilders, NFL football players, arm wrestling champions, powerlifters, and professional wrestlers competed among each other. In modern-day competitions, hybrid athletes training specifically for each event dominate the sport. Some notable competitors include Bruce Wilhelm, Bill Kazmaier, Jon Pall Sigmarsson, Magnus ver Magnusson, Jouko Ahola, Zydrunas Savickas, Magnus Samuelsson, Jill Mills, Svend Karlsen, Brian Shaw, Mariusz Pudzianowski, Eddie Hall, and Hafthor Julius Bjornsson. Strength competitions have made their mark on the strength and conditioning community as events and training practices of strength athletes have increased in popularity to where other groups of athletes have integrated these training methods.

The CrossFit games began in 2007, which marked a time where RT was integrated with fitness competition. Although CrossFit training increased in popularity circa 2000, the sport of CrossFit was established in 2007. CrossFit involves an integrated approach to high-intensity interval training targeting all health- and skill-related fitness components. Training and competition consist of contested events that involve Olympic weightlifting, weight training, various strength implements, gymnastics, calisthenics and bodyweight exercises, plyometrics, speed and agility, climbing, loading/carry, and obstacle challenges, and aerobic events. Some notable competitors include James Fitzgerald, Jolie Gentry Macias, Rich Froning Jr., Annie Thorisdottir, Katrin Tanja Davidsdottir, and Mathew Fraser. Likewise, CrossFit training has transcended beyond the sport and its practices have been adopted by other groups of athletes, fitness professionals, and tactical strength and conditioning practitioners.

Weight training for other sports conceptually was not widely accepted initially because of myths and misconceptions associated with RT. Among the first sports to accept RT was track and field throwing in the 1950s. One prominent supporter of RT was four-time Olympic discus gold medal winner, *Al Oerter*. In the early 1930s, Bob Hoffman began promoting weight training for athletes and later encouraged some boxers to train, but very few other athletes followed. American football players helped pave the way in the 1960s and 1970s when the first full-time strength coaches were hired in the late 1960s. In the 1970s, mostly strength and power athletes began RT. A key development in the field was the formation of the National Strength and Conditioning Association (NSCA) in 1978 that began widespread recommendations of RT and was instrumental in dispelling myths and demonstrating benefits both practically and scientifically. From the 1980s on, most athletes and coaches have recommended RT to some extent for all sports.

Strength and Conditioning Today

Currently, RT is a modality of exercise recommended for virtually everyone in some capacity because it has been shown to enhance health, well-being, and performance in clinical, fitness, and athletic populations (11–13). There has been a large increase in the scientific study of RT since the mid-1970s [please see Kraemer et al. (6) for historic review]. Thus, we have seen a dramatic change not only in the perception of RT but also in the total magnitude of individuals who actively participate in RT. Contributing to the increased popularity of RT has been its adoption into general exercise programming by major health organizations including the American College of Sports Medicine (ACSM). The ACSM first recommended RT in 1990 (9). In the 1998, ACSM position stand (10) entitled "The recommended quantity and quality of exercise for developing and maintaining cardiorespiratory and muscular fitness, and flexibility in healthy adults," the initial standard was set for a RT program with the performance of one set (or multiple sets depending on time) of 8–12 repetitions for 8–10 exercises, including one exercise for all major muscle groups, and 10–15 repetitions for older and more frail persons for 2–3 days per week (10). This initial program has been shown to be effective in previously untrained individuals for improving muscular fitness during the first 3–4 months of training. However, it did not address the need for progression or recommendations for different training goals. In 2002 (11) and again in 2009 (12), the ACSM revised the document to include recommendations for progression for novice, intermediate, and advanced trainees with different training goals, *e.g.*, muscle strength, power, hypertrophy, endurance, and motor performance. The 2002 document was well received and the body of scientific literature did support much of practitioner training advice given throughout the years. The 2009 document was updated to expand the recommendations but also was evidence based meaning that every recommendation was given a rating based on the level research supporting it or if it was more practitioner based due to a lack of research. Thus, RT has come a long way to where it is now a scientifically proven and overwhelmingly recommended form of exercise for healthy adults.

Today, S&C has grown tremendously. Nearly all athletes follow an S&C program off-season, preseason, and in-season. Because of the overwhelming evidence demonstrating the importance of S&C for optimal performance, the S&C coach position has increased greatly among all levels of competition from middle and high school to the professional levels. Although not all schools or programs have a true S&C coach on staff, most will at least have an assistant coach in charge of supervising S&C sessions. The increased popularity of S&C has given students an exceptional opportunity to major in an S&C-related field in college and enter a promising career where they have the opportunity to work with athletes of varying background.

Tactical Strength Training and Conditioning

Tactical S&C refers to the training of tactical athletes such as military personnel, special weapons and tactics (SWAT), special operations forces, law enforcement officers, firefighters, and rescue first responders (Fig. 1.9). Tactical S&C programs prepare the individual for prescreening fitness testing, basic training and occupational instruction periods, and for maintaining and improving fitness while on the job. Tactical S&C programs target improvements in muscle strength and power, aerobic and anaerobic endurance, and mobility. Fundamental skills such as sprinting and running, striking, swimming, rolling, climbing, crawling, kneeling, squatting and lunging, pushing/pulling, jumping, landing, vaulting, throwing, carrying, and hand-to-hand combat are emphasized to improve tactical performance in military and law enforcement personnel. Firefighters perform tasks such as carrying heavy equipment, raising ladders, pulling, hoisting, and climbing stairs with hoses, dragging victims, forcible entry with a sledge hammer or axe, ceiling breach and pull maneuver with a pole, and searching for victims which can be specifically trained within a tactical S&C program (14). Comprehensive training for tactical athletes includes the integration of RT with plyometric, speed, agility, flexibility, and aerobic training with specific occupational training. The precise balance is essential to optimize performance and reduce the risk of overtraining and injury.

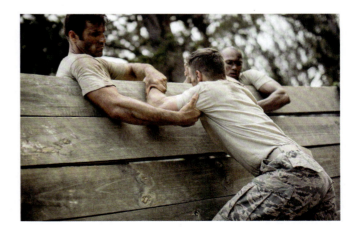

FIGURE 1.9 A soldier in training. (Image from Shutterstock.)

Why Do Individuals Resistance Train?

The goals and benefits of RT are numerous, and individuals train for different reasons (11–13). The Sidebar (Goals Associated with Resistance Training) and Table 1.1 outline basic goals and benefits of RT. Many engage in RT for recreational purposes where the goals are to moderately increase size, endurance, and strength but not to a great extent. Others engage in RT to maximize their muscular strength, power, endurance, or size. Some engage in RT for rehabilitation. Rehabilitation implies an injury or disease occurred, which posed some physical limitation and now the individual trains to strengthen the weakened area. Many individuals engage in RT for prehabilitation, where the primary goal is injury prevention. Competitive strength, power, and endurance athletes engage in RT to enhance athletic performance, and some strength and power athletes compete in lifting sports where maximal performance, or a one repetition-maximum (1 RM) of each exercise determines competitive placing. In season, athletes engage in maintenance training. The goal of maintenance training is to maintain off-season training gains and adaptations as best as possible in season as the emphasis shifts to sport-specific conditioning, practice, and competitions/games. This phase is temporary until the season is completed. However, nonathletes may engage in maintenance training as well depending on their circumstances. Many engage in RT to elicit positive health adaptations to the body, e.g., connective tissue, muscle, nerve, respiratory, and cardiovascular systems and for occupational purposes, e.g., tactical S&C. Lastly, one does not need to train specifically for one goal; rather, many resistance train with multiple goals in mind. This is referred to as integrative training where multiple goals are sought for training purposes.

Benefits of Resistance Training

Health and performance benefits of RT are shown in Table 1.1 (13). Several studies have shown RT to improve multiple facets of health and performance. Collectively, these studies have been conducted in athletes, general fitness, clinical, tactical, or special populations, and children have shown RT is safe and effective for most individuals. These ramifications are critical to optimal athletic performance and to any individual striving to enhance performance of activities of daily living.

Fitness Components

Health-Related Fitness Components

Strength and conditioning programs target multiple levels of fitness. Fitness components may be classified in two

Table 1.1	Benefits of Resistance Training
Health Benefits	**Performance Benefits**
↓ risk factors for disease	↑ muscle power
↓ percent body fat	↑ balance and coordination
↑ dynamic, isometric, and isokinetic muscle strength	↑ speed and agility
↑ muscle hypertrophy	↑ capacity to perform activities of daily living
↑ muscular endurance	↑ vertical jump ability
↑ basal metabolic rate	↑ throwing velocity
↓ blood pressure	↑ kicking performance
↓ blood lipids, LDL cholesterol	↑ exercise economy and time trial performance
↓ resting heart rate	↑ baseball bat swinging velocity
↓ cardiovascular demand to exercise	↑ tennis serve velocity
↑ bone mineral density	↑ wrestling performance
↑ glucose tolerance and insulin sensitivity	↑ cycling and swimming power and performance
↓ age-related muscle atrophy (sarcopenia)	
↓ risk of colon cancer and osteoporosis	
↑ $\dot{V}O_{2max}$	
↑ flexibility	
↓ risk/symptoms of low back pain	

| | Chapter 1 Introduction to Strength Training and Conditioning | **11** |

Sidebar | Goals Associated with Resistance Training

- General fitness and recreation
- Strength training
- Power training
- Muscular endurance training
- Muscle hypertrophy
- Body fat reduction
- Rehabilitation and prehabilitation

- Competitive lifting sports (bodybuilding, strength athletics, powerlifting, weightlifting, CrossFit)
- Athletics
- Occupational and tactical S&C
- Maintenance training
- Physiological adaptations
- Integration training

---

ways: health-related and skill-related fitness components (15). Health-related fitness components are those that are designated as improving health, wellness, and one's quality of life. Improvements in these components can enhance physical performance. Health-related components include muscular strength, muscular endurance, cardiovascular endurance, flexibility, and body composition.

Muscular Strength

Muscular strength may be defined as the maximal amount of force one can generate during a specific movement pattern at a specified velocity of contraction (16). For a dynamic muscle action, it may be assessed in the weight room via a 1 RM lift for a given exercise; *i.e.*, the maximal amount of weight lifted in one all-out effort. In other cases, it may be estimated from submaximal strength performance. This ultimate magnitude of force development may be defined as *absolute muscular strength* as it represents the limit of physical capacity of an individual for a specific exercise. When maximal strength is expressed relative to body mass or lean body mass (the mass of nonfat tissue, *e.g.*, muscle, bone, water, etc.), it is defined as *relative muscular strength*. Relative muscular strength is critical for many athletes who compete in weight classes because the higher the ratio, the more advantageous it is for that athlete.

A high strength-to-mass ratio enables high levels of force production without the addition of substantial mass gains where strength gains exceed increases in body mass. Relative strength measures have been used to compare lifting performances among athletes of different sizes. For example, when weight classes are not used or when the best lifter in a competition among all weight classes is determined, the weight lifted may be divided by the individual's body mass (or lean body mass) to yield a ratio, which can be used comparatively (known as *body mass scaling*). However, simply performing this calculation as is tends to strongly favor athletes of smaller mass. For example, a 165-lb lifter who bench pressed 285 lb would generate a factor value of ~1.73 (285/165). Another lifter weighing 245 lb would have to bench press at least 425 lb in order to beat the 165-lb lifter in direct competition. Attempts have been made to correct for this, *e.g.*, by raising the mass to the two-thirds power using *allometric scaling* or by using height

as a scaling factor, but still certain somatotypes (or types of physiques) may gain advantage. Allometric scaling is theoretically based on the two-thirds law where geometric similarity is sought (17). Geometric similarity suggests that strength measures (two-dimensional) and mass (three-dimensional) conform to the relationship: strength $\times$ (mass$^{2/3}$)$^{-1}$ (17). Although allometric scaling may be more practical than body mass scaling, it still has deficiencies favoring middle-sized athletes (17).

In lifting competitions, the Wilks and Sinclair formulas have been used. The *Wilks formula* (developed by Robert Wilks) used mostly in powerlifting is complex, but typically a conversion table (for men and women) is used based on body mass to obtain a conversion factor, *i.e.*, multiplied by the weight lifted to correct for size differences. For example, an athlete with a body mass of 80.5 kg would generate a factor of 0.68 and an athlete with a body mass of 124 kg would generate a factor of 0.57. If the first athlete lifted 200 kg (0.68 $\times$ 200 kg = 136 kg) in competition and the second athlete lifted 230 kg (0.57 $\times$ 230 kg = 131 kg), the first athlete would place higher. The *Sinclair formula* (18) is a polynomial equation where the coefficients are updated every 4 years (to account for world record totals in each weight class) and primarily used in international weightlifting competitions. The following coefficients will be used through 2020. If the athlete's body mass is ≥ 175.51 kg (men) or 153.56 kg (women), then the Sinclair coefficient = 1. For all other athletes, the Sinclair coefficient is calculated via the following equation: Sinclair coefficient = 10^{AX^2} where $X = \log_{10}(x \cdot b^{-1})$ as x = athlete's body mass and $b = 175.51$ kg (men) or 153.56 kg (women), $A = 0.751945030$ (men) or 0.783497476 (women). The coefficient is then multiplied by the athlete's weightlifting total to calculate the Sinclair total. For example, a male athlete with a body mass of 62 kg would generate a Sinclair coefficient of ~1.43. If his total was 300 kg, then his Sinclair total = 429 kg (300 kg $\times$ 1.43).

Muscular strength is certainly multidimensional and depends on several factors discussed later in this book, *e.g.*, muscle action (concentric, eccentric, isometric), contraction velocity, muscle group and length, joint angle, and other physiological and biomechanical factors concerning the muscular, nervous, metabolic, endocrine, and skeletal systems. The ability to develop muscular strength is critical to health and performance especially as one grows older.

Case Study 1.1

A high strength-to-mass ratio is beneficial for athletes.

Questions for Consideration: What types of athletes benefit the most from having a high strength-to-mass ratio? Why might this be the case?

Muscular Endurance

Muscular endurance is the ability to sustain performance and resist fatigue. The intensity (or difficulty of exercise) of muscle activity plays a role. *Submaximal muscular endurance* is characterized by the ability to sustain low-intensity muscular activity for an extended period of time. *High-intensity (or strength) endurance* is the ability to maintain high-intensity muscular activity over time. For example, it entails the ability to run repeated sprints with similar times or perform a specific number of repetitions for a resistance exercise over a number of sets despite a rest interval in between sets. Another common term used is *local muscular endurance*. Local muscular endurance is defined by the ability to sustain exercise; however, the term *local* specifically refers to the muscle groups involved in that exercise. Overall, increasing muscular endurance is important for good posture, health, and injury prevention and aids in optimizing sports performance (13).

Cardiovascular Endurance

Cardiovascular endurance is the ability to perform prolonged aerobic exercise at moderate to high exercise intensities. Cardiovascular endurance is highly related to functioning of the lungs, heart, and circulatory system and the capacity of skeletal muscle to extract oxygen and thereby sustain performance. The key measure of cardiovascular endurance or aerobic capacity is maximal oxygen uptake or $\dot{V}O_{2\,max}$. A moderately high to high $\dot{V}O_{2\,max}$ is a critical component for success in endurance athletes, and possessing a good aerobic base can enhance recovery from anaerobic exercise as well. Cardiovascular endurance is essential to good health and reducing risk factors for disease, as well as improving self-image, cognitive functioning, and stress management.

Flexibility

Flexibility is the ability of a joint to move freely through its ROM. Enhanced joint flexibility can reduce risk for certain types of injury, improve muscle balance and function, increase performance, improve mobility and posture, and reduce the incidence of low back pain (13). The best ways to increase flexibility are to perform exercises in a full ROM and engage in a proper stretching program, preferably at the end of an aerobic/anaerobic workout when the muscles are thoroughly warmed up or as a part of a flexibility/mobility/corrective exercise workout.

Body Composition

Body composition refers to the proportion of fat and fat-free mass throughout the body. Fat-free mass (or lean body mass) consists of bone, muscle, water, and other nonfat tissues. Healthy body composition involves minimizing the fat component while maintaining or increasing the lean body mass component. An individual with an excessive amount of body fat may be considered obese and may be at greater risk for disease and other debilitating conditions. The most effective way to enhance body composition is to eat properly and exercise regularly. Strength training, as well as other forms of anaerobic training, is effective for enhancing body composition as it increases lean body mass (muscle and bone components) while reducing fat. A common term used to describe tissue growth is hypertrophy, especially with respect to muscle growth where the term *muscle hypertrophy* is commonly used. Aerobic training plays a large role in reducing fat mass and a lesser role in enhancing lean tissue mass. Body composition plays a key role in those sports where weight classes are used (wrestling, weightlifting), where athletes have to overcome their own body mass for success (high jump, gymnastics, endurance sports), or where athletic competition is based on physique development (bodybuilding).

Skill-Related Components of Fitness

Skill-related components of fitness include power, speed, agility, balance and coordination, and reaction time. These components are essential to athletic performance and the ability to perform activities of daily living. Skill-related components may be developed in a variety of ways including RT, sprint/interval training, agility training and plyometrics, and through sport-specific practice.

Power

Power is the rate of performing work. Because power is the product of force and velocity, there is a strength component to power development (strength at low-to-high velocities of contraction). The optimal expression of muscle power is reliant upon correct exercise technique. Although at times the terms *power* and *strength* are used interchangeably, this is not correct. Power has a time component; thus, if two athletes have similar maximal strength, the one who expresses strength at a higher rate (higher velocity or shorter period of time) will have a distinct advantage during performance of anaerobic sports. In addition, power has been described in terms of strength. For example, terms such as *speed strength* and *acceleration strength* have been used to define force development across a spectrum of velocities. *Starting strength* is a term used to describe power production during the initial segment of movement. *Rate of force development* (a term used primarily in scientific publications) describes the time needed to reach a threshold level of force or the amount of force produced per second. The velocity component of the power equation indicates that high contraction velocities (or at least the intent to contract at maximal velocities even against a heavy resistance) of muscle contraction are imperative. Therefore, power development is multidimensional, involving enhancement of both force and velocity components. Muscle power may be enhanced via RT, speed, agility, and plyometric training, and through sport-specific practice/conditioning.

Speed

Speed is the capacity of an individual to perform a motor skill as rapidly as possible. Speed is an integral component of sport. For example, linear running speed may be defined by its three distinct phases: (a) acceleration, (b) maximum speed, and (c) deceleration. The *acceleration* phase is characterized by an increase in speed and is reliant upon strength, power, and reaction time. The *maximum speed* phase is characterized by the individual's attainment of his or her fastest speed and how long he or she can maintain it, *e.g.*, speed endurance. The *deceleration* phase is a result of fatigue and is characterized by the individual involuntarily decreasing speed after maximum speed has been attained. Speed may be enhanced by a combination of methods including nonassisted and assisted sprint training, strength and power training, plyometrics, technique training, and sport-specific practice.

Agility

Agility is the ability of an individual to change direction rapidly without a significant loss of speed, balance, or bodily control. Being agile requires a great deal of power, strength, balance, coordination, quickness, speed, anticipation, and neuromuscular control. Agility is a critical component to any sport that requires rapid changes of direction, decelerations, and accelerations. Agility training is comprised of predetermined drills (*closed drills*) and drills that force the athlete to anticipate, adjust, and react explosively (*open drills*). Likewise, agility can be enhanced by plyometrics, multidirectional agility and reactive drills, strength and power training, balance training, and sport-specific practice.

Balance and Coordination

Balance is the ability of an individual to maintain equilibrium. It requires control over the athlete's center of gravity and allows him or her to maintain proper body position during complex motor skill performance. Balance can be enhanced by strength and power training, plyometrics, flexibility, sprint and agility training, specific balance training (with unstable equipment, unilateral exercises, exercises with small base supports, and combination exercises), and through sport-specific practice.

Gross motor coordination refers to the ability of an individual to perform a motor skill with good technique, rhythm, and accuracy. Critical elements to coordination include balance, spatial awareness, timing, and motor learning. Likewise, coordination can be improved by similar training methods. Sport-specific practice is very important as repetitive exposure to different motor patterns is essential to improving motor coordination.

Reaction Time

Reaction time is the ability to respond rapidly to a stimulus. Reaction time is critical to sports performance. The quicker an athlete reacts to a stimulus, the more likely success will be obtained. Some athletic skills require less than half-second response times, *i.e.*, hitting a 90+-mph fastball in baseball. The ability to react quickly is paramount and can be used to separate athletes of different caliber. Reaction time may be improved by explosive exercise (power, sprint, agility, quickness training) and sport-specific practice.

Keys to Success: The Training Program

The key ingredient to training responses and subsequent adaptations is the program (11,12). A training program is a composite of several variables that may be manipulated in different ways to achieve a desired effect. Although specific recommendations and guidelines for program design will be discussed in subsequent chapters, it is important to define these variables with other terminology. These variables include

- Muscle Action: refers to the type of muscular contraction. An *eccentric* (ECC) muscle action involves muscle lengthening and is sometimes described as a negative component of each repetition. ECC muscle actions produce higher levels of force, are very conducive to muscle growth, and make an athlete more susceptible to muscle damage and soreness. A *concentric* (CON) muscle action involves muscle shortening and is sometimes described as a positive component of each repetition. An *isometric* (ISOM) muscle action involves force development with no noticeable change in joint angle or muscle length. In comparison, greatest muscle force is produced during ECC muscle actions, followed by ISOM and CON actions. CON and ECC muscle actions are considered to be *dynamic* muscle actions because force production throughout the ROM is variable. However, some authors prefer to use the term *isotonic*. Isotonic implies that equal tension is produced throughout the ROM. Although the weight lifted is constant throughout the ROM, the amount of force (or torque) developed is not. Therefore, *dynamic muscle action* (sometimes called dynamic constant external resistance) is a more appropriate and accurate term. The term isoinertial has been used because it assumes the mass lifted is constant.
- Repetition: a complete movement cycle including an ECC and CON muscle action, *e.g.*, lifting the weight up and down during RT. May also refer to a single ISOM contraction.

- Set: a specified group or number of repetitions, *i.e.*, three sets of 10 repetitions.
- Volume: the total amount of work performed during a workout. Represented by the total duration, length covered, or number of sets of exercise. During RT, *volume load* represents the number of sets × the number of repetitions × the resistance used.
- Intensity: describes the magnitude of loading (or weight lifted) during resistance exercise, *e.g.*, 90% of 1 RM is high intensity. Some have defined intensity as representing the magnitude of difficulty associated with training. The latter is more representative of *perceived exertion*, and thus the most widely accepted definition of intensity relates to loading.
- Frequency: a term used to describe the number of training sessions per week or day. It also has been used to describe the number of times per week a muscle, muscle group, or specific exercise is performed.
- Exercise Selection: the exercises selected or chosen to be performed during a workout or throughout a training program.
- Exercise Order: the sequence in which exercises are performed.
- Rest Periods or Intervals: the amount of rest taken between sets and exercises. This term may also be used to define the amount of rest taken in between reps within a set.
- Repetition Velocity: the velocity at which reps are performed.

Competitive Forms of Resistance Training

Many individuals engage in RT for competitive purposes. RT competitions have been popular since the late 1800s. Currently, there are numerous local, state, national, and international competitions, as well as federations, in which an athlete can participate. The competitive RT sports include bodybuilding, weightlifting, powerlifting, strength (Strongman, Strongwoman) competitions, and CrossFit. As one might expect, the level of dedication, motivation, and training is much higher as one embarks on a competitive career.

Bodybuilding

Bodybuilding is a competitive sport in which athletes compete on stage in a physique contest where they are judged subjectively by a panel of judges who assign points based on their aesthetic appearance. Although weights are not lifted during a bodybuilding competition, RT is an essential component of training for bodybuilding competition. Following a precompetition training period accompanied by strict dieting, bodybuilders will attempt to maximize muscle size and minimize

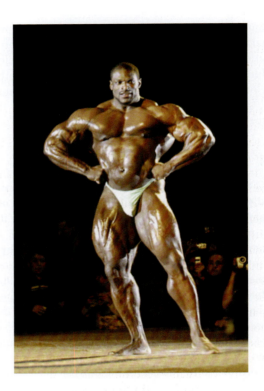

FIGURE 1.10 A bodybuilder.

body fat and dehydrate to maximize their appearance. Critical to bodybuilding is the presentation of the physique. Following a period of performing compulsory poses (most muscular, front double biceps, lat spread, etc.), or prejudging, bodybuilders pose on stage to music in a choreographed posing routine. They are judged on presentation as well as their physiques. Bodybuilding training is aimed at maximizing muscular hypertrophy, symmetry, shape, and definition while maintaining low levels of body fat. Muscular strength may be a goal but is secondary to hypertrophy. Several bodybuilders (Fig. 1.10) use RT to enhance muscle size; thus, strength gains may be considered a by-product and not the primary goal. However, some bodybuilders include strength training to enhance their muscle growth. This has been helpful for those bodybuilders in attaining large amounts of muscle hypertrophy due to heavier loading required for strength training. Bodybuilding workouts typically consist of multiple exercises per muscle group for moderate to heavy loads for rep ranges from few to many with little rest between sets. These workouts are aimed at maximizing muscular development in all facets, hence a wide spectrum of intensity, volume, exercises, and techniques are used. Off-season training focuses on improving size and strength, whereas precompetition is devoted to size maintenance while reducing body fat, weight, and water. Several individuals include bodybuilding training for competition purposes; however, others use it to enhance appearance, performance, and health in a noncompetitive manner.

Weightlifting

Weightlifting (Fig. 1.11) was actually the first true competitive lifting sport to develop historically (19). It is the only lifting sport, *i.e.*, included in the Olympics. Unlike bodybuilding, weightlifting is a performance sport where athletes place based on how much weight they lift relative to their weight class (there are seven weight classes for women and eight for men). The sport of weightlifting involves two competitive lifts, the *snatch* and *clean and jerk* (although others have been used throughout its >150-yr history). The snatch, clean and jerk, and their variations (referred to as the *Olympic lifts*) are the most technically demanding and complex resistance exercises in existence. Thus, good coaching is mandatory. Weightlifters normally begin competitive training at an early age. Hence, the initial phases of training are dedicated to learning proper form and technique, whereas subsequent years are dedicated to improving lift performance, strength, and power. Performance of these competition lifts requires total body coordination, power, and speed. Therefore, weightlifters are extremely well-conditioned athletes. Heavyweight records for the snatch and clean and jerk are ~484 and 581 lbs, respectively, in men and ~341 and 425 lb in women. Because the Olympic lifts require a high degree of balance, coordination, strength, power, and speed, these exercises form the foundation of RT for anaerobic strength and power athletes. Much of the training programs of weightlifters will be developed around these two lifts and will include variations of these (hang clean, drop snatch), basic strength exercises (squat, deadlift), and assistance exercises (lunge, Romanian deadlift). Weightlifting programs normally consist of high load, low reps with long rest periods between sets. The quality of each repetition is critical as explosive lifting speeds are used. As with strength/power programs, periodized training cycles to peak performance for each competition are used. USA Weightlifting, a very prominent weightlifting organization and governing body of Olympic weightlifting in the United States, offers various coaching certifications as well as the E-magazine *USA Weightlifting*.

Powerlifting

Powerlifting (Fig. 1.12) is a competitive lifting sport involving maximal performance of three competition lifts: *squat*, *bench press*, and *deadlift*. In addition, other types of competitions have evolved based on inclusion of only a few of these lifts (bench press competitions), or in some cases other exercises have been included (strict barbell curl). Placing is based on maximum lifting performance over three trials for each exercise. Judges play a critical role to standardize a technique, *e.g.*, assure parallel position attained in squat, sufficient pause length used in the bench press, rhythmic ascent of the bar during the deadlift (no "hitching"), and will either allow or discard the trial. Like weightlifters, powerlifters compete in weight classes; thus, a high strength-to-mass ratio is desirable, especially for light to middle weights. Male super heavyweight records for the bench press and deadlift now exceed 1,000 lb and the squat >1,200 lb. The record for female powerlifters for the bench press is ~600 lb; records exceed 680 lb in the deadlift and 850 lb in the squat. Powerlifting performance has been greatly enhanced by the use of specialized equipment such as bench press shirts, squat suits, erector shirts, and wraps; thus, lifting records in supportive apparel may exceed "raw" records (those without specialized apparel) by more than 200–300 lb. Multiple federations exist and each has slightly different rules regarding gear. The major publication that covers an array of subjects from competitions to training and nutrition advice was *Powerlifting USA* (from 1977 to 2012 in print). Powerlifting training encompasses focusing on the structural lifts plus additional assistance exercises for low to moderate repetition number with gradual periodized increase in intensity as the competition approaches.

Strength Competitions

Modern-day strength competitions consist of six to eight events in which an athlete will score a specific amount of points based on how the athlete performs (or what place the athlete attains) (20). After all events have been completed, the leading scorer will win the competition. The events epitomize maximal dynamic and ISOM strength, grip strength and

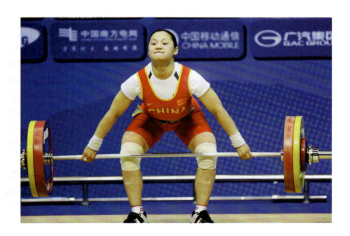

FIGURE 1.11 A weightlifter.

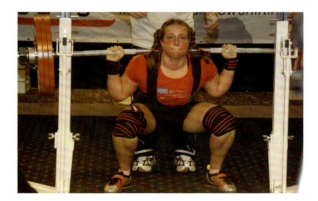

FIGURE 1.12 A powerlifter.

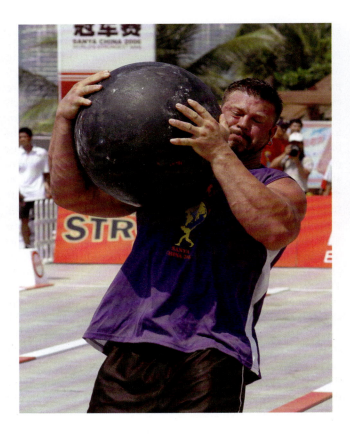

FIGURE 1.13 A strength competitor.

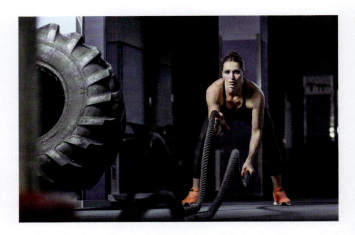

FIGURE 1.14 A strength/fitness competitor. (Image from Shutterstock.)

endurance, power, strength endurance, and perhaps a high degree of pain tolerance and determination (Fig. 1.13). Events commonly contested include the farmer's walk (180–375 lb per arm), tire flipping (450–900 lb), various loading (220–360 lb objects) medleys, barrel loading, various deadlifts (*e.g.*, silver dollar, car), car walk (~800 lb), duck walk (400 lb), log press (185–305 lb) or other overhead lifting, crucifix (isometric holding), Hercules hold, stone circle or Conan wheel, keg toss, truck/plane pulling, stone lifting (Atlas/McGlashen stones, 220–365 lb or more) and carries (*e.g.*, Husafell stone ~385 lb), incline press for reps, various squatting or backlifts, yoke walk (~904 lb), caber toss, carry and drag (anchor, weights), Fingal fingers, bar bending, power stairs (with 400–600 lb objects), Thomas Inch dumbbell lift, refrigerator carry, and tug-of-war. Training for strength competitions is very rigorous and multidimensional as multiple components of fitness need to be maximized to perform well across all of the events. Various federations have been formed over the years, with the *World's Strongest Man or Woman* still the epitome of international strength athletics competition.

Strength/Fitness Competitions

Strength/fitness competitions, *e.g.*, CrossFit, National Pro Grid League, involve an integrated approach consisting of contested events that involve Olympic weightlifting, weight training, various strength implements, gymnastics, calisthenics and bodyweight exercises, plyometrics, speed and agility, climbing, loading/carry, and obstacle challenges, and aerobic events (Fig. 1.14). Competitions are multiple-day consisting of up to 15 events. Events are named and may consist of single or multiple exercises performed maximally based on time, weight lifted, and rep or round totals, Some contested exercises include handstand walks, push-ups, glute-ham sit-ups, pull-ups, rope climbing, overhead squats, power cleans, snatches, rowing, swimming, running, cycling, 1 RM lifts, burpees, thrusters, sled pushing, sprints/hurdles/agility drills, hammering, wall ball, push jerks, carries, kettle bell swings, squats, pistol squats, deadlift, shoulder presses, box jumps, farmer's walk, muscle-ups, and tire flips. Individual and team competitions are contested. These competitions are very rigorous and competitors need to be very well-rounded fitness-wise with muscle strength, power, speed, mobility/agility, and muscle and cardiovascular endurance.

Competitive Lifting Modes and Performance

When comparing the different competitive lifting modes, a high degree of training specificity is observed especially in the classic lifting modes. Best power clean and snatch performances are observed in Olympic weightlifters. Weightlifters produce very high power outputs during Olympic lifting (21). This is a major reason why weightlifting exercises are included in training programs of strength/power athletes. Upon examination of maximal 1 RM strength during the multiple-joint competitive lifts of the squat, bench press, and deadlift, powerlifters and strength competitors hold the majority of records. Many strength competitors evolve from a powerlifting background. Olympic weightlifters also score very well on the squat and deadlift. McBride et al. (22) showed similar maximal squat performance among Olympic weightlifters and powerlifters of similar size. However, weightlifters produced more force, velocity, power, and greater heights during the vertical jump and jump squat assessments, thereby showing superiority of weightlifting training for enhancing jumping performance. Powerlifting performance is enhanced to a substantial degree by training accessories (suits, belts, wraps, shirts) many Olympic weightlifters do not use or use to a lesser extent. "Raw" performance of these lifts may be similar when athletes are matched for size. Many times weightlifters do not emphasize the bench press for fear it may limit shoulder ROM for the snatch and power clean. Thus, powerlifters and some bodybuilders may score better on this exercise. Some bodybuilders who also prioritize strength training ("power bodybuilders") score well on these three lifts, better than those bodybuilders who view strength gains as merely a by-product of bodybuilding training. Interestingly, an early study from Sale and MacDougall (23) showed that powerlifters and bodybuilders possessed similar maximal isokinetic strength for most single-joint exercises tested. Bodybuilders may score well on other single-joint exercises as some powerlifters either do not routinely perform them or do not emphasize them. Because of their training principles, bodybuilders tend to score very well on strength-endurance type of events or display a much lower fatigue rate than powerlifters during various lifting tasks with short rest intervals (24).

Strength and strength/fitness competition training may have the highest degree of diversity of fitness component enhancement given the integrated nature of these training modes. Athletes in these sports often train using a hybrid approach, or combining several modalities to maximize muscle strength, power, mobility, and cardiovascular and local muscular endurance. CrossFit training has been shown to increase aerobic capacity, lean body mass, and reduce percent body fat (25). CrossFit training prepares the body for the rigors of the different types of workouts (26). Bellar et al. (26) reported that one's aerobic capacity and anaerobic power (determined by a Wingate test) were associated with success in a CrossFit workout involving performance of as many reps as possible in 12 minutes of medicine ball throws, kettle bell swings, and burpee pullups. Strength competitors often use a multimodal approach. Winwood et al. (27) eloquently characterized strongman competitor training and found 100% reported using traditional resistance exercises (*e.g.*, squat and deadlift), 80% reported using a periodized approach, 74% reported targeting muscle hypertrophy, 97% reported using maximal strength training, 90% reported using power training methods (including 88% reporting using Olympic lifts, 20% reported using ballistic RT, and 54% reported using lower-body plyometrics), 90% reported using aerobic and anaerobic conditioning methods, and more than 80% reported routinely targeting strength events such as using tire flips, log clean and press, stone lifting, and farmer's walk implements in training. Thus, these hybrid approaches can be successful at improving several fitness components and serve as an attractive alternative training method for athletes from a variety of sports.

The Strength and Conditioning Profession

The S&C professional position has evolved to be one of the most critical coaching positions. The fundamental responsibility of the S&C professional is to design, implement, and supervise sports conditioning programs. Strength and conditioning professionals may work in various settings including middle or high schools, colleges or universities, professional sports teams, health and fitness facilities, and sports complexes and can run or assist with S&C camps, workshops, and clinics. In addition, personal trainers have filled a role in the S&C field as many upper-level and elite athletes have hired personal trainers for one-on-one specialized training. The roles and responsibilities of the S&C coach have increased over the years owing to the importance of improving conditioning to optimize performance and reduce the risk of injury. Thus, complete preparation is paramount for a student planning on becoming a competent professional in the S&C field. Critical concepts such as education, proficiencies required for the field, the importance of holding professional memberships and certifications, and knowledge gained through practical experience are discussed next. In addition, the duties and responsibilities of the S&C coach are outlined.

Education and Proficiencies

Education in the S&C field is gained via three major ways: (a) scholarly study, (b) personal experience, and (c) professional practice. *Scholarly study* entails content knowledge gained through taking college courses; reading scholarly books, journals, and articles; personal research; self-study; viewing videos; and attending conferences, workshops, and seminars (which are also excellent avenues for networking within the field). The S&C professional should at least have a B.S. or B.A. degree in an exercise-related field, *e.g.*, Exercise Physiology or Science, Kinesiology, Physical Education, Athletic Training, and Health and Human Performance. Some colleges and universities offer a major in S&C. Students take several courses in Biology, Physiology, Chemistry, Health, Mathematics and Statistics, Nutrition, and Exercise Science and Training/Testing that are vital in acquiring the underlying knowledge needed in the field. Most S&C jobs require at least a B.S. or B.A. degree. Some higher-level jobs may require a master's degree in an exercise-related field. A master's degree offers more in-depth knowledge in human physiology, greater specialization in coursework, *e.g.*, Biomechanics, Exercise Science, and other fields, and introduces students to research (for those students who had limited undergraduate research experiences). Another advantage of graduate training is that the student may serve as a graduate assistant or volunteer in the S&C program. This can lead to full-time employment at that facility or is valuable experience for obtaining a position elsewhere upon graduation. Some S&C positions can be difficult to attain, so serving as an assistant (or intern and volunteer) initially can be an excellent means of gaining entry into the field, especially if the student works with an established S&C coach. A competent S&C professional should have an extensive library of scholarly material, which is constantly updated with new texts and articles to keep abreast of current information. Doctoral training is not usually necessary unless an academic position is sought.

Personal experience is the education gained by playing sports, training, and observations of other athletes and coaches training/instructing. The S&C coach should have an extensive background in exercise (RT, speed and agility, plyometric, flexibility, and aerobic training). One must "practice what they preach" in the S&C field. It is very difficult to instruct athletes on proper technique if one has limited or no experience with the exercise or drill. Thus, competent S&C professionals exercise regularly and should have an extensive background performing all of the modalities they will be instructing.

Professional practice refers to the knowledge gained once the individual attains the position and is working in the S&C field. Education gained in the field is unique and in many instances is not directly learned from taking courses or reading textbooks. For example, this is the knowledge gained through interacting with athletes, staff, coaches, parents, and administrators, hands-on experience in training and testing, and the experiences of supervising or working in a facility (equipment maintenance, accidents, facility issues, staff issues, organization and planning, etc.). Professional practice experience (along with success) is critical and may be viewed by many as the key component to resume development.

Proficiency is defined as advancement in knowledge, skill, or expertise in a particular area of interest. Strength and conditioning professionals must be proficient in several areas. That is, they must have at least a rudimentary knowledge base in pertinent areas of S&C. The Sidebar (Strength and Conditioning Professional Proficiencies) depicts several proficiencies desired by a competent S&C professional.

In addition, S&C professionals must possess other skills that transcend directly into successful coaching or training. For example, the S&C professional should have excellent organizational and time management skills to handle the rigors of training a large number of athletes at various times of day, keeping training logs of all athletes, designing workout schedules around athletic competitions and practices, and perhaps supervising a staff of employees, graduate assistants, and interns. He or she should have the ability to motivate athletes to train hard and correctly follow procedures. The S&C coach should have good interpersonal, communication, and teaching skills that are mandatory for quality instruction. In addition, the S&C coach should always be well prepared, cautious, and hands-on when instructing. Because the S&C coach works within a team of professionals catering to athletes, *e.g.*, athletic trainers, physical therapists, nutritionists,

Sidebar	Strength and Conditioning Professional Proficiencies
Anatomy and physiology	Weight training and Olympic lifting
Kinesiology	Plyometric training
Sports endocrinology	Aerobic endurance training
Bioenergetics and metabolism	Speed, agility, quickness, and mobility training
Neuromuscular physiology	Balance and functional training
Connective tissue physiology	Power and ballistic training
Biomechanics and motor learning	Strength training
Cardiorespiratory physiology	Bodyweight training
Environmental physiology	Metabolic/high-intensity interval training
Immune function	Flexibility and myofascial release
Sport psychology	Muscle endurance and hypertrophy training
Sports nutrition	Implement training
Supplements and ergogenic aids	Sport-specific demands and conditioning
Overtraining and detraining	Advanced program design
Periodization	Exercise technique and spotting
Recovery	Performance/postural assessment
Weight loss/body fat reduction	Injury prevention
CPR administration and first aid	Facility design and management
Special populations (children, older adults, clinical)	Equipment use and maintenance
Warm-ups/cooldowns	Organization and administration
Corrective exercise	Risk management and liability

doctors, head and assistant coaches, etc., he or she must constantly communicate with staff on the athlete's health and performance status. Leadership is a critical component as the S&C coach must set the example for athletes to follow. Lastly, the S&C coach should be dedicated and willing to work long hours.

Memberships and Certifications

Holding memberships in professional organizations is an important component of professionalism. Membership has many benefits, including access to educational resources, dissemination of current knowledge, networking, career resources and job advertisements, conferences and seminars, certification information, scholarships and grants, merchandise, and in some cases liability insurance. There are several organizations that serve the S&C profession in numerous ways. Many of these serve the Exercise Science or related fields (Athletic Training, Physical Therapy, Sports Medicine, Nutrition, and Personal Training) in general. However, some of the most popular and influential organizations targeting the S&C profession include the ACSM, NSCA, Collegiate Strength and Conditioning Coaches Association (CSCCa), National Academy of Sports Medicine (NASM), USA Weightlifting, and the International Sport Sciences Association (ISSA).

Unlike some other professional occupations, *e.g.*, physical therapy, S&C does not require licensure. However, obtaining credible certifications increases the education and marketability of the S&C professional. Strength and conditioning professionals either obtain a specific S&C certification or become certified in a related field, *e.g.*, personal trainer, health and fitness instructor, and/or exercise specialist. The ACSM offers several clinical and specialty certifications. Some common certifications for the S&C professional may be the ACSM Certified Personal Trainer (ACSM-CPT), ACSM Certified Exercise Physiologist (ACSM-EP), and ACSM Certified Group Exercise Instructor (ACSM-GEI). The NSCA offers the Certified Strength and Conditioning Specialist (CSCS), Tactical Strength and Conditioning Facilitator (TSAC-F), Certified Personal Trainer (NSCA-CPT), and the Certified Special Population Specialist (CSPS). The CSCS certification is most popular and widely regarded as the "gold standard" of S&C certifications. It requires at least an undergraduate degree (or a college senior in good standing) and current CPR certification. USA Weightlifting offers the Sports Performance Coach Certification, which is excellent for coaching the Olympic lifts and variations. They also offer the Advanced Sports Performance certification plus a few advanced coaching certifications. CSCCa offers the Strength and Conditioning Coach

Sidebar — Potential Duties of a Strength and Conditioning Professional

- Design and implement all S&C training programs: this includes developing yearly training plans—programs designed to increase strength, power, endurance, aerobic capacity, flexibility, balance and coordination, speed, agility, hypertrophy, and reduce body fat
- Supervise athletes during training hours: the coaches office/desk should be in clear view of the entire facility
- Monitor athlete's technique and correct errors
- Assist in spotting athletes during RT when necessary
- Supervise and schedule all performance testing
- Ensure all safety procedures are being used
- Oversee purchase and maintenance of equipment and possibly design of a facility
- Budget allocation
- Facility uptake (cleaning), inspection, and maintenance
- Data collection: storage and examination of all training logs, evaluations, equipment manuals, and health history documents
- When applicable, travel with sport teams and supervise pregame warm-ups
- Instruct and educate athletes on injury prevention, proper nutrition, recovery practices, and use of supplements and banned substances
- Design and enforce facility rules and regulations and have them posted in plain view of athletes
- Staff training, development, and creation of job listings/criteria for new staff hires

- Delegate duties to other staff including assistant coaches, graduate assistants, interns, and volunteers
- Risk management and minimize potential litigation
- Oversee staff meetings and develop staff working schedules
- Control the training environment including music type and volume
- Design athlete's training schedules: organize different groups of athletes into scheduled time slots
- Motivate athletes to train maximally
- Prepare training sheets and other documents to be used in the facility including sign-in sheets, health history forms, and rules and regulations
- Post or distribute educational information that can benefit athletes and perhaps post a motivational "leader board" depicting athlete's weight room accomplishments
- Communicate with other coaches, athletic trainers, physical therapists, doctors, nutritionists, and staff regarding the status of athletes
- Maintain certification CEUs and keep abreast with the latest research and information
- Develop and post emergency procedures and place them (along with pertinent phone numbers and locations) in plain view
- Ensure staff has CPR and first aid certification
- Attend professional conferences and meetings

Certified (SCCC) plus an advanced certification. NASM offers the Performance Enhancement Specialization (NASM-PES), Certified Personal Trainer (NASM-CPT), and the Corrective Exercise Specialization (NASM-CES). Other organizations offer certifications as well. Once certified, practitioners must maintain certification by generating continuing education units (CEUs). Each certification and organization is specific regarding the number of CEUs needed in a given time span. CEUs can be attained in various ways, but self-study, attending conferences, publishing articles, awards and achievements, experience, and taking courses are just a few ways to earn CEUs. These ensure that the S&C professional is continuing to educate herself or himself and keep current with up-to-date information. It is recommended that S&C professionals obtain at least one major certification upon entering the field.

Duties, Roles, and Responsibilities

The S&C professional will have numerous duties and responsibilities depending on if the individual is the S&C director or head strength coach, an assistant S&C coach, or facility staff employee (28). The Sidebar (Potential Duties of a Strength and Conditioning Professional) depicts several potential duties and responsibilities of the S&C professional. As defined by the NSCA, "certified strength and conditioning specialists are professionals who practically apply foundational knowledge to assess, motivate, educate, and train athletes for the primary goal of improving sport performance. They conduct sport-specific testing sessions, design and implement safe and effective S&C programs, and provide guidance for athletes in nutrition and injury prevention" (29).

SUMMARY POINTS

- ◆ Strength training is an essential component to improving health and maximizing performance. Virtually all health- and skill-related components of fitness are enhanced when specifically targeted through proper program design.
- ◆ Scoring highly on various measures of physical fitness can separate athletes of different caliber.
- ◆ Examination of the history of S&C is important for the practitioner as it magnifies the accomplishments of many pioneering individuals in the field and perhaps may provide insight into future S&C trends.
- ◆ The key ingredient to RT responses and subsequent training adaptations is proper design of the training program.
- ◆ Competitive forms of RT include weightlifting, bodybuilding, powerlifting, strength competitions, and strength/fitness competitions, *e.g.*, CrossFit.
- ◆ Education in S&C is gained through scholarly study, personal experience, and professional practice.

REVIEW QUESTIONS

1. The maximal amount of force one can generate during a specific movement pattern at a specified velocity of contraction is
   a. Muscle endurance
   b. Muscle power
   c. Muscle strength
   d. Body composition

2. A competitive sport where lifters place based on the amount of weight they lift in the snatch and clean and jerk is
   a. Bodybuilding
   b. Weightlifting
   c. Powerlifting

3. A Greek strongman whose training program was ascribed as being the first known example of using progressive overload was
   a. Milo of Crotona
   b. Galen
   c. Michel de Montaigne
   d. Dudley Sargent

4. The Dynamic Tension philosophy and training course was developed by which legendary strongman?
   a. Louis Cyr
   b. Thomas Inch
   c. Eugen Sandow
   d. Charles Atlas

5. The individual most responsible for increasing the popularity of bodybuilding in the United States from the 1940s to present day is
   a. Joe Weider
   b. Bob Hoffman
   c. Bernarr McFadden
   d. Hopton Hadley

6. The ability of an athlete to change direction rapidly without a significant loss of speed, balance, or bodily control is
   a. Speed
   b. Power
   c. Agility
   d. Balance

7. RT can
   a. Increase bone mineral density
   b. Increase local muscle endurance
   c. Decrease percent body fat
   d. All of the above

8. The first lifting sport to develop in the late 1800s was bodybuilding.
   a. T
   b. F

9. During early times a relationship existed between the medical/scientific communities and fascination with muscular strength and development.
   a. T
   b. F

10. The "health lift" (partial deadlift) was an exercise first promoted by George Barker Windship.
    a. T
    b. F

11. Ben Franklin was a well-known proponent of dumbbell RT during the late 1700s.
    a. T
    b. F

12. The first weight training magazine published was *Iron Man* in the 1930s.
    a. T
    b. F

13. The "Father of American Weightlifting" was Bob Hoffman.
    a. T
    b. F

14. Certification is a critical component to becoming a competent strength and conditioning professional.
    a. T
    b. F

REFERENCES

1. Hoffman J. *Norms for Fitness, Performance, and Health.* Champaign (IL): Human Kinetics; 2006. 220 p.
2. Sierer SP, Battaglini CL, Mihalik JP, Shields EW, Tomasini NT. The National Football League combine: performance differences between drafted and nondrafted players entering the 2004 and 2005 drafts. *J Strength Cond Res.* 2008;22:6–12.
3. Garstecki MA, Latin RW, Cuppett MM. Comparison of selected physical fitness and performance variables between NCAA Division I and II football players. *J Strength Cond Res.* 2004;18:292–7.
4. Fleisig GS, Barrentine SW, Zheng N, Escamilla RF, Andrews JR. Kinematic and kinetic comparison of baseball pitching among various levels of development. *J Biomech.* 1999;32:1371–5.
5. Fair JD. *Muscletown USA: Bob Hoffman and the Manly Culture of York Barbell.* University Park (PA): The Pennsylvania State University Press; 1999. 804 p.
6. Kraemer WJ, Ratamess NA, Flanagan SD, Shurley JP, Todd JS, Todd TC. Understanding the science of resistance training: an evolutionary perspective. *Sports Med.* 2017;47:2415–35.
7. Stoppani J. *Encyclopedia of Muscle and Strength.* Champaign (IL): Human Kinetics; 2006. p. 1–7.
8. Todd T. The myth of the muscle-bound lifter. *NSCA J.* 1985;7: 37–41.
9. American College of Sports Medicine. Position Stand: the recommended quantity and quality of exercise for developing and maintaining cardiorespiratory and muscular fitness, and flexibility in healthy adults. *Med Sci Sports Exerc.* 1990;22:265–74.
10. American College of Sports Medicine. Position Stand: the recommended quantity and quality of exercise for developing and maintaining cardiorespiratory and muscular fitness, and flexibility in healthy adults. *Med Sci Sports Exerc.* 1998;30:975–91.
11. American College of Sports Medicine. Progression models in resistance training for healthy adults. *Med Sci Sports Exerc.* 2002;34:364–80.
12. American College of Sports Medicine. Progression models in resistance training for healthy adults. *Med Sci Sports Exerc.* 2009; 41:687–708.
13. Kraemer WJ, Ratamess NA, French DN. Resistance training for health and performance. *Curr Sports Med Rep.* 2002;1:165–71.
14. Abel MG, Sell K, Dennison K. Design and implementation of fitness programs for firefighters. *Strength Cond J.* 2011;33:31–42.
15. Fahey TD, Insel PM, Roth WT. *Fit and Well: Core Concepts and Labs in Physical Fitness and Wellness.* 6th ed. Boston (MA): McGraw-Hill; 2005. p. 28–37.
16. Knuttgen HG, Kraemer WJ. Terminology and measurement in exercise performance. *J Appl Sport Sci Res.* 1987;1:1–10.
17. Stone MH, Sands WA, Pierce KC, Carlock J, Cardinale M, Newton RU. Relationship of maximum strength to weightlifting performance. *Med Sci Sports Exerc.* 2005;37:1037–43.
18. Sinclair RG. Normalizing the performances of athletes in Olympic weightlifting. *Can J Appl Sport Sci.* 1985;10:94–8.
19. Drechsler A. *The Weightlifting Encyclopedia: A Guide to World Class Performance.* Whitestone (NY): A is A Communications; 1998. p. 1–15.
20. Waller M, Piper T, Townsend R. Strongman events and strength and conditioning programs. *Strength Cond J.* 2003;25:44–52.
21. Garhammer J. Power production by Olympic weightlifters. *Med Sci Sports Exerc.* 1980;12:54–60.
22. McBride JM, Triplett-McBride T, Davie A, Newton RU. A comparison of strength and power characteristics between power lifters, Olympic lifters, and sprinters. *J Strength Cond Res.* 1999;13:58–66.
23. Sale DG, MacDougall JD. Isokinetic strength in weight-trainers. *Eur J Appl Physiol Occup Physiol.* 1984;53:128–32.
24. Kraemer WJ, Noble BJ, Clark MJ, Culver BW. Physiologic responses to heavy-resistance exercise with very short rest periods. *Int J Sports Med.* 1987;8:247–52.
25. Smith MM, Sommer AJ, Starkoff BE, Devor ST. CrossFit-based high-intensity power training improves maximal aerobic fitness and body composition. *J Strength Cond Res.* 2013;27:3159–72.
26. Bellar D, Hatchett A, Jusge LW, Breaux ME, Marcus L. The relationship of aerobic capacity, anaerobic peak power and experience to performance in CrossFit exercise. *Biol Sport.* 2015;32:315–20.
27. Winwood PW, Keogh JWL, Harris NK. The strength and conditioning practices of strongman competitors. *J Strength Cond Res.* 2011;25:3118–28.
28. Epley B, Taylor J. Developing a policies and procedures manual. In: Baechle TR, Earle RW, editors. *Essentials of Strength Training and Conditioning.* 3rd ed. Champaign (IL): Human Kinetics; 2008. p. 569–88.
29. National Strength and Conditioning Association. *Strength and Conditioning Professional Standards and Guidelines.* Colorado Springs (CO): NSCA; 2009.

CHAPTER 2

Biomechanics of Force Production and Performance

OBJECTIVES

After completing this chapter, you will be able to:

◆ Understand basic biomechanics and the biomechanics of the neuromuscular system in relation to strength and power performance

◆ Understand how muscle force and torque vary depending on its length and contraction velocity

◆ Understand how acute changes in a pennate muscle's angle of pennation may limit force production, but how chronic increases resulting from muscle hypertrophy can be advantageous for strength and power increases

◆ Understand the principles of torque and leverage and how altering moment arm length affects joint force production and speed

◆ Understand how force/torque varies throughout full joint range of motion and the ramifications this has for weight training performance

◆ Understand how friction affects force production and sports performance

◆ Understand the principles of stability and how performance is altered via changes in the body's center of gravity

◆ Understand how mass, inertia, momentum, and impulse affect performance

◆ Understand how lifting performance can be enhanced via various training accessories

Biomechanics is the science of applying the principles of mechanics to biological systems. Basic knowledge of biomechanics is critical to strength and conditioning coaches, practitioners, and athletes to improve technique and efficiency, athletic performance, the quality of coaching, prevent injuries (see Sidebar: General Factors Associated with Injuries), and understand the underlying factors associated with performance enhancement. Biomechanical concepts apply to all motor skills performed in sports as well as all training modalities. There are several physiological and biomechanical properties of the human body (*e.g.*, within the skeletal, neuromuscular, metabolic, endocrine, and connective tissue systems) that affect one's acute level of performance and subsequent long-term improvements concomitant to training. Several mechanical properties of skeletal muscle are discussed in this chapter as well as basic biomechanical concepts that affect exercise performance.

Basic Biomechanics

Biomechanics is a field that studies all aspects of motion, from the description of the motion to the underlying causes of motion. The branch that deals with the forces and torques that cause motion is **kinetics** whereas the description of motion, *e.g.*, position, distance and displacement, speed and velocity, acceleration, is known as **kinematics**. **Motion** is the process of changing position. Critical to studying the biomechanics of exercise and sport is the application of each concept to the type(s) of motion involved. **Linear motion** is produced by *centric* [resultant force applied through object's center of gravity (COG)] and *eccentric* (resultant force applied off the object's COG) force application. Linear motion occurs when all points on a body or object move the same distance, at the same time, and in the same direction, thereby yielding a straight (*rectilinear motion*) or curved (*curvilinear motion*) pathway. An example of rectilinear motion would be the straight pathway of an athlete taken during a 40-yard dash. Curvilinear motion may be exemplified by the airborne pathway of an athlete during a long jump or may be seen during the up/down trajectory of a barbell during exercises such as the bench press and squat. Figure 2.1 depicts the curvilinear trajectory of the barbell during performance of the snatch with three different loads in elite Olympic weightlifters. Loading was shown to affect the trajectory primarily in the vertical bar displacement (1).

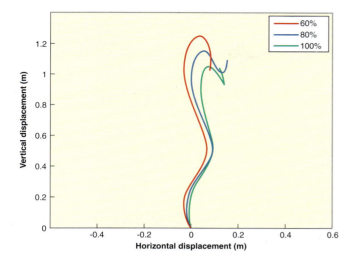

FIGURE 2.1 Bar trajectories observed during the snatch exercise in elite Olympic weightlifters. Three loads (60%, 80%, and 100% of 1 RM) were analyzed. Data show less vertical bar displacement with increasing load. (Reprinted from Hadi G, Akkus H, Harbili E. Three-dimensional kinematic analysis of the snatch technique for lifting different barbell weights. *J Strength Cond Res.* 2012;26:1568–1576, Figure 4.)

Angular (rotary) motion is the product of eccentric forces and *force couples* (forces in equal and opposite directions). It occurs when all points on a body or object move in circular patterns around the same axis. Some examples of angular motion include any single-joint action of the body (*e.g.*, elbow flexion, knee extension), total-body activities such as cartwheels, somersaults, and swinging motions such as driving a golf ball or hitting a baseball or softball, and rotation of an object such as a soccer ball as it acts as a projectile. Angular motion of bodily segments can produce linear and angular motion of the entire body. Angular kinetic and kinematic variables have similar analogs to linear motion. A critical difference is that leverage and moment arms are seen with angular motion (described later in this chapter) which is why we see exercises or sports motor skill performances made easier or more difficult by limb repositioning or changing the location of loading. An understanding of the type of motion present is critical to understanding how the underlying biomechanical principles affect motion and subsequent performance. Lastly, motion is governed in part by the Laws of Motion proposed by *Sir Isaac Newton* also discussed throughout this chapter. The Sidebar depicts some of the key biomechanical variables affecting sport and exercise performance discussed here and in subsequent chapters.

 Muscle Actions

Skeletal muscles produce force in three different ways. Muscle shortening is a *concentric* (CON) muscle action, while muscle lengthening is an *eccentric* (ECC) muscle action. A muscle action characteristic of no noticeable change in muscle length or joint position is an *isometric* (ISOM) muscle action. Greatest muscle force is produced during ECC muscle actions, followed by ISOM and CON actions in a manner specific to velocity and

---

Sidebar — General Factors Associated with Injuries

Injuries are often multifactorial and could result from several factors. The following Sidebar presents some basic factors involved with injury:

- Loading—the magnitude, duration, location and direction, frequency, and variability of loading related to tissue deformation
- Impact/contact forces and velocity of the body or other objects during collisions with opponents, ground, or other obstacles. Related to the level of contact adaptation of the athlete
- Overuse—related to the volume and intensity of training/practice and competition, individual's recovery ability, nutritional and hydration practices, training status and skill level, and technical breakdowns (especially during times of fatigue)
- Structural vulnerabilities or predispositions to injury. Genetics may contribute to certain types of vulnerabilities (related to strength/stiffness of connective tissues) that could relate to injury risk. A history of previous injuries or pain in a certain bodily region could play a role.
- Muscle strength and length imbalances and postural deficits
- A lack of flexibility may play a role for certain types of injuries.
- Age and gender. Some injuries are more common as one ages and some injuries are seen at higher rates in men or women (*i.e.*, women have up to an 8-times greater risk of a major knee injury than men).
- Environmental factors, *e.g.*, ground contact (turf, grass, floor, surface stability), footwear, weather, etc.
- Equipment failure
- Psychological and physical stress
- Drug use, *e.g.*, anabolic steroids
- Anthropometric factors such as bodyweight, height, and limb lengths
- Accidents

> **Sidebar — General Biomechanical Factors Affecting Performance**
>
> **General Biomechanics and Performance**
>
> **Kinesiology**—joint arthrology (function and movement), skeletal muscle anatomy and function, planes of motion and axes of rotation, center of gravity and stability principles
>
> Laws of motion, gravity, and basic dimensions (length, time, mass/inertia)
>
> *Linear Motion Variables:*
> - Force components and pressure
> - Friction
> - Mass/inertia
> - Position
> - Distance and displacement
> - Speed and velocity
> - Acceleration and deceleration
> - Tangential kinematics
> - Centripetal kinetics and kinematics
> - Projectile motion
> - Impulse and momentum
> - Elasticity and collisions
> - Work and power
> - Potential and kinetic energy
>
> *Angular Motion Variables:*
> - Torques, moment arms, and leverage
> - Friction
> - Moment of inertia
> - Position
> - Distance and displacement
> - Speed and velocity
> - Acceleration and deceleration
> - Impulse
> - Momentum
> - Work
> - Rotational energy
> - Power

joint range of motion. ECC muscle actions are particularly important for strength and hypertrophy gains. All three muscle actions are commonly used in training and motor skill performance. However, CON and ECC actions predominate during agonist-prescribed movements, whereas ISOM actions play a key role in joint stabilization and maintenance of static bodily positions. CON and ECC muscle action velocities can be controlled by specialized dynamometers. Velocity-controlled CON and ECC muscle actions are isokinetic, and isokinetic devices enable strength testing or training at slow, moderate, and/or fast velocities.

The Influence of Muscle Length

Skeletal muscle length plays a substantial role in force production. It is clear that muscle strength is range of motion specific, and a number of factors contribute this difference including muscle length. This concept has been termed the muscle *length-tension relationship*. Figures 2.2 and 2.3 depict isometric strength at various sarcomere lengths. This parabolic curve indicates that greatest tension is produced in the middle slightly past resting muscle length. This sarcomere (the functional component of a muscle fiber) length indicates optimal interaction of the maximal number of muscle contractile proteins (actin and myosin). Figure 2.2 depicts the *active* length-tension relationship where passive elements (and subsequently the whole muscle) are not considered. When examining total muscle tension, both active and passive elements contribute, with active elements contributing greatly from short to moderate lengths and passive elements contributing greatly at moderate to longer lengths. At shorter muscle lengths, there is overlap of the actin filaments, which reduces actin and myosin interaction. Because muscle tension is proportionate to the number of cross-bridges formed, shorter lengths geometrically pose a problem reducing active muscle tension. Theoretically (as shown in Fig. 2.2), at longer muscle lengths, a similar phenomenon may occur where cross-bridge formation is reduced. In this case, myosin filaments cannot reach as many actin filaments. However, the passive neuromuscular elements need to be considered, as shown in Figure 2.3, where at longer lengths they contribute highly to the rebound of muscle tension. Tension developed within the tendon, cross-bridges, and structural proteins (*series elastic component*) and from the muscle fascia (*parallel elastic component*) increases. Although cross-bridge interaction is minimal at long muscle lengths, tension rebounds mostly due to resistance to stretch from tendons and skeletal muscle fascia along with some tension produced within the contractile and structural proteins.

Another consideration in examining the muscle's strength potential relates to the number of joints it spans. A multiarticular muscle initiates movements at more than one joint. Although multiarticular muscles are advantageous for many elements of movement (*i.e.*, efficiency), there are a few notable disadvantages. One is *active insufficiency*. This refers to the inability of a muscle to generate sufficient force due to its

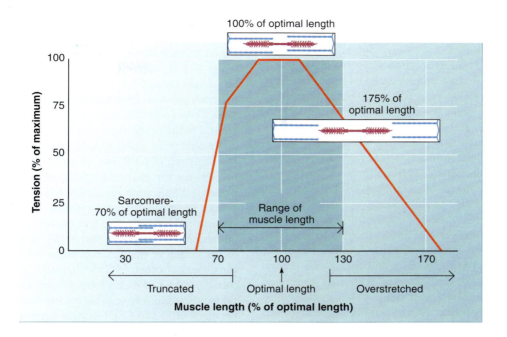

FIGURE 2.2 The active muscle length-tension relationship. Muscle tension is proportional to the number of cross-bridges formed between actin and myosin filaments. Here, the passive elements are minimal. Tension is greatest in the middle segment of the curve but lessens as cross-bridge numbers decrease at both shorter and longer muscle lengths. (Adapted from Premkumar K. *The Massage Connection: Anatomy and Physiology*. 2nd ed. Baltimore (MD): Lippincott Williams & Wilkins; 2004. Figure 4.8.)

positioning and length relative to the other joint it spans. For example, if one were to measure the strength of the hamstring muscles during knee flexion, then the position of the hip needs to be accounted for as the hamstrings collectively flex the knee but also extend the hip. The hamstrings contract more forcefully when the hip is flexed as it functions in a stronger segment of its length-tension curve. As a result, most lying leg curl machines in the gym have a declination in the angle of the padding support for the thighs to allow some hip flexion when performing the exercise (compared to some older machine designs that were straight throughout). A second disadvantage is *passive insufficiency*. This refers to the inability to reach full ROM of both joints. Let us stay with hamstrings for another example. When one bends over (flexing the hips), often the knees flex to reduce tension in the hamstrings that are being stretched to their ROM limits. Flexing the hips while the knees are extended lengthens the hamstrings and, depending on one's flexibility, could limit bending ROM unless the knees flex to alleviate the stress. Thus, both the strength and ROM of a multiarticular muscle depends on the relative position of each joint.

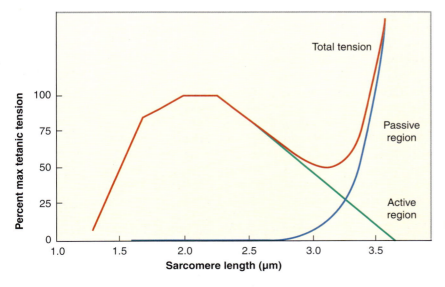

FIGURE 2.3 The passive muscle length-tension relationship. This relationship is similar to Figure 2.2 with the exception that the passive elements contribute greatly to longer muscle lengths.

Stretch-Shortening Cycle

Human movement that begins with a windup or countermovement results in a more powerful action when the movement is reversed. An ECC phase that precedes a CON phase results in a more forceful CON action especially during the initial phase on CON action. This phenomenon is known as the stretch-shortening cycle (SSC) and allows the athlete to develop large force and power outputs. The ECC phase involves a "preloading" effect of the musculotendinous unit to the extent of which may depend on the muscle involved (*i.e.*, mono- vs. biarticular), range of motion or amplitude of movement, level of effort, and velocity of movement (2). The subsequent reversal of action is potentiated presumably due to the combined effects of a few contributory mechanisms (2). The SSC is thought to consist of residual force enhancement or potentiation, utilization of the muscle stretch reflex (see Chapter 4), and the muscle-tendon complex's ability to store elastic energy within its series and parallel elastic components. The stretch reflex is initiated by a specific sensory receptor, the *muscle spindle*, which responds to both the magnitude and rate of muscle length change. It has also been suggested that the ECC action augments neural stimulation, muscle contractility, and length-tension properties, and stimulates the "active state" of muscle (*i.e.*, fraction of available actin binding sites) where cross-bridge formation augmented during the ECC phase may contribute to performance seen during the CON phase (3). The resultant effect is that the SSC can enhance performance by an average of 15%–20% (4). The SSC is most prominent in fast-twitch (FT) muscle fibers (as FT fiber motion is faster resulting in greater elastic energy storage) and is highly trainable via high-velocity plyometric, sprint, agility, and resistance training (RT).

The SSC has often been studied in comparing exercises such as a countermovement vertical jump (CMJ) to a squat jump (SJ) (with no countermovement) or by examining the effect a pause or a lack of a negative phase may have on an exercise such as the bench press. Jump height and power are greater during a CMJ (2). In fact, comparisons of jump height or power between the two jumps have led to the development of assessments targeting SSC utilization. Using jump height (m) or peak power (W), the *pre-stretch augmentation percent* (PSA) is calculated via [(CMJ − SJ)/SJ] × 100. The *eccentric utilization ratio* (EUR) is calculated via CMJ/SJ. *Reactive strength (RS)* has been calculated via CMJ − SJ. The *reactive strength index modified* (RSImod) is calculated via CMJ height/time to takeoff. Higher values are indicative of higher SSC activity, and all have been used to assess various training programs and shown to vary between athletes of different sports (5,6). For example, Suchomel et al. (6) reported PSA values of ~0.5%–6.8% (peak power) and ~12.5%–25% (peak height); EUR values of ~1.12–1.25 (jump height) and ~1.01–1.06 (peak power); RS values of ~25–180 W and ~0.03–0.05 (m); and RSImod values of ~0.2–0.43 in Division I male and female tennis, soccer, volleyball, and baseball athletes. Likewise, bench press performance is best when an ECC phase is utilized prior to the CON phase. Wilson et al. (7) showed a continuum in performance where maximal bench press strength was greatest with a standard "touch and go" bench press, followed by a bench press with a short and long pause (>1 s), while the lowest values was seen when no ECC phase was included. It appears that most of the augmentation of bench press performance occurs during the early stage of the CON action with SSC augmentation decreasing during the latter end of the range of motion (8).

Critical to SSC performance is that the CON action follows the ECC action right away if maximal CON force and power outputs are the goals. Any pause between the ECC and CON phases (or initiating an action without a countermovement) results in attenuated performance. In musculotendinous tissues, stored elastic energy can be lost as heat energy over time. Subsequently, force and power can be reduced in proportion to the length of the pause between muscle actions. It may be possible that other SSC mechanisms can be attenuated by a pause or a lack of ECC phase. Maximizing SSC activity entails performing ballistic muscle actions with minimal time lapse between ECC and CON muscle actions. Minimizing contact time with the ground is critical to plyometric training to maximize SSC activity. However, some athletes (powerlifters) benefit from including a CON-only repetition or pause between ECC and CON actions at various points in training because competition necessitates it. Some view limiting the elastic response via a CON-only repetition or a pause repetition as a way to target CON strength especially during the initial segment of the CON repetition. Hence, an integrated approach is typically used by these strength athletes. Lastly, SSC activity is reduced following periods of high-intensity static stretching (9). Muscle stiffness enhances SSC function; therefore, static stretching that reduces stiffness can lessen force and power production by 3%–10% (9).

The Role of Velocity on Muscle Force Production

The velocity of dynamic muscle contraction plays a critical role in the magnitude of force produced. This nonlinear *force-velocity relationship* for a single-joint movement is shown in Figure 2.4. Skeletal muscle fibers produce force to match external loading, *i.e.*, increasing velocity of shortening during light loading and decreasing velocity of shortening with greater loading. For CON muscle actions, greatest force is produced at slower velocities of contraction, whereas less force is produced at fast velocities of contraction. Thus, force increases as velocity slows and decreases as velocity increases. A similar relationship between force and velocity can be seen during multiple-joint movements although more linearity in the shape of the curve is present (10). For example, the CON phase of a one-repetition maximum (1 RM) bench press is performed at a slow velocity. Although the individual provides as much force as possible, the overall net

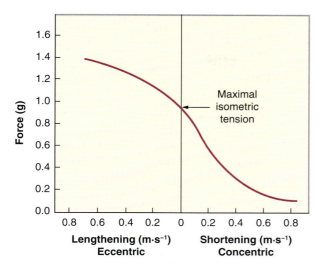

FIGURE 2.4 The force-velocity relationship.

velocity is slow due to the high external load. Peak ISOM force at optimal muscle lengths occurs at 0 m·s⁻¹ (no movement) with a value that is larger than peak CON force. Deviations from the muscle's optimal length alter the force-velocity relationship. The force disparity appears related to the number of muscle cross-bridges formed once again. Actin filaments slide rapidly at fast velocities, thereby making it more difficult for myosin to form cross-bridges with actin (11). As cross-bridge cycling rate increases, less cross-bridges remain intact at any given time. However, cross-bridge formation is enhanced at slow velocities and during ISOM actions where the cross-bridge cycling rate is low. The result is greater force production. On the contrary, muscle force increases as velocity increases during ECC actions. Loading greater than the peak ISOM force level causes muscle fibers to lengthen. Additional loading increases the lengthening velocity. Thus, muscle force increases as lengthening velocity increases because the fibers are contracting as they are lengthening and greater force is present during ECC actions. Strength and power training has the ability to shift the curve over time to indicate that greater force can be produced at each specific velocity (12,13).

 ## Muscle Architecture

Muscle architecture is a strong predictor of skeletal muscle's force-generation and motion capacity. It refers to the length, number, and geometric arrangement of muscle fibers relative to the muscle's line of pull, as well as muscle thickness. The muscle's line of pull dictates the direction of motion of the joint that ensues as muscle fibers shorten. Architectural features of skeletal muscle include the length of fascicles, fibers (and subsequent number of serial sarcomeres), and the arrangement of muscle fibers (more information on skeletal muscle is found in Chapter 5). Long fibers with a higher number of sarcomeres in series elicit higher contraction velocities, whereas a larger number of sarcomeres in parallel (*i.e.*, affecting muscle fiber diameter) is conducive to stronger forces of contraction. Muscle myofibrils may consist of 1,000 to more than 200,000 sarcomeres in series depending on the muscle, size, and activity level. Thus, muscles with higher numbers of sarcomeres in series have the ability to shorten over a large displacement during a specific unit of time compared to a muscle with a lower number of serial sarcomeres; hence, contraction velocity augmentation is an attribute of long fibers. See Myths & Misconceptions: Intentionally Slow Lifting Velocities with Submaximal Loads Are the Best Way to Train for Maximal Strength Based on the Force-Velocity Relationship.

Muscle Fiber Arrangement

The arrangement of skeletal muscle fibers plays an important role in their ability to produce force, power, and speed. Two general fiber arrangements are shown, pennate and nonpennate muscles (Fig. 2.5). Each specific muscle may have a tendency toward one type of arrangement although a combination of both arrangements may be seen (17). Nonpennate muscles have their fibers run parallel to the muscle's line of pull. Various types of nonpennate muscles exist. *Longitudinal (strap)* muscles, *e.g.*, sartorius and rectus abdominis, are long in length. *Quadrate (quadrilateral)* muscles, *e.g.*, rhomboids, are flat, four-sided nonpennate muscles. *Fan-shaped (radiate, triangular)* muscles, *e.g.*, pectoralis major, gluteus medius, have fibers that radiate from a narrow point of attachment at one end to a broader point of attachment at the opposite end. *Fusiform* muscles, *e.g.*, biceps brachii and brachioradialis, are rounded, spindle-shaped muscles that taper at both ends. Nonpennate muscles have longer fiber lengths and are typically fewer in number. Thus, nonpennate muscle fiber arrangement is more advantageous for range of motion (ROM) and speed of contraction. Although nonpennate muscles' force-producing capacity can increase with muscle growth, *e.g.*, an increase in its *anatomical cross-sectional area*, they are designed more efficiently for optimizing muscle fiber ROM and contraction velocity.

Pennate muscle fibers (from the Latin "penna" meaning "feather") are arranged obliquely to the central tendon, or line of pull. A *unipennate* muscle, *e.g.*, tibialis posterior, has one column of fibers that are arranged at an angle to the line of pull. A *bipennate* muscle, *e.g.*, rectus femoris, has a long central tendon with fibers extending diagonally in pairs from either side in two columns. A *multipennate* muscle, *e.g.*, deltoid, has more than two columns of fibers converging on a tendon to form one muscle. The pennate muscle arrangement, *e.g.*, shorter fibers oriented at an angle, is advantageous for strength and power production but not as much for velocity of contraction and ROM.

The Angle of Pennation

The *angle of pennation* refers to the angle between the fibers and fascicles and its longitudinal axis. This angle in the resting

Myths & Misconceptions
Intentionally Slow Lifting Velocities with Submaximal Loads Are the Best Way to Train for Maximal Strength Based on the Force-Velocity Relationship

When examining the velocity of the external load as it is lifted during resistance exercise, some have argued that intentionally lifting a weight slowly is the best way to maximize strength and point to the force-velocity relationship as supporting evidence. However, the missing elements in this argument are the magnitude of external loading and the effort level given by the individual and how this impacts the velocity of motion. When maximal effort is given by the athlete against a submaximal external load, the net velocity of movement is fast, but this is not the case during maximal loading where the net velocity is slow. The force-velocity relationship assumes that muscles are CON contracting maximally at a given velocity when examining the total system (14). This can be seen when isokinetic strength testing or when 1 RM strength testing is performed. During submaximal loading, intentionally slow velocities occur when the individual purposely limits contraction velocity. Albeit intentionally slow velocities may pose a potent stimulus for endurance and hypertrophy training, slow velocities with submaximal loads are not conducive to maximal strength and power training. The underlying factor is that the individual must purposely slow contraction velocity when lifting a submaximal weight, and this in turn limits the neuromuscular response (less recruitment and firing rate of activated muscle fibers).

Research has shown that the amount of weight lifted (15) or repetitions performed with a given weight, force (14,16), and neural responses (16) are lower when a weight is intentionally lifted at a slower velocity. Motion of the external load is governed by Sir Isaac Newton's Second Law of Motion (*Law of Acceleration*) where *force = mass × acceleration*. When mass is held constant, greater force produces higher acceleration. As Schilling et al. (14) have addressed, the required force to lift a slowly moving weight is just slightly larger than the weight itself as the velocity is slightly higher than 0 m·s^{-1}. Greater force is needed to accelerate the weight to a higher velocity. The justification of using intentionally slow repetitions (for maximal strength improvements) with submaximal weights is not supported by the force-velocity relationship. In contrast, greater acceleration (from higher force application) seen during the initial CON segment of the repetition lessens the need for high levels of force to continue or maintain the momentum of the weight as the lift progresses. This brings into question the level of effort needed when loads are decelerated during the latter stage of the range of motion with traditional repetitions and warrants discussion of the benefits of ballistic repetitions and ROM-specific training discussed later in this textbook in Chapter 12.

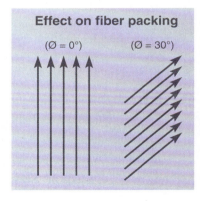

FIGURE 2.5 Muscle architecture. Pennate and nonpennate muscle arrangements are shown. Shown above as the legend is below the picture is the effect of pennation angle on fiber packing density. More fibers can be located in a given volume when their arrangement is oblique. Geometrically, this has a positive effect on strength and power production. A nonpennate muscle has angle near 0°. (Fiber packing from Oatis CA. *Kinesiology: The Mechanics and Pathomechanics of Human Movement*. Baltimore (MD): Lippincott Williams & Wilkins; 2004, cites back to Adapted with permission from Lieber RL. *Skeletal Muscle Structure, Function, and Plasticity: The Physiological Basis of Rehabilitation*. 3rd ed. Baltimore (MD): Lippincott Williams & Wilkins; 2009. Adapted from Lieber Figure 1.21—copyright returned to author 2017.)

state may be low (near 0° in nonpennate muscles) or high (>30°) depending on the muscle and the athlete's level of muscle mass (18–20). The angle of pennation (and subsequent changes) has great functional significance but also serves as part of a complex strategy (with fascicle length changes) to produce and transmit force between skeletal muscle and connective tissues. The mechanical behavior is dependent on the specific muscle involvement as well as the contraction type, velocity (in some cases), joint angle, and the intensity. The role of the angle of pennation needs to be discussed in terms of acute active muscular contractions versus its quantification at rest following a period of training. Acutely, the angle of pennation may increase largely to account for muscle contraction. As a muscle shortens, fibers must shorten to accommodate the change in muscle belly shape. Muscle fiber rotation takes place which makes the fibers more oblique (changing contraction leverage) thereby decreasing the fraction of force directed along the muscle's line of action. Fiber rotation decreases a muscle's output force but increases output velocity by allowing the muscle to function at a higher *gear ratio* (ratio of muscle fiber velocity to whole muscle velocity) (21). The larger the angle of pennation, the smaller amount of force transmitted to the tendon. The oblique orientation of pennate muscle fibers means that only the component of fiber force oriented along the line of action can contribute to the rotational force.

Increased angles of pennation have been reported during isometric and ECC muscle actions (compared to resting levels) (22).

The increased angle of pennation appears to help produce space within the muscle. Although the oblique angle may limit force transmission longitudinally on its surface [i.e., force component × cosine of the pennation angle (COS θ) for a 30° angle would yield ~13% reduction] (11), the greater *packing density* of fibers helps contribute to higher levels of force production and appears to offset the aforementioned limitation. Geometrically, a pennate muscle enables greater fiber number per cross-sectional area. Shorter fiber length coupled with greater fiber packing density yields greater force and power production compared to nonpennate muscles of similar volume. This oblique fiber orientation can be advantageous over time when an athlete trains because a chronic increase in the angle of pennation at rest corresponds to muscle hypertrophy. The magnitude of force generation is determined by the number (volume) and arrangement of fibers. The short, oblique nature of the fibers makes it difficult to precisely quantify cross-section or volume. Hence, the *physiologic cross-sectional area* (PCSA; sum total of all fiber cross-sections in a plane perpendicular to fiber orientation) is used to estimate muscle CSA. Because there is a positive relationship between a muscle's PCSA and its force potential, an increase in a muscle's angle of pennation accommodates growth thereby increasing strength and power potential.

$$\text{PCSA}\left(\text{cm}^2\right) = \frac{\text{muscle mass}(g) \cdot \text{cosine } \theta}{\rho\left(g \cdot \text{cm}^{-3}\right) \cdot \text{fibre length}(\text{cm})}$$

The equation for PSCA estimation accounts for muscle mass, COS θ, muscle density (ρ; 1.05 g·cm^{-3} for fixed mammalian muscle), and fiber length (11). Thus, increasing muscle mass and the angle of pennation relative to fiber length can increase PCSA. PCSA is proportional to isometric force capacity, e.g., PCSA × 22.5 N·cm^{-2} = estimation of maximal isometric force (11). Figure 2.6 depicts PCSA values from lower extremity muscles (17). Based on PCSA, some of the stronger lower-extremity muscles include the soleus, vastus lateralis, gluteus medius, and gluteus maximus, whereas muscles such as the sartorius, gracilis, and semitendinosus with small PCSAs favor contraction velocity.

Training-induced changes in the pennation angle are often discussed with potential changes in muscle thickness and fascicle length and are thought to govern, in part, some performance improvements. In fact, significant architectural changes may take place within the first 2 weeks of a training program (23). An increased angle of pennation enables more sarcomeres arranged in parallel and for muscle fibers to shorten less for a given velocity due to fiber rotation thereby favoring its length-tension relationship (13). However, the increased angle of pennation could result in slower contraction velocities. A number of longitudinal (18,24–27) and cross-sectional studies (19,28) have shown that RT (resulting in muscle growth) increases a muscle's angle of pennation in the resting state over time. Ballistic RT (jump squats with 0%–30% of 1 RM) and bodyweight squat jump training (29) may also increase vastus lateralis pennation angle (12). Positive relationships between muscle thickness and pennation angle have been reported (30), and competitive Olympic weightlifters have been shown to have larger resting pennation angles in the vastus lateralis compared to other resistance-trained adults (28). The increase in pennation angle is muscle-specific (i.e., varies from one muscle to another) and occurs regionally within each segment (i.e., slightly varies when examining proximal, mid, or distal regions of the muscle) of hypertrophied muscle (25,30). The muscle action plays a role in the adaptation process. Eccentric-only training has been shown to increase (31), not change (26,32,33), or decrease (23) pennation angles, whereas CON training results in an increase (23). However, these studies reporting a lack of change or decrease in pennation angle following ECC training showed significant increases in fascicle length of 16%–34%. In contrast, flexibility training may only have trivial effects on muscle pennation angle (34), and sprint training and resisted sprint training have been shown to decrease muscle pennation angle by 3%–6% (35) indicating this architectural change could favor velocity of contraction.

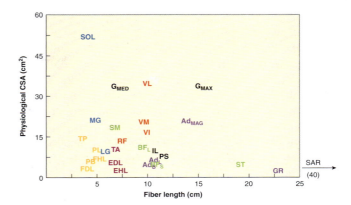

FIGURE 2.6 PCSA and Fiber Length of Lower Extremity Muscles. Ad$_B$, adductor brevis; Ad$_L$, adductor longus; Ad$_{MAG}$, adductor magnus; BF$_L$, biceps femoris, long head; BFS, biceps femoris, short head; EDL, extensor digitorum longus; EHL, extensor hallucis longus; FDL, flexor digitorum longus; G$_{MAX}$, gluteus maximus; G$_{MED}$, gluteus medius; GR, gracilis; FHL, flexor hallucis longus; IL$_{PS}$, iliopsoas; LG, lateral gastrocnemius; MG, medial gastrocnemius; PEC, pectineus; PB, peroneus brevis; PL, peroneus longus; RF, rectus femoris; SAR, sartorius; SM, semimembranosus; SOL, soleus; ST, semitendinosus; TA, tibialis anterior; TP, tibialis posterior; VI, vastus intermedius; VL, vastus lateralis; VM, vastus medialis. (Reprinted from Lieber RL, Ward SR. Skeletal muscle design to meet functional demands. *Phil Trans R Soc B*. 2011;366:1466–1476, Figure 4.)

Muscle Fascicle Length

Muscle fibers are arranged in parallel within a larger structure known as a fascicle (Chapter 5). Fascicle length is another muscle architectural component of interest. Similar to pennation angle, fascicle length tends to decrease with muscle shortening.

Chronic changes in fascicle length appear to be a significant muscular adaptation to training (29,36). Increases in fascicle length affect the force-velocity and force-length relationships. The increase in fascicle length may result from greater serial sarcomere number and/or perhaps increased tendon stiffness and has also been implicated as a potential mechanism affecting injury risk. This was shown previously where soccer players with short fascicle lengths in the biceps femoris (long head) muscle and lower ECC muscle strength were at greater risk of injury (37).

Some studies have shown greater fascicle lengths in athletes with large levels of muscle hypertrophy (38), perhaps suggesting that increasing fascicle length may be a mechanism contributing to hypertrophy. Studies have shown increases in fascicle length during traditional and ballistic RT (27,29,31,36), whereas some studies have reported no changes in fascicle length with smaller levels of muscle hypertrophy (20,39). Likewise, increases in fascicle length have been shown to be muscle specific as well as regional within each muscle (*i.e.*, variations seen from observations of proximal, mid, or distal regions) (25). Muscle actions trained plays a substantial role as studies have shown increases in fascicle length more so during ECC-only than CON-only training (23), while CON-only could lead to a decrease in fascicle length (23). In addition, ECC training at longer muscle lengths may induce greater fascicle lengthening than ECC training at shorter lengths (40). Use of the Nordic hamstring exercise (which involves ECC loading of the hamstrings) has increased in popularity, and it has been shown to result in increased biceps femoris (long head) fascicle lengths (41).

Sprint/plyometric training has been shown to increase fascicle length for selected lower-extremity muscles during short-term training periods (35,42). Among comparisons in athletes, soccer players have shorter fascicle lengths in the vastus lateralis and gastrocnemius muscles than swimmers (43), and sprinters have larger fascicle lengths than distance runners in the same muscles (44). It is thought that greater fascicle lengths favor high contraction velocity (greater running speed). In support, fascicle length correlates highly with vertical jump power, and sprint running, swimming, and cycling performance (45–48). Lastly, flexibility training may have only a trivial effect on muscle fascicle length as increases, decreases, and no changes have been shown (34).

Torque and Leverage

A force can be defined as a push or pull that has the ability to accelerate, decelerate, stop, or change the direction of an object. Forces are described by their magnitude, direction, and point of application.

Torque (also known as moment) is the rotation caused by a force about a specific axis and is the product of force and moment arm length. The net force may be centric, eccentric, or multiple forces may result in force couples. Centric and eccentric forces can produce linear motion, and eccentric forces and force couples can produce angular motion. A moment arm (or lever arm) is the perpendicular distance between the force's line of action and the fulcrum, but it may also be the perpendicular distance between the resistance and fulcrum. Two types of moment arms exist in human motion. A moment arm is formed between the point of muscle attachment and the center of the joint or instantaneous joint center (*moment arm of force or force arm*), and a moment arm is formed between the joint center and where the loading is concentrated (*moment arm of resistance or resistance arm*). Because it is an angular kinetic variable, torque is dependent upon not only the force applied but also the leverage involved. Figure 2.7 depicts an example where an individual pulls at two different angles with the same net force. The torque generated differed because the moment arm length and the rotational force perpendicular to the axial line changed.

Numerous examples can be seen in sports and exercise. A RT example is the side lateral raise. If the athlete selects 20-lb dumbbells to perform this exercise, one can see that the exercise is more difficult or easy by repositioning the arms. With the elbows extended, the exercise is more difficult than if the athlete flexes the elbows. If we assume muscle force to be similar in both cases, less torque is generated to lift the dumbbells with the elbows flexed because the resistance arm is smaller. The athlete can perform more repetitions with the elbows flexed. It is not uncommon to see individuals instinctively bend their arms when this exercise becomes more difficult. The same can be seen with other exercises such as flys, reverse flys, and leg raises. Here, limb repositioning by maintaining straight limb positions makes the exercise more difficult per unit of loading used. The moment arm of resistance can be manipulated in many ways to alter exercise performance. In some cases, it is advisable

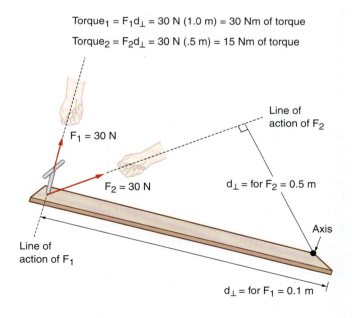

FIGURE 2.7 Torque generation at two angles of force application.

to decrease the resistance arm. For example, athletes and the population in general have been taught to lift objects off of the floor as close to the body as possible (and by using as much lower-extremity muscle involvement as possible). A reason is to decrease the resistance arm between the load and the lumbar spine axis. Greater torque is placed on the lumbar spine when objects are lifted further away from the body. Given the nature and high incidence of low-back pain and injury, reducing spinal torque often is recommended. In RT, this may be seen during the performance of exercises such as the dead lift, bent-over row, or pulls during shrugs, cleans, and snatches where pulling the bar close to the body is critical. It may also be seen during those exercises which require carrying objects.

The human body acts as a system of levers (Fig. 2.8). A *lever* is used to overcome a large resistance and is used to enhance speed and ROM. A lever is made up of a *fulcrum* (pivot point), *resistance*, and *force*. The distance from the fulcrum to the concentration of the resistance is the *resistance arm*, whereas as the distance from the fulcrum to the concentration of the force is the force or *effort arm*. The relative location of each determines what type of lever is present. A *first-class lever* (e.g., open chain cervical extension) has its fulcrum lie between the force and resistance. Speed and ROM are maximized with this type of lever and force is secondary. A *second-class lever* (e.g., standing plantar flexion onto the toes) has its resistance lie between the fulcrum and force. An advantage with this type of lever is augmented force. A *third-class lever* (e.g., open-chain elbow flexion) has its force lie between the fulcrum and resistance. Similar to a first-class lever, a third-class lever is more advantageous for speed and ROM and not as much for force.

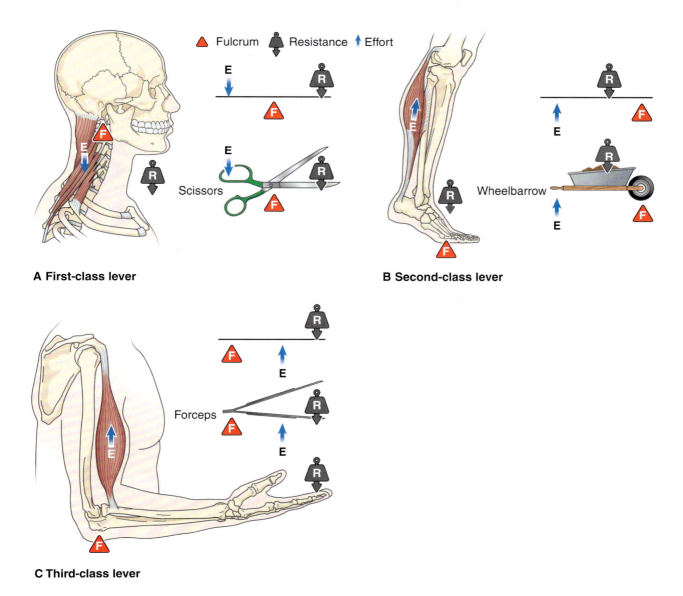

FIGURE 2.8 Three classes of levers. (Reprinted from Cohen BJ, Taylor JJ. *Memmler's The Human Body in Health and Disease*. 11th ed. Baltimore (MD): Wolters Kluwer Health; 2009. Figure 8.8.)

Most single-joint movements in the human body operate via third-class levers. Levers can change based on the relative positions of the force, fulcrum, and resistance. For example, abduction of the hip while standing in an erect position (in an open chain) exemplifies a third-class lever. However, if that same leg were to remain firmly planted on the ground during hip abduction, it would cause rotation of the body to the same side. In doing so, hip abduction in this closed-chain position exemplifies a first-class lever as the resistance encountered is now the weight of the body as opposed to weight of limb in the open-chain position. As mentioned previously, standing plantar flexion onto the toes exemplifies a second-class lever. However, if one were to perform a seated plantar flexion exercise with an elastic band providing resistance to the toes, this would exemplify a first-class lever. Complicating the matter is that leverage changes throughout the ROM of a movement as the lengths of the force and resistance arms vary and that much of human movement involves multiple-joint actions where a combination of lever systems play a role.

As a leverage system, bones act as levers, joints act as fulcrums, and contracting skeletal muscles act as the force where the muscle is inserted into the bone. Weight (or the concentration of the weight) of each segment plus external loading both act as the resistance. A term used to describe a lever's potential for force production is *mechanical advantage*. Mechanical advantage is the ratio of the moment arm of muscle force (effort arm) to the moment arm of resistance (resistance arm). A value of 1 indicates balance between the effort and resistance arms. A value >1 indicates a mechanical advantage where the torque created by the effort force is magnified, whereas a value <1 indicates a mechanical disadvantage (although it would be an advantage for speed and ROM) where a larger effort force is needed to overcome the resistance (49). First-class levers in the human body operate mostly at values similar to or <1 indicating a mechanical disadvantage under certain conditions during motion (49). Third-class levers pose mechanical disadvantages (<1) and are more suitable for greater joint angular velocities as the resistance arm is larger than the effort arm. However, a second-class lever provides a mechanical advantage (>1) as the effort arm is larger than the resistance arm. Most skeletal muscles produce single-joint movements that operate at a mechanical disadvantage thereby requiring muscles to produce additional force in order to overcome a resistance. Based on lever systems, it appears that the human body was designed to produce motion at higher speeds at the expense of the large force applications. A proportional relationship exists between the force and resistance components. If the resistance increases, greater force or a larger force arm is needed to produce comparable torque to produce or balance movement. Likewise, greater force or force arm length allows a larger resistance to be overcome. From an exercise perspective, manipulating mechanical advantage can be used to increase efficiency of exercise or to intentionally make an exercise more difficult. In Chapter 14, we will discuss bodyweight exercise and how leverage can be manipulated during different exercise variations to increase the difficulty or training stimulus.

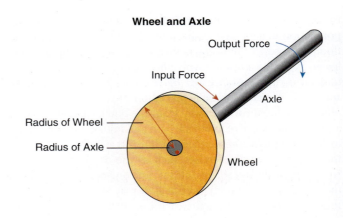

FIGURE 2.9 Mechanical advantage of a wheel/axle system.

Lever systems are one type of machine found in the musculoskeletal system. A *machine* is used to increase mechanical advantage. Two others are wheel/axles and pulleys. An object that acts as a "wheel" secured to an axle rotates in response to a tangential force (Fig. 2.9). The centers of the wheel and axle correspond to the fulcrum. The mechanical advantage >1 when the radius of the wheel is larger than the axle. The mechanical advantage of this system is shown in the following equation:

$$MA = \frac{r_w}{r_a}$$

MA = mechanical advantage

r_w = radius of the wheel (moment arm from the motive force)

r_a = radius of the axle (moment arm for the resistive force)

It can be seen that mechanical advantage can increase by increasing the radius of the wheel, decreasing the radius of the axle, or both. An example seen in the human body is internal or external rotation of the glenohumeral joint of the shoulder. The humerus acts as the axle, whereas the distance from the humerus to the fingertips acts as the wheel. When flexing the elbow to 45° (from the anatomical position) prior to rotation, the radius of the "wheel" increases and so does mechanical advantage.

Pulleys change the direction of the force application. Increasing the axle number increases the mechanical advantage of the pulley. There are several examples of anatomical pulleys within the human body. The patella acts as a pulley to increase the mechanical advantage of the quadriceps muscles during knee extension. Some bones of the ankle and foot region act as axles for the tendons of lower-extremity muscles. For example, the peroneus longus tendon is redirected around the lateral malleolus of the ankle assisting in the performance of eversion and plantar flexion of the ankle and foot regions. In addition, pulleys are seen in some RT machines. For example, pulleys can be seen on a lat pulldown machine. The individual pulls downward on the bar yet the weight stack is lifted upward due

Chapter 2 Biomechanics of Force Production and Performance

Moment Arms and Tendon Insertion

The location of a muscle's tendon insertion into bone is another factor contributing to strength expression. The distance from the joint center to the point of tendon insertion represents the moment arm of muscle force, or the effort arm. A tendon inserted slightly further away from the joint poses more of a mechanical advantage for torque production, whereas insertion closer to the joint is more advantageous for speed. An athlete with a longer force arm has the ability to lift more weight but at the expense of speed. For a given amount of muscle shortening, a muscle that has a tendon inserted closer to the joint will experience a greater change in ROM than a muscle with its tendon inserted farther from the joint. Greater ROM covered in the same period of time reflects greater joint angular velocity. Consequently, a baseball or tennis player might benefit more from a smaller moment arm of force, whereas a powerlifter would benefit more from a larger moment arm of force. Great variability exists between different muscles, which affects the strength and velocity of joint action. For example, the brachioradialis has the largest moment arm and mechanical advantage of the elbow flexor muscles. Thus, it is a key contributor to elbow flexion strength especially when the forearm is pronated in the midrange position. Tendon insertion is a genetic factor contributing to strength that does not change with training.

Case Study 2.1

Michael is a S&C coach who is strength testing athletes from various sports. Michael is using the 1 RM bench press assessment to test upper-body maximal strength. One athlete, a basketball player, who is 6′8″ and weighs 220 lb, maxes out at 225 lb. Another athlete, a wrestler, who is 6′0″ and weighs 220 lb, also maxes out at 225 lb.

Question for Consideration: What mechanically can be deduced from the performance data of both athletes?

Moment Arms and Bodily Proportions

An athlete's stature plays an important role in performance. Longer limbs create a longer resistance arm that can reduce mechanical advantage. However, a longer resistance arm yields greater velocity. This is advantageous for sports such as basketball, volleyball, and pitching in baseball. Longer limb lengths contribute to greater stride length in running and stroke length

and frequency in swimming (50). Limb length is a genetic attribute that is not coached but increases the likelihood of success in some sports. However, in lifting sports, a longer moment arm of resistance makes it difficult to lift a great deal of weight for some exercises.

Proportions contribute, in part, to the success an individual will have in athletics. As previously discussed, limb lengths affect moment arm sizes and leverage can be gained or lost depending on bodily proportions. Although bodily proportions are stable in adulthood, an athlete can modify technique and/or train specifically to accommodate or compensate for genetic structural attributes. Relative proportion is an area of interest to coaches as certain anthropometric variables have been linked to sporting success. Some commonly used variables include (a) *crural index* ([ratio of leg length/thigh length] × 100); (b) *brachial index* ([ratio of forearm length/arm length] × 100]; (c) *trunk to upper or lower extremity index*; (d) *lower limb to trunk ratio*; and (e) *seated height to stature index*. As Ackland and de Ridder (51) have pointed out:

- Tennis players with long limbs have an advantage with high-velocity shots, whereas players with shorter limbs need to play with more agility to compensate.
- Elite swimmers tend to have a larger stature depending on the event. Sprinters have displayed a higher brachial index, arm span, and lower leg and foot length compared to middle-distance and distance swimmers. Freestyle and backstroke swimmers tend to have longer limbs, and butterfly swimmers tend to have longer trunks.
- Gymnasts tend to have shorter statures with a low crural index and lower limb/trunk ratio.
- Weightlifters and powerlifters tend to have long trunks, low crural index, low lower limb/trunk ratio, low brachial index, and high sitting height/stature ratio.
- Sprinters tend to have a low lower limb/trunk ratio with an average-to-high crural index compared to middle-distance runners.
- High and triple jumpers tend to have a high lower limb/trunk ratio and a high crural index.
- Discus and javelin throwers tend to have longer arms with normal trunk lengths.
- Cyclists tend to have a high crural index that increases mechanical advantage during pedaling.
- Sports such as baseball and football are more variable based on the diversity of different positions.
- Basketball and volleyball players tend to be tall and have long upper and lower limbs, and a high crural index.
- Wrestlers and judo athletes tend to have a low lower limb/trunk ratio and a low crural index to assist in maintaining a low COG.

Human Strength Curves

An athlete's level of muscular strength varies on the position within the ROM, *e.g.*, peak torque and force varies depending on joint position. This concept can be illustrated by

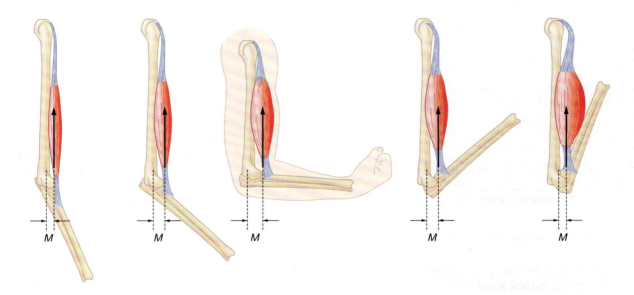

FIGURE 2.10 Effort arm changes during elbow flexion.

examining any weight training exercise. There are areas that feel easier, and there is a point where the exercise is most difficult. The area of greatest difficulty where the velocity of the weight slows down is known as the sticking region. Sticking regions may not be seen during low-intensity repetitions; however, they do become apparent during high-intensity lifts or when fatigue is substantial (52). At this point, it is very tempting for the athlete to break form and cheat the weight to its full repetition completion. However, proper technique must be emphasized, and weight selection should consider this weak link for a given exercise.

There are several physiological and biomechanical factors that contribute to human strength curves. Some factors are addressed in this and subsequent Chapters 4 and 5 including neural activation, muscle cross-sectional area, muscle length, and architecture. Perhaps the most significant of these factors is the changes in length of the moment arm of muscle force that takes place throughout full joint ROM. Figure 2.10 depicts moment arm of muscle force changes of the biceps brachii that take places during elbow flexion. The moment arm of force is largest in the middle of the ROM near an elbow angle of 90°. The force arm decreases in length as the arm is flexed or extended toward the limits of the ROM. Graphically, this kinetic pattern yields a parabolic-shaped joint angle-torque curve known as an *ascending-descending torque curve* (Fig. 2.11). Starting from full elbow extension, muscle torque is low but gradually increases to a peak at or near 90° (the ascending segment). Beyond this point, muscle torque gradually decreases until full joint flexion (the descending segment). Although peak ISOM torque may vary slightly among different joint actions, single-joint movements are depicted as ascending-descending torque curves (53,54).

The strength, or force, curves for multiple-joint actions differ. They tend to be somewhat more linear (as linear motion is produced), and either ascend or descend on a joint angle-force curve. An *ascending strength curve* is one where overall net force is lowest initially but gradually increases as the exercise progresses (Fig. 2.12). Many pushing exercises such as the

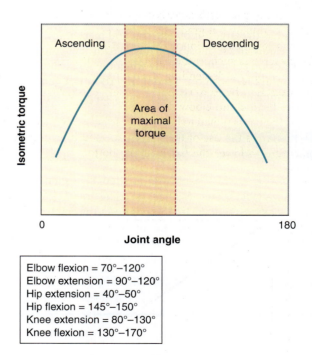

FIGURE 2.11 Ascending-descending strength (torque) curve. The values depict areas of maximal strength determined by several studies. (Redrawn from Kraemer WJ, Fry AC, Ratamess NA, French DN. Strength testing: development and evaluation of methodology. In: Maud PJ, Foster C, editors. *Physiological Assessments of Human Performance*. 2nd ed. Champaign (IL): Human Kinetics; 2006. p. 119–150.)

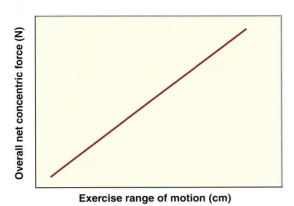

FIGURE 2.12 Ascending strength (force) curve.

squat, bench press, and shoulder press exemplify an ascending strength curve. In the barbell squat, the exercise is most difficult at the parallel bottom position (or lower) but easiest at the very top near full knee and hip extension. The difference in the amount of weight lifted between a parallel and a quarter squat is of great significance as this value can be in excess of 200 lb or more in some athletes. This is why it is common to see athletes not descend to the parallel position when the squat exercise becomes more difficult with fatigue or heavy loading.

A *descending strength curve* is one where the overall net force is greatest initially but gradually decreases as the exercise progresses to its final position within the ROM (Fig. 2.13). Many pulling exercises such as the barbell row, pull-up, and lat pull-down exemplify a descending strength curve. In the lat pull-down exercise, the exercise is easiest at the top position (full shoulder flexion and elbow extension) but becomes more difficult as the bar is pulled to below chin level. Hence, a common mistake seen is the use of the lower back and hips to generate momentum to lower the bar near the bottom position of the exercise.

Action/Reaction Forces and Friction

An *action force* is the force (a push or pull) applied by an individual to an object with the intent to accelerate, decelerate, stop, maintain, or change the direction of the object. Muscular contraction, in addition to the effects of gravity, produces action forces in sports and exercise. However, a *reaction force* is produced in response to the action. In his Third Law of Motion, Sir Isaac Newton has stated "for every action there is an equal and opposite reaction." That is, the reactive force is equal and opposite of the action force. During weight training, a reactive force is seen by the barbell in response to the action force provided by the lifter. Critical to our discussion is that the response may differ even though the forces are equal and opposite. When the lifter applies the force to the barbell, the reactive force is equal; however, the barbell does move. Thus, similar forces can lead to dissimilar results in that the object with less mass, stability, and/or leverage may move despite the similar underlying kinetics.

Ground reaction forces are critical to most motor skills and exercises. The ground supplies an equal and opposite force in response to a force applied to the ground by the athlete during locomotion. The ground reaction force enables the athlete to run. Action/reaction forces consist of three components corresponding to each plane of motion:

- F_x — indicates the medial-to-lateral or side-to-side component
- F_y — indicates the anterior-posterior or forward-backward component
- F_z — indicates the vertical or perpendicular component, which is typically the largest of the three components.

For each directional component, there are also corresponding angular motion components or *moments* (M_x, M_y, and M_z shown in Fig. 2.14). Figure 2.15 depicts a typical vertical

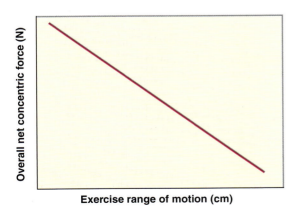

FIGURE 2.13 Descending strength (force) curve.

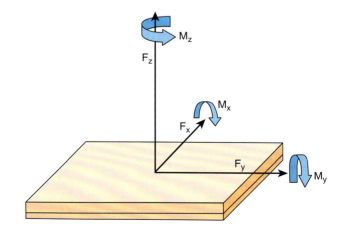

FIGURE 2.14 Ground reaction force and moment components.

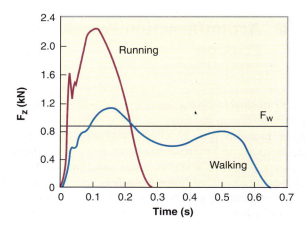

FIGURE 2.15 Ground-reaction force (F_z) curves. The important components to view are the forces (peaks and slopes) and the time. The foot is in contact with the ground for less time in running than walking. Data demonstrate increased ground reaction forces with increasing speeds of running and walking. Ground-reaction force curve shows two distinct segments (the curves are more visible during running). The first rise in force (or peak) is known as the *peak impact force*, which depicts force produced upon the foot landing on the ground especially when striking close to the heel. The second rise (or peak) is known as the *peak propulsion force*, which is the peak force produced during acceleration as the individual's center of gravity moves forward during push-off. The slopes of the curves represent the rate of impact loading and the rate of propulsion. These curves are important for helping to design athletic shoes in sports. F_w indicates the force of bodyweight.

ground reaction force (F_z)-time curve observed during running and walking. Reaction forces are seen in other conditions as well and range from a magnitude slightly greater than one's bodyweight to more than 10 times one's bodyweight for intense ballistic movements with respect to the vertical force component (F_z). The shape of the curve will differ from one activity to another. For example, the running curve shown in Figure 2.15 is considerably different than that observed during a vertical jump as the vertical jump involves countermovement, propulsion, takeoff, and landing phases. The shape of the running force-time curve can vary significantly and may be influenced by a number of factors such as the velocity, running style (rearfoot, midfoot, and forefoot striking pattern), stride length, technique, footwear, ground surface and inclination, fatigue, and level of conditioning. For example, several studies have investigated the mechanics of running barefoot (or using *minimalist shoes* [shoes designed to mimic barefoot running via thin soles, reduced cushioning, lack of arch support, and reduced weight]) versus wearing athletic shoes. Collectively, research has shown that running barefoot tends to yield more of a forefoot or midfoot striking pattern compared to running in shoes and that the loading rates seen during running are higher with shoes (55). Thus, ground reaction force data provide critical information that can influence coaching and training, as well as influence athletic shoe design. See Sidebar: Forces and Loading Vectors.

Force platforms have been instrumental in recording ground reaction force data from a number of different motor skills and exercises. They can be mounted in the ground, mounted into a piece of equipment (*i.e.*, such as leg press sled), and some are portable and can be used in many locations. They consist of force transducers (*i.e.*, strain gauges or piezoelectric) located within the corners of the top plate that enable accurate assessment of force, moments, center of pressure, velocity, and power. The technology used has been adapted to be used for sport-specific assessment. For example, *pressure insoles* can be placed within athletic shoes to determine pressures encountered during walking, running, jumping, or many athletic skills and exercises. Force transducers can be placed within sport-specific equipment such as blocking sleds in football or within boxing manikins mounted to a wall to measure the forces of different punches (56). In addition, *accelerometers* and *global positioning system* (GPS) units have been used for several testing purposes but have been instrumental in examining the effects of impact during collisions in sports such as football and rugby (57,58).

Action forces applied to an object or another body will be higher if stable contact is made between the two objects. These action/reaction forces are considered perpendicular (F_z), but there needs to be a sufficient parallel force (F_x, F_y) present to create stability between the two surfaces in contact. This resultant parallel force is known as friction. Friction acts to oppose relative motion of these two surfaces in terms of linear and angular motion. That is, friction causes stability at the point of contact and prevents one object from sliding past the other up to a point. The maximum frictional force is the product of the reactive force and a dimensionless quantity known as the *coefficient of friction*, which is a numerical representation of the two contact surfaces. There are different types of friction. Here, dry

Sidebar Forces and Loading Vectors

During RT, the human body can be loaded at multiple angles in multiple directions. A *loading vector* refers to the direction that the resistance is applied to the body. Figure 2.16 depicts the basic loading vectors encountered during RT (59). The loading vector needs to match the movement trained. Changing the loading vector changes muscle activation and performance of the exercise. For example, the barbell squat provides resistance in the axial direction. Thus, performing this exercise increases strength mostly in that longitudinal direction. Pushing a sled provides resistance to the body in the anteroposterior direction. This may increase strength in a direction more specifically to an athlete who encounters

(*Continued*)

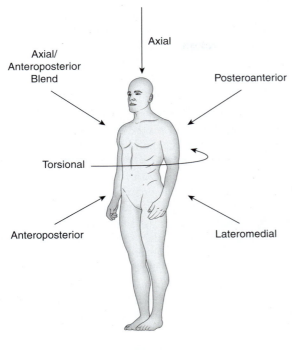

The 6 Primary Load Vectors in Sports and the Weight Room

FIGURE 2.16 Loading vectors.

and must overcome an opponent directly, *e.g.*, American football. Rotating the body can change the loading vector. For example, performing a standing chest press with bands or on a cable machine directly targets the pectoralis major, deltoid, triceps, and core musculature in an anteroposterior direction. However, performing the same exercise (with the hands together) from a rotated position of the body (90°) reduces the loading on the chest musculature but greatly increases loading of the core musculature in a lateromedial direction (an anti-rotational exercise known as the *Pallof press*). Free weights supply a resistance mostly downward due to the effects of gravity and, depending on the position of the body (*i.e.*, upright, prone, supine, angled), may not adequately load the body in all directions. For example, performing standing external shoulder rotations with a dumbbell (while the humerus is located next to the trunk in the anatomical position) loads the deltoid muscles mostly with little resistance to the rotator cuff muscles. However, using dumbbells while the body is supine or by changing the starting position to where the humerus is abducted to 90° changes, the loading vector to more directly target the external rotators of the shoulder. Elastic bands, cables, and machines can be used to help target directions limited by free weights alone. Thus, S&C programs should target exercises that stress all loading vectors.

friction is discussed, but friction also occurs between objects and fluid mediums such as air and water. The main types of friction are static, dynamic, and rolling friction. *Static friction* acts between two objects not moving relative to each other where there is sufficient stability between the contact surfaces. *Dynamic (sliding) friction* acts between two surfaces moving relative to each other, resulting in sliding. *Rolling friction* is the frictional component seen between a circular object such as wheel or ball and the surface. Figure 2.17 demonstrates the relationship between static and dynamic frictional forces once the static force is overcome and movement ensues. The coefficients of static friction values are largest in comparison but also transient as they are affected by a number of environmental factors. For example, Newton et al. (60) have shown that the coefficient of friction was 36% higher on a new wrestling mat compared to an old mat, that the coefficient of friction was 23%–28% lower in old wrestling shoes compared to new shoes, and that perspiration (saline) decreased the coefficient of friction between the mat and shoe by 14%.

Numerous examples of friction can be seen in athletics, and its importance is great from maximizing performance to injury prevention. Friction is critical for all RT exercises. For the bench press, static friction between the lifter's back and bench, feet and floor, and hands and bar are important for stability and lifting performance. For the dead lift, static friction between the lifter's feet and floor and hands and bar are important for lifting performance. Greater friction equals better performance or weight lifted. This is why powerlifters and weightlifters use chalk on their hands and on their backs (powerlifters) as chalk increases the coefficient of static friction. In addition, knurling on a bar enhances friction and improves gripping. Static friction plays critical roles in sports as well. Static friction between a player's feet and the ground is essential and has been a major consideration when examining shoe design. Greater force and

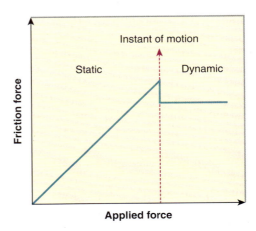

FIGURE 2.17 The relationship between static and dynamic frictional forces.

power can only be produced when the individual is in the most stable position. However, with greater stability, an accompanying increased joint loading may ensue which could increase the risk of certain types of injuries (61,62). Static friction is important when gripping an object whether it is a baseball, basketball, tennis racquet, or football. Some exercise devices (weighted sled) rely on frictional forces to provide resistance to the trainee, and these differ based on the type of sled, loading, surface texture, and the speed of movement. For example, Andre et al. (63) reported static friction coefficients of 0.47–0.39 and dynamic friction coefficients of 0.35–0.31 during sled pulls of increasing weight (up to 136 kg). The coefficients decreased in response to greater loading possibly reflecting the compressive nature of the surface and its interaction with the bottom of the sled. Cross et al. (64) reported values of 0.34–0.38 for sled pulling but found the values differed with speed of movement. These values (multiplied by the vertical force or weight [in Newtons] of the sled) correspond to the horizontal force component that needs to be overcome during the exercise. That is, the static component represents the force necessary to start the sled moving and the dynamic component represents the force encountered once the sled is moving. However, some sports strive for much lower dynamic friction coefficients, *e.g.*, 0.003–0.007 for ice skating and 0.05–0.20 for skiing. Skiers and skaters perform much better and achieve better times when the coefficient of sliding friction is ultralow between the skis/skates and the ground/ice.

Stability

Stability is the ability of an object or individual to resist changes in equilibrium. Maintaining a stable position is critical to the expression of maximal strength and power. However, instability increases the activity of stabilizer muscles and forms the basis for training on unbalanced surfaces. Stability is reliant to a great extent on manipulation of the COG. The COG is the point at which the weight is concentrated. The COG is multiplanar, meaning it has longitudinal, side-to-side, and front-to-back orientations. Thus, the COG can move side to side when limbs are abducted or the trunk is laterally flexed, can be lowered by flexing the trunk, hips, or knees; can be raised by lifting the arms; can shift from front to back or vice versa during sagittal plane movements; and may occur outside of the body during pike or hyperextended bodily positions. Motion changes the COG in one or more planes, and manipulation of the COG is crucial to maintaining and optimizing stability. Relevant to the COG is an imaginary line that connects the COG to the ground known as the *line of gravity*. As the COG changes, so potentially can the line of gravity, and manipulating the line of gravity affects an object's stability.

Of significance to stability is the object's weight, level of friction, and size of the base support. The *base support* is an area within the lines connecting the outer perimeter of the parts of the body in contact with the ground. For example, a sprinter in 4-point stance would have a larger base support than an individual standing in an upright position with a shoulder-width stance (2-point stance). The size of the base support can be manipulated to increase stability. Increasing the size of the base support leads to greater stability. For example, postural stability is greater when an individual performs the squat with a wide stance versus a narrow stance. Thus, stability is governed by general principles:

- *Greater stability is seen when the COG is lower*, as is the case with a football player or wrestler who maintains a low position to increase the likelihood of success.
- *Greater stability is present when the line of gravity is aligned equidistantly within the base support*, when weight is not shifted from side to side or front to back; stability is greater when the line of gravity is centralized.
- *Greater stability is observed when the base support is wide*, increasing the width of the stance or the number of contact points with ground enhances stability.
- *Greater stability is observed in objects with larger mass*; objects larger in mass possess greater stability.
- *Greater stability is observed when the level of friction is greater*; when the coefficient of friction increases, greater stability is present.
- *Stability decreases when external loading is applied to the upper body*; external loading to the upper extremities raises the COG and reduces stability.

Mass and Inertia

Mass is the amount of matter an object takes up, whereas *inertia* is the resistance of an object to changing its motion. Newton's First Law of Motion states that "a body at rest will remain at rest, while a body in motion will remain in uniform motion unless it is compelled to change that state by forces impressed." Thus, inertia resists changes in motion. In linear motion, objects with larger mass and inertia have more stability. Mass is a critical element to many sports especially those that have weight classes. For some sports, increasing mass can be advantageous especially in the form of muscle mass increases, *e.g.*, football. However, sports with weight classes or sports where the athlete must overcome mass for success (high jumper, pole-vaulter, and gymnast) limit the amount of mass an athlete may be willing to gain. For these sports, a high *strength-to-mass ratio* is important. A high strength-to-mass ratio indicates that the athlete produces a high level of force (or power for the *power-to-mass ratio*) with less or similar body mass. A 10% increase in strength with only a 2% increase in body mass could be advantageous for many athletes. Thus, an athlete who competes in weight classes or against gravity could theoretically perform better with strength increases while maintaining a similar mass. Additional mass could be problematic for athletes such as gymnasts or jumpers as the individual has to overcome more inertia to accelerate, potentially resulting in less distance or height jumped. Small mass increases could be beneficial if performance is enhanced. However, some athletes have to weigh the advantages and disadvantages of mass gains via trial and error to possibly increase mass slightly but not too much to limit performance. Training can be designed to enhance strength and power while minimizing mass gains.

In angular motion, mass is still critical. However, the distribution of mass is a major factor of consideration. The angular kinetic analog to mass or inertia is the *moment of inertia*. The moment of inertia is the property of an object to resist changes in angular motion and is the product of the object's mass and a measure of mass distribution about an axis of rotation known as the *radius of gyration*, *e.g.*, moment of inertia (I_a) = mass (m) × radius of gyration (r)^2. The radius of gyration is the distance from the axis of rotation to where the object's mass is concentrated. Because the radius of gyration is a squared term, a small change yields a large change in the moment of inertia. Changing an object's center of mass changes the moment of inertia. Some examples of decreasing the moment of inertia in sports are "choking up" in baseball or softball to increase bat velocity; flexing the hips, knees, and trunk in diving or gymnastics to facilitate aerial rotations; and flexing the knee during the swing phase in sprinting to enhance leg angular velocity by decreasing the moments of inertia about the hip joint. For RT, increasing the moment of inertia places greater tension on the muscles (performing a torso rotation with the arms straight rather than bent) as it becomes more difficult to start and stop the movement and requires greater muscle activation.

Momentum and Impulse

Newton's Second Law of Motion (*i.e.*, *Law of Acceleration*) states that "the change of motion of an object is proportional to the force impressed and is made in the direction of the line of action." In linear terms, the Law of Acceleration (where Force = mass × acceleration; $F = ma$) could be rewritten to yield two additional biomechanical variables. If we substitute the equation for acceleration (Δvelocity/time) and multiply both sides by time to remove the denominator, we end up with an equation $F \times T = m \times \Delta v$. The left side of the equation ($F \times T$) is linear *impulse*, whereas the right side of the equation ($m \times \Delta v$) is linear *momentum* yielding the impulse-momentum relationship. Impulse represents the level of force applied over time (N seconds) and causes and is equal to changes in momentum. It graphically represents the integrated area under the force-time curve. Increasing force and/or time in which it is applied increases impulse. Momentum can be increased by increasing either the mass or the velocity. Increasing linear momentum can be advantageous especially with *collisions*. A football player who increases mass (via an off-season S&C program) and maintains or increases velocity can generate more linear momentum at the point of contact with an opponent. There are many examples in sports where decreasing momentum is positive. For example, catching a ball decreases ball momentum, blocking or tackling decreases an opponent's momentum, and landing from a jump. Protective equipment reduces momentum and lessens the peak force absorbed by an athlete. Protective equipment, *e.g.*, pads, helmets, mats, changes the impulse curves by lengthening the time of force distribution (while reducing the peak force absorbed) throughout the body segment or entire body during contact. For weight training, linear momentum can be increased or decreased by manipulating the repetition velocity for a given submaximal load during a multiple-joint exercise. Changes in momentum are proportional to the force applied. A large force application can increase impulse throughout the remainder of the exercise. This may assist in helping the lifter overcome the sticking region of the concentric phase during high-intensity sets. Another way to utilize momentum during lifting is to involve more muscle groups not directly targeted by the exercise, or "cheating". Although "cheating" is often regarded as improper and counterproductive, a recent computer-simulated study indicated that some (but not too much) additional angular momentum applied to the beginning segment of each repetition of the lateral raise exercise may provide a novel hypertrophic stimulus due to additional loading used and increased muscle time under tension (65). Some argue that the generation of too much momentum can reduce muscle development as lower momentum generated requires a longer period of force application. The choice is based on training goals as increasing momentum (primarily through faster lifting velocities) may play a greater role in strength and power development with submaximal lifting intensities.

Angular motion analogs are seen for momentum and impulse as well. Angular impulse is equivalent to torque × time, and angular momentum is the product of angular velocity and the moment of inertia. Similar to linear momentum, maximizing angular momentum necessitates the optimal combination of angular velocity and the moment of inertia. Swinging a baseball and softball bat can be used to illustrate this point. Mass distribution and the radius of gyration can be altered by modifying the size and type of bat used, arm positioning, and by where the individual holds the bat. Choking up on a bat reduces the moment of inertia to make the bat easier to swing. However, choking up on the bat historically has not been a method used commonly by power hitters (although some modern-day notable Major League Baseball players have successfully hit home runs while choking up on the bat). Less angular momentum is generated upon contact with the ball yielding less velocity of the ball after it is struck. When a player "extends the arms," the ball generally travels farther and faster. The moment of inertia is increased at minimal expense to angular velocity thereby increasing angular momentum. Thus, an athlete with the power to swing a heavier (or more concentrated) bat at a fast velocity presents a greater power hitting threat at the plate. Naturally, a number of additional factors to bat velocity and momentum affect how fast and far a ball will travel after it is struck by the bat. For example, the pitched ball velocity and mass of the ball, type of bat (*i.e.*, aluminum, wood), *coefficient of restitution* (*i.e.*, measure of elasticity) of the ball and bat, mass distribution of the bat, the angle of ball strike (*i.e.*, "launch angle"), hit location on the bat (*center of percussion* or "sweet spot" generates the highest velocity), ball spin, and wind resistance all affect the quality of the hit. A similar scenario is presented in golf where the driver (longest club resulting in a longer radius of gyration) yields farther ball distances upon contact. Some sports depend on increasing and decreasing angular momentum during performance. For example, a discus thrower will spin fast initially to use a larger moment of inertia to maximize the time of torque application. After this phase, the moment of inertia is reduced to maximize angular velocity before release.

 ## Body Size

An athlete's body size is an influential factor for maximal force production. In general, the larger the body size, the larger the force potential. However, this only applies relative to muscle mass as a positive relationship exists between muscle mass and absolute force production. Several coaches and practitioners have used relative strength measures to compare athletes of different sizes in lifting events (see Chapter 1). Body mass scaling clearly favors smaller individuals. As body size increases, body mass increases to a greater extent than muscle strength. Larger athletes have a higher absolute segment of their body mass in the form of bone mass or nonmuscle mass that does not contribute directly to greater muscle force production. In addition, potential reductions in leverage (larger moment arms of resistance in taller athletes) could limit the maximal amount of weight lifted. Other scaling methods, *e.g.*, allometric scaling, tend to favor middle-weight individuals. Perhaps the best solution is to use weight classes and compare absolute performances when possible.

 ## Other Kinetic Factors in Strength and Conditioning

Intra-Abdominal and Intrathoracic Pressures

Intra-abdominal pressure (IAP) is the pressure developed within the abdominal cavity during contraction of deep trunk muscles and the diaphragm. The abdominal cavity contains a large fluid element that provides great stability (Fig. 2.18). This element has been described as a fluid ball that assists in stabilizing the vertebral column and reducing compressive forces on spinal disks. This fluid component is structurally greater than the support seen in gaseous environments such as the thoracic cavity, *e.g.*, *intrathoracic pressure* (ITP) (66). IAP pushes against the spine and helps keep the torso upright, which is important for preventing lower-back injuries

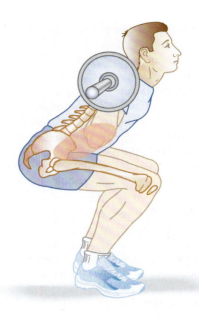

FIGURE 2.18 Intra-abdominal pressure. (Reprinted with permission from Harman E. Biomechanics of resistance exercise. In: Baechle T, Earle R, editors. *Essentials of Strength Training and Conditioning*. 3rd ed. Champaign (IL): Human Kinetics; 2008. 85 p.)

especially during exercises involving high-intensity trunk flexion, extension, and jumping (66,67) and during fatiguing back extension exercises (68). IAP tends to be high during hip/spine extension exercises such as the dead lift and during exercises that involve exertion while the hips are flexed such as the leg press and low pulley row (66). An exercise such as the bench press may result in higher ITP than IAP due to reactive forces from the diaphragm as the high forces produced by the upper body musculature in response to weight forces air toward the diaphragm (66). Both IAP and ITP have been shown to increase with heavier loads lifted (66,69). A study has shown that increasing IAP by up to 60% increased spinal stiffness up to 31% (70). Thus, methods used to increase IAP and ITP play a role in increasing postural stability and reducing risks of injury. Greater postural stability is essential for the optimal expression of strength and power.

Ways to Increase Intra-Abdominal Pressure

Because higher IAP provides a protective effect against lumbar spinal injuries, increasing IAP has important training ramifications. There are three ways to increase IAP during exercise and training: (a) trunk contraction and subsequent trunk muscle training, (b) breath holding, and (c) lifting belts. Contraction of abdominal (transversus abdominis, rectus abdominis, and external and internal obliques) and lumbar (erector spinae, paraspinal) muscles contribute greatly to the development of IAP (71). This technique, *i.e.*, *abdominal bracing*, is a more widely recommended technique than compressing just the transversus abdominis via "hollowing." Bracing should be performed during any exercise but should be emphasized during exercises which require greater spinal stability. In fact, a recent study has shown that bracing solely as a primary mode of training (*i.e.*, 5 sets of 10 repetitions performed 3 times per week for 8 weeks) can increase trunk muscle strength, power, maximal IAP, the rate of IAP generation, and internal oblique muscle thickness (72). Contraction and subsequent strengthening of the diaphragm via diaphragmatic breathing and muscles of the pelvic floor may also contribute to trunk stability as these structures form the upper and lower areas of the abdominal compartment (73). Consistent core training allows athletes to develop greater IAP and increase the rate of IAP development (74). Athletes with stronger trunk flexion strength (than untrained control subjects) can generate higher levels of IAP (75).

Breath holding, *e.g.*, a *Valsalva maneuver*, also results in an increased IAP at a level higher than what is seen during RT with normal breathing patterns (66). Air cannot escape the lungs and the glottis is closed, thereby creating torso rigidity. Although negative side effects are associated with the Valsalva maneuver (see Chapter 9), breath holding may be reflexive and has been shown to result in increased spine stability, high levels of IAP, and the IAP elevation may be more prominent in RT individuals (66,69,76). This is why many experienced lifters temporarily hold their breath during the most difficult area (sticking region) of a heavy exercise. Valsalva maneuvers are unavoidable at RT intensities of at least 80% of maximal strength and during sets where muscular exhaustion is rapidly approaching (69). Brief Valsalva maneuvers may be seen during ballistic, high power exercise as well. The use of Valsalva maneuvers in conjunction with remote muscle contraction and jaw clenching via mouth guards, *e.g.*, a phenomenon referred to as *concurrent activation potentiation*, has been shown to augment back squat and jump squat performance by 3%–32% (77). Thus, Valsalva maneuvers do have ergogenic benefits during strength and power activities despite the cardiovascular demands. Lastly, weight lifting belts increase IAP (78,79). However, caution must be used as overuse of lifting belts can actually weaken muscles and make it more difficult for core musculature to generate IAP over time.

Lifting Accessories

Lifting accessories have been developed to reduce the risk of injury and increase the efficiency of RT. Although these accessories provide substantial joint support and reduce injury risk, most strength athletes use them for their ergogenic potential. For example, many athletes use lifting straps and gym chalk to enhance grip during performance of heavy pulling exercises. Other training accessories are commonly used and are discussed in this section.

Lifting Belts

Many different types of lifting belts are sold on the market. Athletes use belts for support and for the assumed lower risk of back injuries. Lifting belts augment IAP during lifting by 13%–40% and reduce compressive forces on the back by ~6% (79). During performance of a near-maximal squat, belts were shown to increase the magnitude of IAP, peak rate of IAP, and IAP over time compared to performing the same exercise with no belt (80). Belts allow athletes to use more weight, perform more reps, and perform faster reps during exercises such as the squat and dead lift (78). The magnitude depends on the type and tightness of the belt as tighter belts are more supportive. Quadriceps muscle activity increases during the back squat when belts are used. In contrast, core muscle activation is lower with belt use as muscle activity was greater by 8%–24% in the rectus abdominis, 13%–44% in the external obliques, and 12%–23% in the erector spinae without a belt during the squat (79). It is important to recognize that belts should not be overused as they limit potential core strength development. It is recommended that lifting belts be used only during performance of exercises that involve trunk flexion/extension (squats, dead lift, bent-over row) with maximal or near-maximal weights. Powerlifters and strength athletes commonly use belts in competition but are used to a lesser extent by competitive weightlifters during performance of the Olympic lifts. Intense core training allows the musculature to increase strength and IAP-generating capacity, thus reducing the need to use a belt. Lastly, belts should only be used during a set and should be loosened or removed between sets as they reduce blood flow back to the heart and increase blood pressure (76).

Wraps

Some athletes use various types of wraps (or sleeves) on their knees, elbows, or wrists. Knee wraps can enhance performance of exercises involving knee extension by providing support that resists knee flexion and increasing the mechanical advantage. Elastic energy may be stored and used in addition to elastic force during the ascent phase of an exercise such as the squat and leg press. The magnitude may be dependent upon the type of wraps used, wrapping technique, the angle of knee flexion during wrapping, and tightness of the wraps. Thick, heavy wraps long in length with sufficient elasticity wrapped very tightly are thought to provide the most support. Some athletes anecdotally claim increased squat lifts of 50 lb or more. Gomes and colleagues (81) reported up to a 22% augmentation in maximal isometric squat force with use of knee wraps. Research indicates that wearing knee wraps during back squats reduces horizontal bar displacement and eccentric phase duration, increases vertical impulse, and power (82). They may lessen vastus lateralis muscle activity (compared to no wraps with the same loading) due to a mechanical carryover effect of the wraps (83). Elbow wraps are effective for reducing elbow pressure and enhancing performance of extension exercises (bench press, shoulder press). Wrist wraps reduce pressure on the wrist by limiting joint flexion and extension and allow for greater stability during exercises using heavy weights. Likewise, wraps should not be overused in order to maximize muscular involvement in the exercise.

Weightlifting Shoes

Different types of footwear have been used during RT. Although athletic shoes are acceptable under most conditions, weightlifting shoes may be advantageous for exercises such as the Olympic lifts and squats. Weightlifting shoes are designed with stiff, noncompressible soles, raised heels (~2.0–2.5 cm) relative to the forefoot, outsole with a high coefficient of friction, and metatarsal straps (to support the transverse arch) thereby assisting the lifter with balance and stability. During the back squat, they are purported to reduce forward lean and allow the lifter to maintain a more upright posture. One two-dimensional study showed that wearing weightlifting shoes produces less trunk forward displacement and a greater foot segment angle by ~3.5° (due to stiff sole and raised heel) compared to athletic shoes (84). However, a three-dimensional study failed to report significant kinematic differences between weightlifting and athletic shoes other than greater peak dorsiflexion angles with athletic shoes (85). Southwell and colleagues (86) compared squatting in weightlifting and athletic shoes but also during a barefoot condition in trained weightlifters and reported that greater moments at the knee were seen with both shoes and greater moments at the hip were seen barefoot. Barefoot squatting also produced less knee flexion but greater hip flexion ROM (and forward lean) during descent compared to athletic and weightlifting shoes. No differences were reported for spinal compression and shear force for any footwear condition. However, both shod conditions resulted in deeper squats compared to barefoot squatting. Another study reported more upright posture while squatting in weightlifting shoes that helped enable greater depth only in experienced lifters (87). Thus, it is unclear as to how much of a benefit weightlifting shoes may provide beyond athletic shoes but a more upright posture and better depth may be critical for advanced lifting goals. Barefoot or flat shoes such as *dead lift slippers* appear advantageous for stability and ROM enhancement during deadlifting.

Bench Press Shirts

A bench press shirt is very tight, supportive gear that several powerlifters use during competition and during the final stages of precompetition training to maximize performance and reduce the risk of injury. Bench press shirts can enhance 1 RM strength greatly. Although research is lacking, gains of at least 25–50 lb are expected, with some elite lifters suggesting increases of >100 lb. The amount of increase is dependent on the type (polyester, denim, canvas; single or double layer) and tightness of shirt used, biomechanics of the lifter, and prior experience of bench press shirt use. These shirts tend to provide the greatest support near full descent where the bar is close to the chest and favors lifters who use wide grips. One study found that bench press shirts enable the lifter to maintain a more efficient bar trajectory primarily in a vertical plane (88). Bench press shirts are tight enough to potentially cause bruising and require assistance from one or two experienced individuals to put on in a systematic manner. Powerlifters tend to start with a basic single-layer polyester shirt and progress with training. The tighter the shirt, the greater the support gained by the lifter. Athletes need to train with and accustom themselves to bench press shirts in order to maximize bench press performance. It is recommended that powerlifters use the shirt several times during the precompetition preparation phase.

The Slingshot

Given the difficulty of putting on and using a bench press shirt without trained assistants, another alternative has been developed. The "Slingshot" was developed by elite powerlifter Mark Bell. It consists of two elbow sleeves connected together medially so it can be applied anteriorly to both arms beyond the lifter's elbows. The stiff connecting fabric drapes across the chest during the exercise and restricts frontal plane movement of the arms thereby increasing the load lifted and reducing stress to the shoulders. It has been estimated that it could add 10%–15% to one's 1 RM bench press. A recent study showed that the Slingshot could add ~20.7 kg to a 1 RM bench press (89).

Lifting Suits

Lifting suits include super suits, briefs, and erector shirts. *Super suits* (or squat suits) and briefs are tight compression garments used primarily by powerlifters to enhance stability and performance of the squat and dead lift. The super suits extend from the upper quadriceps area to the upper abdomen with straps that are placed over the shoulders (similar to a singlet). Greater support is gained as the lifter descends and it assists the lifter in the "up" phase through the sticking region. The material stretches and stores elastic energy during descent and subsequently releases the elastic energy in addition to the elastic force developed during the ascent phase. Some lifters estimate at least a 50- to 60-lb increase in the squat, whereas some experienced lifters estimate >150 lb. The magnitude is dependent upon experience with the equipment and quadriceps and lumbar extension strength during the top of the ROM where the suit is less supportive. Blatnik et al. (90) showed that super suits increased velocity and power during the concentric phase of squats in elite powerlifters. Escamilla (91) stated that individuals with knee wraps and suits lifted an average of ~13% more weight than without. The mean total time needed to complete a repetition was almost half a second less when suits and wraps were used (2.82 s with gear; 3.29 s without gear). Erector shirts are the opposite of the bench press shirt in that the majority of the support is in the core. Lifters use erector shirts to maintain an erect posture during the squat and dead lift.

SUMMARY POINTS

- Biomechanics is a field that studies all aspects of motion, from the description of the motion (kinematics) to the underlying causes of motion (kinetics).
- Skeletal muscles produce greater force during ECC actions, followed by ISOM and CON actions.
- A relationship between muscle length and force exists where muscles are strongest near resting sarcomere lengths (where the optimal number of myofilament cross-bridges are formed) but weaken as the muscle shortens. At longer lengths, passive elements become more engaged and enhance muscle force production.
- When maximal intensity contractions are used, greatest muscle force is produced at slow velocities, whereas less force is produced at fast velocities.
- Muscle architectural changes, *e.g.*, in a pennate muscle's angle of pennation and/or fascicle length, take place during training that enhances muscular strength.
- Strength and speed performance is based, in part, upon stature, leverage, and mechanical advantage, *e.g.*, the ratio of the moment arm of force to the moment arm of resistance.
- Torque production changes throughout joint ROM. An ascending-descending curve is seen with single-joint movements, an ascending curve is seen with pushing movements, and descending curves are seen with pulling movements.
- Friction is a critical component to force production and stability.
- The development of intra-abdominal pressure is important for relieving spinal stress during lifting.
- Various lifting accessories have been developed that can reduce the risk of injury but also can significantly enhance lifting performance.

REVIEW QUESTIONS

1. A muscle action characteristic of muscle shortening is a(n) _____ muscle action
   a. Eccentric
   b. Concentric
   c. Isokinetic
   d. Isometric

2. The biceps brachii is an example of a(n) _____ muscle
   a. Pennate
   b. Fusiform
   c. Quadrilateral
   d. Triangular

3. The shoulder press exercise displays a(n)
   a. Ascending-descending strength curve
   b. Ascending strength curve
   c. Descending strength curve
   d. Isometric strength curve

4. During isokinetic maximal strength testing, which of the following velocities would result in the greatest muscle torque produced?
   a. $30°\cdot s^{-1}$
   b. $90°\cdot s^{-1}$
   c. $150°\cdot s^{-1}$
   d. $300°\cdot s^{-1}$

5. Muscle tension is reduced at short muscle lengths primarily because
   a. The stretch-shortening cycle is maximally engaged
   b. Actin filaments are extended excessively thereby making it difficult to reach a large number of myosin heads
   c. Actin filaments slide past each other thereby reducing the number of active sites available to bind with myosin heads
   d. No actin-myosin cross-bridges can be formed

6. The perpendicular distance between the force's line of action to the fulcrum is known as a(n)
   a. Torque
   b. Mechanical advantage
   c. Inertia
   d. Moment arm

7. Which of the following scenarios would decrease an individual's stability?
   a. Increasing the level of friction between the feet and the ground
   b. Lowering the size of the base support
   c. Lowering the center of gravity
   d. Increasing the mass of the individual

8. The branch of biomechanics that deals with the forces that cause motion is kinetics.
   a. T
   b. F

9. Stretch-shortening cycle activity is highest in slow-twitch muscle fibers.
   a. T
   b. F

10. The lower extremity muscle with the largest PCSA is the sartorius.
    a. T
    b. F

11. Muscle hypertrophy can increase the angle of pennation at rest in a pennate muscle.
    a. T
    b. F

12. Increasing the length of the resistance arm increases mechanical advantage.
    a. T
    b. F

13. Choking up on a baseball bat increases the moment of inertia.
    a. T
    b. F

REFERENCES

1. Hadi G, Akkus H, Harbili E. Three-dimensional kinematic analysis of the snatch technique for lifting different barbell weights. *J Strength Cond Res*. 2012;26:1568–76.
2. Van Hooren B, Zolotarjova J. The difference between countermovement and squat jump performance: a review of underlying mechanisms with practical applications. *J Strength Cond Res*. 2017;31:2011–20.
3. Bobbert MF, Casius LJR. Is the effect of a countermovement on jump height due to active state development? *Med Sci Sports Exerc*. 2005;37:440–6.
4. Newton RU. Biomechanics of conditioning exercises. In: Chandler TJ, Brown LE, editors. *Conditioning for Strength and Performance*. Philadelphia, PA: Lippincott Williams & Wilkins; 2008. p. 77–93.
5. McGuigan MR, Doyle TL, Newton M, Edwards DJ, Nimphius S, Newton RU. Eccentric utilization ratio: effect of sport and phase of training. *J Strength Cond Res*. 2006;20:992–5.
6. Suchomel TJ, Sole CJ, Stone MH. Comparison of methods that assess lower-body stretch-shortening cycle utilization. *J Strength Cond Res*. 2016;30:547–54.
7. Wilson GJ, Elliott BC, Wood GA. The effect on performance of imposing a delay during a stretch-shorten cycle movement. *Med Sci Sports Exerc*. 1991;23:364–70.
8. Perez-Castilla A, Comfort P, McMahon JJ, Pestana-Melero FL, Garcia-Ramos A. Comparison of the force-, velocity-, and power-time curves between the concentric-only and eccentric-concentric bench press exercises. *J Strength Cond Res*. 2020;34(6):1618–24.
9. Power K, Behm D, Cahill F, Carroll M, Young W. An acute bout of static stretching: effects on force and jumping performance. *Med Sci Sports Exerc*. 2004;36:1389–96.
10. Jaric S. Force-velocity relationship of muscle performing multijoint maximum performance tasks. *Int J Sports Med*. 2015;36:699–704.
11. Lieber RL. *Skeletal Muscle Structure and Function: Implications for Rehabilitation and Sport Medicine*. Baltimore, MD: Williams and Wilkins; 1992.
12. Cormie P, McGuigan MR, Newton RU. Adaptations in athletic performance after ballistic power versus strength training. *Med Sci Sports Exerc*. 2010;42:1582–98.
13. Cormie P, McGuigan MR, Newton RU. Developing maximal neuromuscular power: part 1—biological basis of maximal power production. *Sports Med*. 2011;41:17–38.
14. Schilling BK, Falvo MJ, Chiu LZF. Force-velocity, impulse-momentum relationships: Implications for efficacy of purposely slow resistance training. *J Sports Sci Med*. 2008;7:299–304.
15. Keeler LK, Finkelstein LH, Miller W, Fernhall B. Early-phase adaptations of traditional-speed vs. superslow resistance training

on strength and aerobic capacity in sedentary individuals. *J Strength Cond Res*. 2001;15:309–14.
16. Keogh JWL, Wilson GJ, Weatherby RP. A cross-sectional comparison of different resistance training techniques in the bench press. *J Strength Cond Res*. 1999;13:247–58.
17. Lieber RL, Ward SR. Skeletal muscle design to meet functional demands. *Phil Trans R Soc Lond B Biol Sci*. 2011;366:1466–76.
18. Aagaard P, Andersen JL, Dyhre-Poulsen P, et al. A mechanism for increased contractile strength of human pennate muscle in response to strength training: changes in muscle architecture. *J Physiol*. 2001;534:613–23.
19. Kawakami Y, Abe T, Fukunaga T. Muscle-fiber pennation angles are greater in hypertrophied than in normal muscles. *J Appl Physiol*. 1993;74:2740–4.
20. Kawakami Y, Abe T, Kuno SY, Fukunaga T. Training-induced changes in muscle architecture and specific tension. *Eur J Appl Physiol Occup Physiol*. 1995;72:37–43.
21. Azizi E, Brainerd EL, Roberts TJ. Variable gearing in pennate muscles. *Proc Natl Acad Sci U S A*. 2008;105:1745–50.
22. Reeves ND, Narici MV. Behavior of human muscle fascicles during shortening and lengthening contractions in vivo. *J Appl Physiol*. 2003;95:1090–6.
23. Timmins RG, Ruddy JD, Presland J, Maniar N, Shield AJ, Williams MD, Opar DA. Architectural changes of the biceps femoris long head after concentric or eccentric training. *Med Sci Sports Exerc*. 2016;48:499–508.
24. Kanehisa H, Nagareda H, Kawakami Y, et al. Effects of equivolume isometric training programs comprising medium or high resistance on muscle size and strength. *Eur J Appl Physiol*. 2002;87:112–9.
25. Pelzer T, Ullrich B, Pfeiffer M. Periodization effects during short-term resistance training with equated exercise variables in females. *Eur J Appl Physiol*. 2017;117:441–54.
26. Reeves ND, Maganaris CN, Longo S, Narici MV. Differential adaptations to eccentric versus conventional resistance training in older humans. *Exp Physiol*. 2009;94:825–33.
27. Seynnes OR, de Boer M, Narici MV. Early skeletal muscle hypertrophy and architectural changes in response to high-intensity resistance training. *J Appl Physiol*. 2007;102:368–73.
28. Storey A, Wong S, Smith HK, Marshall P. Divergent muscle functional and architectural responses to two successive high intensity resistance exercise sessions in competitive weightlifters and resistance trained adults. *Eur J Appl Physiol*. 2012;112:3629–39.
29. Coratella G, Beato M, Milanese C, et al. Specific adaptations in performance and muscle architecture after weighted jump-squat vs. body mass squat jump training in recreational soccer players. *J Strength Cond Res*. 2018;32:921–9.
30. Ema R, Wakahara T, Miyamoto N, Kanehisa H, Kawakami Y. Inhomogeneous architectural changes of the quadriceps femoris induced by resistance training. *Eur J Appl Physiol*. 2013;113:2691–703.
31. Blazevich AJ, Cannavan D, Coleman DR, Horne S. Influence of concentric and eccentric resistance training on architectural adaptation in human quadriceps muscles. *J Appl Physiol*. 2007;103:1565–75.
32. Franchi MV, Atherton PJ, Reeves ND, et al. Architectural, functional and molecular responses to concentric and eccentric loading in human skeletal muscle. *Acta Physiol (Oxf)*. 2014;210:642–54.

33. Potier TG, Alexander CM, Seynnes OR. Effects of eccentric strength training on biceps femoris muscle architecture and knee joint range of movement. *Eur J Appl Physiol.* 2009;105:939–44.

34. Freitas SR, Mendes B, LeSant G, Andrade RJ, Nordez A, Milanovic Z. Can chronic stretching change the muscle-tendon mechanical properties? A review. *Scand J Med Sci Sports.* 2018;28:794–806.

35. Luteberget LS, Rasstad T, Seynnes O, Spencer M. Effect of traditional and resisted sprint training in highly trained female handball players. *Int J Sports Physiol Perform.* 2015;10:642–7.

36. Alegre LM, Jimenez F, Gonzalo-Orden JM, Martin-Acero R, Aguado X. Effects of dynamic resistance training on fascicle length and isometric strength. *J Sports Sci.* 2006;24:501–8.

37. Timmins RG, Bourne MN, Shield AJ, Williams MD, Lorenzen C, Opar DA. Short biceps femoris fascicles and eccentric knee flexor weakness increase the risk of hamstring injury in elite football (soccer): a prospective cohort study. *Br J Sports Med.* 2016;50:1524–35.

38. Kearns CF, Abe T, Brechue WF. Muscle enlargement in sumo wrestlers includes increased muscle fascicle length. *Eur J Appl Physiol.* 2000;83:289–96.

39. Blazevich AJ, Gill ND, Deans N, Zhou S. Lack of human muscle architectural adaptation after short-term strength training. *Muscle Nerve.* 2007;35:78–86.

40. Guex K, Degache F, Morisod C, Sailly M, Millet GP. Hamstring architectural and functional adaptations following long vs short muscle length eccentric training. *Front Biol.* 2016;7:340. doi: 10.3389/phys.2016.00340.

41. Presland JD, Timmins RG, Boune MN, Williams MD, Opar DA. The effect of Nordic hamstring exercise training volume on biceps femoris long head architectural adaptation. *Scand J Med Sci Sports.* 2018;28:1775–83.

42. Blazevich AJ, Gill ND, Bronks R, Newton RU. Training-specific muscle architecture adaptation after 5-wk training in athletes. *Med Sci Sports Exerc.* 2003;35:2013–22.

43. Kanehisa H, Muraoka Y, Kawakami Y, Fukunaga T. Fascicle arrangements of vastus lateralis and gastrocnemius muscles in highly trained soccer players and swimmers of both genders. *Int J Sports Med.* 2003;24:90–5.

44. Abe T, Kumagai K, Brechue WF. Fascicle length of leg muscles is greater in sprinters than distance runners. *Med Sci Sports Exerc.* 2000;32:1125–9.

45. Kumagai K, Abe T, Brechue WF, Ryushi T, Takano S, Mizuno M. Sprint performance is related to muscle fascicle length in male 100-m sprinters. *J Appl Physiol.* 2000;88:811–6.

46. Mangine GT, Fukuda DH, LaMonica MB, et al. Influence of gender and muscle architecture asymmetry on jump and sprint performance. *J Sports Sci Med.* 2014;13:904–11.

47. Nasirzade A, Ehsanbakhsh A, Ilbeygi S, Sobhkhiz A, Argavani H, Aliakbari M. Relationship between sprint performance of front crawl swimming and muscle fascicle length in young swimmers. *J Sports Sci Med.* 2014;13:550–6.

48. Van der Zwaard S, van der Laarse WJ, Weide G, et al. Critical determinants of combined sprint and endurance performance: an integrative analysis from muscle fiber to the human body. *FASEB J.* 2018;32:2110–23.

49. Hamill J, Knutzen KM. *Biomechanical Basis of Human Movement.* 3rd ed. Philadelphia (PA): Wolters Kluwer Lippincott Williams & Wilkins; 2009. p. 411–61.

50. McArdle WD, Katch FI, Katch VL. *Exercise Physiology: Energy, Nutrition, and Human Performance.* 6th ed. Philadelphia (PA): Lippincott Williams & Wilkins; 2007.

51. Ackland TR, de Ridder JH. Proportionality. In: Ackland TR, Elliott BC, Bloomfield J, editors. *Applied Anatomy and Biomechanics in Sport.* 2nd ed. Champaign (IL): Human Kinetics; 2009. p. 87–101.

52. Elliott BC, Wilson GJ, Kerr GK. A biomechanical analysis of the sticking region in the bench press. *Med Sci Sports Exerc.* 1989;21:450–62.

53. Kraemer WJ, Fry AC, Ratamess NA, French DN. Strength testing: development and evaluation of methodology. In: Maud PJ, Foster C, editors. *Physiological Assessments of Human Performance.* 2nd ed. Champaign (IL): Human Kinetics; 2006. p. 119–50.

54. Kulig K, Andrews JG, Hay JG. Human strength curves. *Exerc Sports Sci Rev.* 1984;12:417–66.

55. Murphy K, Curry EJ, Matzkin EG. Barefoot running: does it prevent injuries? *Sports Med.* 2013;43:1131–8.

56. Smith MS, Dyson RJ, Hale T, Janaway L. Development of a boxing dynamometer and its punch force discrimination efficacy. *J Sports Sci.* 2000;18:445–50.

57. Broglio SP, Surma T, Ashton-Miller JA. High school and collegiate football athlete concussions: a biomechanical review. *Ann Biomed Eng.* 2012;40:37–46.

58. Gabbett TJ, Jenkins DG, Abernethy B. Physical demands of professional rugby league training and competition using microtechnology. *J Sci Med Sport.* 2012;15:80–6.

59. Contreras B. Force vector training. https://bretcontreras.com/load-vector-training-lvt/

60. Newton RU, Doan B, Meese M, Conroy B, Black K, Sebastianelli W, Kraemer W. Interaction of wrestling shoe and competition surface: effects on coefficient of friction with implications for injury. *Sports Biomech.* 2002;1:157–66.

61. Dragoo JL, Braun HJ. The effect of playing surface on injury rate: a review of the current literature. *Sports Med.* 2010;40:981–90.

62. Xiao X, Hao W, Li X, Wan B, Shan G. The influence of landing mat composition on ankle injury risk during a gymnastic landing: a biomechanical quantification. *Acta Bioeng Biomech.* 2017;19:105–13.

63. Andre MJ, Fry AC, Bradford LA, Buhr KW. Determination of friction and pulling forces during a weighted sled pull. *J Strength Cond Res.* 2013;27:1175–8.

64. Cross MR, Tinwala F, Lenetsky S, Samozino P, Brughelli M, Morin JB. Determining friction and effective loading for sled sprinting. *J Sports Sci.* 2017;35:2198–203.

65. Arandjelovic O. Does cheating pay: the role of externally supplied momentum on muscular force in resistance exercise. *Eur J Appl Physiol.* 2013;113:135–45.

66. Harman EA, Frykman PN, Clagett ER, Kraemer WJ. Intra-abdominal and intra-thoracic pressures during lifting and jumping. *Med Sci Sports Exerc.* 1988;20:195–201.

67. Cholewicki J, Juluru K, McGill SM. Intra-abdominal pressure mechanism for stabilizing the lumbar spine. *J Biomech.* 1999;32:13–7.

68. Essendrop M, Schibye B, Hye-Knudsen C. Intra-abdominal pressure increases during exhausting back extension in humans. *Eur J Appl Physiol.* 2002;87:167–73.

69. Hackett DA, Chow CM. The Valsalva maneuver: its effect on intra-abdominal pressure and safety issues during resistance exercise. *J Strength Cond Res.* 2013;27:2338–45.

70. Hodges PW, Eriksson AE, Shirley D, Gandevia SC. Intra-abdominal pressure increases stiffness of the lumbar spine. *J Biomech.* 2005; 38:1873–80.

71. Cresswell AG, Grundstrom H, Thorstensson A. Observations on intra-abdominal pressure and patterns of abdominal intra-muscular activity in man. *Acta Physiol Scand.* 1992;144:409–18.

72. Tayashiki K, Maeo S, Usui S, Miyamoto N, Kanehisa H. Effect of abdominal bracing training on strength and power of trunk and lower limb muscles. *Eur J Appl Physiol.* 2016;116:1703–13.

73. Park H, Han D. The effect of the correlation between the contraction of the pelvic floor muscles and diaphragmatic motion during breathing. *J Phys Ther Sci.* 2015;27:2113–5.

74. Cresswell AG, Blake PL, Thorstensson A. The effect of an abdominal muscle training program on intra-abdominal pressure. *Scand J Rehabil Med.* 1994;26:79–86.

75. Kawabata M, Shima N, Hamada H, Nakamura I, Nishizono H. Changes in intra-abdominal pressure and spontaneous breath volume by magnitude of lifting effort: highly trained athletes versus healthy men. *Eur J Appl Physiol.* 2010;109:279–86.

76. McGill SM, Norman RW, Sharratt MT. The effect of an abdominal belt on trunk muscle activity and intra-abdominal pressure during squat lifts. *Ergonomics.* 1990;33:147–60.

77. Ebben WP, Kaufmann CE, Fauth ML, Petushek EJ. Kinetic analysis of concurrent activation potentiation during back squats and jump squats. *J Strength Cond Res.* 2010;24:1515–9.

78. Lander JE, Hundley JR, Simonton RL. The effectiveness of weight-belts during multiple repetitions of the squat exercise. *Med Sci Sports Exerc.* 1992;24:603–9.

79. Lander JE, Simonton RL, Giacobbe JKF. The effectiveness of weight-belts during the squat exercise. *Med Sci Sports Exerc.* 1990;22:117–26.

80. Harman EA, Rosenstein RM, Frykman PN, Nigro GA. Effects of a belt on intra-abdominal pressure during weight lifting. *Med Sci Sports Exerc.* 1989;21:186–90.

81. Gomes WA, Serpa EP, Soares EG, et al. Acute effects on maximal isometric force with and without knee wrap during squat exercise. *Int J Sports Sci* 2014;4:47–9.

82. Lake JP, Carden PJC, Shorter KA. Wearing knee wraps affects mechanical output and performance characteristics of back squat exercise. *J Strength Cond Res.* 2012;26:2844–9.

83. Gomes WA, Brown LE, Soares EG, et al. Kinematic and sEMG analysis of the back squat at different intensities with and without knee wraps. *J Strength Cond Res.* 2015;29:2482–7.

84. Sato K, Fortenbaugh D, Hydock DS. Kinematic changes using weightlifting shoes on barbell back squat. *J Strength Cond Res.* 2012;26:28–33.

85. Whitting JW, Meir RA, Crowley-McHattan ZJ, Holding RC. Influence of footwear type on barbell back squat using 50, 70, and 90% of one repetition maximum: a biomechanical analysis. *J Strength Cond Res.* 2016;30:1085–92.

86. Southwell DJ, Petersen SA, Bleach TAC, Graham RB. The effects of squatting footwear on three-dimensional lower limb and spine kinetics. *J Electromyogr Kinesiol.* 2016;31:111–8.

87. Legg HS, Glaister M, Cleather DJ, Goodwin JE. The effect of weightlifting shoes on the kinetics and kinematics of the back squat. *J Sports Sci.* 2017;35:508–15.

88. Silver T, Fortenbaugh D, Williams R. Effects of the bench press shirt on sagittal bar path. *J Strength Cond Res.* 2009;23:1125–8.

89. Dugdale JH, Hunter AM, DiVirgilio TG, MacGregor LJ, Hamilton DL. Influence of the "Slingshot" bench press training aid on bench press kinematics and neuromuscular activity in competitive powerlifters. *J Strength Cond Res.* 2019;33:327–36.

90. Blatnik JA, Skinner JW, McBride JM. Effect of supportive equipment on force, velocity, and power in the squat. *J Strength Cond Res.* 2012;26:3204–8.

91. Escamilla R. The use of powerlifting aids in the squat. *Powerlifting USA.* 1988;12:14–5.

CHAPTER 3

Basic Nutrition

OBJECTIVES

After completing this chapter, you will be able to:

- Discuss the importance of proper nutrition in optimizing health and performance
- Discuss the functions of macro- and micronutrients and their roles in health and performance
- Discuss the importance of hydration in maintaining health and achieving optimal performance
- Discuss the importance of the microbiome and probiotics
- Discuss the rationale, benefits, and recommendations for sports supplements
- Discuss some basic pre- and postworkout/competition nutritional strategies

Nutrition is the science that studies the relationship of nutrient consumption to optimal health, development, and performance. It involves the ingestion, digestion, absorption, and metabolism of nutrients. Food, beverages, and sport supplements are the carriers of nutrients. Nutrition and athletic performance are closely linked. In fact, training, diet/nutrition, and recovery are all equally important when it comes to optimizing athletic performance (Fig. 3.1). A deficit in one, *e.g.*, nutrition, will have negative ramifications upon the others. *Proper nutrition* entails utilizing a diet that supplies essential nutrients needed to carry out normal tissue growth and repair, while providing the energy needs of the athlete to meet the demands of training and competition. In contrast, *malnutrition*, *e.g.*, improper nutrition caused by inadequate, excessive, or imbalanced nutrient intake, poor nutrient absorption, and abnormal metabolism, may compromise recovery, adaptation, and ultimately athletic performance (1). Failure to consider nutrition as an integral component of the S&C program will increase health risks and result in poor performances. Well-nourished athletes perform better, recover more quickly from soreness and injuries, and derive more performance-improving benefits from training. A number of dietary strategies can work in athletes. In some ways, diets are like training programs in that each individual athlete will respond to a specific plan. As training programs differ between off-, pre-, and in-season periods, the athlete's personal nutrition plan will change to accommodate the differences in activity. Comfort is gained with experimental progress and the registered dietician or nutrition counselor will develop plans that work best for them within a guise of scientific nutritional guidelines. Thus, nutritional programs should be individualized and tailored to the needs and environment of the athlete. In this chapter, basic nutrition is discussed with the aim of helping the coach and athlete understand key nutritional strategies related to improving exercise performance and health.

Nutrients

Nutrients are substances found in food that provide energy, regulate metabolism, are needed for growth and repair of body tissue, and are needed for maintenance of life. *Macronutrients* are large nutrients including carbohydrates, proteins, fats, and water. In addition, alcohol may be considered a macronutrient as it supplies 7 kcal·g^{-1} of energy, but these are viewed as "empty" calories with little nutritional value plus the depressant effects are detrimental to the athlete. *Micronutrients* are smaller nutrients such as vitamins and minerals. Both types are needed in quantities to satisfy the training demands of the athlete. Athletes require nutrients from multiple sources as no single food contains all required nutrients. Obtaining nutrients from food and beverages is the primary goal. Over the years, recommendations for selecting foods and servings have been updated. For example, in 1992, the Food Guide Pyramid was used as a guide where recommendations included suggested servings from dairy (2–3 servings), fruits (2–4 servings), vegetables

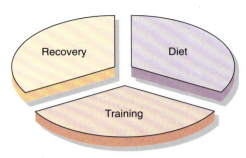

FIGURE 3.1 Components to building the complete athlete.

(3–5 servings), grains (6–11 servings), and meat (2–3 servings) sources predominately with fats, oils, and sweets consumed sparingly. In 2005, the MyPyramid Food Guidance System was introduced and further expanded upon the Food Guide Pyramid. In 2011, MyPlate (Fig. 3.2) was introduced updating the dietary guidelines for Americans and used in present day.

Nutrient balance is critical to optimal sports nutrition. Nutrient deficiencies can result in malnutrition or poor health and performance. In addition, some nutrients biochemically work in synergy whereby a deficiency in one nutrient could impact the biochemistry of another. The best strategy for maintaining nutrient balance is to eat a wide variety of foods, regularly consume fresh fruits and vegetables, avoid intake of few foods day after day, and consume nutritional supplements when necessary. Some athletes may be deficient in certain nutrients, and supplementation can help correct the deficiency. With the rigors of off-season training, and in-season training, practice, and competition, the nutrient needs of the athlete increases greatly. In order to get adequate dietary intake of all essential nutrients, athletes must increase the amount of food and beverages consumed as athletes have greater nutritional needs than the average individual. This may be a difficult task especially during the midst of heavy training, practice, and a competition schedule. Added time constraints from school and/or work may exist thereby leaving the athlete some degree of difficulty in maintaining a consistent meal plan. Training, practice, and competition, especially in hot, humid weather, have another potential antagonizing effect of reducing the athlete's appetite.

Energy nutrients provide fuel for cellular work. Carbohydrates, proteins, and fats provide carbon used for energy production. Energy is measured in *kilocalories*, *e.g.*, the heat required to increase the temperature of 1 g of water by 1°C. Often, the term "calorie" is used synonymously with kilocalorie (kcal) in nutrition because they represent 1,000 times the calorie unit used in physics. Caloric balance is determined by intake versus output. If the athlete consumes more kcals than expended than body weight can increase. Likewise, if the athlete expends more energy than kcals consumed, then a decrease in body weight may occur. Therefore, maintaining an energy-balanced state or deviating from it only slightly is an important strategy for both body weight and body composition maintenance. The term "empty calories" is used to describe food or beverages with little nutritional value consisting mostly of sugars, fats or oils, or alcohol-containing beverages. Athletes involved in moderate levels of intense training or high volume training may expend 600–1,200 kcal or more per hour during exercise; or 2,000–7,000 kcal·d^{-1} for a 50–100 kg athlete (2). Some elite athletes may expend >12,000 kcal·d^{-1}, and this value could be higher depending on the intensity and volume of training as well as the size of the athlete (2). It can be very difficult for athletes to meet these energy demands solely through consuming a well-balanced diet. Analysis of the diets of some athletes have revealed a susceptibility to negative energy intake which could lead to immunosuppression, loss of lean tissue mass, reduced quality of sleep, inadequate recovery and risk of overtraining, and psychological stress (2–4). Thus, the use of nutrition supplements has been commonly used to help meet energy and nutrient demands.

Dietary Reference Intakes

The Institute of Medicine has published the **Dietary Reference Intakes** (DRI) to establish the most recent nutrient needs of the population. It was introduced in 1997 to extend the recommended dietary allowance (RDA). The objective is to provide a template of acceptable nutrient intake levels for the average healthy person. The macro- and micronutrient needs of athletes may vary given the extensive training and competition demands. It comprises five categories of nutrient intake measures:

- *Recommended dietary allowance* (RDA) — the average daily nutrient intake sufficient to meet the requirements of 97.5% of the healthy population in each life stage and sex.
- *Estimated average requirement* (EAR) — average daily nutrient intake estimated to meet the requirements of 50% of the healthy population in each life stage and sex.

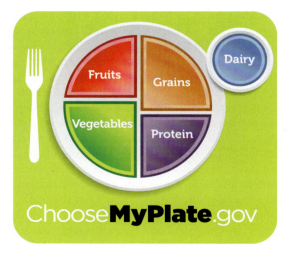

FIGURE 3.2 MyPlate. (Reprinted from https://www.choosemyplate.gov/)

- *Adequate intake* (AI) — the recommended average daily intake based on estimations when RDA values are not established.
- *Tolerable upper intake level* (UL) — highest average daily nutrient intake likely to not pose a health risk in 97.5% of the healthy population in each life stage and sex.
- *Acceptable macronutrient distribution range* (AMDR) — recommended macronutrient intake as a percentage of daily energy intake, *e.g.*, 45%–65% kcal from carbohydrates, 20%–35% kcal from fats, and 10%–35% kcal from protein (5).

Carbohydrates

Carbohydrates, which are categorized as monosaccharides, disaccharides, and oligosaccharides/polysaccharides, are macromolecules consisting of carbon, hydrogen, and oxygen atoms. *Monosaccharides* are basic 6-carbon carbohydrate units that consist of glucose, fructose, and galactose. Although monosaccharides are the simplest form of carbohydrates, only glucose can be used by muscles for energy. Therefore, fructose and galactose must be converted to glucose in the liver prior to use. *Disaccharides* consist of two monosaccharides. Both di- and monosaccharides are considered simple sugars based on their structures and ease of breakdown. Disaccharides include sucrose (glucose-plus-fructose), lactose (glucose-plus-galactose), and maltose (glucose-plus-glucose). Sucrose is the most commonly consumed disaccharide in the United States, as it is contained in table sugar and honey. Lactose is mostly found in milk, and maltose is found in breakfast cereals. *Oligosaccharides* consist of 3–9 monosaccharides, while *polysaccharides* consist of more than 10 monosaccharides (Fig. 3.3).

Polysaccharides include starch, glycogen, and fiber and can be digestible (starch, dextrins, and glycogen) or indigestible (cellulose, hemicellulose, pectin, gums, and mucilages). Starch is a complex carbohydrate found in abundance in grain products (*e.g.*, pasta, cereal, rice, and bread), and corn. *Glycogen* is the stored form of carbohydrates in humans and is very important for rapid use of glucose during high-intensity exercise. Most glycogen is stored in skeletal muscle (300–500 g). However, some glycogen (75–100 g) is stored in the liver (*e.g.*, values seen in the average 70 kg male), which is crucial to increasing blood sugar levels during exercise. Fiber (both soluble and insoluble) is indigestible, so the intake of fiber enhances the excretion of fats and other substances that can have a negative impact on health (*i.e.*, cholesterol) and improves blood sugar control. Diets higher in fiber (25–35 g·d^{-1}) may reduce hunger as well as the risk of gastrointestinal disease, cardiovascular disease, and various forms of cancer. The DRI for fiber ranges from 21 to 29 g·d^{-1} for women and 30 to 38 g·d^{-1} in men depending on age (6). Good food sources of fiber include fruits, vegetables, legumes, nuts, beans, and grain products.

Carbohydrates perform many functions critical to optimal performance and athletic success (Table 3.1). Blood glucose level reaches its peak ~1 hour after a meal and returns

Table 3.1 Functions of Carbohydrates

- Major source of energy for optimal exercise performance and stored energy in the form of glycogen
- The predominant source of energy for the central nervous system
- Maintenance of cell structure and integrity
- Enhance function of the immune system
- Structural component of genetic material (DNA and RNA)
- Regulate lipid metabolism, amino acid metabolism, and protein synthesis and breakdown by stimulating the secretion of the anabolic hormone *insulin*
- Increased thermogenesis

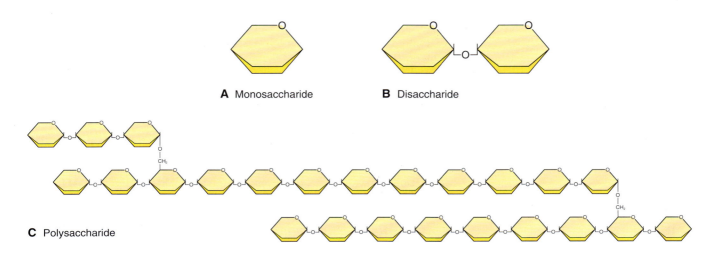

FIGURE 3.3 A–C. Structure of carbohydrates.

to premeal levels about 2 hours after in healthy individuals (7). Carbohydrates provide 4 kcal·g^{-1} of energy in the human body. The average carbohydrate intake in the United States is 200–300 g·d^{-1} (800–1,200 kcal) and fiber is 10–15 g·d^{-1} (8). However, athletes require greater carbohydrate intake to meet the demands of training while maximizing recovery. The recommended intake of carbohydrate as percentage of total caloric intake is 45%–65% of total calories for athletes (8) largely in the form of complex carbohydrates. However, this recommendation can be flexible as athletes may perform well on a wide spectrum of dietary carbohydrate intakes. Often, athletic carbohydrate intake recommendations are relative to body mass. Athletes participating in moderately intense training (2–3 h·d^{-1}, 5–6 d training frequency) may require 5–8 g CHOs kg body mass^{-1}·d^{-1} and those athletes participating in intense, high-volume training (3–6 h·d^{-1}, possible multiple workouts per day, 5–6 d training frequency) may require 8–10 g CHOs kg body mass^{-1}·d^{-1} to maintain glycogen stores (2,9). Others have recommended high carbohydrate intake in endurance athletes, i.e., 8–12 g CHOs kg body mass^{-1}·d^{-1} (5,6,10). It has been recommended that strength and power athletes consume 4–7 g CHOs kg body mass^{-1}·d^{-1} (5,6,10,11). The American College of Sports Medicine (12) recommends that athletes consume 3–12 g CHOs kg body mass^{-1}·d^{-1} to perform optimally and recover in between workouts (12). However, the range is dependent on the intensity and volume of exercise as well as other environmental factors where the recommendations are as follows (12):

- 3–5 g·kg BM·d^{-1} for low-intensity exercise
- 5–7 g·kg BM·d^{-1} for moderate-intensity exercise (~1 h·d^{-1})
- 6–10 g·kg BM·d^{-1} for moderate- to high-intensity endurance training (1–3 h·d^{-1})
- 8–12 g·kg BM·d^{-1} for extreme exercise of 4–5 h·d^{-1}

Adequate carbohydrate intake on the days leading up to competition is important for maximizing muscle glycogen stores. Proper intake ensures that muscle glycogen is restored from previous workouts, especially if the athlete tapers prior to the competition. A high carbohydrate diet or "carbo loading" increase muscle and liver glycogen content for ~3 days after loading more so than a normal diet (see Chapter 8). The consumption of carbohydrates within hours of endurance training/competition is important for increasing blood-sugar levels and possibly glycogen content (depending on the timing, type, amount, etc.). Carbohydrate supplementation during endurance events of at least moderate intensity or during long competitions lasting at least 90 minutes appears to positively affect sports performance. Carbohydrate supplementation during prolonged exercise can maintain blood sugar levels, spare muscle and liver glycogen, and promote glycogen synthesis (i.e., during rest periods between intermittent bouts or periods of low-intensity activity), in addition to assisting with hydration (see Chapter 17). Carbohydrates consumed can be used at a rate of ~1.0–1.1 g·min^{-1} (2). Different types of carbohydrates are oxidized at different rates in skeletal muscle such that combinations of glucose and sucrose or maltodextrin and fructose (with a ratio of 1.0–1.2 maltodextrin to 0.8–1.0 fructose) promote

greater rates of oxidation than individual carbohydrates (2). Post exercise or competition, carbohydrate intake is aimed at restoring muscle and liver glycogen and augmenting recovery (see Chapter 8). Thus, for acute carbohydrate loading strategies prior to and during exercise, the ACSM recommends the following (12):

- 7–12 g·kg BM·d^{-1} for 1 day prior to competition for events <90 minutes
- 10–12 g·kg BM·d^{-1} for 36–48 hours prior to competition for events >90 minutes
- 1–4 g·kg BM for 1–4 hours before exercise longer than 60 minutes
- None needed during brief exercise <45 minutes
- Small amounts during intense exercise 45–75 minutes
- 30–60 g·h^{-1} during 1–2.5 hours of endurance or "stop and go" exercise
- Up to 90 g·h^{-1} during ultra-endurance events >2.5–3 hours

The Glycemic Index and Glycemic Load

The **glycemic index** (GI) is a reference system tested in isolation (based on a standardized amount of glucose) pertaining to the elevation in blood sugar and insulin in response within a 2-hour period to dietary food and beverage consumption. The **glycemic load** (GL) is based on the total carbohydrate content of a serving of food instead of on a standardized glucose reference point. The GL equals the GI multiplied by the carbohydrate content. The GL has low, medium, and high classifications. The GI has important ramifications for the time of food consumption prior to, and/or during, exercise, as well as for appetite control. The index consists of averaged values based on high-, moderate-, and low-index foods. For example, glucose has an index value of 100. This value indicates that a rapid increase in blood glucose will occur. Foods with a high GI (>70) result in rapid elevations in blood sugar (Table 3.2). The potential advantage to the athlete here is that the rapid increase in blood glucose is readily available for "quick" energy during exercise or for immediate postexercise recovery with high rates of glycogen resynthesis. The disadvantage is that consuming high GI foods separate from exercise may cause high insulin spikes, rapid fluctuations in blood sugar concentrations, hunger sensations, and fatigue. Some examples of high-glycemic foods include pancakes, baked potatoes, pretzels, and some fruit bars and cereals. Moderate-glycemic foods (56–69) increase blood sugar at a slower rate than high-index foods and beverages. Some examples of moderate-glycemic foods include doughnuts, muffins, candy bars, and rice. Low-glycemic foods (<55) raise blood-sugar levels more slowly than moderate- and high-index foods. Some examples include legumes, some fruits and vegetables, and yogurt. Although some studies indicated that a low GI meal consumed before exercise could enhance exercise performance more so than high GI meals, meta-analyses comparing low versus high GI meals 30–240 minutes prior to endurance exercise showed slight or no additional benefit of the low GI meal on exercise performance (14,15). Thus, findings

Chapter 3 Basic Nutrition 51

Table 3.2	High, Medium, and Low Glycemic Index Foods	
High Glycemic Index (>70)	**Medium Glycemic Index (56–79)**	**Low Glycemic Index (<55)**
Glucose	All-bran cereal	Fructose
Pancakes	Grapes	Apple
Waffles	Oatmeal	Applesauce
Maple syrup	Honey	Cherries
Corn syrup	Cranberry juice cocktail	Banana
Jelly beans		Kidney beans
Bagel	Ice cream	Baked beans
Candy	Sucrose	Navy beans
Toasted corn cereals	Rice	Peanuts
Toasted oat cereals	Whole-grain rye bread	Chick-peas
Crisped rice cereals	Corn	Lentils
Crackers	Pineapple	Dates
Molasses	Sweet potatoes	Figs
Potatoes	French fries	Peaches
Raisins	Popcorn	Oranges
Taco shells	Potato chips	Pears
Fruit bars		Strawberries
Water melon		Grapefruit
White bread		Plums
Whole wheat bread		Juices
Sports drinks		Milk
		Yogurt
		Spaghetti noodles
		Carrots
		Tomato soup

Data from Atkinson FS, Foster-Powell K, Brand-Miller JC. International tables of glycemic index and glycemic load values: 2008. *Diabetes Care*. 2008;31:2281–3. Ref. (13).

Sidebar: Carbohydrates and Sports Drinks

Carbohydrates are a major component of many sports drinks consumed during exercise. Sports drinks may provide carbohydrates to maintain blood sugar, delay fatigue, assist with recovery during rest periods or following exercise, and helps maintain adequate hydration. The rate of CHO digestion, intestinal absorption, and hepatic metabolism dictate CHO availability (18). The type and concentration of carbohydrates are two major considerations when selecting a sports drink. Both affect the *osmolality* (*i.e.*, ratio of solutes to fluid) of the beverage. A *hypotonic* solution has an osmolality less than bodily tissue leading to fluid uptake, whereas a *hypertonic* solution has an osmolality greater than bodily tissue leading to fluid efflux. Increased osmolality decreases gastric emptying rate and a hypotonic solution with low-to-moderate glucose concentrations increases fluid absorption through the small intestine (11). Maltodextrins (glucose polymers) increase the carbohydrate content without much increase in osmolality and may improve taste. Most sports drinks contain a combination of glucose, sucrose and glucose polymers, and fructose which is better than individual sugars (11). Too high of a carbohydrate content can delay gastric emptying. The majority of sports drinks contain ~6%–8% carbohydrate in solution which may be ideal as it is low enough to avoid inhibiting fluid absorption but high enough to increase endurance performance (8,11). The ingestion of CHO at 30–80 g·h^{-1} (6%–8% solution) has been shown to improve endurance performance parameters by ~2%–54% compared to a placebo (18). The sport drink should also be palatable to encourage drinking especially in hot, humid conditions. From a hydration perspective, sport drinks provide advantages over water as sports drinks have flavor and good taste, provide electrolytes, amino acids, and other nutrients in addition to the CHO content (8).

have been inconsistent (possibly due to methodological differences) where some studies have shown better endurance performance with low GI versus high GI carbohydrates, while others showed no differences (16). It appears that GI may not have a major effect on endurance performance when matched for macronutrient and energy content (12). Thus, a mixed approach could be beneficial as athletes commonly consume multiple foods as opposed to only one. Although use of the GI may be controversial at times, it gives coaches and athletes an indication of the response time for certain foods. Different athletes have different responses to food. For instance, people who exercise regularly are more tolerant of high GI foods than untrained individuals. The glycemic effect of the meal is diurnal. For example, low GI foods play less of a role in glycemic control when consumed in the evening than in the morning (17). Athletes interested in lowering either weight or body fat levels may consider consuming foods with a medium to low GI prior to exercise and consume higher GI foods/beverages during and immediately following exercise or competition (especially if exercising twice per day) to have quick elevations in blood sugar, delay fatigue, and increase the rate of recovery.

Protein

Protein is a large macronutrient made up of *amino acids* attached via peptide bonds and constitutes ~22% of skeletal muscle mass. Each amino acid has the same fundamental structure consisting of a central carbon atom bonded to an amino

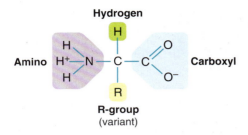

FIGURE 3.4 Amino acid structure.

group (NH$_2$), to a carboxyl group (COOH), and to a hydrogen atom (Fig. 3.4). The R-group is what makes the amino acid unique. The nitrogen component of protein makes it unique in comparison to carbohydrates and fats. Nitrogen must be removed if protein is used as an energy source or stored as fat. Measuring nitrogen balance can serve as a measure of protein metabolism. *Positive nitrogen balance* occurs when more nitrogen is retained than excreted (anabolism), while *negative nitrogen balance* occurs when more nitrogen is excreted than retained (catabolism). Positive nitrogen balance is indicative of enhanced protein synthesis at the whole body level. A protein consists of a specifically sequenced chain of more than 100 amino acids linked together. Of the 20 amino acids that have been identified, nine are "essential" and 11 are "nonessential" (Table 3.3). *Nonessential* amino acids can be produced within the body, whereas *essential* amino acids must be obtained through the diet. Of the nonessential amino acids, arginine, cysteine, glycine, glutamine, proline, serine, and tyrosine may be considered *conditionally essential* because their synthesis can be limited under certain pathophysiological conditions and stress. The structure and folding of a protein dictates its function and is dependent upon the biochemical interaction of amino acids within the chain. The *primary structure* is the sequence of amino acids. The secondary structure is hydrogen bonding. The *tertiary structure* is the protein's shape. The *quaternary structure* is the number of polypeptides or proteins attached as side chains. Many proteins have been identified, each with specific functions. Proteins serve as the building blocks of bodily tissue and perform a number of critical functions within the human body. Table 3.4 presents basic functions of proteins. In addition, individual amino acids can perform a multitude of functions as well.

Protein quality is determined by the presence and distribution of essential amino acids. Food sources consisting of protein may be classified as complete or incomplete. *Complete proteins* contain all of the essential amino acids in adequate quantities and include meat, poultry, fish, dairy products, and soy protein. *Incomplete proteins* lack one or more essential amino acids and include vegetables, grains, and nuts. Complete proteins are more efficient (*i.e.*, better absorption and utilization) and should be included in the athlete's diet. Proteins from animal sources are of the highest quality based on rating scales. Common ratings scales used are as follows:

- **Protein-efficiency ratio** (PER) — measure of weight gained by a test animal divided by the total protein consumed during the test period [*PER = gain in body mass (g)/protein intake (g)*].
- **Biological value** (BV) — measure of the proportion of absorbed protein from a consumed food that is incorporated into total body protein [*BV = (nitrogen retained/nitrogen absorbed) × 100*].
- **Protein digestibility–corrected amino acid score** (PDCAAS) — based on amino acid requirements and the ability to digest it [*PDCAAS = (mg of limiting amino acid in 1 g of test protein/mg of same amino acid in 1 g of reference protein) × digestibility %*].
- **Digestible indispensable amino acid score** (DIAAS) — accounts for different amino acid digestibility [*DIAAS % = 100 × [(mg of digestible dietary indispensable amino acid in 1 g of dietary protein)/(mg of the same dietary indispensable amino acid in 1 g of the reference protein)*].

Protein requirements for athletes may be more than double of that recommended for nonathletes. The RDA for a healthy adult is 0.8 g·kg^{-1}·body mass^{-1}, and 10%–35% of total kcal intake should be nutrient-dense protein sources to ensure adequate protein signaling for protein synthesis (11). This intake value is suboptimal for athletes and individuals who routinely exercise. Factors such as the intensity, volume, and frequency of training, novelty of the training stimulus, carbohydrate availability, and presence of an energy deficit influence the magnitude of protein needed. The current daily protein intake recommendations for athletes range from 1.2 to 2.2 g·kg^{-1} of body mass (11). Strength and power athletes, as well as athletes training to increase or maximize muscle hypertrophy, consume protein at the higher end of this range. Protein intakes of 1.4–2.2 g·kg^{-1} of body mass per day during resistance training (RT) result in positive

Table 3.3	Essential and Nonessential Amino Acids
Essential	**Nonessential**
Leucine	Alanine
Isoleucine	Arginine
Valine	Asparagine
Histidine	Aspartic acid
Methionine	Cysteine
Phenylalanine	Glutamic acid
Threonine	Glutamine
Tryptophan	Glycine
Lysine	Proline
	Serine
	Tyrosine

Amino acids in italics indicate branched-chain amino acids.

Table 3.4	Functions of Protein and Amino Acids

- Enzymes — proteins act as enzymes which catalyze reactions in the human body.
- Transport and storage — proteins are involved in transporting molecules (e.g., hormones, oxygen, etc.) in the blood and storing molecules within the cells. Proteins located within the cell membrane regulates passage in (and how much) and out of the cell.
- Energy — certain amino acids may be used for energy (~5%–10% of energy) during times of nutrient deprivation or strenuous endurance exercise where carbohydrate and fat sources are limited. The carbon in protein provides the same amount of energy per unit of weight as carbohydrates (4 kcal·g^{-1}).
- Hormones and receptors — proteins act as hormones in the human body. Some important protein hormones involved in increasing muscle size and strength are insulin, insulin-like growth factor 1, and the growth hormone superfamily. Proteins act as receptors which are necessary to mediate the hormonal response as well as other physiological signaling.
- Immune system function — many immune cells are proteins which help the body fight disease and improve recovery ability.
- Nerve transmission — some amino acids form neurotransmitters which are necessary for proper nerve function.
- Mechanical support — certain proteins (e.g., collagen) are essential to maintaining strength of tendons, ligaments, bones, skin, organs, etc.
- Muscle function — proteins form the contractile unit which enables muscles to contract and produce force. Structural proteins are necessary to stabilize these proteins as well as the muscle itself. Protein is needed to build and maintain muscle tissue.
- Acid-base balance — proteins can buffer acids to preserve blood and muscle pH.
- Fluid balance — protein helps control the fluid balance between the blood and surrounding tissues.

nitrogen balance (11,19). Higher protein intake is needed in athletes making weight or who participate in weight-controlled sports. Endurance athletes benefit from increased protein intake as intake levels of at least 1.2–1.4 g·kg^{-1} of body mass have been recommended (11). Higher protein intake is thought to be important early in training when increases in muscle hypertrophy are greater, while a somewhat reduced intake may suffice for maintenance (12,20). It is recommended that athletes involved in moderate amounts of intense training consume 1.2–2.0 g·kg^{-1} of body mass, while athletes involved in high volume, intense training consume 1.7–2.2 g·kg^{-1} of body mass of protein per day (2). The ACSM has recommended a range of 1.2–2.0 g·kg^{-1} of body mass in athletes (12). Others have recommended higher protein intakes in resistance-trained athletes (>3.0 g·kg^{-1} of body mass) in combination with RT to optimize changes in body composition (2). In cases of energy restriction or sudden inactivity resulting from injury, the ACSM recommends daily protein intakes as high as 2.0 g·kg^{-1} of body mass or higher (12), while others have recommended 2.3–3.1 g·kg^{-1} of lean body mass (LBM) to maximize retention of LBM (2).

It is recommended that daily protein intake goals be met with a meal plan providing a regular spread of moderate amounts of high-quality protein across the day and following strenuous training sessions (12); e.g., every 3–4 hours with an absolute dose of 20–40 g (2,19). It has been suggested that there is a limit to how much protein (i.e., ~20–25 g) can be absorbed per meal. However, other studies have shown that 40–70 g may be utilized; therefore, relative protein per meal amounts of

0.45–0.55 g·kg^{-1}·meal^{-1} across a minimum of four meals in order to reach a minimum of 1.3–2.2 g·kg^{-1}·d^{-1} has been recommended (20,21). It is recommended that the majority of protein be consumed via food (2,12). However, there may be difficulty in obtaining sufficient protein solely from meals. Hence, protein supplements are commonly used. Protein supplements may be beneficial when inadequate dietary intake is observed. A number of studies investigated effects of protein supplementation on strength performance where some have shown no ergogenic performance augmentation, while some have shown strength increases with higher protein intake (19). Reviews of the literature shown that protein supplementation of at least 15–25 g may have small to moderate effects on muscle strength (19). A meta-analysis has shown that protein supplementation augmented increases in muscle strength and hypertrophy during RT and was more effective in resistance-trained individuals (22). However, protein supplementation beyond intakes of 1.62 g·kg^{-1}·d^{-1} from those intakes studied produced no further gains in LBM (22).

Proteins differ based on their source, amino acid composition, and the method of processing or isolation. Determining the effectiveness of a protein is accomplished via quality (i.e., availability of amino acids), digestibility (i.e., protein utilization), absorption, and metabolic activity assessed on aforementioned rating scales (2,23). Supplements mostly contain mixtures of protein from whey, casein, milk and egg, and soy sources. The branched-chain amino acids (BCAAs), mostly leucine, have been regarded as key nutrients increasing protein synthesis and augmenting recovery following a workout.

It has been recommended that the acute protein dose include 700–3,000 mg of leucine or more plus an array of other essentials amino acids (2,24).

The timing of protein intake relative to the workout period is important with respect to optimizing recovery and, in some cases, training-related adaptations. Consumption of protein or various forms of amino acids in the hours before or during exercise maximizes muscular signaling, protein synthesis, and muscle repair (19). Amino acid uptake into muscle is greatest when blood flow increases so consuming a supplement in close proximity to a workout is important to maximize amino acid uptake. Supplementing before the workout increases amino acid delivery to a greater extent than supplementing following the workout. Consuming protein (and carbohydrates) right after a workout may lead to an earlier increase in protein synthesis especially if the athlete is fasted or consumed few nutrients prior to training (25). The consumption of 20–30 g of protein (before or after RE) increases protein synthesis (19). The immediate postexercise period has been viewed as an "anabolic window" for nutrient ingestion as some studies have shown greater muscle protein synthesis and hypertrophy when nutrients were consumed closer to, rather than further from, the workout (25). However, it appears the value of this postexercise period is largely dependent on when the preworkout meal or meals were consumed, the size and composition of the meal(s), and total protein intake throughout the day (19,25). One study showed similar strength, and hypertrophy increases when similar magnitudes of protein (25 g + 1 g of CHO) were consumed prior to or following a workout over 10 weeks of RT (26). A meta-analysis showed that consuming protein within 1 hour post RE had a small but significant effect on increasing muscle hypertrophy (with no effect of muscle strength) compared to consumption >2 hours later. However, the effect disappeared after controlling for total protein intake. It was concluded that total protein intake was the strongest predictor of muscular hypertrophy, and protein timing played a minor role (27). Thus, timing may not play a major role when a high-protein diet is used with frequent meal intervals (*i.e.*, 3-hour) daily (19). However, consuming protein (with carbohydrates) following a workout (and maintaining AI throughout the recovery period) appears to be an effective strategy to enhance recovery when athletes are fasted or consumed low amounts of protein prior to the workout. Lastly, some recent evidence indicates that consuming 30–40 g of protein (casein) 30 minutes prior to sleep increases muscle protein synthesis, recovery, and metabolism; thus, suggestive that a final protein dose prior to sleep could potentially be beneficial for recovery (19,28).

One concern with very high levels of protein intake (and supplementation) is potential risk for metabolic, cardiac, renal, bone, and liver diseases. In some cases, high protein intakes may be seen in anabolic steroid users. The use of anabolic drugs (*e.g.*, synthetic steroids, testosterone, and growth hormone) may increase protein requirement. It is unclear, though, by how much, as science has not addressed this issue adequately. Therefore, drug-free athletes should not mimic the dietary strategies of an athlete who uses anabolic drugs because he will then run the risk of consuming too much protein. Studies have shown that consumption of 2.5–3.3 $g \cdot kg^{-1} \cdot d^{-1}$ of protein in healthy resistance-trained individuals for 1 year produced no harmful effect on blood lipids or markers of kidney and liver function (29). Protein supplementation within the recommended range appears safe and effective. Any intake beyond this level could increase the risk of problems such as compromised kidney function and bone mineral loss.

Lipids

Lipids are fatty substances that do not dissolve in water. Lipids come in the form of oils (liquid at room temperature), fats (solid at room temperature), and other compounds such as sterols and phospholipids. Lipids perform several functions critical to health and performance. *Glycerides*, the most common form of lipid, consist of a molecule of glycerol, which is bound to either one (*monoglyceride*), two (*diglyceride*), or three (*triglyceride*) fatty acids. Triglycerides account for ~90%–95% of the lipids consumed by humans (Fig. 3.5). Most fatty acids have ~12–28 carbon atoms but some have less. Fatty acids may be saturated or unsaturated, with saturation referring to the number of hydrogen atoms bound to carbons in the fatty acid chain (Fig. 3.6).

Therefore, **saturated fats** contain no double bonds and hold the maximum number of hydrogen atoms. They are solid at room temperature and are found in higher concentrations in meat, poultry, butter, cheese, whole milk, cream, cookies, crackers, chips, and baked foods. A **trans fatty acid** (which has a slightly different configuration than a saturated fatty acid) is an artificial fat found commonly in partially hydrogenated oils in many foods such as desserts, margarine, shortening, snack foods, and fried foods. Trans fatty acids may increase low-density lipoprotein (LDL) levels and increase the risk for heart

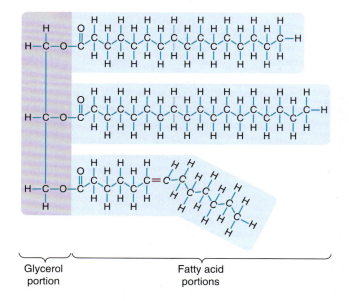

FIGURE 3.5 Triglyceride structure.

Stearic acid
$C_{18}H_{36}O_2$
Saturated fat

Oleic acid
$C_{18}H_{34}O_2$
Monosaturated fat

Linoleic acid
$C_{18}H_{32}O_2$
Polysaturated fat

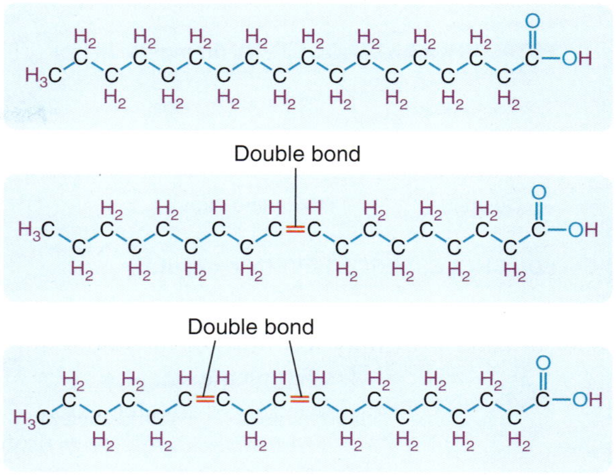

FIGURE 3.6 Saturated and unsaturated fat structure.

disease, stroke, and cancer. **Unsaturated fats** contain double bonds, which reduce the number of bound hydrogen atoms, and tend to be liquid at room temperature (*e.g.*, various oils). *Monounsaturated fatty acids* (MUFAs) contain one double bond, while *polyunsaturated fatty acids* (PUFAs) contain two or more double bonds. MUFAs lower blood cholesterol level while maintaining high-density lipoprotein (HDL) cholesterol (found in olive, safflower, sunflower, and canola oil, nuts). PUFAs lower blood cholesterol level and are associated with vitamin E (found in vegetable oil, nuts, and seeds). The length of the fatty acid chain also plays a key role in its function. Fatty acids with <6 carbons are *short-chain fatty acids*. Fatty acids with 6–12 carbons are considered *medium-chain fatty acids*. The most abundant fatty acids are *long-chain fatty acids*, which contain >12 carbons.

Transport of lipids is important once they are consumed through the diet. Short- and medium-chain fatty acids may be absorbed directly into the blood, but long-chain fatty acids (in addition to cholesterol and other phospholipids) need to be grouped together in the liver for transportation (*e.g.*, the formation of a *lipoprotein* which is a complex consisting of cholesterol, lipids, and protein). Four types of lipoproteins exist in the human body. **Chylomicrons** have the highest amount of fat attached to the protein carrier and are very atherogenic. They remain in the blood until they are converted to LDLs. **Very low-density lipoproteins** (VLDL) are made in the liver from cholesterol and triglycerides and then converted to LDLs. These are highly atherogenic and associated with heart disease. **Low-density lipoproteins** contain a high proportion of cholesterol (*e.g.*, "bad cholesterol") and tend to be more atherogenic with more regularity. **High-density lipoproteins** carry lipids away from storage to the liver for metabolism and/or excretion, they contain more protein (and less cholesterol), and protect against cardiovascular disease (*e.g.*, "good cholesterol"). Cholesterol is a steroid precursor (*i.e.*, a molecule needed to synthesize steroids) that also plays other significant roles in the human body. However, elevated cholesterol is a risk factor for cardiovascular disease in men and women (30). Reference data for some blood lipids is shown in Figure 3.7.

Essential fatty acids are not manufactured in the human body so they must be consumed in the diet in foods such as fish, shellfish, leafy vegetables, and walnuts. The essential fatty acids include linoleic acid and α-linolenic acid. *Linoleic acid* is an unsaturated omega-6 fatty acid and is important for bone strength, hair and skin growth, and normal neurologic function, and may lower the risk for heart disease (1). It is found in corn, sunflower, safflower, and soybean oils, pecans, Brazil nuts, and many other nuts. *Linolenic acid* is an unsaturated omega-3 fatty acid and is important for reducing inflammation, healthy cell membranes, and improved cardiovascular function (1). It is consumed as α-linolenic acid, eicosapentaenoic acid (EPA), and docosahexaenoic acid (DHA), and the three forms are found in flaxseed, soybeans, pumpkin seeds, walnuts, canola oil, fish, fish oil, and marine foods. Supplementation with omega-3 fatty acids has positive health benefits (*e.g.*, reduced risk of cardiovascular disease, reduced LDL and triglycerides, and inflammation) but do not appear to have any ergogenic effect on athletic performance at doses of $3–6 \text{ g·d}^{-1}$ (31). However, fish-oil supplementation may reduce exercise-induced bronchoconstriction in elite athletes, possibly due to an anti-inflammatory effect (32).

Phospholipids are essential components of biological membranes, playing important roles in intracellular signaling, acting as antioxidants, and enhanced insulin sensitivity (33). Phospholipids consist of a glycerol backbone and a phosphate head group typically located at the *sn-3* position. The simplest phospholipid is phosphatidic acid (PA), and others include phosphatidylethanolamine, phosphatidylserine, phosphatidylinositol, phosphatidylglycerol, phosphatidylcholine, lysophospholipids, and sphingolipids. Many foods contain phospholipids but animal-based sources contain abundance. Phospholipid supplementation may take place in various forms from individual supplements to supplements with an assortment of phospholipids (*e.g.*, lecithin, Krill oil). PA is present naturally in the diet but at low levels in vegetables. A critical function of PA is its role in partially mediating protein synthesis via activation of the mammalian target of rapamycin (mTOR) pathway (see Chapter 5). Studies have examined PA supplementation of $250–750 \text{ mg·d}^{-1}$ with some showing no ergogenic

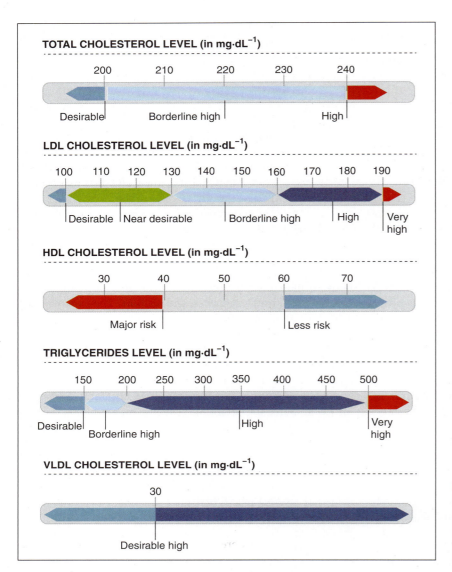

FIGURE 3.7 Reference values for selected blood lipids. (From Reference Ranges for Blood Lipids. Understanding what your cholesterol level means [Internet]. Available from: http://www.cholesterolmenu.com/cholesterol-levels-chart/. Accessed September 2020.)

potential but a few showed small enhancing effects on strength and LBM (33). Studies examining other phospholipid supplements have been equivocal showing no effects to minimal effects mostly on endurance performance despite increasing phospholipid concentrations in the blood (33).

Lipids perform a number of critical functions in the human body (Table 3.5). Adequate dietary fat intake (mostly in the form of unsaturated fats with sufficient amount [at least 3 g] of omega-3 fatty acids) is essential for an athlete, despite fat being demonized as something to be avoided at all costs. The generally accepted healthy range of fat intake for physically active people is between 20% and 35% of total daily calories. The prevailing thought among some athletes has been to keep fat intake low. However, reducing fat intake to below 15% of daily caloric intake may have negative consequences on endurance performance, testosterone concentrations, and reduce fat usage during exercise (2,11). The ACSM recommends that athletes be discouraged from dietary fat intakes of <20% of energy intake but recommend saturated fat intakes of <10% of energy intake (12). In addition, some athletes may benefit from fat intake >35%. Trans fatty acid consumption should be kept to a minimum.

There has been a great deal of attention given to high-fat, high-protein, and low-carbohydrate diets in both the athletic and nonathletic communities. Different diets exist based on relative fat, protein, and carbohydrate intake as well as food choices. Some diets are very low CHO (<20%) such as the **ketogenic diet** and Atkins diet, while some are low CHO (20%–40%) such as the Zone diet and South Beach diet. Because of low carbohydrate intake, the liver converts fat into fatty acids and ketone bodies (mostly acetoacetate, beta-hydroxybutyric acid, and acetone), which replaces glucose as an energy source (a process known as *ketosis* resulting in 0.5–5.0 mM of circulating ketones) (34). Typically, a ketogenic diet may compromise ~60%–70% fat, 5%–15% carbohydrate (or <50 g·d^{-1}), and 15%–25% protein (*i.e.*, 1.2–2.0 g·kg^{-1} of body mass)

Table 3.5	Functions of Lipids

- Provide energy: lipids are the most concentrated macronutrient energy source. One gram of fat equals 9 kcal·g^{-1} and provides more than 12 times the energy as 1 g of carbohydrate. Adipose tissue provides a large store of energy (e.g., subcutaneous body fat).
- Provide essential fatty acids: lipids provide essential fatty acids (i.e., linoleic acid, linolenic acid) necessary for bodily growth and function.
- Transport fat soluble vitamins: vitamins A, D, E, and K are fat-soluble vitamins; therefore, fat is necessary for absorption of these vitamins.
- Structural components: lipids makeup cell membranes, nerve coverings, some hormones (e.g., cholesterol is a precursor of testosterone), and other substances vital to normal function.
- Thermal insulation: body fat is essential to maintain normal body temperature.
- Protection of vital organs: essential body fat acts like a "shock absorber" as it surrounds major organs and protects these organs from damage during movement. Essential fat constitutes about 3%–4% in men and ~12% in women.
- Flavor: lipids add flavor to food to improve taste.
- Satiety control: lipids create a sense of "fullness" because it stays in the stomach longer than other energy nutrients.

(11,34). A review of the literature has shown fat intake ranges of 55%–84%, carbohydrate intake ranges of <2%–22%, and protein intake ranges of 15%–41% on high-fat, low-carbohydrate diets (35). Polyunsaturated fats may not be well tolerated at the high levels required so saturated and monounsaturated fats may be more suitable (34). High-fat, low-CHO diets have been shown to increase HDLs; decrease triglycerides, hepatic fat, chronic inflammation, appetite, and body weight (fat loss); and increase insulin and leptin sensitivity (35,36).

High-fat diets have been used mostly by endurance athletes in an attempt to increase endurance during long-duration, low-to-moderate intensity aerobic exercise, although some strength and power athletes have consumed high-fat diets. The rationale is based on attempts to spare muscle glycogen, increase fat usage, and improve endurance performance. A high-fat diet can reduce glycogen use and increase fat use to a much greater degree during exercise, but it also reduces muscle glycogen and increases muscle triglyceride levels prior to exercise. It is clear from the literature that substrate availability and use is dramatically altered with high-fat diets. Research studies have shown positive, negative, and no effects on endurance performance on non–calorie-restricted high-fat diets depending on the level of the athlete (11,35). While endurance performance may improve during moderate-intensity exercise, performance during high-intensity endurance exercise (>80% of VO_{2max}) is compromised following consumption of a high-fat diet (11). A meta-analysis showed that 10 of 12 studies reported no change or decrease in VO_{2max} while training on a high-fat, low-CHO diet (35). Other studies have shown no consistent improvement in strength and power performance while consuming a high-fat, low-CHO diet (35). It was concluded that high-fat, low-CHO diets may reduce body mass and percent body fat while maintaining LBM but does not augment endurance performance presumably due to limited CHO availability and that a combined high-fat, low-CHO diet and RT will pose no harm to developing strength and power (35). Thus, high-fat, low-CHO diets may have some limitations in maximizing performance. If an endurance athlete decides to consume a high-fat, low-CHO diet, a strategy suggested might be to habitually ingest a high-fat diet for several weeks to months prior to competition to increase fat metabolism and then subsequently increase carbohydrate consumption in the days prior to the competition (11).

Water

Water is a macronutrient that carries nutrients to cells and carries waste products away from cells. It serves as a lubricant, aids in digestion and absorption of food, helps build and repair cells, and helps maintain body temperature. Lean tissue is >70% water, and about 60% of total body weight is water (8). Recommendations for water intake per day vary. The general AI for water intake is 2.7 L·d^{-1} in women and 3.7 L·d^{-1} in men (6). All sources of fluid in food and beverages are considered part of this recommendation (6). Hydration in athletes is a critical concept and extends the intake guidelines depending on the intensity, volume, and duration of training as well as other environmental factors. Fluid intake and hydration for athletes during exercise are discussed in Chapter 17.

Vitamins and Minerals

Micronutrients (i.e., vitamins and minerals) are needed in small amounts in the human body (μg to mg per day). **Vitamins** are organic compounds essential for numerous bodily reactions to take place (Fig. 3.8). They act as cofactors in many metabolic reactions and most need to be consumed in the diet for an individual to reach the RDA value (Table 3.6). Thirteen vitamins are classified based on their solubility as either water- or fat-soluble. Water-soluble vitamins, which include the B vitamins and vitamin C, play major roles in energy metabolism and immune function. Fat-soluble vitamins, which include vitamins A, D, E, and K, are potent antioxidants and assist in recovery between workouts and practices. **Minerals** are inorganic compounds found in nature that are also essential to

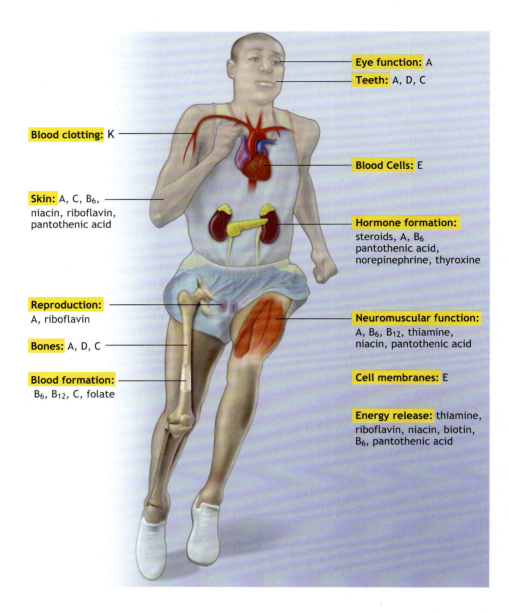

FIGURE 3.8 Basic functions of vitamins. (Reprinted from McArdle WD, Katch FI, Katch VL. *Exercise Physiology: Energy, Nutrition, and Human Performance.* 6th ed. Philadelphia (PA): Lippincott Williams & Wilkins; 2007. p. 123–228. Ref. (37).)

normal human functioning (Table 3.7). Seven minerals are macrominerals (sodium, chloride, potassium, calcium, magnesium, phosphorus, and sulfur), because they are required in larger quantities. Others are microminerals required in small (trace) amounts.

The amount of vitamins and minerals consumed in the diet is critical to an athlete. Although vitamins and minerals are plentiful in food, vitamin/mineral content can be lost because of the way foods are processed, stored, and cooked. For example, cutting, cooking, freezing, heating, drying, and canning foods can reduce their nutritional value. Not only are some athletes' diets deficient in vitamin- and mineral-rich foods such as fruits and vegetables, but exercise stresses several metabolic pathways and training results in adaptations that increase the need for some micronutrients on a daily basis (12). Studies in athletes show greater micronutrient turnover with high levels of physical activity, which results in additional loss of nutrients. Athletes, who restrict energy intake, rely on extreme weight loss practices, eliminate one or more food groups from their diet, or have poor nutritional diets benefit from micronutrient supplementation (12). This often occurs with calcium, vitamin D, iron, and some antioxidants (12). Considering most young athletes' poor food selection and limited time for proper food preparation, vitamin/mineral supplementation appears very appealing. The rationale for micronutrient supplementation is to correct deficiencies that may lead to performance reductions and other health consequences. Vitamin/mineral supplements are not ergogenic if sufficient amounts of micronutrients are consumed in the diet. A deficiency may develop if an athlete only eats certain foods, has too low of a total caloric intake, or has a reduced ability to absorb vitamins/minerals due to other factors such as illness or drug or alcohol use. The best strategy to make certain that an adequate

Chapter 3 Basic Nutrition   **59**

Table 3.6 — Vitamin Functions, Intake, Deficiency, and Food Sources

Vitamin	Functions	RDA/AI/DRI Intake	Sources	Deficiency
Thiamin (B_1)	• Carbohydrate, fat, and protein metabolism • Nerve conduction	1.1 (F)–1.2 (M) mg·d^{-1} UL = ND *Athletes: 1.5–3.0 mg·d^{-1} (0.5 mg·d^{-1} per 1,000 kcal)*	Seeds, legumes, pork, ham, enriched/fortified grains and cereals, liver, nuts, potatoes	Beriberi (heart disease, weight loss, neurological failure), weakness, depression, confusion
Riboflavin (B_2)	• Oxidation of carbohydrates and fats • Endurance • Hormone production • Normal eye function • Healthy skin	1.1 (F)–1.3 (M) mg·d^{-1} UL = ND *Athletes: 1.1 mg·d^{-1} per 1,000 kcal*	Milk, liver, whole and enriched grains and cereals, meat, eggs, green leafy vegetables, beans	Swollen tongue, sensitivity to light, fatigue, dermatitis, oral sores, eye damage
Niacin (B_3)	• Oxidation of carbohydrates and fats • Electron transport (energy reactions) and endurance • Blood flow to skin	14 (F)–16 (M) mg·d^{-1} UL = 35 mg·d^{-1} *Athletes: 14–20 mg·d^{-1}*	Meat, poultry, liver, fish, turkey, nuts, grains, milk, eggs, foods high in tryptophan	Pellagra (diarrhea, dermatitis, dementia), weakness, lethargy
Pyridoxine (B_6)	• Coenzyme in protein, fat, and CHO metabolism • Neurotransmitter formation • Formation of hemoglobin and RBCs	1.5 (F)–1.7 (M) mg·d^{-1} UL = 100 mg *Athletes: ≥1.5–2.0 mg·d^{-1}*	Meat, liver, poultry, fish, grains and cereals, bananas, green leafy vegetables, potatoes, legumes	Nausea, weakness, anemia, convulsions, depression, headaches, immunosuppression
Folic acid	• Coenzyme in formation of DNA and RBCs	400 µg·d^{-1} (M&F) UL = 1,000 µg·d^{-1} *Athletes: ≥400 µg·d^{-1}*	Meat, green leafy vegetables, liver, grains and cereals, potatoes, legumes, nuts, fruit	Fatigue, anemia, gastrointestinal problems
Cobalamin (B_{12})	• Coenzyme in protein, fat, and CHO metabolism • Maintenance of nerve cells • Formation of DNA and RBCs	2.4 µg·d^{-1} (M&F) UL = ND *Athletes: ≥2.4–2.5 µg·d^{-1}*	Meat, fish, poultry, liver, eggs, cereals, dairy products	Anemia, fatigue, nerve damage, ↑ homocysteine
Pantothenic acid (B_5)	• Coenzyme in metabolism	5 mg·d^{-1} (M&F) UL = ND *Athletes: ≥5 mg·d^{-1}*	Meat, poultry, liver, eggs, dairy products, grains, legumes, vegetables	Fatigue, tingling in feet and hands, weakness
Biotin (vitamin H)	• Gluconeogenesis and fatty acid synthesis • Gene expression	30 µg·d^{-1} (M&F) UL = ND *Athletes: ≥30 µg·d^{-1}*	Nuts, soybeans, milk, eggs, green leafy vegetables	Depression, skin irritation, weakness

(Continued)

Table 3.6	Vitamin Functions, Intake, Deficiency, and Food Sources (*Continued*)			
Vitamin	**Functions**	**RDA/AI/DRI Intake**	**Sources**	**Deficiency**
Vitamin C (ascorbic acid)	• Antioxidant and immune system • Collagen formation • Wound healing • ↓ Muscle damage • Iron absorption • Carnitine synthesis • Norepinephrine and epinephrine synthesis • Steroid hormone synthesis	75 (F)–90 (M) mg·d^{-1} UL = 2,000 mg *Athletes: ≥100–200 mg·d^{-1}, possibly more under stressful conditions*	Citrus fruits, green peppers, green vegetables, fruit juices, sports drinks	Muscle weakness, fatigue, infections, overtraining, ↑ risk of injury, anemia, bleeding gums, scurvy, slow wound healing, bruising
Vitamin A (retinoids, beta carotene)	• Vision • Growth and differentiation, gene expression • Reproduction • Immune function • Antioxidant • Bone strength • Healthy skin	700 (F)–900 (M) μg·d^{-1} UL = 3,000 μg·d^{-1} *Athletes: ≥700–900 μg·d^{-1}*	Carrots, green leafy vegetables, spinach, tomatoes, oranges, apricots, broccoli, cantaloupe, mango, sweet potatoes, liver, fish, dairy products, eggs	Night blindness, dry skin, rough mucous membranes, poor immune function, impaired growth and wound healing
Vitamin D (ergocalciferol, cholecalciferol [D$_3$])–converts a skin compound 7-dehydrocholesterol into vitamin D	• Acts like a steroid hormone • Calcium absorption • Phosphorus absorption • Mineralization of bone • Muscle function and anabolism • Anti-inflammation • Gene expression, cell differentiation	5–15 (M&F) μg·d^{-1} (600 IU) — plus sunlight (UV light) exposure so recommendation varies UL = 50 μg·d^{-1} *Athletes: ≥15–20 μg·d^{-1}, 1,000–2,000 IU*	Liver, fish, eggs, oils, margarine, cereal and dairy products (fortified with vitamin D), sunlight exposure	Rickets in children, osteomalacia and osteoporosis, poor bone mineralization, muscle aches and weakness
Vitamin E (α-tocopherol)	• Powerful antioxidant • Involved in immune function • Possible ↓ muscle damage	15 (M&F) mg·d^{-1} UL = 1,000 mg *Athletes: ≥15 mg·d^{-1}*	Nuts, liver, eggs, vegetable and seed oils, whole grains	Anemia, RBC hemolysis, muscle and nerve damage, inflammation
Vitamin K (phylloquinone K$_1$, menaquinone, menadione)	• Blood clotting • Glycogen and bone formation • Protein synthesis	90 (F)–120 (M) μg·d^{-1} UL = ND *Athletes: ≥90–120 μg·d^{-1}*	Liver, eggs, green leafy vegetables, tea, cheese, butter	Bleeding

M - males; F - females; UL - upper limit; ND - not determined; UV - ultraviolet

From Battista RA. Nutrition and human performance. In: *ACSM's Resources for the Personal trainer*. Philadelphia, PA: Wolters Kluwer, 2018; Benardot D. *ACSM's Nutrition for Exercise Science*. Philadelphia, PA: Wolters Kluwer; 2019; Kang J. *Nutrition and Metabolism in Sports, Exercise and Health*. New York, NY: Routledge, 2012, pp. 20-109.

Table 3.7   Mineral Functions, Intake, Deficiency, and Food Sources

Mineral	Functions	RDA/AI/DRI Intake	Sources	Deficiency
Calcium	• Structure of bones and teeth • Blood coagulation • Nerve impulse transmission • Muscle contraction • Regulates some enzyme activity • Intracellular signaling • Acid-base control	1,000–1,200 (MF) mg·d^{-1} UL = 2,500 mg·d^{-1} *Athletes: ≥1,300–1,500 mg·d^{-1}*	Dairy products, egg yolks, beans, peas, dark green vegetables, cauliflower, canned fish, some beverages (orange juice) fortified with calcium	↓ Bone density, ↑ risk of osteoporosis, stress fractures, muscle dysfunction, weakness, cramps
Chloride	• Fluid balance • Nerve function • Component of digestive enzymes, gastric acids	2,300 (MF) mg·d^{-1} UL = 3,500 mg·d^{-1} *Athletes: ≥2,300 mg·d^{-1}*	Table salt, canned foods, meat, fish	Muscle weakness, lethargy, loss of appetite, cramps
Chromium	• Augment insulin action — *glucose tolerance factor*	25 (F)–35 (M) µg·d^{-1} UL = ND *Athletes: 30–35 µg·d^{-1}*	Whole-grain foods, meat, nuts, legumes, eggs, cheese, mushrooms, asparagus	Glucose intolerance, fatigue, craving for sweets
Copper	• Component of enzymes involved in iron absorption, energy metabolism, neurotransmission, connective tissue formation, immune, CV function	900 (MF) µg·d^{-1} UL = 10 mg·d^{-1} *Athletes: ≥900 µg·d^{-1}*	Meat, fish, poultry, liver, eggs, nuts, legumes, bananas, cocoa, whole grains	Anemia
Fluoride	• Promotes the formation of bone in teeth	3 (F)–4 (M) mg·d^{-1} UL = 10 mg *Athletes: 3–4 mg·d^{-1}*	Seaweed, milk, eggs, tea, drinking water, toothpaste	Dental problems
Iodine	• Component of thyroid hormones triiodothyronine and thyroxine	150 (MF) µg·d^{-1} UL = 1,100 µg·d^{-1} *Athletes: ≥150 µg·d^{-1}*	Saltwater fish, iodized salt, dairy products, bread	↓ Metabolic rate, goiter
Iron	• Involved in oxygen transfer to cells (hemoglobin in blood; myoglobin in muscle; cytochromes) • Component of some enzymes • DNA synthesis • Protects antioxidants and enhances immune system	8 (M)–18 (F) mg·d^{-1} UL = 45 mg·d^{-1} *Athletes: 15–18 mg·d^{-1}*	Liver, eggs, meat, poultry, seafood, oysters — *heme iron* Bread, legumes, nuts, green leafy vegetables, broccoli, dried fruit, fortified cereals — *nonheme iron*	Microcytic anemia, weakness, loss of energy, fatigue
Magnesium	• Cofactor for >300 enzymes • Carbohydrate and fat metabolism • Protein synthesis • Fluid balance • Bone structure • Membrane stability • Cardiovascular function • Muscle contractions and nerve function	320 (F)–420 (M) mg·d^{-1} UL = 350 mg supplement *Athletes: ≥350–450 mg·d^{-1}*	Green leafy vegetables, fruits, whole-grain products, milk, seafood, nuts, yogurt, chocolate, legumes	Muscle weakness, fatigue, cramps, muscle spasms, nausea, poor performance
Manganese	• Component of enzymes involved in energy and bone metabolism • Immune function	1.8 (F)–2.3 (M) mg·d^{-1} UL = 11 mg·d^{-1} *Athletes: 2.0–2.5 mg·d^{-1}*	Grains, peas, beans, nuts, leafy vegetables, and bananas	Reduced growth, poor wound healing

(Continued)

Table 3.7   Mineral Functions, Intake, Deficiency, and Food Sources (*Continued*)

Mineral	Functions	RDA/AI/DRI Intake	Sources	Deficiency
Molybdenum	• Component of enzymes in CHO and fat metabolism	45 (MF) µg·d⁻¹ UL = 2,000 µg·d⁻¹ *Athletes: ≥45 µg·d⁻¹*	Liver, grains, beans, peas, milk, nuts	Rarely deficient
Phosphorous	• Structure of bones and teeth • Component of ATP and other energy-yielding compounds • Part of vitamin B coenzymes • Part of DNA and RNA • Component of cell membranes • Cell growth and repair • Formation of 2,3-diphosphoglycerate • Phosphorylation reactions • Acid-base balance	700 (MF) mg·d⁻¹ UL = 4,000 mg·d⁻¹ *Athletes: 1,250–1,500 mg·d⁻¹*	Meat, eggs, fish, milk, cheese, grains, nuts, legumes, soft drinks	Muscle weakness, cramps, weak bones
Potassium	• Nerve conduction • Muscle contraction • Establishment of membrane potentials • Fluid balance • Maintenance of heart rate • Acid-base balance • Protein and CHO metabolism	4,700 (MF) mg·d⁻¹ UL = ND *Athletes: ≥4,700 mg·d⁻¹ (more with sweat loss)*	Meat, fish, milk, yogurt, fruits, vegetables, potatoes, bananas, bread	Muscle cramps, loss of appetite, irregular heart beat
Selenium	• Antioxidant — part of glutathione peroxidase • Works in synergy with vitamin E	55 (MF) µg·d⁻¹ UL = 400 µg·d⁻¹ *Athletes: ≥55 µg·d⁻¹*	Meat, liver, poultry, fish, seafood, dairy products, nuts, grains	Immune dysfunction, fatigue, impaired recovery, cardiac problems, and potentially cancer
Sodium	• Maintains blood volume, fluid balance, blood pressure regulation • Muscle contraction • Nerve transmission • Acid-base balance • Cell membrane function	1,500 (MF) mg·d⁻¹ UL = 2,300 mg·d⁻¹ *Athletes: ≥1,500 mg·d⁻¹ (more with sweat loss)*	Meat, fish, bread, canned foods, sauces, many processed canned foods and "junk" foods, soup, table salt, sport drinks	Dizziness, muscle cramps, nausea, loss of appetite, seizures
Sulfur	• Acid-base balance • Component of some amino acids (methionine, cysteine) — protein synthesis • Connective tissue structure	ND — part of sulfur-containing amino acids intake recommendations	Animal sources	Synonymous with protein deficiency
Zinc	• Immune system — antioxidant • Wound healing • Protein synthesis • Energy metabolism • Cell membrane stability • Component of >300 enzymes	8 (F)–11 (M) mg·d⁻¹ UL = 40 mg·d⁻¹ *Athletes: ≥11–15 mg·d⁻¹*	Beef, shellfish, oysters, red meats, eggs, liver, whole-grain cereals, nuts, legumes	Impaired growth and immune function, ↓ work and power, ↑ muscle damage, poor wound healing

M - males; F - females; UL - upper limit; ND - not determined; UV - ultraviolet

From Battista RA. Nutrition and human performance. In: *ACSM's Resources for the Personal trainer.* Philadelphia, PA: Wolters Kluwer, 2018; Benardot D. *ACSM's Nutrition for Exercise Science.* Philadelphia, PA: Wolters Kluwer; 2019; Kang J. *Nutrition and Metabolism in Sports, Exercise and Health.* New York, NY: Routledge, 2012, pp. 20-109.

amount of all the vitamins is consumed is to eat a wide variety of foods and consume plenty of fresh fruits and vegetables daily. Given that nutrients work in synergy, a multivitamin/mineral approach is recommended rather than individual micronutrients (unless a clinical need requires it).

Most studies examining vitamin supplementation in athletes have shown no to minimal effects of athletic performance when a deficiency is not present. This is especially true with the B vitamins. Some of the more commonly studied vitamins include vitamins C, E, D, and some of the B vitamins. Although most studies do not show ergogenic effects of vitamin C and E supplementation, supplementation with these vitamins have been shown in some studies to produce health-promoting effects such as enhanced immune function and reduced muscle damage (31). These antioxidant-related functions could have indirect benefits to the athlete regarding recovery and maintaining health in order to train maximally. Some recent studies have examined ergogenic effects of vitamin D supplementation. Three meta-analyses examining 4–12 weeks of vitamin D supplementation of doses ranging from 600 to 5,000 $IU \cdot d^{-1}$ of D_3 showed that blood concentrations of 25-hydroxyvitamin D increased. One of the studies concluded D_3 supplementation had a significant effect on lower body muscle strength but had no effect on upper body strength and power (38), another showed positive improvements in muscle strength (39), and one study showed no effect on muscle strength (40). Thus, a balanced diet is recommended but athletes who are in weight-controlled sports, kilocalorie deficits, or those with other predisposing concerns could benefit from a multivitamin supplement.

Some of the more commonly studied minerals regarding athletic performance and supplementation are calcium, sodium and chloride, potassium, phosphorus, magnesium, iron, zinc, chromium, and selenium. Little is gained via supplementation unless a deficiency is present. The ACSM has recommended that an individualized multivitamin/mineral supplement regimen may be appropriate in cases where there are deficiencies or in athletes who are following an energy-restricted diet or unable to consume sufficient variation in dietary selections (12).

Calcium supplementation may help increase fat metabolism but supplementation does not appear to provide an ergogenic effect on exercise performance (2,41). However, there is a greater risk of low bone mineral density and bone damage especially in athletes who consume hypocaloric diets and those female athletes with menstrual dysfunction (12). Thus, calcium intakes of 1,500 $mg \cdot d^{-1}$ and 1,500–2,000 $IU \cdot d^{-1}$ of vitamin D are needed to optimize bone health in these athletes (12). The **electrolytes** sodium, chloride, and potassium are the major minerals (mostly sodium) lost in sweat during exercise, and electrolyte loss is exacerbated in hot, humid environments. Sodium loss in sweat may range from 0.2 to 12.5 $g \cdot L^{-1}$ (6). Thus, consuming additional sodium in the diet or supplying additional electrolytes prior to, during, and following exercise via a sport drink is a recommended strategy to combat dehydration and electrolyte loss. Athletes must be careful to not over drink water (at higher amounts than sweat rate and urinary losses) as this could lead to **hyponatremia**, a condition where blood sodium levels fall below 130 $mmol \cdot L^{-1}$ (6,12). Some symptoms

include nausea, vomiting, headache, confusion, delirium, and potentially much more life-threatening symptoms. Thus, the presence of electrolytes in fluid helps retain fluid balance and maintain appropriate electrolyte concentrations in the blood.

Phosphorous, in the form of sodium phosphate, has been used for supplementation purposes. The results have been equivocal where phosphate loading (4 $g \cdot d^{-1}$) increased VO_{2max}, exercise time to exhaustion, 2,3-DPG concentrations, and improved markers of cardiovascular function in endurance athletes in some studies, but had no effect on aerobic performance or power in others (1,2,31). Supplementation with magnesium (250–500 $mg \cdot d^{-1}$) reduced muscle damage, increased muscle strength and power, and improved endurance in a few studies in untrained individuals with unknown magnesium status (31). However, other studies have shown no such effects, probably because the athletes in these studies were not deficient in magnesium. The consensus appears to be that magnesium supplementation has minimal effect on endurance performance beyond correcting a deficit (2). Some data indicate possibly a small strength enhancing effect, but further research is needed to confirm ergogenic potential in athletes (41,42).

The most common nutrient deficiency in the world is iron deficiency. Iron deficiency first begins with depletion, followed by marginal deficiency, and anemia (6). **Anemia** is a condition where weakness and fatigue occurs as a result of a reduced ability to deliver oxygen to tissues from reduced RBCs and hemoglobin. Iron deficiency can reduce athletic performance and is far more common in female athletes, especially in endurance athletes. Factors contributing to the deficiency include limited intake from *heme* (iron found in hemoglobin, myoglobin in meat products that is easiest to absorb) food sources, reduced kilocalorie intake, vegetarian diets, periods of rapid growth, altitude training, menstrual blood loss, gastrointestinal bleeding, hemolysis from foot-to-ground contact, injury, blood donation, or increased losses in sweat, urine, and feces from training (12). It has been shown that 25%–44% of female runners were deficient in iron, while only 4%–13% of male runners were iron deficient (31). Iron requirements for female athletes may be increased by up to 70% of the average requirement (12). Thus, iron supplementation may be an attractive alternative for iron-deficient athletes if dietary intake is insufficient. In addition, iron absorption is increased by vitamin C, so nonheme sources of iron may show better absorption capacity if the athletes consumes sufficient fruits and vegetables (11). In most cases, iron supplementation in athletes with only a mild deficiency or none at all has shown no ergogenic effects (2). However, many benefits are seen in athletes with iron-deficient anemia (2). Studies have shown significant elevations in iron content in the blood (*i.e., ferritin* — an indirect blood marker of iron status), as well as ergogenic effects such as improvements in exercise time to exhaustion, increased VO_{2max}, and reduced blood lactate concentrations with iron supplementation (31). Blood tests are commonly used to determine iron content, and serum ferritin levels of <10–35 $ng \cdot mL^{-1}$ may necessitate increased dietary intake and/or iron supplementation (12). Supplementation is not necessary for athletes who are not deficient in iron.

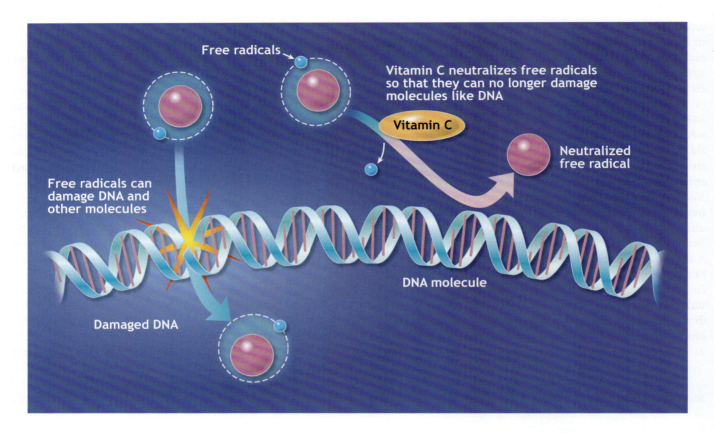

FIGURE 3.9 Free radicals and antioxidants. (Reprinted from McArdle WD, Katch FI, Katch VL. *Exercise Physiology: Energy, Nutrition, and Human Performance*. 6th ed. Philadelphia (PA): Lippincott Williams & Wilkins; 2007. p. 123–228.)

Dietary intake of zinc may be deficient in some groups of athletes especially endurance athletes, athletes who need to compete in weight classes, and athletes with high-carbohydrate, low-protein, and low-fat diets (31). Zinc supplementation can benefit athletes who have a deficiency by improving immune function, reducing free radical damage, and improving muscle strength, endurance, and exercise tolerance (31). Supplementation with 25 mg·d^{-1} of zinc can reduce training-induced immunosuppression (2). Zinc supplementation is not necessary for athletes who consume a balanced diet with adequate protein intake (and consumption of animal products). Supplementation with chromium picolinate (most absorbable form) showed some equivocal results where a few early studies showed increases in LBM and fat loss with 200 µg·d^{-1} (31). The majority of subsequent well-controlled studies with 200–800 µg·d^{-1} have shown no effect on lean tissue mass, fat mass, or muscle strength in several groups of athletes (2,31).

Antioxidants

Antioxidants, such as vitamins A, E, C, and selenium, play major health-promoting roles in the human body. Antioxidants protect cell membranes from oxidative damage. Atoms are "grounded" when every electron in the outer shell has a complimentary pair. A **free radical** has at least one unpaired reactive electron and will steal electrons from cell membranes (*e.g.*, *lipid peroxidation*), known as a *reactive oxygen species* (ROS) in relation to oxygen, which causes damage. The most common ROS are superoxide anion, hydroxyl radical, singlet oxygen, and hydrogen peroxide. Up to 5% of oxygen consumed becomes damaging free radicals and damage occurs when free-radical production exceeds the body's control ability (*i.e.*, *oxidative stress*). Antioxidants provide control for this process. Exercise increases free-radical production, which ultimately could lead to tissue damage, injury, and fatigue. Antioxidants protect tissues by donating an electron to the free radical, thereby rendering it harmless (Fig. 3.9). Oxidative stress occurs in all athletes, but the magnitude may be worse in lesser-trained individuals (12). Dietary antioxidant intake is critical to up-regulating the body's antioxidant defense system. The three major enzymes that are used to neutralize free radicals are *superoxide dismutase (SOD)*, *catalase*, and *glutathione peroxidase*. Consumption of antioxidants from dietary sources or through supplementation helps the body increase the ability to neutralize free radicals. A good strategy for athletes is to consume dietary sources of antioxidants and, if necessary, a balanced antioxidant formula to limit free-radical damage and improve health (43). Athletes at greatest risk for poor antioxidant intakes are those who restrict energy intake, follow a chronic low-fat diet, or limit dietary intake of fruits, vegetables, and whole grains (12). Supplementation is not ergogenic for athletic performance per se but may help in reducing tissue oxidative damage.

Energy availability (EA) is defined as dietary intake minus exercise energy expenditure relative to LBM (44). A healthy value of EA reflecting energy balance is estimated to occur at ~45 kcal·kg LBM^{-1}·d^{-1}, whereas values ≤30 kcal·kg LBM^{-1}·d^{-1} are associated with symptoms of the triad or RED-S (44,45 Sidebar below). Factors such as moderate-to-severe energy restriction to make a weight or for appearance, eating disorders (*anorexia nervosa*, *bulimia nervosa*, *binge-eating disorder*) or abnormal behaviors (*i.e.*, use of laxatives, enemas, and diuretics), poor dietary choices or limited types of foods consumed (*i.e.*, vegetarian), and excessive energy expenditure from exercise to further reduce body weight or fat can result in energy deficiency (1,44). Strong evidence shows that triad/RED-S symptoms occur in sports emphasizing leanness (44). Epidemiological studies examining the prevalence in female athletes have shown the following: 25%–62% of female athletes showed some evidence of eating disorders; 22%–69% showed some evidence of primary or secondary amenorrhea; 22%–50% showed evidence of osteopenia while 0%–13% showed evidence of osteoporosis; with 1.2%–4.3% of female athletes showing simultaneous evidence of all three factors (44).

Screening and diagnosis of RED-S in susceptible athletes is challenging but should be undertaken as part of a routine assessment program possibly during a preseason or preparticipation examination, annual checkup, or when athletes display menstrual issues, eating disorders, or recurrent injuries (44,45). Screening may include patient history profiles, physical examinations, and laboratory testing. Treatment recommendations include a multicomponent approach involving increased energy intake and/or reduced energy expenditure, nutrition counseling, and psychological counseling for eating disorders with input from physicians, registered dietician, mental health practitioner, athletic trainers, strength coaches and fitness trainers, coaching staff, and parents and family members (44). Treatment noncompliance may result in the athlete being limited from training/practice and competitions (44).

Sports Supplements

In 1994, Congress passed the Dietary Supplement Health and Education Act (DSHEA) defining a supplement as "a product

Sidebar: The Female Athlete Triad — Relative Energy Deficiency in Sport

The examination of energy deficiency in mostly female athletes emerged from discussions and observations of the female athlete triad. The **female athlete triad** referred to the interrelationships between energy availability, menstrual function, and bone mineral density and was thought to have major implications in eating disorders, *secondary amenorrhea* (the absence of menstrual cycles for >90 d), and osteoporosis (44). Figure 3.10 shows the classic paradigm depicting a continuum to where low energy availability was more likely to lead to lower BMD and menstrual dysfunction (amenorrhea, oligomenorrhea). In 1992, the female athlete triad was recognized, and in 1997, the ACSM published its first Position Stand that was later updated in 2007. Since, a broader and more comprehensive term has evolved, *e.g.*, **Relative energy deficiency in sport** (RED-S) (Fig. 3.11 panel A). RED-S extends the female athlete triad by acknowledging a broader array of issues such as endocrine, gastrointestinal, renal, neuro-psychiatric, musculoskeletal, immune, metabolic, hematological, and cardiovascular dysfunction resulting from the excessive energy deficiency (44,45). Notwithstanding the primary importance of these negative health ramifications, RED-S may also lead to an array of performance-related issues ultimately limiting athletic performance (Fig. 3.11 panel B).

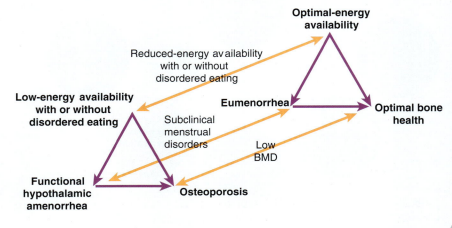

FIGURE 3.10 The female triad. (Reprinted from ACSM position state: the female athlete triad. *Med Sci Sports Exerc*. 2007;39(10):1867–82. doi: 10.1249/mss.0b013e318149f111.)

(*Continued*)

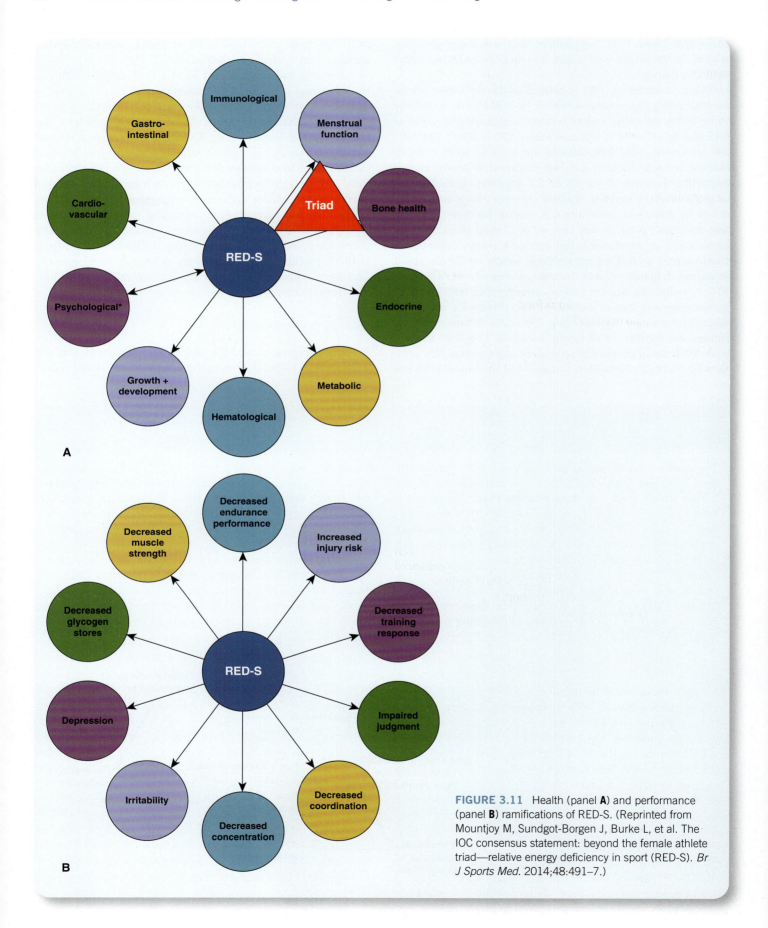

FIGURE 3.11 Health (panel **A**) and performance (panel **B**) ramifications of RED-S. (Reprinted from Mountjoy M, Sundgot-Borgen J, Burke L, et al. The IOC consensus statement: beyond the female athlete triad—relative energy deficiency in sport (RED-S). *Br J Sports Med*. 2014;48:491–7.)

(other than tobacco) intended to supplement the diet that bears or contains one or more of the following dietary ingredients: a vitamin, a mineral, an herb or other botanical, an amino acid, a dietary substance for use by man to supplement the diet by increasing the total daily intake, or a concentrate, metabolite, constituent, extract, or combination of these ingredients." Although this document highlighted the importance of supplements for improving health and reducing the risk factors for disease — as well as the importance of the supplement industry as an integral part of the economy — it also made it easier for supplement manufacturers to market their products. Prior to this document, federal legislation passed in 1993 limited the jurisdiction of the Food and Drug Administration (FDA) for regulating the quality, safety, and testing of nutrition supplements. The result has been a dramatic increase in sport-supplement marketing and sales. It has been estimated that 37%–89% of athletes internationally have used sports supplements (12). Sports supplements are classified as food products in the United States, so there is no need for FDA approval before selling products to consumers.

A number of nutrients have been sold as supplements either alone or as multinutrient supplements. Sports supplements may be found in many forms such as tablets, capsules, softgels, gelcaps, liquids, bars, or powders only intended for oral consumption. Several of these have been discussed in this chapter as well as other chapters in this textbook. Although it is beyond the scope of this book to discuss each one in detail, Table 3.8 depicts many of these supplements and classifies them based on whether there is strong evidence regarding efficacy, limited to mixed evidence, or little to no evidence. The important concept for the athlete is to try to get maximum nutrients from the diet. Macro- and micronutrient supplements may help if they correct a deficiency or they are used to meet a high demand of training, practice, competition, travel, environmental stress, etc. difficult to attain with dietary intake. Only few supplements have consistently enhanced various elements of athletic performance beyond deficiency correction, and the effects are relatively short term, far inferior to the effects seen by several banned performance-enhancing drugs, which often possess a dose-response relationship (31).

Microbiome, Microbiota, and Probiotics

The **microbiota** refers to the diverse ecosystem of bacteria, archaea, viruses, protists, and fungi living in the gut, whereas the **microbiome** consists of the genomes from all of these microorganisms (49). The number of genes in all of the trillions of microbes in the microbiome is 200 times greater than the human genome. The microbiota hosts digestion, metabolism, and immune function. The microbiome plays a major role in every aspect of human health and performance and is affected by many factors including diet, stress, exercise, aging, drug use, infant delivery and feeding, and geography (11,49). It appears the microbiome may impact nutritional preference and the foods we consume and is positively affected by exercise (11). Dietary soluble fermentable fibers are the preferred food source for the microbiota where they are fermented and

Table 3.8	Efficacy of Various Sports Supplements	
Evidence		
Strong	**Limited or Mixed**	**Little to None**
Protein and essential amino acids	BCAAs	Prohormones
	Quercetin	Ribose
β-HMB	Taurine	Inosine
Creatine	Glycerol	Boron
β-Alanine	Citrulline	Medium-chain triglycerides
Sodium bicarbonate and phosphate	Citrus aurantium	Arginine (NO₂)
	Betaine	Agmatine sulfate
Caffeine	L-carnitine	Alpha-ketoglutarate
Carbohydrates	L-Alanyl-L-glutamate	Alpha-ketoisocaproate
Sports drinks/water	Arachidonic acid	Chromium
	Phosphatidic acid	Chrysin
	Nitrates	Conjugated linoleic acid
	Phosphate	D-Aspartic acid
	Adenosine-5′-triphosphate	Ecdysterones
	Coenzyme Q10	Gamma oryzanol
		GH releasers
		Sodium citrate
		Fenugreek extract
		Glutamine
		Phospholipids (phosphatidylcholine, phosphatidylserine, phosphatidylglycerol, phosphatidylinositol, phosphatidyl-ethanolamine)
		Ornithine-alpha-ketoglutarate
		Tribulus terrestris
		Isoflavones
		Sulfo-polysaccharides (myostatin inhibitors)
		Vanadyl sulfate
		Zinc-magnesium aspartate

Adapted from References (2,9,12,33,46–48).

metabolized into short-chain fatty acids, acetate, propionate, and butyrate (11). Exercise increases microbiota diversity and butyrate-producing bacteria levels which have been shown to correlate with aerobic fitness (11).

Nutritional strategies used to modulate the microbiota via prebiotic, probiotic, and symbiotic supplements have been implemented. **Prebiotics** are undigested dietary fibers that reach the gut and are fermented to support the microbiota. **Probiotics** are live bacteria (*i.e.*, "good bacteria") and yeasts that have healthy beneficial effects in the digestive system. A **symbiotic** is a combination of both. Some studies have shown that certain probiotics can assist with symptoms of upper respiratory tract illness and improve gastrointestinal function in endurance athletes, and enhance recovery following resistance training (11). Active individuals, including athletes, show health-promoting bacterial species, increased microbiome diversity, increased metabolic pathways, and fecal metabolites that are associated with higher levels of fitness (49). Probiotic strains show differences in their ability to inhabit the gastrointestinal tract and induce health-promoting benefits (49). Protein intake (especially whey) is strong modulator microbiota diversity, and a high CHO and fiber intake in athletes is associated with the abundance of the *Prevotella* strain (49). A growing number of supplements containing probiotics targeting health and performance in athletes are available in the form of capsules, tablets, powder, liquids, and in nutrition bars and yogurt (49). In a recent position stand (49), it was concluded that probiotic supplementation can improve exercise performance in athletes. Specifically, the discrete strain is critical as single-strain supplements have shown minimal effects, while supplementation with multistrain probiotics was shown to increase VO_{2max}, training load, and time to exhaustion in some studies but not all. It was also concluded that probiotic supplementation can reduce muscle damage and increase recovery from RE, but equivocal results in regard to body composition changes (49). Thus, these growing lines of research may hold promise in uncovering another source of nutritional ergogenics for athletes. It is important for the athlete or coach to identify specific strains, within a multistrain supplement, scientifically shown to enhance health and performance. Some strains showing benefit for health and performance include *Lactobacillus acidophilus* (LA14) and (SPP), *Lactobacillus fermentum* (PCC) and (VRI-003), *Bifidobacterium longum* (BL05), *Bacillus coagulans* (BC30), *Bifidobacterium breve* (BR03), *Streptococcus thermophilus* (FP4), *Lactobacillus plantarum* (TWK10), *Lactobacillus rhamnosus* (IMC 501), *Lactobacillus paracasei* (IMC 502), *Lactobacillus delbrueckii bulgaricus*, *Bifidobacterium bifidum*, and others (49).

 Practical Considerations

Designing a meal plan involves determining the needed amount of energy intake per day, calculating recommended amounts of macro- and micro-nutrients per day, selecting appropriate food sources, partitioning nutrients across meals and snacks or nutrient timing, and maintaining appropriate hydration. The athlete should try to obtain adequate nutrient intake through dietary food and beverage consumption. When necessary, sports supplements may be used to consume appropriate nutrient intake. The recommended intakes have been discussed in this chapter and in other chapters (*i.e.*, hydration strategies). Here, some strategies or tips are given to help the athlete with pre- and posttraining or competition nutrient intake.

Precompetition Strategies

The precompetition strategy begins days before the competition and ultimately depends on the metabolic responses of the sport, environment (*e.g.*, altitude, temperature, humidity), training volume and intensity and/or tapering strategy, and the need to make weight (*e.g.*, wrestling) or lose weight (*e.g.*, bodybuilding). Major goals of precompetition strategy are to maximize carbohydrate intake (for glycogen stores), maintain or protein intake to maintain LBM as much as possible (especially while consuming a hypocaloric diet), optimize micronutrient intake, consume sports supplements when needed, and maximize hydration levels. For endurance athletes, an increase in fat intake in days prior to competition may help as well. Some suggested strategies for preexercise nutrition include (1,8,10,12) the following:

- The preexercise meal should focus on providing carbohydrates (1–4 g·kg body mass^{-1}) regardless of the GI and fluids. The athlete should consume a high-carbohydrate, low-fat meal 3–4 hours before exercising or competition to allow adequate digestion time. A light carbohydrate snack or sport drink could be consumed after the meal and before exercise, provided that large amounts are not consumed at one time. If the meal is 2 hours before, then intake of 1 g·kg body mass^{-1} is good. Meals should be smaller the closer to the event they are consumed (*e.g.*, 0.5 g·kg body mass^{-1} if consumed 1 h before).
- Consuming only familiar foods and foods that are well tolerated by the gastrointestinal system.
- Energy intake should be at a level to allow the athlete make it at least most, if not all, the way through the workout or competition. The ability to consume fluids or energy bar/snack during breaks in the competition will help.
- The athlete should try to prevent feelings of hunger, or hypoglycemia.
- The athlete should avoid foods high in fiber or foods that may cause gas (*e.g.*, broccoli, cauliflower).
- The athlete should consume fluids (with CHOs, amino acids, and electrolytes) at least 5–10 mL·kg^{-1}·body weight^{-1} at least 2–4 hours prior and continue fluid intake each hour and 10–20 minutes prior to the competition. Fluids should be flavored to improve thirst and encourage fluid intake.

- Cutting fluids to make weight may result in a significant fluid deficit which could be difficult to correct between weigh-in and the start of competition.
- Cold fluids or ice slurries before exercise can help prior to exercise on hot, humid days.
- Fat content should be low right before as it could slow down gastric emptying.
- A moderate amount of protein can be consumed.
- For those athletes who consume sports supplements, consuming a multipurpose preworkout supplement with micronutrients, thermogenics such as caffeine, and other nutrients (*i.e.*, nitrates, acid-base buffers) could be helpful.

During Exercise or Competition

Nutrient intake during exercise or competition is mostly designed to maintain hydration and provide CHOs, amino acids, and electrolytes. The makeup of the sport is critical. Sports such as football, basketball, and baseball allow many opportunities to consume fluids throughout. Fluid stations are available at fixed intervals during distance running. Thus, opportunity dictates the fluid intake strategy during competition. It is important to have athletes practice hydration strategies with similar intervals prior to competition, so there is familiarity. Some suggested strategies for nutrition during exercise and competition include (1,5,8,10,12) the following:

- Fluids should be readily available to all athletes and each athlete should have a bottle or method of ensuring intake during event. This may not be an issue for sports where coaches and athletic training staffs provide fluids for the athletes.
- Fluid intake should match sweat loss to where weight is maintained or <2% of body weight is lost. It helps if athletes know their sweat rate prior to competition which range from 0.3 to >2.4 $L \cdot h^{-1}$. Thus, ~200–500 mL every 10–15 minutes is good but could be higher depending on body size, sweat rate, exercise intensity, and environmental conditions.
- Ingestion of cold beverages helps to reduce core temperature and improve performance in the heat. The beverage should taste good to increase palatability and fluid intake.
- Overdrinking water that leads to hyponatremia should be avoided.
- Consumption of CHOs may not have a significant impact on very brief exercise (<45 min) performance so may not be needed however should be consumed with more sustained and higher intensity exercise (45–75 min and beyond) in the form of sport drinks or a mouth rinse (*e.g.*, contact of CHO with mouth can stimulate the brain and CNS to enhance perceptions of well-being). If food can be consumed, a high GI easily digestible CHO source is good (*i.e.*, bananas, breads, energy bar).
- The carbohydrate target should be ~30–60 $g \cdot h^{-1}$, or up to 90 $g \cdot h^{-1}$ for exercise >2.5 hours in duration.
- The fluid should contain 6%–8% CHO solution and electrolytes. Typical electrolyte losses in sweat are 920–1,840 $mg \cdot L^{-1}$ of sodium, 1,065–2,485 $mg \cdot L^{-1}$ of chloride, and 156–312 $mg \cdot L^{-1}$ of potassium. Athletes who are not acclimatized to heat nor have high sweat rates may lose more electrolytes (especially sodium) during exercise. Many sport drinks contain 80–160 mg of sodium and 18–46 mg of potassium per 8 oz of fluid, or 336–670 mg and 76–195 $mg \cdot L^{-1}$.

Post Exercise or Competition

The postexercise meal is designed to replenish fluids lost (and not consumed during exercise), repair skeletal muscle tissue, and maximize recovery of glycogen stores. The timing is critical especially if the athlete has another training session or competition soon thereafter. Some suggested strategies for nutrition during the postexercise and competition period include (1,5,8,10,12) the following:

- Consuming 1.0–1.5 $g \cdot kg$ body mass^{-1} of CHOs soon after completion (within 30–60 min) of workout or competition is important to enhance muscle glycogen recovery. This prime "window" takes advantage of the rapid, non–insulin-dependent first phase of glycogen resynthesis. This intake should be repeated every 2 hours for 4–6 hours. Sports drink or supplements can be used here if the athlete has reduced hunger in order to obtain the required nutrients. Delayed consumption can reduce glycogen resynthesis so the earlier the intake the better.
- For slower repletion (if the athlete does not need to rapidly recover for another training session or competition within the next day or two), the individual should consume 8–10 $g \cdot kg^{-1}$ of body mass of CHOs over a 24-hour period.
- Many high GI CHOs are beneficial post exercise to achieve rapid glycogen resynthesis.
- Athletes should drink ~1.5 L of water/sports drink per kg of body mass or ~600 mL per pound of weight lost during exercise. This should be consumed within 2 hours of completion to return to normal body weight prior to the next exercise session.
- Athletes should consume at least 0.2–0.5 $g \cdot kg$ body mass^{-1} of high-quality protein (*e.g.*, casein, whey, egg) every 3–5 hours in multiple meals. The first bolus of protein (along with CHOs) should be consumed soon after completion of the workout or competition. At least 20–30 g (with approximately half coming from essential amino acids and 2–3 g of leucine) but a larger amount may be taken especially by strength/power athletes striving to increase muscle strength and hypertrophy. Many protein supplements or shakes enable the consumption of a larger amount of protein post exercise.
- For subsequent meals consumed every 3–4 hours, protein intake should match the desired distribution. For example, a 100–kg athlete who targets 1.7 $g \cdot kg$ BM$^{-1} \cdot d^{-1}$ would consume ~170 $g \cdot d^{-1}$. This total can be broken down per meal so if the athlete consumed 4–5 meals (or snacks and supplements) then they would consume ~30–40 $g \cdot meal^{-1}$.
- Micronutrient and fat intake should max targeted goals for subsequent postexercise meals.

SUMMARY POINTS

- Nutrition is the science that studies the relationship of nutrient consumption to optimal health, development, and performance. Nutrition, recovery, and training are all equally important to the athlete.
- Nutrients are needed for growth and repair of body tissue, and maintenance of life. Macronutrients include carbohydrates, proteins, fats, and water; and micronutrients include vitamins and minerals.
- Carbohydrates perform a multitude of functions including serving as a major source of energy.
- Proteins serve as hormones, receptors, enzymes, transporters, building blocks of tissue, acid-base balance, immune cells, and as a last resort energy source.
- Fats serve as an energy source, source of essential fatty acids, transporter for certain vitamins, insulation, and structural components.
- Vitamins and minerals are involved in multitude of biochemical reactions involved in health and performance.
- Probiotics are live bacteria and yeasts that have healthy beneficial effects in the digestive system.
- Designing a meal plan for athletes involves determining the needed amount of energy intake per day, calculating recommended amounts of macro- and micro-nutrients per day, selecting appropriate food sources, partitioning nutrients across meals and snacks or nutrient timing, and maintaining appropriate hydration.

REVIEW QUESTIONS

1. Carbohydrates, fats, and protein are considered
   a. Micronutrients
   b. Macronutrients
   c. Vitamins
   d. Minerals

2. Monosaccharides, disaccharides, oligosaccharides, and polysaccharides are
   a. Carbohydrates
   b. Proteins
   c. Fats
   d. Probiotics

3. Vitamins A, D, E, and K are
   a. Electrolytes
   b. Macronutrients
   c. Water-soluble vitamins
   d. Fat-soluble vitamins

4. A mineral that forms a critical structural component of hemoglobin is
   a. Iodine
   b. Magnesium
   c. Potassium
   d. Iron

5. The electrolyte in highest concentration in sweat is
   a. Calcium
   b. Sodium
   c. Potassium
   d. Iron

6. The female triad was used to describe the link between low energy intake, menstrual dysfunction, and weakened bones.
   a. T
   b. F

7. The branch-chained amino acids include glutamine, arginine, and proline.
   a. T
   b. F

8. The glycemic index is a reference system (based on a standardized amount of glucose) pertaining to the elevation in blood sugar and insulin in response to food and beverage consumption.
   a. T
   b. F

9. High-density lipoproteins carry lipids away from storage to the liver and protect against cardiovascular disease.
   a. T
   b. F

10. The ketogenic diet is an example of a high-carbohydrate, low-fat diet.
    a. T
    b. F

REFERENCES

1. Benardot D. *ACSM's Nutrition for Exercise Science*. Philadelphia (PA): Wolters Kluwer; 2019.
2. Kerksick CM, Wilborn CD, Roberts MD, et al. ISSN exercise & sports nutrition review update: research & recommendations. *J Int Soc Sports Nutr.* 2018;15:38.
3. Clark N. *Nancy Clark's Sports Nutrition Guidebook*. Champaign (IL): Human Kinetics; 2014.
4. Jeukendrup AE. Periodized nutrition for athletes. *Sports Med.* 2017;47(Suppl 1):51–63.
5. Hertzler S, Carlson-Phillips A. Basic nutrition for tactical populations. In: Alvar B, Sell K, Deuster PA, editors. *NSCA's Essentials of Tactical Strength Training and Conditioning*. 4th ed. Champaign (IL): Human Kinetics; 2017. p. 69–99.
6. Spano M. Basic nutrition factors in health. In: Haff G, Triplett T, editors. *Essentials of Strength Training and Conditioning*. 4th ed. Champaign (IL): Human Kinetics; 2016. p. 175–200.

7. American Diabetes Association. Postprandial blood glucose. *Diabetes Care*. 2001;24:775–8.

8. Battista RA. Nutrition and human performance. In: Battista RA, editors. *ACSM's Resources for the Personal Trainer*. Philadelphia (PA): Wolters Kluwer; 2018.

9. Kerksick CM, Arent S, Schoenfeld BJ, et al. International society of sports nutrition position stand: nutrient timing. *J Int Soc Sports Nutr*. 2017;14:33.

10. Spano M. Nutrition strategies for maximizing performance. In: Haff G, Triplett T, editors. *Essentials of Strength Training and Conditioning*. 4th ed. Champaign (IL): Human Kinetics; 2016. p. 201–24.

11. Kraemer WJ, Fleck SJ, Deschenes MR. Nutrition and environment. In: *Exercise Physiology: Integrating Theory and Application*. 2nd ed. Philadelphia (PA): Wolters Kluwer; 2015.

12. American College of Sports Medicine, American Dietetic Association, Dietitians of Canada. Joint position stand. Nutrition and athletic performance. *Med Sci Sports Exerc*. 2016;48(3):543–68.

13. Atkinson FS, Foster-Powell K, Brand-Miller JC. International tables of glycemic index and glycemic load values: 2008. *Diabetes Care*. 2008;31:2281–3.

14. Burdon CA, Spronk I, Cheng HL, O'Connor HT. Effect of glycemic index of a pre-exercise meal on endurance exercise performance: a systematic review and meta-analysis. *Sports Med*. 2017;47:1087–101.

15. Heung-Sang Wong S, Sun FH, Chen YJ, Li C, Zhang YJ, Ya-Jun Huang W. Effect of pre-exercise carbohydrate diets with high vs low glycemic index on exercise performance: a meta-analysis. *Nutr Rev*. 2017;75:327–38.

16. Ormsbee MJ, Bach CW, Baur DA. Pre-exercise nutrition: the role of macronutrients, modified starches and supplements on metabolism and endurance performance. *Nutrients*. 2014;6:1782–808.

17. Gibbs M, Harrington D, Starkey S, Williams P, Hampton S. Diurnal postprandial responses to low and high glycaemic index mixed meals. *Clin Nutr*. 2014;33:889–94.

18. Orrù S, Imperlini E, Nigro E, et al. Role of functional beverages on sport performance and recovery. *Nutrients*. 2018;10:1470.

19. Jäger R, Kerksick CM, Campbell BI, et al. International Society of Sports Nutrition Position Stand: protein and exercise. *J Int Soc Sports Nutr*. 2017;14:20.

20. Phillips SM, Van Loon LJ. Dietary protein for athletes: from requirements to optimum adaptation. *J Sports Sci*. 2011;29(Suppl 1):S29–38.

21. Schoenfeld BJ, Aragon AA. How much protein can the body use in a single meal for muscle-building? Implications for daily protein distribution. *J Int Soc Sports Nutr*. 2018;15:10.

22. Morton RW, Murphy KT, McKellar SR, et al. A systematic review, meta-analysis and meta-regression of the effect of protein supplementation on resistance training-induced gains in muscle mass and strength in healthy adults. *Br J Sports Med*. 2018;52:376–84.

23. Hoffman JR, Falvo MJ. Protein—which is best? *J Sports Sci Med*. 2004;3(3):118–30.

24. Norton LE, Layman DK. Leucine regulates translation initiation of protein synthesis in skeletal muscle after exercise. *J Nutr*. 2006;136(2):533S–7S.

25. Aragon AA, Schoenfeld BJ. Nutrient timing revisited: is there a post-exercise anabolic window? *J Int Soc Sports Nutr*. 2013;10:5.

26. Schoenfeld BJ, Aragon A, Wilborn C, Urbina SL, Hayward SE, Krieger J. Pre-versus post-exercise protein intake has similar effects on muscular adaptations. *Peer J*. 2017;5:e2825.

27. Schoenfeld BJ, Aragon AA, Krieger JW. The effect of protein timing on muscle strength and hypertrophy: a meta-analysis. *J Int Soc Sports Nutr*. 2013;10:53.

28. Snijders T, Trommelen J, Kouw IWK, Holwerda AM, Verdijk LB, van Loon LJC. The impact of pre-sleep protein ingestion on the skeletal muscle adaptive response to exercise in humans: an update. *Front Nutr*. 2019;6:17.

29. Antonio J, Ellerbroek A, Silver T, et al. A high protein diet has no harmful effects: a one-year crossover study in resistance-trained males. *J Nutr Metab*. 2016;2016:9104792.

30. Peters SA, Singhateh Y, Mackay D, Huxley RR, Woodward M. Total cholesterol as a risk factor for coronary heart disease and stroke in women compared with men: a systematic review and meta-analysis. *Atherosclerosis*. 2016;248:123–31.

31. Ratamess NA. *Coaches Guide to Performance-Enhancing Supplements*. Monterey (CA): Coaches Choice Books; 2006.

32. Mickleborough TD, Murray RL, Ionescu AA, Lindley MR. Fish oil supplementation reduces severity of exercise-induced bronchoconstriction in elite athletes. *Am J Respir Crit Care Med*. 2003;168:1181–9.

33. Ratamess NA. Emerging ergogenic aids for strength/power development. In: Hoffman JR, editor. *Dietary Supplementation in Sport and Exercise: Evidence, Safety and Ergogenic Benefits*. 1st ed. New York (NY): Routledge Press; 2019. p. 255–78.

34. Volek JS, Kraemer WJ, Fleck SJ, Deschenes MR. Formulating a ketogenic diet. In: *Exercise Physiology: Integrating Theory and Application*. 2nd ed. Philadelphia (PA): Wolters Kluwer; 2015.

35. Kang J, Ratamess NA, Faigenbaum AD, Bush JA. Ergogenic properties of ketogenic diets in normal-weight individuals: a systematic review. *J Am Coll Nutr*. 2020;39(7):665–675. doi: 10.1080/07315724.2020.1725686.

36. Ludwig DS, Willett WC, Volek JS, Neuhouser ML. Dietary fat: from foe to friend? *Science*. 2018;362:764–70.

37. McArdle WD, Katch FI, Katch VL. *Exercise Physiology: Energy, Nutrition, and Human Performance*. 6th ed. Philadelphia (PA): Lippincott Williams & Wilkins; 2007. p. 123–228.

38. Zhang L, Quan M, Cao ZB. Effect of vitamin D supplementation on upper and lower limb muscle strength and muscle power in athletes: a meta-analysis. *PLoS One*. 2019;14:e0215826.

39. Chiang CM, Ismaeel A, Griffis RB, Weems S. Effects of vitamin D supplementation on muscle strength in athletes: a systematic review. *J Strength Cond Res*. 2017;31:566–74.

40. Han Q, Li X, Tan Q, Shao J, Yi M. Effects of vitamin D3 supplementation on serum 25(OH)D concentration and strength in athletes: a systematic review and meta-analysis of randomized controlled trials. *J Int Soc Sports Nutr*. 2019;16:55.

41. Heffernan SM, Horner K, De Vito G, Conway GE. The role of mineral and trace element supplementation in exercise and athletic performance: a systematic review. *Nutrients*. 2019;11:696.

42. Zhang Y, Xun P, Wang R, Mao L, He K. Can magnesium enhance exercise performance? *Nutrients*. 2017;9(9):946.

43. Huang D. Dietary antioxidants and health promotion. *Antioxidants (Basel)*. 2018;7:9.

44. Nattiv A, Loucks AB, Manore MM, et al. American College of Sports Medicine position stand. The female athlete triad. *Med Sci Sports Exerc*. 2007;39:1867–82.

45. Mountjoy M, Sundgot-Borgen J, Burke L, et al. The IOC consensus statement: beyond the Female Athlete Triad—Relative Energy Deficiency in Sport (RED-S). *Br J Sports Med*. 2014;48:491–7.

46. Campbell B. Performance-enhancing substances and methods. In: Haff G, Triplett T, editors. *Essentials of Strength Training and Conditioning*. 4th ed. Champaign (IL): Human Kinetics; 2016. p. 225–48.

47. Kang J. *Nutrition and Metabolism in Sports, Exercise and Health*. New York (NY): Routledge; 2012. p. 20–109.

48. Lockwood C. Overview of sports supplements. In: Antonio J, Kalman D, Stout J, et al., editors. *Essentials of Sports Nutrition and Supplements*. Totowa, NJ: Human Press; 2008. p. 459–540.

49. Jäger R, Mohr AE, Carpenter KC, et al. International Society of Sports Nutrition Position Stand: probiotics. *J Int Soc Sports Nutr*. 2019;16:62.

PART II

Physiological Responses and Adaptations

CHAPTER 4
Neural Adaptations to Training

OBJECTIVES

After completing this chapter, you will be able to:

- Describe the central and peripheral nervous systems
- Describe the anatomy and functions of neurons
- Describe the major sites of adaptation within the brain and spinal cord
- Define a motor unit and discuss how changes in recruitment, firing rate, and firing patterns affect muscular strength and power
- Describe changes that take place at the neuromuscular junction in response to training
- Describe the roles of sensory receptors, especially Golgi tendon organs and muscle spindles
- Describe how training variables can affect the neural responses and training adaptations
- Discuss the role of the autonomic nervous system during exercise

---

The nervous system is extremely important for modulating acute exercise performance and the subsequent training adaptations. Nerves provide the major lines of communication between the brain and bodily tissues including skeletal muscles. They ensure that the message or signal travels to the appropriate location. From a training perspective, the nervous system is critical for motor learning and the acquisition of skill. Optimal expressions of performance can only be seen when the exercise or motor skill technique is proper. The magnitude (or strength) of the signal is critical in determining the final output, which could be the expression of muscular strength, endurance, and power. This quantity is termed *neural drive* and an increase in neural drive is critical to the individual striving to maximize performance. The increase in neural drive is thought to occur via increases in *agonist* (*i.e.*, those major muscles involved in a specific movement or exercise) muscle recruitment, firing rate, and the timing/pattern of discharge during high-intensity muscular contractions. A reduction in inhibitory mechanisms is thought to occur. Although it is not exactly clear how these mechanisms coexist, it is clear that neural adaptations are complex and may precede changes in skeletal muscle size.

Functional Organization of the Nervous System

The nervous system is one major control system contained within the human body (the other being the endocrine system). It has the ability to receive sensory information (pain, pressure, hot/cold temperatures, joint position, muscle length), integrate this information in appropriate places, and control the output or response (voluntary and involuntary) from every tissue, gland, and organ. It also controls our emotions, personality, and other cerebral functions.

The nervous system is composed of two major divisions, the central and peripheral nervous systems (Fig. 4.1). The *central nervous system* (CNS) consists of the brain and spinal cord. The *peripheral nervous system* consists of two major divisions: the sensory and motor divisions. Thirty-one pairs of spinal nerves enter or exit the posterior (sensory) and anterior (motor) roots of the spinal cord, respectively. The *sensory nervous system* detects various stimuli and conveys this information afferently to the CNS. The *motor nervous system* consists of two major divisions: the somatic and autonomic nervous systems (ANS). The *somatic nervous system* conveys information from the CNS efferently (*e.g.*, away from CNS) to skeletal muscle ultimately leading to muscle contraction (and fatigue). The ANS consists of nerves conveying efferent information to smooth muscle, cardiac muscle, and other glands, tissues, and organs. The ANS consists of the *sympathetic* and *parasympathetic* nervous systems, both of which are essential for preparing the body for the stress of exercise and returning the body back to normal resting conditions. Training may elicit adaptations along the neuromuscular chain initiating in the higher brain centers and continuing down to the level of individual muscle fibers.

75

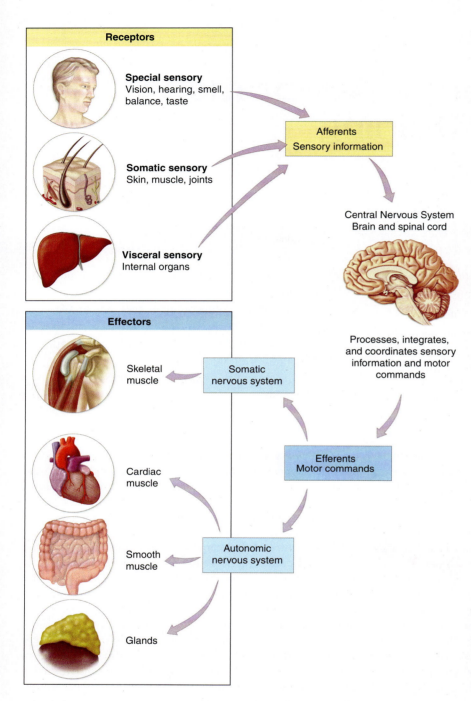

FIGURE 4.1 Divisions of the nervous system. The central (brain and spinal cord) and peripheral (sensory and motor) nervous systems are shown. (Reprinted From Premkumar K. *The Massage Connection: Anatomy and Physiology.* Baltimore (MD): Lippincott Williams & Wilkins; 2004.)

Aerobic training imposes specific neural demands although the pattern of neural activation appears less complex than anaerobic, high-intensity training where high levels of muscle strength, power, and speed are required.

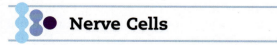

Nerve Cells

Nervous tissue comes in two forms: (a) *supporting cells* and (b) *neurons*. Supporting cells play key stability roles throughout the CNS. Neurons are the actual nerve cells with the ability to communicate with other tissues and nerves. Sensory neurons tend to be unipolar, whereas motor neurons are multipolar (Fig. 4.2). Neurons possess several key features. *Dendrites* receive input from other nerve cells. The *cell body* contains the organelles responsible for protein synthesis, transport, energy metabolism, and packaging and plays the critical role in integrating stimuli from other neurons from within the CNS to determine if and how much stimuli will make its way to skeletal muscle. *Axons* are long processes that are responsible for communicating with target tissues. The *axon hillock* is the area where the action potential is initiated once the critical threshold

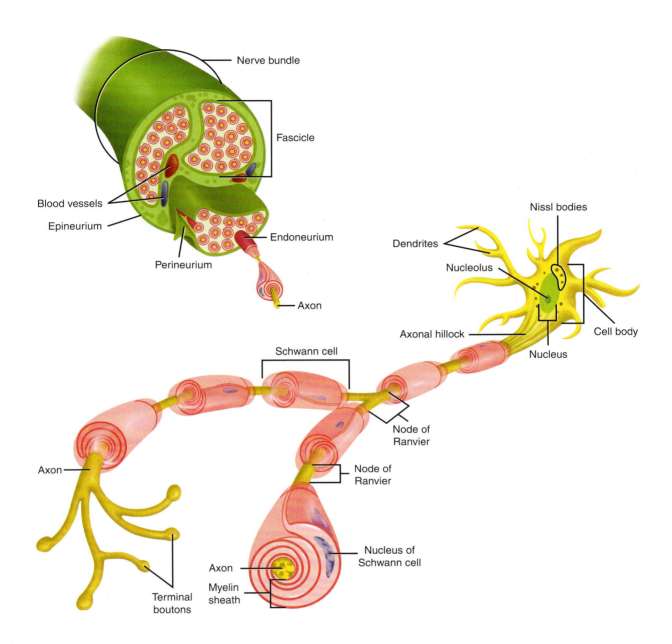

FIGURE 4.2 Motoneuron anatomy. The peripheral nerve bundle (collection of axons) and key structures of the motoneuron such as the dendrites, cell body, axon, axon hillock, myelin sheath, and nodes of Ranvier are shown. (From Eroschenko VP. *di Fiore's Atlas of Histology, with Functional Correlations*. 9th ed. Baltimore (MD): Lippincott Williams & Wilkins; 2000.)

is reached. *Myelin sheath* (fatty tissue) is wrapped around the axons, which greatly increases the speed of transmission. The end of the axon branches and is known as the *presynaptic terminal* where it forms a synapse with the target tissue.

Neural Communication

Nerves communicate with other nerves and tissue via generation of an electrical current (signal) called the *action potential*. The action potential (Fig. 4.3) consists of three major events: (a) integration, (b) propagation, and (c) neurotransmitter release.

Integration occurs within the cell body (within the CNS) and determines whether or not the action potential will be sent to the target tissue. The cell body integrates charges from other neurons (excitatory, inhibitory) known as postsynaptic potentials, *e.g.*, excitatory (EPSP) or inhibitory (IPSP) postsynaptic potentials. If the threshold voltage is reached, the action potential will travel in all-or-none fashion to the end of the nerve terminal. Propagation is brought about by ion movement (sodium and potassium) down the axon at the Nodes of Ranvier via a process called *saltatory conduction*. This drives the electrical current rapidly down the axon to the terminal. The presence

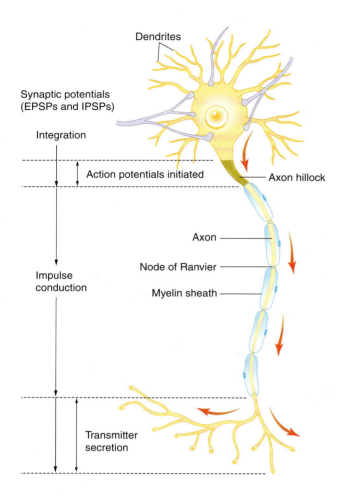

FIGURE 4.3 The action potential. The dendrites receive information from other neurons and interneurons in the spinal cord. The resultant messages (excitatory postsynaptic potential [EPSP] and inhibitory postsynaptic potential [IPSP]) are integrated in the cell body and an action potential is produced if the threshold voltage is reached. This recruitment threshold is critical and dependent on motor unit type, *e.g.*, high-threshold fast-twitch units or low-threshold slow-twitch units. The action potential is propagated down the axon to the terminal where neurotransmitters are released to allow communication with target tissues, *i.e.*, skeletal muscle. (From Cohen BJ. *Medical Terminology*. 4th ed. Philadelphia (PA): Lippincott Williams & Wilkins; 2003.)

of myelin sheath greatly accelerates this process. At the nerve terminal, calcium influx increases mediating the release of neurotransmitters (chemical signaling molecules, *acetylcholine* at the neuromuscular junction [NMJ]), thereby allowing communication to take place with the target tissue. Acetylcholine (Ach) binds to receptors on the postsynaptic membrane and produces end-plate potentials ultimately leading to the depolarization of skeletal muscle fibers. One Ach vesicle produces a miniature end-plate potential (MEPP), which is the smallest level of depolarization that can be induced in skeletal muscle. This entire process occurs at a very fast speed with reference to motor neurons stimulating skeletal muscles, thereby enabling several action potentials to be conducted in a second.

Higher Brain Centers

The brain contains billions of neurons each with the ability to communicate with nearly 10,000 others (Fig. 4.4). Ultimately, the brain controls nearly all aspects of human bodily function from psychological/emotional factors to motor performance. Although complete discussion of the brain is beyond the scope of this text, some critical areas need to be mentioned because they serve as potential sites of adaptations to training. The *brainstem* (consisting of the medulla oblongata, midbrain, pons, and reticular formation) contains neuronal centers that control cardiac heart rate and force of contraction, blood pressure, blood vessel diameter, breathing, hearing, vision, sleep, and consciousness. The *diencephalon* (consisting of the thalamus, hypothalamus, and pineal body or epithalamus) is the major relay area of the brain (thalamus) and control center for sleep (pineal body). The *hypothalamus* is the major link between the nervous and endocrine systems because it is an endocrine gland under neural control. It releases several hormones that either cause or inhibit the release of hormones from the anterior pituitary, ultimately controlling *homeostasis*, autonomic control, body temperature, emotions, and essentially most functions within the body. The *cerebrum* is the largest part of the brain, with 75% of the neurons within the nervous system located in the outermost region of the cerebrum known as the *cerebral cortex*. Although many areas of the cerebral cortex have important functions, critical areas include the *primary sensory area* (where sensory information is integrated), the *premotor cortex* (where a voluntary muscle contraction begins and also a memory bank for skilled motor activities), and the *primary motor cortex* (where voluntary muscle contraction is controlled). The *supplementary motor area* (SMA) lies above the premotor cortex and is involved in the planning and coordination of complex movements. The *posterior parietal cortex* is an association cortex thought to be involved in transforming multisensory information into motor commands and motor planning. The *cerebellum* integrates sensory information and coordinates skeletal muscle activity, *e.g.*, it provides a blueprint of how the motor skill should be performed. Lastly, the *basal ganglia* is involved with planning and control of muscle function, posture, and controlling unwanted movements.

Neural responses and adaptations begin in the brain and may occur at multiple central and peripheral locations extending to the muscle fiber level. Acute exercise and chronic aerobic and anaerobic training have been shown to positively affect cognition, memory, and has been successful in treating various neurodegenerative disorders (1). Exercise has been suggested to increase the synthesis and release of neurotransmitters (*e.g.*, dopamine, serotonin, acetylcholine, and norepinephrine) and neurotrophins, which function to increase neuroplasticity, angiogenesis and cerebral blood flow and oxygenation, myelination, and neurogenesis (1). Neurogenic responses occur both centrally and peripherally

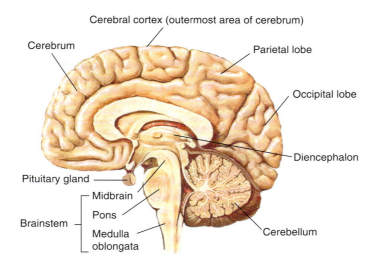

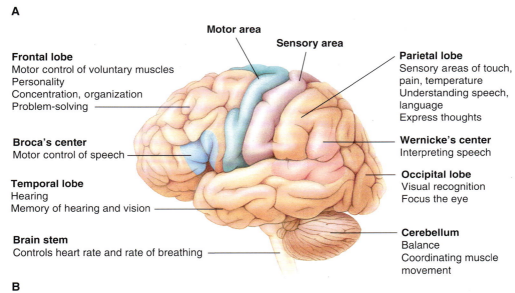

FIGURE 4.4 The brain. **A.** Image shows the anatomy of the brain. Key areas of the brain such as the medulla oblongata, cerebrum, cerebellum, cerebral cortex, diencephalon, primary motor area, and sensory area are identified. (From Bickley LS, Szilagyi P. *Bates' Guide to Physical Examination and History Taking*. 8th ed. Philadelphia (PA): Lippincott Williams & Wilkins; 2003.) **B.** Image shows the various areas of the brain and their control over body systems and function.

(*e.g.*, axon regeneration and reinnervation following injury) in response to exercise, electrical stimulation, and androgens and estrogens (2). Neurotrophins such as brain-derived neurotrophic factor (BDNF), vascular endothelial growth factor (VEGF), neurotrophin-3 (NT3), nerve growth factor (NGF), glial cell line-derived neurotrophic factor (GDNF), insulin-like growth-factor-1 (IGF-1), epidermal growth factor (EGF), and fibroblast growth factor (FGF-2) are shown to increase in response to exercise (1,3). BDNF (a protein consisting of 252 amino acids that functions specifically through binding to its tropomyosin receptor kinase B [TrkB] receptor is involved in neuronal protection and survival, synaptogenesis, neurite expression, and dendrite and axonal growth and remodeling) appears most responsive to acute exercise possibly in an intensity-dependent manner (3,4). In fact, both aerobic and resistance exercise have been shown to acutely elevate BDNF for up to 1 hour postexercise (3). A recent study showed the BDNF response greater during a hypertrophy-based RE protocol compared to a strength protocol (5) although similar increases have been reported between high-intensity, low-volume RE and low-intensity, high-volume RE (6). In addition, chronic resistance training (RT) may augment the acute response to RE (6). However, most studies show that neither training modality appears to produce chronic resting elevations in the blood (3) although sprinters have been shown to have higher basal values than untrained subjects (7).

The ability to induce neuroplasticity to motor learning and increase/modulate neural drive to agonist and antagonist muscles begins in the higher brain centers, *i.e.*, motor cortex. Motor learning results in functional organization of the cerebral cortex. Cortical adaptations are paramount for enhanced coordination, motor learning, skill acquisition, strength, power, and speed. In fact, visualization training (*i.e.*, performing mental contractions or visualizing lifting weights without actually lifting them) has been shown to result in significant strength increases in untrained individuals (8,9). The uses of technologies including electroencephalography, transcranial magnetic stimulation, and various imaging techniques (often in conjunction with electromyography) have provided some insight to cortical responses and adaptations to training. *Electroencephalography* (EEG) is used to quantify electrical activity of the brain noninvasively with surface electrodes applied to the scalp. Movement-related cortical potentials (MRCPs) are generated prior to and during muscle contraction. Acutely, MRCPs are seen prior to muscle contraction in a biphasic manner: a "readiness potential" is seen ~600–1200 ms prior to contraction indicating depolarization of the premotor area/SMA and a subsequent phase is seen ~400 ms prior to contraction indicating depolarization of the primary motor cortex (10). The magnitude of sensorimotor cortex/SMA MRCP has been shown to correlate to with elbow flexion force and rate of force development (RFD) (11), increase during fatigue (10), and higher in ECC than CON actions (12). In direct comparison, Flanagan et al. (13) reported that cortical activity increased the most during a high-volume squat protocol, compared to strength and power protocols. A progressive increase was seen over the course of six sets during the high-volume and strength protocols indicating that acute fatigue may influence the cortical response (13). The motor cortex appears to be a critical area controlling antagonist muscle cocontraction as reduced antagonist muscle cortical potentials during isometric actions of varying force have been seen in strength-trained subjects compared to endurance-trained subjects (14).

Chronic training-induced cortical adaptations may take place in a muscle-specific manner as early as the first workout. *Corticomuscular coherence*, or the synchronization of neural activity in the cortex with muscle function, may be modulated by the types of activity performed and may differ between dominant and nondominant limbs. In fact, RT subjects and ballet dancers have been shown to have less coherence during sustained submaximal contractions compared to untrained control subjects (15). Falvo et al. (16) examined 3 weeks of unilateral leg press RT and reported attenuated MRCPs at relative submaximal contractions. Both studies suggest a "fine-tuning CNS strategy" where the cortical response to long-term specific submaximal muscle recruitment patterns is less, or more efficient, following RT that increases muscle strength and RFD.

Transcranial magnetic stimulation (TMS) involves applying a magnetic field noninvasively to selectively target specific areas of the brain. The magnetic field generator is connected to a pulse generator where a single- or paired-pulse stimulus is applied. The stimuli invoke action potentials along the corticospinal pathways and cause a motor response also measured in conjunction with electromyography. TMS generates critical information regarding cortical responses including the motor-evoked potential (MEP), motor threshold, and the cortical silent period (CSP). MEP amplitude represents cortical activity. Motor thresholds represent membrane excitability of neurons in the motor cortex; a higher threshold represents reduced cortical excitability, whereas lower threshold represents increased cortical excitability, *e.g.*, commonly seen during motor learning. CSP represents corticospinal inhibition. As reviewed by Kidgell et al. (17), RT (in 19 studies reviewed) has been shown to result in decreased MEP amplitude in 4 studies, not change MEP amplitude in 5 studies, and increase MEP amplitude in 10 studies (by a range of 0.7%–34%). They concluded that short-term RT may increase MEP amplitude; however, it appears to have no effect on motor threshold. In addition, all studies reported corresponding strength increases ranging from 8% to 87%. However, the majority of studies have shown reduced CSP duration ranging from 3 to 25 ms and reduced short-interval intracortical inhibition. Thus, the authors suggested that a key cortical adaptation to RT may be reduced corticospinal inhibition via targeting of specific inhibitory $GABA_B$ sensitive intracortical neurons, thereby increasing neural drive (17). Lastly, RT has been shown to increase white matter, subcortical gray matter, axon density, and myelination (18). These collective findings demonstrate that the motor cortex is a potential site for enhanced neural drive during training.

Descending Corticospinal Tracts

The descending corticospinal (or *pyramidal*) tracts are a large collection of axons linking the cerebral cortex to the spinal cord. The motor pathway is characterized by neurons in the brain (primarily in the motor areas) forming synapses with other nerves that eventually make their way down the spinal cord to the exact anterior root of exit for innervation of skeletal muscle. Two common tracts are the lateral and anterior tracts. Neurons of the descending tracts are referred to as *upper motor neurons*. A substantial proportion of potential neural changes are thought to take place in the spinal cord along the descending corticospinal tracts. Untrained individuals display limited ability to maximally recruit all of their muscle fibers. A study by Adams et al. (19) showed that only 71% of muscle mass was activated during maximal effort in untrained individuals. It is believed that a limitation in this central drive reduces strength and power and much of the inhibition originates from these descending corticospinal tracts (20). However, training can greatly reduce this deficit (21–23), thereby showing a greater potential to recruit a larger percent of one's muscle mass with training.

Motor Units

The functional unit of the nervous system is the *motor unit*. A motor unit consists of a single alpha motor nerve and all of the muscle fibers it innervates (Fig. 4.5). Cell bodies and dendrites are located within the spinal cord (to receive excitatory and inhibitory signals from other neurons), whereas axons extend beyond the spinal cord and innervate skeletal muscles in the periphery. Motor neurons may innervate only a few muscle fibers for small muscles (for greater coordination and control) and >1000 for large trunk and limb muscles (for greater force and power). Greater force is produced when excitatory signals increase, inhibitory signals decrease, or a combination of both. When maximal force and power is desired from a muscle, all available motor units must be activated. This generally results from an increase in recruitment, rate of firing, synchronization of firing, or a combination of these factors in agonist muscles. The amplitude of the *compound muscle action potential*, i.e., a measure of motor unit electrical current, has been shown to increase by more than 23% during RT (24) indicating a chronic increase in the number of activated motor units and muscle fibers. Motor unit control strategies have been shown to differ in the vastus lateralis muscle of strength-versus endurance-trained individuals primarily due to differences in type I and II fiber compositions (25).

Recruitment

Recruitment refers to the voluntary activation of motor units during effort. Motor units are recruited and decruited in an orderly progression based on the *size principle* (Fig. 4.6), which states that motor units are recruited in succession from smaller (slow-twitch [ST] or type I) to larger (fast-twitch [FT] or type II) units based on each activation threshold and firing rate (26). Small units are recruited first for more intricate control, and larger units are recruited later to supply substantial force for high-intensity contractions. The activation threshold is the most critical determinant of motor unit recruitment especially among units of similar size. Force and power production may vary greatly because most muscles contain a range of type I and II motor units. Thus, type II motor units are not recruited unless there is a high force, power, agility, and speed requirement, or they are needed to attempt to maintain force output via replacing fatigued motor units. Interestingly, the ability of type II motor units for recruitment is based on previous activation history. Once a motor unit is recruited, less activation is needed for it to be re-recruited (27). This has important ramifications for acute strength and power performance as type II motor units are more readily recruited. Both aerobic and anaerobic forms of training recruit type I and II motor units as evidenced by specific fiber-type adaptations seen within each motor unit type. It appears that the intensity of exercise and level of fatigue are critical to the recruitment strategies used during exercise.

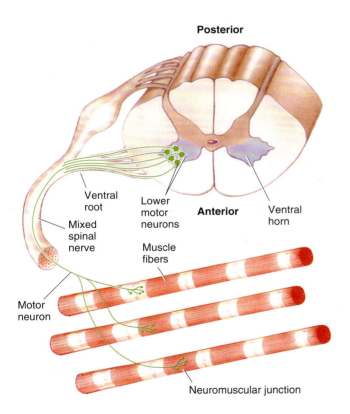

FIGURE 4.5 The motor unit. The motor unit consists of an alpha motoneuron and all of the muscle fibers it innervates. (From Bear M, Conner B, Paradiso M. *Neuroscience, Exploring the Brain.* 2nd ed. Baltimore (MD): Lippincott Williams & Wilkins; 2000.)

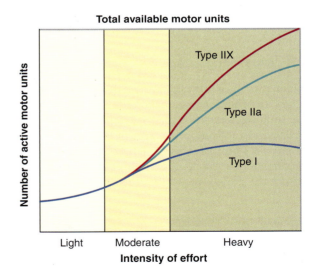

FIGURE 4.6 The size principle. Motor units are recruited under most conditions based on their size where smaller (ST) units are recruited first and larger (FT) units may be recruited later if a substantial amount of force or power is required. (From McArdle WD, Katch FI, Katch VL. *Exercise Physiology: Nutrition, Energy, and Human Performance.* 7th ed. Baltimore (MD): Lippincott Williams & Wilkins; 2010.)

Motor unit recruitment may increase to replace fatigued motor units or units with depleted glycogen during exercise (28). Likewise, motor units are decruited (inactivated) in the reverse order where type II motor units relax first. Type II motor units are also characterized by greater action potential amplitude. A recent study has shown that RT increases motor unit AP amplitude only in type II motor units (29). The increased AP amplitude correlated with muscle hypertrophy indicating that the increased muscle size and sarcolemma area following RT necessitated greater AP amplitude (29).

Selective Recruitment

Under normal conditions, 84%–90% of motor units are recruited in accordance with the size principle (30). However, variations in the timing of motor unit recruitment occur. *Selective recruitment*, or the preferential earlier recruitment of type II motor units, can occur during change in direction of exerted forces (31) and explosive muscle actions (32). The threshold for type II motor unit recruitment may be lower during ballistic muscle actions (33); thus, earlier activation of type II motor units may contribute to selective recruitment. Selective recruitment, or earlier-onset type II motor unit activation, may be of great benefit high-velocity power training. In addition, altered recruitment orders have been reported in individuals maintaining a specific level of force in the presence of pain (34). That is, discharge rates of type I motor units may decrease and be replaced by higher-threshold motor units to maintain a certain level of force while experiencing pain (34). It does appear that the nervous system may attempt to augment motor unit recruitment strategies under certain circumstances to improve or maintain muscle performance.

Muscle Mass Activation

The amount of muscle mass activated to lift a specific amount of weight depends on the magnitude of muscle hypertrophy. A training adaptation that takes place is that the level of muscle mass activation per unit of loading may decrease when muscle size increases. A larger muscle does not require as much neural activation to lift a standard weight as it did before the growth took place (because the muscle fibers themselves are larger and stronger and therefore require less stimuli to produce a certain level of force). A landmark study by Ploutz et al. (35) showed that less quadriceps muscle tissue was activated to lift a standard pretraining load after 9 weeks of RT (3–6 sets × 12 reps) that resulted in a 5% increase in muscle size. Thus, progressive overload during training is mandatory in order to continually activate an optimal amount of muscle mass. See Myths and Misconceptions: Lifting Light Weights at Slow Velocities Optimally Stimulates Muscle Fiber Activation.

Postactivation Potentiation

Activated motor units stay facilitated for a period of time following use. Maximal or near-maximal muscle contractions elicit a *postactivation potentiation* (PAP) (*e.g.*, where force exerted is augmented by previous intense contraction) for subsequent muscle contractions occurring within several seconds to a few minutes (36–38). That is, when an individual performs a moderately high to high-intensity contraction, there is a window of time following where it is easier to recruit type II motor units and subsequently produce higher levels of force and RFD. During this time, lifting a certain amount of weight may feel lighter or jumping a certain height may seem easier. Ultimately, acute strength and power may be enhanced (39). A recent meta-analysis has shown that at least 3 minutes of rest between the PAP stimulus and max vertical jump is needed to maximize performance (40). PAP appears dependent upon neural and muscular factors such as increased motor unit activity, increased phosphorylation of the light chains on myosin increasing calcium sensitivity and subsequent cross-bridge formation, and temporary reductions in skeletal muscle pennation angles. PAP is more prominent in explosive power athletes (41) and highly related to type II muscle fiber content (42), although endurance athletes demonstrate PAP (37). Some examples of how PAP has been shown to enhance athletic performance include

1. Swinging a weighted bat or performing a max isometric contraction in the early swing position prior to stepping in the batter's box for a baseball of softball player (43);
2. Performing a few sets of squats prior to testing for max vertical jump performance (40,44);

Myths & Misconceptions
Lifting Light Weights at Slow Velocities Optimally Stimulates Muscle Fiber Activation

Some have postulated that lifting light weights at slow velocities can maximally recruit all available motor units during an exercise. However, research has shown that motor unit recruitment is intensity dependent. Greater numbers of muscle fibers are recruited only when needed and the need is high during the lifting of heavy weights. There appears to be a unique neural activation pattern consequent to heavy lifting, which may help explain why 1 RM strength increases are most specific to heavy RT in trained lifters. Thus, heavy RT is effective for maximally recruiting type II motor units.

3. Performing a squat with 90% of 1 RM can augment subsequent squat repetition performance with 70% of 1 RM by 13% (or ~6 reps during the first set) and maximal isometric force by 9% (45);
4. Performing near maximum lunge and arm stroke contractions can improve 50-m swim sprint performance (46);
5. Performing kicks with elastic resistance improved roundhouse kick velocity by 3.3% in martial artists (47);
6. Performing augmented eccentric loading via weighted drop jumps (with up to 30% of body mass) 2–6 minutes prior increased max vertical jump height and power with the largest effect seen with 20% of body mass (48);
7. Performing jump squats with 11.2 kg loading can augment 20- and 40-m sprint times (49);
8. Performing pause box squats with elastic bands (4 sets of 2 reps) augmented broad jump performance with the largest PAP effect seen in stronger individuals (50);
9. Warming-up with a heavy shot augmented shot performance by nearly 2% (51); and
10. Using a weighted vest as part of a warm-up prior to speed or agility events (52).

PAP also serves as a mechanism of training to be targeted for advanced techniques such as complex training (discussed later in this book). The majority of studies have shown a high-intensity PAP conditioning activity can augment various types of performance. Thus, use of PAP as part of a warm-up may be an effective strategy to maximize acute athletic performance. The critical element is to use a PAP protocol that does not elicit fatigue.

Case Study 4.1

Steve is an athlete who is preparing to maximally test his vertical jump. He was told he might enhance his vertical jump height by utilizing a loaded warm-up. In this case, the loaded warm-up refers to a scenario where PAP can be used to augment performance. Steve approaches you for advice on how he can design a warm-up to augment performance.

Question for Consideration: What would you advise him to do?

Firing Rate

Firing rate refers to the number of times per second a motor unit discharges. Firing rate is affected by the muscle action and the nerve's conduction velocity as conduction velocities are higher in type II motor units. Conduction velocity tends to be higher in power athletes compared with endurance athletes (53) possibly due to a larger contingent of type II motor units in power athletes and can increase in response to training (54).

In fact, RT, continuous endurance, and high-intensity interval training can increase conduction velocity (54). Increases in conduction velocity have been attributed to increased recruitment, muscle fiber size, type II fibers, and enhanced sodium-potassium pump activity (54). At rest, motor units have low firing rates; however, a positive relationship exists between the amount of force produced and firing rate (23,55,56). Force production from a single motor unit can increase by 3–15 times when firing rate is increased from minimum to maximum stimulation (57). It appears a systematic motor control pattern exists between motor unit recruitment and discharge rates during submaximal and maximal muscular efforts and that the ability to improve both is brought about via anaerobic training.

Advances in technology have enabled the examination of motor unit mean firing rates from surface EMG signal decomposition. Stock and Thompson (56) reported that mean firing rates in the vastus lateralis and rectus femoris muscles may decrease or not change during submaximal (50% of MVC) absolute and relative isometric contractions following 10 weeks of deadlift RT. Motor unit discharge variability significantly affects force variation and a recent study showed that RT, but not endurance training, significantly reduced discharge rate variability in the vastus lateralis and medialis muscles (58). Low-threshold motor units recruited early during sustained force production may achieve higher mean firing rates than motor units recruited subsequently to maintain force (25). The role of increasing firing rate (vs. recruitment) depends on muscle size as some, especially smaller muscles, rely more on increasing rate to enhance force and power production, whereas larger muscles rely more on recruitment (59) and may depend upon the muscle action, *i.e.*, dynamic versus isometric (23). Anaerobic training enhances the firing rates of recruited motor units especially at higher force levels (33,60,61). High firing rates at the onset of ballistic muscle contraction are especially critical to increasing the RFD (60). Two consecutive motor unit discharges with short interspike intervals (*i.e.*, <5 ms) seen mostly early during contractions are known as *doublets*. Doublets lead to increased force production and RFD possibly due to increased calcium release from the sarcoplasmic reticulum within the muscle fibers. A large increase in the number of doublets in muscles of trained athletes has been shown and thought to reflect an increase in the speed of contraction after training (33). Endurance athletes have been shown to achieve higher mean firing rates during low levels of force production than strength-trained individuals (25).

Motor Unit Synchronization

Synchronization occurs when two or more motor units fire at fixed time intervals. Although motor units typically fire asynchronously, it is thought motor synchronization may be advantageous for bursts of strength or power needed in a short period of time. Greater motor unit synchronization has been shown following RT (62–64), is muscle-specific (65), and greater in strength-trained individuals especially at higher force levels (65). Although it is unclear as to the exact role synchronization plays during training, the bursts of grouped motor unit discharges may be advantageous for the timing of force production and may not be advantageous for the overall level of force produced.

Antagonist Muscle Activation

The cocontraction of *antagonist* muscles during movement increases joint stability, movement coordination, and reduces the risk of injury. However, there are occasions when cocontraction can be counterproductive because it may counteract the effects of agonist muscles. Muscle group, velocity and type of muscle action, intensity, joint position, and injury status affect the magnitude of antagonist cocontraction (66). Neural adaptations of antagonist musculature may take place with training that benefit performance enhancement. For sprint or plyometric training, the timing of coactivation may change, *i.e.*, it is higher during the precontact phase with the ground but less during propulsion or acceleration phases (67). During RT, studies have shown no change in antagonist cocontractions (61,68,69) and reductions (22,70,71). A recent study found reduced antagonist muscle cocontraction following 12 weeks of RT; however, the reduction did not significantly relate to agonist muscle strength increases (72). Thus, cocontraction of antagonist musculature appears to be a mechanism in place when there is a lack of familiarity with the exercise and the magnitude of decrease may be minor compared with the improvements in strength.

Communication with Skeletal Muscle: The Neuromuscular Junction

The nerve and muscle are not continuous, meaning there is a gap between the two (Fig. 4.7). A chemical messenger must be released in order for the action potential to reach the muscle. The chemical messenger is called a *neurotransmitter*, and there are several excitatory and inhibitory neurotransmitters found at synapses between neurons and other neurons, tissues, and organs. The key neurotransmitter released between a motor nerve and skeletal muscle is *acetylcholine*. When the action potential reaches the terminal, neurotransmitters are ultimately released into the space (*cleft*) where they bind to specific receptors on muscle and spread the action potential to muscle. The NMJ refers to the nerve terminal, space, and muscle fiber membrane.

Critical to training adaptations is the nerve terminal (also called *presynaptic terminal*). The NMJ in type I motor units tends to be less complex than type II (73), which is not surprising since type II units are advantageous for strength and power. Aerobic training results in greater presynaptic nerve terminal area, increased number of nerve terminal branches, increased perimeter of nerve terminal, and increased average length of individual nerve terminals (74). However, NMJ changes are much more pronounced during high-intensity training because the terminal branches become more dispersed, longer, asymmetrical, and irregularly shaped (74). RT may result in greater terminal area and greater dispersion of acetylcholine receptors (75). These changes in the NMJ that expand surface area and enable greater acetylcholine release are conducive to enhanced neural drive to skeletal muscle, thereby potentially increasing force and power production.

Sensory Nervous System

The sensory nervous system contains receptors that send information to the CNS via afferent pathways. Sensory receptors pick up various stimuli such as pain, hot/cold temperatures, and pressure. Proprioceptors are important because they pick up information concerning muscle length, joint position, movement, and tension. Although several types of sensory receptors function within the human body, two proprioceptors critical to exercise and sports performance are the Golgi tendon organs (GTOs) and muscle spindles.

Golgi Tendon Organs

GTOs are encapsulated proprioceptors located at the muscle-tendon junction (Fig. 4.8). Each capsule encloses collagen fibers attached to skeletal muscle fibers with nerve (Ib) endings intertwined between collagen fibers. Because of their location, their primary role is to convey information regarding muscle tension to the CNS. They also provide the nervous system with information on the state of muscle contraction and their afferent nerve fibers form a reflex network that helps regulate movement. As muscle tension increases, so does the amount of stretch to the GTOs collagen fibers and subsequent activation of the Ib afferent nerve. Once a threshold level of tension is attained, GTO activity increases greatly and its response is to cause agonist muscle relaxation (or fatigue) via inhibition and antagonist muscle excitation. GTOs may be considered to be a defense mechanism to protect the body from excessive damage. This may help explain why untrained individuals are only able to voluntarily recruit a smaller portion of their muscle mass in large muscle groups. However, their role inhibits performance to some extent. Although not sufficiently studied, many experts believe that gradual training reduces GTO sensitivity, which enables many neural adaptations to take place, *e.g.*, recruitment, rate, synchronization, and less antagonist cocontraction.

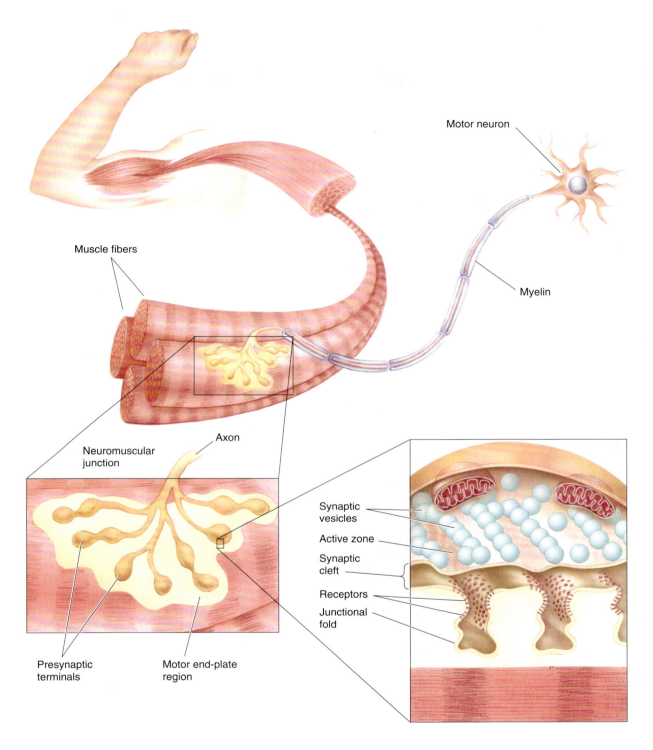

FIGURE 4.7 The motor neuron and neuromuscular junction (NMJ). The NMJ marks the end of the axon and forms a synapse with skeletal muscle. Synaptic vesicles migrate to the terminal membrane and release neurotransmitters into the synaptic cleft via exocytosis where they bind to receptors on the surface of the sarcolemma membrane. (From Bear MF, Connors BW, Paradiso MA. *Neuroscience, Exploring the Brain*. 2nd ed. Baltimore (MD): Lippincott Williams & Wilkins; 2001.)

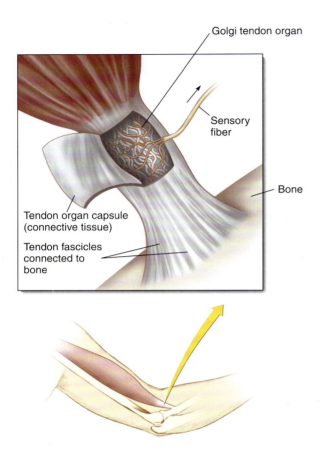

FIGURE 4.8 Golgi tendon organ. Golgi tendon organs are located in the muscle-tendon junction and respond to tension. (Reprinted from Premkumar K. *The Massage Connection: Anatomy and Physiology.* Baltimore (MD): Lippincott Williams & Wilkins; 2004.)

Muscle Spindles

Muscle spindles are encapsulated proprioceptors (Fig. 4.9) located within muscle fibers (*i.e.*, intrafusal fibers). They consist of two components called nuclear chain and nuclear bag fibers. Muscle spindles respond to the magnitude of change in muscle length, the rate of change of length, and convey information to the CNS via the Ia afferent nerve regarding static changes in muscle length or joint angle. Unlike GTOs, muscle spindles enhance human performance. Muscle spindles are critical because they initiate the stretch reflex. The *stretch reflex* is a monosynaptic reflex (a sensory nerve directly synapses with motor nerve in spinal cord) where muscle force production is enhanced when the muscle is previously stretched. A reflex itself is an involuntary response and reflects a time component because more force is produced in a short period of time. When a muscle is stretched (*i.e.*, from repeated contractions), information is sent from the muscle spindles to the spinal cord where a potent agonist muscular response ensues. The stretch reflex enhances muscular performance, efficiency, and is trainable via intense modalities of training such as aerobic and anaerobic interval, RT, plyometrics, speed, and agility training.

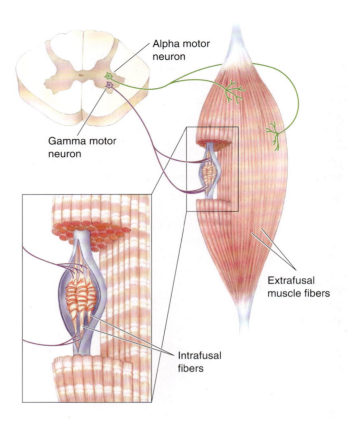

FIGURE 4.9 Muscle spindle. Muscle spindles are located within muscle fibers and respond to changes in length. (From Bear MF, Connors BW, Paradiso MA. *Neuroscience, Exploring the Brain.* 2nd ed. Baltimore (MD): Lippincott Williams & Wilkins; 2001.)

Reflex Potentiation

Potentiation of spinal reflexes and motor neuron excitability has been measured by examining the magnitude of pre-to-post training changes in the evoked Hoffman reflex (H-reflex) and its variant the V-wave (although the H-reflex may be more sensitive to motor neuron excitability and altered presynaptic inhibition). These are typically measured by electrical stimulation and/or voluntary contraction of a muscle group at various stimulus intensities. The secondary waves produced represent reflexive responses and these responses are quantified (and possibly normalized as a ratio compared to the maximal muscle response [M-wave or M_{max}]) and compared to pretraining values. Training can enhance reflex potentiation in a variety of ways. RT can increase reflex potentiation by more than 15% mostly in the form of V-wave changes (reflective of enhanced descending neural drive to the motor neuron pool) and H-reflex values recorded at higher stimulus intensities (76–80). Strength-trained athletes (weightlifters, bodybuilders) have greater reflex potentiation in the soleus muscle compared to untrained individuals (81). Enhanced reflex potentiation is associated with increases in RFD and power (77). Endurance athletes have been shown to have higher H-reflex excitability at rest (more so than power athletes) indicative of reflex potentiation at lower contraction levels (80). One study compared 3 weeks of endurance training to RT and showed that RT led to significant increases (~55%) in V/M_{max} ratio, whereas endurance training led to increased low-level H-reflex excitability, thereby showing each training modality improved different components of reflex potentiation (80). Increased reflex potentiation of the soleus muscle has also been shown following 4 weeks of plyometric training (82) but further improvements could be limited in already well-trained athletes (83). Thus, aerobic and anaerobic forms of training appear to have the ability to improve various components of reflex function.

Training Studies

Most studies examining changes in neural function with training have used *electromyography* (EMG). EMG quantifies the level of electrical activity from the surface of a skeletal muscle. An increase in EMG reflects greater neural activation; however, the precise mechanism(s) (increased recruitment, rate, and synchronization) cannot be determined using basic surface EMG. Most studies have shown increases in EMG with some showing no change following RT despite increases in muscle strength of >70% in some studies (84). This includes increased neural drive specific to concentric (CON), eccentric (ECC), and isometric (ISOM) RT. Training status is critical as trained individuals may show limited potential for further neural adaptation during short-term RT (85). Training is initially characterized by neural adaptations, *e.g.*, increased motor learning and coordination (86,87). A recent study has shown that increased agonist muscle neural drive, along with quadriceps muscle volume and pretraining strength, accounted for 60% of the variance in muscle strength increases following 12 weeks of RT (72). When muscle hypertrophy takes place, declines in EMG occur at a fixed level (88) because muscle fibers are capable of providing more tension. Beyond this point, it has been suggested that training exhibits an interplay between neural and hypertrophic mechanisms (Fig. 4.10) for strength and power improvements (66). That is, lifters must specifically stress the nervous system in training when hypertrophy occurs, *i.e.*, by lifting heavier weights or fast lifting velocities. Advanced weightlifters show limited potential for further neural adaptations over the course of 1 year (89). Plyometric training and ballistic RT, *i.e.*, loaded jump squats, has been shown to increase lower-body muscle EMG following training (90); however, the increased neural drive may be considerably less in trained athletes where muscle morphological and architectural changes may play a larger role in strength and power improvements (91). A few studies examining plyometric training have shown that neural drive during preactivation prior to ground contact and muscle activity of the plantar flexors may increase with greater neural drive potential seen in lower extremity muscles when plyometric training is combined with RT (92). Interestingly, performing the same plyometric training program on a 15° incline compared to flat ground increased medial gastrocnemius neural activation during propulsion to a greater extent (93).

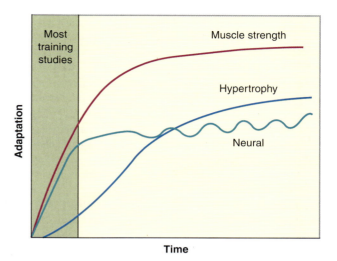

FIGURE 4.10 Contributions of neural and hypertrophic adaptations to resistance training. Neural adaptations predominate as the major mechanism for strength increases early in training. Muscle hypertrophy takes places after the first few weeks of training and becomes the major mechanism for further strength increases as training advances. The *shaded area* denotes a time frame examined by most studies. Thus, the remaining segment is theoretical and based partly on some cross-sectional data. It appears that there is interplay between neural and hypertrophic factors during advanced RT. That is, muscle hypertrophy lessens the need for optimal neural activation unless progressive overload is applied. Progressive overload in the form of high-intensity loading and/or fast lifting velocities are needed to optimally stimulate the nervous system with advanced training. (Based on information from Sale DG. Neural adaptations to strength training. In: Komi PV, editor. *Strength and Power in Sport*. 2nd ed. Malden (MA): Blackwell Science; 2003. p. 281–314.)

Case Study 4.2

William is a 20-year-old, healthy man who has no previous weight training experience. He begins a progressive weight training program and he realizes his strength has improved over the course of his first six workouts. For example, his bench press weight increased 10 lb and he is now performing 12 reps on the bent-over row with a weight he initially was only able to lift for 8 reps. William is amazed yet surprised he got stronger without any noticeable changes in muscle size.

Questions for Consideration: What mechanisms may have accounted for William's strength increase in the absence of noticeable muscle growth?

The training program dictates the pattern of adaptation. EMG, or neural activation, has been shown

- To be higher for high-intensity muscular effort versus lower-intensity muscular effort (94–96).

- To be higher on a set-by-set basis for the leg press exercise during a strength training (multiple sets of 1 RM repetitions) protocol compared to hypertrophy (5 sets of 10 reps with 80% of 1 RM loading) (96).
- To be higher during ballistic or explosive resistance exercise compared to slower velocities (39,94,95,97). However, EMG may be lower during the last segment of the CON phase during fast repetitions due to deceleration of the bar (95).
- To be greater primarily during the early phase of contraction following explosive ISOM training (69).
- To be higher for CON versus ECC muscle actions when matched for intensity (98).
- To be affected by the resistance exercise sequence and subsequent fatigue from exercises performed prior (99).
- To increase as fatigue ensues in CON and ECC muscle actions during submaximal or hypertrophy-designed resistance exercise presumably to compensate for fatigued motor units, termed by some as *neuromuscular inefficiency* (96,97,100–102). This may also be seen on a set-to-set basis within performance of a specific exercise where EMG may be higher during each rep of the 3rd or 5th sets compared to the 1st (96).
- To be reduced following a workout compared to preworkout, *e.g.*, a fatigue-induced state from training, especially following strength or power workouts compared to hypertrophy workouts (100,103).
- To be lower for high-volume, high-intensity training (*i.e.*, overreaching) but return to baseline during "tapering" (*i.e.*, reduced training volume) (104,105).
- To be increased following periods of electrical muscle stimulation (106).
- To be higher in selected lower extremity muscles during the propulsive phase of sprinting at increasing speeds (107).
- To be reduced during periods of detraining (94).

See Myths and Misconceptions: Performing Repetitions with Light to Moderate Loading at an Intentionally Slow Velocity Yields Similar Neuromuscular Responses to Heavier Loading at Moderate to Fast Velocities.

Collectively, these studies show that EMG increases or is higher when the intensity is high, the lifting velocity is fast, and CON muscle actions are used. Training programs targeting the nervous system are ones that emphasize heavy weight lifting and explosive movements such as plyometrics, ballistic RT, speed, and agility training. Fatigue is another factor affecting neural responses and adaptations to training. With submaximal exercise (*e.g.*, performing a 10-repetition set), EMG increases as the set progresses. This is thought to reflect greater motor unit recruitment to replace fatigued units as the set duration increases. However, the fatigue associated with a complete workout is high and results in a lower EMG response if assessed immediately after the workout ends. Fatigue limits motor unit activation to some extent; subsequently, EMG responses are lower. Therefore, recovery after a workout is critical before the next training session to restore maximal neural function.

Unilateral versus Bilateral Training

Training with one or two limbs simultaneously affects neural adaptations to training. *Cross education*, first reported by Scripture and colleagues in 1894 (108), refers to strength and endurance gained in the nontrained limb during unilateral training. Several studies have shown an average strength increase of up to 22% with a mean increase of nearly 8% compared to pretraining in the untrained limb (109) where strength increases of more than 30% in the nontrained limb have been reported (110). The strength increase is accompanied by greater EMG activity in the trained and nontrained limbs (86,110–112); endurance may increase in the untrained limb as well (113), with minimal ergogenic adaptations (*i.e.*, muscle hypertrophy) peripherally to the nontrained muscle group. The cross education effect may be more prominent during eccentric RT (114) and when high-intensity (>85% of maximal voluntary contractile force [MVC]) unilateral RT is used compared to moderate intensity (110). The contralateral limb strength improvements are thought to occur via motor learning in the brain (*i.e.*, *bilateral-access hypothesis*) and through *cross-activation* where unilateral contractions stem from bilateral cortical activity in the contralateral and ipsilateral motor cortices whereby a spill-over of neural activity to the untrained limb manifests (114). The practical ramification is that training only one limb at a time induces a novel stimulus to the nervous system. Adaptations are carried over to the opposite limb. In addition, some studies have shown that unilateral training can prevent muscle atrophy associated with injury or immobilization in the nontrained (114). Thus, unilateral training may be useful in improving functional performance and very useful for injured individuals because a partial training effect may be gained by the injured (nontrained) limb during a time of immobilization or greatly reduced activity.

In reference to unilateral and bilateral training, a range of motion–specific bilateral deficit has been shown. The *bilateral deficit* refers to the maximal force produced by both limbs contracting bilaterally (together) is smaller than the sum of the limbs contracting unilaterally. *Bilateral facilitation* refers to greater maximal force generation when both limbs contract together. Although neural inhibition during bilateral contractions has been proposed as a potential influencing factor, studies have been equivocal where reduced agonist neural drive and no differences (compared to unilateral contractions) have been reported (115). No differences during antagonist muscle EMG have been reported as well (115) making it difficult to ascertain mechanisms contributing to the strength differences. Unilateral training increases unilateral strength to a greater extent and bilateral training increases bilateral strength to a greater extent (and bilateral facilitation) with a corresponding greater specific EMG response (116–118). The bilateral deficit is seen especially in lesser-trained individuals because it is reduced with bilateral training. Practically, it is important to include unilateral and bilateral exercises in a training program.

Myths & Misconceptions
Performing Repetitions with Light to Moderate Loading at an Intentionally Slow Velocity Yields Similar Neuromuscular Responses to Heavier Loading at Moderate to Fast Velocities

Some have stated that performing an intentionally slow lifting velocity (longer than 3–5-s CON and ECC phases) produces similar neuromuscular responses to either heavier loading with a moderate velocity (1–2-s CON and ECC phases) or lighter loading with explosive velocity (<1-s CON and ECC phases). However, this is not the case. Intentionally slowing the repetition velocity limits motor unit recruitment and results in less muscular force and power. This was shown in a study by Keogh et al. (97). They compared several aspects of bench press performance. Three comparisons were made between standard heavy weight training (HWT; 6 reps performed with a 6 RM load or 80%–85% of 1 RM), super-slow (SS) training (5-s CON phase, 5-s ECC phase with 55% of 1 RM for 5–6 reps), and ballistic bench press (BBP) training (6 explosive reps where the bar was released at the end of each repetition with 30% of 1 RM). It is important to note that in order to perform the SS reps in 10 seconds, a significant weight reduction was needed. They measured force and power characteristics as well as EMG activity of the pectoralis major and triceps brachii muscles. Figure 4.11 shows the EMG results during the CON muscle actions from this study. For the pectoralis major muscle, HWT produced much higher EMG activity than SS and BBP. For the triceps brachii muscle, HWT and BBP produced much higher EMG than SS. These results showed that for each muscle, HWT produced much greater neural activation than SS and for the triceps brachii, ballistic reps with less weight produced higher neural activation than SS. Therefore, faster lifting velocities produce a greater neural response to resistance exercise than intentionally slow velocities.

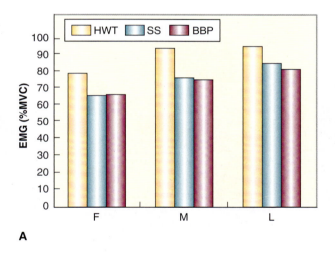
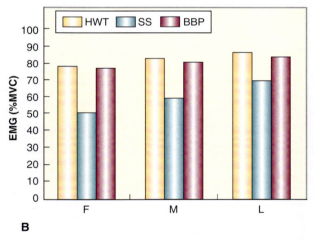

FIGURE 4.11 Neuromuscular responses to heavy weight training (HWT), super-slow training (SS), and ballistic bench press training (BBP). **A.** Pectoralis major EMG data (expressed as a percent of maximal voluntary effort). **B.** Triceps brachii EMG data (expressed as a percent of maximal voluntary effort). F, first repetition; M, middle repetition; L, last repetition. (Data from Keogh JWL, Wilson GJ, Weatherby RP. A cross-sectional comparison of different resistance training techniques in the bench press. *J Strength Cond Res.* 1999;13:247–58.)

Autonomic Nervous System

The ANS is a branch of the peripheral nervous system highly involved in bodily control (Fig. 4.12). Target tissues of autonomic nerves include cardiac muscle, smooth muscle, and other glands, organs, and tissues. The ANS controls such functions such as heart rate and force of contraction, respiration rate, digestion, blood pressure and flow, and fuel mobilization, to name a few. The sympathetic branch (also called the "fight or flight" system) prepares the body for stress or exercise by increasing heart rate and force of contraction, increasing breathing rate, increasing blood glucose and muscle glycogen breakdown, fat mobilization, increasing blood pressure, redirecting blood flow toward

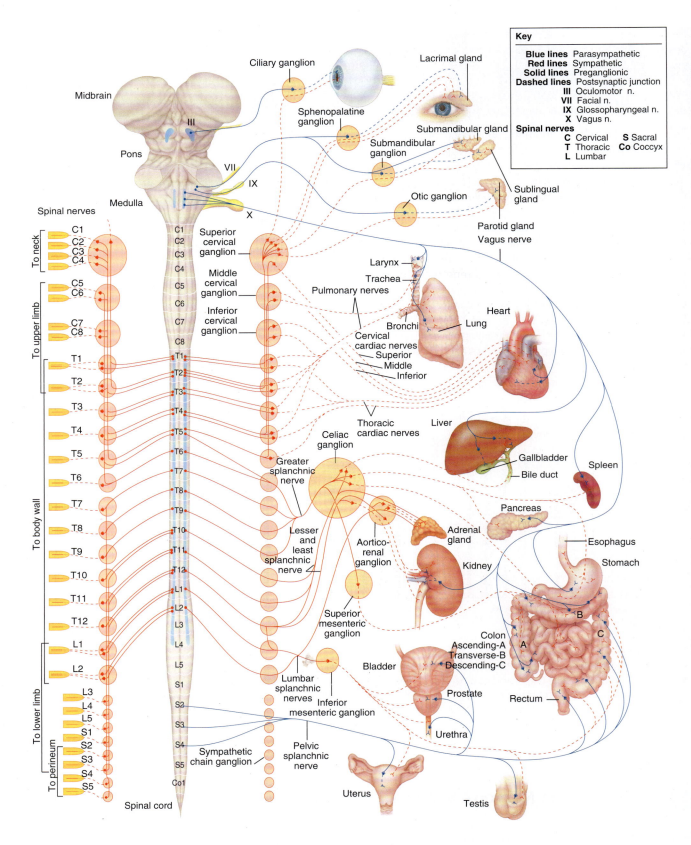

FIGURE 4.12 Autonomic nervous system. The sympathetic and parasympathetic nervous systems are shown in this figure. (Asset provided by Anatomical Chart Co.)

skeletal muscle, and pupil dilation for enhanced performance. The parasympathetic branch has the opposite effect by returning the body back to normal (or *homeostasis*). Several facets of the ANS are enhanced through aerobic and anaerobic training, as well as the target tissues and organs (several of which are discussed in other chapters). Ultimately, these changes enhance acute exercise performance and increase recovery postexercise.

SUMMARY POINTS

◆ Training may elicit adaptations along the neuromuscular chain initiating in the higher brain centers and continuing down to the level of individual muscle fibers.
◆ Cerebral adaptations are important for technique enhancement, coordination, and strength and power increases.
◆ Greater agonist muscle motor unit recruitment, firing rates, synchronization, antagonist coactivation, and reflex potentiation enhance muscular strength, power, speed, endurance, and performance.
◆ Neural activation is highest during high-intensity and ballistic muscular efforts and is lower during times of overreaching and detraining.

REVIEW QUESTIONS

1. An athlete is performing a 1 RM bench press to evaluate the off-season conditioning program. His previous best was 280 lb. After a warm-up, he attempts 315 lb and is unable to lift the weight. Which of the following mechanisms was most responsible for this failure?
   a. Increase in muscle spindle activity
   b. Increase in Golgi tendon organ activity
   c. Decrease in Golgi tendon organ activity
   d. Decrease in antagonist muscle cocontraction

2. The preferential or early activation of FT motor units during explosive exercise is known as
   a. Action potential
   b. Motor unit synchronization
   c. Cross education
   d. Selective recruitment

3. The part of the neuron that receives information from other neurons is a
   a. Node of Ranvier
   b. Dendrite
   c. Axon
   d. Myelin sheath

4. After 10 weeks of RT, an athlete comes into the lab and performs a strength test while connected to an EMG system.

His strength increases and subsequently his maximal EMG response increases as well. The increase in EMG may have resulted from
   a. Greater motor unit recruitment
   b. Higher firing rates
   c. Motor unit synchronization
   d. All of the above

5. Unilateral training that results in a strength increase in the nontrained limb is known as
   a. Motor unit
   b. Bilateral deficit
   c. Cross education
   d. Size principle

6. Which of the following is true regarding EMG changes/responses to training?
   a. EMG is higher during low- versus high-intensity contractions
   b. EMG does not change over the course of a resistance exercise set
   c. EMG is higher during fast versus intentionally slow velocity contractions (using a standard load)
   d. EMG is higher during ECC versus CON muscle actions (using a standard load)

7. The CNS consists of the brain and spinal cord.
   a. T
   b. F

8. Based on the size principle, FT motor units are recruited before ST motor units.
   a. T
   b. F

9. The parasympathetic nervous system helps prepare the body for the stress of exercise by increasing heart rate, blood pressure, and skeletal muscle force of contraction.
   a. T
   b. F

10. The bilateral deficit refers to the maximal force produced by both limbs contracting together is smaller than the sum of the limbs contracting individually.
    a. T
    b. F

11. Muscle hypertrophy increases the need to recruit additional motor units in order to lift a standard amount of weight.
    a. T
    b. F

12. Cocontraction of antagonist skeletal muscles is an important mechanism to increase joint stability and reduce the risk of injury.
    a. T
    b. F

REFERENCES

1. Portugal EMM, Cevada T, Monteiro-Junior RS, et al. Neuroscience of exercise: from neurobiology mechanisms to mental health. *Neuropsychobiology*. 2013;68:1–14.

2. Sabatier MJ, English AW. Pathways mediating activity-induced enhancement of recovery from peripheral nerve injury. *Exerc Sport Sci Rev*. 2015;43:163–71.

3. Knaepen K, Goekint M, Heyman EM, Meeusen R. Neuroplasticity – exercise-induced response of peripheral brain-derived neurotrophic factor: A systematic review of experimental studies in human subjects. *Sports Med*. 2010;40:765–801.

4. Huang T, Larsen KT, Ried-Larsen M, Moller NC, Andersen LB. The effects of physical activity and exercise on brain-derived neurotrophic factor in healthy humans: a review. *Scand J Med Sci Sports*. 2014;24:1–10.

5. Marston KJ, Newton MJ, Brown BM, Rainey-Smith SR, Bird S, Martins RN, Peiffer JJ. Intense resistance exercise increases peripheral brain-derived neurotrophic factor. *J Sci Med Sport*. 2017;20:899–903.

6. Church DD, Hoffman JR, Mangine GT, et al. Comparison of high-intensity vs. high-volume resistance training on the BDF response to exercise. *J Appl Physiol*. 2016;121:123–8.

7. Correia PR, Scorza FA, Gomes da Silva S, Pansani A, Toscano-Silva M, de Almeida AC, Arida RM. Increased basal plasma brain-derived neurotrophic factor levels in sprint runners. *Neurosci Bull*. 2011;27:325–9.

8. Ranganathan VK, Siemionow V, Liu JZ, Sahgal V, Yue GH. From mental power to muscle power—gaining strength by using the mind. *Neuropsychologia*. 2004;42:944–56.

9. Yue G, Cole KJ. Strength increases from the motor program: comparison of training with maximal voluntary and imagined muscle contractions. *J Neurophysiol*. 1992;67:1114–23.

10. Lattari E, Arias-Carrion O, Monteiro-Junior RS, et al. Implications of movement-related cortical potential for understanding neural adaptations in muscle strength tasks. *Int Arch Med*. 2014;7:9.

11. Siemionow V, Yue GH, Ranganathan VK, Liu JZ, Sahgai V. Relationship between motor activity-related cortical potential and voluntary muscle activation. *Exp Brain Res*. 2000;133:303–11.

12. Fang Y, Siemionow V, Sahgal V, Xiong F, Yue GH. Distinct brain activation patterns for human maximal voluntary eccentric and concentric muscle actions. *Brain Res*. 2004;1023:200–12.

13. Flanagan SD, Dunn-Lewis C, Comstock BA, Maresh CM, Volek JS, Denegar CR, Kraemer WJ. Cortical activity during a highly-trained resistance exercise movement emphasizing force, power or volume. *Brain Sci*. 2012;2:649–66.

14. Dal Maso F, Longcamp M, Amarantini D. Training-related decrease in antagonist muscles activation is associated with increased motor cortex activation: evidence of central mechanisms for control of antagonist muscles. *Exp Brain Res*. 2012;220:287–95.

15. Ushiyama J, Takahashi Y, Ushiba J. Muscle dependency of corticomuscular coherence in upper and lower limb muscles and training-related alterations in ballet dancers and weightlifters. *J Appl Physiol*. 2010;109:1086–95.

16. Falvo MJ, Sirevaag EJ, Rohrbaugh JW, Earhart GM. Resistance training induces supraspinal adaptations: evidence from movement-related cortical potentials. *Eur J Appl Physiol*. 2010;109: 923–33.

17. Kidgell DJ, Bonanno DR, Frazer AK, Howatson G, Pearce AJ. Corticospinal responses following strength training: a systematic review and meta-analysis. *Eur J Neurosci*. 2017;46:2648–61.

18. Palmer HS, Haberg AK, Fimland MS, et al. Structural brain changes after 4 wk of unilateral strength training of the lower limb. *J Appl Physiol*. 2013;115:167–75.

19. Adams GR, Harris RT, Woodard D, Dudley G. Mapping of electrical muscle stimulation using MRI. *J Appl Physiol*. 1993;74:532–7.

20. Carroll TJ, Riek S, Carson RG. The sites of neural adaptation induced by resistance training in humans. *J Physiol*. 2002;544: 641–52.

21. Del Olmo MF, Reimunde P, Viana O, Acero RM, Cudeiro J. Chronic neural adaptation induced by long-term resistance training in humans. *Eur J Appl Physiol*. 2006;96:722–8.

22. Pensini M, Martin A, Maffiuletti MA. Central versus peripheral adaptations following eccentric resistance training. *Int J Sports Med*. 2002;23:567–74.

23. Pucci AR, Griffin L, Cafarelli E. Maximal motor unit firing rates during isometric resistance training in man. *Exp Physiol*. 2006;91:171–8.

24. Duez L, Qerama E, Fuglsang-Frederiksen A, Bangsbo J, Jensen TS. Electrophysiological characteristics of motor units and muscle fibers in trained and untrained young male subjects. *Muscle Nerve*. 2010;42:177–83.

25. Herda TJ, Siedlik JA, Trevino MA, Cooper MA, Weir JP. Motor unit control strategies of endurance- versus resistance-trained individuals. *Muscle Nerve*. 2015;52:832–43.

26. Henneman E, Somjen G, Carpenter DO. Excitability and inhabitability of motoneurons of different sizes. *J Neurophysiol*. 1965;28:599–620.

27. Gorassini M, Yang JF, Siu M, Bennett DJ. Intrinsic activation of human motor units: reduction of motor unit recruitment thresholds by repeated contractions. *J Neurophysiol*. 2002;87:1859–66.

28. Osborne MA, Schneider DA. Muscle glycogen reduction in man: relationship between surface EMG activity and oxygen uptake kinetics during heavy exercise. *Exp Physiol*. 2006;91:179–89.

29. Pope ZK, Hester GM, Benik FM, DeFreitas JM. Action potential amplitude as a noninvasive indicator of motor unit-specific hypertrophy. *J Neurophysiol*. 2016;115:2608–14.

30. Somjen G, Carpenter DO, Henneman E. Responses of motoneurons of different sizes to graded stimulation of supraspinal centers of the brain. *J Neurophysiol*. 1965;28:958–65.

31. Ter Haar Romeny BM, Dernier Van Der Goen JJ, Gielen CCAM. Changes in recruitment order of motor units in the human biceps muscle. *Exp Neurol*. 1982;78:360–8.

32. Nardone A, Romano C, Schieppati M. Selective recruitment of high-threshold human motor units during voluntary isotonic lengthening of active muscles. *J Physiol*. 1989;409:451–71.

33. Van Cutsem M, Duchateau J, Hainut K. Changes in single motor unit behaviour contribute to the increase in contraction speed after dynamic training in humans. *J Physiol*. 1998;513:295–305.

34. Tucker K, Butler J, Graven-Nielsen T, Riek S, Hodges P. Motor unit recruitment strategies are altered during deep-tissue pain. *J Neurosci*. 2009;29:10820–6.

35. Ploutz LL, Tesch PA, Biro RL, Dudley GA. Effect of resistance training on muscle use during exercise. *J Appl Physiol*. 1994;76:1675–81.

36. Hamada T, Sale DG, MacDougall JD, Tarnopolsky MA. Postactivation potentiation, fiber type, and twitch contraction time in human knee extensor muscles. *J Appl Physiol*. 2000;88: 2131–7.

37. Hamada T, Sale DG, MacDougall JD. Postactivation potentiation in endurance-trained male athletes. *Med Sci Sports Exerc.* 2000;32:403–11.

38. Hamada T, Sale DG, MacDougall JD, Tarnopolsky MA. Interaction of fibre type, potentiation and fatigue in human knee extensor muscles. *Acta Physiol Scand.* 2003;178:165–73.

39. Häkkinen K, Komi PV, Alen M. Effect of explosive type strength training on isometric force- and relaxation-time, electromyographic and muscle fibre characteristics of leg extensor muscles. *Acta Physiol Scand.* 1985;125:587–600.

40. Dobbs WC, Tolusso DV, Fedewa MV, Esco MR. Effect of postactivation potentiation on explosive vertical jump: a systematic review and meta-analysis. *J Strength Cond Res.* 2019;33(7):2009–18.

41. Chiu LZ, Fry AC, Weiss LW, Schilling BK, Brown LE, Smith SL. Postactivation potentiation response in athletic and recreationally trained individuals. *J Strength Cond Res.* 2003;17:671–7.

42. Seitz LB, Trajano GS, Haff GG, Dumke CC, Tufano JJ, Blazevich AJ. Relationships between maximal strength, muscle size, and myosin heavy chain isoform composition and postactivation potentiation. *Appl Physiol Nutr Metab.* 2016;41:491–7.

43. Gilmore SL, Brilla LR, Suprak DN, Chalmers GR, Dahlquist DT. Effect of high-intensity isometric potentiating warm-up on bat velocity. *J Strength Cond Res.* 2018;33:152–8.

44. Hoffman JR, Ratamess NA, Faigenbaum AD, Mangine GT, Kang J. Effects of maximal squat exercise testing on vertical jump performance in American college football players. *J Sports Sci Med.* 2007;6:149–50.

45. De Freitas CM, Rossi FE, Colognesi LA, et al. Postactivation potentiation improves acute resistance exercise performance and muscular force in trained men. *J Strength Cond Res.* 2019. [ahead-of-print].

46. Cuenca-Fernández F, Ruiz-Teba A, López-Contreras G, Arellano R. Effects of 2 types of activation protocols based on postactivation potentiation on 50-m freestyle performance. *J Strength Cond Res.* 2020;34:3284–92.

47. Aandahl HS, Von Heimburg E, Van den Tillaar R. Effect of postactivation potentiation induced by elastic resistance on kinematics and performance in a roundhouse kick of trained martial arts practitioners. *J Strength Cond Res.* 2018;32:990–6.

48. Bridgeman LA, McGuigan MR, Gill ND, Dulson DK. The effects of accentuated eccentric loading on the drop jump exercise and the subsequent postactivation potentiation response. *J Strength Cond Res.* 2017;31:1620–6.

49. Creekmur CC, Haworth JL, Cox RH, Walsh MS. Effects of plyometrics performed during warm-up on 20 and 40 m sprint performance. *J Sports Med Phys Fitness.* 2017;57:550–5.

50. Seitz LB, Mina MA, Haff GG. Postactivation potentiation of horizontal jump performance across multiple sets of a contrast protocol. *J Strength Cond Res.* 2016;30:2733–40.

51. Judge LW, Bellar DM, Craig BW, Gilreath EL, Cappos SA, Thrasher AB. Influence of postactivation potentiation on shot put performance of collegiate throwers. *J Strength Cond Res.* 2016;30:438–45.

52. Faigenbaum AD, McFarland JE, Schwerdtman JA, Ratamess NA, Kang J, Hoffman JR. Dynamic warm-up protocols, with and without a weighted vest, and fitness performance in high school female athletes. *J Athl Train.* 2006;41:357–63.

53. Kamen G, Kroll W, Zignon ST. Exercise effects upon reflex time components in weight lifters and distance runners. *Med Sci Sports Exerc.* 1981;13:198–204.

54. Martinez-Valdes E, Farina D, Negro F, Del Vecchio A, Falla D. Early motor unit conduction velocity changes to high-intensity interval training versus continuous training. *Med Sci Sports Exerc.* 2018;50:2339–50.

55. Monster AW, Chan H. Isometric force production by motor units of extensor digitorum communis muscles in man. *J Neurophysiol.* 1977;40:1432–43.

56. Stock MS, Thompson BJ. Effects of barbell deadlift training on submaximal motor unit firing rates for the vastus lateralis and rectus femoris. *PLoS One.* 2014;9:1–18.

57. Enoka RM. Morphological features and activation patterns of motor units. *J Clin Neurophysiol.* 1995;12:538–59.

58. Vila-Cha C, Falla D. Strength training, but not endurance training, reduces motor unit discharge rate variability. *J Electromyogr Kinesol.* 2016;26:88–93.

59. DeLuca CJ, LeFever RS, McCue MP, Xenakis AP. Behaviour of human motor units in different muscles during linearly varying contractions. *J Physiol.* 1982;329:113–28.

60. Aagaard P. Training-induced changes in neural function. *Exerc Sport Sci Rev.* 2003;31:61–7.

61. Aagaard P, Simonsen EB, Andersen JL, Magnusson P, Dyhre-Poulsen P. Increased rate of force development and neural drive of human skeletal muscle following resistance training. *J Appl Physiol.* 2002;93:1318–26.

62. Felici F, Rosponi A, Sbriccoli P, Filligoi C, Fattorini L, Marchetti M. Linear and non-linear analysis of surface electromyograms in weightlifters. *Eur J Appl Physiol.* 2001;84:337–42.

63. Milner-Brown HS, Stein RB, Lee RG. Synchronization of human motor units: possible roles of exercise and supraspinal reflexes. *Electroencephalogr Clin Neurophysiol.* 1975;38:245–54.

64. Semmler JG, Sale MV, Meyer FG, Nordstrom MA. Motor-unit coherence and its relation with synchrony are influenced by training. *J Neurophysiol.* 2004;92:3320–31.

65. Fling BW, Christie A, Kamen G. Motor unit synchronization in FDI and biceps brachii muscles of strength-trained males. *J Electromyogr Kinesiol.* 2009;19:800–9.

66. Sale DG. Neural adaptations to strength training. In: Komi PV, editor. *Strength and Power in Sport.* 2nd ed. Malden (MA): Blackwell Science; 2003. p. 281–314.

67. Kellis E, Arabatzi F, Papadopoulos C. Muscle co-activation around the knee in drop jumping using the co-contraction index. *J Electromyogr Kinesiol.* 2003;13:229–38.

68. Seger JY, Thorstensson A. Effects of eccentric versus concentric training on thigh muscle strength and EMG. *Int J Sports Med.* 2005;26:45–52.

69. Tillin NA, Pain MTG, Folland JP. Short-term training for explosive strength causes neural and mechanical adaptations. *Exp Physiol.* 2012;97:630–41.

70. Carolan B, Cafarelli E. Adaptations in coactivation after isometric resistance training. *J Appl Physiol.* 1992;73:911–7.

71. Häkkinen K, Kallinen M, Izquierdo M, et al. Changes in agonist-antagonist EMG muscle CSA and force during strength training in middle-aged and older people. *J Appl Physiol.* 1998;84: 1341–9.

72. Balshaw TG, Massey GJ, Madsen-Wilkinson TM, et al. Changes in agonist neural drive, hypertrophy and pre-training strength all contribute to the individual strength gains after resistance training. *Eur J Appl Physiol.* 2017;117:631–40.

73. Sieck GC, Prakash YS. Morphological adaptations of neuromuscular junctions depend on fiber type. *Can J Appl Physiol.* 1997;22:197–230.

74. Deschenes MR, Maresh CM, Crivello JF, Armstrong LE, Kraemer WJ, Covault J. The effects of exercise training of different intensities on neuromuscular junction morphology. *J Neurocytol.* 1993;22:603–15.

75. Deschenes MR, Judelson DA, Kraemer WJ, et al. Effects of resistance training on neuromuscular junction morphology. *Muscle Nerve.* 2000;23:1576–81.

76. Aagaard P, Simonsen EB, Andersen JL, Magnusson P, Dyhre-Poulsen P. Neural adaptation to resistance training: changes in evoked V-wave and H-reflex responses. *J Appl Physiol.* 2002;92: 2309–18.

77. Holtermann A, Roeleveld K, Engstram M, Sand T. Enhanced H-reflex with resistance training is related to increased rate of force development. *Eur J Appl Physiol.* 2007;101:301–31.

78. Sale DG, McComas AJ, MacDougall JD, Upton, ARM. Neuromuscular adaptation in human thenar muscles following strength training and immobilization. *J Appl Physiol.* 1982;53:419–24.

79. Sale DG, MacDougall JD, Upton ARM, McComas AJ. Effect of strength training upon motoneuron excitability in man. *Med Sci Sports Exerc.* 1983;15:57–62.

80. Vila-Cha C, Falla D, Correia MV, Farina D. Changes in H reflex and V wave following short-term endurance and strength training. *J Appl Physiol.* 2012;112:54–63.

81. Sale DG, Upton ARM, McComas AJ, MacDougall JD. Neuromuscular functions in weight-trainers. *Exp Neurol.* 1983;82:521–31.

82. Voigt M, Chelli F, Frigo C. Changes in the excitability of the soleus muscle short latency stretch reflexes during human hopping after 4 weeks of hopping training. *Eur J Appl Physiol.* 1998;78:522–32.

83. Alkjaer T, Meyland J, Raffalt PC, Lundbye-Jensen J, Simonsen EB. Neuromuscular adaptations to 4 weeks of intensive drop jump training in well-trained athletes. *Physiol Rep.* 2013;1:1–11.

84. Ratamess NA, Izquierdo M. Neuromuscular adaptations to training. In: Schwellnus, M, editor. *The Olympic Textbook of Medicine in Sport.* Hoboken, NJ: Wiley-Blackwell, 2008.

85. Marshall PWM, McEwen M, Robbins DW. Strength and neuromuscular adaptation following one, four, and eight sets of high intensity resistance exercise in trained males. *Eur J Appl Physiol.* 2011;111:3007–16.

86. Narici MV, Roi GS, Landoni L, Minetti AE, Cerretelli E. Changes in force, cross-sectional area and neural activation during strength training and detraining of the human quadriceps. *Eur J Appl Physiol.* 1989;59:310–9.

87. Rutherford OM, Jones DA. The role of learning and coordination in strength training. *Eur J Appl Physiol.* 1986;55:100–5.

88. Moritani T, deVries HA. Neural factors versus hypertrophy in the time course of muscle strength gain. *Am J Phys Med.* 1979;58:115–30.

89. Häkkinen K, Komi PV, Alen M, Kauhanen H. EMG muscle fibre and force production characteristics during a 1 year training period in elite weight-lifters. *Eur J Appl Physiol.* 1987;56:419–27.

90. McBride JM, Triplett-McBride T, Davie A, Newton RU. The effect of heavy- vs. light-load jump squats on the development of strength, power, and speed. *J Strength Cond Res.* 2002;16:75–82.

91. Ullrich B, Pelzer T, Pfeiffer M. Neuromuscular effects to 6 weeks of loaded countermovement jumping with traditional and daily undulating periodization. *J Strength Cond Res.* 2018;32:660–74.

92. Markovic G, Mikulic P. Neuro-musculoskeletal and performance adaptations to lower-extremity plyometric training. *Sports Med.* 2010;40:869–96.

93. Kannas TM, Kellis E, Amiridis IG. Incline plyometrics-induced improvement of jumping performance. *Eur J Appl Physiol.* 2012;112:2353–61.

94. Häkkinen K, Alen M, Komi PV. Changes in isometric force-and relaxation-time, electromyographic and muscle fibre characteristics of human skeletal muscle during strength training and detraining. *Acta Physiol Scand.* 1985;125:573–85.

95. Sakamoto A, Sinclair PJ. Muscle activation under varying lifting speeds and intensities during bench press. *Eur J Appl Physiol.* 2012;112:1015–25.

96. Walker S, Davis L, Avela J, Häkkinen K. Neuromuscular fatigue during dynamic maximal strength and hypertrophic resistance loadings. *J Electromyogr Kinesiol.* 2012;22:356–62.

97. Keogh JWL, Wilson GJ, Weatherby RP. A cross-sectional comparison of different resistance training techniques in the bench press. *J Strength Cond Res.* 1999;13:247–58.

98. Komi PV, Kaneko M, Aura O. EMG activity of leg extensor muscles with special reference to mechanical efficiency in concentric and eccentric exercise. *Int J Sports Med.* 1987;8(Suppl):22–9.

99. Soncin R, Pennone J, Guimaraes TM, Mezencio B, Amadio A, Serrao JC. Influence of exercise order on electromyographic activity during upper body resistance training. *J Hum Kinet.* 2014;44:203–9.

100. McCaulley GO, McBride JM, Cormie P, Hudson MB, Nuzzo JL, Quindry JC, Triplett NT. Acute hormonal and neuromuscular responses to hypertrophy, strength and power type resistance exercise. *Eur J Appl Physiol.* 2009;105:695–704.

101. Pincivero DM, Gandhi V, Timmons MK, Coelho AJ. Quadriceps femoris electromyogram during concentric, isometric, and eccentric phases of fatiguing dynamic knee extensions. *J Biomech.* 2006;39:246–54.

102. Tesch PA, Dudley GA, Duvoisin MR, Hather BM, Harris RT. Force and EMG signal patterns during repeated bouts of concentric or eccentric muscle actions. *Acta Physiol Scand.* 1990;138:263–71.

103. Benson C, Docherty D, Brandenburg J. Acute neuromuscular responses to resistance training performed at different loads. *J Sci Med Sport.* 2006;9:135–42.

104. Häkkinen K, Kauhanen H. Daily changes in neural activation, force-time and relaxation-time characteristics in athletes during very intense training for one week. *Electromyogr Clin Neurophysiol.* 1989;29:243–9.

105. Häkkinen K, Kallinen M, Komi PV, Kauhanen H. Neuromuscular adaptations during short-term "normal" and reduced training periods in strength athletes. *Electromyogr Clin Neurophysiol.* 1991;31:35–42.

106. Hortobagyi T, Maffiuletti NA. Neural adaptations to electrical stimulation strength training. *Eur J Appl Physiol.* 2011;111:2439–49.

107. Mero A, Komi PV. Electromyographic activity in sprinting at speeds ranging from sub maximal to supramaximal. *Med Sci Sports Exerc.* 1987;19:266–74.

108. Scripture EW, Smith TL, Brown EM. On the education of muscular control and power. *Yale Psychological Library.* 1894;2:114–9.

109. Munn J, Herbert RD, Gandevia SC. Contralateral effects of unilateral resistance training: a meta-analysis. *J Appl Physiol.* 2004;96:1861–6.

110. Fimland MS, Helgerud J, Solstad GM, Iversen VM, Leivseth G, Hoff J. Neural adaptations underlying cross-education after unilateral strength training. *Eur J Appl Physiol.* 2009;107:723–30.

111. Shima SN, Ishida K, Katayama K, Morotome Y, Sato Y, Miyamura M. Cross education of muscular strength during unilateral resistance training and detraining. *Eur J Appl Physiol*. 2002;86: 287–94.

112. Weir JP, Housh TJ, Weir LL. Electromyographic evaluation of joint angle specificity and cross-training after isometric training. *J Appl Physiol*. 1994;77:197–201.

113. Yuza N, Ishida K, Miyamura M. Cross transfer effects of muscular endurance during training and detraining. *J Sports Med Phys Fitness*. 2000;40:110–7.

114. Hendy AM, Lamon S. The cross-education phenomenon: brain and beyond. *Front Physiol*. 2017;8:1–9.

115. Kuruganti U, Murphy T, Pardy T. Bilateral deficit phenomenon and the role of antagonist muscle activity during maximal isometric knee extensions in young, athletic men. *Eur J Appl Physiol*. 2011;111:1533–9.

116. Häkkinen K, Kallinen M, Linnamo V, Pastinen UM, Newton RU, Kraemer WJ. Neuromuscular adaptations during bilateral versus unilateral strength training in middle-aged and elderly men and women. *Acta Physiol Scand*. 1996;158:77–88.

117. Kuruganti U, Parker P, Rickards J, Tingley M, Sexsmith J. Bilateral isokinetic training reduces the bilateral leg strength deficit for both old and young adults. *Eur J Appl Physiol*. 2005;94: 175–9.

118. Taniguchi Y. Lateral specificity in resistance training: the effect of bilateral and unilateral training. *Eur J Appl Physiol*. 1997;75: 144–50.

CHAPTER 5: Muscular Adaptations to Training

OBJECTIVES

After completing this chapter, you will be able to:
- Discuss the differences between cardiac, smooth, and skeletal muscles
- Describe the various roles skeletal muscles play within the human body
- Describe the gross anatomy of skeletal muscle
- Diagram the organization of a myofibril
- Describe the processes involved in skeletal muscle contraction
- Distinguish between different fiber types and discuss the importance of fiber types on performance
- Understand the importance of genetics to muscular adaptations to training
- Discuss factors and pathways that influence muscle hypertrophy
- Describe structural changes to skeletal muscle and discuss how they enhance muscular performance

---

Muscles perform a multitude of functions in the human body. There are three types of muscles: cardiac, smooth, and skeletal. Cardiac muscle is found in the heart. It contracts involuntarily with strong force and is responsible for creating a rhythmic pressure head and moving blood throughout the body. Smooth muscle is found in the walls of hollow organs and blood vessels. It contracts involuntarily resulting in a squeezing-type phenomenon where constriction takes place. The focus of this chapter is skeletal muscle. Skeletal muscle is larger, constitutes nearly 40% of body mass and up to 75% of all bodily proteins, contracts voluntarily, contracts and relaxes rapidly, and contains multiple *nuclei* (which is critical to the exercise adaptation process). Skeletal muscle performs several important functions including movement, production of body heat, posture maintenance, and assists with communication. Lastly, rhythmic skeletal muscle contraction enables ventilation to occur.

 ## Roles of Skeletal Muscles

Contraction of skeletal muscles produces tension and acts on bones to produce movement. The size of skeletal muscle is determined mostly by the number and size of its muscle fibers. The human body contains more than 660 skeletal muscles. Muscles are attached to bones in two general locations. The *proximal* attachment, or attachment closest to the midline, is known as the origin. The *distal* attachment, or attachment farther from the midline, is known as the insertion. Some muscles may have multiple points of origin or insertion. A muscle (tendon) must cross a joint in order for movement to occur. Several muscles' points of origin and insertion may span only one joint (*e.g.*, vastus lateralis). These muscles are *uniarticular* because they produce movement at one joint. Some muscles' origins and insertions span two joints. These muscles are *multiarticular* because they produce movement about two joints (*e.g.*, hamstrings). A muscle will shorten when it contracts, thereby pulling on its ends at the origin and insertion. However, movement may take place at one end as the other end may be held fixed by stabilizer muscle contraction and/or by the mass of the skeletal attachment point. Many times movement will take place at the point of insertion; however, movement may take place at the origin as well. One example is the *psoas* muscle group of the hip. When an individual is standing, contraction of the psoas muscle will flex the hip by raising the thigh (movement at the insertion). However, when lying supine with the lower body stable, contraction of this muscle will produce hip flexion by lifting up on the trunk (*e.g.*, a sit-up), thereby causing movement at the point of origin.

When a muscle contracts to perform a specific movement, it is known as an agonist. In contrast, a muscle that opposes agonist movement is known as an antagonist. For example, lifting a weight during elbow flexion, the biceps brachii is an agonist muscle whereas the triceps brachii is an antagonist muscle. Antagonist muscles must relax to some degree to allow agonist movement to take place. Antagonist muscle cocontraction plays a key role in stabilizing the joint, decelerating agonist movement, and reducing the risk of joint injury. When a muscle contracts to stabilize either the point of origin or insertion for a corresponding muscle, it is known as a stabilizer or fixator. When a muscle contracts to eliminate one movement of a multiarticular muscle, it is known as a neutralizer. For example, the hamstrings muscle group is a knee flexor and hip extensor. When only hip extension takes place, the quadriceps muscles will contract to eliminate or minimize knee flexion. When only knee flexion takes place, the hip flexors will contract to eliminate or minimize hip extension. Muscles can function under any of these roles depending on the situation. Human movement is predicated upon a complex recruitment strategy of muscle activation to allow the best and most efficient motion patterns to take place.

Skeletal Muscle Gross Anatomy

The structure of skeletal muscle is shown in Figure 5.1. Skeletal muscle is designed to generate high levels of force efficiently and to have these forces effectively transmitted to bone. Muscular structures are stacked in parallel. That is, smaller units are arranged in parallel to form larger units, and these units are stacked in parallel to form still larger units, etc. The most basic structural units of skeletal muscle are the myofilaments. Myofilaments are composed primarily of the contractile proteins *actin* and *myosin*, as well as a number of structural/cytoskeletal proteins and barrier proteins. The myofilaments form the basic functional unit of muscle, the sarcomere. Sarcomeres are stacked in series to form a myofibril. Myofibrils are stacked in parallel to form muscle fibers (the muscle cells). A muscle fiber may have a diameter of 10–100 μm on average while the length may range up to 30 cm. Groups of muscle fibers form

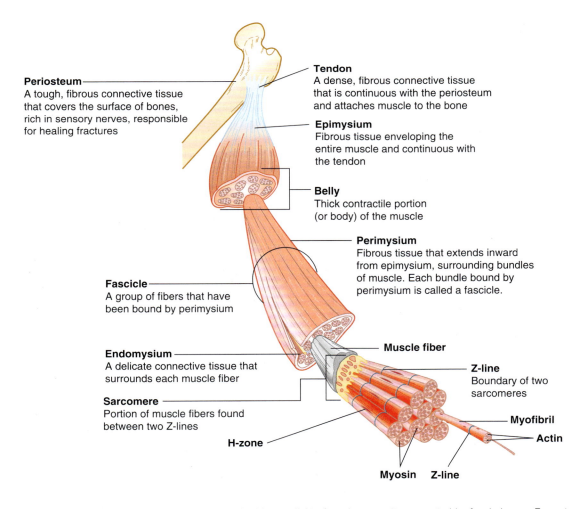

FIGURE 5.1 Skeletal muscle anatomy. Smaller units are stacked in parallel to form larger units separated by fascia layers. Force transmission is efficient from shortening of the sarcomeres and cross-bridge cycling of the myofilaments to the endomysium, perimysium, epimysium, tendons, and ultimately to bone. (Asset provided by Anatomical Chart Co.)

fascicles that are separated by fascia known as *endomysium*. Groups of fascicles form the muscle belly that is separated by fascia known as *perimysium*. The muscle belly is surrounded by fascia known as the *epimysium*. At the polar regions of muscle, tendons are located. The tendon connects muscle to bone. Fascia (endomysium, perimysium, and epimysium) located throughout the muscle assists in transferring forces produced by the shortening sarcomeres to the tendons and then ultimately to bone. These connective tissue sheaths help contribute to the elastic component of skeletal muscle. Fascia (especially the endomysium) also assists in stabilizing blood vessels and nerves surrounding muscle fibers. Thus, a continuum of tissues involved in muscle contraction exists and force transmission from basic proteins to fascia to strong tendons.

Muscle Fiber Organization

The organization of a skeletal muscle fiber is shown in Figure 5.2. Surrounding the muscle fiber (beneath the endomysium) is the cell membrane, also known as the sarcolemma. The sarcolemma encloses the fiber and regulates what enters and exits. It is important for propagating the action potential along the periphery of the fiber. The sarcolemma contains an outer plasma membrane and an inner basement membrane that is associated with structures of the basal lamina. Extending from openings in the sarcolemma to the interior of the fiber are transverse tubules (T tubules). The T tubules propagate the action potential deeper into the muscle fiber. Surrounding the myofibrils is the liquid cytoplasm (sarcoplasm) of the muscle fiber. The sarcoplasm contains enzymes, fat, glycogen, mitochondrion (site of aerobic energy production), multiple nuclei, and other organelles. The sarcoplasmic reticulum is a latticework of conductile tissue that penetrates deep into the muscle fiber allowing propagation of the action potential. It surrounds the myofilaments and carves them into myofibrils. On either side of the T tubules lies an extension of the sarcoplasmic reticulum known as the terminal cisternae or lateral sacs that are storage houses for calcium. The two terminal cisternae and the associated T tubule are collectively known as a *triad*. The nucleus contains the muscle fiber's genetic material and is especially important for initiating processes involved in protein synthesis. The muscle fiber has many peripherally located nuclei. Each nucleus controls a specific domain, known as the *myonuclear domain*, and the subsequent protein synthesized. Protein expression appears mostly uniform along adjacent domains within the same muscle fiber, thereby creating balance in the geometric proportion of proteins synthesized. Myonuclei number increases to accommodate muscle hypertrophy as each domain may be limited in its ability to produce proteins beyond ceiling limits.

Functional Unit of a Muscle Fiber: The Sarcomere

The sarcomere spans from one *Z line* to the next adjacent Z line and is the functional unit of the muscle fiber. A sarcomere on average is ~2.5 μm and is arranged in series with other sarcomeres within a myofibril. Figure 5.3 depicts the sarcomere and its constituents. Sarcomeres consist of contractile proteins and structural proteins that maintain the alignment of the contractile proteins, contribute to muscle elasticity, and assist in transmitting force longitudinally and laterally from the sarcomeres throughout the muscle. Ultimately, many proteins are expressed in isoforms that are specific to the muscle fiber type. Anchored to each Z line are the actin filaments. Several structural proteins anchor and structurally stabilize actin and the Z line including proteins such as *nebulin*, *myopalladin*, *filamin*, and *α-actinin*. Filamin (*Filamin-C*) may also act as a mechanical force sensor capable of stimulating anabolic pathways within skeletal muscle in response to training (1). Actin and its associated proteins make up the thin filament. The M line represents the central region of the sarcomere. The thick filaments consist of myosin and its associated proteins. Myosin is anchored (to the M line) and stabilized by structural proteins including the proteins *titin*, *M-protein*, *myomesin*, and *myosin-binding protein C*. Titin is a large elastic protein that spans half of the sarcomere and also stabilizes myosin to the Z line. Cross section of a myofibril shows that a myosin filament has the opportunity to interact with any of six actin filaments surrounding it. Both actin and myosin are key proteins involved in muscle contraction. However, muscle contraction would be highly limited without the structural and cytoskeletal proteins maintaining stability of the sarcomere and proper orientation of the myofilaments. Under a microscope, areas of the sarcomere housed predominantly by actin stain very light (*isotropic*) and are referred to as the I band. Areas of the sarcomere housed predominantly by myosin stain dark (*anisotropic*) and are referred to as the A band. Alternating light and dark bands from sequential sarcomeres give the muscle fiber a striated or striped appearance.

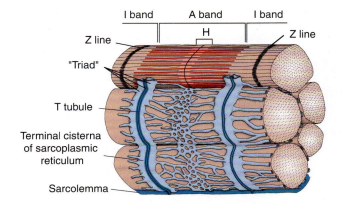

FIGURE 5.2 Muscle fiber organization. Key structures such as the sarcolemma, T tubules, and sarcoplasmic reticulum are shown. The conductile structures shown are important for propagating the action potential throughout the muscle fiber and mobilizing calcium from its intracellular storage site. (From Rubin R, Strayer DS. *Rubin's Pathology: Clinicopathologic Foundations of Medicine*. 5th ed. Philadelphia (PA): Lippincott Williams & Wilkins; 2008.)

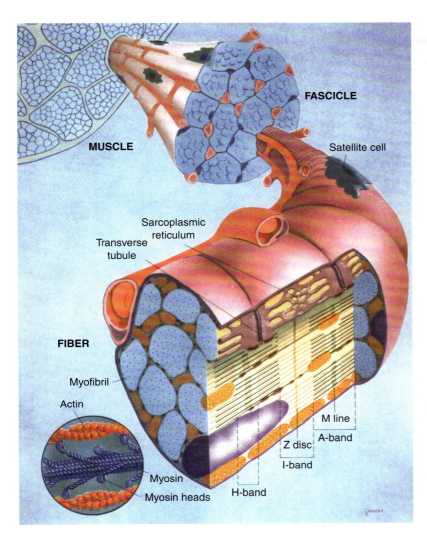

FIGURE 5.3 Structure of the sarcomere. The sarcomere spans from a Z line (disc) to an adjacent Z line (disc). The A band represents area comprised of the thick filaments. The I band represents area comprised of the thin filaments. The centrally located H zone (band) disappears during full muscle shortening. Sarcomeres are arranged in series spanning the length of the myofibril. (From Rubin E, Farber JL. *Pathology*. 3rd ed. Philadelphia (PA): Lippincott Williams & Wilkins; 1999.)

The area surrounding the M line is devoid of actin filaments and is known as the *H zone*. This area may be thought of as a spacer as it will disappear during full sarcomere shortening.

The Myofilaments

The myofilaments (shown in Fig. 5.4) are actin and myosin that account for nearly 85% of the protein content of the myofilaments. Actin is structured in a helical chain. Each strand of actin (known as fibrous or *F actin*) comprises a chain of ~200 smaller monomers (known as globular or *G actin*). A segment on G actin has a very high binding affinity to myosin. This region is known as an *active site* on actin. At rest, this area is not exposed but rather is covered by a barrier and protective protein known as *tropomyosin*. Tropomyosin consists of two coiled strands that lie in the groove of the F-actin helix that is associated with another critical protein, *troponin*. Each tropomyosin strand binds to seven successive actin subunits and has two troponin binding sites. Troponin (Tn) consists of three major subunits: TnI, TnC, and TnT. TnI is the subunit that binds to actin. TnC is the subunit with high affinity for the mineral calcium. TnT is the subunit that binds to tropomyosin. We will discuss the roles of these proteins in a moment during our discussion of muscle contraction. Myosin is a large protein known as a "molecular motor" due to its involvement in muscle contraction. It is composed of two heavy chains that form a helix. Each heavy chain binds two light chains, an *essential* and a *regulatory* light chain. The chain (part of the heavy chain and the light chains) complexes form two globular regions shaped like golf clubs known as *myosin heads*. One light chain is important for regulating the activity of a key metabolic enzyme myosin ATPase in the myosin head. The tail of myosin forms the thick filament backbone, whereas the two heads (head region) have actin-binding sites and form cross-bridges with actin during muscle contraction. The *hinge region* (at the neck) allows for mobility of the myosin heads.

Muscle Contraction: The Sliding Filament Theory

The *sliding filament* theory or model of muscle contraction was proposed by Hugh Huxley and Andrew Huxley in the early 1950s. It was so named because the underlying principle was that the thick and thin filaments slide past each other without changing length (although the sarcomere shortens).

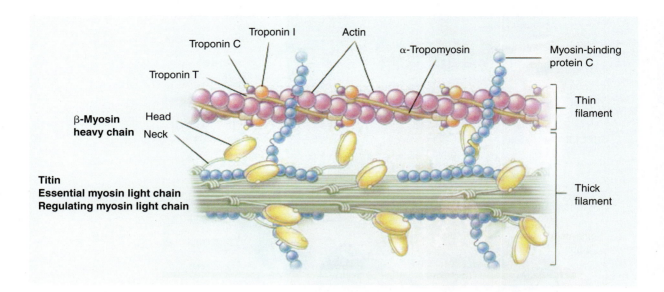

FIGURE 5.4 The myofibrillar proteins. The key contractile proteins actin and myosin and barrier proteins troponin (I [actin], C [calcium], and T [tropomyosin] subunits) and tropomyosin are shown. Myosin-binding proteins myosin-binding protein C and titin are also shown. (Reprinted with permission from Nabel EG. Cardiovascular disease. *N Engl J Med*. 2003;349:60–72, Fig. 3.)

Subsequent research has shown that the myofilaments rotate during shortening. Ultimately, sarcomere shortening in series leads to shortening of the muscle fibers and muscle belly leading to movement and force generation. Muscle contraction occurs in stages: (a) excitation-contraction coupling, (b) cross-bridge cycling, and (c) relaxation.

Excitation-Contraction Coupling

The electrical signal propagated along the motor nerve must be propagated throughout the muscle fibers. Skeletal muscle contains conductile tissue able to propagate the action potential throughout at a high speed. The action potential first propagates along the sarcolemma. Neurotransmitters (acetylcholine) released from the motor nerve bind to receptors and open adjacent sodium channels, initiating the spread of depolarization throughout the sarcolemma. From the sarcolemma, the action potential spreads through the T tubules and sarcoplasmic reticulum where calcium is stored in the terminal cisternae. The goal of the electrical discharge, or *excitation*, is to mobilize calcium. Calcium concentrations are low in the sarcoplasm at rest. An increase in calcium initiates subsequent events of muscle contraction. Depolarization causes a conformational change in voltage-sensitive channel proteins (*dihydropyridine [DHP]* and *ryanodine* receptors), thereby opening and allowing calcium from the SR to diffuse into the sarcoplasm. Once in the sarcoplasm, calcium rapidly binds to troponin (TnC) that triggers a conformational change in the protein configuration. That is, binding of calcium to TnC laterally shifts tropomyosin off of the actin active site (via TnT). The active site of actin is now exposed and will immediately bind to a myosin head forming a cross-bridge (also called an *actomyosin* complex). Troponin-tropomyosin complex can be viewed as a barrier protein complex that inhibits muscle contraction. However, once it is removed, cross-bridges can form and muscle contraction can take place. Therefore, one can view *excitation-contraction coupling* as a mechanism where electrical discharge at the muscle level leads to chemical events stimulating muscle contraction.

Cross-Bridge Cycling

Figure 5.5 depicts the events involved in cross-bridge cycling. Formation of the cross-bridge is only an initial step. For muscle contraction to proceed, numerous cross-bridges need to form until the sarcomere shortens as each cross-bridge only contributes a small magnitude to the sliding motion of the filaments. The term for multiple cross-bridge formation is *cross-bridge cycling*. Cross-bridge cycling can most simply be described by events analogous to a "tug-of-war" where the competitors are analogous to myosin (or the thick filament), their arms analogous to myosin heads, and the rope analogous to the thin filament. The goal of cross-bridge cycling is for the centrally stabilized myosin filaments to pull the structurally stabilized thin filaments inward toward the M line to shorten the sarcomere. When an actomyosin cross-bridge is formed, myosin is weakly bound to actin initially prior to movement of the myosin head. The release of P transforms the cross-bridge into a high-force state and subsequently initiates a powerful motion. This cyclical movement is referred to as the *power stroke* and is analogous to a tug-of-war participant pulling the rope inward. ADP is released at the end of the power stroke as the cross-bridge remains in a position of strength. The power stroke involves a pivot of the myosin head. However, this motion of the myosin head is not complete. Rather, the myosin head must disengage and bind to another active site on actin further upstream. This is referred to as *cross-bridge cycling* as myosin

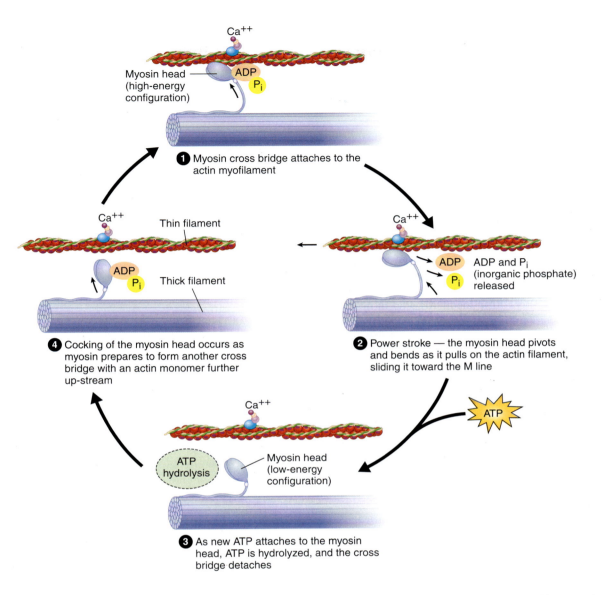

FIGURE 5.5 Cross-bridge cycling. (Adapted from Kraemer WJ, Fleck SJ, Deschenes MR. *Exercise physiology: Integrating Theory and Application.* Baltimore (MD): Wolters Kluwer Health; 2012.)

heads form multiple cross-bridges with actin until sarcomere shortening ceases. This process occurs asynchronously. That is, there are always cross-bridges formed (keeping tension on the thin filaments) while other myosin heads and actin monomers are disengaged. In our tug-of-war example, there is no part of the competition where all participants on a team will let go of the rope at the same time to switch hand position. That would result in losing tension on the rope and the competition. The same applies here. Myosin heads rotate asynchronously as cross-bridges form and subsequently detach. ATP binding at the conclusion of the power stroke quickly causes dissociation of the cross-bridge and the myosin lever arm is recocked to the prepower stroke position. ATP hydrolysis follows and enables formation and oscillation of a new cross-bridge. Energy released from ATP hydrolysis yields ADP and P. ADP and P bound to the myosin head changes its conformational state and helps increase myosin's leverage and properly direct the myosin head toward actin. Myosin ATPase (in the head of myosin) splits ATP for energy enabling the head of myosin to detach and subsequently bind to another exposed active site on actin further upstream. Cross-bridge formation and cycling continue (while calcium concentrations are elevated in the sarcoplasm) until relaxation takes place. Subsequently, cross-bridge cycling rotates the filaments and pulls the thin filaments in sliding past the thick filaments, thereby causing muscle contraction. All muscle fibers within a motor unit will be activated accordingly, and motor unit recruitment, rate, and firing patterns will depend upon the amount of force and power needed.

As previously discussed in Chapter 2, muscle force production is predicated upon sarcomere length where optimal interaction of actin and myosin proteins (*i.e.*, formation of cross-bridges) yields a peak in force centrally when viewing it active length-tension relationship curve. However, force increases at longer lengths passively, which may conflict with traditional applications of the sliding filament theory. Recently, the roles of structural proteins and connective tissue components have been implicated to play a significant role in this increased passive force seen at longer muscle lengths and during eccentric muscle actions. The protein titin has been the target of several investigations. It has been termed a "third filament" owing to its proposed role in passive muscle force production (2,3). Titin (initially known as *connectin*) is the largest known sarcomeric protein (>1 μm in length) and third in abundance that spans from the M line to the Z line (see Fig. 5.6) (4). Initially thought to stabilize myosin in the A-band region, titin's roles have expanded since its region extending to the Z line has been proposed to act as a "spring" and increase passive force production (2) and potentially act as a mechanosensor to skeletal muscle loading (1). Structurally, titin consists of an elastic I-band region with tandem immunoglobulin (Ig) domains, an N2A region, and a PEVK (proline, glutamate, valine, and lysine) segment and a supportive A-band region consisting of Ig and fibronectin domains. It has been proposed that titin may increase sarcomeric force by reducing its resting length or increasing stiffness during lengthening via binding to actin at the N2A region in the presence of calcium and rotating along with the myofilaments where the PEVK region is stretched (3). These processes have been described as a "winding filament" hypothesis where cross-bridge force and rotation is linked to titin force (3). Although still debated in the scientific community, this hypothesis would help partly explain the greater force and low-energy cost seen during eccentric muscle actions.

Relaxation

Relaxation begins with a reduction in neural stimuli. As force requirements decrease, action potentials along the motor nerve will decrease. This will reduce action potentials through the muscle fiber and remove the stimulus for calcium mobilization. In the sarcoplasm, calcium is restored by the actions of energy-requiring protein "pumps" located in the SR (*calcium ATPase pumps, SERCA proteins*). The barrier proteins return to their resting configuration blocking the actin active sites, and the myofilaments return to their resting state.

Skeletal Muscle's Graded Responses

The contraction of muscle in response to a stimulus is known as a twitch. Multiple twitches are needed as tension requirements increase. The effect of multiple twitches is known as summation. When multiple motor units are activated thereby contributing to force development, it is known as *spatial summation*. When a motor unit increases its frequency of discharge to increase force, it is known as *temporal summation*. Both types of summation increase force and power production dramatically. Tetanus refers to maximal force production (graphically depicted as a plateau or flat line) when summation is peaked.

Skeletal Muscle Mechanotransduction: Costameres

Human biological tissue capable of adapting to overload must be able to couple mechanical stimuli to biochemical signaling. This process is known as *mechanotransduction* and occurs in many tissue types including skeletal muscle. Skeletal muscle modeling of mechanotransduction involves tissue deformation in response to the intensity and volume of loading, sensing of stimulus magnitude, integrating the input with output processes, and increasing the level of intracellular signaling leading to the anticipated outcome. The response appears to be mediated by a number of systems or pathways communicating with each other to enable tissue adaptation appropriate and proportional to the level of overload. In order for muscles to effectively

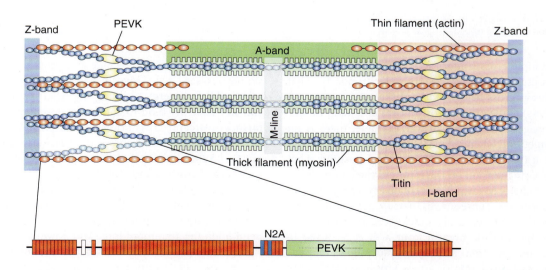

FIGURE 5.6 The structure of titin. (Reprinted from Rassier DE. Sarcomere mechanics in striated muscles: from molecules to sarcomeres to cells. *Am J Physiol Cell Physiol.* 2017;313:C134–45.)

transmit force, the cytoskeleton must be tethered to the cell membrane. Skeletal muscle contains linkage proteins known as *costameres* ("rib-like"), which anchor M lines and Z lines to the cell membrane, while some are also present parallel to the long axis of the myofibril. These protein connections allow the membrane to move in unison with the sarcomeres during contraction and allowing force to be transmitted laterally from myofibril to myofibril, across the membrane to the extracellular matrix, and ultimately to the tendon (5). Approximately 75% of muscle force produced is transmitted laterally through the sarcolemma versus 20%–30% transmitted longitudinally from sarcomere to sarcomere (5). Several key costameric proteins such as α-actinin and *desmin* are shown in Figure 5.7 (6). These proteins form complexes that reinforce the membrane, link the contractile apparatus to the extracellular matrix, and link mechanotransduction force-related deformation to intramuscular signaling leading to muscular adaptations. The extracellular matrix consists of *laminin* and collagen fibrils that give it strength to mediate high forces produced within skeletal muscles. The cell membrane consists of major complexes including the *dystroglycans*, *sarcoglycan*, *integrin*, and *ankyrin* (not shown) complexes, which are linked to other networks of proteins such as *vinculin*, *talin*, *dystrophin*, *syntrophin*, and *spectrin* that form links for force transmission and sarcomere stability. Costamere proteins appear sensitive to and may be up-regulated in response to consistent mechanical, electrical, and chemical stimuli. The integrin complex functions as a key signal transducer via signaling of the proteins focal adhesion kinase (FAK) and integrin-linked kinase (ILK). Integrins (and sarcoglycans and dystroglycans) sense mechanical stress and activate intracellular signal transduction pathways, leading to changes in gene transcription and cytoskeletal reorganization. Changes in the dystrophin-associated protein complex may take place during resistance training (RT) (7). FAK and ILK respond to increased muscle overload and play key roles in mediating intracellular hypertrophic signaling and myogenesis (8). For example, FAK may stimulate the phosphatidylinositol-3 kinase (PI3), Akt, and mammalian target of rapamycin (mTOR) pathways (discussed later in this chapter), thereby increasing protein synthesis and possibly muscle hypertrophy (8). Integrins may act as sensors for cell swelling, thereby stimulating protein synthesis (1). Several, but not all, studies have shown aerobic and anaerobic exercise may increase FAK phosphorylation (8). RT has been shown to up-regulate FAK, vinculin, and integrin content, and these changes correlated to type I muscle hypertrophy (9). It appears mechanical loading may activate the *Hippo family* of proteins, which may help mediate training-induced hypertrophy (10).

Skeletal Muscle Characteristics and Adaptations

Skeletal muscle adapts to exercise in various and specific ways. Training up-regulates the activity of numerous genes that enhance muscle function. Skeletal muscle can enlarge (hypertrophy) when subjected to stress demanding greater force

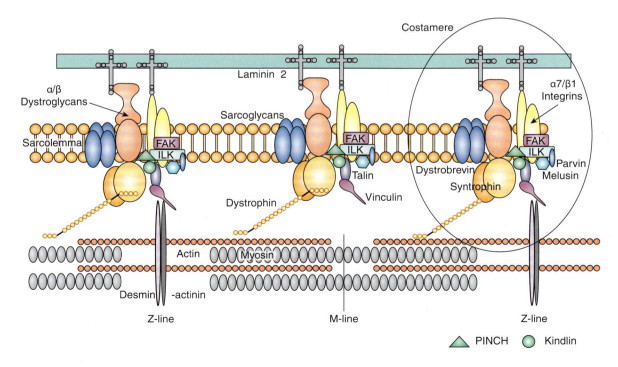

FIGURE 5.7 The costamere proteins. FAK, focal adhesion kinase; ILK, integrin-linked kinase; PINCH, particularly interesting cysteine- and histidine-rich protein. (Reprinted from Jaka O, Casas-Fraile L, Lopez de Munain A, Saenz A. Costamere proteins and their involvement in myopathic processes. *Expert Rev Mol Med*. 2015;17:e12. doi: 10.1017/erm.2015.9.)

Sidebar: Genetics and Muscle Performance

Genetics is the branch of biology that focuses on the study of genes, variation, and heritability. *Genes* are specific segments of a deoxyribonucleic acid (DNA) molecule that contain the instructions or "blueprint" (*i.e., genotype*) that code for proteins ultimately determining an individual's makeup (*i.e., phenotype*) (Fig. 5.8). Genes are organized within *chromosomes* and come in pairs. Humans possess 22 paired chromosomes plus the sex chromosomes (x, y) and the location of the gene is known as a locus. Humans have two copies of each gene from both parents. Different forms of the same gene are called *alleles*. A chromosome is made from tightly packed strands of DNA wrapped around proteins (histones) forming structures known as *chromatids*. Two chromatids join together to form a chromosome. Each strand of DNA is bonded to a second strand via hydrogen bonding between base pairing (adenine-thymine, guanine-cytosine) to a double helix. DNA is found mostly in the nucleus but also in the mitochondria. DNA is replicated and transcribed into messenger ribonucleic acid (mRNA). An *exon* is a region of the gene that will encode a part of the RNA produced after the *introns* (noncoding regions) have been removed via splicing. The message encoded by mRNA is read in three-letter codons, initiating with a "start" codon and concluding with a "stop" codon, which code for specific amino acids. Most amino acids can be coded by more than one codon. Transfer RNA (tRNA) reads mRNA and facilitates translation by transporting the amino acids, thereby sequencing them into peptides, polypeptides, or proteins in the ribosomes.

The human genome contains more than 3 million base pairs (>99% similar between individuals) and 20,000–25,000 genes that encode a host of proteins. These small differences contribute to each individual's unique features or their phenotypic expression. Phenotypic expression reflects not only genetics but also the influence of environmental factors. Several genes encode for proteins that directly have some effect on athletic performance beyond that of just the muscular system. These genes are known as *candidate genes*. Although humans have these genes, the ways they are expressed directly affects development in all health- and skill-related fitness components. *Epigenetics* is the study of biological mechanisms that activate or repress gene expression that does not involve change in DNA sequence (*i.e.*, mostly through DNA methylation or histone modification) such as aging, diet, exercise, disease, drugs, and environmental chemicals. Variations in DNA sequence affect gene expression. Different alleles or *polymorphisms* present variations of gene expression that will affect phenotype. The major types of polymorphisms identified include (a) insertions and deletions; (b) DNA duplication (copy number); (c) repeat patterns; and (d) single nucleotide polymorphisms (SNPs), which are the most common (11). Human studies have shown more than 200 genetic variations exists affecting performance (11,12). Thus, all physiologic systems and training adaptations discussed in this textbook are affected by genetics. Many genetics studies involve heritability where the proportion of variance observed between individuals within a specific population for a given trait can be explained by genetic influences. For example, some heritability studies have shown that genetics may explain 45%–80% of the variation in lean body mass (LBM), 70%–90% in muscle size, 22%–83% in various types of

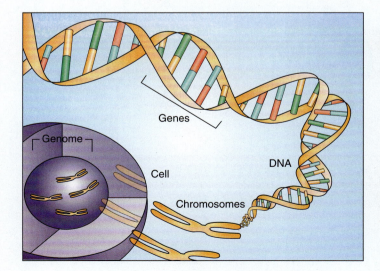
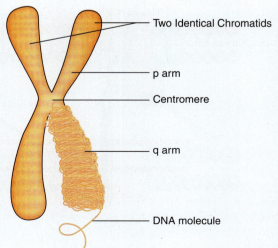

FIGURE 5.8 Chromosomes, genes, and DNA.

(Continued)

muscle strength, and 45%–50% in fiber types (11,13). The heritability status for athletic performance (independent of the sport) has been estimated to be ~66% (14). To illustrate, genetics may be a major contributor to "responder" or "non-responder" status when it comes to training. If two trainees (with similar training experience) complete the same 10-week RT program and LBM increases by 0.8 kg in one individual and by 2.6 kg in the other individual, research suggests that between 50% and 80% of this difference could be explained by genetic factors, leaving the remaining segment related to environmental factors. Other studies involve candidate-gene associations where the relationships between specific genotypes and performance measures are examined. Several candidate genes for performance have been identified. The following are just a few examples of candidate genes shown to have one or more polymorphisms associated with muscle strength, power, LBM, speed, endurance, or linked to some aspect of injury prevention (11–15): *ACTN3*, α-actinin-3; *ACE*, angiotensin converting enzyme; *APOE*, apolipoprotein E; *AR*, androgen receptor; *COL1A1, COL1A2*—collagen type 1 alpha 1 and 2; *CTNF*, ciliary neurotrophic factor; *FST*, follistatin; *IGF-1, IGF-2*, insulin-like growth factor-1 and 2; *GR*, glucocorticoid receptor; *HIF1α*, hypoxia-inducible factor 1α; *IL-6*, interleukin-6; *MSTN*, myostatin; *NO3*, endothelial nitric oxidase synthase 3; *PPARα*, peroxisome proliferator-activated receptor alpha; and *VDR*, vitamin D receptor. It is important to note that strength, hypertrophy, endurance (muscular and cardiovascular), flexibility, power, and speed phenotypes present quantified traits by several variants rather than isolated effects of a few.

The other key element is epigenetic gene expression. Gene expression is influenced by a number of factors including exercise and training. Ultimately, gene expression changes mediate many training adaptations. Increased or decreased expression of a gene will influence the amount of protein produced and subsequently the phenotype of the individual. Aerobic and anaerobic exercise can alter the expression of several genes as part of the process of adaptation. Roth et al. (16) have shown that 9 weeks of unilateral RT of the knee extensors resulted in the differential expression of 69 genes (many muscle-related structural and metabolic genes) measured 48–72 hours after the last workout. Significant gene expression alterations take place following resistance exercise, *i.e.*, 4 and 24 hours post, with the response shown to be sex specific (17). Some gene expression differences (especially with known regulators of anabolic signaling, muscle cytoskeleton) were shown, and the overall response was prolonged in men (*i.e.*, still altered at 24 hours post) potentially leading to a greater hypertrophic response (17). Interestingly, some genes involving mitochondrial structure and oxidative phosphorylation were down-regulated (17). Aerobic exercise has been shown to increase gene expression (18). Catoire et al. (18) reported increased gene expression in 938 genes immediately following acute aerobic exercise (single-leg cycling). Interestingly, they reported significant changes in expression of 516 genes in the nonexercised leg as well (18).

production. Fiber-type and architectural transitions can occur, increasing one's force, power, and endurance. Changes in skeletal muscle enzyme activity, substrate content, receptor content, capillary and mitochondrial density, and protein content also enhance athletic performance. Several of these changes are discussed in the next section while a few are discussed in subsequent chapters in relation to other physiological systems.

Muscle Fiber Formation and Repair

Aerobic and anaerobic exercise (especially exercise with a potent ECC component) has the ability to produce significant muscle damage when the stimulus is novel or unaccustomed (and of significant volume and intensity). The damage response is greatest initially but is lessened over time as a protective effect (19–23) possibly due to several factors including motor unit recruitment differences, stiffness changes, the addition of serial sarcomeres, altered expression of inflammatory mediators, or up-regulation of protective proteins. For example, RE has been shown to up-regulate the content of a few (*i.e.*, HSP27, HSP70, αB-crystallin) *heat shock proteins* (*e.g.*, proteins that protect muscle fibers from damage during stress) possibly indicative of an adaptational strategy to resist future exercise-induced damage and a more efficient *remodeling* of muscle tissue (24).

Thus, the repair of damaged muscle and possible formation of new muscle fibers are critical to normal muscle function.

Muscle fibers must be remodeled to replace old or damaged muscle fibers. The process of muscle fiber formation and regeneration is known as myogenesis. *Satellite cells* (stem cells located in a niche between the basal lamina and sarcolemma that are quiescent at rest) are released, migrate to the area of fiber formation, fuse to existing muscle fibers, and provide myonuclei to the muscle fiber (Fig. 5.9). Satellite cells may also self-renew to maintain the quiescent population upon activation. Satellite cell activity is controlled by a complex interplay of local and systemic factors such as a number of growth factors, myokines, Wnt/β-catenin signaling, androgens, nitric oxide, and Notch signaling (25) as well as by external factors such as protein intake and exercise (26). Satellite cells proliferate (increase in number) and differentiate into more functional cells called *myoblasts*. Myoblasts proliferate, differentiate, fuse to existing fibers to donate nuclei, and form a multinucleated *myotube*. Myotubes form the scaffold of the new fiber, and further maturation results in a new muscle fiber. The process of myogenesis is enhanced by several myogenic regulatory transcription factors (MRFs) expressed in a sequence corresponding to satellite cell proliferation, differentiation, and myofiber formation including *Pax-7, MyoD, Myf5, MRF4,* and *myogenin* but is inhibited by the

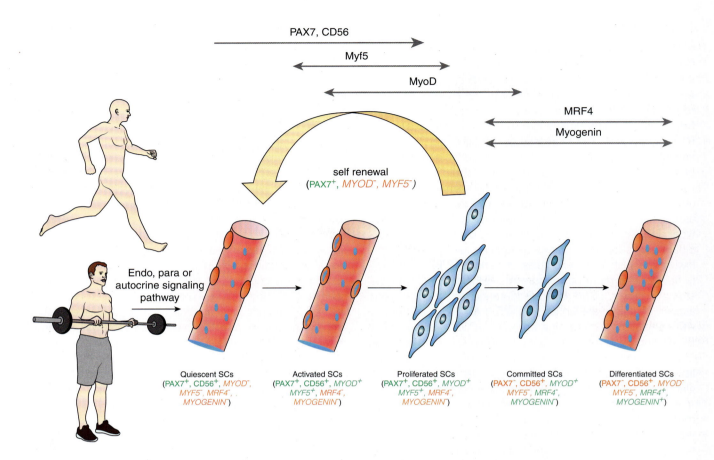

FIGURE 5.9 Myogenesis and satellite cell activation. (Reprinted from Bazgir B, Fathi R, Valojerdi MR, Mozdziak P, Asgari A. Satellite cells contribution to exercise mediated muscle hypertrophy and repair. *Cell J*. 2017;18:473–84.)

protein *myostatin*. These transcription factors may also increase gene expression of several contractile and structural proteins and subsequently contribute to fiber-type plasticity, *i.e.*, greater expression of MRFs is associated with fast-twitch fiber population. Up-regulation of myogenic factors is thought to contribute to training-induced muscle hypertrophy, repair of damaged muscle, and training-induced fiber-type plasticity.

Myostatin is a member of the transforming growth factor-β (TGF-β) superfamily that acts as a negative regulator of muscle growth and muscle fiber-type expression. Myostatin binds to the activin-type IIB receptor (which is inhibited by protein *follistatin*), may blunt anabolic signaling (*i.e.*, mTORC1 pathway discussed later in this chapter), and is involved in catabolic signaling and gene expression via *Smad* transcription factors (25,27). Myostatin may limit myogenic proliferation and differentiation by suppressing MyoD and can increase satellite cell self-renewal (as opposed to differentiation) (28). Thus, myostatin may directly promote skeletal muscle catabolism or limit myogenesis, in either case a scenario is imposed limiting skeletal muscle size. Myostatin has been of interest to scientists since it was discovered that animals not expressing or possessing mutations of the myostatin (MSTN) gene had extremely large muscle mass.

A number of studies have shown that exercise can increase myogenesis in a fiber-type–specific manner. Aerobic and high-intensity interval exercise increases satellite cell content acutely with some data indicating larger responses at higher intensities (28,29). Satellite cell increases may not be accompanied by hypertrophy during aerobic training indicating that the primary role may be muscle repair and regeneration (27,29). An acute bout of eccentric RE increases satellite cell content within 1 hour postexercise, peaks ~72 hours postexercise (27), but also concentric-only RT can increase satellite cell content in type I and II fibers (26). Resistance and combined RE and plyometrics increase satellite cell numbers significantly up to 96 hours postexercise with some studies showing an intensity and volume dependency (28,30–32). Long-term RT, sprint training, and simultaneous aerobic and RT increase satellite cell content (28,30,32–34), and powerlifters have higher numbers of satellite cells and myonuclei than control subjects (35). Twelve weeks of low-intensity RT (15.5% of 1 RM) increased satellite cell content by 18% versus a 32% increase following moderate-intensity RT (70% of 1 RM) (36). Six weeks of heavy RT (6–10 reps, 80%–85% of 1 RM) increased satellite cell content (and hypertrophy) in all fiber types more than slow-velocity training (6–10 reps, 40%–60% of 1 RM, 10-s CON: 4-s ECC) and endurance training (20–30 reps, 40%–60% of 1 RM) (37). The acute RE satellite cell increase may be augmented with chronic RT (34). Lastly, trainees deemed as "responders" to RT incur greater increases in fiber area, myonuclei per fiber, and satellite cell content (38).

Satellite cell activation contributes to training-induced muscle hypertrophy although some muscle hypertrophy may occur in the absence of myonuclear accretion. Satellite cells are incorporated into muscle fibers and contribute myonuclei, which expands its growth potential by maintaining an appropriate myonuclei to cytoplasm ratio (*i.e.*, known as the *myonuclei domain theory*). In fact, elite powerlifters with much greater muscle size have a similar myonuclear domain to control subjects (35). It is thought that each myonuclei domain comprises ~2,000 μm^2 per nucleus (or higher in responders to RT) (38) limiting muscle growth; thus, expansion of the myonuclei pool stimulates a considerable magnitude of training-induced hypertrophy (28). Correlations have been shown between satellite cell content and muscle fiber size during RT (30,32). A meta-analysis showed that myonuclear addition may occur when hypertrophy is ≤10% but is more consistent with higher levels of hypertrophy (≥22%), thereby showing the threshold of growth needed to induce myonuclear accretion may be lower than previously thought (39). Upon detraining-induced atrophy, myonuclei number may remain despite the smaller fiber size and lead to a faster "retraining route" of hypertrophy once training reconvenes, *e.g.*, a concept known as *muscle memory* (40). The myonuclear increase seen during RT is reduced in the presence of low testosterone (41).

Several (42–47), but not all (48), studies have shown acute RE up-regulates myogenesis markers (myogenin, MyoD) within a few hours (up to 24–48 hours) postexercise. The acute response to a workout may be enhanced by chronic RT (34,45). Endurance exercise poses a modest effect on these responses (49), but high-intensity interval exercise may augment the response. Long-term studies (12–16 weeks) have shown RT up-regulates or does not alter myogenic marker expression over time (45,50,51). Acutely, the percent of satellite cells coexpressing myostatin in type I and II muscle fibers may decrease following RE (27,30). Reductions in myostatin and *p27^kip* (a protein that inhibits cell cycle initiation) have been shown 6 hours following RE (47), and myostatin mRNA is reduced from 45 minutes to 48 hours following RE (52). Chronically myostatin expression may decrease following RT (43,45,53) or not change (30,33), and the response may depend on age (54). In older men, it may take at least three workouts to see myostatin down-regulation (54). Long-term RT may not affect the expression of follistatin or the activin type IIb receptor (54,55); however, activin type Iib receptor expression may decrease 1 hour after a workout in older men (45). Low-to-moderately high-intensity aerobic training may reduce myostatin protein content (56). Thus, changes in myogenic markers appear to be part of a larger strategy allowing for the recovery of skeletal muscle following exercise and potential increased muscle size accompanying training if a threshold of exercise intensity and volume is utilized beyond one's current level of adaptation.

Gene Expression and MicroRNAs

MicroRNAs are small (~18–25 bp) noncoding RNAs that regulate mRNA expression post-transcriptionally. MicroRNA biogenesis begins in the nucleus, translocates to the cytoplasm, and is incorporated into a protein complex (*RNA-induced silencing complex*) where it can bind to target mRNAs and destabilize or degrade them blocking the translation of genes. One microRNA can target up to thousands of genes and one gene may be targeted by multiple microRNAs (57). More than 1,800 microRNAs have been identified in the human genome (58). Muscle-specific microRNAs are known as myomiRs. Some commonly studied myomiRs are miR-1, miR-16, miR-23, miR-133a, miR-133b, miR-206, miR-208, miR-221, miR-222, miR-378, miR-486, and miR-494 (59,60). MyomiRs are expressed uniformly throughout muscle in both fiber types, although there are a few confined only to slow-twitch fibers (59,61). MyomiRs respond to exercise and appear to play major roles in subsequent gene expression, protein synthesis/degradation, myogenesis, angiogenesis, and muscle fiber-type plasticity. Exercise has been shown to down-regulate more myomiRs than those myomiRs that are up-regulated (62). Some myomiRs have been shown to inhibit anabolic signaling via IGF-1/IRS-1 and mTOR pathways (60).

Resistance exercise decreases expression of some myomiRs (*i.e.*, miR-1, miR-133a, miR-133b, miR-206) (57,59,61), and these reductions are thought to help mediate, in part, increased protein synthesis commonly seen for 2–3 days following a workout. The reductions appear larger if RE is preceded by high-intensity interval exercise (63). In a cross-sectional study, D'Souza et al. (35) investigated the myomiR profiles of elite powerlifters compared to recreationally active men. They found 12 myomiRs were differentially expressed. Five of these (miR-486, miR-499a, miR-126, miR-133a, and miR-1) were higher in controls than powerlifters, whereas miR-15a, miR-16, miR-23a, miR-23b, miR-30b, miR-206, and miR451a were elevated in powerlifters. This profile was thought to play key roles in mediating differences in fiber type, protein turnover, muscle remodeling, and angiogenesis between groups (35). In another study comparing responders to nonresponders, 85 myomiRs were differentially expressed 3–6 hours after a workout and 102 myomiRs were differentially expressed chronically following 12 weeks of RT (64). Twenty-six of these were differentially expressed in high versus low responders (64).

Endurance exercise may down-regulate some myomiRs while up-regulating a few (59). Nielsen et al. (65) showed increased miR-1 and miR-133a following one endurance workout that was attenuated after 12 weeks of endurance training. In addition, resting myomiRs were reduced at rest following the training period but reverted back to pretraining levels after 14 days of detraining (65). MyomiR changes following aerobic exercise are thought to help mostly mediate changes in angiogenesis and mitochondrial biogenesis (59).

Some microRNAs can be packaged and exported into circulation where they can be taken up by target tissues and inhibit transcription of target genes (60). Some studies have investigated the potential for examining *circulating microRNAs* from blood sampling as a measure of anabolic status of muscle following RE. The responses appear equivocal as data support the predictive nature (60), but other studies have found differential responses between specific muscle myomiR changes and circulating microRNA responses (58). Thus, microRNAs appear to play major roles in mediating the anabolic status of skeletal muscle and help explain, in part, differential responses between responders and nonresponders.

Muscle Fiber Types

Muscle fibers reflect the type of stimulation they receive from the nervous system. This was shown many years ago by early classic cross-innervation studies in animals. Muscle fiber phenotypes reflect a combination of heritability and activity level. Two general fiber-type classifications exist based on muscle's contractile and metabolic properties: *slow twitch* (ST) and *fast twitch* (FT). ST (type I) fibers are predominantly endurance fibers, whereas FT (type II) fibers are strength/power fibers. Each fiber type has distinct characteristics leading to its force/endurance profile, and every muscle in the human body contains a mosaic of fiber types (Table 5.1). Within these major classifications, muscle fibers exist on a continuum. Intermediate

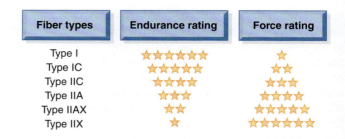

FIGURE 5.10 Fiber-type continuum with force and endurance ratings. (Based on data from Staron RS. The classification of human skeletal muscle fiber types. *J Strength Cond Res.* 1997;11(2):67.)

fibers exist such that there are six fiber-type subclassifications based on myosin ATPase histochemical staining. Figure 5.10 depicts the fiber-type intermediates. Because fiber types operate on a continuum, the type I fibers possess the least generated force, power, and speed capacity but are highest in endurance, whereas the type II fiber has the least endurance but the greatest strength, power, and shortening velocity. Other fibers lie somewhere in between on a continuum. The continuum (I, IC, IIC, IIAC, IIA, IIAX, and IIX) exists concomitant to immunohistochemical or single-fiber SDS-PAGE determination of myosin heavy chain (MHC) expression, *i.e.*, MHCI, IIA, IIX, and fibers coexpressing multiple isoforms (66,67). Muscle fibers are composed of proteins that express isoforms characteristic of that fiber type. Isoform-specific protein expression relates to the force, speed, power, and endurance qualities of the motor unit.

Fiber Types in Athletes

Skeletal muscle is composed of ST and FT fibers. The ratio of the two assists in determining the muscle's functional capacity to a certain extent. Each muscle will have a distinct ratio and may favor one type or the other; the gastrocnemius muscle is predominantly FT in many individuals (but not some endurance athletes), whereas the soleus muscle is predominantly ST. Endurance athletes (*e.g.*, long- and middle-distance runners, cyclists) display larger percentages of type I fibers, whereas strength/power athletes (*e.g.*, sprinters, throwers, weightlifters, jumpers) display larger percentages of type II fibers (68). Häkkinen et al. (69) showed that the percentage of FT fibers in the vastus lateralis muscles of powerlifters, bodybuilders, and wrestlers were 60%, 59%, and 42%, respectively. Other reviews have shown endurance athletes to have 18%–25% of type II fibers in the same muscle (70). In a review of studies, Tesch and Alkner (71) compared fiber-type composition of various strength athletes. For the vastus lateralis muscle, powerlifters possessed ~55%–56% FT fibers, bodybuilders had ~45%–48% FT fibers, and weightlifters had ~54%–62% FT fibers. Bodybuilders possess a relatively higher percentage of ST fibers and lower type II/type I area ratios than weightlifters, powerlifters, and other power athletes (68). Powerlifters have a significantly higher FT fiber percent in the vastus lateralis than control subjects and shown to have reduced levels

Table 5.1	Muscle Fiber-Type Characteristics	
Characteristic	**Slow Twitch**	**Fast Twitch**
Motor nerve size	Smaller	Larger
Nerve conduction velocity	Slower	Faster
Nerve recruitment threshold	Lower	Higher
Size	Smaller	Larger
Contraction speed	Slower	Faster
Type of myosin	Slower	Faster
Myosin ATPase activity	Lower	Higher
Sarcoplasmic reticulum development	Poor	Great
Troponin affinity for calcium	Poor	Great
Force	Lower	Higher
Muscle efficiency	Great	Poor
Fatigability	Lower	Higher
Anaerobic energy stores	Lower	Higher
Relaxation time	Slower	Faster
Glycolytic enzyme activity	Lower	Higher
Glycogen stores	Moderate	Higher
Endurance	Higher	Lower
Triglyceride stores	Higher	Lower
Myoglobin	Higher	Lower
Aerobic enzyme activity	Higher	Lower
Capillary density	Higher	Lower
Mitochondrial density	Higher	Lower

of miR-499a, which is known to be linked to higher FT fiber percent (35). A single-fiber case study of an elite world champion sprint runner showed that the vastus lateralis muscle contained 24% MHCIIX, 34% MHCIIA, 29% MHCI, 4.5% MHCI/IIA, and 8.5% MHCIIA/IIX (67). They also showed that the MCHIIX fibers were 50% faster and 78% more powerful than the MHCIIA fibers (67). This athlete possessed much higher IIX content than any others measured in the literature and his single-fiber FT power values were the highest reported to date (67). Thus, elite athletes may pose a unique scenario in viewing muscle fiber composition. Muscle fiber-type composition is one attribute that may lead athletes toward participation in certain sports.

Fiber-Type Transitions

Although the proportions of type I and II fibers are genetically determined to some extent, transitions have been shown to occur. The pattern of muscle stimulation leads to specific intramuscular signaling, which ultimately increases gene expression of proteins corresponding to a fiber type. The most common pattern seen is the type IIX to IIA transition, which has been shown across multiple training modalities, e.g., RT, sprint, plyometric, and endurance training. Changes in MHC content (IIX to IIA) can occur within the first few workouts (72,73) that precede changes in fiber types. With RT, transitions take place from IIX to IIA (38,50,72,74–76) (Fig. 5.11). Type IIX fibers are considered reservoir fibers that tend to transform into a more oxidative form upon training (i.e., to an intermediate fiber type IIAX to IIA) (77). The advantage of this transition is unclear but could be related to enhanced force produced over time. Although type IIX fibers are the strongest, fastest, and most powerful of all fiber types (67), their fatigability may limit their true potential when performing some strength/power tasks. Thus, the transition appears to be beneficial for certain types of strength/power performances. However, having a higher IIX population could be highly advantageous for a short-term, explosive athlete like a sprinter (67). It is important to note that type IIX fibers are not readily recruited (based on the size principle; see Chapter 4). The intensity of exercise needs to be high to consistently activate this fiber type. This was shown by Holm et al. (78) who showed reductions in MHCIIX (from 7% to 3%) following 12 weeks of RT with 70% of 1 RM versus no change in MHCIIX percent following low-intensity training (15.5% of 1 RM). Once activated consistently through training, however, recruitment of these fibers may lead to segmental transitions of some IIX to type IIAX and subsequently to IIA fibers. Detraining results in an increase in type IIX fibers and a reduction in type IIA fibers, with a possible overshoot (i.e., a larger percentage seen after detraining than before training) of type IIX fibers (79). Complete reversal (i.e., type IIA to IIX transitions) of training-induced fiber-type transitions can be seen after 32 weeks of detraining with half of the benefits lost by 16 weeks of detraining (74). Reducing RT volume by 2/3 was enough to maintain fiber composition; however, reducing volume to 1/9 of the original resulted in a partial reversal (IIA to IIX) in fiber composition (74).

Moderate- to high-intensity aerobic training has produced similar fiber-type transitions (80,81). In a review, McComas (70) reported reduced type IIX percentages and slight increases in type IIA and I populations in nearly all studies examined. The magnitude of type IIX fiber percent reduction is greater following RT than endurance training (75). Simultaneous aerobic and RT result in a reduction in MHCIIX (82). Sprint training produces similar IIX to IIA transitions (83,84). Plyometric training has been shown to decrease type IIX populations and increase type IIA populations in some, but not all, studies (85).

Recent scientific advances have shown the importance of genetics and intramuscular signaling in fiber-type transitions. Ahmetov et al. (86) reported 14 gene polymorphisms that are associated with fiber-type composition. Several of these are associated with type I fiber expression (i.e., ACE I, ACTN3 577X, HIF1A Pro582, etc.), whereas some are associated with type II fiber expression (i.e., ACE D, ACN3 R577, HIF1A 582Ser, etc.). These polymorphisms help explain baseline fiber-type composition and the fiber-type transitions that take place during training. The pattern of muscle activation contributes greatly to the transitional state of muscle fibers to a more oxidative phenotype. Fiber transitions ultimately involve the up-regulation of certain genes while repressing other genes. Figure 5.12 depicts intramuscular signaling via endurance exercise. Muscle contraction increases activation of the calcium/calmodulin/calcineurin pathway ultimately leading to increased expression of slow-twitch genes via activation of nuclear factor of activated T cells (NFAT) (87). Activation of the calcium/calmodulin-dependent

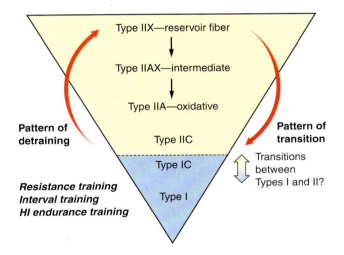

FIGURE 5.11 Fiber-type transitions with training and detraining. Resistance training, interval training, and high-intensity endurance training have been shown to reduce type IIX population with a concomitant increase in type IIA fiber percent. Type IIAX fiber changes may reflect fibers in transition (to type IIA). Detraining produces the opposite direction of transition. This theoretical *dotted line* reflects the potential transformation of a type II fiber to a type I fiber or vice versa.

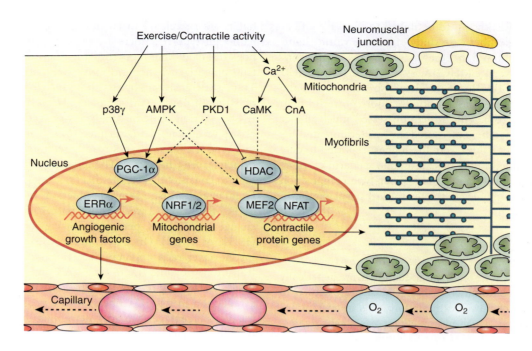

FIGURE 5.12 Endurance exercise intramuscular signaling. (Reprinted from Yan Z, Okutsu M, Akhtar YN, Lira VA. Regulation of exercise-induced fiber type transformation, mitochondrial biogenesis, and angiogenesis in skeletal muscle. *J Appl Physiol*. 2011;110:264–74.)

protein kinases (CaMK) inhibits the *class II histone deacetylases* (HDACs, which represses target genes), thereby stimulating the *myocyte enhancer factor 2* (MEF2) proteins leading to expression of slow-twitch genes (87). Figure 5.12 also depicts activation of *AMP-activated protein kinase* (AMPK; a kinase sensitive to metabolic stress and energy turnover that helps coordinate anabolic versus catabolic signaling in muscle fibers) and p38γ mitogen-activated protein kinase, which activates *peroxisome proliferator-activated receptor γ coactivator 1α* (PGC-1α). Activation of this pathway through PGC-1α leads to angiogenesis (capillary formation) and mitochondrial biogenesis, both of which are characteristic of more oxidative fiber types (87). Different isoforms of PGC-1α exist and some are up-regulated in response to RE (52). *Reactive oxygen species* (chemically active molecules containing oxygen that increase in response to the oxidative stress of exercise) may activate PGC-1α indirectly via AMPK and MEF2 may activate PGC-1α (25). It has been suggested that some MRFs such as MyoD and myogenin may assist in regulation of fiber-type specific gene expression.

Of interest to exercise scientists has been the capacity to transform between muscle fiber types, *e.g.*, transformations from a type I to type II fiber or vice versa. Most fiber-type transitions shown occur within each population (*e.g.*, from a type IIX to IIA). However, there have been a few studies that have shown a significant change in type I and type II muscle fiber populations as a result of training (74). Some methods have been criticized in these studies making it difficult to conclusively state if these changes occurred. Cross-sectional comparisons of different athletes have shown substantial differences in type I and II populations for a given muscle especially when strength/power athletes are compared to endurance athletes or to control subjects (35). However, the effects of genetics make interpretation of cross-sectional studies more difficult. Were these athletes genetically gifted with this fiber-type variation, did training affect these percentages, or both? Since heritability studies show that genetics may contribute to 45%–50% of the variation in fiber types between individuals, it is likely epigenetic factors such as training can cause a shift between major fiber types. Based on the fact that fiber types function on a continuum, it seems plausible that fiber conversion is a possibility. The identification of transitional hybrid fiber types (*i.e.*, type IC and IIC fibers) has supported this contention. Extreme forms of training at higher levels, *e.g.*, cross-country running versus powerlifting, would benefit from fiber transitions and this could help explain some of the large differences in fiber types seen in these athletes. However, further research is needed to analyze transitions in major fiber types.

Muscle Hypertrophy

An increase in muscle size, *e.g.*, muscle hypertrophy, is a common adaptation to overload. There is a positive relationship between a muscle's size and its force potential; thus, a larger muscle is a stronger muscle. Muscle hypertrophy can result from an increase in *protein synthesis*, a decrease in protein breakdown, or a combination of both. Although skeletal muscle constantly undergoes remodeling, which involves protein catabolism (*i.e.*, > 280 g·d^{-1} in the average 70 kg man), a net gain in proteins synthesized over time can result in an increased number of sarcomeres in parallel and in series leading to greater muscle size. Exercise is catabolic (*i.e.*, protein synthesis is inhibited and breakdown is augmented during exercise) especially when nutrient consumption is minimal. The major catabolic pathways in skeletal muscle include the *ubiquitin-proteasomal* pathway (with associated E3 ligases such as *atrogin I* and *muscle specific ring finger 1* [MURF-1], *calpain-calcium* dependent (*i.e.*, calpains-1, -2, and -3) pathway, *lysosomal autophagy,* and *caspsases* (88). These pathways act in an integrated manner to degrade proteins and other cellular components for normal remodeling or at accelerated rates during and following exercise (88). Protein breakdown increases following RE especially in untrained subjects or during unaccustomed exercise but becomes less pronounced in trained individuals (88). Several catabolic molecules (*i.e.*, calpain-1, calpain-2, Murf-1, atrogin-1) and cell apoptosis genes/proteins (*caspase-3, Bax/ Bcl-2*) are elevated (in a fiber-type specific manner) within 4 hours (and some extending to 24 hours) following a RE workout (89). Although catabolic gene expression does not necessarily equate to increased protein breakdown in all cases, it is clear the initial phase of exercise recovery involves catabolism via activity of these pathways. However, rates of protein synthesis exceed breakdown provided adequate feeding or protein intake takes place to where net protein balance favors anabolism for 24–48 hours following a workout (88). See Myths and Misconceptions: Muscles Grow While the individual Is in the Gym Lifting Weights.

One thing that is quite clear is that muscle hypertrophy is a complex process involving a multitude of factors. Several intercommunicating pathways converge to modulate the amount of protein synthesized relative to the protein degraded based on the training stimulus and other known factors discussed in this chapter. Exercise increases gene expression, mRNA expression, translational efficiency (*i.e.*, amount of protein synthesized per unit of RNA) and capacity (*i.e.*, total number of ribosomes), and synthesis of skeletal muscle proteins through multiple pathways and ribosome biogenesis. It has been suggested that translational factors may be more critical in postexercise protein synthesis increases than transcriptional factors (90). RE stimulates gene expression leading to greater myofibrillar protein synthesis, whereas endurance exercise increases gene expression of mitochondrial proteins (91). Endurance exercise increases postexercise protein synthesis (by 22%–84%) but to a lesser extent than RE (92). Protein (mixed, myofibrillar, and sarcoplasmic) synthesis increases by 30%–350% following a RE workout (within 1 hour) and may be elevated up to 48 hours after an acute bout of RE (92,93) provided protein is consumed. The post-RE elevated protein synthesis time window appears shorter in trained individuals than untrained. Mixed and myofibrillar protein synthesis rates may increase within 4 hours post-RE with the response dependent upon intensity and volume load where sets are terminated at failure (94). In previously untrained individuals, elevated rates of protein synthesis following RE are thought to be indicative of greater remodeling and recovery from excessive muscle dam-

age (91). The protein synthesis post-RE increases become lessened over time with accommodation to the same RT program (91,95). Damas et al. (96) found that the protein synthesis increase seen at 24–48 hours after RE was significantly higher after the 1st week than the 3rd or 10th weeks of RT. When the protein synthesis values were expressed relative to muscle fiber damage (*i.e.*, Z-line streaming), no differences were seen between the responses indicating that much of the early higher protein synthesis was needed to repair damaged muscle tissue. The protein synthesis increases seen at weeks 3 and 10 (but not week 1) strongly correlated with muscle fiber hypertrophy. The authors concluded that initial protein synthesis augmentation during RE may be directed toward tissue remodeling, whereas increases seen weeks later are more directed toward muscle hypertrophy (96). Enhanced postworkout protein synthesis depends on several factors including protein intake and amino acid availability from nutrient intake, the timing of nutrient intake (before, during, or immediately after a workout), the intensity and volume of the workout (mechanical and metabolic stress), and hormonal and growth factor responses (97). Although measures of acute protein synthesis provide some indication of muscle anabolic status, correlations to hypertrophy have not always been shown, thereby showing the response is generated for other purposes beyond that of just muscle growth.

Muscle growth results in a proportional greater size and number of actin/myosin filaments and the addition of sarcomeres, which is highly important for strength and power development. Although neural adaptations predominate early, hypertrophy becomes increasingly important as RT continues. Changes in muscle proteins take place within a couple of workouts (76). However, a longer period of time is needed to demonstrate significant muscle growth and this is only provided the workout stimulus surpasses one's own threshold of conditioning. Some studies have shown increased muscle hypertrophy within 2 weeks of RT (32,33). However, it is thought that hypertrophy this early may be due to cell swelling–induced increased size via muscle damage (91). It has been suggested that 8–12 workouts may elicit modest hypertrophy of 3%–4%, whereas more than 18 workouts (over 6–10 weeks) may lead to higher levels of hypertrophy (~7%–10%) (95). Men and women experience increases in muscle size during training. Relative increases may be similar (50). However, men experience more absolute hypertrophy (68,98) predominantly due to higher concentrations of the hormone *testosterone*. Increases in protein synthesis may be similar between men and women 2 hours following a workout, and sex may not influence baseline protein synthesis or protein breakdown either (90). It has been suggested that acute protein synthesis data obtained early in training are independent of sex and do not play a role in the sexual dimorphism seen in muscle hypertrophy (90). Thus, there is a need for long-term studies examining a more distinct time line of protein metabolism especially in trained subjects who routinely vary their programs. The novelty of changing the RE stimulus could have

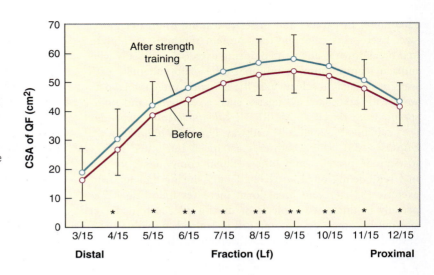

FIGURE 5.13 Muscle growth in the quadriceps muscles following resistance training. This figure shows greater muscle hypertrophy toward the middle of muscle (the belly) and is less approaching the tendon areas. Muscle fiber area measurements are based on MRI data where the proximal and distal ends approach the polar ends of the muscle and the fractions illustrate the slice area of the measurement. The *asterisks* indicate the fractions of the muscle where significant increases took place. (Adapted from Häkkinen K, Pakarinen A, Kraemer WJ, Häkkinen A, Valkeinen H, Alen M. Selective muscle hypertrophy, changes in EMG and force, and serum hormones during strength training in older women. *J Appl Physiol.* 2001;91:569–80.)

impact on long-term training adaptations in men and women but has not been adequately addressed. Lastly, muscle growth typically occurs in higher magnitude along the muscle belly in a nonuniform manner with the most significant increase seen centrally toward the area of largest circumference (Fig. 5.13) (99). Research indicates that segments of the muscle mostly highly activated during a resistance exercise may experience higher levels of muscle hypertrophy when that exercise is chronically performed (100).

Ribosome Biogenesis

Ribosomes bind mRNA and tRNA to synthesize peptides, polypeptides, and proteins. Ribosome biogenesis is the process of forming ribosomes in the nucleolus and consists of ribosomal DNA transcription, processing, maturation, and assembly of rRNAs and ribosomal proteins (101). Ribosomes (80S) consist of a large (60S) and small subunit (40S) with a few ribosomal RNAs and several ribosomal proteins linked (102). There are approximately few thousand ranging up to 14,000 ribosomes per µm^3 making up close to 20% of cell volume (101). Measurement of ribosome biogenesis involve assessment of muscle total RNA (a proxy measure of ribosome content since ~85% of RNA in muscle fibers is ribosomal) or specific expression of ribosomal subunits (101,102). An increase in ribosome number or total RNA content per unit of tissue (*e.g.*, *translational capacity*) occurs and may be an important factor in mediating muscle hypertrophy (101). Total RNA and preribosomal RNA increase during hypertrophy (possibly through enhanced mTOR and MAPK pathway signaling) (101,102). Stec et al. (103) reported acute increases in some ribosomal markers 24 hours post-RE mostly in young (compared to older) individuals; however, they also reported significant increases in total RNA in older moderate and extreme responders following 4 weeks of RT (104). Similar results were seen in young men after 12 weeks of RT where no changes in total RNA were found in low responders but increases were shown in moderate and high responders (105). Another study showed that 3 months of RT increased total RNA (and a few other ribosomal subunits) in the vastus lateralis muscle, which positively correlated to increased muscle thickness and leg volume (106). The acute response of selected ribosomal biogenic markers increases early in RT but become lessened over time (107). Thus, cumulated bouts of RE may lead to increased ribosomal biogenesis, which appears to play a role in mediating increased protein synthesis and muscle hypertrophy.

Myths and Misconceptions
Muscles Grow While Lifting Weights in the Gym

Some have postulated that muscles grow mostly while the athlete is working out. Although the stimulus for muscle growth is the workout, muscles actually grow during the recovery period. Part of the misconception is due to the fact the muscle blood flow increases during RE leading to a "muscle pump." The pump temporarily increases the size of the muscles. Rather, protein breakdown is high during and immediately following the workout but muscle protein synthesis is elevated for up to 24–48 hours following the workout. Consistent training over time where there is a pattern of breakdown and synthesis leads to greater net protein deposition. Greater protein accretion leads to muscle hypertrophy and an increase in muscle cross-sectional area (CSA). Thus, muscles grow during recovery and not during the act of lifting weights.

Muscle Hypertrophy and Signaling Pathways

Skeletal muscle hypertrophy may be signaled through multiple pathways. Some pathways and intermediates have been discussed already in this chapter (*e.g.*, myogenesis and satellite cells, myostatin, integrins, and FAK), and hormonal control will be discussed in Chapter 7. In addition to mediating muscle contraction and fiber-type plasticity, calcium-calmodulin binding is thought to dephosphorylate NFAT, causing it to translocate to the nucleus increasing gene transcription (108). Calcium may play a role in muscle growth via interactions with myogenic factors, mTOR, and MAPK proteins (108). Here, signaling via the Wnt/β-catenin, mTOR, and MAPK pathways as well as growth factor influences is discussed.

Canonical *wingless-type MMTV integration site family* (Wnt) binding to Frizzled receptors leads to a cascade of events that increases the transcription factor β-catenin. β-Catenin translocates to the nucleus, binds to DNA response elements (T-cell factor/lymphoid enhancer factor 1, TCF/LEF), increases transcription, and activation of muscle satellite cells, thereby establishing a role for mediating muscle growth. Wnt/β-catenin pathway gene expression and protein content increase following 8 weeks of RT and power training, with power training producing more potent changes (109).

One of the most widely recognized anabolic pathways in skeletal muscle is the *mammalian target of rapamycin (mTOR)* pathway. mTOR is a serine/threonine kinase that integrates input in a synergistic manner from upstream regulators such as insulin, insulin-like growth factor-1 (IGF-1), androgens, growth factors, integrins/FAK, and amino acids and amino acid derivatives such as leucine and β-HMB. The phospholipid phosphatidic acid (PA) plays a role in partially mediating protein synthesis via activation of the mTOR pathway (Fig. 5.14). mTOR pathway is sensitive to oxidative stress, mechanical stimuli, and energy levels (110). Although part of a complex signaling process, the mTORC1 pathway appears more relevant for anabolic signaling compared to mTORC2 (110). mTORC1 consists of mTOR and several other coregulatory proteins. mTORC1 is regulated upstream by the *tumor suppressor tuberous sclerosis complex (TSC1/TSC2)*, which inhibits Rheb (GTPase activating protein) and subsequently mTORC1. TSC1/2 is inhibited by the upstream regulators MAPK ERK1/2 and Akt. Growth factor receptor binding activates *class 1 phosphoinositide-3 kinase (PI3K)* and *protein kinase B (Akt)*, which inhibits TSC1/2, glycogen synthase kinase 3β (GSK3β), and the catabolic protein FOX01 and activates mTORC1 (111). Myostatin signaling reduces Akt and decrease mTOR signaling (110). mTORC1 controls protein synthesis via increasing ribosomal binding to mRNA and

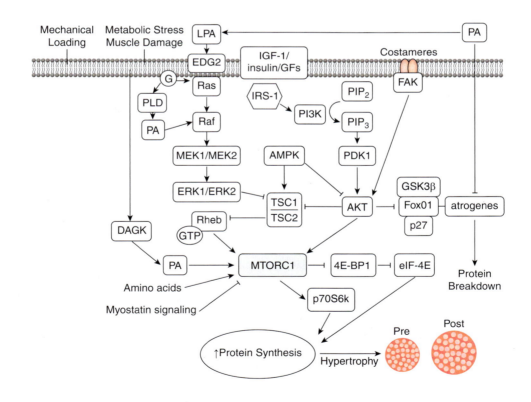

FIGURE 5.14 mTOR pathway signaling. Muscle mechanotransduction increases synthesis of PA via diacylglycerol kinase (DAGK). PA may bind to Raf or mTORC1 and activates mTORC1, which stimulates downstream phosphorylation of p70S6K increasing protein synthesis. Activated mTORC1 phosphorylates 4EBP1, releasing it from eIF4E increasing protein synthesis. PA in blood may enter muscle and inhibit atrogenes. PA may be hydrolyzed to lysophosphatidic acid (LPA), activate endothelial differentiation gene (EDG2) receptor, and mitogen-activated protein kinase (MEK) and extracellular regulated kinase (ERK) pathways. ERK1/2 inhibits TSC1/2 putting the Rheb in its GTP-bound state where it activates mTORC1. IGF-1/insulin receptor binding increases AKT.

up-regulation (translation efficiency) by activating *p70 ribosomal S6 kinase 1 (p70^{S6K})* and inhibiting *4E-binding protein 1 (4EBP1)*, which releases the translating initiating factor eIF-4E. Lastly, mTOR signaling is inhibited by *5' AMP-activated protein kinase (AMPK)* via multiple mechanisms. AMPK is an intracellular sensor of ATP (via AMP accumulation) consumption, key regulator of skeletal muscle metabolism, largely involved in glucose and fat oxidation, protein degradation, and autophagy, *i.e.*, the process of degrading and recycling defective cellular constituents such as organelles (112). Endurance, sprint, high-intensity interval, and concurrent RE and endurance exercise increase isoforms of AMPK (*e.g.*, AMPKα1, AMPKα2) in a volume- and intensity-dependent manner (63,112,113) with subsequent increase in PGC-1α mRNA (113). AMPK-mediated responses to endurance exercise are thought to have some negative impact on muscle hypertrophy via increased catabolic atrogene stimulation and reduced mTOR signaling (112). RE has no effect or acutely increases phosphorylation of AMPK (63,114).

Since 1999, several studies have examined mTOR signaling during RT and its relationship to muscle hypertrophy (115). RE increases phosphorylation of p70S6K 30 minutes to 5 hours postexercise (31,114,116–118) as well as phosphorylated mTOR and S6 (31,94,114), PI3K, Akt (31,94), and 4E-BP1 (31,94,118) with a timeline corresponding to increased protein synthesis. The response to RE appears higher than the response to combined RE and plyometric exercise in Olympic weightlifters (31). Some studies have shown that p706SK phosphorylation may be sensitive to RE volume in untrained subjects (94,114), whereas similar responses have been shown between high-intensity low volume and moderate-intensity, high volume RE protocols in trained subjects (119). The response appears greater following a 5 × 10 protocol than a 15 × 1 protocol (116), see Interpreting Research: Molecular Signaling and Resistance Exercise. However, the acute response may be lessened with chronic RT and attenuated in older subjects (107). Phosphorylation of p70S6K correlates to increased muscle hypertrophy (115,117). Concurrent RE and aerobic exercise appears to induce similar mTOR pathway signaling compared to RE alone (63).

Mitogen-activated protein kinase (MAPK) molecules are key divergent signaling proteins involved in muscle hypertrophy and endurance adaptations (Fig. 5.15). They are stimulated by mechanical forces, oxidative stress, growth factors, and cytokines and may interact with mTOR pathway intermediates. *Mitogen-activated protein kinase 1* (MEK1) activates *extracellular signal-regulated kinase 1 and 2* (ERK1/2), which activates other downstream nuclear transcription factors including *mitogen- and stress-activated protein kinase 1* (MSK1) and *signal transducer and activator of transcription* 1 (STAT1). MAPK proteins also include the stress-activated protein kinases *c-JunN-terminal kinase* (JNK) and *p38 MAPK* (with four isoforms), which activate downstream factors such as *transcription factor 2* (ATF2), *p53*, and c-Jun. Up-regulation of MAPK proteins is thought to increase gene expression and muscle hypertrophy during RT and increase fatty acid uptake and oxidation, increase glucose uptake and oxidation,

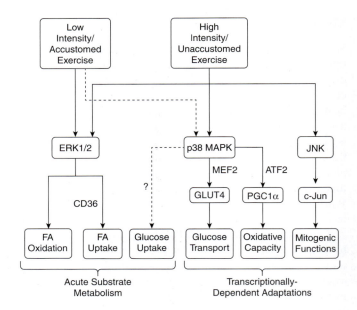

FIGURE 5.15 MAPK pathway signaling.

and increase oxidation capacity during endurance exercise (120). The most studied MAPK proteins are MEK1, ERK1/2, JNK, and p38 MAPK. Endurance and sprint exercise acutely increase phosphorylation of p38 MAPK and ERK1/2 in an intensity-dependent manner (120). Various MAPK protein phosphorylations are increased during RT or within 30 minutes to 1 hour following acute RE (94,114,116,121). One study showed that MAPK phosphorylation increased 2–3-fold during performance of 15 sets of 3 reps (with 85% of 1 RM) of clean pulls in Olympic weightlifters (122). Some studies have shown greater increases in MAPK proteins following high- versus low-intensity RT although a few studies have shown no differences (121). RE volume load may augment the response (116), but not all studies have reported a volume effect. A study by Gonzalez et al. (121) showed similar MAPK protein response in the vastus lateralis 1 hour postexercise (for just a few proteins including STAT1 and JNK) between training with 70% of 1 RM for 4–6 sets of 10–12 reps versus 90% of 1 RM for 4–6 sets of 3–5 reps. Phosphorylation of MAPK proteins may increase following RT overreaching; however, the opposite may occur during overtraining (123). Lastly, resting ERK 1/2 may be lower at rest in well-trained weightlifters and powerlifters (124).

Myokines are *cytokines* (*e.g.*, a broad category of small proteins that are critical to cell signaling) that are produced and released by muscle fibers. Cytokines were initially thought to modulate communication between neuroendocrine and the immune systems. Since, they have been shown to have autocrine, paracrine, and endocrine (systemic) functions actively involved in muscle fiber regeneration, cell signaling, hypertrophy, and a whole slew of functions across a number of tissues. Skeletal muscle has been considered as a secretory organ capable of affecting other tissues by releasing myokines into circulation. Exercise increases the secretion

> ## Interpreting Research
> ### Molecular Signaling and Resistance Exercise
>
> Hulmi JJ, Walker S, Ahtiainen JP, Nyman K, Kraemer WJ, Häkkinen K. Molecular signaling in muscle is affected by the specificity of resistance exercise protocol. *Scand J Med Sci Sports*. 2012;22:240–48.
>
> Hulmi et al. (116) compared a maximal strength protocol (leg press; 15 sets of 1 RM loading with 3-minutes rest intervals) to a traditional hypertrophic protocol (leg press; 5 sets of 10 RM loading [80% of 1 RM] with 2-min rest intervals) in a fed state. Muscle biopsies were obtained from the vastus lateralis muscle 0.5 hours before and following each protocol. Maximum isometric force decreased significantly more following the 5 × 10 protocol (~45%) compared to the 15 × 1 protocol (~21%), and blood lactate values were higher following the 5 × 10 protocol. They reported that p70[S6K] phos-
>
> phorylation (at Ser[424]/Thr[421]) ribosomal protein S6 and p38 MAPK (β and γ) were increased following both protocols but significantly higher following the 5 × 10 protocol (p38 MAPK γ only). They also reported that phosphorylation of ERK1/2 increased only after the 5 × 10 protocol. mTOR phosphorylation remained unchanged 30 minutes following both protocols. These results showed that a traditional "hypertrophic" protocol resulted in greater blood lactates and fatigue but augmented MAPK and mTOR signaling 30 minutes following a workout. These results suggest that the interaction of volume and intensity (as opposed to intensity alone) may be critical to postexercise anabolic and endurance muscular signaling.

of myokines including the interleukins IL-6, IL-8, IL-10, and IL-15, IL-1 receptor antagonist (IL-1ra), leukemia inhibitory factor (LIF), hepato growth factor (HGF), fibroblast growth factor (FGF), decorin, and vascular endothelial growth factor (VEGF) (125,126). Studies have shown increased concentrations of pro-inflammatory cytokines (*i.e.*, IL-6) in blood following intense exercise, followed by an elevation in anti-inflammatory cytokines (*i.e.*, IL-10, IL-1ra). Skeletal muscle is the main source of circulating IL-6 following exercise and the response is higher when muscle glycogen content is reduced (127). These responses are important for mediating the immune responses to promote muscle regeneration. RE and intense exercise potentially leading to muscle damage increases the myokines response (125). Myokines that remain local may bind to receptors and facilitate satellite cell proliferation and differentiation (*i.e.*, IL-6, LIF, TGF-β, decorin) and induce muscle fiber hypertrophy (*i.e.*, IL-6, IL-15, TGF-β, decorin, VEGF) (125,126,128). VEGF is essential for angiogenesis in support of muscle hypertrophy (128). Interestingly, although IL-6 is pro-inflammatory, responds to hypertrophic overload, and mediates satellite cell activity, potential catabolic roles in muscle atrophy have also been discussed demonstrating the pleiotropic nature of this cytokine (129).

Muscle Hypertrophy and Fiber Types

Muscle growth occurs in both ST and FT muscle fibers (30,34,130), and higher relative RT intensities are associated with muscle hypertrophy (68). However, absolute growth potential is higher in FT fibers (7,34,106,130,131). Fry (68) reported that relative training intensity accounts for ~18% of the variation seen in type I fiber hypertrophy, whereas it accounts for ~35% of variance seen in type II fiber hypertrophy. As FT fibers are known for their strength and power, it is not

surprising that they increase in size to a greater extent and are more reliant upon high training intensity for maximal hypertrophy. Tesch et al. (132) showed that the size of vastus lateralis FT fibers in athletes was 118%–144% larger than untrained individuals, whereas ST fiber size was only 55%–78% greater. A recent study showed significant muscle hypertrophy of type II fibers within 2 weeks of RT; however, type I fiber increases did not occur until week 12 of a 12-week RT program (32). A review of the literature shows that the growth potential of FT fibers is much larger than that of ST fibers at all RT intensities but especially when the RT intensity is ≥60% of 1 RM (133). Interestingly, type IIA and IIAX fiber areas are significantly larger than type IIX fibers in bodybuilders (134). This indicates that these fibers may be more specifically targeted with bodybuilding training as some were transitioned originally from IIX. However, ST fiber hypertrophy appears similar to FT hypertrophy with RT intensities of <50% of 1 RM indicating that low-load RT to muscular failure may be a more specific stimulus to ST fiber development (133). ST fibers increase in size to a certain extent (133) but, because of their vital role in muscular endurance, too much hypertrophy may be counterproductive.

Other Factors Influencing Muscle Hypertrophy

Several factors influence the magnitude of muscle growth. Training to maximize muscle hypertrophy involves targeting mechanical and metabolic stress factors associated with muscle growth. *Mechanical factors* focus on the tension/force produced by muscle fibers and the subsequent mechanotransduction (discussed previously in this chapter) to increased protein synthesis. These include the type of muscle actions trained, the intensity and volume of training, and muscle damage to some extent. *Metabolic stress factors* focus on hypoxia, restricted blood flow (and subsequent reactive hyperemia), and muscle metabolism during training. Both mechanical and metabolic stress factors elicited by a training session done for hypertrophy may influence muscle gene expression, protein synthesis, growth factor expression, and anabolic/catabolic hormonal responses. Lastly, *nutritional factors* play a significant role in supporting these factors. This includes diet, supplement use, and perhaps anabolic drug use. Important factors influencing muscle growth include

- *Muscle Action*: Muscle hypertrophy results from CON, ECC, and ISOM training (135). Greater gains in muscle size are seen when ECC muscle actions are used or emphasized in training (136). A study by Vikne et al. (137) compared 12 weeks of CON-only training to ECC-only training in resistance-trained men and showed that types I and II fiber area changed by −2% and 5%, respectively, following CON-only training but increased by 25% and 40%, respectively, following ECC-only training. Similar findings were obtained from Hortobagyi et al. (131) who trained subjects for 12 weeks and found ECC-only trained increased type II fiber area 10 times more than CON-only training. The importance of ECC muscle actions, or muscle lengthening, has been noted for several years especially in animal studies where muscles exposed to chronic stretch hypertrophied or maintained mass during immobilization. Mechanical stretch on muscle fibers increases protein synthesis and the number of sarcomeres in series, and with the added tension (and potential for muscle damage) from loaded ECC actions, presents a potent stimulus for muscle growth.
- *Training Program*: The training program is a composite of acute program variables that can be varied to alter the stimulus. Long-term increases in muscle hypertrophy are best accomplished by systematic training variation that targets the mechanical and metabolic stress factors leading to hypertrophy. Muscle hypertrophy training comprises numerous intensity/volume schemes seen across the entire muscle strength-endurance spectrum. The interaction of the exercise selection and sequence, intensity, volume and volume load, contraction duration, rest intervals, velocity, set termination point, and frequency form the stimulus that, when is beyond one's current threshold point of adaptation, can induce muscle growth over time. A number of systematic reviews and meta-analyses have been published recently examining the effects of different program variables on muscle hypertrophy. The interaction of intensity and volume is critical to the stimulus. Although low-intensity RT (*i.e.*, ~16% of 1 RM) may produce muscle hypertrophy, it has been shown to be inferior compared to heavier (70% of 1 RM) loading (78). Analysis of the literature revealed that intensities ≥60% of 1 RM produces greater rates of hypertrophy for the quadriceps and elbow flexor muscle groups (135). Fry (68) reported that intensity accounted for 18%–35% of the variance in RT-induced fiber hypertrophy and suggested that 80%–95% of 1 RM may be an ideal range for long-term muscle hypertrophy (mostly in type II fibers) especially in competitive lifters. This was shown by Mangine et al. (138) who compared a traditional hypertrophy program (4 sets of 10–12 reps with 70% of 1 RM, 1-min rest intervals) to a strength program (4 sets of 3–5 reps with 90% of 1 RM, 3-min rest intervals) in resistance-trained men and reported both groups increased muscle hypertrophy but the strength training group experienced larger gains in a few measures. In contrast, Schoenfeld et al. (139) reported similar muscle hypertrophy of the arms but superior hypertrophy in the thigh favoring the hypertrophy program (compared to strength training) in resistance-trained men. Schoenfeld et al. (140) reported similar hypertrophy between volume-equated hypertrophy versus strength training programs in trained men. All of these studies showed the high-intensity programs increased maximal strength to a greater extent. Thus, a range of intensities elicit significant muscle growth provided repetitions are performed to failure or near failure. Volume and volume load affect the magnitude of muscle hypertrophy. Some studies have shown greater muscle hypertrophy with higher volumes of RT (33,98), especially when single-set programs are compared to multiple-set RT (141,142). Volume is not an independent variable but must be viewed in context with other variables. Although increasing RT volume may be productive, at some point volume may be too great, which is why the periodization of both volume and intensity appears to be the key training strategy. A wide range of rest intervals can be used for hypertrophy training. Short rest intervals target metabolic stress hypertrophic factors and long rest intervals (with heavier loading and augmented repetition performance) target mechanical factors with some carryover between. Although some data indicate longer rest intervals produce more hypertrophy (143), a range of rest intervals can be effectively used based on the goals of each set (144). Research shows that training each muscle group 2–3 times per week may produce more hypertrophy than 1 day (135,145).
- *Metabolic Stress*: Metabolic stress during exercise results in metabolite accumulation (*i.e.*, lactate, inorganic phosphate, H^+) resulting from high-energy usage and tissue hypoxia. Exercise programs that target glycolysis, *e.g.*, large muscle mass, low to moderate to high intensity, high volume, short rest intervals, and blood flow restriction, result in high levels of metabolic stress. See Sidebar: Blood Flow Restriction Training. Metabolic stress is thought to increase muscle hypertrophy via increased muscle fiber recruitment, anabolic hormone activity, cell swelling and muscle hydration, increased myokines production, and increased ROS (146,147). ROS include oxygen radicals and nonradical oxidizing agents generated during exercise via oxygen metabolism. Although ROS concentrations increase during exercise leading to oxidative stress, they can increase intracellular signaling of hypertrophic pathways such as MAPK and by mediating the transcription of heat shock proteins (147). The fluid content of skeletal muscle plays a role in

muscle hypertrophy. Studies show that increased cellular hydration decreases protein breakdown and increases protein synthesis (148). The increased fluid pressure against the fiber cytoskeleton and sarcolemma is thought to activate integrin-associated osmosensors to increase protein synthesis (146,147). Cell swelling may be seen with osmotic changes due to muscle damage, metabolite accumulation, increased glycogen and phosphagen stores, and with supplemental *creatine*. Creatine supplementation increases cellular hydration, leads to initial weight gain, and increases muscle growth during training.

- *Nutritional Factors*: Carbohydrate and protein intake affect protein synthesis. Carbohydrates increase the synthesis and secretion of the potent anabolic hormone insulin. Insulin plays a role in regulating muscle mass in addition to its metabolic roles. It has been recommended that an athlete consume ~55%–65% of calories from carbohydrates at levels approaching 6 g CHO·kg^{-1} body mass per day (149). Protein is a macronutrient made up of amino acids. Out of the 20 identified amino acids, 9 are essential and 11 are nonessential. Nonessential amino acids are produced within the body,

whereas essential amino acids must be obtained through the diet. Muscle growth and recovery necessitate the amount of protein synthesized be greater than the amount broken down. Protein intake (amino acid availability) should be high when training to increase muscle size. Studies have shown that athletes require higher protein intake (in a range of 1.7–2.2 g·kg^{-1} of body mass of protein per day) depending on the intensity, volume, and frequency of training (149,150). Protein supplementation is recommended if the athlete does not consume an adequate amount from the diet (149,150). Protein supplements contain various amounts of protein (from various sources) per serving. Protein and/or amino acid intake before, during, or immediately after a workout very important for increasing protein synthesis and enhancing recovery prior to the next workout. Lastly, a few supplements and anabolic drugs increase muscle growth. Anabolic drugs (*e.g.*, anabolic steroids, testosterone esters, hGH, testosterone enhancers) have potent muscle-building effects and are very effective for increasing muscle hypertrophy (149,151). However, these are banned for use for health and athletic purposes.

Sidebar   Blood Flow Restriction Training

Blood flow restriction training (BFRT) has increased in popularity in the past decade. It involves continuously restricting blood flow to the limbs distally via wraps, tourniquets, or inflatable cuffs during aerobic exercise or low-load (10%–50% of 1 RM) RT. The resultant acute effect is reduced reps per level of light loading compared to resistance exercise with no occlusion (152). Factors such as the cuff width and tension affect the level of vascular occlusion, and these are related to the size of the targeted muscle groups. Often, a tolerable occlusion pressure is used initially and increased as the training program progresses. Scott et al. (153) have recommended occlusion pressures ranging from 120 to 210 mm Hg based on thigh circumference, *e.g.*, increased pressure with larger circumferences. The rationale is to increase metabolic stress during exercise via hypoxia, thereby creating an augmented hypertrophic response compared to similar exercise or loading paradigms without blood flow restriction. Increased accumulation of metabolites, ROS, cellular swelling, fiber recruitment, hormonal, intramuscular anabolic (*i.e.*, mTOR) and myogenic signaling, and protein synthesis are thought to mediate augmented muscle hypertrophy (153–155). Studies have shown that BFRT with light loads produces comparable muscle hypertrophy (but less strength gains) compared to high-load RT (156–160). One meta-analysis showed that BFRT 2–3 days per week produced greater effect sizes for strength and hypertrophy increases compared to low-intensity RT with no occlusion (161). Another meta-analysis showed that BFRT increased muscle strength by a range of 6%–40%

(mean = 14.4%) and muscle hypertrophy by a range of 1%–17% (mean = 7.2%) and was not affected by cuff width or pressure (162). Another meta-analysis showed that strength improvements were greater when 20%–30% of 1 RM were used compared to <20% of 1 RM (163). Limb muscle hypertrophy is most evident while trunk muscle augmentation is minimal during BFRT. Yasuda et al. (164) compared 6 weeks of bench press training (3 × 10 reps, 75% of 1 RM) to BFRT (100 to 160 mm Hg) with 30% of 1 RM (30 reps for the 1st set and 15 reps for last 3 sets) and showed bench press 1 RM increased more (by 19.9%) in the high-intensity group versus 8.7% in BFRT. Triceps brachii and pectoralis major muscle CSA increased 8%–17% in the high-intensity group and 4.9%–8.3% in BFRT showing heavy bench press training increased muscle size in both muscles but BFRT mostly increased triceps brachii CSA. In a follow-up study, Yasuda et al. (165) examined a combined high-intensity and BFRT group and showed that adding one session of heavier training to BFRT produced similar strength increases to high-intensity–only training. Muscle CSA increased the most following heavy training, although increases were shown in the other training groups. Given the number of studies in the area, it has been recommended that loads of 20%–40% of 1 RM be used for 50–80 reps per exercise for single- and multiple-joint exercises with 30–45 seconds rest intervals in between sets 2–4 days per week (153). The highest number of reps may be performed during the 1st set and fatigue may result in fewer reps during subsequent sets.

Case Study 5.1

Michael is a college track and field athlete who has just completed his first full year of serious and consistent RT. Over the course of the year, Michael's bodyweight increased from 165 to 178 lb. In addition, his body fat decreased from 12.1% to 11.2%. Based on these assessments, Michael's coach calculates that he gained 13.1 lb of lean tissue mass. Much of this gain in lean tissue mass was attributed to muscular hypertrophy.

Questions for Consideration: Based on our previous discussions of skeletal muscle, what mechanisms may have contributed to Michael's muscle growth? What types of fiber composition changes may have been expected?

Muscle Hypertrophy and Other Training Modalities

Sprint and power training increases muscle size to a lesser extent than RT (166). Linossier et al. (167) found type II fiber hypertrophy after 9 weeks of high-intensity cycle ergometry training. Häkkinen et al. (168) found greater muscle fiber area after 24 weeks of plyometric training compared to before training. Sprint, agility, and plyometric training require high levels of force and power; thus, FT muscle fiber recruitment is high. Fiber transitions and muscle growth occur. Bodyweight training may induce muscle hypertrophy in previously untrained subjects as Kikuchi and Nakazato (169) reported 9.5%–18.3% increases in triceps brachii and pectoralis major muscle thickness following 8 weeks of push-up training. When combined with weight training, gains in muscle size are more substantial from sprint, agility, and plyometric training (170). Aerobic training results in no change (82), reduced (75,171), or small increases in muscle size (172). Reductions in muscle size occur mostly in type I and IIC fiber populations (75). The few studies that have shown some hypertrophy during aerobic training reported small increases in type I and II fibers as well as the whole muscle level (172). The response is likely related to the initial training status of the individual and the intensity of aerobic training as sedentary or deconditioned muscle may be more responsive. High-intensity interval exercise may provide greater overload to muscle, thereby eliciting a hypertrophic effect (173). Simultaneous RT and aerobic training results in substantial increases in muscle CSA (75,82). In comparison to RT alone, concurrent training attenuates, augments, or produces similar increases in lower-body muscle hypertrophy (174). A meta-analysis showed smaller (but insignificant) hypertrophic effect sizes for concurrent training compared to RT alone and significant negative correlations were found between effect sizes for muscle hypertrophy and the frequency of aerobic training ($r = -0.26$) and the average duration of each aerobic workout ($r = -0.75$) (174). Regarding the sequence, a meta-analysis showed the sequence (aerobic or RE first) may not compromise increases in lower body hypertrophy (175). Thus, muscle hypertrophy occurs during concurrent training but caution may be needed if the aerobic training is high in volume and frequency.

Hyperplasia

Hyperplasia is thought to involve longitudinal splitting of existing muscle fibers (new fiber development), subsequently resulting in an increased number of muscle cells. Hyperplasia has been suggested to occur via increased satellite cell proliferation following muscle damage (70). Hyperplasia was first shown in animals (176). A meta-analysis of studies in animals showed increases (mean of 15% across all studies) in muscle fiber number accompanying greater muscle size with the technique used for fiber counting, type of animal, and type of overload used affecting fiber number (177). Increases in fiber size (~31%) were double that of increased fiber number (177). However, it has been controversial in humans. Bodybuilders and powerlifters have shown greater number of muscle fibers than untrained individuals (178,179). However, it was not known if this was a result of training or genetics as other research has shown similar muscle fiber number between strength athletes and untrained controls (180). Split muscle fibers have been shown in power lifters, but these have been attributed to branching resulting from defect regeneration (181). Although some data indicate the potential for hyperplasia in humans (182), it is still not known conclusively if it is a viable mechanism leading to muscle fiber growth. If hyperplasia does occur, it may represent an adaptation to RT when certain muscle fibers reach a theoretical upper limit in cell size. Large increases in muscle size over years of training or use of anabolic drugs where one's level of muscle mass may surpass the drug-free potential pose interesting scenarios testing the viability of hyperplasia as a mechanism of adaptation. In these cases, hyperplasia may seem possible due to large increases in muscle size where the human body may be viewed as possessing secondary mechanisms to take muscle growth to higher levels. However, if hyperplasia does occur, it is thought to be secondary with hypertrophy accounting for the greater increase in muscle size.

Structural Changes to Muscle

Structural changes to skeletal muscle enhance performance. We have previously discussed several components of skeletal muscle with regard to muscle contraction. The structures discussed, proteins, and enzymes all have the ability to adapt to training enabling muscle to increase its strength, power, size, and endurance. RT increases the number of myofibrils, the density of the sarcoplasm, sarcoplasm reticulum, and T tubules, and *sodium-potassium ATPase pump activity* (130,178,183–185) with the increase in Na^+-K^+-ATPase pump activity correlated to increased muscle endurance (185). As protein synthesis increases, proteins are synthesized relative to their distribution within muscle fibers to maintain optimal proportions. Actin-to-myosin ratio remains constant, structural proteins increase in proportion, and sarcomere length remains constant although sarcomere number increases. Endurance training decreases calcium kinetics and increases Na^+-K^+-ATPase pump activity (184,186,187). Exercise results in a rise in plasma potassium, in part, due to fatigue-related reductions in Na^+-K^+-ATPase pump activity. Endurance training increases resting Na^+-K^+-ATPase pump activity more so than RT, and endurance-trained individuals display a smaller rise in plasma potassium concentrations during exercise indicative of fatigue resistance (188). Other studies have shown specific isoforms of Na^+-K^+-ATPase pumps increase as a result of endurance and interval training in a fiber-type specific manner (189–191), thereby reflecting a training-induced adaptation capable of increasing muscle endurance. Endurance training decreases *SERCA1a proteins* (*i.e.*, key proteins involved in calcium reuptake into the SR in skeletal muscle) and calcium uptake by 13%–40% (192). However, sprint training and speed endurance training improves calcium kinetics (*i.e.*, SERCA1), which may assist in speed development and endurance (189,193).

Other Changes to Skeletal Muscle

Other changes may take place within skeletal muscle that improves performance. These changes are discussed in other chapters (because different physiological systems interact within skeletal muscle) but need to be mentioned here. Sprint and RT increase anaerobic substrate content, alter enzyme activity, and increase a muscle's buffer capacity. Aerobic training increases the activity of aerobic enzymes. RT up-regulates anabolic hormone receptors. Aerobic training increases mitochondrial and capillary density; however, RT decreases these variables. Connective tissue within skeletal muscle increases in capacity, which helps support strength development and hypertrophy. Lastly, the length of fascicles and muscle fiber orientation may change in response to sprint and RT, which favor force production and power.

SUMMARY POINTS

- Skeletal muscles play several important roles upon contraction, including agonist, antagonist, stabilizer, and neutralizer functions.
- Skeletal muscle is designed such that structures are stacked in parallel, *i.e.*, smaller units are arranged in parallel to form larger units and so on, to increase force production and transmission to tendons and bones.
- The functional unit of muscle fibers is the sarcomeres. Sarcomeres contain actin and myosin, as well as other structural proteins, critical to muscle contraction.
- Muscle contraction consists of a series of events beginning with spreading the action potential throughout each muscle fiber, mobilization of calcium, cross-bridge formation and cycling (theoretically similar to a "tug-of-war"), and culminating in relaxation.
- Genetics play a critical role in training responses and adaptations; certain candidate genes have been identified to help identify responders and nonresponders to training.
- Myogenesis is the process by which new muscle fibers are formed (as part of remodeling and regeneration after injury) and contributes to muscle hypertrophy.
- Muscle fibers are either slow twitch (ST) or fast twitch (FT). ST fibers are high in endurance, whereas FT fibers are strength/power fibers. The relative distribution of each type within each muscle is an attribute that points athletes toward competing and succeeding in certain sports.
- Fiber-type transitions occur during resistance, sprint, and endurance training. Type IIX (reservoir fibers) percents decrease with a concomitant increase in the percent of type IIA and/or type IIAX fibers.
- Muscle hypertrophy increases in response to anaerobic training and appears related to the training intensity and volume, muscle actions used (especially ECC muscle actions), fiber type, nutritional intake, metabolite formation, and the water content of muscle.
- Muscle hypertrophy is a complex, multifactorial phenomenon that involves in several intercommunicating mechanisms/pathways that ultimately results in greater net protein deposition.
- Hyperplasia has been shown to occur in animals, but its influence on muscle growth in humans is debatable at the current time.
- Structural changes in skeletal muscle occur in response to training. These include increases in the number of myofibrils, the density of the sarcoplasm, sarcoplasm reticulum, and T tubules, and sodium-potassium ATPase pump activity.
- Other adaptations in skeletal muscle include increased buffer capacity, anaerobic substrate content, altered enzyme activity, increased connective tissue strength, anabolic hormone receptor up-regulation, increased fascicle length and fiber orientation, and, in some cases (aerobic training), increased mitochondrial and capillary density.

REVIEW QUESTIONS

1. A muscle that opposes agonist movement is known as a(n)
   a. Fixator
   b. Antagonist
   c. Stabilizer
   d. Origin

2. A structural barrier protein that needs to be displaced in order for muscle contraction to occur is
   a. Titin
   b. Myosin
   c. Tropomyosin
   d. Actin

3. An untrained individual begins a 10-week resistance training program. Which of the following fiber-type transitions would be expected in this individual after 10 weeks of training?
   a. Type IC to type I
   b. Type IIA to type IIX
   c. Type IIX to type IIA
   d. Type IIX to type I

4. The longitudinal splitting of muscle fibers resulting in an increase in muscle fiber number is
   a. Myogenesis
   b. Hyperplasia
   c. Hypertrophy
   d. Myoblast

5. Which of the following statements is true concerning muscle hypertrophy and training?
   a. Metabolites may play a direct or indirect role in muscle growth
   b. Concentric muscle actions are most critical to muscle growth
   c. Type I fibers hypertrophy to the greatest extent
   d. Tension plays a minimal role in muscle growth

6. Which of the following proteins has an inhibiting effect on muscle growth?
   a. Myostatin
   b. Myosin
   c. Actin
   d. Myogenin

7. Fast-twitch muscle fibers have _____ compared to slow-twitch fibers.
   a. Slower myosin
   b. Lower cross-sectional area
   c. Greater capillary density
   d. Greater glycogen stores

8. Myofibrils stacked in parallel form muscle fascicles.
   a. T
   b. F

9. The process of muscle fiber generation is known as myogenesis.a. T
   a. F

10. Endurance training leads to substantial muscle hypertrophy.
    a. T
    b. F

11. Blood flow restriction training using light to moderate loading has been shown to produce increases in muscle hypertrophy.
    a. T
    b. F

12. Consistent progressive resistance training leads to a greater net amount of protein content within skeletal muscle.
    a. T
    b. F

REFERENCES

1. Wackerhage H, Schoenfeld BJ, Hamilton DL, Lehti M, Hulmi JJ. Stimuli and sensors that initiate skeletal muscle hypertrophy following resistance exercise. *J Appl Physiol.* 2019;126:30–43.

2. Herzog W. The multiple roles of titin in muscle contraction and force production. Biophys Rev. 2018;10:1187–99.

3. Hessel AL, Lindstedt SL, Nishikawa KC. Physiological mechanisms of eccentric contraction and its applications: a role for the giant titin protein. *Front Physiol.* 2017;8:1–14.

4. Rassier DE. Sarcomere mechanics in striated muscles: from molecules to sarcomeres to cells. *Am J Physiol Cell Physiol.* 2017;313:C134-45.

5. Bloch RJ, Gonzalez-Serratos H. Lateral force transmission across costameres in skeletal muscle. *Exerc Sport Sci Rev.* 2003;31:73–8.

6. Jaka O, Casas-Fraile L, Lopez de Munain A, Saenz A. Costamere proteins and their involvement in myopathic processes. *Expert Rev Mol Med.* 2015;17:e12. doi: 10.1017/erm.2015.9.

7. Kosek DJ, Bamman MM. Modulation of the dystrophin-associated protein complex in response to resistance training in young and older men. *J Appl Physiol.* 2008;104:1476–84.

8. Graham ZA, Gallagher PM, Cardozo CP. Focal adhesion kinase and its role in skeletal muscle. *J Muscle Res Cell Motil.* 2015;36:305–15.

9. Li R, Narici MV, Erskine RM, et al. Costamere remodeling with muscle loading and unloading in healthy young men. *J Anat.* 2013;223(5):525–36. doi: 10.1111/joa.12101.

10. Watt KI, Goodman CA, Hornberger TA, Gregorevic P. The hippo signaling pathway in the regulation of skeletal muscle mass and function. *Exerc Sport Sci Rev.* 2018;46:92–6.

11. Puthucheary Z, Skipworth JRA, Rawal J, Loosemore M, Van Someren K, Montgomery HE. Genetic influences in sport and physical performance. *Sports Med.* 2011;41:845–59.

12. Eynon N, Hanson ED, Lucia A, Houweling PJ, Garton F, North KN, Bishop DJ. Genes for elite power and sprint performance: *ACTN3* leads the way. *Sports Med.* 2013;43:803–17.

13. Garatachea N, Lucia A. Genes, physical fitness and ageing. *Ageing Res Rev.* 2013;12:90–102.

14. Guth LM, Roth SM. Genetic influence on athletic performance. *Curr Opin Pediatr.* 2013;25:653–8.

15. Tan LJ, Liu SL, Lei SF, Papasian CJ, Deng HW. Molecular genetic studies of gene identification for sarcopenia. *Hum Genet.* 2012;131:1–31.

16. Roth SM, Ferrell RE, Peters DG, et al. Influence of age, sex, and strength training on human muscle gene expression determined by microarray. *Physiol Genomics.* 2002;10:181–90.

17. Liu D, Sartor MA, Nader GA, et al. Skeletal muscle gene expression in response to resistance exercise: sex specific regulation. *BMC Genomics.* 2010;11:1–14.

18. Catoire M, Mensink M, Boekschoten MV, et al. Pronounced effects of acute endurance exercise on gene expression in resting and exercising human skeletal muscle. *PLoS One.* 2012;7:1–10.

19. Chen TC. Effects of a second bout of maximal eccentric exercise on muscle damage and electromyographic activity. *Eur J Appl Physiol.* 2003;89:115–21.

20. Howatson G, Van Someren K, Hortobagyi T. Repeated bout effect after maximal eccentric exercise. *Int J Sports Med.* 2007;28:557–63.

21. Mair J, Mayr M, Muller E, et al. Rapid adaptation to eccentric exercise-induced muscle damage. *Int J Sports Med.* 1995;16:352–6.

22. Nosaka K, Sakamoto K, Newton M, Sacco P. The repeated bout effect of reduced-load eccentric exercise on elbow flexor muscle damage. *Eur J Appl Physiol.* 2001;85:34–40.

23. Nosaka K, Newton MJ, Sacco P. Attenuation of protective effect against eccentric exercise-induced muscle damage. *Can J Appl Physiol.* 2005;30:529–42.

24. Paulsen G, Hanssen KE, Ronnestad BR, et al. Strength training elevates HSP27, HSP70, and αB-crystallin levels in musculi vastus lateralis and trapezius. *Eur J Appl Physiol.* 2012;112:1773–82.

25. Hoppeler H. Molecular networks in skeletal muscle plasticity.

26. *J Exp Biol.* 2016;219:205–13.

27. Farup J, Rahbek SK, Riis S, Vendelbo MH, de Paoli F, Vissing K. Influence of exercise contraction mode and protein supplementation on human satellite cell content and muscle fiber growth. *J Appl Physiol.* 2014;117:898–909.

28. Snijders T, Nederveen JP, McKay BR, Joanisse S, Verdijk LB, van Loon LJC, Parise G. Satellite cells in human skeletal muscle plasticity. *Front Physiol.* 2015;6:1–21.

29. Bazgir B, Fathi R, Valojerdi MR, Mozdziak P, Asgari A. Satellite cells contribution to exercise mediated muscle hypertrophy and repair. *Cell J.* 2017;18:473–84.

30. Joanisse S, Snijders T, Nederveen JP, Parise G. The impact of aerobic exercise on the muscle stem cell response. *Exerc Sport Sci Rev.* 2018;46:180–7.

31. Bellamy LM, Joanisse S, Grubb A, et al. The acute satellite cell response and skeletal muscle hypertrophy following resistance training. *PLoS One.* 2014;9:1–10.

32. Lim CH, Luu TS, Phoung LQ, Jeong TS, Kim CK. Satellite cell activation and mTOR signaling pathway response to resistance and combined exercise in elite weight lifters. *Eur J Appl Physiol.* 2017;117:2355–63.

33. Snijders T, Smeets JSJ, van Kranenburg J, Kies AK, van Loon LJC, Verdijk LB. Changes in myonuclear domain size do not precede muscle hypertrophy during prolonged resistance-type exercise training. *Acta Physiol (oxf).* 2016;216:231–9.

34. Hanssen KE, Kvamme NH, Nilsen TS, et al. The effect of strength training volume on satellite cells, myogenic regulatory factors, and growth factors. *Scand J Med Sci Sports.* 2013;23:728–39.

35. Nederveen JP, Snijders T, Joanisse S, et al. Altered muscle satellite cell activation following 16 wk of resistance training in young men. *Am J Physiol Regul Integr Comp Physiol.* 2017;312:R85–92.

36. D'Souza RF, Bjornsen T, Zeng N, et al. MicroRNAs in muscle: characterizing the powerlifter phenotype. *Front Physiol.* 2017;8:1–12.

37. Mackey AL, Holm L, Reitelseder S, et al. Myogenic response of human skeletal muscle to 12 weeks of resistance training at light loading intensity. *Scand J Med Sci Sports.* 2011;21:773–82.

38. Herman-Montemayor JR, Hikida RS, Staron RS. Early-phase satellite cell and myonuclear domain adaptations to slow-speed vs. traditional resistance training programs. *J Strength Cond Res.* 2015;29:3105–14.

39. Petrella JK, Kim J, Mayhew DL, Cross JM, Bamman MM. Potent myofiber hypertrophy during resistance training in humans is associated with satellite cell-mediated myonuclear addition: a cluster analysis. *J Appl Physiol.* 2008;104:1736–42.

40. Conceicao MS, Vechin FC, Lixandrao M, et al. Muscle fiber hypertrophy and myonuclei addition: a systemtic review and meta-analysis. *Med Sci Sports Exerc.* 2018;50:1385–93.

41. Gundersen K. Muscle memory and a new cellular model for muscle atrophy and hypertrophy. *J Exp Biol.* 2016;219:235–42.

42. Kvorning T, Kadi F, Schjerling P, et al. The activity of satellite cells and myonuclei following 8 weeks of strength training in young men with suppressed testosterone levels. *Acta Physiol (oxf).* 2015;213:676–87.

43. Bickel CS, Slade J, Mahoney E, Haddad F, Dudley GA, Adams GR. Time course of molecular responses of human skeletal muscle to acute bouts of resistance exercise. *J Appl Physiol.* 2005;98: 482–8.

44. Drummond MJ, Fujita S, Takashi A, Dreyer HC, Volpi E, Rasmussen BB. Human muscle gene expression following resistance exercise and blood flow restriction. *Med Sci Sports Exerc.* 2008;40:691–8.

45. Haddad F, Adams GR. Selected contribution: acute cellular and molecular responses to resistance exercise. *J Appl Physiol.* 2002;93:394–403.

46. Hulmi JJ, Ahtiainen JT, Kaasalainen T, et al. Postexercise myostatin and activin IIb mRNA levels: effects of strength training. *Med Sci Sports Exerc.* 2007;39:289–97.

47. Psilander N, Damsgaard R, Pilegaard H. Resistance exercise alters MRF and IGF-I mRNA content in human skeletal muscle. *J Appl Physiol.* 2003;95:1038–44.

48. Wilborn CD, Taylor LW, Greenwood M, Kreider RB, Willoughby DS. Effects of different intensities of resistance exercise on regulators of myogenesis. *J Strength Cond Res.* 2009;23:2179–87.

49. Bamman MM, Ragan RC, Kim JS, et al. Myogenic protein expression before and after resistance loading in 26- and 64-yr-old men and women. *J Appl Physiol.* 2004;97:1329–37.

50. Coffey VG, Shield A, Canny BJ, Carey KA, Cameron-Smith D, Hawley JA. Interaction of contractile activity and training history on mRNA abundance in skeletal muscle from trained athletes. *Am J Physiol Endocrinol Metab.* 2006;290:E849–55.

51. Kosek DJ, Kim JS, Petrella JK, Cross JM, Bamman MM. Efficacy of 3 days/wk resistance training on myofiber hypertrophy and myogenic mechanisms in young vs. older adults. *J Appl Physiol.* 2006;101:531–44.

52. Willoughby DS, Rosene JM. Effects of oral creatine and resistance training on myogenic regulatory factor expression. *Med Sci Sports Exerc.* 2003;35:923–9.

53. Schwarz NA, McKinley-Bernard SK, Spillane MB, et al. Effect of resistance exercise intensity on the expression of PGC-1α isoforms and the anabolic and catabolic signaling mediators, IGF-1 and myostatin, in human skeletal muscle. *Appl Physiol Nutr Metab.* 2016;41:856–63.

54. Roth SM, Martel GF, Ferrell RE, Metter EJ, Hurley BF, Rogers MA. Myostatin gene expression is reduced in humans with heavy-resistance strength training: a brief communication. *Exp Biol Med.* 2003;228:706–9.

55. Dalbo VJ, Roberts MD, Sunderland KL, et al. Acute loading and aging effects on myostatin pathway biomarkers in human skeletal muscle after three sequential bouts of resistance exercise. *J Gerontol.* 2011;66:855–65.

56. Hulmi JJ, Kovanen V, Selanne H, Kraemer WJ, Häkkinen K, Mero AA. Acute and long-term effects of resistance exercise with or without protein ingestion on muscle hypertrophy and gene expression. *Amino Acids.* 2009;37:297–308.

57. Hittel DS, Axelson M, Sarna N, Shearer J, Huffman KM, Kraus WE. Myostatin decreases with aerobic exercise and associates with insulin resistance. *Med Sci Sports Exerc.* 2010;42:2023–9.

58. Margolis LM, Rivas DA. Potential role of microRNA in the anabolic capacity of skeletal muscle with aging. *Exerc Sport Sci Rev.* 2018;46:86–91.

59. D'Souza RF, Markworth JF, Aasen KMM, Zeng N, Cameron-Smith D, Mitchell CJ. Acute resistance exercise modulates microRNA expression profiles: combined tissue and circulatory targeted analyses. *PLoS One.* 2017;12:1–15.

60. Kirby TJ, McCarthy JJ. MicroRNAs in skeletal muscle biology and exercise adaptation. *Free Radic Biol Med.* 2013;64:95–105.

61. Margolis LM, Lessard SJ, Ezzyat Y, Fielding RA, Rivas DA. Circulating microRNA are predictive of aging and acute adaptive responses to resistance exercise in men. *J Gerontol A Biol Sci Med Sci.* 2017;72:1319–26.

62. McCarthy JJ, Esser KA. MicroRNA-1 and microRNA-133a expression are decreased during skeletal muscle hypertrophy. *J Appl Physiol.* 2007;102:306–13.

63. Silva GJJ, Bye A, Azzouri H, Wisloff U. MicroRNAs as important regulators of exercise adaptation. *Prog Cardiovasc Dis.* 2017;60:130–51.

64. Fyfe JJ, Bishop DJ, Zacharewicz E, Russell AP, Stepto NK. Concurrent exercise incorporating high-intensity interval or continuous training modulates mTORC1 signaling and microRNA expression in human skeletal muscle. *Am J Physiol Regul Integr Comp Physiol.* 2016;310:R1297–311.

65. Ogasawara R, Akimoto T, Umeno T, Sawada S, Hamaoka T, Fujita S. MicroRNA expression profiling in skeletal muscle reveals different regulatory patterns in high and low responders to resistance training. *Physiol Genomics.* 2016;48:320–4.

66. Nielsen S, Scheele C, Yfanti C, et al. Muscle specific microRNAs are regulated by endurance exercise in human skeletal muscle. *J Physiol.* 2010;588:4029–37.

67. Staron RS. The classification of human skeletal muscle fiber types. *J Strength Cond Res.* 1997;11:67.

68. Trappe S, Luden N, Michev K, Raue U, Jemiolo B, Trappe TA. Skeletal muscle signature of a champion sprint runner. *J Appl Physiol.* 2015;118:1460–6.

69. Fry AC. The role of resistance exercise intensity on muscle fibre adaptations. *Sports Med.* 2004;34:663–79.

70. Häkkinen K, Alen M, Komi PV. Neuromuscular, anaerobic, and aerobic performance characteristics of elite power athletes. *Eur J Appl Physiol Occup Physiol.* 1984;53:97–105.

71. McComas AJ. *Skeletal Muscle: Form and Function.* Champaign (IL): Human Kinetics; 1996.

72. Tesch PA, Alkner BA. Acute and chronic muscle metabolic adaptations to strength training. In: Komi PV, editor. *Strength and Power in Sport.* 2nd ed. Boston (MA): Blackwell Science; 2002. p. 265–80.

73. Fry AC, Allemeier CA, Staron RS. Correlation between percentage fiber type area and myosin heavy chain content in human skeletal muscle. *Eur J Appl Physiol.* 1994;68:246–51.

74. Harber MP, Fry AC, Rubin MR, Smith JC, Weiss LW. Skeletal muscle and hormonal adaptations to circuit weight training in untrained men. *Scand J Med Sci Sports.* 2004;14:176–85.

75. Bickel CS, Cross JM, Bamman MM. Exercise dosing to retain resistance training adaptations in young and older adults. *Med Sci Sports Exerc.* 2011;43:1177–87.

76. Kraemer WJ, Patton JF, Gordon SE, et al. Compatibility of high-intensity strength and endurance training on hormonal and skeletal muscle adaptations. *J Appl Physiol.* 1995;78:976–89.

77. Staron RS, Karapondo DL, Kraemer WJ, et al. Skeletal muscle adaptations during early phase of heavy-resistance training in men and women. *J Appl Physiol.* 1994;76:1247–55.

78. Campos GE, Luecke TJ, Wendeln HK, et al. Muscular adaptations in response to three different resistance-training regimens: specificity of repetition maximum training zones. *Eur J Appl Physiol.* 2002;88:50–60.

79. Holm L, Reitelseder S, Pedersen TG, et al. Changes in muscle size and MHC composition in response to resistance exercise with heavy and light loading intensity. *J Appl Physiol.* 2008;105:1454–61.

80. Andersen JL, Aagaard P. Myosin heavy chain IIX overshoot in human skeletal muscle. *Muscle Nerve.* 2000;23:1095–104.

81. O'Neill DS, Zheng D, Anderson WK, Dohm GL, Houmard JA. Effect of endurance exercise on myosin heavy chain gene regulation in human skeletal muscle. *Am J Physiol.* 1999;276:R414–9.

82. Short KR, Vittone JL, Bigelow ML, et al. Changes in myosin heavy chain mRNA and protein expression in human skeletal muscle with age and endurance exercise training. *J Appl Physiol.* 2005;99:95–102.

83. Putnam CT, Xu X, Gillies E, MacLean IM, Bell GJ. Effects of strength, endurance and combined training on myosin heavy chain content and fibre-type distribution in humans. *Eur J Appl Physiol.* 2004;92:376–84.

84. Allemeier CA, Fry AC, Johnson P, Hikida RS, Hagerman FC, Staron RS. Effects of sprint cycle training on human skeletal muscle. *J Appl Physiol.* 1994;77:2385–90.

85. Jacobs I, Esbjornsson M, Sylven C, Holm I, Jansson E. Sprint training effects on muscle myoglobin, enzymes, fiber types, and blood lactate. *Med Sci Sports Exerc.* 1987;19:368–74.

86. Markovic G, Mikulic P. Neuro-musculoskeletal and performance adaptations to lower-extremity plyometric training. *Sports Med.* 2010;40:859–95.

87. Ahmetov II, Vinogradova OL, Williams AG. Gene polymorphisms and fiber-type composition of human skeletal muscle. *Int J Sport Nutr Exerc Metab.* 2012;22:292–303.

88. Yan Z, Okutsu M, Akhtar YN, Lira VA. Regulation of exercise-induced fiber type transformation, mitochondrial biogenesis, and angiogenesis in skeletal muscle. *J Appl Physiol.* 2011;110:264–74.

89. Tipton KD, Hamilton DL, Gallagher IJ. Assessing the role of muscle protein breakdown in response to nutrition and exercise in humans. *Sports Med.* 2018;48:S53–64.

90. Yang Y, Jemiolo B, Trappe S. Proteolytic mRNA expression in response to acute resistance exercise in human single skeletal muscle fibers. *J Appl Physiol.* 2006;101:1442–50.

91. Dreyer HC, Fujita S, Glynn EL, et al. Resistance exercise increases leg muscle protein synthesis and mTOR signaling independent of sex. *Acta Physiol (Oxf).* 2010;199:71–81.

92. McGlory C, Devries MC, Phillips SM. Skeletal muscle and resistance exercise training; the role of protein synthesis in recovery and remodeling. *J Appl Physiol.* 2017;122:541–8.

93. Poortmans JR, Carpentier A, Pereira-Lancha LO, Lancha A. Protein turnover, amino acid requirements and recommendations for athletes and active populations. *Braz J Med Biol Res.* 2012;45:875–90.

94. Phillips S, Tipton K, Aarsland A, Wolf S, Wolfe R. Mixed muscle protein synthesis and breakdown after resistance exercise in humans. *Am J Physiol.* 1997;273:E99–107.

95. Burd NA, West DWD, Staples AW, et al. Low-load high volume resistance exercise stimulates muscle protein synthesis more than high-load low volume resistance exercise in young men. *PLoS One.* 2010;5:1–10.

96. Damas F, Libardi CA, Ugrinowitsch C. The development of skeletal muscle hypertrophy through resistance training: the role of muscle damage and muscle protein synthesis. *Eur J Appl Physiol.* 2018;118:485–500.

97. Damas F, Phillips SM, Libardi CA, et al. Resistance training-induced changes in integrated myofibrillar protein synthesis are related to hypertrophy only after attenuation of muscle damage. *J Physiol.* 2016;594:5209–22.

98. Kraemer WJ, Ratamess NA. Fundamentals of resistance training: progression and exercise prescription. *Med Sci Sports Exerc.* 2004;36:674–8.

99. Peterson MD, Pistilli E, Haff GG, Hoffman EP, Gordon PM. Progression of volume load and muscular adaptation during resistance exercise. *Eur J Appl Physiol.* 2011;111:1063–71.

100. Häkkinen K, Pakarinen A, Kraemer WJ, Häkkinen A, Valkeinen H, Alen M. Selective muscle hypertrophy, changes in EMG and force, and serum hormones during strength training in older women. *J Appl Physiol.* 2001;91:569–80.

101. Wakahara T, Miyamoto N, Sugisaki N, et al. Association between regional differences in muscle activation in one session of resistance exercise and in muscle hypertrophy after resistance training. *Eur J Appl Physiol.* 2012;112:1569–76.

102. Figueiredo VC, McCarthy JJ. Regulation of ribosome biogenesis in skeletal muscle hypertrophy. *Physiology (Bethesda).* 2019;34:30–42.

103. Wen Y, Alimov AP, McCarthy JJ. Ribosome biogenesis is necessary for skeletal muscle hypertrophy. *Exerc Sport Sci Rev.* 2016;44:110–5.

104. Stec MJ, Mayhew DL, Bamman MM. The effects of age and resistance loading on skeletal muscle ribosome biogenesis. *J Appl Physiol.* 2015;119:851–7.

105. Stec MJ, Kelly NA, Many GM, Windham ST, Tuggle SC, Bamman MM. Ribosome biogenesis may augment resistance training-induced myofiber hypertrophy and is required for myotube growth in vitro. *Am J Physiol Endocrinol Metab.* 2016;310:E652–61.

106. Mobley CB, Haun CT, Roberson PA, et al. Biomarkers associated with low, moderate, and high vastus lateralis muscle hypertrophy following 12 weeks of resistance training. *PLoS One.* 2018;13:1–20.

107. Reidy PT, Borack MS, Markofski MM, et al. Post-absorptive muscle protein turnover affects resistance training hypertrophy. *Eur J Appl Physiol.* 2017;117:853–66.

108. Brook MS, Wilkinson DJ, Mitchell WK, et al. Synchronous deficits in cumulative muscle protein synthesis and ribosomal biogenesis underlie age-related anabolic resistance to exercise in humans. *J Physiol.* 2016;594:7399–417.

109. Tu MK, Levin JB, Hamilton AM, Borodinsky LN. Calcium signaling in skeletal muscle development, maintenance and regeneration. *Cell Calcium.* 2016;59:91–7.

110. Leal ML, Lamas L, Aoki MS, et al. Effect of different resistance-training regimens on the WNT-signaling pathway. *Eur J Appl Physiol.* 2011;111:2535–45.

111. Yoon MS. mTOR as a key regulator in maintaining skeletal muscle mass. *Front Physiol.* 2017;8:1–9.

112. Hornberger TA. Mechanotransduction and the regulation of mTORC1 signaling in skeletal muscle. *Int J Biochem Cell Biol.* 2011;43:1267–76.

113. Thomson DM. The role of AMPK in the regulation of skeletal muscle size, hypertrophy, and regeneration. *Int J Mol Sci.* 2018;19:1–20.

114. Gibala MJ, McGee SL, Garnham AP, Howlett KF, Snow RJ, Hargreaves M. Brief intense interval exercise activates AMPK and p38 MAPK signaling and increases the expression of PGC-1α in human skeletal muscle. *J Appl Physiol.* 2009;106:929–34.

115. Terzis G, Spengos K, Mascher H, et al. The degree of p70S6K and S6 phosphorylation in human skeletal muscle in response to resistance exercise depends on the training volume. *Eur J Appl Physiol.* 2010;110:835–43.

116. Baar K, Esser K. Phosphorylation of p70(S6K) correlates with increased skeletal muscle mass following resistance exercise. *Am J Physiol.* 1999;276:C120–7.

117. Hulmi JJ, Walker S, Ahtiainen JP, Nyman K, Kraemer WJ, Häkkinen K. Molecular signaling in muscle is affected by the specificity of resistance exercise protocol. *Scand J Med Sci Sports.* 2012;22:240–8.

118. Mitchell CJ, Churchward-Venne TA, Bellamy L, et al. Muscular and systemic correlates of resistance training-induced muscle hypertrophy. *PLoS One.* 2013;8:1–10.

119. Moore DR, Atherton PJ, Rennie MJ, Tarnopolsky MA, Phillips SM. Resistance exercise enhances mTOR and MAPK signaling in human muscle over that seen at rest after bolus protein ingestion. *Acta Physiol.* 2011;201:365–72.

120. Gonzalez AM, Hoffman JR, Townsend JR, et al. Intramuscular anabolic signaling and endocrine response following high volume and high intensity resistance exercise protocols in trained men. *Physiol Rep.* 2015;3:1–15.

121. Kramer HF, Goodyear LJ. Exercise, MAPK, and NF-KB signaling in skeletal muscle. *J Appl Physiol.* 2007;103:388–95.

122. Gonzalez AM, Hoffman JR, Townsend JR, et al. Intramuscular MAPK signaling following high volume and high intensity resistance exercise protocols in trained men. *Eur J Appl Physiol.* 2016;116:1163–670.

123. Galpin AJ, Fry AC, Chiu LZF, Thomason DB, Schilling BK. High-power resistance exercise induces MAPK phosphorylation in weightlifting trained men. *Appl Physiol Nutr Metab.* 2011;37:80–7.

124. Nicoll JX, Fry AC, Galpin AJ, et al. Changes in resting mitogen-activated protein kinases following resistance exercise overreaching and overtraining. *Eur J Appl Physiol.* 2016;116:2401–13.

125. Galpin AJ, Fry AC, Nicoll JX, Moore CA, Schilling BK, Thomason DB. Resting extracellular signal-regulated protein kinase 1/2 expression following a continuum of chronic resistance exercise training paradigms. *Res Sports Med.* 2016;24:298–303.

126. Hoffmann C, Weigert C. Skeletal muscle as an endocrine organ: the role of myokines in exercise adaptations. *Cold Spring Harb Perspect Med.* 2017;7:1–22.

127. Kanzleiter T, Rath M, Gorgens SW, et al. The myokines decorin is regulated by contraction and involved in muscle hypertrophy. *Biochem Biophys Res Commun.* 2014;450:1089–94.

128. Pedersen BK. Muscle and their myokines. *J Exp Biol.* 2011;214:337–46.

129. Huey KA. Potential roles of vascular endothelial growth factor during skeletal muscle hypertrophy. *Exerc Sport Sci Rev.* 2018;46:195–202.

130. Munoz-Canoves P, Scheele C, Pedersen BK, Serrano AL. Interleukin-6 myokine signaling in skeletal muscle: a double-edge sword? FEBS J 2013;280:4131-48.

131. MacDougall JD, Sale DG, Moroz JR, Elder GC, Sutton JR, Howald H. Mitochondrial volume density in human skeletal muscle following heavy resistance training. *Med Sci Sports.* 1979;11:164–6.

132. Hortobagyi T, Hill JP, Houmard JA, Fraser DD, Lambert NJ, Israel RG. Adaptive responses to muscle lengthening and shortening in humans. *J Appl Physiol.* 1996;80:765–72.

133. Tesch PA, Thorsson A, Essen-Gustavsson B. Enzyme activities of FT and ST muscle fibers in heavy-resistance trained athletes. *J Appl Physiol.* 1989;67:83–7.

134. Grgic J, Schoenfeld BJ. Are the hypertrophic adaptations to high and low-load resistance training muscle fiber type specific? *Front Physiol.* 2018;9:1–6.

135. Kesidis N, Metaxas TI, Vrabas IS, et al. Myosin heavy chain isoform distribution in single fibres of bodybuilders. *Eur J Appl Physiol.* 2008;103:579–83.

136. Wernbom M, Augustsson J, Thomee R. The influence of frequency, intensity, volume and mode of strength training on whole muscle cross-sectional area in humans. *Sports Med.* 2007;37:225–64.

137. Dudley GA, Tesch PA, Miller BJ, Buchanan MD. Importance of eccentric actions in performance adaptations to resistance training. *Aviat Space Environ Med.* 1991;62:543–50.

138. Vikne H, Refsnes PE, Ekmark M, Medbo JI, Gundersen V, Gundersen K. Muscular performance after concentric and eccentric exercise in trained men. *Med Sci Sports Exerc.* 2006;38:1770–81.

139. Mangine GT, Hoffman JR, Gonzalez AM, et al. The effect of training volume and intensity on improvements in muscular strength and size in resistance-trained men. *Physiol Rep.* 2015;3:1–17.

140. Schoenfeld BJ, Contreras B, Vigotsky AD, Peterson M. Differential effects of heavy versus moderate loads on measures of strength and hypertrophy in resistance-trained men. *J Sports Sci Med.* 2016;15:715–22.

141. Schoenfeld BJ, Ratamess NA, Peterson MD, Contreras B, Sonmez GT, Alvar BA. Effects of different volume-equated resistance training loading strategies on muscular adaptations in well-trained men. *J Strength Cond Res.* 2014;28:2909–18.

142. Krieger JW. Single vs. multiple sets of resistance exercise for muscle hypertrophy: a meta-analysis. *J Strength Cond Res.* 2010;24:1150–9.

143. Radaelli R, Fleck SJ, Leite T, et al. Dose-response of 1, 3, and 5 sets of resistance exercise on strength, local muscular endurance, and hypertrophy. *J Strength Cond Res.* 2015;29:1349–58.

144. Buresh R, Berg K, French J. The effect of resistive exercise rest interval on hormonal response, strength, and hypertrophy with training. *J Strength Cond Res.* 2009;23:62–71.

145. Henselmans M, Schoenfeld BJ. The effect of inter-set rest intervals on resistance exercise-induced muscle hypertrophy. *Sports Med.* 2014;44:1635–43.

146. Schoenfeld BJ, Ogborn D, Krieger JW. Effects of resistance training frequency on measures of muscle hypertrophy: a systematic review and meta-analysis. *Sports Med.* 2016;46:1689–97.

147. Schoenfeld BJ. The mechanisms of muscle hypertrophy and their application to resistance training. *J Strength Cond Res.* 2010;24:2857–72.

148. Schoenfeld BJ. Potential mechanisms for a role of metabolic stress in hypertrophic adaptations to resistance training. *Sports Med.* 2013;43:179–94.

149. Waldegger S, Busch GL, Kaba NK, et al. Effect of cellular hydration on protein metabolism. *Miner Electrolyte Metab.* 1997;23:201–5.

150. Ratamess NA. *Coaches Guide to Performance-Enhancing Supplements.* Monterey (CA): Coaches Choice Books; 2006.

151. Ratamess NA. Amino acid supplementation: what can it really do for you? *Pure Power.* 2004;4:38–42.

152. Hoffman JR, Ratamess NA. Medical issues of anabolic steroids: are they over-exaggerated? *J Sports Sci Med.* 2006;5:182–93.

153. Wernbom M, Augustsson J, Thomee R. Effects of vascular occlusion on muscular endurance in dynamic knee extension exercise at different submaximal loads. *J Strength Cond Res.* 2006;20:372–7.

154. Scott BR, Loenneke JP, Slattery KM, Dascombe BJ. Exercise with blood flow restriction: an updated evidence-based approach for enhanced muscular development. *Sports Med.* 2015;45:313–25.

155. Pearson SJ, Hussain SR. A review on the mechanisms of blood-flow restriction resistance training-induced muscle hypertrophy. *Sports Med.* 2015;45:187–200.

156. Takarada Y, Nakamura Y, Aruga S, Onda T, Miyazaki S, Ishii N. Rapid increase in plasma growth hormone after low-intensity resistance exercise with vascular occlusion. *J Appl Physiol.* 2000;88:61–5.

157. Madarame H, Neya M, Ochi E, Nakazato K, Sato Y, Ishii N. Cross-transfer effects of resistance training with blood flow restriction. *Med Sci Sports Exerc.* 2008;40:258–63.

158. Rooney KJ, Herbert RD, Balwave RJ. Fatigue contributes to the strength training stimulus. *Med Sci Sports Exerc.* 1994;26:1160–4.

159. Shinohara M, Kouzaki M, Yoshihisa T, Fukunaga T. Efficacy of tourniquet ischemia for strength training with low resistance. *Eur J Appl Physiol.* 1998;77:189–91.

160. Smith RC, Rutherford OM. The role of metabolites in strength training I A comparison of eccentric and concentric contractions. *Eur J Appl Physiol.* 1995;71:332–6.

161. Takarada Y, Tsuruta T, Ishii N. Cooperative effects of exercise and occlusive stimuli on muscular function in low-intensity resistance exercise with moderate vascular occlusion. *Jpn J Physiol.* 2004;54:585–92.

162. Loenneke JP, Wilson JM, Marin PJ, Zourdos MC, Bemben MG. Low intensity blood flow restriction training: a meta-analysis. *Eur J Appl Physiol.* 2012;112:1849–59.

163. Lixandrao ME, Ugrinowitsch C, Berton R, et al. Magnitude of muscle strength and mass adaptations between high-load resistance training versus low-load resistance training associated with blood-flow restriction: a systematic review and meta-analysis. *Sports Med.* 2018;48:361–78.

164. Slysz J, Stultz J, Burr JF. The efficacy of blood flow restricted exercise: a systematic review and meta-analysis. *J Sci Med Sport.* 2016;19:669–75.

165. Yasuda T, Ogasawara R, Sakamaki M, Bemben MG, Abe T. Relationship between limb and trunk muscle hypertrophy following high-intensity resistance training and blood flow-restricted low-intensity resistance training. *Clin Physiol Funct Imaging.* 2011;31:347–51.

166. Yasuda T, Ogasawara R, Sakamaki M, Ozaki H, Sato Y, Abe T. Combined effects of low-intensity blood flow restriction training and high-intensity resistance training on muscle strength and size. *Eur J Appl Physiol.* 2011;111:2525–33.

167. Ross A, Leveritt M. Long-term metabolic and skeletal muscle adaptations to short-sprint training: implications for sprint training and tapering. *Sports Med.* 2001;31:1063–82.

168. Linossier MT, Dormois D, Geyssant A, Denis C. Performance and fibre characteristics of human skeletal muscle during short sprint training and detraining on a cycle ergometer. *Eur J Appl Physiol.* 1997;75:491–8.

169. Häkkinen K, Alen M, Komi PV. Changes in isometric force-and relaxation-time, electromyographic and muscle fibre characteristics of human skeletal muscle during strength training and detraining. *Acta Physiol Scand.* 1985;125:573–85.

170. Kikuchi N, Nakazato K. Low-load bench press and push-up induce similar muscle hypertrophy and strength gain. *J Exerc Sci Fit.* 2017;15:37–42.

171. Perez-Gomez J, Olmedillas H, Delgado-Guerra S, et al. Effects of weight lifting training combined with plyometric exercises on physical fitness, body composition, and knee extension velocity during kicking in football. *Appl Physiol Nutr Metab.* 2008;33:501–10.

172. Kraemer WJ, Nindl BC, Ratamess NA, et al. Changes in muscle hypertrophy in women with periodized resistance training. *Med Sci Sports Exerc.* 2004;36:697–708.

173. Grgic J, McIlvenna LC, Fyfe JJ, et al. Does aerobic training promote the same skeletal muscle hypertrophy as resistance training? A systematic review and meta-analysis. *Sports Med.* 2019;49:233–54.

174. Osawa Y, Azuma K, Tabata S, et al. Effects of 16-week high-intensity interval training using upper and lower body ergometers on aerobic fitness and morphological changes in healthy men: a preliminary study. *Open Access J Sports Med.* 2014;5:257–65.

175. Wilson JM, Marin PJ, Rhea MR, et al. Concurrent training: a meta-analysis examining interference of aerobic and resistance exercises. *J Strength Cond Res.* 2012;26:2293–307.

176. Eddens L, van Someren K, Howatson G. The role of intra-session exercise sequence in the interference effect: a systematic review with meta-analysis. *Sports Med.* 2018;48:177–88.

177. Gonyea W, Ericson GC, Bonde-Peterson F. Skeletal muscle fiber splitting induced by weight lifting exercise in cats. *Acta Physiol Scand.* 1977;99:105–9.

178. Kelley G. Mechanical overload and skeletal muscle fiber hyperplasia: a meta-analysis. *J Appl Physiol.* 1996;81:1584–8.

179. MacDougall JD, Sale DG, Elder GC, Sutton JR. Muscle ultrastructural characteristics of elite powerlifters and bodybuilders. *Eur J Appl Physiol.* 1982;48:117–26.

180. Tesch PA, Larsson L. Muscle hypertrophy in bodybuilders. *Eur J Appl Physiol.* 1982;49:301–6.

181. MacDougall JD, Sale DG, Alway SE, Sutton JR. Muscle fiber number in biceps brachii in body builders and control subjects. *J Appl Physiol.* 1984;57:1399–403.

182. Eriksson A, Lindstrom M, Carlsson L, Thornell LE. Hypertrophic muscle fibers with fissures in power-lifters; fiber splitting or defect regeneration? *Histochem Cell Biol.* 2006;126: 409–17.

183. McCall GE, Byrnes WC, Dickinson A, Pattany PM, Fleck SJ. Muscle fiber hypertrophy, hyperplasia, and capillary density in college men after resistance training. *J Appl Physiol.* 1996;81: 2004–12.

184. Alway SE, MacDougall JD, Sale DG. Contractile adaptations in the human triceps surae after isometric exercise. *J Appl Physiol.* 1989; 66:2725–32.

185. Green HJ, Ballantyne CS, MacDougall JD, Tarnopolsky MA, Schertzer JD. Adaptations in human muscle sarcoplasmic reticulum to prolonged submaximal training. *J Appl Physiol.* 2003;94:2034–42.

186. Medbo JI, Jebens E, Vikne H, Refsnes PE, Gramvik P. Effect of strenuous strength training on the Na-K pump concentration in skeletal muscle of well-trained men. *Eur J Appl Physiol.* 2001;84:148–54.

187. Green HJ, Barr DJ, Fowles JR, Sandiford SD, Ouyang J. Malleability of human skeletal muscle Na$^+$-K$^+$-ATPase pump with short-term training. *J Appl Physiol.* 2004;97:143–8.

188. Madsen K, Franch J, Clausen T. Effects of intensified endurance training on the concentration of Na,K-ATPase and Ca-ATPase in human skeletal muscle. *Acta Physiol Scand.* 1994;150:251–8.

189. Fraser SF, Li JL, Carey MF, et al. Fatigue depresses maximal in vitro skeletal muscle Na+-K+-ATPase activity in untrained and trained individuals. *J Appl Physiol.* 2002;93:1650–9.

190. Skovgaard C, Almquist NW, Bangsbo J. Effect of increased and maintained frequency of speed endurance training on performance and muscle adaptations in runners. *J Appl Physiol.* 2017;122:48–59.

191. Wyckelsma VL, McKenna MJ, Serpiello FR, et al. Single-fiber expression and fiber-specific adaptability to short-term intense exercise training of Na+-K+-ATPase α- and β-isoforms in human skeletal muscle. *J Appl Physiol.* 2015;118:699–706.

192. Wyckelsma VL, Levinger I, Murphy RM, et al. Intense interval training in healthy older adults increases skeletal muscle [³H] ouabain-binding site content and elevates Na+, K+-ATPase α2 isoform abundance in type II fibers. *Physiol Rep.* 2017;5:1–13.

193. Stammers AN, Susser SE, Hamm NC, et al. The regulation of sarco(endo)plasmic reticulum calcium-ATPases (SERCA). *Can J Physiol Pharmacol.* 2015;93:843–54.

194. Ortenblad N, Lunde PK, Levin K, Andersen JL, Pedersen PK. Enhanced sarcoplasmic reticulum Ca(2+) release following intermittent sprint training. *Am J Physiol.* 2000;279:R152–60.

CHAPTER 6

Connective Tissue Adaptations to Training

OBJECTIVES

After completing this chapter, you will be able to:

◆ Identify the types of stresses and subsequent strain that lead to connective tissue adaptations

◆ Understand the internal and external features of a bone

◆ Discuss how bones hypertrophy in response to loading

◆ Discuss ways to alter training programs to target increased bone strength and size

◆ Describe the components of connective tissue structures and understand adaptations to exercise training

◆ Discuss the functions of cartilage and subsequent responses and adaptations to exercise

Increases in muscle size, strength, endurance, and power can only be maximized when the supporting structures adapt proportionally. That is, increases in connective tissue (CT) size, strength, and durability need to take place in order to accommodate changes in skeletal muscle performance. CT structures include bones, tendons, ligaments, fascia, and cartilage. Adaptations in CT resulting from training are critical for how muscle force is transmitted to bone, joint stability, and injury prevention. This chapter discusses various types of CT structures and concurrent adaptations to training.

Stimuli for Connective Tissue Adaptations

Before discussing CT, it is important to overview terminology associated with loading, which initiates the adaptation process. CT can only adapt when it is progressively overloaded by increasing stress. Mechanical stress is defined by the internal force observed divided by the cross-sectional area (CSA) of the CT structure. By definition, less mechanical stress is placed on CT when the CSA (denominator in the equation) increases per level of force encountered. Thus, CT increases tolerance for loading by increasing size and/or by altering structural properties. These have important ramifications for injury prevention

in sports and force transmission from muscle to bone. CT adaptations must take place to accommodate changes in muscle performance. However, CT adaptations take place at a slower rate compared to skeletal muscle. This could be of concern early in training as muscular adaptations precede CT changes temporally. Too much stress may increase the risk of injury. In addition, after injury has occurred, CT has longer recovery rates compared to skeletal muscle.

Types of Stress

Stress relates to the force applied to CT. The three most common types of stress associated with CT are tension, compression, and shear stresses. *Tension* stresses result in pulling forces on the tissue. Stretching or elongation occurs as is the case with tendons during muscle contraction. *Compression* stresses result in pushing the structure inward or compressing its longitudinal length. Some examples include the spine when performing the squat exercise or the humerus (upper arm bone) when performing a push-up. *Shear* stresses result in skewing where force is encountered obliquely. Examples include scissors during cutting and the knee during a knee extension exercise. Shear stresses tend to be more injurious when encountered athletically. In some cases, a twisting effect, or *torsion*, is seen. The result of stress is deformation to CT. Deformation leads to adaptation and is proportional to the level of stress encountered.

Stress-Strain Relationship

As stress is the level of force encountered by a tissue, strain is the magnitude of deformation that takes place in proportion to the amount of stress applied. Two types of strain are shown in CT, linear and shear. *Linear strain* results from compressive and tensile stresses where the tissue (tendons, ligaments) changes length, and the quantification of linear strain is expressed as a percentage relative to resting length. *Shear strain* results in bending of the tissue (bone) and is quantified by the angle of deformation. For circular-type tissues (cartilage), another type of strain can be seen. When a tissue is compressed, its longitudinal height decreases, but it laterally expands. The ratio of strain in the longitudinal direction to strain in the lateral direction is known as Poisson ratio. This is a useful measure to examine compression in articular cartilage and intervertebral disks (where too great of a strain can lead to a rupture).

The stress-strain relationship for a tendon is shown in Figure 6.1 and for multiple CT structures in Figure 6.2. In Figure 6.1, stress is shown on the Y-axis, whereas strain (%) is shown on the X-axis. At complete rest, there is a small degree of slack in the tendon fibers. Upon low level of muscle contraction, the tendon elongates to its normal length and is denoted as the *toe region* on the graph. With greater stress, there is a proportional increase in strain depicted as the *linear* (or *elastic*) *region* on the graph. If the level of stress is too high, injury can result as denoted as the *failure region* on the graph, which may occur at 4%–10% strain depending on the tendon. Upon elongation as a result of stress, the tendon can return to its normal length when the stress is removed. The magnitude and rate of loading may affect the shape of the stress-strain curve. The property of CT to return to its original length after being stretched is elasticity. However, chronic stretching to a tissue can cause transient or permanent deformation where the tissue remains at least partially elongated and does not return entirely to its original length. This property is known as plasticity. There are times where plasticity is good (tendons in response to chronic flexibility training) or bad (ligaments in response to damage over time).

The slope of the line in the linear region is representative of the CT stiffness. *Stiffness* is defined as the resistance to a change in length and is directly related to the CT structure, *e.g.*, CSA, collagen and other protein, glycosaminoglycan, and proteoglycan content. The ratio of stress to strain (*Young modulus*: the product of stiffness and the original length-to-CSA ratio) increases as stiffness increases. Subsequently, stiffness is reduced when the slope is gradual and the modulus is low. Physiologic strain varies between different tendons and ligaments. In tendons, regional differences within the same tendon occur where the region closest to the bone is much stiffer than the myotendinous junction where tendon collagen fibers are woven with skeletal muscle fibers. In fact, high-tension, slow-velocity injury is most likely to occur at the bone-tendon junction, whereas high-tension fast-velocity injuries are likely to occur at the tendon belly. Tendon size and stiffness shows great disparity within the body depending on its regional location. The Achilles (calcaneal) tendon is much thicker, stronger, and tolerable of stress and has much greater stiffness and elastic modulus than the extensor carpi radialis brevis tendon (1). Stiffness may vary based on joint position. Figure 6.2 shows that compact (cortical) bone is stiffer than spongy (cancellous) bone, and both are much stiffer than tendons. In general, ligaments are less stiff than tendons, and cartilage has the lowest stiffness of the CT structures.

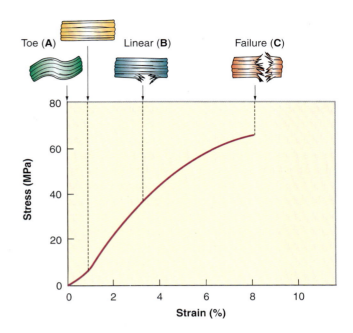

FIGURE 6.1 The stress-strain relationship in a ruptured Achilles tendon. The three distinct regions are (**A**) toe region, (**B**) linear region, and (**C**) failure region.

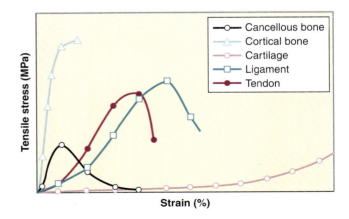

FIGURE 6.2 The stress-strain relationships of bones, tendons, ligaments, and cartilage. (Redrawn from Hamill J, Knutzen KM. *Biomechanical Basis of Human Movement*. 3rd ed. Philadelphia (PA): Wolters Kluwer Lippincott Williams & Wilkins; 2009. p. 411–61)

Skeletal System
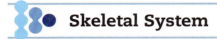

The skeletal system consists of 206 bones, 177 of which are involved in human voluntary movement (Fig. 6.3). The skeletal system is divided into two major subdivisions: axial and appendicular. The *axial skeleton* consists of 80 bones of the skull and trunk (vertebral column, ribs, sternum, sacrum, and coccyx), whereas the *appendicular skeleton* consists of 126 bones of the limbs, shoulder, and pelvic girdle. The skeletal system plays several important roles in human function. It provides support, area for muscular attachment, and protection to several organs. Bones provide leverage and produce movement upon skeletal muscle contraction. Bones provide a storage site for minerals in times where dietary intake may be low. Bones assist in acid-base balance and act as a reservoir for growth factors, lipids, and cytokines. Lastly, bones produce red blood cells from red marrow, which are essential for transporting oxygen.

Bone Anatomy

Bones exist in five forms. *Long bones* (femur, humerus) contribute greatly to human height and limb lengths. *Short bones* (carpals and tarsals of hands and feet) are typically found in areas where mobility is critical. *Flat bones* (ribs, scapula, bones of the skull, and sternum) are especially important for protection. *Irregular bones* (vertebrae) are uniquely shaped because they perform a multitude of functions. *Sesamoid bones* (patella) help create a more favorable line of pull for muscles that span their surface area.

To understand how bones adapt to exercise, it is important to examine the anatomy of a bone. Figure 6.4 depicts the anatomy of a long bone. The polar ends of the bone are known as the *epiphyses*. Growth plates (epiphyseal plates) are located here and are the sites of longitudinal bone growth during the developmental years. The long region of the bone is known as the shaft or *diaphysis*. The narrow region between the diaphysis and epiphyses is the *metaphysis*, which also contains growth

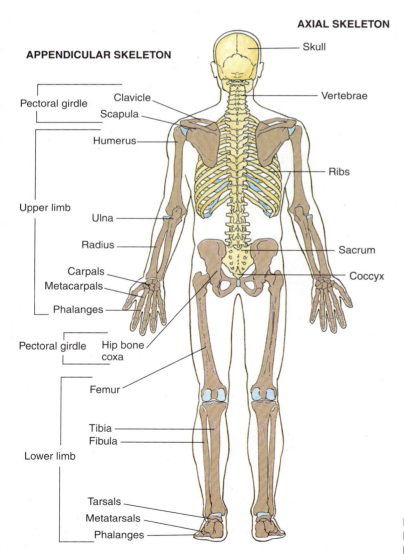

FIGURE 6.3 The axial and appendicular skeletons. (From Moore KL, Agur AMR. *Essential Clinical Anatomy*. 2nd ed. Baltimore (MD): Lippincott Williams & Wilkins; 2004.)

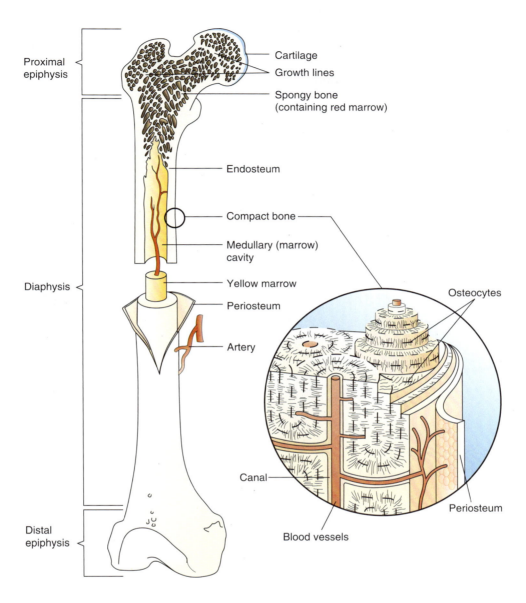

FIGURE 6.4 Anatomy of a long bone (femur). (From Smeltzer SC, Bare BG. *Textbook of Medical-Surgical Nursing.* 9th ed. Philadelphia (PA): Lippincott Williams & Wilkins; 2000.)

plates during development. Long bones consist of two types of bone: compact and spongy. *Compact (cortical) bone* is located on the perimeter and is much denser and stronger than *spongy (trabecular) bone*, which is located within and especially in the epiphyses and helps give bone its pliability. Compact bone is ~5%–10% porosity versus 50%–90% porosity seen in spongy bone. The ratio of each within a bone dictates the degree of strength and pliability of the bone. For example, the ratios of compact-to-spongy bone are ~25:75 in vertebra, 50:50 in the femoral head, and 95:5 in the diaphysis of the radius (2). The outermost layer of the bone is the *periosteum*. The periosteum consists of two layers of importance. The outermost layer provides a firm base for CT attachment. The innermost layer secretes cells involved in bone remodeling. The *endosteum* is the innermost layer that surrounds the medullary cavity, which also secretes cells involved in bone remodeling. The medullary cavity houses bone marrow.

The internal anatomy of a long bone is shown in Figure 6.5. The layer of compact bone is highly organized. Compact and spongy bones are composed of basic structural units known as osteons. The *osteon* in compact bone resembles a concentric layer of a mineralized matrix with a central canal that provides a conduit for nerves and blood vessels. A cellular look shows the mature bone cells, the *osteocytes*, as well as the surrounding bone matrix comprise osteons, which are ~0.2 mm in diameter. Osteons are aligned parallel to the bone axis and contain lamellae (concentric layers of bone), which surround the central (haversian) canal. Collagen fibers within the lamellae are oriented in longitudinal, perpendicular, and oblique directions. Lamellae in spongy bone are more irregular as the trabeculae

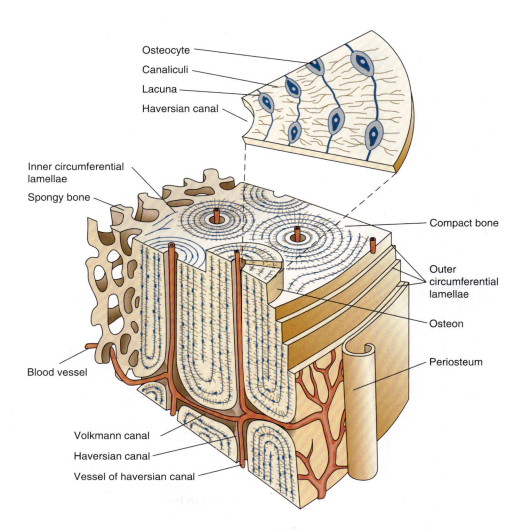

FIGURE 6.5 Internal anatomy of a long bone. (From Porth CM. *Pathophysiology Concepts of Altered Health States*. 7th ed. Philadelphia (PA): Lippincott Williams & Wilkins; 2005.)

osteons are composed of a network of plates and rods known as packets. Below, it is shown that the osteocyte is housed within the *lacunae* (space) and is surrounded by canaliculi. The *canaliculi* act similar to a capillary bed in that nutrients are dispersed throughout thereby supplying the osteocyte. Canaliculi play a major role in how bones adapt to loading as they deform during fluid movement, which stimulates the osteocytes. The area surrounding the osteocyte is known as the *bone matrix*. The bone matrix consists of an organic (~35%) and inorganic (~65%) region. The organic region consists primarily of protein, most of which is in the form of collagen, which helps give bone strength and pliability. Collagen (mostly type I) comprises ~85%–90% of the bone matrix protein, while the remaining 10%–15% is composed by glycosaminoglycans (*e.g.*, decorin, aggrecan), glycoproteins (*e.g.*, alkaline phosphatase, osteonectin), osteopontin, bone sialoprotein, osteocalcin, and several others (2). Collectively, these proteins are involved in matrix organization and stability, mineralization, and remodeling. The inorganic region consists of minerals and specialized cells that help ossify bone known as *hydroxyapatites*. Hydroxyapatites (calcium-phosphate based) are the primary mineral component found primarily between collagen fibers. The inorganic region is important for giving bone its stiffness and compression strength. Overall, bone consists of ~25%–30% of its content in water.

Bone Remodeling

Bone remodeling is the process where packets of old bone is catabolized and replaced by new bone, whereas *bone modeling* is the process by which bone adapts to mechanical loading. Bone is constantly broken down and built up again. Remodeling takes place in four general phases: (a) activation, (b) resorption, (c) reversal, and (d) formation (Fig. 6.6). Activation involves the recruitment and activation of catabolic bone cells known as *osteoclasts*. Osteoclasts are derived from the monocyte-macrophage cell cycle lineage, which first is formed in an inactive parent form known as a preosteoclast (or pro-osteoclast). Activated osteoclasts bind to the bone matrix and digest the mineralized region via acids and enzymes

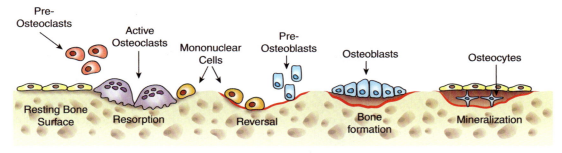

FIGURE 6.6 The bone remodeling cycle. (Redrawn from internet image available at https://www.orthopaedicsone.com/display/Clerkship/Describe+the+process+of+bone+remodeling)

(*i.e.*, tartrate-resistant acid phosphatase, cathepsin K, gelatinase, and matrix metalloproteinase), thereby breaking down bone (2). Osteoclast activation is under the control of *receptor activator of NF-κB ligand* (RANKL; cytokine required for osteoclast formation) and other cytokines such as *macrophage colony-stimulating factor 1* (CSF-1; cytokine required for proliferation and differentiation of osteoclast precursors), *osteoprotegerin* (and its ratio to RANKL), TNF-α, IL-1 and IL-6, growth factors, hormones, physical activity, and nutrients. Osteoprotegerin (OPG) is a protein that acts as a decoy receptor and binds RANKL with high affinity to inhibit receptor activation and thus inhibits osteoclast differentiation and bone resorption. The *OPG* gene is a target of canonical Wnt/β-catenin signaling to reduce bone catabolism (3). Resorption lasts ~2–4 weeks per remodeling cycle.

Reversal comprises the transition between bone resorption and formation. Bone formation is brought about by specialized activated cells known as *osteoblasts*. Activated osteoblasts are derived first from mesenchymal stem cells and subsequently from the osteochondral progenitor cell (OPC) lineage to the inactive preosteoblast (or pro-osteoblast). Osteoblasts are activated via specific hormones and growth factors (such as *bone morphogenetic proteins*), and critical to OPC proliferation and osteoblast differentiation is canonical Wnt/β-catenin signaling and other transcription factors such as runt-related transcription factor 2 (RUNX2) and osterix (SP7). Control of bone growth is accomplished, in part, through regulation of osteoblast differentiation. *Sclerostin* (a product of the *SOST* gene that is expressed in osteocytes) is a protein that regulates OPC proliferation, osteoblast differentiation, and regulation of mineralization genes, thereby regulating bone mass increases (Fig. 6.7). It inhibits Wnt/β-catenin–induced signaling. The absence of sclerostin leads to exaggerated bone formation, and the *SOST* gene is regulated by cytokines, growth factors, and hormones (3). It appears that sclerostin acts to regulate the magnitude of bone growth via negative feedback. Preosteoblasts are recruited to the area of resorption, bind to the matrix forming an osteoid of bone lining cells, and secrete a collagen-rich ground substance (to help form the bone matrix), noncollagen proteins, and regulate mineralization that aids in bone formation once they are activated. They are secreted by the periosteum and endosteum and secrete *osteocalcin*, which serves as a blood marker for bone metabolism. Osteoblasts secrete an enzyme known as *bone alkaline phosphatase* (involved in bone mineralization), which has been used as a blood marker of bone metabolism. It has been shown that numerous microRNAs play critical roles in the differentiation of osteoclasts and osteoblasts (4). Bone formation takes ~4–6 months to complete. The product is an osteon that is located within compact or spongy bone. Compact bone has a

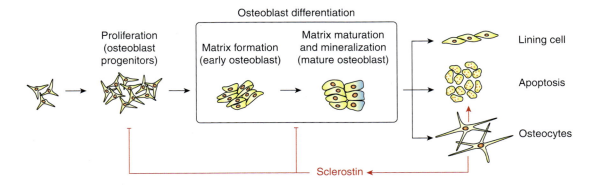

FIGURE 6.7 Osteoblast differentiation and sclerostin. (From https://www.semanticscholar.org/paper/Osteocyte-derived-sclerostin-inhibits-bone-its-role-Dijke-Krause/1148c1b3662ddfe42b8a9b1e19d92d200686c6eb)

slow turnover rate of ~2%–3% per year, whereas spongy bone turnover rate is much higher (2).

As shown in Figure 6.7, differentiated osteoblasts may form bone lining cells, die (apoptosis; ~50–70% of osteoblasts), or terminally differentiate to the mature bone cell known as the osteocyte subsequently becoming entrapped in the matrix. Osteocytes account for 90%–95% of all bone cells and have a very long lifespan of decades compared to other types of cells. They have integral proteins (*connexins*) that maintain gap junctions that allows direct cell-to-cell communication (2). Critical to the osteocyte is its role in mechanotransduction where it acts as a sensor for mechanical loading (discussed later in this chapter).

Bone Growth

Bones grow in both length and width. Longitudinal bone growth occurs during our developmental years and occurs primarily in two ways. Bone growth resulting from CT membranes is known as *intramembranous ossification*, whereas growth from cartilage is known as *endochondral ossification*. After the first few years of life, bones continue to develop mostly by endochondral ossification. Longitudinal bone growth takes place at the growth plate. The epiphyses enlarge by growth of cartilage and bone replacement as the diaphysis extends. Each bone has its own rate of metabolism; therefore, some bones fully reach their final length by age 18–20 (*i.e.*, femur, tibia), and some may take as long as 25 years (*i.e.*, some bones of the spine and thorax) of age. Changes in longitudinal length are supported by changes in bone width or *appositional growth*.

Of interest to discussion of adaptations to exercise is the process by which skeletal loading increases bone size and strength. Bone strength is determined by its mass and stiffness. An increase in bone CSA allows bone to tolerate greater loading (Fig. 6.8). Muscle strength and size gains increase the force exerted on the bones. Stronger forces of contraction and ground reaction forces increase the mechanical stress (and strain) on bone, and bone must increase its size to accommodate larger muscles. The elements critical to bone stiffness are the collagen content and the magnitude of mineralization. Bone responds to loading intracellularly by a general process known as *mechanotransduction* or the transduction of a mechanical force into a local cellular signal. In this model, mechanical loading applied to bone causes deformation or bending of the bone. Bending is proportional to the magnitude and rate of loading applied, thereby demonstrating the importance of exercise intensity. Bending may occur as a result of direct compressive loading to the skeletal system or by forces associated with tendons pulling during muscular contraction. Deformation to bone causes fluids to move within the bone increasing the fluid flow shear stress, hydrostatic pressure (5), and creates electrical charges resulting from ion movement. In order for this model to be effective, a sensor is needed to perceive this stimulus. The sensor in bone is mostly the osteocyte (although new evidence suggests that osteoblasts and osteoclasts may be mechanosensitive as well), which has the ability to control osteoblast and osteoclast activity in response to loading (5).

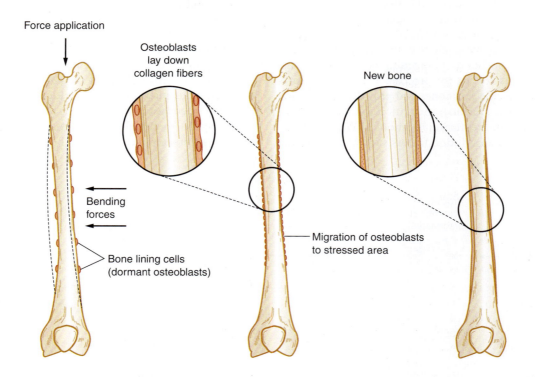

FIGURE 6.8 Model for bone adaptation to loading.

The osteocyte is thought to be activated via integrins (which link the cytoskeleton to the extracellular matrix and increases focal adhesion kinase–induced signaling), cilia, calcium channels, and G-protein–coupled receptors (5). That is, deformation of the osteocyte membrane via activation of these components increases intracellular signaling. Intracellular signaling pathways are thought to be mediated by calcium, ATP, nitric oxide, Wnt/β-catenin, and prostaglandins. In fact, there are anabolic pathways seen in bone also seen in skeletal muscle (*e.g.*, MAPK, mTOR). The main result is to increase gene transcription and translation of proteins ultimately leading to bone deposition and structural changes. A number of genes are targeted via mechanosensitive signaling, including those modulating the expression of sclerostin, RANKL, OPG, and several other growth factors and mineralizing proteins (5). Down-regulation of the *SOST* gene and sclerostin appear critical to mechanotransduction (3). Ultimately, collagen fibers form a scaffold, hydroxyapatites migrate, and osteoblasts reach the targeted area resulting in bone ossification. Although these processes are engaged quickly, measurable bone growth is very slow and may take at least 6–8 months (6).

Bone Adaptations to Exercise

Exercise poses a potent stress to the skeletal system whereby changes in bone mass, shape, and microarchitecture may take place. A significant number of studies have shown that long-term training increases bone mass and strength (7). However, the stress must reach a certain level in order for bones to adapt. The term **minimal essential strain** is defined as the minimal threshold stimulus (volume and intensity) that is needed for new bone formation (8). If the exercise stimulus does not reach this threshold, then there is no need for bones to adapt favorably. In fact, some studies that have shown no effect of training on bone mass used low training intensities (6). The minimal essential strain depends upon an athlete's training status and age as individuals with lower bone mass may be responsive to a lower stimulus, whereas trained individuals may require higher magnitude and rates of loading (7). Exercise needs to be of sufficient intensity and volume to elicit increases in bone mass, bone mineral content, and bone mineral density (BMD). Total body and regional BMD are commonly used to study bone adaptations. However, bone strength can increase independently of changes in BMD (6). Bones can become stronger at a much larger rate and magnitude (via architectural changes) than the potential increases seen in BMD. An increase in BMD of 5% may increase bone strength by 65% (9). It has been suggested that the minimal essential strain is approximately one-tenth of the force required to fracture bone. Certain exercises are better than others for increasing BMD, and bones tend to adapt more favorably in regions under higher strain. Dynamic, high-intensity loading to the skeletal system is paramount. This appears to be the case in athletes and trained populations but was also shown in postmenopausal women with low bone mass where heavy resistance training (RT) was superior for increasing BMD and was well tolerated (no injuries or adverse events)

by trainees (10). Weight-bearing exercise is more effective than non–weight-bearing exercise for increasing BMD as loading magnitude and rate are higher when an individual has to bear his or her bodyweight. Lifting and contact sports, and sports/activities requiring explosive running/jumping ground reaction forces (plyometrics, sprint, and agility) are excellent means to increase BMD, whereas swimming is less effective because of the buoyancy of water decreasing stress on the skeletal system. Several RT and plyometric training studies have shown increased whole-body and regional BMD (11,12). A review of 18 studies examining 5–24 months of plyometric training in children, adolescents, and women showed that plyometric training increased bone mass by 1%–8% in the children and adolescents and by 1%–4% in premenopausal women (13). In 2004, the American College of Sports Medicine (ACSM) (6) published a position stand recommending the following training guidelines for increasing bone mass:

- Weight-bearing endurance exercises, activities that involve jumping, and RT
- Moderate to high exercise intensities
- Endurance exercise frequency of 3–5 days per week, RT frequency of 2–3 days per week
- Exercise for 30–60 minutes per day involving multiple training modalities (RT, endurance training)

Research shows a positive relationship between BMD in various sites and muscle mass and strength (14,15). Stronger individuals tend to have higher BMD values than less-fit populations. Many groups of athletes (*i.e.*, weightlifters, powerlifters, boxers, soccer, football, volleyball, track and field jumpers, sprinters, and hurdlers) have higher BMD than age-matched untrained populations (6,15–17). Resistance-trained athletes have higher BMD in the lumbar spine and proximal femur than age-matched sedentary individuals (14,17). A case study examining a male powerlifting world record holder in the back squat showed the highest recorded lumbar spine BMD (18). Another case study examining 48- and 54-year-old female powerlifters (with >30 years of experience) showed remarkably high total body BMD and lumbar spine and femur BMD compared to age- and gender-matched norms (19). Olympic weightlifters have greater regional BMD of the vertebrae (by 13%–42%), femoral neck/trochanter (by 12%–24%), tibia (by 9%–12%), and radius (by 10%) compared to untrained controls (20). Contact sport athletes, *e.g.*, martial artists, have higher total body BMD than long-distance runners and swimmers (21), and water polo athletes (22). National Football League (NFL) football players have high bone mineral content and spine BMD (23) and NCAA Division I football players may increase total body bone mineral content and BMD over the course of 1 year and throughout their careers (*i.e.*, year 4 compared to year 1) (24). Endurance runners have higher lower-limb BMD than controls but not in the upper body or lumbar spine (16). Power athletes have higher lumbar spine BMD than middle-distance and distance runners (16). Endurance cyclists have 8%–10% less lumbar spine BMD than age-matched controls (25). Soccer players have been shown to have greater total body and regional

BMD, and cortical bone CSA and thickness, trabecular volume and number in the tibia compared to resistance-trained non-athletes (26).

Bones typically have a longer adaptational period compared to soft tissues. Historically, BMD changes were seen after 6 months of training (12,27) and only if an individual trains beyond their current minimal essential strain. However, some recent studies have shown small, but significant, increases in whole-body and regional (*i.e.*, lumbar spine, femoral neck) bone mineral content and BMD within 9 weeks of RT and/or plyometric training (11). Other studies have shown small regional increases in BMD within 7–8 weeks of army basic training in women (28) and high-intensity interval training in untrained men and women (29). Thus, it appears bones may adapt positively sooner than once thought if the program is challenging.

The quantitative deposition of bone is a long process. The initial bone growth processes begin after the first few workouts. Bone metabolic markers in the blood can be measured to investigate potential increases in activation of bone anabolic processes as they are predictive of long-term changes in BMD. Common markers of bone metabolism include (30) the following:

- Bone alkaline phosphatase (BAP)—enzyme involved in bone mineralization and an indicator of osteoblast activity
- Osteocalcin—secreted by osteoblasts and thought to serve as a marker of osteoblast activity: binds to hydroxyapatites during mineralization and may act like a hormone for other metabolic functions
- N- and C-terminal propeptides of type I collagen (PINP, PICP)—enzymes involved in collagen formation
- Tartrate-resistant acid phosphatase 5b (TRAP)—indicator of osteoclast number and marker of bone resorption
- Deoxypyridinoline and hydroxylysylpyridinoline (DPD, PYR)—markers of osteoclast activity
- C- and N-terminal cross-linking telopeptide of type I collagen (CTX, NTX)—by-products of bone collagen breakdown
- C-terminal cross-linked telopeptide of type I procollagen (ICTP)—by-product of bone collagen breakdown

Acute intense exercise has the ability to alter blood concentrations of markers of bone formation and resorption (from hours to days following), although the response is highly variable (30). Bone formation markers (osteocalcin, BAP, PICP) and resorption markers (ICTP, CTX, PYR, TRAP) have shown variable responses where both types were shown to increase, decrease, or do not change following various types of resistive and aerobic exercise depending on the time course (30). The tendency from most studies is resorption markers tend to increase with a variable formation marker response (30). Long-term training studies have shown more consistent elevations in formation markers (30). Baseline osteocalcin concentrations are related to whole-body bone mineral content, BMD, lean mass, and muscle strength (11). High-intensity anaerobic exercise can elevate osteocalcin concentrations (31,32). Weightlifters have higher osteocalcin concentrations (by 35%) than age-matched control subjects (33). Resistance training elevates osteocalcin (and BAP) (34,35) and the magnitude is affected by protein intake (36,37), although no changes in BAP have been reported (12). U.S. Army basic training increases serum BAP, ICTP, and TRAP by 10%–28% (28). Combined RT and plyometric training (for 9 weeks) increased serum osteocalcin by 45% and 27% in men and women, respectively (11). Both RT and plyometric training independently increased baseline osteocalcin after 6 months and 1 year of training and reduced CTX after 6 months of training (12). High-intensity RT and low-intensity RT with blood flow restriction for 6 weeks increase serum BAP (21%–23%), reduce CTX, and increase the ratio of BAP/CTX in older men (38). RT may have no chronic effect on TRAP (12). The mechanisms of bone growth are engaged within the first few workouts but take several months before measurable changes are seen.

Training has the ability to alter bone signaling molecules. Mechanical loading negatively regulates *SOST* gene expression, as do androgens and estrogens (3). In fact, segments of compact bone that are more heavily stressed in training and exhibit higher bone formation also show a reduction in the number of sclerostin-positive osteocytes (3). One year of RT or plyometric training has been shown to reduce baseline serum sclerostin concentrations by 9.5% and 4.5%, respectively (39). U.S. Army basic training (8 weeks) in women may decrease serum sclerostin by 5%–7% (28). See Interpreting Research: Bone Mineral Density Changes Following 1 Year of Training.

Interpreting Research
Bone Mineral Density Changes Following 1 Year of Training

Cussler EC, Lohman TG, Going SB, et al. Weight lifted in strength training predicts bone change in postmenopausal women. *Med Sci Sports Exerc*. 2003;35:10–7.

Although it has long been speculated that heavier weights yield greater increases in BMD, very little long-term research has been conducted to explore this phenomenon. Cussler et al. (40) studied postmenopausal women over the course of 1 year of RT, *i.e.*, eight exercises, two sets of 6–8 repetitions (70%–80% of 1-RM), and 3 days per week. They measured BMD before and after 1 year of RT. They found a linear relationship between changes in BMD in site-specific regions and the amount of weight lifted during training. The weights lifted in the squat exercise showed the highest relationship to BMD increases in the femur. This study demonstrated the importance of lifting progressively heavier loads when training to increase BMD.

Training to Increase Bone Size and Strength

Training programs designed to stimulate bone growth need to incorporate specificity of loading, speed and direction of loading, volume, proper exercise selection, progressive overload, and variation (6–8). Although the scientific study of program differentiation on bone growth is limited, the following general recommendations may be helpful:

- Multijoint exercises (squats, power cleans, dead lifts, bench press) are preferred because they enable the individual to lift greater loads. Exercises should also target key areas such as the lumbar and thoracic spine and hip/femur area as well as the upper extremities.
- Loading should be high with moderate to low volume (10 repetitions and less) with multiple (at least 2–3) sets per exercise. Although moderate loading may have some efficacy in lesser-trained populations, heavier loading is needed with progression to higher levels of training status.
- Fast velocities of contraction are preferred as force is proportional to acceleration, and increasing the force requirement on skeletal muscles produces greater stress on bone.
- Rest intervals should be moderate to long in length (at least 2–3 min) to accommodate greater loading during each set.
- Most studies showing increased BMD used frequencies of 2–3 days per week with some as high as 6 days per week for RT, plyometric, or combined training.
- Variation in the training stress is important for altering the stimuli to bone.

Case Study 6.1

Brenda is a 35-year-old woman who has been weight training for 5 years. A primary goal she wanted to attain was to increase her bone mass to prevent osteoporosis as she ages. At a recent checkup, her physician ordered a bone scan to assess her BMD. It was reported that her BMD did not change in the past 5 years (since the last time she had the test performed). Brenda is confused because she had joined a health club and was working out consistently over the past 5 years. Thus, she anticipated increasing her BMD to some extent. Upon examination of her program, Brenda exercised aerobically 1 day per week and worked out with weights 2 days per week during this time period. Her cardiovascular exercise consisted of stationary cycling for 20 minutes and her weight training consisted of predominantly machine-based exercises for three sets of 10–15 repetitions with loads corresponding to ~30%–45% of her maximal potential. She has performed this same training routine for the majority of the 5 years with little change to the intensity, volume, and exercise selection.

Question for Consideration: What advice would you give to Brenda regarding how she could change her program to more effectively target bone growth?

Components of Dense Connective Tissue

Ligaments connect articulating bones together across a joint, whereas tendons attach muscles to bones. Although many tendons' main function is to transmit force to bones (and store elastic energy), some smaller tendons mainly function to facilitate motion. Tendons and ligaments are dense fibrous CT structures composed of predominantly water (60%–70% of content), stem cells (*i.e.*, tendon stem cells), *fibroblasts* (cells that synthesize components of the *extracellular matrix*) and *fibrocytes* (mature cells that make up ~20% of tissue volume), elastin, collagen, and ground substances. Collagen fibers, elastin, water, and the ground substances comprise the extracellular matrix (ECM), which makes up ~80% of tissue volume. Ground substances fill the space between cells and fibers and help provide structural stability to CT. Ground substances include structural glycoproteins (fibronectin, tenascin-C, fibrillins), proteoglycans (decorin, biglycan, aggrecan), and small amounts of glycosaminoglycans (chondroitin sulfate, hyaluronic acid, dermatan sulfate). Ground substances provide support and spacing between cells and the ECM and bind collagen and help with fiber aggregation.

Elastin is a protein that gives CT its elastic quality, whereas collagen is the strongest, most abundant (20%–25% of total protein) protein in the human body. Elastin comprises 20%–30% of ECM protein content in ligaments but only ~2% in tendons. Collagen provides great tensile strength, which is why it is found in tissues requiring support and strength. There are many types of collagen. Type I is found in skin, bones, tendons, and ligaments, whereas type II is found in cartilage. Tendons and ligaments also possess small amounts of collagen types III, V, VII, IX, X, XI, XII, and XIV with regional differences seen between different tendons and ligaments. Collagen comprises ~70%–80% of ECM protein content in ligaments and >86% in tendons giving tendons greater strength and stiffness. On average, tendons, ligaments, bone, and skeletal muscle have ~677, 510, 307, and 59 nmol·g^{-1} wt of collagen, respectively, demonstrating that tendons are highest in collagen (41). Fibrils in ligaments tend to display a random (longitudinal and oblique) weaving pattern to better tolerate shear loading, whereas tendon fibrils display an organized pattern along the long axis to better tolerate tensile loading.

Figures 6.9 and 6.10 show a collagen fiber and assembly of collagen molecules. Collagen provides strength primarily for two reasons. It is structured in parallel to form larger components. Collagen molecules are as follows: (a) self-assembled or polymerized to microfibrils, (b) microfibrils aggregate to form fibrils, (c) fibrils are stacked in parallel to form fibers, and (d) fibers form a collagen bundle that forms the structure of tendons and ligaments. Connective tissue surrounds the collagen fibers, *e.g.*, endotendon, and the entire tendon, *e.g.*, *epitendon* and *paratendon*. Collagen fiber number and diameter vary between different tendons (42). The fibril is the load-bearing unit. The second major reason is its structure. The collagen

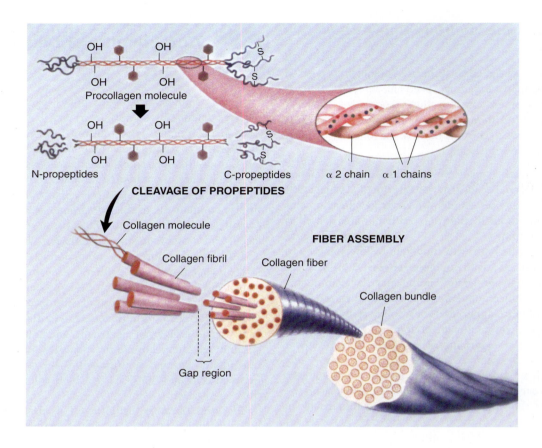

FIGURE 6.9 Structure of collagen.

molecule (or *tropocollagen*) is activated from its parent molecule, *procollagen*, and consists of a triple helix of three chains of >1,400 amino acids in each. Collagen consists mostly of three amino acids, proline (~25%), hydroxyproline (~25%), and glycine (~33%). These amino acids are essential because they help form very tight hydrogen bonds in between collagen molecules. These bonds are called cross-links and provide great strength to the collagen fibers similar to what may be seen in a rope. Cross-links may be formed enzymatically (via *lysyl oxidase*) or nonenzymatically. Collagen molecules are arranged in series and in parallel to form microfibrils. Collagen turnover (the net change in collagen content from synthesis and degradation) is important for determining CT strength and is highly related to stretch and loading (41). Tendon collagen synthesis rate has been estimated at ~2%–3% per 24 hours (41). See Myths and Misconceptions: Resistance Training Will Stunt Bone Growth in Children and Adolescents.

Tendons have a higher proportion of collagen, whereas ligaments possess a higher proportion of elastin. In fact, the collagen content in tendons and ligaments are both higher than bone and much higher than skeletal muscle (41). Tendons provide great strength and passive energy absorption, whereas ligaments tend to be more pliable. Tendon compliance is critical to muscle contraction as they increase the functional range of the muscle-tendon complex. The muscle-tendon complex must be compliant for elastic energy storage and use but also display a degree of stiffness for force transmission. Tendons elongate under force production, store elastic energy, and release the elastic energy during subsequent muscle shortening. It has been shown that stored and released elastic energy from the Achilles (calcaneal) tendon contributes ~6% and 16%, respectively, to the total external work produced during walking and jumping (53). Some elastic energy is lost as heat via a process known as *hysteresis*. A compliant tendon may store and utilize more elastic energy. Tendons produce elastic force when stretched with a magnitude dependent on the stiffness and magnitude of length increase. Muscle-tendon stiffness has been associated with strength and power assessments (54) and changes (or reductions) in *electromechanical delay* (EMD; the time between muscle activation and force production) (55). Reductions in EMD are thought to enhance muscle performance during exercise. Absolute muscle-tendon stiffness is higher in men than in women. Tendon metabolism is slower because of poor circulation. CTs that surround and separate different organizational levels within skeletal muscle are referred to as *fascia*. Fascia contains bundles of collagen fibers arranged in different planes to provide resistance to forces from different directions. Fascia within skeletal muscle converges to form a tendon through which the force of muscle contraction is transmitted to bone.

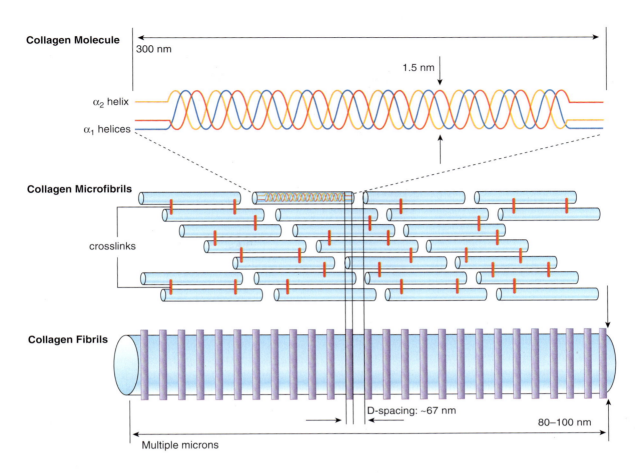

FIGURE 6.10 Collagen arrangement. (Available at https://www.researchgate.net/figure/Model-of-hierarchical-structure-of-collagen-fibrils-Three-helical-two-a-1-one-a-2_fig1_319489789)

Myths & Misconceptions
Resistance Training Will Stunt Bone Growth in Children and Adolescents

One common myth and misconception is RT will stunt a child's growth. However, this is not the case. Of primary concern for a child or adolescent is that the epiphyseal (growth) plates have not fully ossified. Depending on the bone in question, growth plates completely ossify between the ages of 18 and 25 years but occur a few years earlier in females compared to males. A concern exists that a growth plate injury can occur to a child via trauma or overuse. In general, most injuries (fractures) occurring to growth plates will have full recovery provided that blood flow is adequate during healing. Although growth can be temporarily stunted during the injury period, bone metabolism will increase higher than normal following this period resulting in bone growth reaching its normal level (a phenomenon known as *catch-up growth*). Although some growth plate injuries are very serious and pose potential growth problems, full recovery is seen in most cases. Resistance training is a very safe form of exercise for children and adolescents provided that it is supervised and proper recommendations are followed. Although some injuries to children and adolescents have occurred during RT, these were mostly the result of lack of supervision leading to very poor technique, loading, or accidents (43–45). Research has shown that RT in children and adolescents is very safe when properly supervised and has concluded that RT does not negatively impact growth and maturation (43–47). In fact, position stands developed by the National Strength and Conditioning Association and Canadian Society for Exercise Physiology and International Consensus Statement on Youth RT recommend RT as a safe, effective, and worthwhile exercise modality in children and adolescents (43,48,49). Although there is no minimal age requirement (children should be mature enough to be able to listen and follow directions), children as young as 6 years of age have participated safely in RT programs. Some recommendations (43–45,48) include the following:

- Beginning with low to moderate intensities for 6–15 repetitions with gradual increase to higher intensities or loads (by 5%–10%) as technique improves
- 1–4 sets per exercise

- 1–3 sets of 3–6 repetitions for upper and lower body power exercises
- 2–3 nonconsecutive days per week
- Single- and multijoint exercises including weightlifting derivatives

A multiple-modality approach to RT is recommended for children and adolescents. In addition to free weights, machines, and associated equipment, other modalities are shown to be safe and effective for improving fitness in these populations. For example, *integrative neuromuscular training* (INT) has emerged as an effective strategy to improve health- and skill-related fitness components in children and adolescents (50). It is characterized by intermittent bouts of multimodal activities designed to increase fitness and fundamental movement skills. INT involves the integration of weight training with multiple modalities of equipment that provides resistance to the young trainee. For example, it was shown that use of battling ropes and medicine balls are safe, well-tolerated, and an effective means of increasing the cardiometabolic stimulus of resistance exercise (51,52). Thus, RT in all forms can be safe for participation by children and adolescents provided that proper instruction, supervision, and technique-driven progression are utilized.

Tendon, Ligament, and Fascial Adaptations to Training

The major stimulus for growth of tendons, ligaments, and fascia is mechanical loading, which leads to a cascade of events leading to changes in the cytoskeleton, ECM, gene transcription, protein synthesis, and potential hypertrophy. These processes are analogous to the mechanotransduction of skeletal muscle and bone previously discussed. Stretching of the cytoskeleton in response to a threshold level of loading appears to be the stimulus leading to region-specific greater net collagen synthesis, ECM components, and CT growth in a dose-response manner (41,56). CT cells (*i.e.*, fibroblasts, fibrocytes, or tenocytes) deformed in response to loading increase intracellular signaling via cell-ECM coupling via adhesion molecules (integrins), which act as a sensor to the mechanical stimulus. Integrins provide a mechanical pathway by which force can be transmitted from the outside to the inside. Fibrocytes communicate and transmit force between cells via gap junctions formed by protein networks, *e.g.*, *cadherins* and *connexins*. Internally, cadherins are linked to catenin proteins ultimately connecting the junctional proteins to the actin cytoskeleton (57). The linked ECM-cellular components create a mechano-signaling network that increases gene transcription and up-regulates components of the ECM. Fibrocytes respond by secreting cytokines and growth factors (*e.g.*, transforming growth factor-β1 [TGF-β1], connective tissue growth factor [CTGF], plasma-derived growth factor [PDGF], vascular endothelial growth factor [VEGF], IL-1, IL-6, and IGF-1), which stay local in an autocrine/paracrine manner and bind to receptors on fibrocytes, increase intracellular signaling, and subsequently increase gene transcription and collagen synthesis (mostly type I and some type III) and production of ground substances (see Fig. 6.11) (42,58,59). Mechanical loading increases the proliferation and differentiation of tendon stem cells under normal (*i.e.*, nonovertraining or injurious) conditions (42). The degree of adaptation is proportional to the intensity of exercise. Regional adaptations within a tendon take place in response to overload

---

Sidebar   Tendon Responses and Adaptations to Training

Adaptation

Increased tendon strength, thickness, and CSA
Increased tendon stiffness and stiffness at high strain rates (Young modulus)
Increased elastic energy storage
Increased MMPs and TIMPs
Increased gene transcription, expression of growth factors, PICP and PINP (markers of collagen synthesis)
Increased collagen gene transcription and synthesis and reduced collagen degradation
Increased number and size of collagen fibrils
Increased lysyl oxidase activity and cross-linking
Increased tendon stem cell proliferation and differentiation
Increased number of fibroblasts and fibrocytes
Increased up-regulation of cytoskeletal and junctional proteins (*i.e.*, actin, cadherin, connexin) and ECM remodeling
Increased glycosaminoglycans, glycoproteins (*i.e.*, tenascin-C), and proteoglycans
Increased tendon blood flow
Decreased adhesions and inflammatory mediators

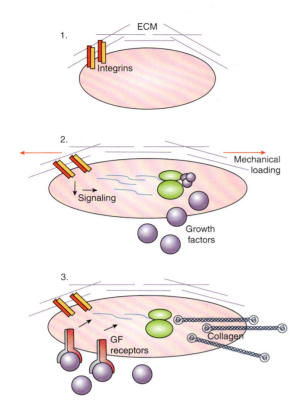

FIGURE 6.11 Tendon response to mechanical loading. *1* represents the resting state; *2* represents mechanical loading, mechanotransduction, intracellular signaling, and up-regulation of growth factors; *3* represents GF-receptor interaction and signaling leading to increased collagen synthesis. (Redrawn from Heinemeier KM, Kjaer M. In vivo investigation of tendon responses to mechanical loading. *J Musculoskelet Neuronal Interact.* 2011;11:115–23.)

with respect to CSA and ECM components. The Sidebar: Tendon Responses and Adaptations to Training depicts common responses and adaptations shown in CT in response to acute exercise and chronic training.

The sites where CT can increase strength are (a) at the junctions between the tendon/ligament and bone surface, *e.g.*, the *enthesis*; (b) within the body of the tendon/ligament; (c) the myotendinous junction; and (d) in the network of fascia within skeletal muscle. Tendon CSA differs along its length. Regional differences exist in those areas of tendons experiencing great mechanical loading increase stiffness and size more so than other regions, *i.e.*, the proximal and distal regions (57). The collagen content varies throughout regions of the tendon consistent with regions of higher loading. The myotendinous junction tends to be the weak link in force-related strain. The collagen content at the myotendinous junction is unique, consisting of types I, III, VI, XII, and XXII (which functions more like a linkage protein rather than a fibril component to stabilize sarcomeric binding) (60). It appears preferential hypertrophy of the tendon occurs at the periphery rather than the deeper segments (59). Muscle hypertrophy necessitates structural and/or CSA changes to tendons to accommodate the larger force

output. The increase in tendon stiffness and potential hypertrophy displays a pattern of progression that is initiated early to accommodate muscle performance changes. However, several positive training-induced tendon adaptations may be reversed (*e.g.*, reduced collagen synthesis, collagen dysplasia, excessive stiffness, reduced MMP-mediated remodeling, and reduced elasticity) with use of anabolic-androgenic steroids (42).

Exercise initiates the processes of tendon adaptations. Acute exercise (aerobic and anaerobic) initially results in collagen degradation; however, subsequent days following collagen synthesis rate increases significantly (41,57). Collagen turnover is critical to the remodeling process. Acute exercise increases the concentrations of *metalloproteinases* (*i.e.*, MMP-9, MMP-2), which are a family of proteolytic enzymes that break down collagen and components of the ECM (56). The actions of MMPs are inhibited by *tissue inhibitors of matrix metalloproteinases* (*i.e.*, TIMP-1, TIMP-2). Both MMPs and TIMPs are acutely elevated during and following exercise in a coordinated manner that augments repair of damaged collagen and ECM remodeling (61). TIMPs may serve as regulators of collagen degradation.

Type I collagen synthesis may be elevated during chronic training (41,56). It has been suggested that training initially results in increased type I collagen turnover to allow for organizational restructuring of the tissue and prolonged training results in an increase in tendon CSA (41,56). The increased collagen synthesis is less pronounced in women compared to men possibly due to the effects of higher estradiol concentrations in women (57). Tendons hypertrophy following as little as 12 weeks of RT (62), and runners have shown larger Achilles tendon CSA than untrained, age-matched sedentary individuals (41). Tendon CSA may increase up to 10% following 12–14 weeks of RT in young and older adults (63). A cross-sectional study examining resistance-trained individuals with a mean of 6–12 years of experience (who did or did not use anabolic steroids) showed patellar tendon CSA that was 19%–34% larger than and stiffness that was 21%–70% greater in anabolic steroid users compared to controls (64). Heavy RT may increase fibril density in individuals with patellar tendinopathy (65), and eccentric training has been used effectively to treat tendinopathies (66). Tendon stiffness (force transmitted per unit of strain) increases as a result of RT (56,67) and may comprise enhanced collagen cross-linking and organizational restructuring changes leading to increased tendon strength initially in the absence of hypertrophy. Kubo et al. (68) showed a 15%–19% increase in Achilles tendon stiffness following 8 weeks of RT. Of great importance is the intensity as heavy loads (70%–85% of 1-RM) increase tendon stiffness but light loads (20% of 1-RM or moderate elastic band training) may not (68–70). A review of the literature indicated that RT with ≥70% of MVC is of sufficient intensity to increase tendon stiffness and CSA (63). Achilles and patellar tendon stiffness and Young modulus (a mechanical property that is used as a measure of stiffness) may increase following 12–14 weeks of RT by 9%–83% in older adults and by 15%–45% in young adults (63). Interestingly, the response to training may be more prominent in men than in women (71). Decreased Achilles tendon stiffness (nearly 50%)

has been shown within 1 month of RT detraining to the point where it approached pretraining values (following a 3-month program) (72).

Endurance training (running) increases calf muscle-tendon stiffness by 19% (55). Muscle-tendon stiffness correlates with running economy in distance runners (73). However, tendon adaptations to plyometric training have shown contrasting results where some studies showed increased stiffness but others showed decrease despite performance improvements (13,55,74). It is possible that muscles and tendons may adapt differently regarding stiffness as Foure et al. (75) showed that plyometric training decreased muscle stiffness but increased Achilles tendon stiffness. Considering the components of elastic energy (SE) and elastic force (Force$_E$) (see equations below), increases in stiffness and/or muscle-tendon compliance could increase power performance.

$$SE = \frac{1}{2}k\Delta x^2 (k \text{ — stiffness constant}; x \text{ — change in length})$$

$$Force_E = kx (k \text{ — stiffness constant}; x \text{ — length change})$$

The combined effects of both ultimately affect performance rather than viewing stiffness independently. Reductions in tendon hysteresis have been shown following plyometric training (75). Flexibility training produces equivocal findings regarding changes in muscle-tendon stiffness. A review of the literature showed four studies found decreases in tendon stiffness following 3–6 weeks of flexibility training, whereas three studies reported increases (76). The authors reported trivial effects of flexibility training on muscle and tendon stiffness and suggested that increased stretch tolerance was the key factor for flexibility enhancement (76). Other studies have shown reduced muscle stiffness with no changes in tendon stiffness indicating that flexibility training may not decrease tendon stiffness (77). However, acute static stretching can reduce tendon stiffness temporarily contributing to increased joint ROM seen during exercise.

Tendon adaptations appear affected to some extent by hormones such as estradiol, androgens, growth hormone (GH), and IGF-1. Six weeks of training plus administration of recombinant human GH produced larger increases in patellar tendon stiffness and CSA than with a placebo in elderly men (78). Lastly, collagen synthesis in skeletal muscle increases during training, indicating adaptations taking place within fascia to accommodate skeletal muscle growth (56). Increased type I collagen synthesis occurs in the perimysium (56) and type XIV collagen content in the endomysium near the muscle-tendon junction following RT (60). See Interpreting Research: Tendon Growth and Resistance Training Loading.

Cartilage Adaptations to Training

Cartilage is composed of fluid (60%–80%), type II collagen (with small amounts of other types), chondrocytes, electrolytes, and other ground substances. Chondrocytes comprise ~10% of the volume of articular cartilage. Proteoglycans comprise ~30% of the dry weight of articular cartilage and are most concentrated deep in cartilage near the subchondral bone. Collagen comprises ~60%–70% of the articular cartilage dry weight. *Articular (hyaline) cartilage* is the type that covers the ends of long bones at joints and is found within the growth plate. *Fibrous cartilage* is found within intervertebral disks, menisci, and at the point of insertion into bone for tendons and ligaments. *Elastic cartilage* is flexible and found in the ear. Articular and fibrous cartilages are the types central to adaptations resulting from exercise as collectively they provide a smooth surface for joint motion, act as a shock absorber, and assist in providing strength to tendon and ligament attachments to bone. Articular cartilage has great strength (despite being relatively thin) due to the magnitude and arrangement of collagen fibers in the superficial, middle, and deep layers. When cartilage is compressed its stiffness increases to resist loading. Unique to cartilage is that it lacks its own blood supply and must receive its nutrients from *synovial fluid*. Thus, cartilage injuries have very long recovery periods and oftentimes require surgery. The process by which cartilage is perfused with synovial fluid highly depends upon physical activity. Compression and decompression of cartilage creates a pressure gradient by which synovial fluid may be absorbed into cartilage. Thus, articular cartilage acts like a sponge in relationship to fluid movement relative to loading

Interpreting Research
Tendon Growth and Resistance Training Loading

Kongsgaard M, Reitelseder S, Pedersen TG, et al. Region specific patellar tendon hypertrophy in humans following resistance training. *Acta Physiol.* 2007;191:111–21.

Kongsgaard et al. (62) examined patellar tendon CSA before and following a RT program. Subjects trained for 12 weeks using unilateral knee extensions. One group trained with heavy weights, whereas another group trained with light weights. After RT, maximal strength increased by 15% in the heavy weight group but did not significantly increase in the light weight group (~6%). Quadriceps muscle CSA increased (by 6%) in the heavy weight group. Light weight training increased proximal patellar tendon CSA and heavy weight training increased proximal and distal tendon CSA. Patellar tendon stiffness increased only after heavy weight training. The results showed that RT increased tendon CSA and that the changes were more comprehensive following heavy weight training.

and unloading, and moderate exercise creates a suitable environment for nutrient exchange and waste removal.

Cartilage deformation is a natural occurrence to most types of exercise. Mechanical loading for 4 hours can acutely reduce articular cartilage thickness by up to 57% with only ~1/3 of the deformation taking place during the first 8 minutes (79). Performing six sets of 50 bodyweight squats can reduce patellar cartilage volume by a mean of 6% with full recovery taking place 90 minutes postexercise (79). Running and vertical landings from jumps may reduce patellar, tibial, and femoral cartilage volume and thickness by 2.2%–9.6% (80,81). The deformation appears dose-dependent and enables the release of certain biomarkers from the ECM into synovial fluid and ultimately into circulation where they can be measured. Studies have shown increased serum concentrations of *cartilage oligomeric matrix protein* (COMP; a noncollagen glycoprotein that binds to type II collagen to help stabilize articular cartilage) by 14%–32% and *lubricin* (a proteoglycan that reduces friction during movement) by 31%–36% immediately following intense running and cycling, walking, vertical drop landings, and lower-body resistance exercise but returns to or near baseline within 30 min post (81–83). Another marker, *hyaluronan* (a glycosaminoglycan that helps stabilize the matrix), increases following exercise of rising intensity or does not change following walking or acute resistance exercise (83). Elevations of COMP are indicative of increased cartilage metabolism and turnover, transport from joint to blood, decreased cartilage volume, but can also reflect tissue damage. Elevations in lubricin may reflect increased joint lubrication during exercise.

Chondrocytes are mechano-sensitive cells thought to adapt to exercise. Animal studies have shown that aerobic exercise can increase articular cartilage thickness (25). Although significant relationships between cartilage volume and activity level have been shown in children, studies in trained adult populations have been conflicting (79). A trend for greater patellar cartilage thickness was shown in weightlifters and bobsledders, and larger joint surface areas have been shown in endurance athletes (79). Other studies have shown that regular exercise can preserve knee cartilage volume and thickness, increase proteoglycan content, and reduce cartilage defects (83). It is unclear if exercise training can increase cartilage thickness in adults or restore lost cartilage thickness in osteoarthritic populations. It appears that training may maintain cartilage thickness (and prevent age/hypoactivity declines) or produce structural changes to the articular surfaces that assist in improving joint stability and load absorption over time.

A major concern regarding articular cartilage is the potential for joint degeneration. With aging, it appears that unloading via minimal exercise or excessive loading may lead to articular cartilage degeneration. Degeneration of articular cartilage can result in a pathological condition known as osteoarthritis. Moderate exercise appears to reduce cartilage degradation. For example, long-time runners have shown no greater prevalence for osteoarthritis compared to sedentary age-matched controls (84,85). However, joint injuries, excessive mechanical stress, and highly repetitive intense exercise upon injured or improperly healed joints pose a scenario where joint degeneration may ensue (86). Athletes from sports requiring great impact loading, *e.g.*, football, soccer, baseball, ice hockey, tennis, have been shown to be more susceptible to osteoarthritis primarily due to past injury (86,87). Buckwalter and Martin (86) have suggested that athletes most susceptible to joint degeneration are those with abnormal joint anatomy, previous joint injury and/or surgery, joint instability, heavy bodyweight, inadequate muscle strength, or altered muscle innervation. Regardless of the individual's past training regimen, it appears that moderate-to-vigorous exercise may be the best way to safeguard cartilage from age-related degeneration.

SUMMARY POINTS

◆ Stress is the level of force placed upon CT, and strain quantifies the magnitude of deformation resulting from stress. Strain is a potent stimulus for CT adaptations to training.
◆ Bone remodeling is a cycle of catabolic and anabolic activities. Chronic training above the minimal essential strain results in remodeling favoring bone anabolism, or growth, via mechanotransduction.
◆ Bone mineral density increases during training are typically greater during weight-bearing exercise, explosive exercise, and high-intensity contact sports.
◆ Recommendations for increasing BMD during RT include multiple joint (especially free weight) exercises of high intensity for 10 repetitions or less performed with high levels of force and/or velocity.
◆ Tendons, ligaments, and fascia adapt to training favorably by increasing stiffness or CSA in order to accommodate greater muscle size and force production. CT adaptations take place at a slower rate compared to skeletal muscle.
◆ Cartilage adaptations to training are less clear and appear related to the duration, intensity, and volume of training, as well as an individual's injury history. The most critical concern may be the effect of training on prevention of cartilage degeneration.

REVIEW QUESTIONS

1. According to the ACSM, which of the following is recommended for enhancing bone mineral density in adults?
   a. Non–weight-bearing activities, low to moderate intensity, 15–30 minutes per day
   b. Non–weight-bearing activities, high intensity, 30–60 minutes per day
   c. Weight-bearing activities, low to moderate intensity, 15–30 minutes per day
   d. Weight-bearing activities, high intensity, 30–60 minutes per day

2. An untrained individual begins a weight-training program. What would be the expected increase in BMD during the first 4 months?

   a. <1%–2%
   b. 5%–10%
   c. 15%–20%
   d. 25%–30%

3. The protein that gives CT an abundance of strength is

   a. Elastin
   b. Collagen
   c. Osteon
   d. Endosteum

4. A joint pathology characterized by degeneration of articular cartilage is

   a. Osteoporosis
   b. Osteogenesis
   c. Osteoarthritis
   d. Osteoblast

5. Which of the following statements is true concerning CT adaptations to exercise?

   a. Connective tissue structures rapidly adapt to training at a pace quicker than skeletal muscle
   b. Connective tissue growth will only take place if the individual trains consistently beyond his or her minimal threshold level of strain
   c. Activities that are non–weight bearing and low in intensity are most effective for eliciting CT growth
   d. None of the above

6. Loading on the spine from placing a loaded barbell on the shoulders in preparation for performing the squat exercise is an example of a(n) _____ stress

   a. Shear
   b. Tensile
   c. Compressive
   d. Torsion

7. The property of CT to return to its original length after being stretched is elasticity.

   a. T
   b. F

8. Bone cells that help build up bone are osteoclasts.

   a. T
   b. F

9. The mature bone cell is known as an osteocyte.

   a. T
   b. F

10. The magnitude of changes in BMD are due, in part, to the level of strain encountered during exercise.

   a. T
   b. F

11. Injuries to articular cartilage heal relatively quickly because of the cartilage's great blood supply.

   a. T
   b. F

12. An elevation in a blood biomarker such as osteocalcin indicates bone anabolism may be taking place despite no noticeable changes in BMD.

   a. T
   b. F

REFERENCES

1. Enoka RM. *Neuromechanics of Human Movement*. 3rd ed. Champaign (IL): Human Kinetics; 2002. p. 132–5.
2. Clarke B. Normal bone anatomy and physiology. *Clin J Am Soc Nephrol*. 2008;3:S131–9.
3. Delgado-Calle J, Sato AY, Bellido T. Role and mechanism of action of sclerostin in bone. *Bone*. 2017;96:29–37.
4. Zhao X, Xu D, Li Y, et al. MicroRNAs regulate bone metabolism. *J Bone Miner Metab*. 2014;32:221–31.
5. Uda Y, Azab E, Sun N, Shi C, Pajevic PD. Osteocyte mechanobiology. *Curr Osteoporos Rep*. 2017;15:318–25.
6. American College of Sports Medicine. Position stand: physical activity and bone health. *Med Sci Sports Exerc*. 2004;36:1985–96.
7. Guadalupe-Grau A, Fuentes T, Guerra B, Calbet JAL. Exercise and bone mass in adults. *Sports Med*. 2009;39:439–68.
8. Ratamess NA. Adaptations to anaerobic training programs. In: Baechle TR, Earle RW, editors. *Essentials of Strength Training and Conditioning*. 3rd ed. Champaign (IL): Human Kinetics; 2008; p. 93–119.
9. Burr DB, Robling AG, Turner CH. Effects of biomechanical stress on bones in animals. *Bone*. 2002;30:781–6.
10. Watson SL, Weeks BK, Weis LJ, Harding AT, Horan SA, Beck BR. High-intensity resistance and impact training improves bone mineral density and physical function in postmenopausal women with osteopenia and osteoporosis: the LIFTMOR randomized controlled trial. *J Bone Miner Res*. 2018;33:211–20.
11. Guadalupe-Grau A, Perez-Gomez J, Olmedillas H, et al. Strength training combined with plyometric jumps in adults: sex differences in fat-bone axis adaptations. *J Appl Physiol*. 2009;106: 1100–11.
12. Hinton PS, Nigh P, Thyfault J. Effectiveness of resistance training or jumping-exercise to increase bone mineral density in men with low bone mass: a 12-month randomized, clinical trial. *Bone*. 2015;79:203–12.
13. Markovic G, Mikulic P. Neuro-musculoskeletal and performance adaptations to lower-extremity plyometric training. *Sports Med*. 2010;40:859–95.
14. Conroy BP, Kraemer WJ, Maresh CM, et al. Bone mineral density in elite junior Olympic weightlifters. *Med Sci Sports Exerc*. 1993;25:1103–9.
15. Wittich A, Mautalen CA, Oliveri MB, Bagur A, Somoza F, Rotemberg E. Professional football (soccer) players have a markedly greater skeletal mineral content, density, and size than age-and BMI-matched controls. *Calcif Tissue Int*. 1998;63:112–7.
16. Bennell KL, Malcolm SA, Khan KM, et al. Bone mass and bone turnover in power athletes, endurance athletes, and controls: a 12-month longitudinal study. *Bone*. 1997;20:477–84.

17. Sabo D, Bernd L, Pfeil J, Reiter A. Bone quality in the lumbar spine in high-performance athletes. *Eur Spine J*. 1996;5:258–63.

18. Dickerman RD, Pertusi R, Smith GH. The upper range of lumbar spine bone mineral density? An examination of the current world record holder in the squat lift. *Int J Sports Med*. 2000;21:469–70.

19. Walters PH, Jezequel JJ, Grove MB. Case study: bone mineral density of two elite senior female powerlifters. *J Strength Cond Res*. 2012;26:867–72.

20. Storey A, Smith HK. Unique aspects of competitive weightlifting: performance, training and physiology. *Sports Med*. 2012;42:769–90.

21. Matsumoto T, Nakagawa S, Nishida S, Hirota R. Bone density and bone metabolic markers in active collegiate athletes: findings in long-distance runners, judoists, and swimmers. *Int J Sports Med*. 1997;18:408–12.

22. Andreoli A, Monteleone M, Van Loan M, et al. Effects of different sports on bone density and muscle mass in highly trained athletes. *Med Sci Sports Exerc*. 2001;33:507–11.

23. Dengel DR, Bosch TA, Burruss TP, et al. Body composition and bone mineral density of National Football League players. *J Strength Cond Res*. 2014;28:1–6.

24. Trexler ET, Smith-Ryan AE, Mann JB, Ivey PA, Hirsch KR, Mock MG. Longitudinal body composition changes in NCAA Division 1 college football players. *J Strength Cond Res*. 2017;31:1–8.

25. Saaf RB. Effect of exercise on adult cartilage. *Acta Orthop Scand Suppl*. 1950;7:1–83.

26. Nilsson M, Ohlsson C, Mellstrom D, Lorentzon M. Sport-specific association between exercise loading and the density, geometry, and microstructure of weight-bearing bone in young adult men. *Osteoporos Int*. 2013;24:1613–22.

27. Chilibeck PD, Calder A, Sale DG, Webber CE. Twenty weeks of weight training increases lean tissue mass but not bone mineral mass or density in healthy, active young women. *Can J Physiol Pharmacol*. 1996;74:1180–5.

28. Hughes JM, Gaffney-Stomberg E, Guerriere KI, et al. Changes in tibial bone microarchitecture in female recruits in response to 8 weeks of U.S. Army Basic Combat Training. *Bone*. 2018;113:9–16.

29. Ravnholt T, Tybirk J, Jorgensen NR, Bangsbo J. High-intensity intermittent "5-10-15" running reduces body fat, and increases lean body mass, bone mineral density, and performance in untrained subjects. *Eur J Appl Physiol*. 2018;118:1221–30.

30. Banfi G, Lombardi G, Colombini A, Lippi G. Bone metabolism markers in sports medicine. *Sports Med*. 2010;40:697–714.

31. Creighton DL, Morgan AL, Boardley D, Brolinson PG. Weight-bearing exercise and markers of bone turnover in female athletes. *J Appl Physiol*. 2001;90:565–70.

32. Woitge HW, Friedmann B, Suttner S, Farahmand I, Muller M, Schmidt-Gayk H, et al. Changes in bone turnover induced by aerobic and anaerobic exercise in young males. *J Bone Miner Res*. 1998;13:1797–804.

33. Karlsson MK, Vergnaud P, Delmas PD, Obrant KJ. Indicators of bone formation in weight lifters. *Calcif Tissue Int*. 1995;56:177–80.

34. Fujimura R, Ashizawa N, Watanabe M, et al. Effect of resistance exercise training on bone formation and resorption in young male subjects assessed by biomarkers of bone metabolism. *J Bone Miner Res*. 1997;12:656–62.

35. Menkes A, Mazel S, Redmond RA, et al. Strength training increases regional bone mineral density and bone remodeling in middle-aged and older women. *J Appl Physiol*. 1993;74:2478–84.

36. Ballard TLP, Clapper JA, Specker BL, Binkley TL, Vukovich MD. Effect of protein supplementation during a 6-mo strength and conditioning program on insulin-like growth factor I and markers of bone turnover in young adults. *Am J Clin Nutr*. 2005;81:1442–8.

37. Ratamess NA, Hoffman JR, Faigenbaum AD, Mangine G, Falvo MJ, Kang J. The combined effects of protein intake and resistance training on serum osteocalcin concentrations in strength and power athletes. *J Strength Cond Res*. 2007;21:1197–203.

38. Karabulut M, Bemben DA, Sherk VD, et al. Effects of high-intensity resistance training and low-intensity resistance training with vascular restriction on bone markers in older men. *Eur J Appl Physiol*. 2011;111:1659–67.

39. Hinton PS, Nigh P, Thyfault J. Serum sclerostin decreases following 12 months of resistance-or jump-training in men with low bone mass. *Bone*. 2017;96:85–90.

40. Cussler EC, Lohman TG, Going SB, et al. Weight lifted in strength training predicts bone change in postmenopausal women. *Med Sci Sports Exerc*. 2003;35:10–7.

41. Kjaer M, Langberg H, Miller BF, et al. Metabolic activity and collagen turnover in human tendon in response to physical activity. *J Musculoskelet Neuronal Interact*. 2005;5:41–52.

42. Guzzoni V, Selistre de Araujo HS, Marqueti RC. Tendon remodeling in response to resistance training, anabolic androgenic steroids and aging. *Cells*. 2018;7:1–8.

43. Faigenbaum AD, Kraemer WJ, Blimkie J, et al. Youth resistance training: Updated position statement paper from the National Strength and Conditioning Association. *J Strength Cond Res*. 2009;23:S60–79.

44. Faigenbaum A, Lloyd R, MacDonald J, Myer G. *Citius, altius, fortius:* beneficial effects of resistance training for young athletes. *Br J Sports Med*. 2016;50:3–7.

45. Faigenbaum AD, Myer G. Resistance training among youth athlete: Safety, efficacy and injury prevention effects. *Br J Sports Med*. 2010;44:56–63.

46. Falk B, Eliakim A. Resistance training, skeletal muscle and growth. *Pediatr Endocrinol Rev*. 2003;1:120–7.

47. Malina RM. Weight training in youth—growth, maturation, and safety: an evidence-based review. *Clin J Sport Med*. 2006;16:478–87.

48. Behm DG, Faigenbaum AD, Falk B, Klentrou P. Canadian Society for Exercise Physiology position paper: resistance training in children and adolescents. *Appl Physiol Nutr Metab*. 2008;33:547–61.

49. Lloyd R, Faigenbaum A, Stone M, et al. Position statement on youth resistance training: the 2014 international consensus. *Br J Sports Med*. 2014;48:498–505.

50. Myer GD, Faigenbaum AD, Ford KR, et al. When to initiate integrative neuromuscular training to reduce sports-related injuries and enhance health in youth? *Curr Sports Med Rep*. 2011;10:155–66.

51. Faigenbaum A, Kang J, Ratamess N, et al. Acute cardiometabolic responses to a novel training rope protocol in children. *J Strength Cond Res*. 2018;32:1197–206.

52. Faigenbaum A, Kang J, Ratamess N, et al. Acute cardiometabolic responses to medicine ball interval training in children. *Int J Exerc Sci*. 2018;11:886–99.

53. Magnusson SP, Narici MV, Maganaris CN, Kjaer M. Human tendon behaviour and adaptation, *in vivo*. *J Physiol*. 2008;586:71–81.

54. Driss T, Lambertz D, Rouis M, Jaafar H, Vanderwalle H. Musculotendinous stiffness of triceps surae, maximal rate of force development, and vertical jump performance. *Biomed Res Int*. 2015;2015:797256.

55. Grosset JF, Piscione J, Lambertz D, Perot C. Paired changes in electromechanical delay and musculo-tendinous stiffness

56. Kjaer M, Magnusson P, Krogsgaard M, et al. Extracellular matrix adaptation of tendon and skeletal muscle to exercise. *J Anat.* 2006;208:445–50.

57. Kjaer M, Langberg H, Heinemeier K, et al. From mechanical loading to collagen synthesis, structural changes and function in human tendon. *Scand J Med Sci Sports.* 2009;19:500–10.

58. Heinemeier KM, Kjaer M. In vivo investigation of tendon responses to mechanical loading. *J Musculoskelet Neuronal Interact.* 2011;11:115–23.

59. Svensson RB, Heinemeier KM, Couppe C, Kjaer M, Magnusson SP. Effect of aging and exercise on the tendon. *J Appl Physiol.* 2016;121:1353–62.

60. Jakobsen JR, Mackey AL, Knudesn AB, Koch M, Kjaer M, Krogsgaard MR. Composition and adaptation of human myotendinous junction and neighboring muscle fibers to heavy resistance training. *Scand J Med Sci Sports.* 2017;27:1547–59.

61. Astill BD, Katsma MS, Cauthon DJ, et al. Sex-based difference in Achilles peritendinous levels of matrix metalloproteinases and growth factors after acute resistance exercise. *J Appl Physiol.* 2017;122:361–7.

62. Kongsgaard M, Reitelseder S, Pedersen TG, Holm L, Aagaard PL, Kjaer M, et al. Region specific patellar tendon hypertrophy in humans following resistance training. *Acta Physiol (Oxf).* 2007;191:111–21.

63. McCrum C, Leow P, Epro G, Konig M, Meijer K, Karamanidis K. Alterations in leg extensor muscle-tendon unit biomechanical properties with ageing and mechanical loading. *Front Physiol.* 2018;9:1–7.

64. Seynnes OR, Kamandulis S, Kairaitis R, et al. Effects of androgenic-anabolic steroids and heavy strength training on patellar tendon morphological and mechanical properties. *J Appl Physiol.* 2013;115:84–9.

65. Kongsgaard M, Ovortrup K, Larsen J, et al. Fibril morphology and tendon mechanical properties in patellar tendinopathy. Effects of heavy slow resistance training. *Am J Sports Med.* 2010;38:749–56.

66. Camargo PR, Alburquerque-Sendin F, Salvini TF. Eccentric training as a new approach for rotator cuff tendinopathy: Review and perspectives. *World J Orthop.* 2014;5:634–44.

67. Kubo K, Yata H, Kanehisa H, Fukunaga T. Effects of isometric squat training on the tendon stiffness and jump performance. *Eur J Appl Physiol.* 2006;96:305–14.

68. Kubo K, Kanehisa H, Fukunaga T. Effects of resistance and stretching training programmes on the viscoelastic properties of human tendon structures in vivo. *J Physiol.* 2002;538:219–26.

69. Eriksen CS, Svensson RB, Gylling AT, et al. Load magnitude affects patellar tendon mechanical properties but not collagen or collagen cross-linking after long-term strength training in older adults. *BMC Geriatr.* 2019;19:1–15.

70. Kubo K, Komuro T, Ishiguro N, et al. Effects of low-load resistance training with vascular occlusion on the mechanical properties of muscle and tendon. *J Appl Biomech.* 2006;22:112–9.

71. Westh E, Kongsgaard M, Bojsen-Moller J, et al. Effect of habitual exercise on the structural and mechanical properties of human tendon, in vivo, in men and women. *Scand J Med Sci Sports.* 2008;18:23–30.

72. Kubo K, Ikebukuro T, Maki A, Yata H, Tsunoda N. Time course of changes in the human Achilles tendon properties and metabolism during training and detraining in vivo. *Eur J Appl Physiol.* 2012;112:2679–91.

73. Saunders PU, Pyne DB, Telford RD, Hawley JA. Factors affecting running economy in trained distance runners. *Sports Med.* 2004;34:465–85.

74. Foure A, Nordez A, McNair P, Cornu C. Effects of plyometric training on both active and passive parts of the plantarflexors series elastic component stiffness of muscle-tendon complex. *Eur J Appl Physiol.* 2011;111:539–48.

75. Foure A, Nordez A, Cornu C. Plyometric training effects on Achilles tendon stiffness and dissipative properties. *J Appl Physiol.* 2010;109:849–54.

76. Freitas SR, Mendes B, LeSant G, et al. Can chronic stretching change the muscle-tendon mechanical properties? A review. *Scand J Med Sci Sports.* 2018;28:794–806.

77. Blazevich AJ, Cannavan D, Waugh CM, et al. Range of motion, neuromechanical, and architectural adaptations to plantar flexor stretch training in humans. *J Appl Physiol.* 2014;117:452–62.

78. Boesen AP, Dideriksen K, Couppe C, et al. Effect of growth hormone on aging connective tissue in muscle and tendon: gene expression, morphology, and function following immobilization and rehabilitation. *J Appl Physiol.* 2014;116:192–203.

79. Eckstein F, Hudelmaier M, Putz R. The effects of exercise on human articular cartilage. *J Anat.* 2006;208:491–512.

80. Kersting UG, Stubendorff JJ, Schmidt MC, Bruggermann GP. Changes in knee cartilage volume and serum COMP concentration after running exercise. *Osteoarthritis Cartilage.* 2005;13:925–34.

81. Niehoff A, Muller M, Bruggermann L, et al. Deformational behavior of knee cartilage and changes in serum cartilage oligomeric matrix protein (COMP) after running and drop landing. *Osteoarthritis Cartilage.* 2011;19:1003–10.

82. Roberts HM, Moore JP, Griffith-McGeever CL, Fortes MB, Thom JM. The effect of vigorous running and cycling on serum COMP, lubricin, and femoral cartilage thickness: a pilot study. *Eur J Appl Physiol.* 2016;116:1467–77.

83. Roberts HM, Moore JP, Thom JM. The effect of aerobic walking and lower body resistance exercise on serum COMP and hyaluronan, in both males and females. *Eur J Appl Physiol.* 2018;118:1095–105.

84. Lane NE, Michel B, Bjorkengren A, et al. The risk of osteoarthritis with running and aging: a five year longitudinal study. *J Rheumatol.* 1993;20:461–8.

85. Puranen J, Ala-Ketola L, Peltokallio P, Saarela J. Running and primary osteoarthritis of the hip. *Br Med J.* 1975;2:424–5.

86. Buckwalter JA, Martin JA. Sports and osteoarthritis. *Curr Opin Rheumatol.* 2004;16:634–9.

87. Thelin N, Holmberg S, Thelin A. Knee injuries account for the sports-related increased risk of knee osteoarthritis. *Scand J Med Sci Sports.* 2006;16:329–33.

CHAPTER 7: Endocrine System Responses and Adaptations

OBJECTIVES

After completing this chapter, you will be able to:

- Define a hormone and explain autocrine, paracrine, and endocrine hormonal actions
- Identify and explain the types of hormones that play key roles in exercise performance
- Discuss general functions of various hormones and relate these to their importance for acute exercise performance and chronic training adaptations
- Discuss how hormones are released, travel through circulation, bind to specific receptors, and their cellular signaling properties
- Discuss how acute hormonal responses and changes in signaling during training contribute to performance enhancement and physiologic adaptations

---

The endocrine system is a major system of control in the human body. Along with the nervous system, the endocrine system plays a role in a multitude of physiologic processes. It helps the body maintain normal function, prepares the body for exercise, mediates several adaptations, and is involved to some extent in every system. The actions help facilitate exercise performance and mediate chronic adaptations to training. The endocrine system operates by releasing a chemical messenger, transporting the chemical to specific target tissues, and eliciting a chain of intracellular signaling events leading to the desired function. The chemical messenger is a hormone. Hormones come in various types and perform a multitude of functions. Most hormones are released from *endocrine glands*, although some are released from nerve, muscle, cardiac, fat cells, and other tissues. Figure 7.1 depicts major endocrine glands.

Hormonal signaling is part of a complex system involving thousands of molecules in some cases. Signaling is part of a communication process that involves many cellular actions. To make an analogy, hormone signaling is like playing a team sport. All players on the team have distinct roles and responsibilities during each play. Some roles may be primary, while some may be secondary. The success of the play depends on how well the team executes and communicates in an integrative manner to carry out the team objectives. Thus, the entirety of the team (each player's contribution) must be considered when accurately determining the success of the play. Hormones work in a similar manner. All stages from production, release, transportation, tissue uptake, and intracellular signaling must be considered in an integrative manner to accurately portray the effects of the hormone-receptor interaction. Thus, viewing only a small fraction of the signaling chain may underrepresent the entirety of the hormonal actions. Science has shown the great complexity of hormonal signaling as strides have been made in cell biology and biochemistry.

 ## Hormone Actions

When released, hormones act as signal molecules and may regulate the cells that released them, adjacent cells, or enter circulation and systemically travel throughout the body. When a hormone is produced by cells and acts upon the same cells that produced it, this is known as an *autocrine* action. Some hormones are produced by cells, released by these cells, and then regulate activity of adjacent cells. This action is known as a *paracrine* action. When released, most hormones enter general circulation where they travel systemically to specific target tissues, *e.g.*, an *endocrine* action.

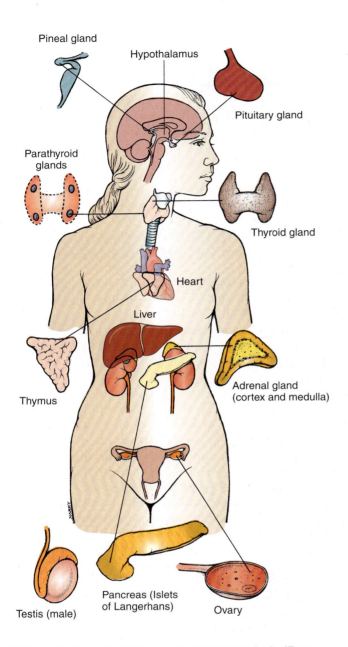

FIGURE 7.1 Major endocrine glands in the human body. (From *Stedman's Medical Dictionary*. 27th ed. Baltimore (MD): Lippincott Williams & Wilkins; 2000.)

Role of Releasing Hormones

Some hormones cause the release of other hormones and are referred to as releasing hormones. For example, the *hypothalamus* is a segment of the brain that acts as an endocrine gland. It provides a link between the nervous and endocrine systems. The hypothalamus synthesizes and releases neurohormones that are transported to the pituitary gland (anterior segment). The hypothalamus releases the hormones *corticotrophin-releasing hormone* (CRH), *gonadotropin-releasing hormone* (GnRH), *growth hormone–releasing hormone*, *growth hormone–inhibiting hormone* (somatostatin), *thyrotropin-releasing hormone* (TRH), and *prolactin-inhibiting hormone* (PIH) that control the release of other hormones including the growth hormone superfamily (GH), follicle-stimulating hormone (FSH), luteinizing hormone (LH), adrenocorticotropic hormone (ACTH), thyroid-stimulating hormone (TSH), prolactin, and β-endorphins. For example, GnRH neurons are highly regulated by neuropeptides (neurokinin-B, dynorphin-A, phoenixins) that ultimately affect the amount of GnRH and subsequent LH and FSH released. The most commonly studied neuropeptide(s) is the **kisspeptin** family. Kisspeptins are neuropeptides produced from the *KISS1* gene thought to play a significant role in the onset of puberty. The arcuate nucleus and anteroventral periventricular nucleus release kisspeptins from specific neurons, and they bind to KISS1 receptors on GnRH neurons leading to hormonal release. Reduced kisspeptin signaling has been linked to obesity and hypogonadism, and kisspeptin signaling is known to be affected by nutritional factors and stress (1).

The posterior pituitary releases two hormones in response to stimuli, *antidiuretic hormone* (ADH or vasopressin [AVP]) and *oxytocin*. Unlike the anterior pituitary, the posterior pituitary does not require releasing hormones to secrete these hormones. Hormones released from the pituitary travel to all tissues to elicit specific physiologic actions. Some of these hormones (FSH, LH, GnRH, TSH, GH, and ACTH) cause the release of other hormones from endocrine glands.

Types of Hormones

Hormones come in three major forms. Steroid hormones are made of three 6-carbon cyclohexane rings (A, B, and C rings) and one 5-carbon cyclopentane ring (D ring). All steroids are synthesized from *cholesterol* via synthetic pathways consisting of many intermediates, some of which are biologically active. Steroids are synthesized as needed, released into circulation via diffusion; bind to transport protein; arrive at the target tissue; diffuse through the cell membrane; and bind to a specific cytoplasmic- or nuclear-bound receptor within the cell. Common steroids include androgens (testosterone [TE]), estrogens, mineralocorticoids (aldosterone), glucocorticoids (cortisone), progesterone, vitamin D, and prostaglandins. Anabolic steroids, a common type of steroids used/abused by athletes, are just one type, as steroids have other applications, including anti-inflammation, fluid balance, and sex characteristics.

Peptide hormones are proteins of various sizes. Small chains (<20 amino acids) are *peptides*, and large chains (up to 100 amino acids) are *polypeptides*. Peptide hormones are the direct product of mRNA translation, cleavage from larger parent molecules, and/or other postsynthesis modifications. The quantity and sequence of amino acids determine the function of each hormone, although some partial sequences of amino acids (isoforms) may have biologic significance. Several hormones are peptides/proteins, including glucagon, leptin, atrial natriuretic

Chapter 7 Endocrine System Responses and Adaptations **147**

peptide, insulin, insulin-like growth factor-1 (IGF-1), and the superfamily of GH molecules. Peptides are prone to degradation, so pharmaceuticals (insulin and 22-kD GH) need direct routes into circulation (injection), although oral alternatives such as specific secretagogues have been studied. Peptides/proteins are synthesized in advance and stored in secretory vesicles, released via exocytosis, circulate bound to transport proteins, and bind to specific receptors on the cell membranes of target tissues to engage second messenger intracellular signaling systems. They are lipophobic and cannot pass through cell membranes, so receptors need to be external for binding.

A third type is an amine hormone. These have an amine (NH_2) group at the end of the molecule. Because they are derived from amino acids, amines may be classified as protein hormones. Amines include epinephrine, norepinephrine, and dopamine (collectively known as *catecholamines*). Catecholamines are synthesized in advance from the amino acid tyrosine, sometimes phenylalanine (via conversion to tyrosine), and tryptophan and stored in secretory vesicles until release. Similar to peptides, amines must bind to a surface-bound receptor on the target tissue. Catecholamines can act as neurotransmitters in the autonomic nervous system.

Endocrine Glands and Hormonal Functions

Several glands release hormones into circulation. Figure 7.1 depicts major endocrine glands including the hypothalamus, pituitary, thyroid, parathyroid, heart, liver, adrenals, pancreas, kidneys, testes, and ovaries. Skeletal muscle has the capacity to produce certain hormones. There are a multitude of hormones functioning within the human body. Table 7.1 presents some major hormones and their functions. Several hormones released can alter the concentrations and potency of other hormones. The endocrine system is quite complex where there are multiple levels of control and interaction between numerous tissues, cells, and other hormones.

Table 7.1	Hormones and Related Functions	
Gland	**Hormone**	**Functions**
Anterior pituitary	Growth hormone	Tissue growth, increased amino acid transport and protein synthesis, increased fat mobilization and utilization, release of IGF-1, decreased glucose utilization and glycogen synthesis, increased collagen synthesis and cartilage growth, enhanced immune cell function
	ACTH	Stimulates secretion of glucocorticoids from adrenal cortex
	β-Endorphins	Analgesia
	LH	Produces testosterone (males), ovulation and secretion of sex hormones (females)
	FSH	Spermatogenesis in males, maturation of graafian follicles of ovaries in females
	TSH	Secretion of thyroxine (T4) and triiodothyronine (T3) from thyroid
	Prolactin	Stimulates milk production in mammary glands, secretion of progesterone
	Melanocyte-stimulating hormone (MSH)	Stimulates melanocytes, skin pigmentation
Posterior pituitary	ADH	Increased reabsorption of water in kidneys, arteriole vasoconstriction
	Oxytocin	Stimulates uterine contractions and milk release from mammary glands
Thyroid	T3, T4	Increased BMR and sensitivity to catecholamines, oxygen consumption, protein synthesis, PGC-1α and mitochondrial biogenesis, utilization of lipids, muscle development and differentiation, decrease body fat
	Calcitonin	Decreased blood calcium levels, increased calcium uptake into bone
Parathyroid	Parathyroid hormone (PTH)	Increased osteoclast activity in bone, increased blood calcium, decreased blood phosphates, stimulates vitamin D_3 synthesis
Pancreas	Insulin	Glucose/amino acid transport into cells, protein synthesis, lipid and glycogen synthesis
	Glucagon	Increases blood glucose and glycogenolysis, lipolysis

(Continued)

Table 7.1	Hormones and Related Functions (Continued)	
Gland	**Hormone**	**Functions**
Adrenal cortex	Cortisol	Gluconeogenesis, spares glucose, fat breakdown, proteolysis, inhibits amino acid incorporation into proteins, increases myostatin, increases insulin resistance
	Aldosterone	Sodium and water reabsorption
Adrenal medulla	Catecholamines	"Fight-or-flight" sympathetic response, preparation for stress and exercise
	Peptide F	Analgesia, immune function
Liver	Insulin-like growth factors (IGFs)	Increased protein synthesis, growth, development
	Angiotensin	Vasoconstriction, release of aldosterone, increase blood pressure
Ovaries	Estrogens	Female sex characteristics, egg production, growth, bone formation, increase HDLs
	Progesterone	Female sex characteristics, pregnancy maintenance
Testes	Testosterone (androgens)	Growth, male sex characteristics, protein synthesis, neural stimulation, blood volume
Heart	Atrial natriuretic peptide	Regulates sodium excretion, potassium, fluid volume
Kidney	Renin (enzyme)	Kidney function, fluid balance, blood pressure
	Erythropoietin	Increased red blood cells
Adipose tissue	Leptin	Increased energy expenditure, decreased appetite, reproduction
	Adiponectin	Increased glucose uptake, fatty acid oxidation, insulin sensitivity, energy expenditure, weight loss
	Resistin	Insulin resistance, metabolic syndrome characteristics
Gastrointestinal	Ghrelin	Stimulates appetite, GH
	Neuropeptide Y	Increased food intake, decreased activity
	Peptide YY	Decreased food intake, appetite
	Glucagon-like peptide 1	Decreased food intake, appetite
	Pancreatic polypeptide	Decreased food intake, appetite
	Bombesin	Decreased appetite, increase CCK, gastrin
	Gastrin family; secretin, cholecystokinin (CCK)	Gastric acid secretion, digestion, GI motility

Hormone Activity: Production, Release, and Transportation

The production, release, and transportation of hormones to target tissues are critical for mediating the desired effects. Production depends upon the type of hormone. For example, peptides and amines are synthesized in advance and stored within vesicles until they are needed. Amines are produced from precursor molecules and stored in vesicles until release. Tyrosine is converted to dopamine, norepinephrine, and epinephrine in the adrenal medulla. Dopamine and norepinephrine also act as neurotransmitters. Thyroid hormones are produced in follicular cells of the thyroid gland (with incorporation of iodine) and stored in vesicles until released. Steroids are synthesized from cholesterol (see Fig. 7.2) via several enzymatic reactions as they are released upon completion (they are not stored) via diffusion through the cell membrane. Steroids are synthesized in adrenal glands, ovaries, testes (Leydig cells), and to a lesser extent in other peripheral tissues. Hormonal synthesis/release is modified at several levels for greater control.

Chapter 7 Endocrine System Responses and Adaptations **149**

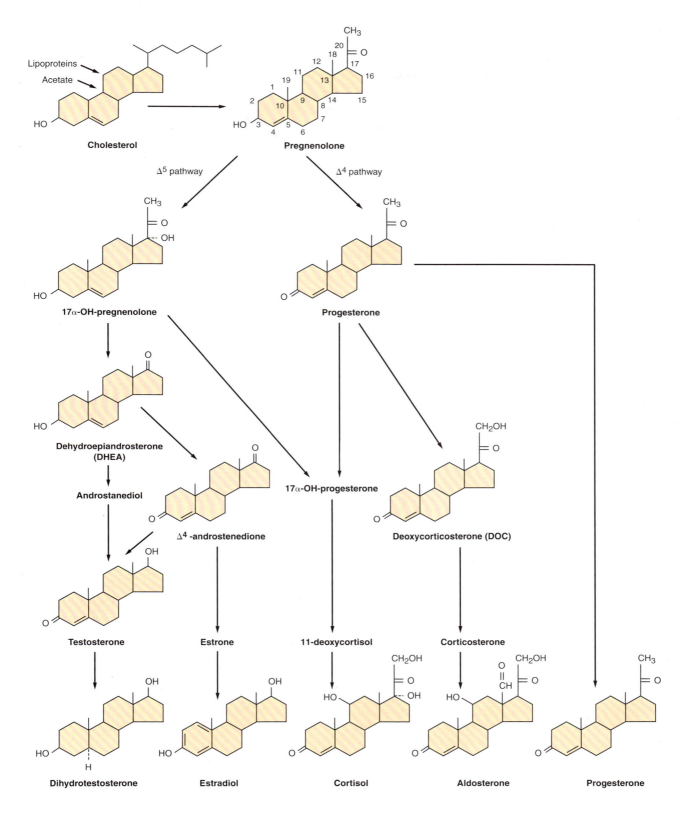

FIGURE 7.2 Steroid biosynthesis. (Reprinted with permission from Greenspan F, Baxter J. *Basic & Clinical Endocrinology*. 4th ed. Norwalk (CT): Appleton and Lange; 1994.)

Hormones must be transported to target tissues. The time a hormone remains active in circulation affects transportation. Some hormones have a short half-life (time it takes for half of the hormone secreted to be degraded) of a few minutes, *e.g.*, catecholamines, thereby limiting interaction with target tissues. However, some hormones have long half-lives of several minutes (peptides, steroids) to hours that increase the likelihood of receptor interaction (assuming the hormone arrives before it is metabolized). Thyroid hormones have half-lives of 1–7 days. Preservation of a hormone is critical. Many hormones are transported via transport (binding) proteins that protect the hormone from metabolism and help deliver the hormone to its receptor. Thyroid hormones (by thyroid hormone–binding globulin), GH molecules (by GH-binding protein), IGF-1 (by IGF-binding proteins), and steroid hormones (by sex hormone–binding globulin [SHBG] for TE mostly, corticosteroid-binding globulin for cortisol and progesterone) are chaperoned by transport proteins, whereas some hormones such as catecholamines and some peptides circulate unbound and partially dissolved in plasma. The hormone-binding protein complex travels in circulation but must dissociate prior to receptor binding, although some recent evidence suggests bound steroid hormones such as TE may enter tissues via networks of internalization proteins found in the cell membrane (*e.g.*, *megalin*). The free hormone binds to its receptor and elicits intracellular signaling.

What Determines Hormonal Concentrations in the Blood?

Several factors affect hormonal concentrations in the blood (Table 7.2). Hormonal concentrations are transient and depend upon several factors including the amount of hormone released, the pattern of release (*pulsatility*), rate of metabolism, quantity of transport proteins, the time of day, and plasma volume shifts (2). Genetics, gender, menstrual cycle, age, diet, and various stimuli (in addition to regulation from other hormones) affect hormone synthesis and secretion rates. For example, men have higher concentrations of TE, whereas women have higher concentrations of estrogens, and the hormonal responses tend to decrease with age for several hormones. The insulin response is highly dependent upon blood sugar levels, whereas hormones such as TE, cortisol, and the GH superfamily are responsive to the stress of exercise. Most hormones are released in periodic pulsatile bursts where the concentration will vary between peaks. The frequency and amplitude of the pulses dictate hormone concentrations and depends on circadian patterns and cellular stimulation. This is true for the GH superfamily that is released in a series of pulses overnight, *i.e.*, ~50% of GH secretion may occur during the third and fourth rapid eye movement (REM) stages of sleep. The quantum of hormone released in a pulse provides enough quantity to maintain physiologic function until the next pulse is released.

Several hormone concentrations vary in circadian patterns depending on the time of day. *Circadian patterns* or rhythms are physiological variations that take place over a 24-hour cycle. The primary circadian endocrine gland operating as an internal "pacemaker" is the hypothalamus (the suprachiasmatic nuclei), which receives information regarding the solar cycle from the retina (3). It coordinates biorhythms via temperature regulation, neural activation, and hormonal secretion (3). It appears that hypothalamic control is part of an integrated system that consists of genes that encode for proteins, which contribute to circadian variation, *e.g.*, *clock genes*. For example, TE in men and cortisol concentrations are highest in the morning but are gradually reduced throughout the day in what some have referred to as an "awakening effect" (4). The rise in cortisol is thought to accelerate metabolism and stimulate proteolysis and gluconeogenesis, whereas the rise in TE is thought to counteract the proteolytic cortisol effects (5). Circadian pattern of hormone secretion is relatively stable; however, under certain conditions (*i.e.*, stress, sleep deprivation), alterations may be seen especially for cortisol (4). Exercise does not affect circadian patterns (other than the immediate period of time that the trainee is working out) under most conditions. However, the effects of hormonal peaks and nadirs have been a topic of interest relating to muscular performance. Diurnal variations in performance have been shown. However, diurnal systemic hormonal changes throughout the day do not appear to play a major role in acute performance. Because TE concentrations in men are highest in the morning and progressively decrease throughout the day, some strength and conditioning professionals have recommended afternoon/early evening workouts to stimulate TE concentrations, *e.g.*, the workout can provide a stimulus to low TE concentrations. Afternoon resistance exercise–induced elevations in TE may be greater than that observed in the morning (6). Morning or afternoon/evening workouts do not appear to alter diurnal TE or cortisol concentrations (7,8). However, Sedliak et al. (8) reported lower cortisol concentrations in the morning during familiar RT morning workouts. The authors suggested that the cortisol reduction may have been due to reduced anticipatory psychological stress seen prior to morning workouts. Resistance exercise (RE) has limited effects on normal TE circadian patterns (8,9) as normal circadian rhythm (within 1 h) is quickly reestablished upon completion of a workout. However, nocturnal circadian patterns may be affected (10). Nindl et al. (11) showed that 22-kD GH pulsatility was higher during the second phase of sleep on a day where high-volume RE was performed. One study showed acute RE in the evening (18:00 h) produced a 14% greater IGFBP-3 response compared to the same RE workout performed in the morning (08:00 h) (12).

Plasma volume shifts occur during exercise. Plasma is the liquid portion of blood. During exercise, fluid lost intracellularly is replaced by extracellular fluid. Coupled with fluid loss to thermoregulation, plasma volume is reduced during exercise. Hormone measurements express the amount of hormone per volume of blood. A higher hormone value will be obtained when fluid volume is reduced despite having the same amount of hormone molecules present (hemoconcentration). In fact, for some hormones such as TE, the majority

Table 7.2 Adult Resting Serum Hormonal Value Ranges

Hormone	Range
LH	
Men	1–9 IU·L^{-1}
Women	<1–80 IU·L^{-1}
Total testosterone	
Men	10–40 nmol·L^{-1}, 3–12 ng·mL^{-1}
Women	<3.5 nmol·L^{-1}; <0.1 ng·mL^{-1}
Free testosterone	
Men	0.30–1.04 nmol·L^{-1}; 9–30 ng·dL^{-1}
Women	0.01–0.07 nmol·L^{-1}; 0.3–1.9 ng·dL^{-1}
DHEA-S	
Men	0.7–12.4 µmol·L^{-1}; 25–460 µg·dL^{-1}
Women	0.4–9.0 µmol·L^{-1}; 15–330 µg·dL^{-1}
Estradiol	
Men	36–147 pmol·L^{-1}; 10–40 pg·mL^{-1}
Women	36–1,285 pmol·L^{-1}; <10–350 pg·mL^{-1}
Progesterone	
Men	<4 nmol·L^{-1}
Women	<3–64 nmol·L^{-1}
Cortisol	50–680 nmol·L^{-1}; 2–25 µg·dL^{-1}
Aldosterone	28–583 pmol·L^{-1}; 1–21 ng·dL^{-1}
Growth hormone (22 kD)	
Men	0–5 µg·L^{-1}
Women	0–10 µg·L^{-1}
IGF-1	
Men	0.45–2.2 units·mL^{-1}; 7–84 nmol·L^{-1}
Women	0.34–1.9 units·mL^{-1}; 7–70 nmol·L^{-1}
Insulin (fasting)	2–20 µU·mL^{-1}
Total triiodothyronine	1.2–3.4 nmol·L^{-1}; 70–200 ng·dL^{-1}
Free triiodothyronine	3.5–6.5 pmol·L^{-1}; 2.3–4.2 pg·mL^{-1}
Total thyroxine	90–250 nmol·L^{-1}; 5.5–12.5 µg·dL^{-1}
Free thyroxine	10–24 pmol·L^{-1}; 0.8–1.8 ng·dL^{-1}

of the potential acute exercise–induced elevation may be explained by plasma volume reductions and reduced clearance (13), whereas hormones such as the GH superfamily and catecholamines are released in greater abundance during exercise. LH-induced TE elevations may take at least 20–30 minutes (14); thus, hormone elevations during exercise may result from a combination of factors separate from production (2,15–17). Corrections for plasma volume shifts ameliorate the elevation. The elevated hormones are thought to expedite receptor interaction (2,15–17).

Sidebar — Circadian Patterns, Muscle Performance, and Training Specificity

Many studies have shown that acute strength and power performance varies throughout the day (3,5,18). Performance is better in the late afternoon and reduced early in the morning. Decrements in strength and power performances

(Continued)

in early morning (*i.e.*, 06:00 and 10:00 h) may be between 3% and 21% compared to the afternoon (*i.e.*, 16:00 and 20:00 h) (18). However, aerobic endurance performance and $\dot{V}O_{2max}$ are equivocal where circadian variations may not be seen. The most likely physiological explanation is circadian changes in core body temperature. Better performances are seen at higher body temperatures; thus, higher body temperature in the afternoon appears to play a significant role. Neural and intramuscular factors, energy metabolism, differences in nutritional intake, insufficient time to recover from sleep inertia, and psychological/motivational factors have been proposed in addition to body temperature variations (3,18). This circadian pattern of strength variance is seen in resistance-trained men as well, although the morning strength nadir was attenuated with consumption of caffeine (3 mg/kg body mass) (19). Although circadian performance differences are well observed, the differential may be reduced or nullified with morning training sessions. Training specificity has been observed when performance testing sessions match the training time of day. This occurs during aerobic and RT (18). Thus, morning training sessions may be an effective way to minimize circadian strength and power fluctuation. Studies have shown similar strength increases independent of morning or afternoon/evening combined RT and aerobic training session times (7). Interestingly, some data support greater vastus lateralis muscle hypertrophy during RT in the afternoon/evening (16:30–19:30) compared to the morning (06:30–09:30) (7). However, other studies have shown similar hypertrophy potential and intramuscular signaling of mTOR and MAPK pathways independent of the time of day (20).

Negative Feedback Control

Hormonal concentrations are controlled by negative feedback systems. A negative feedback system will elevate a hormone when it is low or reduce a hormone when it is elevated. Negative feedback system can be seen with TE. A male athlete who uses anabolic steroids will experience reductions in his own TE production. As a result, testicular shrinkage can occur due to negative feedback inhibition of *endogenous* (produced within one's body) TE production. Negative feedback systems predominate and provide multiple levels of control.

 ## Receptor Interaction

As hormones are messengers, their message would be useless without other molecules' ability to receive the signal and continue the signaling process. The ultimate fate of a hormone is to bind to specific receptors on the target tissue. Receptor binding leads to a cascade of cellular events that leads to the desired function. Receptors for amines and peptides/proteins lie within the cell membrane, whereas steroid and thyroid hormone receptors are mostly located either in the nucleus (thyroid) or cytoplasm (steroids), although membrane-bound receptors produce *nongenomic* effects in addition to genomic effects. Receptors come in different forms but are specific to the hormone they are coupled with via a lock-and-key principle. Theoretically, only one hormone will activate the receptor. However, there are many exceptions. Some molecules that are similar to the hormone may act as a barrier for hormonal interaction, whereas some bind to the receptor with high affinity leading to activation. This cross-reactivity allows more than one hormone or molecule to activate a receptor and leads to the introduction of multiple other pathways of hormonal control. This can be of great value in the pharmaceutical industry where drug analogues are produced. For example, *selective androgen receptor modulators* (SARMs) and *selective estrogen receptor modulators* (SERMs) are classes of drugs that stimulate or inhibit androgen/estrogen signaling independent of the specific hormone. They are used for a multitude of purposes clinically. In addition, receptors may be altered (*i.e.*, phosphorylated, acetylated, methylated, etc.) by other molecules intracellularly, which could increase or decrease their transcriptional capacity. Various amino acid residues may be sites of modification within the receptor. Modifications change the protein folding pattern that affects the receptor's nuclear translocation, binding, and transcriptional activity. Thus, the potential for a hormone receptor to interact with many molecules is vast and shows the great complexity of intracellular hormone signaling. Upon binding to a receptor, second messenger systems are engaged (for membrane-bound receptors) or the nucleus will be activated (for cytoplasmic-nuclear receptors).

Second Messenger Systems

Because some hormones (amines, peptides/proteins) bind to a membrane-bound receptor on the surface of the cell (the *first messenger* of signaling), other molecules must mediate this signal intracellularly. Several *second messengers* are activated and initiate a cascade of events leading to the desired cellular response. The major second messenger systems mediating membrane-bound receptor-hormone binding include the cyclic nucleotides (*e.g.*, cyclic AMP, cyclic GMP — mediate hormones such as glucagon, LH, catecholamines, ANP, TSH, FSH, ACTH), inositol triphosphate (IP3), diacylglycerol (DAG) (*i.e.*, for hormones such as ADH, GnRH, TRH), calcium-mediated signaling, and tyrosine kinases (*e.g.*, 22-kD GH). Many second messenger systems are mediated by guanylyl (G) proteins that can stimulate or inhibit further cellular activity. Figure 7.3 depicts the adenylate cyclase-cyclic AMP second messenger system.

Steroid and Thyroid Hormones

Because steroids are lipophilic, they diffuse through target cell membranes and bind to receptors in the cytoplasm or nucleus

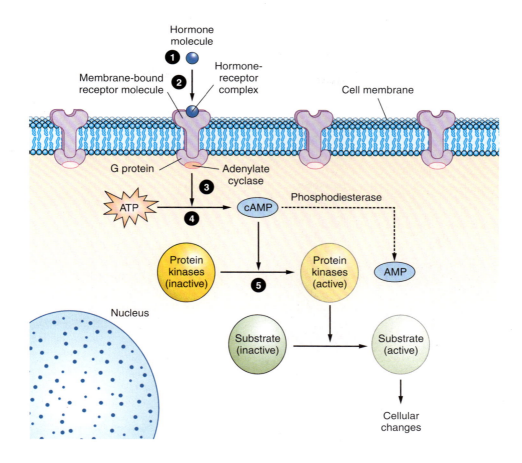

FIGURE 7.3 Adenylate cyclase-cyclic AMP second messenger system. A hormone that binds to its specific membrane-bound receptor can stimulate or inhibit this system. A stimulatory hormone binds to its receptor and activates a stimulating G-protein that activates the enzyme adenylate cyclase to produce cyclic AMP from ATP. Cyclic AMP activates protein kinases (*i.e.*, protein kinase A). Protein kinase A phosphorylates several proteins/substrates yielding numerous cellular effects. An inhibitory hormone activates an inhibiting G-protein to limit these reactions. Cyclic AMP has a short half-life and is rapidly degraded by the enzyme *phosphodiesterase*, which itself is inhibited by caffeine.

(Fig. 7.4). Many steroids bind to receptors in the cytoplasm. Receptors are bound to heat shock proteins in the cytoplasm prior to hormone binding. Heat shock proteins dissociate, and the hormone-receptor complex translocates to the nucleus where it binds to specific response elements on DNA (leading to protein synthesis). Receptors possess transcriptional activation, DNA-binding motifs, and ligand-binding domains. Subsequent folding of the protein complex and binding to the DNA response elements recruit coregulatory proteins that can increase (*i.e.*, coactivators) or reduce (*i.e.*, corepressors) transcription activity. Coactivators interact with the signature motif contained within the ligand-binding domain. For example, the androgen receptor/androgen complex is regulated by more than 300 coregulator proteins and microRNAs. Several coactivators are involved with histone modification and chromatin remodeling to loosen the nucleosomal structure to ease binding. Coactivators assist in the recruitment of RNA polymerase II to the promoter of target genes and enhance assembly of and stabilize the *preinitiation complex* (consisting of RNA polymerase II and other transcription factor proteins) to serve in transcription initiation and elongation and ultimately protein synthesis. The hormone-receptor complex, along with coregulators, acts as a transcriptional factor playing a large role in the potency of the hormonal signaling response. The responses and adaptations of these proteins to training may serve as an interesting area of research. Thus, steroid hormone signaling begins with hormone production and release and culminates with formation of the transcriptional unit. Thyroid hormones (T3, T4) enter the cell membrane via transporter proteins, travel to the nucleus, and bind with two types of thyroid receptors (mostly T3 binds to the α and β isoforms) to stimulate or inhibit gene transcription. Thyroid receptors (nuclear) can bind to corepressor proteins in the absence of hormone binding.

Hormones and Exercise

Exercise presents a potent stimulus for hormonal responses. For resistance training (RT), the manipulation of the acute program variables (intensity, volume, rest intervals, exercise selection and sequence, repetition velocity, frequency) ensures an optimal endocrine response. The level of motor unit recruitment is an essential quality for endocrine-mediated tissue responses

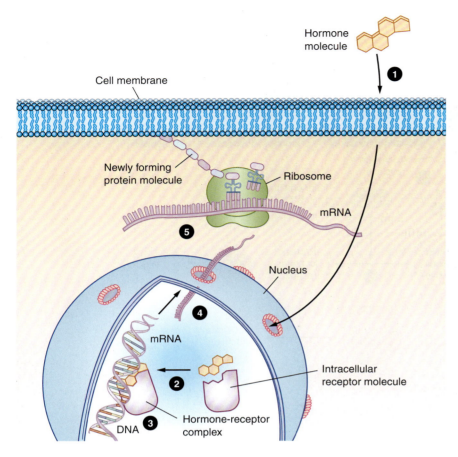

FIGURE 7.4 Steroid hormone action. (From Golan DE, Tashjian AH, Armstrong EJ. *Principles of Pharmacology: The Pathophysiologic Basis of Drug Therapy*. 2nd ed. Baltimore (MD): Wolters Kluwer Health; 2008.)

and adaptations. Intensity, volume and duration, modality, work:rest ratio, and frequency are critical variables for aerobic training and other anaerobic modalities including plyometric, sprint, and agility training. The training program as well as genetic predisposition, gender, fitness level, nutritional intake, and the potential for adaptation all play roles in the hormonal responses. Hormonal responses and adaptations entail four classifications: (a) acute responses during exercise, (b) chronic changes in resting concentrations, (c) chronic changes in the acute response to exercise, and (d) receptor and intramuscular signaling changes.

Testosterone

More than 95% of TE in men is secreted from Leydig cells of the testes, with the remainder produced by the adrenals. In women, ovarian and adrenal production of androgens is the major sources (usually DHEA in the adrenals and androstenedione in the adrenals and ovaries with peripheral conversion to TE) (21). Skeletal muscle contains the necessary enzymes and may have the potential to produce small amounts of androgens as well (22). Most (~98%) of TE travels bound to SHBG (60%) and a protein *albumin* (38%); however, it is mostly the unbound free TE that diffuses into cells and interacts with cytoplasmic- or membrane-bound androgen receptors. Testosterone is a potent hormone. However, some TE is converted to a more potent (about six times that of TE) analyte dihydrotestosterone (DHT) in peripheral tissues via the 5α-*reductase* enzyme. This enzyme is present in skeletal muscle, and circulating DHT can diffuse into muscle cells and bind to receptors with higher affinity than TE. Thus, skeletal muscle does possess DHT in addition to TE and other androgens, although the potency of DHT in muscle remains unknown. It is TE that is the major androgen mediating anabolic processes in men. Testosterone has many ergogenic effects on performance (see the Sidebar: *Ergogenic Effects of Testosterone*). Some TE is aromatized to estrogens, and final metabolism of TE occurs in the liver and kidneys where inactivated metabolites are excreted in urine.

The key to all hormones is the signaling properties. Hormones are messengers that require other molecules to produce a desired effect. There are several ways in which TE regulates skeletal muscle (*e.g.*, mature muscle fiber and satellite cell activity) anabolism or anticatabolism. These are as follows:

- Classic genomic signaling where TE binds to a cytoplasmic androgen receptor (AR), dissociates from heat shock proteins, and the complex translocates to the nucleus to bind to specific androgen response elements on DNA. The AR-TE complex serves as a transcription factor leading to protein synthesis with the help of coactivator proteins and may alter the expression of several genes involved in the regulation of skeletal muscle structure (23).
- Nongenomic effects are thought to be mediated by direct binding to a target molecule, through intracellular

AR activation, through a transmembrane AR receptor (through G-protein second messenger system) or via changes in membrane fluidity (24). Nongenomic signaling may either increase intracellular calcium concentrations (possibly leading to enhanced contractile properties) or stimulate activation of MAPK signaling and mTOR pathway signaling (see Chapter 5 for review). Nongenomic signaling occurs rapidly within seconds to minutes, much faster than classic genomic signaling, which takes hours. Interaction between pathways may occur, and both genomic and nongenomic signaling appear critical to maximizing muscle hypertrophy (25). MAPK signaling may phosphorylate the AR, increasing its transcriptional capacity. Receptors for SHBG are found in muscle membranes. Binding of SHBG to its receptor may influence transcription, but the magnitude of response is currently unclear (26).

- Stimulating the Wnt/β-catenin pathway. The TE-AR complex may inhibit glycogen synthase kinase-3 (GSK-3), which dephosphorylates β-catenin increasing its activity or can chaperone β-catenin to the nucleus where it binds to specific DNA elements. The presence of TE increases AR-β-catenin interaction and transcriptional capacity.
- TE may bind to ARs on satellite cells to increase proliferation and differentiation, *e.g.*, myogenesis, and Notch signaling of satellite cells. TE may increase follistatin and decrease myostatin and its signaling molecules.
- TE may bind to ARs on stem cells (mesenchymal pluripotent cells) to shift their cell lineage to myogenesis instead of adipogenesis.

Sidebar	Ergogenic Effects of Testosterone

- Increases LBM and muscle CSA
- Increases cardiac tissue mass
- Decreases body fat percentage
- Increases ISOM and dynamic muscle strength and power
- Enhances recovery ability between workouts
- Increases protein synthesis
- Increases red blood cell formation, hemoglobin, hematocrit, and endurance
- Increases osteoblast activity and BMD
- Increases lipolysis (fat breakdown) and low-density lipoproteins, decreases high-density lipoproteins, increases adipocyte β-adrenergic receptors, and decreases TG uptake and lipoprotein lipase activity
- Increases neural transmission, neurotransmitter release, BDNF, and regrowth of damaged peripheral nerves
- Increases insulin and leptin sensitivity, mitochondrial function, GLUT4, glycogen synthase and glycogen storage, and MCT1 and MCT4 lactate transporters
- Increases aggression

- TE may be anticatabolic by either decreasing glucocorticoid receptor expression, interfering with cortisol binding, or the AR-TE complex may compete with cortisol-GC complex for binding sites on DNA response elements.
- TE-AR complex may augment of the effects of other anabolic hormones such as the GH superfamily, IGF-1, and mechano-growth factor (MGF).

Acute Systemic Responses to Exercise

TE may be elevated during and immediately following aerobic and RE in men and women (21,27), and during combined aerobic and RE workouts (28). In women, prolonged endurance exercise results in elevations in total TE while the response to RE is elevations or no change (21,29,30). The acute free and total TE response to endurance exercise may take place during the first hour but may then decline further into recovery (31). RE is a potent modality that elevates total and free TE concentrations in men (32–41) if a threshold stimulus consisting of the interaction of volume, muscle mass involvement, rest interval length, and intensity are reached/activated (Fig. 7.5). The acute TE response to RE in women appears limited compared to men (33,42,43). The response may be greater in resistance-trained men than endurance-trained men (44) and may be enhanced with training experience (37,45), although some research showed training status may not affect the acute TE response (46). These elevations are mostly attributed to plasma volume reductions and reduced clearance in the short term, while the adaptations in TE synthesis and secretion capacity over the course of a long workout may be a possibility (2,13). The impact of acute TE elevations during RE is not clear as studies have shown relationships between acute TE elevations and performance improvement, AR content, or muscle hypertrophy (47–50), whereas other studies have not (51–53). It is difficult to parcel out the effects of acute TE elevations because TE signaling needs to be viewed in its entirety from synthesis and release to transcription. RT effects seen in AR content or in other intracellular signaling molecules could increase the efficacy of TE despite a lack of change seen in systemic concentrations. Thus, the magnitude of acute TE elevations during exercise is not clear, although it is thought to, in part, mediate some training adaptations. Several other factors affect the acute TE response. These include the following:

- Exercise selection and muscle mass involvement: acute TE response is greater with large muscle mass exercises (41,47,54,55). Some studies have shown similar TE responses between unilateral and bilateral upper and lower body RE protocols (56,57) and similar responses between CON and ECC muscle actions when matched for relative intensity.
- Intensity and volume interaction: acute TE response is greater with high- versus low-intensity RE, and the response is greater with moderate- to high- versus low-volume workouts (58–62). The interaction between intensity and volume is critical as those programs with a high glycolytic component (*e.g.*, moderate to high intensity, high volume, and short rest intervals like bodybuilding or high-intensity interval

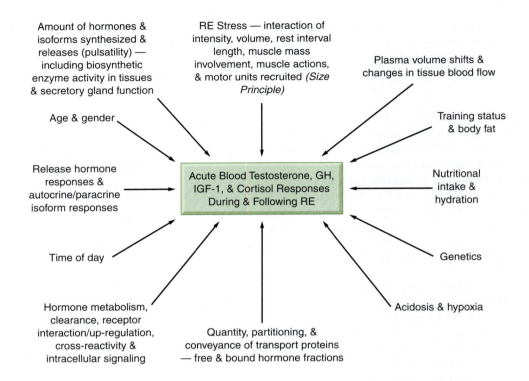

FIGURE 7.5 Factors affecting acute testosterone, cortisol, 22-kD GH, and IGF-1 during and following resistance exercise. (From Kraemer WJ, Ratamess NA, Nindl BC. Recovery responses of testosterone, growth hormone, and IGF-1 after resistance exercise. *J Appl Physiol.* 2017;122:549–58.)

programs) yield substantial TE elevations, even greater than strength training or power training programs with longer rest intervals between sets (59,60,63–65), although some data show no response or no difference between strength and hypertrophy protocols (66,67). Short rest intervals (1 min) elicit a more substantial response than longer rest intervals (2.5 min) at least early in training but may subside as training progresses (68). However, during heavy strength training, short (1 min) and long (3 min) rest intervals produce similar responses with volume equated (69). Low-intensity workouts may not elicit an acute TE response (64).

- Training frequency: acute TE response may be more substantial when training volume is divided into two sessions instead of one (70).
- Acute TE response may be similar between traditional sets structures and cluster sets (71).
- Acute TE is elevated during blood flow restriction RE of the arms and legs (72).
- Performing a RE sequence of multiple-joint to single-joint exercises compared to the reverse sequence appears to produce similar total and free TE response (73,74).
- Nutritional intake: acute TE response is limited with carbohydrate/protein intake before, during, or immediately after a workout (35,38,75,76). Caffeine intake prior to RE may augment the acute TE response in a dose-dependent manner (77).
- Overtraining and dehydration: TE response may be less when athletes are overtrained (78) and dehydrated prior to RE (79).

Chronic Changes in Resting Testosterone Concentrations

Changes in resting TE concentrations during RT have been inconsistent in the absence of clinical issues such as hypogonadism or normal aging, obesity, androgen deprivation therapy (for men with prostate cancer), or polycystic ovary syndrome in women. In fact, resting baseline total and free TE (in addition LH, FSH) may be lower to hypogonadal levels in men who previously used anabolic-androgenic steroids (80). Although some studies show elevations (37,46,81–84), no changes (78,85,86), and reductions (87) in resting TE concentrations after RT, it seems that resting concentrations reflect the current state of muscle such that temporal changes may occur at various stages depending on the volume and intensity of training and timing of measurement relative to the last workout. A study examining elite Olympic weightlifters showed no differences in 1 year of training (78); however, elevations were shown following a 2nd year of training (81). Changes in volume and intensity produce transient changes in resting baseline TE (46,87) but appear to return to a homeostatic level upon adaptation to the change in program design. Short-term (7–10 d) detraining in strength/power athletes may result in elevated TE concentrations (88); however, long-term detraining (>8 wk) results in TE reductions (78,89). Long-term intense, high-volume endurance training (seen in ultra-endurance athletes) in some men produces reduced baseline total and free TE concentrations (with normal LH), a condition known as "*exercise-hypogonadal male condition*"

(90). Symptoms have been seen in other populations such as the military (91). This condition is likely a combination of several factors that may be addressed through training changes and nutritional interventions (91).

Skeletal Muscle Steroidogenesis

Skeletal muscle possesses enzymes to produce TE from precursors such as DHEA (22). Steroidogenic enzyme content and TE concentrations in skeletal muscle are similar between men and women (22). In older men, 12 weeks of RT has been shown to increase skeletal muscle DHEA, free TE, DHT, 3β-HSD, 17β-HSD, 5α-reductase type I content, and AR protein content (92). The increased DHT and free TE were related to increased isokinetic strength, muscle CSA, and power (92). However, RT studies in younger men and women have shown no changes in muscle TE or steroidogenic enzymes (22,93). However, responders to RT were shown to increase 5α-reductase (93). It is possible that increased muscle steroidogenesis may be a mechanism to help counteract TE reductions in older men but not likely in young men.

Interpreting Research
The Importance of Testosterone to Strength Training

Kvorning T, Andersen M, Brixen K, Madsen K. Suppression of endogenous testosterone production attenuates the response to strength training: a randomized, placebo-controlled, and blinded intervention study. *Am J Physiol Endocrinol Metab.* 2006;291:E1325–32.

Kvorning T, Andersen M, Brixen K, Schjerling P, Suetta C, Madesn K. Suppression of testosterone does not blunt mRNA expression of myoD myogenin IGF myostatin or androgen receptor post strength training in humans. *J Physiol.* 2007;578:579–93.

TE deficiencies in humans and animal studies have shown its importance for mediating muscle hypertrophy and strength in trained and nontrained states. For example, administration of an AR antagonist in rats (oxendolone) during 2 weeks of electrical stimulation of the gastrocnemius muscle attenuated 70% of hypertrophy compared to the control condition (94). In humans, Kvorning et al. (48) administered a GnRH analog (goserelin, 3.6 mg administered three times) or a placebo to subjects (with minor previous RT experience) undergoing 8 weeks of RT consisting of 7 exercises stressing major muscle groups for 3–4 sets with 6–10 RM, with 2- to 3-minute rest intervals, and performed 3 days per week. The drug was successful in suppressing total and free TE and DHT. Figure 7.6 displays the strength and lean tissue mass results. The placebo group increased leg mass and strength by 6% and 9% compared to 4% and 2% (not significant) in the goserelin group. The authors concluded that suppression of serum TE below 10% of normal levels strongly attenuates the increase in lean mass and muscle strength and increases fat mass during RT. These results (along with other studies (47)), demonstrate the importance of TE in mediating part of training-induced adaptations in muscle strength and hypertrophy. In a follow-up study using a similar protocol, Kvorning et al. (95) reported that AR mRNA (and myostatin, myoD, and myogenin) did not differ between groups despite differences in TE and differential strength and hypertrophy adaptations.

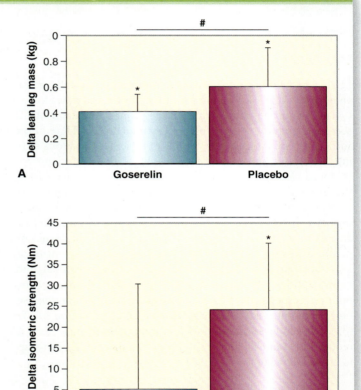

FIGURE 7.6 Strength and lean tissue mass results. Panel A is the change in leg lean tissue mass. Panel B is the change in isometric strength. * indicates a significant longitudinal training effect whereas # indicates a significant difference between conditions. (From Kvorning T, Andersen M, Brixen K, Madsen K. Suppression of endogenous testosterone production attenuates the response to strength training: a randomized, placebo-controlled, and blinded intervention study. *Am J Physiol Endocrinol Metab.* 2006;291:E1325–32.)

Myths & Misconceptions
Resistance Training Will Increase Resting Testosterone Concentrations Incrementally

One misconception is that RT will increase TE in healthy young men at rest over time. Although some elevations in resting TE may take place, these tend to be transient and return to a normal baseline level upon accommodation to training. Resting TE values reflect a diurnal pattern and change throughout the day. Basal TE levels decrease as one ages independent of training status. Thus, an expectation of large resting TE elevations is not warranted. Although elevations in TE at rest may be advantageous to some extent in the short term, long-term elevations could be counterproductive when one views potential negative health risk factors (elevated low-density lipoprotein [LDL] cholesterol, prostate ailments) and receptor desensitization (down-regulation). This has also been shown in women with polycystic ovary syndrome, which produces chronic elevations in androgens. *Receptor down-regulation*, or *tolerance*, is a term used to describe a reduction in receptors from chronic exposure to high levels of hormones or drugs. It takes a larger hormonal output to generate a given response once tolerance develops. Many anabolic steroid users cycle drugs to prevent tolerance and keep receptors primed for adaptation. Thus, it seems beneficial to an athlete to have other changes within the TE signaling cascade rather than chronic TE elevations. TE could potentially have negative side effects at chronically high levels, and it appears that the body safeguards against this.

Luteinizing Hormone

LH is a protein hormone secreted from basophilic cells of the anterior pituitary (under the control of GnRH and other hypothalamic neuropeptides), which is the primary regulator of TE secretion from the testes in men. LH stimulation of TE requires sufficient time (at least 20–30 min) (14), so TE elevations during a workout appear to be the result of other mechanisms (reduced clearance and plasma volume shifts), at least during the first part of the workout. A workout may not induce LH secretion (96), although a delayed response may occur later during recovery (44). Studies have shown no change (78) or an elevation (6) in LH at rest, again reflecting the transient nature of resting hormonal concentrations and the control of LH secretion by GnRH via stimulation from hypothalamic neuropeptides. Resistance-trained men show a more pronounced response than endurance-trained men during exercise (44). Endurance exercise may cause an acute reduction in LH (31). Ultraendurance events (*i.e.*, ultramarathon) may cause a reduced LH (and TE and SHBG) response that could persist up to 1 day following the race (97).

Sex Hormone–Binding Globulin

Circulating TE is mostly bound to SHBG. A change in SHBG concentrations may influence the binding capacity of TE and the availability of free TE. During RT, differential responses (elevations, reductions, and no change) occur (2). Similar to TE, it appears that hypertrophy-driven protocols produce a more substantial elevation compared to strength or power protocols (65). Endurance exercise may increase SHBG in women (98).

Other Androgens (Prohormones)

The synthesis of TE contains many steps involving precursors such as dehydroepiandrosterone (DHEA), androstenedione, and androstenediol. In comparison to TE, these precursors are less potent as evidenced by a lack of ergogenic effects seen with prohormone supplementation (2). Androgens such as DHEA may play a greater role in women because of their lower levels of TE. Women can convert a larger percentage of DHEA to androstenedione and TE and have higher baseline concentrations of androstenedione than men (99). In women, prolonged endurance exercise produces acute elevations in DHEA, DHEA sulfate, and androstenedione concentrations (21). In endurance-trained men, running produces an acute elevation in DHEA sulfate in an intensity/duration dose-dependent manner (31). Elevations in circulating androstenedione and DHEA sulfate in men and women occur during RE (44,99). During RT, elevations, reductions, and no changes have been shown in androstenedione, DHEA, and DHEA sulfate, reflecting the lack of consistency or change in hormonal concentrations at rest (21,89,100,101).

The Androgen Receptor and Androgen Signaling

The androgen receptor (AR) gene is located on the q arm of chromosome X at position 11–12. The AR consists of ~919 amino acids and is found in nearly all tissues in the human body. Truncated versions have been identified. The presence of ARs correlates highly with the functions of androgens. The AR consists of four functional domains: a C-terminal hormone-binding domain, a DNA-binding domain, a hinge region, and an N-terminal transcription activation domain. AR activity may be altered by phosphorylation at several serine residues, methylation, ubiquitination, and acetylation. For example, phosphorylation of serine residue 651 is needed for full transcriptional activity. The goal of AR-DNA interaction is to induce transcription and translation of proteins necessary to fulfill specific functions. AR function is enhanced by coactivators that form a bridge between the DNA-bound AR and the transcriptional machinery and by facilitating hormonal binding. Androgen binding to the AR produces a conformational change in the protein structure that forms a pocket to recruit coactivators. More than 300 coregulators exist, many of which are coactivators. Coactivators augment transcriptional activity and enhance signaling. However, little is known regarding training and up-regulation of coactivators. Androgens have different potencies, in part, due to affinity and binding properties of the AR. Androgen binding stabilizes the AR and greater affinity, and stabilization is seen with DHT more so than TE. Other androgens are weaker relative to TE.

The first exon of the AR contains several regions of repetitive DNA sequences one of which is the CAG (polyglutamine) triplet repeat that begins at codon 58 and extends for >21 repeats. This length varies between 8 and 35 repeats (18–24 is most common). Another is a polyglycine (GGN) repeat in the transactivation region. Genetic polymorphisms yielding a variety of repeats are associated with a variety of conditions including male infertility, prostate and testicular cancer, bone disease, and cardiovascular disease. These could contribute, in part, to responder or nonresponder status when examining training adaptations. Long CAG repeats may interfere with androgen actions, whereas short repeats (CAG and GGN) are associated with increased AR protein expression and androgen action. However, contradictory results have been reported where CAG repeat number was positively related, inversely related, or not related to LBM, TE or free TE concentrations, and muscle strength in young and older men (102–105). Nielsen et al. (103) showed inverse relationships between CAG repeat number and thigh and trunk muscle size to where every reductions in repeats of 10 equaled an increase of muscle size by 4%. Thus, performance phenotypes based on AR candidate gene polymorphisms remain unclear but is an area of research interest.

A variety of studies have attempted to determine major mechanisms involved in responder versus nonresponder status. First, defining a "responder" is difficult, and various classifications have been used. Second, it is difficult to ascertain the level of contribution of various mechanisms because many are integrated and communicate/cross-regulate each other. For example, TE communicates via eight general pathways with multiple levels of interaction in between signaling pathways. Thus, it is quite difficult to minimize the relationships between crosstalk among different anabolic signaling pathways. Morton et al. (93) examined 12 weeks of high- versus low-repetition RT. They separated responders and nonresponders as part of their analysis. In order to minimize the relationships (collinearity) between various anabolic measures, the authors used a principle component analysis and reported that AR protein content is the more important variable in RT-induced androgen-mediated skeletal muscle protein accretion in healthy men. These results show the importance of AR-mediated signaling in mediating some of the RT-induced hypertrophic adaptations.

A number of studies have investigated AR responses and adaptations to RT mostly in the vastus lateralis muscle of the thigh. The following are some of the key findings:

1. The concentration of ARs in skeletal muscle depends on muscle fiber type (high in FT fibers), sex, training status, and androgen concentrations. High TE initially up-regulate ARs by stabilization (preventing catabolism) and through *de novo* protein synthesis.

2. Baseline resting AR protein content (at least 4–5 d following the last workout) does not change during RT (13,93).

3. The initial AR response within 1–2 hours post-RE in a fasted state may be down-regulation or no change when RE is of sufficient volume. Postworkout protein/CHO feeding up-regulates AR content or diminishes the reduction within 1 hour post-RE. The response is similar in young and old men (13,30,40,106).

4. Large acute TE elevations during the workout may contribute to the up-regulation and/or prevent down-regulation in the fasted state (107).

5. More notable up-regulation of AR mRNA and protein is seen ~28 hours post-RE (51). Early studies showed 48 hours post-RE is a time where significant AR up-regulation (by 35%–202%) occurs following a workout or repeated workouts over 3 days (108–110).

6. AR response may lessen over long-term RT or be less in trained men (108).

7. Baseline and acute AR up-regulation correlate to muscle strength and hypertrophy (40,111).

8. AR mRNA and protein up-regulation correlated to total and free TE concentrations in the blood (35,110,112).

9. AR protein content may explain most variance in muscle hypertrophy during RT (113).

10. AR-DNA binding increases during RT — possibly linked to greater β-catenin pathway signaling (114).

11. AR modulates its phosphorylation state to sensitize itself to anabolic signals in the presence of lower androgens. Men have higher baseline AR protein content than women; however, women had greater AR phosphorylation at rest at ser515 and ser81 residues indicating that the AR activity could be augmented independent of ligand binding (115).

Selective Androgen Receptor Modulators

Since 1998, it has been shown that other nonsteroidal molecules can activate the AR. These molecules have been termed SARMs because they bind to the AR and have shown anabolic properties in bone and skeletal muscle. However, unlike other androgens, SARMs produce minimal effects on prostate and secondary sexual organs (116). They have the potential to separate androgenic and anabolic effects and have shown promise in clinical trials for increasing muscle mass. There may be great clinical potential for these molecules but potential for use by athletes as well.

Growth Hormone Superfamily

The anterior pituitary secretes molecules that make up the GH family of pleiotropic polypeptide variants. In fact, GH has been described as "a mixture of several different forms" (117). More than 100 isoforms of GH exist at various levels in the anterior pituitary and the blood. Different isoforms arise at the level of the GH gene, mRNA splice variants, posttranslation processing, metabolism, disulfide linkage aggregation, and glycosylation (118). The most commonly studied GH isoform, the 22-kD molecule, consists of 191 amino acids. Immunoreactive GH is released from the anterior pituitary in a pulsatile manner (especially during slow-wave sleep) for ~3–6 pulses per day under the control of GHRH (peptide required for initiation of GH pulses) and is inhibited by somatostatin; both are hypothalamic hormones. Bioactive GH is released in a nonpulsatile manner. The gastrointestinal hormone ghrelin can regulate (increase) secretion of stored GH to a lesser extent. Factors such as age, sex, sex hormones (at the hypothalamic and pituitary levels), body composition (*i.e.*, obesity reduces the response), sleep quality, nutritional intake, and breathing patterns affect the GH response (118,119). In women, the menstrual cycle affects GH secretion, and use of contraceptives may increase the GH response in women (120). Glucocorticoids may suppress GH secretion. The anterior pituitary contains two types of somatotroph cells: band 1, which contains small molecular forms like the 22-kD GH molecule, and band 2, which contain larger molecular weight isoforms such as bioactive GH aggregates (27). A study in rats showed that RT can alter the spatial distribution in the ventral region of somatotroph cells and increase hypertrophy, secretory content, and oscillatory behavior of these somatotroph cells (121), thus providing evidence that anterior pituitary cells are adaptable to training in addition to regulatory hormones. Other biologically active GH fragments are released, and this superfamily of GH molecules operates in a complex manner in mediating GH-related effects (117). Many anabolic effects of GH are mediated through IGF-1. Upon release, GH circulates, attaches to a binding protein (GH-binding protein), and has a half-life of 20–50 minutes. GH deficiencies are related to a variety of conditions including reduced LBM.

Acute Responses to Exercises

Exercise is a potent stimulus for bioactive and immunoreactive GH secretion, which does not respond in the same manner (118). Exercise can modify the activity and molecular character of GH isoforms in circulation (118,122,123). Although most studies have examined changes in the 22-kD GH molecule, RE and aerobic exercise produce acute elevations in other GH variants (16,17,123,124). Gordon et al. (122) showed that immunoreactive GH increased more so during aerobic exercise than RE in young and older women; however, bioactive GH increased more so following RE in young women only. In that study, the older women had diminished immunoreactive GH responses compared to younger women (122). The GH variant response is affected by muscular strength in women (17). RE elevates 22-kD GH (up to a 20-fold increase) through 30-minute postexercise similarly in men (39,64) and women (64), although resting concentrations of GH are often higher in women (43), and the response is limited when amino acids and carbohydrates are consumed (39,75). When GH samples are treated with glutathione (to reduce aggregation), the acute RE response is higher in women but more prolonged in men (125). During RE (reference to the 22-kD GH):

- GH response depends on exercise selection and amount of muscle mass recruited, muscle actions used (greater response during CON than ECC actions), intensity, volume, rest intervals between sets, and training status (greater elevations based on strength and the magnitude of work performed) (2,126). Higher-volume multiple-set workouts elicit larger GH elevations than single-set workouts (58,127,128). A lower-body RT program produces less of a GH elevation than the same program performed after an upper-body workout (129). The GH response is higher when arms and legs are trained relative to arms only (50).
- Bodybuilding workouts produce larger responses than strength training (59,60,64,66,67), although some of the difference may be attenuated with chronic RT (67). These workouts produce substantial blood lactate responses and high correlations between lactate and GH have been shown (130). For example, Zafeiridis et al. (131) compared a strength (4 sets of 5 repetitions, 88% of 1-RM, 3-min rest intervals), hypertrophy (4 sets of 10 repetitions, 75% of 1-RM, 2-min rest intervals), and an endurance protocol (4 sets of 15 repetitions, 60% of 1-RM, 1-min rest intervals) and showed that the GH response matched total work where the largest response was seen in the endurance protocol.
- The GH response is greater with short versus long rest intervals in between sets (132).
- The addition of a single set of high repetitions with 50% of 1-RM to the end of a strength protocol can augment the GH response (133).
- GH response may be larger in experienced trainees who could exert themselves to a greater extent when workload is greater (134,135).
- Using a multiple-joint to single-joint RE sequence produces a larger acute GH response compared to performing the reverse sequence; the GH response patterned differences in total work between protocols (74).
- Bilateral upper-body RE exercise protocols produce more substantial GH elevations than unilateral upper-body RE (57).
- Acute GH response may be greater following traditional RE sets versus cluster sets (71).
- Blood flow restriction training may augment the GH response to RE comparable to heavier loading (136) especially in legs compared to arms (72).

Chronic Changes in Resting Growth Hormone Concentrations

Consistent exercise does not appear to alter resting GH concentrations. One reason may be that GH needs to be measured over a long period of time because of its pulsatile nature. Several studies examining single GH measures show no changes in resting GH concentrations during RT in men and women (37,82,83). Elite strength and power athletes have similar resting GH concentrations to lesser-trained individuals (46,81). The acute GH response to exercise appears more critical to adaptations, although the independent anabolic role GH plays

Chapter 7 Endocrine System Responses and Adaptations

the intracellular domain of GHR, thereby activating multiple signaling pathways producing different cellular effects (141). Substrates for JAK2 activation include a multitude of proteins including the signal transducers and activators of transcription (STAT) family, which leads to increased nuclear gene transcription. STAT1, 3, 5a, and 5b are all phosphorylated during signaling, but it appears STAT5b is the major mediator of GH signaling. In particular, GH signaling can increase IGF-1 gene expression. In men, GH infusion significantly increased GHR signaling in skeletal muscle and adipose tissue as evidenced by increased phosphorylation of STAT5 but via cross-talk with insulin signaling reduced insulin sensitivity (142). In men and women, GH infusion increased GH signaling (i.e., increased STAT5b phosphorylation, IGF-1, and SOC protein mRNA) within 30 minutes, but STAT5b phosphorylation was greater in women, but no age effect was observed (143). Thus, it appears that elevated GH may increase signaling capacity in skeletal muscle but training effects currently remain unclear.

Insulin-Like Growth Factors

IGFs are structurally related to insulin and mediate many actions of GH. IGFs are small polypeptide hormones (70 and 67 amino acids for IGF-1 and IGF-2, respectively) synthesized from a larger precursor peptide that is posttranslationally processed into its active form that is secreted by the liver or produced in skeletal muscle in response to GH stimulation. IGFs increase cell cycle initiation and progression, satellite cell activation, proliferation, survival, and differentiation; increase myotube size and number of nuclei per myotube; stimulate amino acid uptake and protein synthesis and muscle hypertrophy, neuronal myelinization, axonal sprouting, and damage repair; and reduce chronic inflammatory response. The metabolic effects of IGF-1 include increased free fatty acid utilization and enhancing insulin sensitivity. Of the two, IGF-1 has been extensively studied. IGFs are affected by other hormones including TH and thyroid hormones once again demonstrating hormonal synergism. Local mechanical-stretch mechanisms can activate IGF-1 synthesis in local tissues. Many aspects of IGF-1 biology (IGF-1 bioavailability, sequestration of IGF-1 across IGFBPs and biocompartments, IGF-1 receptor activation) all contribute to its impact. Only 2% of IGF-1 circulates in its free form; most circulate as a binary (20%–25%) or ternary complex (~75%) (144,145). In its binary form, IGF-1 circulates with one binding protein, whereas in its ternary form, IGF-1 circulates with IGFBP-3 and its acid labile subunit (ALS). Because of these critical anabolic functions, IGF genes have been considered a potential target for gene therapies and for gene doping in athletes (146). Some IGF-1 gene variants are associated with greater strength changes during RT (147).

Acute Responses to Exercise

The IGF-1 response to exercise is unclear. Some studies showed acute elevations during aerobic and high-intensity interval

in skeletal muscle is unclear. The exercise-induced elevation correlates with type I and type II muscle fiber hypertrophy (86). Interestingly, GH pulsatility during sleep may be altered following RE where lower GH pulses may be seen early in sleep but greater pulses may be seen later in sleep (11).

Growth Hormone–Binding Protein

About 50% of GH binds to GH-specific binding proteins (GHBPs) that extend its half-life and enhance its effects. The GHBP arises from cleavage of the GH receptor in the liver or wherever the GH receptor exists. Two GHBPs have been identified: a high- and low-affinity GHBP. The high-affinity GHBP has high affinity for the 22-kD GH molecule. Little is known about GHBP and exercise. An elevation in GHBP was shown at rest after 2 weeks of endurance training (137). Aerobic exercise produces elevations in GH and GHBP (138,139). RE (6 sets of squats, 80%–85% of 1-RM, 10 repetitions, 2-min rest intervals) produces elevations of GHBP; however, no differences between resistance-trained and untrained individuals were seen, suggesting RT may not alter GHBP or change GH receptor expression (140). Acute RE may elevate GHBP mostly in obese men as baseline concentrations were still higher compared to lean men (118).

Growth Hormone Receptor Signaling

The GH receptor (GHR) is a class I cytokine receptor consisting of 620 amino acids (encoded by the GHR gene) and is expressed in many tissues, including the liver hepatocytes, skeletal muscle, bone and connective tissues, kidney, and adipose tissue (118). The GHR can release its extracellular domain into the circulation, which produces the circulating GH-binding protein. Direct signaling activity of the GH superfamily is regulated to GH receptor binding and subsequent intracellular second messenger signaling cascades (see Fig. 7.7). GH binds to the GHR extracellular domain where one GH molecule binds two GHRs. The dimerized GHR recruits tyrosine kinases (i.e., Janus kinase [JAK], mostly JAK2), which phosphorylate tyrosine residues in

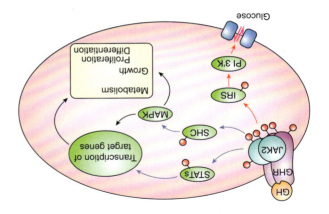

FIGURE 7.7 GH — GH receptor signaling.

exercise (148,149). Studies have shown no change, decreases, and elevations (2,59,60,66,140,145) in IGF-1 during or immediately (up to 30 min) following RE. Similar responses are seen between hypertrophy and strength training protocols (67). Elevations are expected when plasma volume is reduced. However, the lack of change may be attributed to delayed secretion of IGF-1, *i.e.*, 3–9 hours, following GH stimulation, as peak values may not be reached until 16–28 hours after exercise. Despite the anabolic actions of IGF-1, a direct link between RE-induced elevations and muscle strength and hypertrophy is unclear. Some evidence indicates that systemic IGF-1 elevations may act as a "regulator or amplifier" of muscle remodeling (27).

Chronic Changes in Systemic IGF-1 Concentrations

There is not a consistent pattern of change in IGF-1 concentrations during exercise. Because IGF-1 secretion depends upon GH stimulation, resting concentrations are variable due, in part, to the delay in signaling. Reductions in IGF-1 were shown after 11–12 weeks of RT and endurance training (150,151). No changes in resting IGF-1 were shown during short-term RT (37,86,152) and overreaching (87), unless concurrent with carbohydrate/protein supplementation (38). Elevations in IGF-1 may occur during periods of single- and multiple-set RT (153), RT tapering (154), and RT plus protein/amino acid supplementation (155). Resistance-trained men have higher resting IGF-1 concentrations than untrained men (140). A few studies in women have shown elevated resting IGF-1 during long-term RT (83,156). Similar to GH, the measurement of IGF-1 over wider time windows may be more informative.

Muscle IGF-1 Adaptations to Training

Of greater significance may be the training responses of locally produced IGF-1 isoforms. IGF-1 has autocrine/paracrine functions within muscle cells. Three isoforms have been identified, each functioning independently. Two isoforms are similar to circulating IGF-1 (IGF-1Ea and IGF-1Eb), and the third muscle-specific isoform (IGF-1Ec) is known as *mechano growth factor* (MGF) (157). MGF acts independently, is expressed earlier than other IGF-1 isoforms in response to exercise, and may have greater anabolic potency (157). Overloaded muscle and mechanical damage from RT are potent stimuli (158). RE increases IGF-1, IGF-1Ea, and MGF mRNA (109,159,160) for up to 48 hours post, and the effect is greater with protein supplementation (155). IGF-1 and MGF mRNA have increased 2 hours postexercise (but not 6 hours) after a single bout of moderate-intensity RE (65% of 1-RM; 18–20 repetitions) and moderately high-intensity RE (85% of 1-RM; 8–10 repetitions) (161). High-intensity workouts produce great mechanical loading (and a substantial ECC component) and hypertrophy, in part, via up-regulation of muscle IGF-1 and MGF. One study reported increased MGF mRNA 22 hours following high-intensity RE (74% of max) but not following moderate-intensity RE

(54% of max) producing higher metabolic stress (162). Other data show an intensity-dependent increase in muscle IGF-1Ea (163).

Insulin-Like Growth Factor–Binding Proteins

Nearly all circulating IGFs are bound to IGF-binding proteins (IGFBPs 1–6, mostly IGFBP-3). These proteins regulate IGF availability, prolong IGF circulation, and can either stimulate or inhibit IGF-1 biological action. They have generated more consistent responses during RE than systemic IGF-1. Aerobic, sprint, RE, and combined aerobic and RE elevate IGFBP-3 (28,145,148,164,165). Nindl et al. (29) monitored overnight IGF-1 following heavy RE and showed that IGF-1 concentrations remained unchanged but IGFBP-2 increased and ALS decreased suggesting that binding protein partitioning, rather than changes in systemic IGF-1, was critical. Other studies have shown that IGFBP-1 was sensitive to exercise duration but not exercise mode. Nindl et al. (145) failed to report increased IGF-1 receptor phosphorylation during and following RE (despite elevations in IGF-1); however, IGF mRNA content was increased reinforcing the concept that skeletal muscle adaptation may not be dependent on systemic IGF-1 but rather the interplay across biocompartments. Less is known about chronic circulating IGFBP-3 and IGFBP-1. Reductions or no changes occur (2,153) and some have suggested IGFBP-3 (a reduction) may serve as marker of overtraining (166). Other research has shown no changes in IGFBP-3 or IGFBP-1 after 16 weeks of RT (152). No significant changes in IGF-1, IGFBP-1, or IGFBP-3 were found in subjects who were considered extreme responders to 16 weeks of RT versus nonresponders, although a trend was shown where IGFBP-3 in extreme responders tended to be lower than nonresponders (152).

IGF-1 Receptor and Intracellular Signaling

The endocrine, autocrine, and paracrine effects of IGF-1 are mediated through binding to the IGF-1 receptor (IGF-1R), a ligand-activated receptor tyrosine kinase. The *IGF-1R* gene is mapped to chromosome 15q25-26. Two receptor types have been identified (types 1 and 2). IGF-1 binds with greater affinity to type 1 than to type 2 or the insulin receptor, whereas IGF-2 binds with greater affinity to the type 2 receptor (see Fig. 7.8). IGF-1R contains two extracellular IGF-1 binding sites and two transmembrane β subunits that autophosphorylate tyrosine residues, which stimulates intermediates such as the IRS family and Shc proteins. The two main intracellular signaling pathways involve the phosphatidylinositol 3-kinase (PI3)/Akt kinase pathway and the mitogen-activated protein kinase (MAPK)/ERK pathway. A calcium-dependent calcineurin pathway has been identified as well. In addition, IGF-1 may increase cyclin D1 mRNA thereby enhancing proliferation and the myogenic response and inhibit atrogenes. Lastly, IGF-1 interaction with IGF-1R is influenced by other hormone-receptor interactions. IGF-1R phosphorylation may be sensitive to

Chapter 7 Endocrine System Responses and Adaptations

post-RE (161).

Insulin

Insulin is secreted from the Islets of Langerhans (B cells) in the pancreas after modification from its parent molecules, preproinsulin and proinsulin. Proinsulin (86 amino acids) is converted into insulin (51 amino acids) and *C peptide* (31 amino acids). Insulin is secreted in response to glucose intake and has a half-life of 3–5 minutes. Insulin exerts a hypoglycemic effect by increasing tissue uptake of glucose following nutrient consumption but also increases lipogenesis. Insulin increases muscle protein synthesis when adequate amino acid concentrations are available. Insulin concentrations parallel changes in blood glucose, and the response is enhanced when protein/carbohydrates are ingested prior to, during, or following exercise (8,38). Insulin concentrations decrease during prolonged aerobic exercise (167) and RE (61), although some studies have shown elevations post-RE (66,67). Insulin elevations are mostly affected by blood glucose and/or dietary intake rather than exercise levels. Consumption of carbohydrates, amino acids, or combinations of both prior to, during, and/or immediately after exercise is recommended for maximizing insulin's effects on tissue growth.

RE favoring high-volume over high-intensity protocols 1 hour postexercise (66) and moderate-intensity and moderately high-intensity RE has been shown to increase IGF-1R mRNA 2 hours post-RE (161).

Short-term aerobic, anaerobic interval, and RT may have limited impact on resting insulin concentrations. However, several studies have shown long-term aerobic or RT may reduce baseline insulin concentrations especially in older individuals (168). The critical element is that aerobic and anaerobic training improves insulin sensitivity and reduces insulin resistance. *Insulin resistance* is a condition (prominent in obese individuals, elderly, and diabetics) where normal amounts of insulin are inadequate to produce a response. Insulin sensitivity is the opposite. Muscle contraction and hypoxia produce similar muscular effects as insulin performs when it binds to its membrane-bound receptor. Muscle contraction activates glucose transport proteins (known as GLUT proteins, mostly GLUT4) similar to insulin, although the intracellular pathways differ (169). Glucose transporter type 4 (GLUT4) protein, encoded by the *SLC2A4* gene, is one of 14 GLUT proteins; it facilitates glucose transport into adipose tissue, cardiac, and skeletal muscle. Skeletal muscle GLUT4 concentrations correlate with glucose uptake during intense exercise (170). The increase in muscle glucose transport during exercise is primarily due to translocation of GLUT4 from intracellular sites to the sarcolemma and T-tubules. Glucose transport into muscles occurs during exercise independent of insulin, and exercise has a sparing effect on insulin production. It appears that there may be two intracellular pools of GLUT4, one that is recruited primarily by insulin-induced exocytosis and the other by muscle contraction-induced exocytosis/reduced endocytosis (170). GLUT4

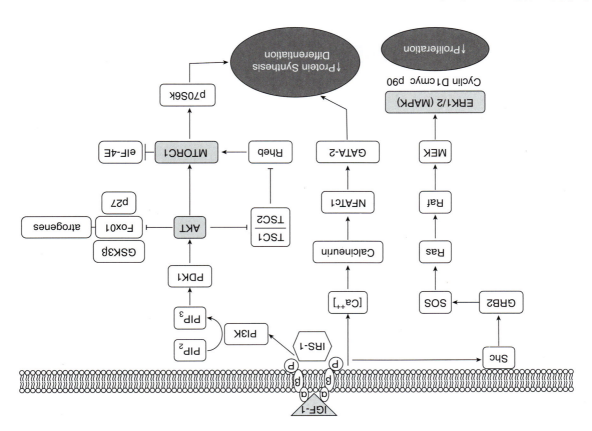

FIGURE 7.8 — IGF-1 receptor signaling.

expression is generally higher in type I fibers by 20%–30%. Regular exercise results in enhanced insulin- and contraction-stimulated glucose transport capacity and a rapid increase in skeletal muscle GLUT4 mRNA and protein levels that lasts for up to 24 hours afterward (170). Repeated exercise tends to produce chronic elevations of GLUT4 (170). RT can increase skeletal muscle GLUT4 (171). See Figure 7.9 (173).

Cortisol

Cortisol is a catabolic glucocorticoid released from the zona fasciculata of the adrenal cortex (with minimal amounts produced in other tissues such as the brain, thymus, skin, and GI tract) in response to stress under the control of CRH and ACTH. Like TE, its release is diurnal where it is highest in the morning and decreases throughout the day. It is synthesized from pregnenolone via P450c17 17α-hydroxylation and a few other intermediate steps. Cortisol accounts for ~95% of all glucocorticoid activity. About 10% of circulating cortisol is free, whereas ~15% is bound to albumin and 75% is bound to

Glucagon

Glucagon is a peptide hormone consisting of 29 amino acids synthesized (from *proglucagon*) in α cells in the islets of Langerhans of the pancreas. The half-life of glucagon is 3–6 minutes until it is removed by the liver and kidneys. Glucagon secretion is inhibited by glucose levels, and when secreted, glucagon stimulates the breakdown of glycogen, increases lipolysis, and increases energy availability. It is the antagonist of insulin.

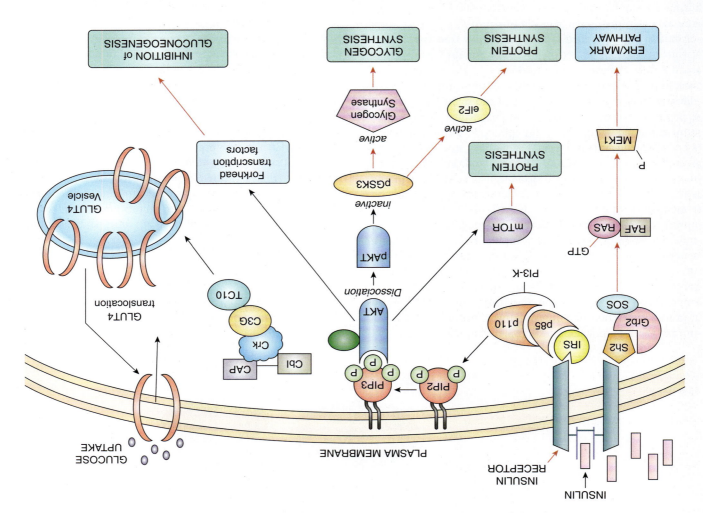

FIGURE 7.9 Insulin signaling. Binding of insulin to its receptor activates a cascade of reactions involving tissue anabolism (ERK/MAPK and mTOR). Insulin binding may stimulate Akt signaling ultimately leading to the increased activation of glycogen synthase leading to glycogen storage. Akt also activates mTOR and forkhead transcription factors, which inhibit gluconeogenesis and lead to GLUT4 translocation to the cell membrane. Another way by which GLUT4 translocation takes place is through casitas B-lineage lymphoma protein (cbl) and adapter protein cap. (From Kumar M, Nath S, Prasad HK, Sharma GD, Li Y. MicroRNAs: a new ray of hope for diabetes mellitus. *Protein Cell.* 2012;3:726–38. Ref. (172).)

It binds to membrane-bound receptors and increases glycogen breakdown via the cyclic AMP second messenger system. Glucagon elevation occurs during exercise as energy demands increase (167).

corticosteroid-binding globulin. Similar to androgens, cortisol diffuses through the cell membrane, and binds to its nuclear receptor (but could also have rapid nongenomic effects), but elicits catabolic effects on skeletal muscle. Cortisol stimulates lipolysis in adipose cells and increases protein degradation and decreases protein synthesis in muscle cells, with greater effects in type II muscle fibers. Glucocorticoids play significant roles in reducing inflammation and modulating immune responses (*i.e.*, immunosuppression via several mechanisms) to exercise and training (174). Glucocorticoid administration can up-regulate myostatin expression and limit muscle growth. Because of its role in tissue remodeling, acute and chronic changes in cortisol during exercise is often studied.

Acute Cortisol Responses to Exercise

Exercise is a potent stimulus for CRH, ACTH, and cortisol elevations especially exercise high in metabolic demand, lactate response, intensity/volume, and that produces increases in creatine kinase and potential muscle damage (174). Aerobic exercise elevates cortisol with the response more prominent as intensity increases (175). The response may be reduced in highly trained endurance athletes who are not overtrained. Large responses may be seen during ultra-endurance events such as triathlons (176). Bobbert et al. (177) studied male marathon runners and divided them into groups based on race time. Runners with the best times had the highest TE/cortisol ratios and runners with the slowest times had the largest cortisol response. Another study found higher cortisol responses in middle-distance runners than marathon runners during intermittent running and the cortisol responses were inversely correlated with $\dot{V}O_{2\,max}$ (178). The high stress of endurance competition produces large elevations in cortisol and is, in part, linked to immunosuppression that follows (179).

Anaerobic exercise produces similar responses, and the response is augmented by dehydration (79). Combined aerobic and RE acutely elevates cortisol concentrations (28) as does intense military training (180). RE elevates cortisol and ACTH (36,37,70) with similar responses in men and women (43). Workouts that elicit the greatest cortisol response elicit the greatest GH and lactate responses. Workouts that are high in volume and moderate to high in intensity and use short rest periods elicit the greatest lactate and cortisol responses with little change during conventional strength/power training sessions (43,63,65–67,130,181). High-volume programs (4–6 sets vs. 2 sets; 6 sets vs. 1 set) produce greater cortisol responses (40,182). Hypertrophy protocols yield greater responses than strength or power training (65). Greater cortisol responses occur during workouts using short (1-min) rest intervals compared to long rest intervals (3 min) (181,183) but are blunted to some extent when carbohydrate supplementation is consumed (38,184) and augmented with a large consumption of caffeine (77). The cortisol responses have been correlated with 24-hour creatine kinase values (43). The sequence of RE may not affect the cortisol response (74). Due to cortisol's catabolic properties, cortisol elevations are necessary for tissue remodeling and recovery.

Chronic Changes in Resting Cortisol Concentrations

Resting cortisol concentrations reflect a long-term training stress and are transient. No change, reductions, and elevations occur during normal strength and power training in men and women (2). Overtraining, resulting from a large increase in volume, elevates cortisol and reduces resting total and free TE concentrations (185) and reduces the TE/cortisol (T/C) ratio that some considered an indicator of the anabolic/catabolic status of skeletal muscle. Some studies have shown increases during RT, whereas some have not (2). Resting cortisol diurnal patterns reflect a multitude of factors in addition to training.

The Glucocorticoid Receptor and Intramuscular Signaling

The catabolic effects of cortisol are mostly mediated through glucocorticoid receptors (GR). The *glucocorticoid receptor (GR)* gene (*NR3C1*) is located on chromosome 5q31-32. It encodes the GR that belongs to the nuclear receptor superfamily of ligand-dependent transcription factors. It contains NH_2-terminal transactivation, DNA-binding, and ligand-binding domains as well as a hinge region. Coactivators, chromatin remodeling enzymes, and RNA polymerase II assist with hormone interaction and transcription processes as previously described for ARs. The GR DNA-binding domain binds to specific DNA sequences in the promoter region of target genes. Cortisol binding to the GR dissociates HSPs, and the cortisol/GR complex is chaperoned to the nucleus via a protein complex along the microtubules. Chromatin remodeling occurs via pioneering transcription factors enabling the hormone/GR complex binding to the genomic target sequence. Several polymorphisms of the *GR* gene have been identified and shown to relate to various health indices. Some polymorphisms are associated with LBM and muscle strength (186,187) and with strength gains during 12 weeks of RT (188). These studies show that some polymorphisms of the GR mediate the sensitivity of cortisol and can partially affect strength and hypertrophy adaptations to RT.

Cortisol/GR interaction increases protein degradation, decreases protein synthesis, decreases transport of amino acids, and causes atrophy, mainly of type II muscle fibers. Of interest is the potential competitive signaling between cortisol/GR and androgens/AR. The homologies of the DNA-binding and ligand-binding domains between the AR and GR are 79% and 50%, respectively, so both AR and GR can competitively bind to the same *cis*-elements on shared response elements (189). Competitive binding mediates, in part, anabolic versus catabolic signaling within muscle. Catabolism may occur in a variety of ways. Cortisol/GR may (a) inhibit the anabolic actions of androgens, insulin, IGF-1, and amino acids (leucine); (b) stimulate major proteolytic pathways (ubiquitin-proteasome, lysosomal [autophagy], and calpain systems); (c) inhibit the PI3/Akt pathway; (d) increase *FOXO* gene expression and activate atrogenes; (e) inhibit mTORC-1; (f) stimulate GSK3 (and decrease β-catenin); (g) inhibit production of muscle IGF-1 isoforms; (h) reduce circulating TE; and (i) increase *myostatin* (*MSTN*) gene expression and mRNA (190,191).

Cortisol and possibly androgen concentrations may determine the level of up- or down-regulation of GC receptor mRNA and protein content. ECC RE up-regulates GC receptor content and protein breakdown 6 and 24 hours post exercise in untrained men (192). The response is attenuated within 3 weeks thereby indicating a protective effect with repeated exposure to ECC exercise (192). However, in RT in men and women, no change was found 10 and 70 minutes following a RE protocol, and women had higher GR content than men in that study (30) but have shown similar content in other studies (115). Willoughby (193) reported higher GR content following 6 and 12 weeks of RT; however, samples were taken in close proximity to training, so the chronic adaptation is difficult to surmise. On the other hand, 6 weeks of intense run training in military cadets induced a 6.3% reduction in GR mRNA (194).

Catecholamines

The chromaffin cells of the adrenal medulla secrete catecholamines (also known as *adrenaline*) that are synthesized from the amino acid *tyrosine* (Fig. 7.10). Epinephrine (~80%) is predominantly secreted with norepinephrine (15%–20%), and dopamine is also secreted. Norepinephrine and dopamine also serve as neurotransmitters in the autonomic nervous system. Catecholamines are secreted in response to cognitive and physical stress (exercise, heat, hypoxia, hypoglycemia) under the control of sympathetic nervous system stimulation, ACTH, and cortisol; reflect the demands of exercise; and are important for increasing force production, muscle contraction rate, energy availability, as well as performing other functions including the augmentation of hormones such as TE. Catecholamine actions are terminated quickly as they bind with low affinity to their membrane-bound receptors (α-1,2 and β-1,2,3 adrenergic), function through second messenger G-protein/cyclic AMP systems, and are dissociated rapidly.

Catecholamine concentrations are increased during aerobic and anaerobic exercise with the magnitude dependent on the muscle mass involved (particularly upper body), posture (upright position yields a higher response), intensity, duration, and caffeine consumption (19,195–197). At a standard submaximal workload, endurance-trained athletes may exhibit a smaller catecholamine response (196). However, some studies have shown that endurance athletes produce a more substantial catecholamine response to exercise (at a similar high relative workload) than untrained individuals (196,197), termed a **sports adrenal medulla**. Similar findings were shown with anaerobic (sprint) training where some studies indicate a greater potential to secrete catecholamines during exercise in trained individuals (197). The acute exercise response may be somewhat blunted in obese individuals (195).

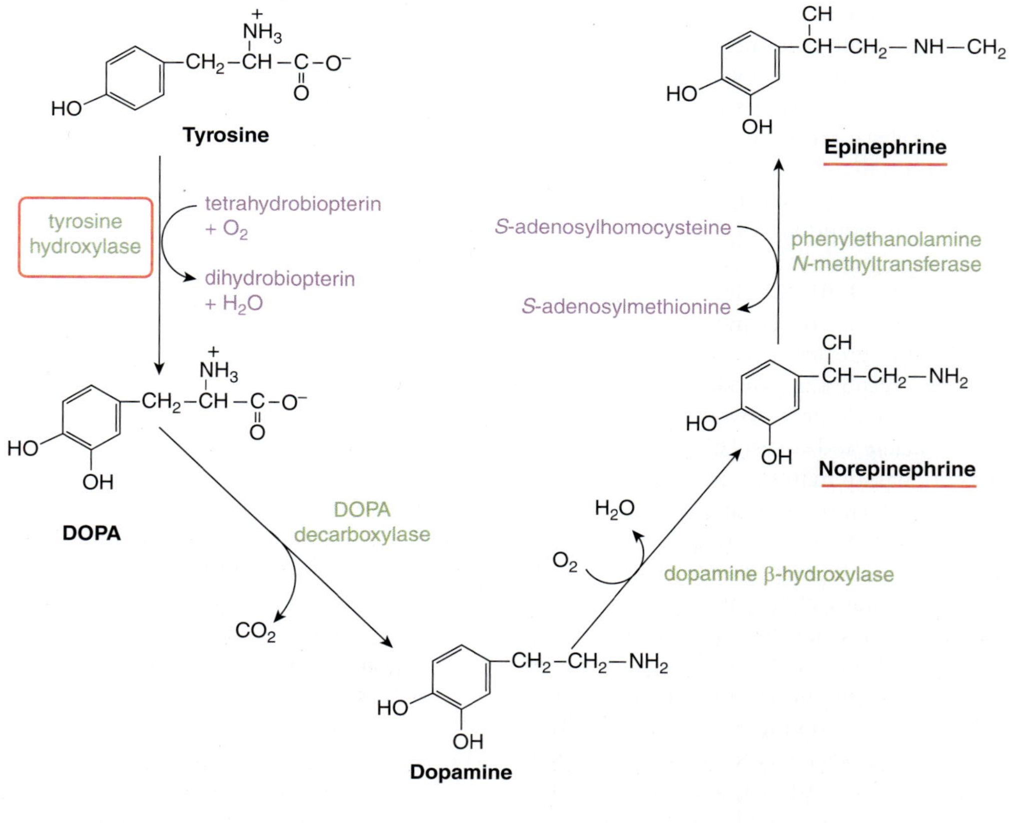

FIGURE 7.10 Catecholamine biosynthesis.

RE increases plasma concentrations of epinephrine (19,36), norepinephrine (19,36), and dopamine (36,181). The magnitude is dependent upon the force of muscle contraction, amount of muscle stimulated, intensity and volume, rest intervals utilized, and level of dehydration (2,79,174). Blood flow restriction of the arms and legs combined with low-intensity RE can increase the norepinephrine response (72). The norepinephrine response to early morning RE may be augmented by caffeine consumption (3 mg/kg body mass) (19). Trained lifters may experience an anticipatory rise in catecholamines to help prepare the body to perform maximally (36,59). Plasma epinephrine and norepinephrine increase in response to high-intensity bodyweight RE and treadmill running; however, the bodyweight protocol yielded a greater epinephrine response (198). Military training increases catecholamine responses but fitter individuals may recover quicker (norepinephrine) following exercise (180). Chronic adaptations are less clear, although it has been suggested that training reduces the catecholamine response (199). Kraemer et al. (200) compared 12 weeks of RT, endurance training, or combined RT and endurance training on the acute catecholamine response to graded exercise every 4 weeks during the 12-week period. They found increased plasma epinephrine and norepinephrine in all training groups each time; however, the combined and endurance groups showed up to 50% elevations, whereas the RT-only group showed a reduced response. The authors concluded that the training modality can alter the acute catecholamine response to graded exercise.

β-Endorphins

β-Endorphin is a 31-amino acid opioid neuropeptide and peptide hormone cleaved in the anterior pituitary from a parent molecule (*proopiomelanocortin*, which gives rise to ACTH and β-*lipotropin*) and also found in hypothalamic neurons. It also acts as a neurotransmitter in the nervous system. It binds to opioid receptors throughout the CNS. β-*Endorphins* act as analgesics, increase relaxation, and enhance immune function. Exercise is a potent stimulus for β-endorphin secretion with the response dependent on the intensity and duration (201). Anaerobic exercise elevates β-endorphins in proportion to blood lactate and ACTH increases (201,202). Aerobic exercise increases β-endorphins with a rise in intensity (203). A threshold intensity and volume may be necessary for elevations (at least 70% of $\dot{V}O_{2\,max}$) (204). β-Endorphin elevations occur during RE in men and women in most (205,206) but not all studies (207). Workouts (bodybuilding-type workouts high in volume, moderate to high intensity, and with short rest intervals) that produce high levels of blood lactate and cortisol also stimulate a rise in β-endorphins (208), although Olympic weightlifting programs increase plasma β-endorphins (45). The elevation has been attributed to the magnitude of muscle mass used, rest interval length, intensity, and volume (2). The rise in β-endorphins may help off-set the acidosis by improving mood state and pain tolerance

(201). Anabolic steroid users have been shown to have higher β-endorphin concentrations compared to other users currently not taking steroids (209).

Thyroid Hormones

The thyroid hormones thyroxine (T4) and triiodothyronine (T3) are released into circulation (under the control of TRH and TSH) where they travel mostly bound to transport proteins (thyroxine-binding globulin, prealbumin, and albumin). Mostly T4 (~20 times more) circulates as it has a longer half-life than T3. T3 and T4 enter cells via transporters. In target tissues, T4 is mostly converted to the more potent T3 via deiodinases. T3 binds to nuclear receptors inducing genomic actions. Two thyroid hormone receptor encoding genes exists termed THRA (chromosome 17 with α1 and α2 isoforms) and THRB (chromosome 3 with β1 and β2 isoforms), which give rise to protein receptors that have different binding affinities for T3 (210). All four isoforms are found in skeletal muscle. Like other steroid hormones, T3 bound to receptors binds to specific thyroid DNA hormone response elements to increase gene transcription especially of proteins involved in energy homeostasis and metabolism. Coactivators and corepressors help or hinder these actions. Thyroid receptor isoforms exist in the nucleus that may have both ligand-dependent and independent actions regulated by coactivators (210). In addition to classic genomic transcription regulation, other mechanisms of action have been identified where thyroid hormone regulation of transcription occurs without binding to thyroid response elements but have other protein interactions (211). Nongenomic actions via membrane binding to other proteins (integrin) have been shown (212).

The thyroid hormones (T3, T4) increase basal metabolic rate, protein synthesis, and augment the actions of catecholamines. In skeletal muscle, thyroid actions include increased MyoD, myosin heavy chain (MHC) IIa, SERCA protein content, GLUT4 expression (and insulin sensitivity), and AMPK activation and fatty acid oxidation (212). They also influence fiber type and PGC-1α signaling (212). The response of thyroid hormones and tissue signaling to exercise and training is not clear. Aerobic exercise elevates T3 and T4 in an intensity-dependent manner (213). However, some studies showed no acute elevations (173). Inconsistent changes have been shown over long-term training periods (214). Intense rowing training decreases in TSH and free T3 as did RT (215). Systemic thyroid hormone concentrations are influenced by energy balance and may be reduced during times of reduced energy availability especially in amenorrheic female athletes (216). The role of thyroid hormones during RT is unclear but may be permissive in its interaction (augmentation) with other hormones, *e.g.*, ARs. Some studies have shown no changes or reductions in resting T4, free T4, T3, and TSH during RT (2,16). Due to the tight control of thyroid hormones, elevations during RT may not be expected. Like other hormones, the whole signaling apparatus of thyroid hormone actions must be viewed in its entirety. However, little is known about intramuscular signaling and exercise or training in humans. Treadmill exercise acutely up-regulates type 2 deiodinases in muscle, increasing T3 conversion and PGC-1α signaling (217). In rats, endurance training above and below the lactate threshold reduced circulating TSH. However, sublactate threshold exercise increase thyroid receptor β1 mRNA and protein content only (and not the other isoforms), whereas supralactate threshold exercise had the opposite effect (218). Thus, exercise positively impacts thyroid hormone signaling, but the full extent is unknown.

Fluid-Regulatory Hormones

Fluid shifts during exercise elicit a hormonal response to restore fluid balance. Acute prolonged exercise increases *plasma osmolality* (the number of molecules relative to fluid volume), plasma sodium and potassium concentrations, and reduces plasma volume (219). AVP (or ADH) is released from the posterior pituitary where it acts on the kidneys and blood vessels to increase fluid reabsorption; sodium, potassium, and chloride reabsorption; and vasoconstriction. Atrial peptide is a 28-amino acid hormone released from the heart in response to increases in blood pressure to induce *natriuresis* (sodium excretion in urine and decrease in blood fluid volume). Renin is a renal enzyme released in response to low blood pressure and reduced renal blood flow that stimulates production of angiotensin I (from angiotensinogen). It is also stimulated by sympathetic nervous system activity. Angiotensin I is converted to angiotensin II via the enzyme angiotensin-converting enzyme (ACE), which stimulates the release of aldosterone from the adrenal cortex (Fig. 7.11). These hormones increase arterial

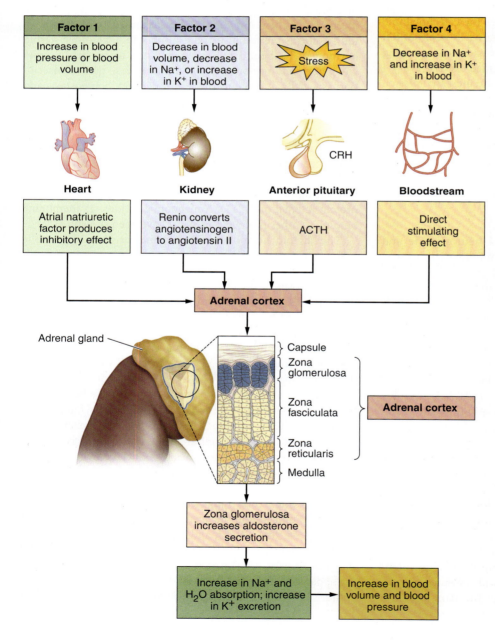

FIGURE 7.11 The renin-angiotensin-aldosterone system.

constriction in addition to aldosterone secretion. Aldosterone secretion is controlled by changes in fluid volume, sodium and potassium content in the blood, stress, cardiac output, and changes in blood pressure, and stimulation from angiotensin II. The resultant effect of aldosterone is to increase sodium retention and fluid volume to increase blood pressure. It stimulates sodium reabsorption in the distal tubules of the kidneys. Aldosterone signaling occurs through the mineralocorticoid receptor, which acts as a ligand-dependent transcription factor regulated by several coactivators. Aldosterone also stimulates the activation of protein kinases and secondary messenger signaling cascades that act independently and modulate its transcriptional action (220).

Fluid homeostasis is critical to exercise performance. Elevations in fluid regulatory hormones such as AVP, atrial peptide, the enzyme renin, aldosterone, and angiotensin II are seen acutely during exercise, with the magnitude dependent on intensity, duration, fitness level, and hydration status (219,221,222). Plasma volume expansion, which accompanies early adaptations to endurance training, may blunt some of the acute fluid regulatory increase seen during aerobic exercise (223). Endurance training poses small reductions to no changes in the fluid regulatory hormone response (224). However, changes in aldosterone signaling are thought to mediate some of the plasma volume expansion seen during endurance training in addition to increased plasma protein content (219,225). A meta-analysis showed that chronic endurance training decreased renin activity but did not affect circulating angiotensin II or aldosterone (226). Thus, it appears that acute responses to exercise are critical in regulating fluid volume rather than long-term effects. This was shown during a marathon where significant elevations in fluid regulatory hormones were reported; however, values returned to baseline within 60 minutes indicative of a short-term effect (219). RE elevates atrial peptide, renin, angiotensin II, and plasma osmolality as early as after the first set (36). Boone et al. (227) compared to a lower-volume, high-intensity strength protocol to a higher-volume, moderate-intensity hypertrophy protocol and reported that only the high-volume hypertrophy protocol elicited acute increases in plasma osmolality, sodium, and aldosterone with a decrease in potassium. As with endurance, it appears that the interaction of RE intensity, muscle mass involvement, volume, and rest intervals pose a stimulus to reduce plasma volume and initiate a hormonal milieu to regulate fluid changes.

Leptin and Appetite Regulating Hormones

Leptin, a product of the *ob* gene in adipose tissue, is a hormone that relays satiety signal to the hypothalamus to regulate energy balance and appetite but is involved in a milieu of bodily responses. Blood leptin concentrations reflect the amount of energy stored in adipose tissue. Obese humans have approximately four times more leptin than lean individuals, and women show higher concentrations than men. Leptin is released in response to intermittent fasting, kilocalorie restriction, and overfeeding and circulates to the brain where it crosses the blood-brain barrier to act with receptors to affect appetite, energy intake and expenditure, thermogenesis, and a number of other actions. Leptin concentrations may be influenced by insulin, glucocorticoids, catecholamines, thyroid hormones, TE, GH, and stimulants. *Leptin resistance* is common in obesity. It develops from gene mutations, altered transport across the blood-brain barrier and receptor signaling (228). A higher concentration of leptin in the blood in obese individuals is the consequence of lack of signaling at the hypothalamic level. Thus, the signal to increase energy expenditure and reduce kilocalorie intake is attenuated and thought to contribute to the effects of obesity.

Exercise may only have a small effect on leptin concentrations independent of percent body fat changes (131,140,229). Studies have shown that low- and high-intensity aerobic exercise, RT, and combined aerobic and RT can reduce serum leptin concentrations (215,230). A meta-analysis examining leptin and training studies showed that chronic aerobic, RT, and combined aerobic and RT (3 weeks to 24 months; 2–7 days per week; 24- to 90-min duration) reduce serum leptin concentrations (230). The changes in leptin were similar in older and younger adults, men, and women, and that changes in percent body fat were associated with the leptin response, although some data indicated leptin reductions independent of percent body fat changes (230). The largest reductions were seen in studies showing significant body fat reductions, and it appeared that the exercise mode and intensity, volume, frequency, and duration were not associated with the leptin reduction (230). Leptin is a critical mediator of several endocrine pathways pertinent to RT. Leptin directly reduces steroidogenesis (231) resulting in lower TE concentrations in obese men.

The effects of acute exercise on other appetite-regulating hormones have been studied. Acylated ghrelin is known to stimulate hunger, whereas peptide YY (PYY), glucagon-like peptide 1 (GLP-1), and pancreatic polypeptide (PP) decrease hunger and food intake. A meta-analysis (232) showed that aerobic exercise such as cycling, running, interval, walking, and swimming (30–120 min, 45%–75% of $\dot{V}O_{2max}$) and RE (45–90 min, 80% of 1-RM, 10–12 repetitions) can decrease the hunger-inducing hormone acylated ghrelin by ~16.5% and increase the hunger-suppressing hormones PPY (by ~8.9%), GLP-1 (by ~13.1%), and PP (by ~15%). These data show that exercise has a positive effect on hormonal regulation of appetite and demonstrate another critical benefit to exercise for weight control.

Estrogens

Estrogens (estradiol or 17β-estradiol, estriol, and estrone) are steroids with long half-lives synthesized and secreted primarily by the ovaries (and adrenals to a lesser extent) in women under the control of LH and FSH but are produced from conversion of androgens in men. Estrogens circulate bound to SHBG or albumin until they reach the target tissue or become metabolized

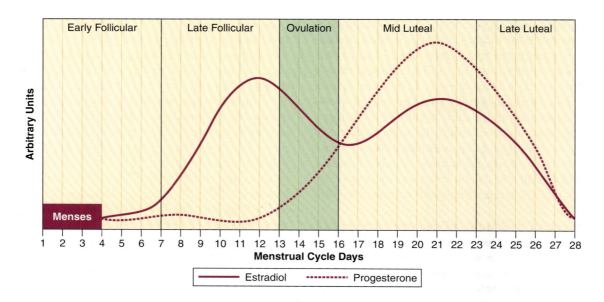

FIGURE 7.12 Menstrual cycle and estradiol and progesterone.

by the liver. Estrogen signaling occurs via α and β estrogen receptor proteins. Estrogens perform many functions, including promoting secondary female characteristics including regulating ovulation and menstruation, reducing bone resorption (and stimulating growth plate closure), enhancing metabolism, increase free fatty acid mobilization, retaining sodium and water, reducing muscle damage, and increasing HDLs (decreasing LDLs). However, estrogens inhibit collagen synthesis (233) that can weaken tendons and ligaments. Susceptibility to injury is a concern for female athletes or males using anabolic steroids.

Estrogen responses to exercise are less clear especially since it is difficult to phase women during the estradiol flux of the menstrual cycle. Aerobic exercise may elevate estradiol in women (234), and elevations have been reported following RE (174). Long-term studies have been conducted in young and older women, athletes, and special populations. Women in precontest dieting/training for fitness competitions (that led to a 12% decrease in bodyweight and 35%–50% decrease in fat mass) were shown to have significantly lower estradiol (in addition to TE, T3, and leptin) that coincided with menstrual irregularities (235). Estradiol returned to normal levels within 3–4 months when regular diet and training ensued (235). This is synonymous with the *female triad* (discussed in Chapter 3) where low kilocalorie intake, high activity, menstrual disturbance, and low bone mineral density are accompanied by reduced levels of estradiol (236). A meta-analysis examining the chronic aerobic and RT in women showed a reduction in total and free estradiol, and the effects were larger in obese women and during training that resulted in weight loss (237). The effect on total estradiol was greater during high-intensity RT (237). Thus, it appears a chronic training response may be lower estradiol concentrations in women. The phase of the menstrual cycle is critical as estradiol levels are low during the follicular phase (days 1–13), but peak value is attained near ovulation (Fig. 7.12). After a short-term reduction, estradiol levels rise and are higher during the luteal phase (days 15–28). Muscle strength, endurance, power, and $\dot{V}O_{2max}$ do not change during various phases of the menstrual cycle (2,238,239). However, prolonged exercise in the heat may be compromised during the mid-luteal phase where body temperature tends to be elevated (238).

SUMMARY POINTS

- The endocrine system is one of two major control systems (along with the nervous system) in the human body.
- The human body contains a multitude of hormones that perform numerous functions.
- Systemic hormones are released into circulation, many bind to transport proteins, travel to the target tissues, and bind to either membrane-bound or cytoplasmic/nuclear receptors to elicit intracellular signaling mechanisms ultimately leading to the target effect.
- Exercise is a potent stimulus eliciting acute hormonal elevations in several key hormones known to enhance exercise performance and subsequent adaptations. The critical element is the signaling process as a whole as each step in signaling plays critical roles in determining the response.
- Chronic changes in resting concentrations for some hormones are not common, but when they do occur, they usually reflect some substantial changes in the training program, nutritional intake, major stress, clinical condition, or recovery activities.

REVIEW QUESTIONS

1. The hormone produced by the liver that is critical to mediating many of the anabolic effects of GH is
   a. Insulin
   b. IGF-1
   c. Cortisol
   d. Glucagon

2. Many side effects associated from excessive TE arise from its conversion into
   a. Estrogens
   b. DHEA
   c. Androstenediol
   d. Cholesterol

3. A major anabolic substance that is produced by muscle cells in response to mechanical stress is
   a. Cortisol
   b. Mechano-growth factor
   c. Insulin
   d. Parathyroid hormone

4. Which of the following hormones plays the most substantial role in fluid volume regulation?
   a. Aldosterone
   b. Leptin
   c. Glucagon
   d. Insulin

5. A hormone known to regulate hunger and energy expenditure is
   a. Leptin
   b. Cortisol
   c. Glucagon
   d. AVP

6. Which of the following hormones does not increase muscle mass?
   a. Insulin
   b. IGF-1
   c. Glucagon
   d. Testosterone

7. LH causes the secretion of cortisol in men.
   a. T
   b. F

8. A negative feedback system is one that will reduce secretion of a hormone if it is already high in concentration.
   a. T
   b. F

9. Because protein hormones have their receptors on the surface of the cell membrane, a second messenger system is needed intracellularly.
   a. T
   b. F

10. Plasma volume reductions have no effect on exercise hormonal concentrations.
    a. T
    b. F

11. An elevation in TE during a workout is an important factor for androgen receptor up-regulation.
    a. T
    b. F

12. Workouts that are low intensity and low volume and use long rest intervals maximize the acute GH response to resistance exercise.
    a. T
    b. F

REFERENCES

1. Clarke H, Dhillo WS, Jayasena CN. Comprehensive review on kisspeptin and its role in reproductive disorders. *Endocrinol Metab*. 2015;30:124–41.
2. Kraemer WJ, Ratamess NA. Hormonal responses and adaptations to resistance exercise and training. *Sports Med*. 2005;35:339–61.
3. Teo W, Newton MJ, McGuigan MR. Circadian rhythms in exercise performance: implications for hormonal and muscular adaptation. *J Sports Sci Med*. 2011;10:600–6.
4. Collomp K, Baillot A, Forget H, Coquerel A, Rieth N, Vibarel-Rebot N. Altered diurnal pattern of steroid hormones in relation to various behaviors, external factors and pathologies: a review. *Physiol Behav*. 2016;164:68–85.
5. Hayes LD, Bickerstaff GF, Baker JS. Interactions of cortisol, testosterone, and resistance training: influence of circadian rhythms. *Chronobiol Int*. 2010;27:675–705.
6. Häkkinen K, Pakarinen A. Serum hormones in male strength athletes during intensive short term strength training. *Eur J Appl Physiol*. 1991;63:191–9.
7. Kuusmaa M, Schumann M, Sedliak M, et al. Effects of morning versus combined strength and endurance training on physical performance, muscle hypertrophy, and serum hormone concentrations. *Appl Physiol Nutr Metab*. 2016;41:1285–94.
8. Sedliak M, Finni T, Cheng S, Kraemer WJ, Häkkinen K. Effect of time-of-day-specific strength training on serum hormone concentrations and isometric strength in men. *Chronobiol Int*. 2007;24:1159–77.
9. Kraemer WJ, Loebel CC, Volek JS, et al. The effect of heavy resistance exercise on the circadian rhythm of salivary testosterone in men. *Eur J Appl Physiol*. 2001;84:13–8.
10. McMurray RG, Eubank TK, Hackney AC. Nocturnal hormonal responses to resistance exercise. *Eur J Appl Physiol*. 1995;72:121–6.
11. Nindl BC, Hymer WC, Deaver DR, Kraemer WJ. Growth hormone pulsatility profile characteristics following acute heavy resistance exercise. *J Appl Physiol*. 2001;91:163–72.
12. Burley SD, Whittingham-Dowd J, Allen J, Grosset JF, Onambele-Pearson G. The differential hormonal milieu of morning versus evening may have an impact on muscle hypertrophic potential. *PLoS One*. 2016;11:e0161500.
13. Ahtiainen JP, Nyman K, Huhtaniemi I, et al. Effects of resistance training on testosterone metabolism in younger and older men. *Exp Gerentol*. 2015;69:148–58.

14. Mendelson C, Dufau M, Catt K. Gonadotropin binding and stimulation of cyclic adenosine 3′:5′-monophosphate and testosterone production in isolated Leydig cells. *J Biol Chem*. 1975;250:8818–23.

15. Kraemer WJ, Mazzetti SA. Hormonal mechanisms related to the expression of muscular strength and power. In: Komi PV, editor. *Strength and Power in Sport*. 2nd ed. Malden (MA): Blackwell Science; 2003. p. 73–95.

16. Kraemer WJ, Ratamess NA. Endocrine responses and adaptations to strength and power training. In: Komi PV, editor. *Strength and Power in Sport*. 2nd ed. Malden (MA): Blackwell Scientific Publications; 2003. p. 361–86.

17. Kraemer WJ, Rubin MR, Häkkinen K, et al. Influence of muscle strength and total work on exercise-induced plasma growth hormone isoforms in women. *J Sci Med Sport*. 2003;6:295–306.

18. Chtourou H, Souissi N. The effect of training at a specific time of day: a review. *J Strength Cond Res*. 2012;26:1984–2005.

19. Mora-Rodriguez R, Pallares JG, Lopez-Samanes A, Ortega JF, Fernandez-Elias V. Caffeine ingestion reverses the circadian rhythm effects on neuromuscular performance in highly resistance-trained men. *PLoS One*. 2012;7:e33807.

20. Sedliak M, Zeman M, Buzgo G, et al. Morphological, molecular and hormonal adaptations to early morning versus afternoon resistance training. *Chronobiol Int*. 2018;35:450–64.

21. Enea C, Boisseau N, Fargeas-Gluck MA, Diaz V, Dugue B. Circulating androgens in women: exercise-induced changes. *Sports Med*. 2011;41:1–15.

22. Vingren JL, Kraemer WJ, Hatfield DL, et al. Effect of resistance exercise on muscle steroidogenesis. *J Appl Physiol*. 2008;105:1754–60.

23. MacLean HE, Chiu WS, Notini AJ, et al. Impaired skeletal muscle development and function in male, but not female, genomic androgen receptor knockout mice. *FASEB J*. 2008;22:2676–89.

24. Michels G, Hoppe UC. Rapid actions of androgens. *Front Neuroendocrinol*. 2008;29:182–98.

25. Basualto-Alarcon C, Jorquera G, Altamirano F, Jaimovich E, Estrada M. Testosterone signals through mTOR and androgen receptor to induce muscle hypertrophy. *Med Sci Sports Exerc*. 2013;45:1712–20.

26. Kahn SM, Hryb DJ, Nakhla AM, Romas NA, Rosner W. Sex hormone-binding globulin is synthesized in target cells. *J Endocrinol*. 2002;175:113–20.

27. Kraemer WJ, Ratamess NA, Nindl BC. Recovery responses of testosterone, growth hormone, and IGF-1 after resistance exercise. *J Appl Physiol*. 2017;122:549–58.

28. Rosa C, Vilaca-Alves J, Fernandes HM, et al. Order effects of combined strength and endurance training on testosterone, cortisol, growth hormone, and IGF-1 binding protein 3 in concurrently trained men. *J Strength Cond Res*. 2015;29:74–9.

29. Nindl BC, Kraemer WJ, Gotshalk LA, et al. Testosterone responses after resistance exercise in women: influence of regional fat distribution. *Int J Sport Nutr Exerc Metab*. 2001;11:451–65.

30. Vingren JL, Kraemer WJ, Hatfield DL, et al. Effect of resistance exercise on muscle steroid receptor protein content in strength-trained men and women. *Steroids*. 2009;74:1033–9.

31. Tremblay MS, Copeland JL, Van Helder W. Influence of exercise duration on post-exercise steroid hormone responses in trained males. *Eur J Appl Physiol*. 2005;94:505–13.

32. Ahtiainen JP, Pakarinen A, Kraemer WJ, Häkkinen K. Acute hormonal and neuromuscular responses and recovery to forced vs maximum repetitions multiple resistance exercises. *Int J Sports Med*. 2003;24:410–8.

33. Häkkinen K, Pakarinen A. Acute hormonal responses to heavy resistance exercise in men and women at different ages. *Int J Sports Med*. 1995;16:507–13.

34. Hooper DR, Kraemer WJ, Focht BC, et al. Endocrinological roles for testosterone in resistance exercise responses and adaptations. *Sports Med*. 2017;47:1709–20.

35. Hulmi JJ, Ahtiainen JP, Selanne H, et al. Androgen receptors and testosterone in men—effects of protein ingestion, resistance exercise and fiber type. *J Steroid Biochem Mol Biol*. 2008;110:130–7.

36. Kraemer WJ, Fleck SJ, Maresh CM, et al. Acute hormonal responses to a single bout of heavy resistance exercise in trained power lifters and untrained men. *Can J Appl Physiol*. 1999;24:524–37.

37. Kraemer WJ, Häkkinen K, Newton RU, et al. Effects of heavy-resistance training on hormonal response patterns in younger vs. older men. *J Appl Physiol*. 1999;87:982–92.

38. Kraemer WJ, Volek JS, Bush JA, et al. Hormonal responses to consecutive days of heavy-resistance exercise with or without nutritional supplementation. *J Appl Physiol*. 1998;85:1544–55.

39. Ratamess NA, Hoffman JR, Ross R, et al. Effects of an amino acid/creatine energy supplement on the acute hormonal response to resistance exercise. *Int J Sport Nutr Exerc Metab*. 2007;17:608–23.

40. Ratamess NA, Kraemer WJ, Volek JS, et al. Androgen receptor content following heavy resistance exercise in men. *J Steroid Biochem Mol Biol*. 2005;93:35–42.

41. Vingren JL, Kraemer WJ, Ratamess NA, et al. Testosterone physiology in resistance exercise and training: the up-stream regulatory elements. *Sports Med*. 2010;40:1037–53.

42. Benini R, Prado Nunes PR, Orsatti CL, Barcelos LC, Orsatti FL. Effects of acute total body resistance exercise on hormonal and cytokines changes in men and women. *J Sports Med Phys Fitness*. 2015;55:337–44.

43. Kraemer WJ, Fleck SJ, Dziados JE, et al. Changes in hormonal concentrations after different heavy-resistance exercise protocols in women. *J Appl Physiol*. 1993;75:594–604.

44. Tremblay MS, Copeland JL, Van Helder W. Effect of training status and exercise mode on endogenous steroid hormones in men. *J Appl Physiol*. 2004;96:531–9.

45. Kraemer WJ, Fry AC, Warren BJ, et al. Acute hormonal responses in elite junior weightlifters. *Int J Sports Med*. 1992;13:103–9.

46. Ahtiainen JP, Pakarinen A, Alen M, et al. Muscle hypertrophy, hormonal adaptations and strength development during strength training in strength-trained and untrained men. *Eur J Appl Physiol*. 2003;89:555–63.

47. Hansen S, Kvorning T, Kjaer M, Szogaard G. The effect of short-term strength training on human skeletal muscle: the importance of physiologically elevated hormone levels. *Scand J Med Sci Sport*. 2001;11:347–54.

48. Kvorning T, Andersen M, Brixen K, Madsen K. Suppression of endogenous testosterone production attenuates the response to strength training: a randomized, placebo-controlled, and blinded intervention study. *Am J Physiol Endocrinol Metab*. 2006;291:E1325–32.

49. Mangine GT, Hoffman JR, Gonzalez AM, et al. Exercise-induced hormone elevations are related to muscle growth. *J Strength Cond Res*. 2017;31:45–53.

50. Ronnestad BR, Nygaard H, Raastad T. Physiological elevation of endogenous hormones results in superior strength training adaptation. *Eur J Appl Physiol*. 2011;111:2249–59.

51. West DWD, Burd NA, Tang JE, et al. Elevations in ostensibly anabolic hormones with resistance exercise enhance neither

51. training-induced muscle hypertrophy nor strength of the elbow flexors. *J Appl Physiol*. 2010;108:60–7.

52. West DWD, Kujbida GW, Moore DR, et al. Resistance exercise-induced increases in putative anabolic hormones do not enhance muscle protein synthesis or intracellular signaling in young men. *J Physiol*. 2009;587:5239–47.

53. Wilkinson SB, Tarnopolsky MA, Grant EJ, Correia CE, Phillips SM. Hypertrophy with unilateral resistance exercise occurs without increases in endogenous anabolic hormone concentration. *Eur J Appl Physiol*. 2006;98:546–55.

54. Shaner AA, Vingren JL, Hatfield DL, et al. The acute hormonal response to free weight and machine weight resistance exercise. *J Strength Cond Res*. 2014;28:1032–40.

55. Volek JS, Kraemer WJ, Bush, JA, et al. Testosterone and cortisol in relationship to dietary nutrients and resistance exercise. *J Appl Physiol*. 1997;8:49–54.

56. Jones MT, Ambegaonkar JP, Nindl BC, Smith JA, Headley SA. Effects of unilateral and bilateral lower-body heavy resistance exercise on muscle activity and testosterone responses. *J Strength Cond Res*. 2012;26:1094–100.

57. Migiano MJ, Vingren JL, Volek JS, et al. Endocrine response patterns to acute unilateral and bilateral resistance exercise in men. *J Strength Cond Res*. 2010;24:128–34.

58. Gotshalk LA, Loebel CC, Nindl BC, et al. Hormonal responses to multiset versus single-set heavy-resistance exercise protocols. *Can J Appl Physiol*. 1997;22:244–55.

59. Kraemer WJ, Gordon SE, Fleck SJ, et al. Endogenous anabolic hormonal and growth factor responses to heavy resistance exercise in males and females. *Int J Sports Med*. 1991;12:228–35.

60. Kraemer WJ, Marchitelli L, Gordon SE, et al. Hormonal and growth factor responses to heavy resistance exercise protocols. *J Appl Physiol*. 1990;69:1442–50.

61. Raastad T, Bjoro T, Hallen J. Hormonal responses to high- and moderate-intensity strength exercise. *Eur J Appl Physiol*. 2000;82:121–8.

62. Schwab R, Johnson GO, Housh TJ, et al. Acute effects of different intensities of weight lifting on serum testosterone. *Med Sci Sports Exerc*. 1993;25:1381–5.

63. Crewther B, Cronin J, Keogh J, Cook C. The salivary testosterone and cortisol response to three loading schemes. *J Strength Cond Res*. 2008;22:250–5.

64. Linnamo V, Pakarinen A, Komi PV, Kraemer WJ, Häkkinen K. Acute hormonal responses to submaximal and maximal heavy resistance and explosive exercises in men and women. *J Strength Cond Res*. 2005;19:566–71.

65. McCaulley GO, McBride JM, Cormie P, et al. Acute hormonal and neuromuscular responses to hypertrophy, strength and power type resistance exercise. *Eur J Appl Physiol*. 2009;105:695–704.

66. Gonzalez AM, Hoffman JR, Townsend JR, et al. Intramuscular anabolic signaling and endocrine response following high volume and high intensity resistance exercise protocols in trained men. *Physiol Rep*. 2015;3:e12466.

67. Mangine GT, Hoffman JR, Gonzalez AM, et al. The effect of training volume and intensity on improvements in muscular strength and size in resistance-trained men. *Physiol Rep*. 2015;3:e12472.

68. Buresh R, Berg K, French J. The effect of resistive exercise rest interval on hormonal responses, strength, and hypertrophy with training. *J Strength Cond Res*. 2009;23:62–71.

69. Scudese E, Simao R, Senna G, et al. Long rest interval promotes durable testosterone responses in high-intensity bench press. *J Strength Cond Res*. 2016;30:1275–86.

70. Häkkinen K, Pakarinen A, Alen M, et al. Neuromuscular and hormonal responses in elite athletes to two successive strength training sessions in one day. *Eur J Appl Physiol*. 1988;57:133–9.

71. Oliver JM, Kreutzer A, Jenke S, et al. Acute response to cluster sets in trained and untrained men. *Eur J Appl Physiol*. 2015;115:2883–93.

72. Madarame H, Sasaki K, Ishii N. Endocrine responses to upper- and lower-limb resistance exercises with blood flow restriction. *Acta Physiol Hung*. 2010;97:192–200.

73. Da Conceicao RR, Simao R, Silveira AL, et al. Acute endocrine responses to different strength exercise order in men. *J Hum Kinet*. 2014;44:111–20.

74. Simao R, Leite RD, Speretta GFF, et al. Influence of upper-body exercise order on hormonal responses in trained men. *Appl Physiol Nutr Metab*. 2013;38:177–81.

75. Hulmi JJ, Volek JS, Selanne H, Mero AA. Protein ingestion prior to strength exercise affects blood hormones and metabolism. *Med Sci Sports Exerc*. 2005;37:1990–7.

76. Schumm SR, Triplett NT, McBride JM, Dumke CL. Hormonal response to carbohydrate supplementation at rest and after resistance exercise. *Int J Sport Nutr Exerc Metab*. 2008;18:260–80.

77. Beaven CM, Hopkins WG, Hansen KT, et al. Dose effect of caffeine on testosterone and cortisol responses to resistance exercise. *Int J Sport Nutr Exerc Metab*. 2008;18:131–41.

78. Häkkinen K, Pakarinen A, Alen M, et al. Relationships between training volume, physical performance capacity, and serum hormone concentrations during prolonged training in elite weight lifters. *Int J Sports Med*. 1987;8(suppl):61–5.

79. Judelson DA, Maresh CM, Yamamoto LM, et al. Effect of hydration state on resistance exercise-induced endocrine markers of anabolism, catabolism, and metabolism. *J Appl Physiol*. 2008;105:816–24.

80. Rasmussen JJ, Selmer C, Ostergren PB, et al. Former abusers of anabolic androgenic steroids exhibit decreased testosterone levels and hypogonadal symptoms years after cessation: a case–control study. *PLoS One*. 2016;11:e0161208.

81. Häkkinen K, Pakarinen A, Alen M, et al. Neuromuscular and hormonal adaptations in athletes to strength training in two years. *J Appl Physiol*. 1988;65:2406–12.

82. Hoffman JR, Ratamess NA, Kang J, et al. Effect of creatine and beta-alanine supplementation on performance and endocrine responses in strength/power athletes. *Int J Sport Nutr Exerc Metab*. 2006;16:430–46.

83. Marx JO, Ratamess NA, Nindl BC, et al. Low-volume circuit versus high-volume periodized resistance training in women. *Med Sci Sports Exerc*. 2001;33:635–43.

84. Staron RS, Karapondo DL, Kraemer WJ, et al. Skeletal muscle adaptations during early phase of heavy-resistance training in men and women. *J Appl Physiol*. 1994;76:1247–55.

85. Häkkinen K, Pakarinen A, Alen M, Komi PV. Serum hormones during prolonged training of neuromuscular performance. *Eur J Appl Physiol*. 1985;53:287–93.

86. McCall GE, Byrnes WC, Fleck SJ, et al. Acute and chronic hormonal responses to resistance training designed to promote muscle hypertrophy. *Can J Appl Physiol*. 1999;24:96–107.

87. Kraemer WJ, Ratamess NA, Volek JS, et al. The effects of amino acid supplementation on hormonal responses to resistance training overreaching. *Metabolism*. 2006;55:282–91.

88. Hortobagyi T, Houmard JA, Stevenson JR, et al. The effects of detraining on power athletes. *Med Sci Sports Exerc*. 1993;25:929–35.

89. Alen M, Pakarinen A, Häkkinen K, Komi PV. Responses of serum androgenic-anabolic and catabolic hormones to prolonged strength training. *Int J Sports Med*. 1988;9:229–33.

90. Hackney AC. Effects of endurance exercise on the reproductive system of men: the "exercise-hypogonadal male condition". *J Endocrinol Invest*. 2008;31:932–8.

91. Hooper DR, Kraemer WJ, Saenz C, et al. The presence of symptoms of testosterone deficiency in the exercise-hypogonadal male condition and the role of nutrition. *Eur J Appl Physiol*. 2017;117:1349–57.

92. Sato K, Iemitsu M, Matsutani K, Kurihara T, Hamaoka T, Fujita S. Resistance training restores muscle sex steroid hormone steroidogenesis in older men. *FASEB J*. 2014;28:1891–7.

93. Morton RW, Sato K, Gallaugher MPD, et al. Muscle androgen receptor content but not systemic hormones is associated with resistance training-induced skeletal muscle hypertrophy in healthy, young men. *Front Physiol*. 2018;9:1373.

94. Inoue K, Yamasaki S, Fushiki T, et al. Androgen receptor antagonist suppresses exercise-induced hypertrophy of skeletal muscle. *Eur J Appl Physiol*. 1994;69:88–91.

95. Kvorning T, Andersen M, Brixen K, Schjerling P, Suetta C, Madesn K. Suppression of testosterone does not blunt mRNA expression of myoD myogenin IGF myostatin or androgen receptor post strength training in humans. *J Physiol*. 2007;578:579–93.

96. Häkkinen K, Pakarinen A, Alen M, et al. Daily hormonal and neuromuscular responses to intensive strength training in 1 week. *Int J Sports Med*. 1988;9:422–8.

97. Kupchak BR, Kraemer WJ, Hoffman MD, Phinney SD, Volek JS. The impact of an ultramarathon on hormonal and biochemical parameters in men. *Wilderness Environ Med*. 2014;25:278–88.

98. Orio F, Muscogiuri G, Ascione A, et al. Effect of physical exercise on the female reproductive system. *Minerva Endocrinol*. 2013;38:305–19.

99. Weiss LW, Cureton KJ, Thompson FN. Comparison of serum testosterone and androstenedione responses to weight lifting in men and women. *Eur J Appl Physiol*. 1983;50:413–9.

100. Aizawa K, Akimoto T, Inoue H, et al. Resting serum dehydroepiandrosterone sulfate level increases after 8-week resistance training among young females. *Eur J Appl Physiol*. 2003;90:575–80.

101. Häkkinen K, Pakarinen A, Kraemer WJ, et al. Basal concentrations and acute responses of serum hormones and strength development during heavy resistance training in middle-aged and elderly men and women. *J Gerontol A Biol Sci Med Sci*. 2000;55:B95–105.

102. Folland JP, McCauley TM, Phypers C, Hanson B, Mastana SS. The relationship of testosterone and AR CAG repeat genotype with knee extensor muscle function of young and older men. *Exp Gerontol*. 2012;47:437–43.

103. Nielsen TL, Hagen C, Wraae K, Bathum L, Larsen R, Brixen K. The impact of the CAG repeat polymorphism of the androgen receptor gene and adipose tissues in 20-29-year-old Danish men: Odense Androgen Study. *Eur J Endocrinol*. 2010;162:795–804.

104. Simmons ZL, Roney JR. Variation in CAG repeat length of the androgen receptor gene predicts variables associated with intrasexual competitiveness in human males. *Horm Behav*. 2011;60:306–12.

105. Walsh S, Zmuda JM, Cauley JA, et al. Androgen receptor CAG repeat polymorphism is associated with fat-free mass in men. *J Appl Physiol*. 2005;98:132–7.

106. Kraemer WJ, Spiering BA, Volek JS, et al. Androgenic responses to resistance exercise: effects of feeding and L-carnitine. *Med Sci Sports Exerc*. 2006;38:1288–96.

107. Spiering BA, Kraemer WJ, Vingren JL, et al. Elevated endogenous testosterone concentrations potentiate muscle androgen receptor responses to resistance exercise. *J Steroid Biochem Mol Biol*. 2009;114:195–9.

108. Ahtiainen JP, Lehti M, Hulmi JJ, et al. Recovery after heavy resistance exercise and skeletal muscle androgen receptor and insulin-like growth factor-1 isoform expression in strength trained men. *J Strength Cond Res*. 2011;25:767–77.

109. Bamman MM, Shipp JR, Jiang J, et al. Mechanical load increases muscle IGF-1 and androgen receptor mRNA concentrations in humans. *Am J Physiol*. 2001;280:E383–90.

110. Willoughby DS, Taylor L. Effects of sequential bouts of resistance exercise on androgen receptor expression. *Med Sci Sports Exerc*. 2004;36:1499–506.

111. Ahtiainen JP, Hulmi JJ, Kraemer WJ, et al. Heavy resistance training and skeletal muscle androgen receptor expression in younger and older men. *Steroids*. 2011;76:183–92.

112. Poole CN, Roberts MD, Dalbo VJ, Sunderland KL, Kerksick CM. Megalin and androgen receptor gene expression in young and old human skeletal muscle before and after three sequential exercise bouts. *J Strength Cond Res*. 2011;25:309–17.

113. Mitchell CJ, Churchward-Venne TA, Bellamy L, et al. Muscular and systemic correlates of resistance training-induced muscle hypertrophy. *PLoS One*. 2013;8:e78636.

114. Spillane M, Schwarz N, Willoughby DS. Upper-body resistance exercise augments vastus lateralis androgen receptor-DNA binding and canonical Wnt/β-catenin signaling compared to lower-body resistance exercise in resistance-trained men without an acute increase in serum testosterone. *Steroids*. 2015;98:63–71.

115. Nicoll JX, Fry AC, Mosier EM. Sex-based differences in resting MAPK, androgen, and glucocorticoid receptor phosphorylation in human skeletal muscle. *Steroids*. 2019;141:23–9.

116. Narayanan R, Mohler ML, Bohl CE, Miller DD, Dalton JT. Selective androgen receptor modulators in preclinical and clinical development. *Nucl Recept Signal*. 2008;6:e010.

117. Kraemer WJ, Dunn-Lewis C, Comstock BA, Thomas GA, Clark JE, Nindl BC. Growth hormone, exercise, and athletic performance: a continued evolution of complexity. *Curr Sports Med Rep*. 2010;9:242–52.

118. Thomas GA, Kraemer WJ, Comstock BA, Dunn-Lewis C, Maresh CM, Volek JS. Obesity, growth hormone and exercise. *Sports Med*. 2013;43:839–49.

119. Chowen JA, Frago LM, Argente J. The regulation of GH secretion by sex steroids. *Eur J Endocrinol*. 2004;151:U95–100.

120. Isacco L, Duche P, Boisseau N. Influence of hormonal status on substrate utilization at rest and during exercise in the female population. *Sports Med*. 2012;42:327–42.

121. Kraemer WJ, Flanagan SD, Volek JS, et al. Resistance exercise induces region-specific adaptations in anterior pituitary gland structure and function in rats. *J Appl Physiol*. 2013;115:1641–7.

122. Gordon SE, Kraemer WJ, Looney DP, Flanagan SD, Comstock BA, Hymer WC. The influence of age and exercise modality on growth hormone bioactivity in women. *Growth Horm IGF Res*. 2014;24:95–103.

123. Nindl BC, Eagle SR, Matheny RW, et al. Characterization of growth hormone disulfide-linked molecular isoforms during post-exercise release vs nocturnal pulsatile release reveals similar milieu composition. *Growth Horm IGF Res*. 2018;42–43:102–7.

124. Hymer WC, Kraemer WJ, Nindl BC, et al. Characteristics of circulating growth hormone in women after acute heavy resistance exercise. *Am J Physiol Endocrinol Metab*. 2001;281:E878–87.

125. Luk HY, Kraemer WJ, Szivak TK, et al. Acute resistance exercise stimulates sex-specific dimeric immunoreactive growth hormone responses. *Growth Horm IGF Res.* 2015;25:136–40.

126. Kraemer WJ, Dudley GA, Tesch PA, et al. The influence of muscle action on the acute growth hormone response to resistance exercise and short-term detraining. *Growth Horm IGF Res.* 2001;11:75–83.

127. Craig BW, Kang H. Growth hormone release following single versus multiple sets of back squats: total work versus power. *J Strength Cond Res.* 1994;8:270–5.

128. Mulligan SE, Fleck SJ, Gordon SE, et al. Influence of resistance exercise volume on serum growth hormone and cortisol concentrations in women. *J Strength Cond Res.* 1996;10:256–62.

129. Spiering BA, Kraemer WJ, Anderson JM, et al. Effects of elevated circulating hormones on resistance exercise-induced Akt signaling. *Med Sci Sports Exerc.* 2008;40:1039–48.

130. Häkkinen K, Pakarinen A. Acute hormonal responses to two different fatiguing heavy-resistance protocols in male athletes. *J Appl Physiol.* 1993;74:882–7.

131. Zafeiridis A, Smilios I, Considine RV, Tokmakidis SP. Serum leptin responses after acute resistance exercise protocols. *J Appl Physiol.* 2003;94:591–7.

132. Bottaro M, Martins B, Gentil P, Wagner D. Effects of rest duration between sets of resistance training on acute hormonal responses in trained women. *J Sci Med Sport.* 2009;12:73–8.

133. Goto K, Sato K, Takamatsu K. A single set of low intensity resistance exercise immediately following high intensity resistance exercise stimulates growth hormone secretion in men. *J Sports Med Phys Fitness.* 2003;43:243–9.

134. Craig BW, Brown R, Everhart J. Effects of progressive resistance training on growth hormone and testosterone levels in young and elderly subjects. *Mech Ageing Dev.* 1989;49:159–69.

135. Hoffman JR, Ratamess NA, Ross R, et al. Effect of a pre-exercise energy supplement on the acute hormonal response to resistance exercise. *J Strength Cond Res.* 2008;22:874–82.

136. Manini TM, Yarrow JF, Buford TW, et al. Growth hormone responses to acute resistance exercise with vascular restriction in young and old men. *Growth Horm IGF Res.* 2012;22:167–72.

137. Roelen CA, deVries WR, Koppeschaar HR, Vervoorn C, Thijssen JH, Blankenstein MA. Plasma insulin-like growth factor-I and high affinity growth hormone-binding protein levels increase after two weeks of strenuous physical training. *Int J Sports Med.* 1997;18:238–41.

138. Betts JA, Stokes KA, Toone RJ, Williams C. Growth-hormone responses to consecutive exercise bouts with ingestion of carbohydrate plus protein. *Int J Sport Nutr Exerc Metab.* 2013;23: 259–70.

139. De Palo EF, Gatti R, Cappellin E, Schiraldi C, De Palo CB, Spinella P. Plasma lactate, GH and GH-binding protein levels in exercise following BCAA supplementation in athletes. *Amino Acids.* 2001;20:1–11.

140. Rubin MR, Kraemer WJ, Maresh CM, et al. Response of high-affinity growth hormone binding protein to acute heavy resistance exercise in resistance-trained and untrained men. *Med Sci Sports Exerc.* 2005;37:395–403.

141. Waters MJ. The growth hormone receptor. *Growth Horm IGF Res.* 2016;28:6–10.

142. Nielsen C, Gormsen LC, Jessen N, et al. Growth hormone signaling in vivo in human muscle and adipose tissue: impact of insulin, substrate background, and growth hormone receptor blockade. *J Clin Endocrinol Metab.* 2008;93:2842–50.

143. Vestergaard PF, Vendelbo MH, Pedersen SB, et al. GH signaling in skeletal muscle and adipose tissue in healthy human subjects: impact of gender and age. *Eur J Endocrinol.* 2014;171:623–31.

144. Nindl BC. Exercise modulation of growth hormone isoforms: current knowledge and future directions for the exercise endocrinologist. *Br J Sports Med.* 2007;41:346–8.

145. Nindl BC, Urso ML, Pierce JR, et al. IGF-I measurement across blood, interstitial fluid, and muscle biocompartments following explosive, high-power exercise. *Am J Physiol Regul Integr Comp Physiol.* 2012;303:R1080.

146. Harridge SDR, Velloso CP. IGF-1 and GH: potential use in gene doping. *Growth Horm IGF Res.* 2009;19:378–82.

147. Kostek MC, Delmonico MJ, Reichel JB, Roth SM, Douglass L, Ferrell RE, Hurley BF. Muscle strength response to strength training is influenced by insulin-like growth factor 1 genotype in older adults. *J Appl Physiol.* 2005;98:2147–54.

148. Copeland JL, Heggie L. IGF-I and IGFBP-3 during continuous and interval exercise. *Int J Sports Med.* 2008;29:182–7.

149. De Palo EF, Antonelli G, Gatti R, Chiappin S, Spinella P, Cappellin E. Effects of two different types of exercise on GH/IGF axis in athletes. Is the free/total IGF-I ratio a new investigative approach? *Clin Chim Acta.* 2008;387:71–4.

150. Izquierdo M, Ibanez J, Gonzalez-Badillo JJ, et al. Differential effects of strength training leading to failure versus not to failure on hormonal responses, strength, and muscle power gains. *J Appl Physiol.* 2006;100:1647–56.

151. Schiffer T, Schulte S, Hollmann W, Bloch W, Struder HK. Effects of strength and endurance training on brain-derived neurotrophic factor and insulin-like growth factor 1 in humans. *Horm Metab Res.* 2009;41(3):250–4.

152. Petrella JK, Kim J, Mayhew DL, Cross JM, Bamman MM. Potent myofiber hypertrophy during resistance training in humans is associated with satellite cell-mediated myonuclear addition: a cluster analysis. *J Appl Physiol.* 2008;104:1736–42.

153. Borst SE, De Hoyos DV, Garzarella L, et al. Effects of resistance training on insulin-like growth factor-I and IGF binding proteins. *Med Sci Sports Exerc.* 2001;33:648–53.

154. Izquierdo M, Ibanez J, Gonzalez-Badillo JJ, et al. Detraining and tapering effects on hormonal responses and strength performance. *J Strength Cond Res.* 2007;21:768–75.

155. Willoughby DS, Stout JR, Wilborn CD. Effects of resistance training and protein plus amino acid supplementation on muscle anabolism, mass, and strength. *Amino Acids.* 2007;32:467–77.

156. Koziris LP, Hickson RC, Chatterton RT, et al. Serum levels of total and free IGF-1 and IGFBP-3 are increased and maintained in long-term training. *J Appl Physiol.* 1999;86:1436–42.

157. Goldspink G. Mechanical signals, IGF-1 gene splicing, and muscle adaptation. *Physiology.* 2005;20:232–8.

158. Goldspink G. Changes in muscle mass and phenotype and the expression of autocrine and systemic growth factors by muscle in response to stretch and overload. *J Anat.* 1999;194:323–34.

159. Hameed M, Orrel RW, Cobbold G, et al. Expression of IGF-1 splice variants in young and old human skeletal muscle after high resistance exercise. *J Physiol.* 2003;547:247–54.

160. Philippou A, Halapas A, Maridaki M, Koutsilieris M. Type I insulin-like growth factor receptor signaling in skeletal muscle regeneration and hypertrophy. *J Musculoskelet Neuronal Interact.* 2007;7:208–18.

161. Wilborn CD, Taylor LW, Greenwood M, Kreider RB, Willoughby DS. Effects of different intensities of resistance exercise on regulators of myogenesis. *J Strength Cond Res.* 2009;23:2179–87.

162. Popov DV, Lysenko EA, Bachinin AV, et al. Influence of resistance exercise intensity and metabolic stress on anabolic signaling and expression of myogenic genes in skeletal muscle. *Muscle Nerve*. 2015;51:434–42.

163. Schwarz NA, McKinley-Barnard SK, Spillane MB, et al. Effect of resistance exercise intensity on the expression of PGC-1α isoforms and the anabolic and catabolic signaling mediators, IGF-1 and myostatin, in human skeletal muscle. *Appl Physiol Nutr Metab*. 2016;41:856–63.

164. Meckel Y, Eliakim A, Seraev M, et al. The effect of a brief sprint interval exercise on growth factors and inflammatory mediators. *J Strength Cond Res*. 2009;23:225–30.

165. Nindl BC, Kraemer WJ, Marx JO, et al. Overnight responses of the circulating IGF-1 system after acute heavy-resistance exercise. *J Appl Physiol*. 2001;90:1319–26.

166. Elloumi M, El Elj N, Zaouali M, et al. IGFBP-3, a sensitive marker of physical training and overtraining. *Br J Sports Med*. 2005;39:604–10.

167. Fry AC, Hoffman JR. Training responses and adaptations of the endocrine system. In: Chandler TJ, Brown LE, editors. *Conditioning for Strength and Human Performance*. Philadelphia (PA): Lippincott Williams & Wilkins; 2008. p. 94–122.

168. Sellami M, Bragazzi NL, Slimani M, et al. The effect of exercise on glucoregulatory hormones: a countermeasure to human aging: insights from a comprehensive review of the literature. *Int J Environ Res Pub Health*. 2019;16:1709.

169. Holloszy JO. Exercise-induced increase in muscle insulin sensitivity. *J Appl Physiol*. 2005;99:338–43.

170. Richter EA, Hargreaves M. Exercise, GLUT4, and skeletal muscle glucose uptake. *Physiol Rev*. 2013;93:993–1017.

171. Stuart CA, Lee ML, South MA, Howell MEA, Stone MH. Muscle hypertrophy in prediabetic men after 16 wk of resistance training. *J Appl Physiol*. 2017;123:894–901.

172. Kumar M, Nath S, Prasad HK, Sharma GD, Li Y. MicroRNAs: a new ray of hope for diabetes mellitus. *Protein Cell*. 2012;3:726–38.

173. Premachandra BN, Winder WW, Hickson R, Lang S, Holloszy JO. Circulating reverse triiodothyronine in humans during exercise. *Eur J Appl Physiol Occup Physiol*. 1981;47:281–8.

174. Fragala MS, Kraemer WJ, Denegar CR, Maresh CM, Mastro AM, Volek JS. Neuroendocrine-immune interactions and responses to exercise. *Sports Med*. 2011;41:621–39.

175. Hill EE, Zack E, Battaglini C, Viru M, Viru A, Hackney AC. Exercise and circulating cortisol levels: the intensity threshold effect. *J Endocrinol Invest*. 2008;31:587–91.

176. Stearns RL, Nolan JK, Huggins RA, et al. Influence of cold-water immersion on recovery of elite triathletes following the ironman world championship. *J Sci Med Sport*. 2018;21:846–51.

177. Bobbert T, Mai K, Brechtel L, et al. Leptin and endocrine parameters in marathon runners. *Int J Sports Med*. 2012;33:244–8.

178. Vuorimaa T, Ahotupa M, Häkkinen K, Vasankari T. Different hormonal response to continuous and intermittent exercise in middle-distance and marathon runners. *Scand J Med Sci Sports*. 2008;18:565–72.

179. Nieman DC. Exercise, upper respiratory tract infection, and the immune system. *Med Sci Sports Exerc*. 1994;26:128–39.

180. Szivak TK, Lee EC, Saenz C, et al. Adrenal stress and physical performance during military survival training. *Aerosp Med Hum Perform*. 2018;89:99–107.

181. Kraemer WJ, Noble BJ, Clark MJ, Culver BW. Physiologic responses to heavy-resistance exercise with very short rest periods. *Int J Sports Med*. 1987;8:247–52.

182. Smilios I, Pilianidis T, Karamouzis M, Tokmakidis SP. Hormonal responses after various resistance exercise protocols. *Med Sci Sports Exerc*. 2003;35:644–54.

183. Kraemer WJ, Clemson A, Triplett NT, et al. The effects of plasma cortisol elevation on total and differential leukocyte counts in response to heavy-resistance exercise. *Eur J Appl Physiol*. 1996;73:93–7.

184. Tarpenning KM, Wiswell RA, Hawkins SA, Marcell TJ. Influence of weight training exercise and modification of hormonal response on skeletal muscle growth. *J Sci Med Sport*. 2001;4:431–46.

185. Fry AC, Kraemer WJ. Resistance exercise overtraining and overreaching. Neuroendocrine responses. *Sports Med*. 1997;23:106–29.

186. Peeters GMEE, van Schoor NM, van Rossum EFC, Visser M, Lips P. The relationship between cortisol, muscle mass and muscle strength in older persons and the role of genetic variations in the glucocorticoid receptor. *Clin Endocrinol (Oxford)*. 2008;69:673–82.

187. Van Rossum EF, Voorhoeve PG, te Velde SJ, et al. The ER22/23EK polymorphism in the glucocorticoid receptor gene is associated with a beneficial body composition and muscle strength in young adults. *J Clin Endocrinol Metabol*. 2004;89:4004–9.

188. Ash GI, Kostek MA, Lee H et al. Glucocorticoid receptor (NR3C1) variants associate with the muscle strength and size response to resistance training. *PLoS One*. 2016;11:e0148112. doi:10.137/journal.pone.0148112.

189. Harada N, Inui H, Yamaji R. Competitive and compensatory effects of androgen signaling and glucocorticoid signaling. *Recept Clin Invest*. 2015;2:e785. doi:10.14800/rci.785.

190. Kuo T, Harris CA, Wang JC. Metabolic functions of glucocorticoid receptor in skeletal muscle. *Mol Cell Endocrinol*. 2013;380:79–88.

191. Schakman O, Kalista S, Barbe C, Loumaye A, Thissen JP. Glucocorticoid-induced skeletal muscle atrophy. *Int J Biochem Cell Biol*. 2013;45:2163–72.

192. Willoughby DS, Taylor M, Taylor L. Glucocorticoid receptor and ubiquitin expression after repeated eccentric exercise. *Med Sci Sports Exerc*. 2003;35:2023–31.

193. Willoughby DS. Effects of heavy resistance training on myostatin mRNA and protein expression. *Med Sci Sports Exerc*. 2004;36:574–82.

194. Silva TS, Longui CA, Rocha MN, et al. Prolonged physical training decreases mRNA levels of glucocorticoid receptor and inflammatory genes. *Horm Res Paediatr*. 2010;74:6–14.

195. Hansen D, Meeusen R, Mullens A, Dendale P. Effect of acute endurance and resistance exercise on endocrine hormones directly related to lipolysis and skeletal muscle protein synthesis in adult individuals with obesity. *Sports Med*. 2012;42:415–31.

196. Kjaer M. Adrenal medulla and exercise training. *Eur J Appl Physiol*. 1998;77:195–9.

197. Zouhal H, Jacob C, Delamarche P, Gratas-Delamarche A. Catecholamines and the effects of exercise, training and gender. *Sports Med*. 2008;38:401–23.

198. Kliszczewicz BM, Esco MR, Quindry JC, et al. Autonomic responses to an acute bout of high-intensity body weight resistance exercise vs. treadmill running. *J Strength Cond Res*. 2016;30:1050–8.

199. Guezennec Y, Leger L, Lhoste F, et al. Hormone and metabolite response to weight-lifting training sessions. *Int J Sports Med*. 1986;7:100–5.

200. Kraemer WJ, Gordon SE, Fragala MS, et al. The effects of exercise training programs on plasma concentrations of proenkephalin Peptide F and catecholamines. *Peptides*. 2015;64:74–81.

201. Schwartz L, Kindermann W. Changes in beta-endorphin levels in response to aerobic and anaerobic exercise. *Sports Med.* 1992;13:25–36.

202. Taylor DV, Boyajian JG, James N, et al. Acidosis stimulates beta-endorphin release during exercise. *J Appl Physiol.* 1994;77:1913–8.

203. Maresh CM, Sokmen B, Kraemer WJ, et al. Pituitary-adrenal responses to arm versus leg exercise in untrained man. *Eur J Appl Physiol.* 2006;97:471–7.

204. Goldfarb AH, Hatfield BD, Armstrong D, Potts J. Plasma beta-endorphin concentration: response to intensity and duration of exercise. *Med Sci Sports Exerc.* 1990;22:241–4.

205. Eliot DL, Goldberg L, Watts WJ, Orwoll E. Resistance exercise and plasma beta-endorphin/beta-lipotrophin immunoreactivity. *Life Sci.* 1984;34:515–8.

206. Walberg-Rankin J, Franke WD, Gwazdauskas FC. Response of beta-endorphin and estradiol to resistance exercise females during energy balance and energy restriction. *Int J Sports Med.* 1992;13:542–7.

207. Kraemer RR, Acevedo EO, Dzewaltowski D, et al. Effects of low-volume resistive exercise on beta-endorphin and cortisol concentrations. *Int J Sports Med.* 1996;17:12–6.

208. Kraemer WJ, Dziados JE, Marchitelli LJ, et al. Effects of different heavy-resistance exercise protocols on plasma β-endorphin concentrations. *J Appl Physiol.* 1993;74:450–9.

209. Hildebrandt T, Shope S, Varangis E, Klein D, Pfaff DW, Yehuda R. Exercise reinforcement, stress, and β-endorphins: an initial examination of exercise in anabolic-androgenic steroid dependence. *Drug Alcohol Depend.* 2014;139:86–92.

210. Vella KR, Hollenberg AN. The actions of thyroid hormone signaling in the nucleus. *Mol Cell Endocrinol.* 2017;458:127–35.

211. Singh BK, Sinha RA, Yen PM. Novel transcriptional mechanisms for regulating metabolism by thyroid hormone. *Int J Mol Sci.* 2018;19:3284.

212. Louzada RA, Carvalho DP. Similarities and differences in the peripheral actions of thyroid hormones and their metabolites. *Front Physiol.* 2018;9:394.

213. Ciloglu F, Peker I, Pehlivan A, et al. Exercise intensity and its effects on thyroid hormones. *Neuro Endocrinol Lett.* 2005;26:830–4.

214. McMurray RG, Hackney AC. Interactions of metabolic hormones, adipose tissue and exercise. *Sports Med.* 2005;35:393–412.

215. Simsch C, Lormes W, Petersen KG, et al. Training intensity influences leptin and thyroid hormones in highly trained rowers. *Int J Sports Med.* 2002;23:422–7.

216. Harber VJ, Petersen SR, Chilibeck PD. Thyroid hormone concentrations and muscle metabolism in amenorrheic and eumenorrheic athletes. *Can J Appl Physiol.* 1998;23:293–306.

217. Bocco BM, Louzada RA, Silvestre DH, et al. Thyroid hormone activation by type 2 deiodinase mediates exercise-induced peroxisome proliferator-activated receptor-γ coactivator-1α expression in skeletal muscle. *J Physiol.* 2016;594:5255–69.

218. Lesmana R, Iwasaki T, Iizuka Y, et al. The change in thyroid hormone signaling by altered training intensity in male rat skeletal muscle. *Endocrine J.* 2016;63:727–38.

219. Rocker L, Kirsch KA, Heyduck B, Altenkirch KU. Influence of prolonged physical exercise on plasma volume, plasma proteins, electrolytes, and fluid-regulating hormones. *Int J Sports Med.* 1989;10:270–4.

220. Thomas W, Harvey BJ. Mechanisms underlying rapid aldosterone effects in the kidney. *Ann Rev Physiol.* 2011;73:335–57.

221. Convertino VA, Keil LC, Bernauer EM, Greenleaf JE. Plasma volume, osmolality, vasopressin, and renin activity during graded exercise in man. *J Appl Physiol.* 1981;50:123–8.

222. Mannix ET, Palange P, Aronoff GR, et al. Atrial natriuretic peptide and the renin-aldosterone axis during exercise in man. *Med Sci Sports Exerc.* 1990;22:785–9.

223. Roy BD, Green HJ, Grant SM, Tarnopolsy MA. Acute plasma volume expansion in the untrained alters the hormonal response to prolonged moderate-intensity exercise. *Horm Metab Res.* 2001;33:238–45.

224. Hespel P, Lijnen P, Van Hoof R, et al. Effects of physical endurance training on the plasma renin-angiotensin-aldosterone system in normal man. *J Endocrinol.* 1988;116:443–9.

225. Convertino VA. Blood volume: its adaptation to endurance training. *Med Sci Sports Exerc.* 1991;23:1338–48.

226. Goessler K, Polito M, Cornelissen VA. Effect of exercise training on the renin-angiotensin-aldosterone system in healthy individuals: a systematic review and meta-analysis. *Hypertens Res.* 2016;39:119–26.

227. Boone CH, Hoffman JR, Gonzalez AM, et al. Changes in plasma aldosterone and electrolytes following high-volume and high-intensity resistance exercise protocols in trained men. *J Strength Cond Res.* 2016;30:1917–23.

228. Gruzdeva O, Borodkina D, Uchasova E, Dyleva Y, Barbarash O. Leptin resistance: underlying mechanisms and diagnosis. *Diabetes Metab Synd Obes.* 2019;12:191–8.

229. Gippini A, Mato A, Peino R, et al. Effect of resistance exercise (body building) training on serum leptin levels in young men. Implications for relationship between body mass index and serum leptin. *J Endocrinol Invest.* 1999;22:824–8.

230. Fedewa MV, Hathaway ED, Ward-Ritacco CL, Williams TD, Dobbs WC. The effect of chronic exercise training on leptin: a systematic review and meta-analysis of randomized controlled trials. *Sports Med.* 2018;48:1437–50.

231. Tena-Sempere M, Manna PR, Zhang FP, et al. Molecular mechanisms of leptin action in adult rat testis: potential targets for leptin-induced inhibition of steroidogenesis and pattern of leptin receptor messenger ribonucleic acid expression. *J Endocrinol.* 2001;170:413–23.

232. Schubert MM, Sabapathy S, Leveritt M, Desbrow B. Acute exercise and hormones related to appetite regulation: a meta-analysis. *Sports Med.* 2014;44:387–403.

233. Hansen M, Miller BF, Holm L, et al. Effect of administration of oral contraceptives in vivo on collagen synthesis in tendon and muscle connective tissue in young women. *J Appl Physiol.* 2009;106(4):1435–43.

234. Consitt LA, Copeland JL, Tremblay MS. Endogenous anabolic hormone responses to endurance versus resistance exercise and training in women. *Sports Med.* 2002;32:1–22.

235. Hulmi JJ, Isola V, Suonpaa M, et al. The effects of intensive weight reduction on body composition and serum hormones in female fitness competitors. *Front Physiol.* 2017;7:689.

236. DeSouza MJ, Nattiv A, Joy E, et al. 2014 female athlete triad coalition consensus statement on treatment and return to play of the female athlete triad. *Br J Sports Med.* 2014;48:289.

237. Ennour-Idrissi K, Maunsell E, Diorio C. Effect of physical activity on sex hormones in women: a systematic review and meta-analysis of randomized controlled trials. *Breast Can Res.* 2015;17:139.

238. De Jonge JAX. Effects of the menstrual cycle on exercise performance. *Sports Med.* 2003;33:833–51.

239. Smekal G, von Duvillard SP, Frigo P, et al. Menstrual cycle: no effect on exercise cardiorespiratory variables or blood lactate concentration. *Med Sci Sports Exerc.* 2007;39:1098–106.

CHAPTER 8

Metabolic Responses and Adaptations to Training

OBJECTIVES

After completing this chapter, you will be able to:
- Discuss adenosine triphosphate (ATP) and understand the major metabolic systems in the human body that resynthesize ATP
- Discuss how training results in substrate and enzymatic changes in the ATP-phosphocreatine, glycolytic, and aerobic energy systems
- Discuss the physiologic effects of metabolic acidosis and how the body buffers acids
- Discuss oxygen consumption and energy expenditure during exercise and understand how one can increase basal metabolic rate through diet and exercise
- Discuss how manipulating training programs affects oxygen consumption during exercise
- Discuss strategies to reduce body fat via exercise and diet

Metabolism is the sum of all chemical reactions in the human body to sustain life. Metabolism involves the breakdown of food and subsequent use for energy production. Energy is defined as the ability to perform work, and human energy requirement will change in proportion to the magnitude (duration and/or intensity) of work being performed. As the first law of thermodynamics states, energy cannot be created or destroyed but can transform from one form to another. *Bioenergetics* refers to this flow of energy transfer within the human body and is concerned mostly with the extraction of energy from carbohydrates (CHOs), fats, and proteins. Although CHOs, fats, and in some instances, proteins are sources of dietary energy, biochemical conversion of these large molecules is necessary to extract chemical energy and transfer energy to form the basis of life-sustaining functions. Although several types of energy are important to human function, chemical energy is needed for several metabolic processes.

A direct application of the first law of thermodynamics to human movement involves the transfer of chemical energy within the bonds of CHOs, fats, and proteins to skeletal muscle contractile proteins; this chemical energy has the ability to be converted to other types of energy such as mechanical (potential, kinetic) energy. Figure 8.1 depicts energy flow via exergonic and endergonic reactions. *Exergonic* reactions result in energy release, whereas *endergonic* reactions result in stored or absorbed energy. Exergonic reactions represent a thermodynamic "downhill" process where ΔG (Gibbs free energy) is negative (as energy is lost) and reactants have a greater driving force to generate and release energy. On the other hand, endergonic reactions represent a thermodynamic "uphill" process where the ΔG is positive as energy is gained, meaning that more energy is required to start the reaction than what is produced. Coupling of endergonic and exergonic reactions is critical in metabolism as investing energy early may be important for releasing energy later in sequence. Understanding bioenergetics is critical to understanding mechanisms of muscular performance and fatigue and is thereby important for developing optimal aerobic and anaerobic training programs.

Adenosine Triphosphate and Metabolic Systems

The human body requires continuous chemical energy to support life and exercise. Large amounts of potential energy from storage or food sources can be transferred to fuel muscle performance. The primary fuel for human movement is the high-energy compound known as adenosine triphosphate (ATP). Figure 8.2 depicts ATP, which is composed of adenine and ribose (adenosine) linked to three phosphates. The bonds that link the outermost two phosphates possess the ability to release

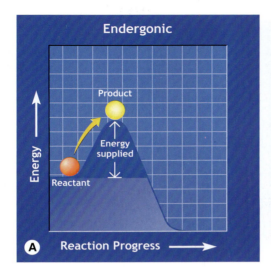
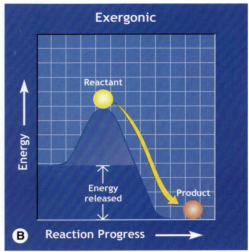

FIGURE 8.1 Endergonic and exergonic reactions. (Reprinted with permission from McArdle WD, Katch FI, Katch VL. *Sports and Exercise Nutrition*. 5th ed. Philadelphia (PA): Wolters Kluwer; 2019.)

chemical energy through hydrolysis. Upon cleavage of the last phosphate bond, energy is released. Hydrolysis of ATP (via ATPase) reaction yields 7.3 kilocalories (kcal) of free energy in addition to *adenosine diphosphate* (ADP) and *free inorganic phosphate* (P_i) (1).

$$ATP + H_2O \rightarrow ADP + P_i + energy$$

The energy liberated transfers to other molecules and is used to perform physiologic work. Energy is liberated aerobically (with oxygen) and anaerobically (without oxygen). Two major anaerobic energy systems include the ATP-phosphocreatine (ATP-PC) and glycolysis systems and one major aerobic energy system.

ATP and Phosphocreatine Systems

There are three ways chemical energy can be utilized very quickly. One way is to use skeletal muscle ATP stores. The human body has a limited capacity to store ATP, *i.e.*, ~80–100 g of ATP at any given time (1), enough to sustain only a few seconds of exercise. Cells must constantly replenish ATP stores, and our metabolic systems are the primary modes. A second way is the phosphocreatine (PC) system. PC (or creatine phosphate) is a high-energy phosphate that provides energy for high-intensity activities lasting up to 5–10 seconds. The PC system is engaged initially during low-intensity activities. Its concentration within skeletal muscle is approximately four to five times greater than stored ATP (2,3) and is more prominent in fast-twitch (FT) than slow-twitch (ST) fibers (4) although highly trained endurance athletes may have higher PC content in ST fibers (5). Maximal rates of PC turnover are ~7–9 mmol·kg^{-1}·s^{-1} dry mass (6), which can be exhausted within 10 seconds. With this rapid turnover rate, the PC system is the predominant energy source for explosive, anaerobic exercise such as sprinting, jumping, and resistance training (RT), and force declines as PC depletes. Because of limited PC stores, the ATP-PC system cannot provide sufficient energy to sustain exercise beyond 10–15 seconds. The PC system operates via the following equation:

$$ADP + phosphocreatine \leftrightarrow ATP + creatine$$

PC rephosphorylates ADP. Substantial free energy is released when the bond between creatine and phosphate is cleaved. Hydrolysis of PC drives ADP to form ATP. This reaction is catalyzed rapidly by *creatine kinase* (CK) (3). CK, because of its location within skeletal muscle fibers, tends to leak into circulation when muscle damage takes place and serves as an indirect marker of muscle damage. CK has several isoforms that identify the source of damage, *i.e.*, skeletal or cardiac muscle, or the brain.

A third way to produce ATP rapidly is from multiple ADP sources. An enzyme *adenylate kinase* (known as *myokinase* in skeletal muscle) catalyzes the following reaction:

$$2\ ADP \leftrightarrow ATP + AMP$$

FIGURE 8.2 Adenosine triphosphate (ATP).

Two ADPs are hydrolyzed to form a molecule of ATP and a molecule of adenosine monophosphate (AMP). The adenylate kinase reaction augments the muscle's ability for rapid energy turnover and produces AMP, which is a potent stimulator of glycolysis (4).

Energy systems operate under the *Law of Mass Action*, which states chemical reactions taking place in solutions progress to the right with the addition of reactants or progress to the left with the addition of products (1). With enzyme-mediated reactions, the rate of product formation is highly influenced by the amount of reactants. For example, greater amounts of ADP formed during exercise increases the rate of the CK and adenylate kinase reactions. This continues until exercise is terminated or performed at an intensity low enough that other metabolic systems can predominate. Having larger amounts of stored substrates shifts the reactions to generate higher ATP resynthesis during high-intensity exercise. This is the rationale for creatine supplementation (see the Sidebar below) where a larger amount of energy can be liberated from the ATP-PC system. All metabolic systems work together in a *continuum* being engaged at all times. However, one system may predominate depending on exercise intensity, duration, and oxygen availability.

Phosphagen Repletion

ATP-PC resynthesis is critical to explosive exercise performance. High-intensity exercise may deplete PC by 60%–80% during the first 30 seconds with up to 70% depletion taking place within 12 seconds (3,6). Longer-duration high-intensity exercise (400-m sprint) may reduce PC by 89% (9). The rate of PC depletion may be higher in trained sprinters versus sprinters who cannot run as fast (10). Acute interval workouts with short (1 min) rest intervals may result in larger PC depletion than interval workouts with long (3-min) rest intervals (13). The greater the PC degradation, the longer the time needed to fully recover PC to preexercise

values. Resynthesis of PC occurs in a biphasic response where there is a faster followed by a slower component, and the rate of PC resynthesis may be affected by the type of recovery (active vs. passive) (6). The half-life of PC resynthesis ranges from 21 to 57 seconds depending on intensity and volume (3,6). Within 90 seconds of recovery, 65% PC repletion may be seen, but <90% repletion occurs within 6 minutes or recovery (3,11). Other critical factors affecting PC resynthesis rates are muscle pH, ADP levels, and oxygen availability. The half-life of PC resynthesis is longer when muscle pH decreases (3). It is thought that accumulation of H^+ inhibits PC resynthesis primarily during the slow component of recovery (3). Oxygen availability and ADP levels are critical during the fast component. ATP used to resynthesize PC is derived from oxidative metabolism, and a faster rate of PC resynthesis in ST compared to FT fibers is seen (3). Thus, the rate of PC resynthesis is dependent upon the oxidative capacity of skeletal muscle. The kinetics of PC resynthesis is important when determining rest intervals for RT and interval training. Less recovery limits PC resynthesis and reduces performance. The resynthesis of PC is related to the recovery of force during maximal repeated sprints, and the rate of PC resynthesis is augmented following high-intensity interval training (12,13).

Training Adaptations

Anaerobic training induces positive adaptations in the ATP-PC and adenylate kinase metabolic systems. Adaptations potentially take place in four general ways: (a) greater substrate storage at rest, (b) greater substrate resynthesis rates during recovery intervals (c) altered enzyme activity, and (d) limited accumulation of fatiguing metabolites. Repeated bouts of high-intensity RT can increase ATP and PC storage via a supercompensation effect (14). An early study by MacDougall et al. (14) showed a 22% increase in resting PC, 39% increase in muscle creatine, and 18% increase in ATP concentrations following 5 months of RT

Sidebar — Creatine Supplementation and Exercise Performance

Creatine is one of the most commonly used supplements by athletes since the early 1990s. The rationale for creatine supplementation derives from two major roles: (a) anaerobic energy metabolism and (b) its ability to act as an osmotic agent. When muscle creatine stores increase via supplementation, this process attracts water to enter the cells (osmosis) causing increased bodyweight and muscle protein synthesis. Creatine is naturally found in foods but is synthesized in the body from the amino acids arginine, glycine, and methionine. Although creatine is absorbed in other tissues, ~95% of creatine is absorbed in skeletal muscle. A specific creatine transporter protein is located within the muscle's cell membrane that helps creatine enter muscle. Creatine supplementation can increase muscle levels of total creatine substantially by ~11%–22%

(7). The majority of muscle creatine elevation occurs within the first few days of supplementation, especially when a loading phase is used. Further supplementation with lower doses can maintain this level. Some individuals are nonresponders, whereas some experience large elevations. There are many creatine supplements available on the market with creatine monohydrate in powder form the most popular. Creatine supplementation increases body mass ranging from 0.6 to 5.2 kg (8) and improves muscle strength, endurance, power, vertical jump height, sprint speed, agility, and sport-specific performance (cycling power, swim performance, skating speed) (7). The benefits of creatine supplementation have extended beyond athletes to clinical populations. Creatine is one of a few sports supplements consistently shown to be ergogenic.

(3–5 sets of 8–10 reps with 2-min rest intervals). Other studies showed increased resting PC concentrations after 5 weeks of RT (15) or no change (16). Sprint training results in no change or a decrease in resting ATP and PC concentrations (17,18). Five weeks of high-intensity interval training with 1- or 3-minute rest intervals did not augment resting muscle PC or ATP concentrations despite the 1-minute workouts producing greater acute PC depletion (13). Trained sprinters may possess a similar resting PC/ATP ratio (despite a higher rate of PC breakdown during exercise) when compared to endurance-trained athletes (19). It appears resting substrate increases may be most prominent during RT with little changes seen during sprint training; however, sprint training appears to augment PC resynthesis rates.

Enzyme changes may occur during training. Two enzymes often studied are CK and adenylate kinase (myokinase). Early studies showed increased activity of CK and myokinase during RT, especially in FT fibers (20,21). However, the magnitude of muscle growth is critical when examining enzyme changes. Enzyme activity is expressed relative to total muscle protein content. No change or a decrease in enzyme activity occurs with training-induced hypertrophy. During muscle hypertrophy, CK may decrease (22–24) or not change, whereas increases (25), no change (16), and decreases (23) in myokinase activity have been shown. Powerlifters and Olympic weightlifters have similar myokinase activity to control subjects, whereas bodybuilders display the highest myokinase activity (26). Myokinase activity may not change or increase up to 20% during sprint and plyometric training of 2–15 weeks (18). Although elite sprinters use PC more rapidly, sprint training does not change CK activity much. A long-term (8-month) combined sprint, plyometric, and RT program showed no change in CK activity as well (27). Metabolic adaptations from sprint training do not appear to be mediated by greater CK activity.

Glycolysis

Glycolysis is the breakdown of CHOs to resynthesize ATP in the cytoplasm. It is another anaerobic metabolic system that can provide energy for high-intensity exercise for up to 2 minutes. Its rate of ATP resynthesis is not as rapid as PC; however, the human body has a larger glycogen supply, so high energy liberation is sustained for a longer period of time. The free energy released in this series of reactions forms ATP and nicotinamide adenine dinucleotide (NADH). The source of CHOs could be blood glucose (derived from consumed CHOs and liver glycogen stores) or muscle glycogen stores. Glycolysis is a series of 10 reactions breaking down the 6-carbon glucose ($C_6H_{12}O_6$) into two 3-carbon pyruvate molecules ($C_3H_4O_3$). The net result is 2 or 3 ATP formed (3 ATP from muscle glycogen, 2 ATP from a molecule of blood glucose) in the following reaction:

$$\text{glucose} + 2\text{ NAD}^+ + 2\text{ ADP} + 2\text{ P}_i \rightarrow 2\text{ pyruvate} + 2\text{ NADH} + 2\text{ H}^+ + 2\text{ ATP} + 2\text{ H}_2\text{O}$$

Figure 8.3 depicts the reactions of glycolysis. The first five steps consume energy (invest), whereas the second half results in the generation and net gain of ATP and NADH. The first step

is the formation of glucose-6-phosphate. For blood glucose, the enzyme *hexokinase* uses ATP to add a phosphate to glucose so it cannot leave the cell (and promotes more glucose uptake into muscle). Remember, glucose must first enter the cell via a glucose transporter (GLUT 4). GLUT 4 (*glucose transporter 4*) is stored in vesicles and translocates to the cell membrane either through insulin-mediated action or via muscle contraction (insulin-independent mechanisms) where it facilitates glucose uptake. Muscle contraction may induce GLUT 4 translocation by activation of 5′-adenosine monophosphate-activated protein kinase (AMPK) and via calcium/calmodulin-dependent protein kinase II (28). The resultant effect is GLUT 4 translocation to the cell membrane in the absence of insulin; thereby sparing insulin and improving insulin sensitivity over time with consistent training (28).

For muscle glycogen, the enzyme *phosphorylase* breaks a molecule of glucose-1-phosphate from glycogen, which will be converted to glucose-6-phosphate (glycogenolysis). This reaction, however, does not require energy. At rest, phosphorylase is inactive (b form) but becomes activated (a form) during exercise in response to greater epinephrine secretion and elevated calcium concentrations (29). Glucose-6-phosphate must then be converted to fructose-6-phosphate (via an *isomerase* enzyme) and to fructose-1,6-biphosphate. The enzyme *phosphofructokinase* (PFK) phosphorylates fructose-6-phosphate and is considered the rate-limiting reaction of glycolysis. The regulation of PFK is critical to the magnitude of energy liberation derived from glycolysis. This reaction also requires energy, so up to this point in glycolysis, we have used (invested) 2 ATPs but have not produced any. These reactions are reversible so glucose could be formed during gluconeogenesis (a process by which glucose is reformed in the opposite direction of glycolysis). From this point, our initial 6-carbon molecule is split via an enzyme, *aldolase*, into two 3-carbon molecules, a dihydroxyacetone phosphate (DHAP) and a glyceraldehyde-3-phosphate (G3P). DHAP is rapidly converted to G3P via an isomerase enzyme. Both 3-carbon G3P molecules undergo a series of reactions (where net ATP will be formed) yielding 1,3-bisphosphoglycerate, 3-phosphoglycerate, and 2-phosphoglycerate. Accompanying these reactions is the formation (generation) of 2 ATP and 2 NADH. We now have formed a net total of 0 ATP for glycolysis to this point (we have used 2 ATP and formed 2 ATP, netting 0 ATP). Phosphoenolpyruvate (PEP) is formed from 2-phosphoglycerate via an enzyme *enolase* and PEP then forms pyruvate via the enzyme *pyruvate kinase*. This reaction produces 2 ATP (one from each PEP molecule) thereby netting 2 ATP formed from glycolysis.

Pyruvate is the end product but can be further modified to meet metabolic demands. If inadequate oxygen is present, pyruvate can be converted into lactate via the enzyme *lactate dehydrogenase* (LDH). This sequence has been called anaerobic or fast glycolysis. This reaction leads to some accumulation of H$^+$ that contributes, in part, to muscle fatigue. Pyruvate can travel to the mitochondria, lose a carbon (forming *acetyl CoA*), and enter the Krebs cycle (aerobic respiration). This is called aerobic or slow glycolysis. The terms *aerobic* and *anaerobic glycolysis* are probably not practical because glycolysis itself is an anaerobic process.

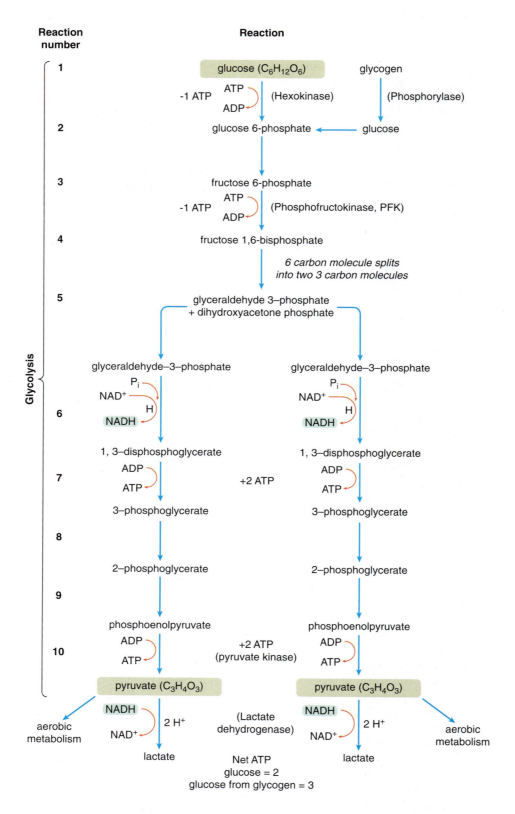

FIGURE 8.3 Glycolysis. (Adapted with permission from Powers SK, Howley ET. *Exercise Physiology: Theory and Application to Fitness and Performance*. 5th ed. New York (NY): McGraw Hill; 2004.)

Control of Glycolysis

Glycolysis can be controlled in several ways. Glycolysis is inhibited by sufficient oxygen levels, *i.e.*, steady-state aerobic exercise or during rest. Glycolysis is stimulated by high concentrations of ADP, P_i, ammonia, and by slight decreases in pH and AMP. Intense exercise results in a marked increase in ATP hydrolysis, thereby yielding higher concentrations of ADP and P_i. Ammonia is a by-product of AMP metabolism, and an increase in ammonia stimulates glycolysis. Glycolysis is inhibited by reductions in pH, increased ATP, PC, citrate, and free fatty acids (FFAs). High ATP and PC levels signify a recovery (or resynthesis) state, thus a further need for glycolysis is reduced. Energy substrates can regulate glycolysis via negative feedback where high concentrations of ATP will limit production. Acidosis (decreased pH) inhibits glycolysis and is a major component of muscle fatigue. Citrate and FFAs are molecules indicative of aerobic metabolism, thereby reflecting adequate oxygen supply/demand.

A substantial portion of glycolysis is regulated through enzyme control. The enzymes hexokinase, PFK, phosphorylase (enzyme that breaks down glycogen), and pyruvate kinase are controlled by other molecules. Enzymes have two major binding areas, a catalytic unit that speeds up reactions and an allosteric unit that binds to regulatory molecules (*i.e.*, hormones, proteins). Negative feedback systems regulate glycolysis via the allosteric unit. For example, hexokinase is inhibited by glucose-6-phosphate. PFK is inhibited by ATP, and H^+ and stimulated by AMP. Pyruvate kinase is inhibited by ATP and acetyl CoA and is stimulated by AMP and fructose-1,6-bisphosphate (4). Phosphorylase is stimulated by hormones (*e.g.*, epinephrine) and is inhibited when another antagonistic enzyme, *glycogen synthase* (enzyme that stores glycogen), is active. This elaborate negative feedback control of glycolysis can stimulate or inhibit key glycolytic enzymes based on the energy needs of the human body.

Glycogen Metabolism

Glycogen plays multiple roles in skeletal muscle but primarily supplies a quick source of glucose, and greater glycogen availability preexercise enhances endurance performance (29). Approximately 5%–15% of muscle glycogen is stored within myofibrils (a preferential site for depletion), 75% is stored between myofibrils, and 5%–15% is stored beneath the sarcolemma (30). Glycogen storage can vary across fiber type where FT fibers may store larger amounts (30). It has been suggested that intermyofibrillar glycogen assists in the release of calcium and intramyofibrillar glycogen preferably powers cross-bridge cycling (and is highly related to fatigue) (31). Glycogen use is most rapid at the beginning of exercise and increases exponentially as intensity increases. On average, humans can store ~500 g (1%–2% of muscle mass) of glycogen in skeletal muscle (depending on body size) and ~80–120 g in the liver. High CHO intake increases muscle glycogen utilization, whereas higher dietary fat intake may spare muscle glycogen (29). Low muscle glycogen concentrations may shift metabolism toward lipid oxidation. During exercise, glycogen breakdown takes place at a high rate in ST and FT fibers depending on recruitment. Liver glycogen breakdown helps maintain blood glucose and provides glucose for muscle uptake. Blood glucose plays an increasing role in ATP turnover as exercise intensity rises as blood flow to working muscles increase (30). Phosphorylase breaks down glycogen and glycogen breakdown takes place during exercise, and the magnitude depends on intensity, volume/duration, and rest intervals. Glycogen depletion in some muscle fibers serves as a stimulus for recruitment of other FT fibers.

Glycogen is a major source of energy for exercise at intensities >50%–60% of VO_{2max} (29), and glycogen depletion causes muscle fatigue during aerobic exercise or repeated, intermittent high-intensity anaerobic exercise of sufficient duration (32). During aerobic exercise, the pattern of glycogen depletion is related to fiber-type recruitment as substantial depletion occurs in ST fibers with secondary depletion occurring in FT fibers (32). During resistance exercise, glycogen breakdown predominates in FT fibers (33) and the rate is intensity dependent (34). For example, Robergs et al. (34) reported glycogenolytic rates of 0.46 and 0.21 mmol·kg wet wt^{-1}·s^{-1}, respectively, in the vastus lateralis muscle during leg extension sets of 70% versus 35% of 1 RM. They reported 38%–39% reductions in muscle glycogen following 6 sets of leg extensions. Interestingly, muscle glycogen increased by 12%–18% during the first 2 hours of recovery despite no nutritional interventions used (34). Intermittent exercise results in partial-to-substantial depletion of glycogen in ST and FT fibers (30). The pattern of glycogen breakdown is similar between trained and untrained individuals (35), and resistance exercise may deplete muscle glycogen by 30%–60% (4,33,34,36) with some cells completely depleting glycogen stores. Initiating a resistance exercise workout with low muscle glycogen may limit up-regulation of some muscle growth factors (37). Sprint exercise of sufficient distance with short recovery intervals leads to high rates of glycogen depletion (especially in FT fibers) (32).

Muscle and liver glycogen repletion is critical to recovery following exercise. It involves many factors such as hormonal action, glucose uptake into muscle cells, and blood flow. Although glycogen resynthesis may occur partially with the absence of nutritional intervention, a critical factor is the amount, type (glucose and sucrose superior to fructose), and timing of CHOs and protein consumed post exercise. An enzyme in promoting glycogen storage is *glycogen synthase*, which is very active following exercise. Glycogen repletion is biphasic, with a rapid early phase during the first hour followed by a slower phase. Most glycogen repletion takes place within the first 6 hours post exercise. The rapid, early phase may be insulin-independent and due to GLUT 4 translocation (38). In addition, high-glycemic index CHOs (plus amino acids) may offer an advantage to glycogen repletion when consumed during this early phase especially when consumed immediately after exercise (38). The second phase of glycogen storage may occur at ~80% slower rate and is characterized by insulin-stimulated muscle glucose uptake and glycogen synthase, but is enhanced by combined CHO and amino acid intake (38). Most, if not all, muscle glycogen can be replenished within 24 hours provided adequate CHO consumption occurs, although repletion can be

Sidebar — Carbohydrate Intake, Muscle Glycogen, and Exercise Performance

CHOs (monosaccharides, disaccharides, and oligosaccharides/polysaccharides) are macromolecules consisting of carbon, hydrogen, and oxygen atoms. CHOs perform many functions including energy liberation, cell structure and integrity, regulation of lipid metabolism, amino acid metabolism, and protein synthesis; enhance immune function; and serve as a structural component of genetic material (7). It is recommended that athletes consume ~55%–65% of their daily caloric intake from CHOs, with the majority from complex CHOs and <10% consumed from simple CHOs (39). The American College of Sports Medicine (ACSM) recommends that athletes consume 6–10 g CHOs·kg body mass^{-1}·d^{-1} to perform optimally and recover in between workouts (39). Studies show *CHO loading* or high-CHO diets (500–650 g of CHOs·d^{-1}; 8–10.5 g of CHO·kg of body mass^{-1} consumed for at least 3 days) increase muscle and liver glycogen content for ~3 days after loading and up to 1.8 times that of a normal diet in men and women (40–43). However, performance may or may not improve depending on the volume and intensity (*i.e.*, performance may increase with long-duration exercise). CHO intake during prolonged exercise helps maintain blood sugar levels, spare muscle and liver glycogen, and promote glycogen synthesis (during rest periods or periods of low-intensity activity). The ACSM recommends that athletes consume ~30–60 g of CHOs·h^{-1} during long-term exercise (39) depending on intensity, size, type of CHOs consumed, and conditioning of the individual. For optimal glycogen repletion following long-duration exercise, CHOs (plus amino acids) should be consumed as soon as possible at ~1.0–1.5 g of CHOs·kg of body mass^{-1} within 30 minutes (38,39). This should be repeated every 2 hours for 4–6 hours. For slower repletion, the individual should consume 8–10 g·kg of body mass^{-1} over a 24-hour period (7).

slowed by muscle damage (4). Restoration of muscle glycogen can exceed normal levels with consistent training via glycogen supercompensation (29).

Training Adaptations

Changes in substrate storage and enzyme activity may occur during training. Training that relies on glycolysis provides a potent stimulus for enhanced glycogen storage. Aerobic training (AT) increases muscle glycogen in FT and ST fibers (32). Steady-state AT and high-intensity interval training can increase resting muscle glycogen (44–47). One study showed 6 weeks of interval AT (10 × 4-min bouts at 90% of VO$_{2max}$ with 2-min rest intervals) increased muscle glycogen content by 59% (46), and Burgomaster et al. (44) showed a 50% increase following 2 weeks of sprint interval training. AT results in a glycogen-sparing effect during low- to moderate-intensity exercise with an increased proportion of energy provided by fat use (45,48), possibly due to reduced phosphorylase activity (30). This glycogen-sparing effect is also seen in the liver following AT (30). Less lactate is produced per given workload as a result of AT or interval training (44,46). Sprint training may not change or increase glycogen content (18). The magnitude depends on how much sprint training affects the glycolytic metabolic system. Longer sprints with short to moderate rest intervals increase reliance upon glycolysis and may pose a more potent stimulus for glycogen storage than short sprints with long rest intervals. RT increases resting glycogen content by up to 112% (14). Bodybuilders have greater glycogen content than untrained individuals (49). RT with light loads with restricted blood flow can increase muscle glycogen more than RT without occlusion (50).

Acute exercise increases non–insulin-dependent GLUT 4 translocation (28). Aerobic training, interval training, and RT have been shown to increase GLUT 4 gene transcription and protein stores, glucose uptake, and decrease insulin resistance (28,46,51). Glycolytic enzyme activity may decrease, not change, or increase during training. Sprint training may increase (16%–49%) or not change PFK activity, increase LDH (9%–20%), and increase phosphorylase (9%–41%) activity (18,52). AT does not increase anaerobic enzyme activity at rest (49) especially since AT induces changes in substrate utilization, *i.e.*, greater fat use versus CHO. During exercise (80% of VO$_{2max}$), AT reduces activation of phosphorylase and reduces glycogen breakdown thereby showing a glycogen-sparing effect (45,53). Trained individuals have a higher activity of glycogen synthase. RT may alter enzyme activity depending on the program and magnitude of hypertrophy. RT programs that stress the ATP-PC system (high weight, low repetitions, and long rest intervals) may show reductions in glycolytic enzyme activity with pronounced hypertrophy (54). Phosphorylase activity may increase (20,55), PFK activity may increase (20) or not change (21,23,55), hexokinase may increase (56), and LDH activity may slightly increase or not change after RT (20,26).

Lactate

Lactate has a negative impact on performance. The production of lactate from pyruvate yields H$^+$, which contributes to muscle fatigue. An accumulation of H$^+$ reduces pH and leads to a rapid onset of fatigue. H$^+$ accumulation causes peripheral fatigue via inhibition of glycolytic enzymes, slowing calcium reuptake, and interference with cross-bridge cycling properties. For many years, the production of lactate via fast glycolysis was thought to be the major pathway for H$^+$ accumulation. However, H$^+$ accumulation results from all metabolic systems, and lactate formation may play a limited role (57). Although the lactate molecule may physically inhibit muscle cross-bridge formation (58), other studies have shown no negative effects (59).

Myths & Misconceptions
Lactate Has No Benefits in the Human Body

Lactate does have benefits. Once produced, lactate will not remain stagnant in skeletal muscles. A large amount is shuttled to adjacent muscle fibers (especially ST) where it can be converted to pyruvate via the reversible LDH catalyzed reaction, or enters circulation (1). Lactate removal is essential for the cell to keep liberating energy via glycolysis. However, a large amount can enter circulation because exercise produces large amounts of lactate that temporarily overwhelm muscle fibers' ability to oxidize it rapidly. The fate of lactate in the blood is short-lived because values typically return to preexercise levels within 1 hour after exercise. Lactate can be taken up by other skeletal (mostly ST fibers) and cardiac muscles and be used as an energy substrate. Lactate in blood can travel to the liver (or kidneys) and be used to form glucose via gluconeogenesis where it can reestablish blood glucose concentrations or replenish liver glycogen. This process is known as the *Cori Cycle*. Lactate is a valuable energy substrate and not a waste product.

The release and uptake of lactate in skeletal and cardiac muscle is dependent upon specific transmembrane transporters known as *monocarboxylate transporters* (MCT) along with chaperone proteins (*e.g.*, basigin). Although many isoforms have been identified, MCT1 and MCT4 are found in skeletal muscle and MCT1 in the heart (60). The MCTs mediate transport for lactate and H+ and assist in pH balance during exercise (61). Lactate transport capacity is greater in ST than FT fibers, and the proportion of ST fibers is related to MCT1 density (61). Lactate uptake from the blood is related to MCT1 content, and training may up-regulate MCT1 and MCT4 expression in skeletal muscle (46,60), although no changes have also been found (12). A recent study showed sprint interval training on a cycle ergometer (with either 1- or 5-min rest intervals) up-regulated MCT1 and *sodium/hydrogen exchanger (NHE)-1* (an antiport membrane protein that transports sodium in a cell while exporting H+ out) similarly (*i.e.*, rest interval length had no effect) but did not alter MCT 4 in women (62). Another study in men showed up-regulation of MCT1, MCT4, basigin, and NHE-1 following interval training (63). These changes took place within the first 2–4 weeks of interval training (63). Maximal speed and speed endurance training have been shown to up-regulate MCT1 but not MCT4, and only speed endurance training up-regulated NHE-1 (64). Thus, it appears that selective up-regulation of lactate/H+ proteins may occur as an adaptation to training to facilitate lactate removal and uptake, as well as regulate pH. It has been suggested that lactate may act as a signaling molecule for MCT1 up-regulation (62). Interestingly, testosterone administration may increase MCT1 and MCT4 content with a concomitant increase in lactate transport capacity (65).

Anaerobic exercise results in an increase in blood lactate concentrations in trained and untrained individuals (Fig. 8.4).

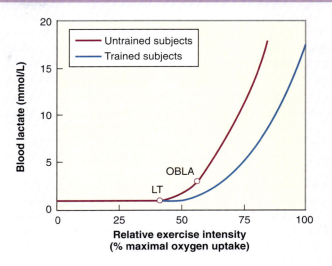

FIGURE 8.4 The lactate threshold. (Reprinted with permission from Cramer JT. Bioenergetics of exercise and training. In: Baechle TR, Earle RW, editors. *Essentials of Strength Training and Conditioning*. 3rd ed. Champaign (IL): Human Kinetics; 2008. p. 21–39.)

At rest, blood lactate values range from 1 to 2 mmol·L^{-1}. Because red blood cells only metabolize glucose, there are low levels of lactate in the blood at rest. As exercise intensity increases (and recruitment of FT fibers increases), blood lactate values increase. This corresponding intensity is known as the lactate threshold. The lactate threshold typically begins ~50%–60% of VO$_{2max}$ in untrained individuals and 70%–80% of VO$_{2max}$ in trained athletes (4). It is thought to reflect the interaction of anaerobic and aerobic energy systems (66). Athletes with high lactate thresholds are capable of excelling at endurance events (66). The blood lactate curve shifts to the right with training at or beyond the lactate threshold indicating that a higher intensity is needed to produce a specific blood lactate level. RT (3–5 sets of 15–20 reps with short rest intervals) and circuit training (8–20 RM with 30-s rest intervals) can increase the lactate threshold (67,68). The second point shown in Figure 8.4 is the onset of blood lactate accumulation (OBLA) and represents the point/intensity where blood lactate values exceed 4 mmol·L^{-1} and increase exponentially. Blood lactate reflects not only production but also the rate of clearance. Endurance athletes possess a higher rate of lactate clearance (69).

The amount of lactate produced depends on the intensity and duration of exercise with the magnitude less in endurance-trained compared to sprint-trained athletes (70). AT and interval training lessen the lactate response to submaximal workloads (46). Blood lactate values in athletes may reach as high as 32 mM immediately following high-intensity exercise (71). During RT, bodybuilding workouts stress the

(Continued)

glycolytic system more than strength/power training. Blood lactate increases during resistance exercise (72–75) with the magnitude greater with high intensities (72,76), large muscle mass exercises (75), high volume (74,77), slow lifting velocities (78), short rest intervals (73), and augmented eccentric loading (76,79). The intensity/volume interaction is critical as larger responses are seen with high-volume, low- to moderate-intensity (multiple sets of 15 reps with 60% of 1 RM) than low-volume, high-intensity (multiple sets of 4 reps with 90% of 1 RM) workouts (80). A reduced lactate response occurs at absolute workloads, but not relative workloads (81) following RT. Powerlifters and weightlifters (but not bodybuilders) exhibit greater increases in blood lactate at an absolute workload during cycling than untrained individuals (82). Bodybuilders possess the ability to train with a higher percent of their 1 RM for multiple sets when short rest intervals are used. Training targeting the glycolytic system induces favorable changes in lactate kinetics.

Metabolic Acidosis and Buffer Capacity

Blood and muscle pH decrease during and immediately following anaerobic exercise (83,84). Muscle pH may drop from 7.1 to 6.4 during exhaustive exercise (83). The drop in pH is less in endurance-trained athletes (70). Reduced blood pH decreases intracellular H^+ efflux and disturbs muscle acid-base balance (85). Acidosis adversely affects energy metabolism and force production so that the onset of fatigue is rapid. Metabolic acidosis may cause fatigue by negatively affecting sodium and potassium movement, reducing calcium kinetics, reducing cross-bridge formation, and inhibiting glycolytic enzymes (71). PFK may be inhibited at a pH of 6.9, and glycogen breakdown may be completely halted at a pH of 6.4 (66). Muscle pH may be maintained by moving H^+ out of the sarcoplasm into the mitochondria or out of the cells (via transporters discussed in the previous section) or improving buffer capacity. Maintaining pH relies upon the cells' ability to extrude protons (H^+) and/or accumulated hydroxide (OH^-) and bicarbonate (HCO_3). An acid is a proton donor, and a base is a proton acceptor. Buffering capacity is the ability to resist changes in pH (71). Several intracellular and extracellular factors contribute to improved skeletal muscle buffer capacity (referred to as either chemical or physiological buffers). These include the following:

- Phosphates (mostly intracellular; *chemical buffer*): Monohydrogen phosphate (HPO_4), CP (~33% of intracellular buffering especially in FT fibers), and P_i.
- Proteins and peptides (intracellular and extracellular; *chemical buffer*): ~50% of intracellular buffering during exercise. Some blood proteins, like hemoglobin, serve as a buffer. Amino acid supplementation results in better buffering capacity during training (86). Associated with protein buffers are the protein-bound histidyl residues, histidine-containing dipeptides, and free histidine. Carnosine accounts for up to 40% of total intracellular buffering capacity (71,87) and is found to be ~20–30 mmol·kg^{-1} dry weight in humans with magnitudes higher in men than women and FT than ST fibers (88). Elevated carnosine is seen in sprinters and rowers compared to endurance athletes and untrained individuals (89). Carnosine (β-alanyl-L-histidine) and β-alanine are used in supplementation. Although oral carnosine supplementation is ineffective at increasing muscle carnosine (as it is metabolized by the enzyme *carnosinase* prior to reaching muscle), β-alanine (the rate-limiting precursor of carnosine) supplementation of 4–6 g·day^{-1} can increase muscle carnosine concentrations by up to 64% after 4 weeks and up to 80% after 10 weeks (88). Four weeks of β-alanine supplementation (4.5–4.8 g·day^{-1}) can augment isokinetic torque, RT volume, muscle endurance, and reduce fatigue (90–92). However, 10 weeks of supplementation with 6.4 g·day^{-1} increased muscle carnosine by 12% but did not augment performance (93). Overall, the literature supports β-alanine as a nutritional supplement. In a position statement, Trexler et al. (88) reported the following: (a) β-alanine generally enhances anaerobic high-intensity exercise lasting 1–4 minutes with greater effects seen during time to exhaustion tasks; (b) β-alanine may improve aerobic exercise duration; (c) β-alanine may increase RT training volume but does not augment strength gains during RT; (d) coingestion of β-alanine with sodium bicarbonate or creatine has modest additive ergogenic benefits; and (e) ingestion of β-alanine as part of a multiingredient supplement may be effective if the supplementation period is sufficient to increase carnosine levels. It has been recommended that a loading phase of 4–6 g in divided doses for ~4 weeks be used to increase muscle carnosine levels when supplementing with β-alanine (88).
- Bicarbonate (extracellular, intracellular; *chemical buffer*): the bicarbonate anion (HCO_3) accepts H^+ to form carbonic acid where it is converted to H_2O and CO_2 by the enzyme *carbonic anhydrase* isozymes. Sahlin (94) suggested that bicarbonate could contribute as much as 15%–18% of total buffer capacity during exercise. Although bicarbonate's role is to buffer extracellular fluid, it indirectly acts as an intracellular buffer by facilitating H^+ flux out of muscle (95). Bicarbonate loading can be an ergogenic aid during exercise (7). Contrasting changes in different carbonic anhydrase isozymes have been reported following high-intensity interval training in men and women so their potential role in adaptation remains unclear (62,63).
- Respiratory and renal buffers: both are *physiological buffers*. Because a rise in CO_2 leads to acidosis, respiratory rate increases (hyperventilation) to expel CO_2 at a higher rate. The kidneys can neutralize acid as the renal tubules expel H^+ from the body.

Training increases the ability to maintain pH or buffer acids in response to exercise. The adaptations may appear at multiple levels from augmenting the movement of protons via up-regulation of lactate or nonlactate coupled transport proteins to buffering the extracellular and intracellular components all of which may enhance force production and endurance. It appears that up-regulation of individual components of pH regulation may occur in response to the type of training stimulus and that a substantial magnitude of the improvement in pH regulation may be lost after 6 weeks of detraining (63). The ability to rapidly move H^+ out of skeletal muscle fibers reduces the likelihood of metabolic or contractile interference. Increasing muscle buffer capacity enables greater tolerance for acidosis. Higher lactate concentrations are seen following anaerobic training with concomitant improvements in performance (95,96). Enhanced buffer capacity prolongs high-intensity exercise performed beyond the lactate threshold. Comparisons of studies measuring buffer capacity are difficult due to differences in techniques used to measure skeletal muscle buffer capacity. These concerns notwithstanding, trained individuals have a greater buffer capacity than untrained individuals (97). Muscle buffer capacity may increase by 16%–44% after 7–8 weeks of sprint training (95,98,99). RT may lessen H^+ accumulation but may not increase buffer capacity in women (67). A few recent studies have shown no changes in nonbicarbonate and nonprotein muscle buffer capacity following high-intensity cycle interval training in men and women (62,63) thereby providing support that other components of pH regulation may lead to performance enhancement.

Aerobic Metabolism

The aerobic, or oxidative, energy system is highly engaged when adequate oxygen is available. In some ways, the term *aerobic* is misleading because oxygen's role is limited until the end where its presence assists indirectly in ATP production. The majority of energy derived aerobically comes from the oxidation of CHOs and fats, with very little from protein under normal conditions (unless the individual has very low kilocalorie intake or has performed a substantial endurance activity). Oxidation reactions donate electrons, whereas reduction reactions accept electrons. The removal of hydrogen is critical as hydrogen atoms possess potential energy stored from food sources, and these electrons are transported and used for ATP synthesis. Aerobic metabolism occurs within the cell's mitochondria (powerhouses of the cell). The mitochondria contain carrier molecules that oxidize electrons from hydrogen and pass them to oxygen via reduction reactions that generate a large amount of ATP (1). The aerobic system provides the primary source of ATP at rest and during low to moderate steady-state exercise. Seventy percent of ATP produced at rest comes from fats, whereas 30% comes from CHOs (4). As exercise intensity increases, so does the percent of ATP liberation from CHOs. High-intensity exercise relies predominantly upon CHO metabolism.

Metabolism of CHOs begins with glycolysis. Remember, the fate of pyruvate was twofold: (a) converted to lactate via LDH or (b) converted to acetyl CoA and CO_2 via *pyruvate dehydrogenase*. Acetyl CoA is capable of being oxidized and can be formed from fat and protein sources, which makes it the common link of these fuel sources. The aerobic system (Fig. 8.5) begins in the mitochondrial matrix with the Krebs cycle (named after Nobel Prize–winning scientist Hans Krebs), which involves reactions (that do not require oxygen) that continue the oxidation of acetyl CoA and produces 2 ATP indirectly. The goals are to oxidize acetyl groups and attach electrons to the carriers NAD^+ and FAD. Acetyl CoA transfers two carbons to oxaloacetate to form the 6-C citrate via *citrate synthase*. Oxaloacetate is further converted into isocitrate (via *aconitase*), α-ketoglutarate (via *isocitrate dehydrogenase*), succinyl CoA (via *α-ketoglutarate dehydrogenase*), and succinate (via *succinyl-CoA-synthetase*). Succinate is converted to fumarate via the enzyme *succinate dehydrogenase (SDH)*. Fumarate is converted to malate (via *fumarase*) and to oxaloacetate (via *malate dehydrogenase [MDH]*). The following reaction describes the Krebs cycle:

$$Acetyl\ CoA + 3\ NAD^+ + FAD + GDP + P_i + 2\ H_2O \rightarrow$$
$$2\ CO_2 + GTP + 3\ NADH + 3\ H^+ + FADH_2 + CoA$$

Remember, two molecules of acetyl CoA enter the Krebs cycle as two pyruvates are produced in glycolysis. The intermediates produced in Figure 8.5 will be doubled. The removal and transport of H^+ via NAD and FAD yields large energy liberation via participation in the *electron transport chain* (ETC) located at the mitochondria's double-layered membrane. Fatty acids can be converted to acetyl CoA via a process known as β-oxidation. Amino acids may enter the Krebs cycle at various sites including conversion to acetyl CoA. Branched-chain amino acids are the major source. Some enzymes of the Krebs cycle are stimulated by ADP concentrations and inhibited by rising ATP and GTP levels.

Overall, six molecules of NADH and two molecules of $FADH_2$ are produced from the Krebs cycle. Most energy is liberated from the *ETC* (Fig. 8.6), which couples reactions between electron donors and acceptors across the inner mitochondrial membrane. ATP synthesis (from ADP) occurs from transferring electrons from NADH and $FADH_2$ to oxygen. Hydrogen atoms are passed along the chain of cytochromes in complexes where they reduce oxygen to form water and a proton-motive gradient to phosphorylate ADP (chemiosmotic hypothesis) (2). Uncoupling proteins (UCP1–UCP5) assist and play a role in thermogenesis and energy expenditure (100).

Energy Yield from Carbohydrates

Generally, 3 ATP will be produced per molecule of NADH and 2 ATP from $FADH_2$. From glucose oxidation, 2 (from blood glucose) or 3 (from stored glycogen) ATP will be produced from glycolysis, 2 ATP will be produced from the Krebs cycle, 12 ATP will be produced from 4 NADH produced from glycolysis and pyruvate conversion to acetyl CoA, and 22 ATP will

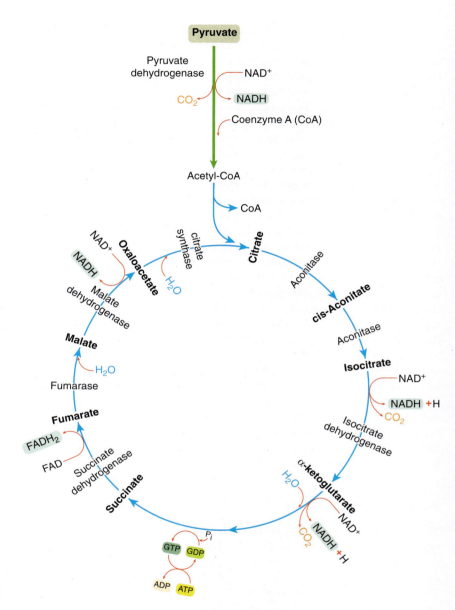

FIGURE 8.5 The Krebs cycle. (Modified from Kraemer WJ, Fleck SJ, Deschenes MR. *Exercise Physiology: Integrating Theory and Application.* Baltimore (MD): Lippincott Williams & Wilkins; 2012.)

be produced from the ETC totaling 38 or 39 ATP. However, the transport of ATP out of the mitochondria into the cytoplasm requires energy therefore yielding a net value of ~32–33 ATP from a molecule of glucose.

Lipid Metabolism

Fat provides a concentrated source of energy with an almost unlimited energy reserve. Fat metabolism predominates at rest and during low- to moderate-intensity exercise. This section briefly discusses fat metabolism from storage, release, transportation and uptake, and mitochondrial entry to β-oxidation and subsequent aerobic metabolism for energy. It is important to note that intramuscular signaling pathways discussed in Chapter 5 appear to play major roles in FFA uptake and lipid metabolism in skeletal muscle and adipocytes. For example, *5′ AMP-activated protein kinase (AMPK)* is an intracellular sensor of ATP consumption and largely involved in glucose and fat oxidation (101). Intramuscular signaling as well as other systemic factors envelops an environment where numerous levels of control are imposed upon lipid metabolism. Potentially, each mechanism in the chain of lipid metabolism may pose a limiting factor to fat oxidation during exercise and be augmented by training, especially aerobic endurance training. However, some mechanisms within the chain appear to play more prominent roles in exercise-enhanced lipid metabolism.

Fats may be metabolized via three major sources: (a) triglycerides stored within skeletal muscle near mitochondria (*e.g., intramuscular triglycerides*) or in between muscle fibers; (b) FFAs in circulation from catabolism in adipose tissue; and (c) circulating triacylglycerols in lipoprotein complexes broken down via *lipoprotein lipase*. Figure 8.7 depicts fat sources, transport, and uses for energy metabolism (1). Approximately 20–40 mmol·kg^{-1} dry muscle of fat may be stored in human skeletal

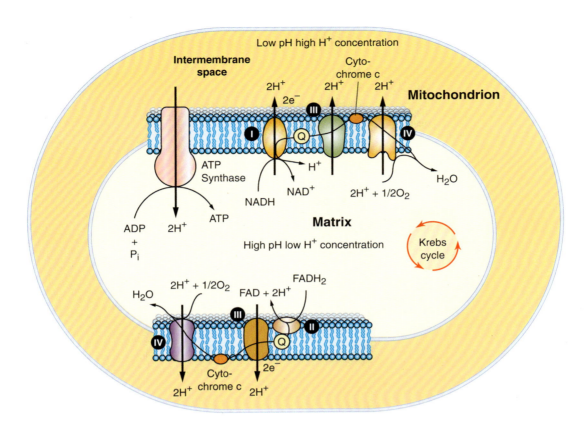

FIGURE 8.6 The electron transport chain. (From Porth CM. *Pathophysiology Concepts of Altered Health States.* 7th ed. Philadelphia (PA): Lippincott Williams & Wilkins; 2005.)

muscle (102). Type I fibers display more prominent intramuscular TG stores than FT fibers (103). Fats, or lipids, are broken down during lipolysis in sequential steps by *adipose triglyceride lipase* (ATGL) and *hormone-sensitive lipase* in adipocytes and skeletal muscle into glycerol and three FFAs (104). Lipase activity plays a critical role in regulating lipolysis. Lipase activity is increased during exercise. Hormones such as epinephrine, norepinephrine, thyroid hormones, growth hormone, and testosterone (via up-regulation of β-adrenergic receptors on adipocytes) can increase lipolysis, whereas insulin is an inhibitor of lipolysis. During exercise, the reduction in insulin and increased catecholamine response may increase FFA release by as much as 400% (105). Caffeine and other stimulants have the ability to increase lipolysis. The reaction catalyzed by lipases is:

$$\text{Triacylglycerol} + 3H_2O \rightarrow \text{glycerol} + 3 \text{ fatty acids}$$

At rest, FFAs are released from adipose tissue two times more than the amount that is oxidized. Large adipocytes have greater baseline lipolytic activity per cell than smaller cell sizes (105). Regional specificity is seen where areas relatively greater in adipocyte size (*i.e.*, gluteal area in women, visceral adipocytes in men) show higher lipolytic activity (105). Glycerol concentrations in adipose tissue increase in response to exercise with responses greater from abdominal than gluteal tissue and more so in women than men thereby showing regional heterogeneity of lipolysis is related to body fat distribution (105).

In adipocytes, FFAs are released and transported in the blood by plasma albumin to skeletal muscle. FFAs are released by albumin and diffused or are transported across the plasma membrane via membrane-associated fatty acid–binding/transport proteins (*e.g.*, plasma membrane–bound fatty acid binding protein [FABP$_{pm}$], fatty acid translocase [FAT/CD36], and fatty acid transport protein [FATP]) (103). FFA delivery to skeletal muscle depends on the quantity of FFAs in the blood as well as increased blood flow to skeletal muscle during exercise (102). Once inside the muscle fiber, FFAs may either reesterify to form intramuscular triglycerides or be metabolized for energy. The FFAs in the cytoplasm are chaperoned by fatty acid-binding protein (FABP$_c$) and are transported to the surface of the outer mitochondrial membrane. The long-chain FFAs subsequently are activated by binding with coenzyme A, converted to a fatty acyl carnitine compound, and transported across the outer mitochondrial membrane bound to carnitine via carnitine palmitoyltransferase I activity (CPT1; which transfers the acyl group of fatty acyl CoA to L-carnitine) (102). Acylcarnitine translocase assists in allowing acylcarnitine passage across the inner mitochondrial membrane as part of a shuttling system. In the mitochondria, carnitine palmitoyltransferase II (CPT2; located on the inner mitochondrial membrane) catalyzes the transfer of the acyl group of carnitine to coenzyme A, and the reformed fatty acyl CoA is metabolized via β-oxidation (102). Short- and medium-chain FFAs may diffuse freely across the mitochondrial membranes. CPT1 activity is considered a rate

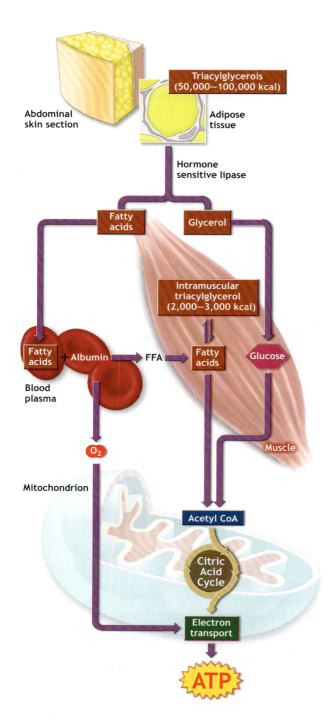

FIGURE 8.7 Fat supply for energy metabolism. (Reprinted with permission from McArdle WD, Katch FI, Katch VL. *Exercise Physiology: Nutrition, Energy, and Human Performance*. 8th ed. Philadelphia (PA): Wolters Kluwer; 2015).

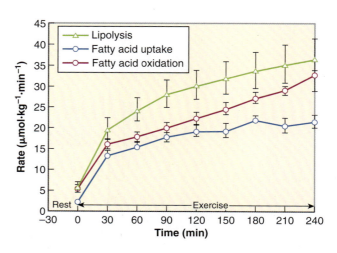

FIGURE 8.8 Rates of lipolysis, FA uptake, and FA oxidation during exercise. (Reprinted with permission from Horowitz JF, Klein S. Lipid metabolism during endurance exercise. *Am J Clin Nutr*. 2000;72(Suppl):558S–63S).

limiting step in fat oxidation and is inhibited by *malonyl-CoA* thereby inhibiting FA metabolism and favoring FA biosynthesis. Malonyl-CoA levels decrease or do not change during exercise (102). Increased AMPK may inhibit the enzyme *acetyl-CoA carboxylase* (ACC; catalyzes the formation of malonyl CoA from acetyl CoA) or increase *malonyl CoA decarboxylase* (enzyme that decarboxylates malonyl CoA to acetyl CoA) thereby reducing malonyl CoA concentrations and promoting lipid metabolism (103).

During aerobic exercise, the rate of lipolysis, plasma FFA concentrations, fatty acid uptake, and FFA oxidation increase as the duration of exercise increases (Fig. 8.8) with the response greater in endurance-trained individuals (103,106). The intensity is a critical factor, as is preexercise diet and potential nutrient intake during exercise. For example, consumption of CHOs may reduce lipid metabolism (103). In contrast, a high-fat diet or low preexercise muscle glycogen may shift emphasis toward lipid metabolism (103). In a fasted state, low level of blood glucose and insulin and elevated catecholamines stimulates greater lipolysis and FFA oxidation (and lower respiratory quotient [RQ]), including intramuscular TG oxidation in type I fibers, during endurance exercise (51,107). During prolonged low- to moderate-intensity aerobic exercise, an increase in FFA delivery to skeletal muscle occurs (102). As exercise intensity increases, release of FFAs from adipose tissue lags behind skeletal muscle uptake; the resultant effect may be no change or a decrease in plasma FFAs (1). The beginning of exercise also produces a transient reduction in plasma FFAs due to increased tissue uptake while an increase will ensue overtime (1,103). During moderate intensity aerobic exercise, 55%–65% of lipid metabolism is provided by plasma FFAs (103). In addition, intramuscular triglyceride stores may provide 15%–35% of the energy contribution with the largest amounts seen in highly trained endurance athletes (1). Reductions of 20%–50% in intramuscular TG stores have been shown during prolonged exercise (1–2 h or more) with larger reductions seen in highly trained populations (103). Rising intensity is a stimulus for glycogen use. In a classic study, Romijn et al. (108) examined fat and CHO metabolism at 25%, 65%, and 85% of VO_{2max}. They showed that FFA oxidation rate was highest during the 65% trial. The contribution of plasma FFAs was highest during the 25% trial and decreased with increases in intensity. Intramuscular triacylglycerol contributions to FFA oxidation were highest during the 65% trial, followed by 85% and minimal at 25%. Lipolysis increased from 25% to 65% of VO$_{2max}$ and was maintained. Large increases in muscle glycogen and plasma glucose contributions to energy expenditure were seen at 85% of VO$_{2max}$. In a follow-up study, they showed that fat oxidation was impaired at 85% VO$_{2max}$ because of, in part, failure of FFA mobilization to increase above resting levels (109). As endurance exercise progresses to longer than 1 hour, fat metabolism contributes a larger percent to energy expenditure as glycogen depletion occurs (1).

Resistance exercise induces a dissimilar type of lipolytic response compared to aerobic exercise given the substantial anaerobic component and subsequent reliance on CHO metabolism. Measurement of plasma glycerol and FFAs has been used to examine lipolysis. However, blood glycerol concentrations may be a better indicator of adipose tissue lipolysis during RE than FFAs due to up-regulated fat oxidation and reesterification of FFAs. Studies have shown elevated glycerol concentrations during and up through 45-minutes post-RE (110–114), increased energy expenditure of 10%–22% during and following RE and increased fat oxidation rates post RE by 49%–75% (112–114), and elevated FFA concentrations post RE (110) but not during RE (111,114). The lipolytic response may be related to the interaction of the intensity and volume of the workout. Enhanced fat oxidation following RE may spare glucose for glycogen replenishment. These data show that RE provides a potent stimulus for lipolysis. Figure 8.9 depicts data from Goto et al. (111) comparing lipolysis during endurance exercise by itself to the same protocol performed 20 and 120 minutes following RE. The orange area depicts the response during endurance exercise, while the pink area consists of the RE time period. Prior RE augmented the glycerol and FFA responses to subsequent endurance exercise performed 20 and 120 minutes afterward. These data show that either modality increases lipolysis during exercise; however, endurance exercise lipolysis was greater when RE was performed first.

Energy Yield from Fats

Fatty acids can enter circulation or be oxidized from muscle stores via β-oxidation (Fig. 8.10). β-Oxidation involves the splitting of 2-carbon acyl fragments from a long chain of fatty acids. Protons are accepted, water is added, ATP phosphorylates the reactions, and acyl fragments form with coenzyme A to yield acetyl CoA (1). Acetyl CoA enters the Krebs cycle and hydrogen released enters the ETC. If an 18-carbon fatty acid is examined, ~147 ATP can be generated per fatty acid. Since there are three fatty acids in a triglyceride, 441 ATP (147 × 3) can be generated. Glycerol can be converted to 3-phosphoglyceraldehyde and enter glycolysis that yields 19 ATP. An 18-carbon triglyceride can yield a total of 460 ATP. Fat breakdown and oxidation is highly dependent on oxygen consumption. β-Oxidation will not proceed if oxygen does not join hydrogen (1). Individuals with high aerobic capacity can oxidize fats at a large rate.

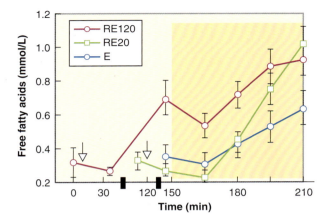

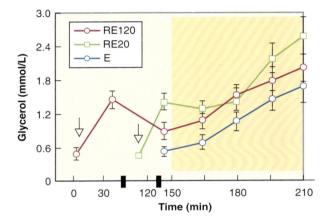

FIGURE 8.9 Glycerol and FFA response to resistance exercise and aerobic exercise following resistance exercise. E, endurance exercise; RE120, endurance exercise performed 120 minutes after RE; RE20, endurance exercise performed 20 minutes after RE. (Reprinted with permission from Goto K, Ishii N, Sugihara S, Yoshioka T, Takamatsu K: Effects of resistance exercise on lipolysis during subsequent submaximal exercise. *Med Sci Sports Exerc*. 2007;39:308–15.)

Aerobic Training Adaptations

AT leads to a milieu of adaptations that increases maximal aerobic capacity (VO$_{2max}$). AT increases the number of capillaries surrounding each muscle fiber and capillary density (number of capillaries relative to muscle CSA) by up to 15% (51,66). Higher capillary content enables greater nutrient and oxygen exchange during exercise, and favors greater reliance on fat metabolism. AT increases the number of mitochondria and mitochondrial density in muscle in proportion to training volume (66). Endurance-trained men may have ~103% greater mitochondrial number and three times greater mitochondrial volume than untrained men (1). Myoglobin (a protein that binds oxygen in muscle and transports it to the mitochondria) is highest in ST fibers and is important for muscle endurance increases. AT may increase myoglobin content up to 80% (66). Krebs cycle, β-oxidation, and electron transport system enzyme activity increases during AT. AT and aerobic interval training increase activities of *SDH, citrate synthase,*

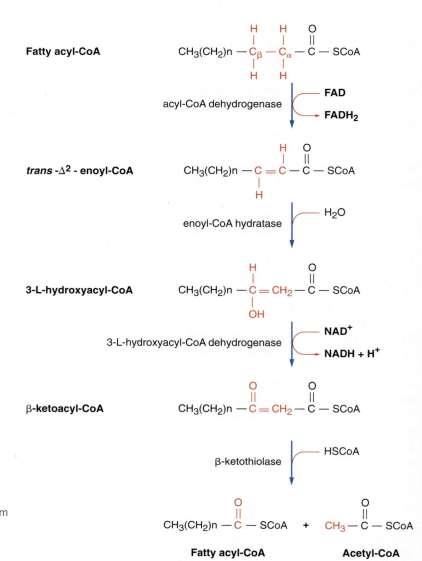

FIGURE 8.10 β-Oxidation and energy yield from fats. (From McArdle WD, Katch FI, Katch VL. *Exercise Physiology: Nutrition, Energy, and Human Performance*. 7th ed. Baltimore (PA): Lippincott Williams & Wilkins; 2010.)

cytochrome C oxidase, *β-hydroxyacyl-CoA dehydrogenase* (β-HAD), and *pyruvate dehydrogenase* (44,46,66). The increased enzyme activity occurs in proportion to the level of training. Kiens (103) has shown a positive relationship between skeletal muscle β-HAD and FFA oxidation rates during exercise. Some evidence indicates that CS and β-HAD increases may be augmented if endurance training is performed in a fasted state (51). AT may induce changes in metabolic substrate availability and use. AT increases muscle glycogen stores at rest and improves the glycogen-sparing effect during exercise (1,32,66). As a result, endurance athletes are better able to utilize FFAs for energy during exercise. Endurance athletes have greater FFA transport through the plasma membrane and within the muscle fiber, intramuscular triglyceride stores at rest, enhanced lipolysis and mobilization of FFAs during exercise, and higher β-oxidation enzymatic activity all resulting in more efficient fat metabolism at rest and during exercise (1,32,66,103). Endurance-trained individuals show higher plasma FFA concentrations, FFA uptake, and FFA oxidation during exercise than lesser-trained or untrained individuals (103). Endurance training may increase $FABP_{pm}$ protein expression in men, FAT/CD36, CPT1, adipose triglyceride lipase (ATGL), and lipoprotein lipase (46,103,104,115).

Anaerobic Training Adaptations

Anaerobic training (resistance, sprint, plyometric, and agility) provides little stimulus to the aerobic energy system as much of the energy demands are met by the ATP-PC and glycolytic systems. An increase in the vascular capacity of muscle is important to maintain perfusion and capillary number per fiber increases during RT (116,117). The capillary-to-fiber ratio may increase 12%–15% during 12 weeks of RT; the increases may start to take place in as little as 2 weeks of RT in type I fibers (by 6%) and 4 weeks in type II fibers (118). The capillary increase may be accompanied by increased hypoxic/vascular protein mRNA and content, *e.g.*, vascular endothelial growth factor (VEGF), VEGF receptor, endothelial nitric oxidase, and HIF-1α

(118,119). Both high-load, moderate-rep and low-load, high-rep RT programs may increase capillary-to-fiber ratio, capillary contacts, and capillary-to-fiber perimeter exchange index similarly (119). Bodybuilders (120) and powerlifters (121) have greater capillary number than untrained individuals. However, capillary density is unaffected by RT and decreases in response to hypertrophy (56,116,118,120–122), which could result in a reduced capacity for oxygen delivery to recruited muscle fibers. Bodybuilders have greater capillary density than powerlifters and Olympic lifters but values are similar to untrained men (49). Mitochondrial density decreases up to 26% in response to RT (123,124) although mitochondrial size may increase in women (56). Myoglobin may not change following 8 weeks of RT (125) to perhaps help preserve oxygen transport during hypertrophy.

Most studies have shown no change or decreases in Krebs cycle and ETC enzyme activity (citrate synthase, MDH, SDH) during RT (20,23,55,56,125,126). However, some studies have shown increased citrate synthase, MDH, cytochrome oxidase, and β-HAD (an enzyme of β-oxidation) activities following RT (56,127,128). Bodybuilders have greater citrate synthase and β-HAD activity than powerlifters and weightlifters (25). Sprint training may increase, decrease, and not change citrate synthase activity and not change or increase SDH activity (18). Most studies that found increased aerobic enzyme activity used long-distance sprints, whereas those that did not used repeated short sprints (18). Sprint training with multiple sets of at least 30-seconds intervals has been shown to increase the activity of hexokinase, PFK, citrate synthase, SDH, and MDH (129).

Energy System Contribution and Athletics

All energy systems are engaged at all times regardless of the activity (Table 8.1). Each system works together to meet the demands of exercise. However, one may predominate based on the intensity, volume/duration, and recovery intervals of exercise. During a 30-second cycle sprint, 28%–40% of energy is liberated from aerobic metabolism, ~45% from glycolysis, and ~17% from ATP-PC system. During a 12-second cycle sprint, 47% of energy is liberated from glycolysis, 22% from ATP-PC, and 31% from aerobic metabolism (6). Table 8.2 depicts the metabolic demands of various sports. Training programs can be designed to target each system by manipulation of the intensity, volume/duration, and rest intervals used. An athlete whose sports require energy from ATP-PC system should target this system specifically with high-intensity, short bouts of explosive exercise to achieve the best results. Metabolic specificity is critical to off-season, preseason, and in-season training of athletes. Interval training allows the athlete to train at higher intensities for periods of time using prescribed rest intervals. The athletes can dedicate a greater proportion of time to high intensities as opposed to continuous training that may limit intensity and depends on fatigue. Work-to-rest ratios are prescribed. A 1:10 ratio indicates that athletes rest 10× longer than the work interval. An explosive bout lasting ~8 seconds requires the athlete to rest ~80 seconds. The work-to-rest ratio can target energy systems such that 1:12 to 1:20 ratios target ATP-PC, 1:3 to 1:5 ratios target fast glycolysis, 1:3 to 1:4 ratios target fast glycolysis and aerobic oxidation, and 1:1 to 1:3 ratios target aerobic oxidation (4).

Case Study 8.1

Nicole is an aerobic athlete who has predominately trained with traditional, continuous aerobic exercise workouts. She had learned from fellow athletes who incorporated interval training into their programs that these individuals improved their race times and attributed their success, in part, to interval training. Nicole has decided to include interval training in preparation for a 10-km race. She has approached you, a prominent strength and conditioning coach, for advice on how to incorporate interval training into her preparatory training program.

Questions for Consideration: What work-to-rest ratio would you prescribe to Nicole to enhance her running program? What type of progression strategy would you suggest Nicole to follow?

Metabolic Demands and Exercise

Exercise metabolism is measured several ways, but the most common method involves indirect calorimetry. Indirect calorimetry involves measurement of oxygen consumption via open-circuit spirometry. Changes in oxygen and CO_2 percentages in expired air are compared to normal inspired ambient air, *e.g.*, 20.93% oxygen, 0.03% CO_2, and 79.04% nitrogen (1).

Table 8.1	Energy System Use	
Duration of Event	Intensity of Event	Primary Energy System(S)
0–6 s	Very intense	Phosphagen
6–30 s	Intense	Phosphagen and fast glycolysis
30 s to 2 min	Heavy	Fast glycolysis
2–3 min	Moderate	Fast glycolysis and oxidative system
>3 min	Light	Oxidative system

Table 8.2 Metabolic Demands of Sports

Sport	Phosphagen System	Anaerobic Glycolysis	Aerobic Metabolism
Baseball	High	Low	—
Basketball	High	Moderate to high	—
Boxing	High	High	Moderate
Diving	High	Low	—
Fencing	High	Moderate	—
Field events	High	—	—
Field hockey	High	Moderate	—
Football (American)	High	Moderate	Low
Gymnastics	High	Moderate	—
Golf	High	—	—
Ice hockey	High	Moderate	Moderate
Lacrosse	High	Moderate	Moderate
Marathon	Low	Low	High
Mixed martial arts	High	High	Moderate
Powerlifting	High	Low	Low
Skiing:			
Cross-country	Low	Low	High
Downhill	High	High	Moderate
Soccer	High	Moderate	Moderate
Strength competitions	High	Moderate to high	Low
Swimming:			
Short distance	High	Moderate	—
Long distance	—	Moderate	High
Tennis	High	Moderate	—
Track (athletics):			
Short distance	High	Moderate	—
Long distance	—	Moderate	High
Ultra-endurance events	Low	Low	High
Volleyball	High	Moderate	—
Wrestling	High	High	Moderate
Weightlifting	High	Low	Low

Note: All types of metabolism are involved to some extent in all activities.

Reprinted with permission from Ratamess NA. Adaptations to anaerobic training programs. In: Baechle TR, Earle RW; National Strength and Conditioning Association, editors. *Essentials of Strength Training and Conditioning.* 3rd ed. Champaign (IL): Human Kinetics; 2008. 95 p.

A metabolic cart can measure each breath and consists of a flow meter, system to analyze expired air, CO_2 and oxygen analyzers, and a computer interface for calculations. Oxygen consumption data can be used to estimate energy expenditure during rest and exercise. Resting energy expenditure provides an estimate of resting metabolic rate. The RQ is a measure of CO_2 produced per unit of oxygen (*e.g.*, RQ = CO_2 produced ÷ O_2 consumed). This gives an indication of fuel usage, *i.e.*, CHO (RQ close to or >1.00), fat (RQ = ~0.70), protein or mixed diet (RQ = ~0.82–0.86). Similar to RQ, the *respiratory exchange ratio* (RER) can be measured. Although RQ assumes that gas exchange results solely from nutrient breakdown, RER reflects more accurately the role of anaerobic exercise metabolism during exhaustive exercise and is calculated the same way as RQ.

Basal Metabolic Rate

Basal metabolic rate (BMR) is the minimal level of energy needed to sustain bodily functions. Control of BMR, and essentially metabolism, is critical to body fat reductions and weight control. BMR represents the individual's total energy expenditure in a day. With aging, BMR decreases approximately 2%–3% per decade, especially in individuals with sedentary lifestyles (1). Total energy expenditure or BMR is composed of resting metabolic rate (RMR; ~60%–75%), the thermic effect of physical activity (15%–30%), and thermic effect of food consumption (~10%). RMR is the energy required to perform normal bodily functions, while the body is at rest and is somewhat similar to BMR although it is measured under less stringent conditions, *e.g.*, does not require a 12-hour fast or 8 hours of sleep. It is the largest single component of total daily caloric expenditure. Manipulation of any or all of these components of BMR can increase energy expenditure thereby resulting in greater kilocalories burned per day. BMR is affected by the following factors:

- *Body mass* — the larger the body size, the higher the BMR. Lean body mass (LBM; or fat-free mass) is a strong component of BMR. This is why RT is important to increasing BMR and reducing body fat. RT increases RMR by up to 9% after 24 weeks, with a larger response seen in men (130). An increase in LBM of 1 lb could increase RMR by 7–10 kcal·day^{-1} (1). RT may or may not preserve LBM and increases RMR during strict dieting, whereas strict dieting alone reduces LBM and RMR (131,132). Because of gender differences in body size, RMR is ~5%–10% higher in men than women (1). Fat tissue has less metabolic activity than muscle mass, so high body fat has a negative impact on BMR.
- *Regular exercise* — regular exercise enhances BMR with the magnitude dependent upon intensity, volume/duration, and muscle mass involvement. AT and RT can increase RMR by 8%–10% (1). Athletes have greater BMR than untrained individuals matched for LBM. A comprehensive progressive program consisting of aerobic and anaerobic exercise is critical to increasing BMR.
- *Diet-induced thermogenesis* — involves the increase in BMR associated with digestion, absorption, and assimilation of nutrients and activation of the sympathetic nervous system in response to meal consumption. Dietary-induced thermogenesis reaches maximum levels ~1 hour after meal consumption (1) but may last up to 6 hours (133). Studies have shown a range of diet-induced thermogenesis augmentations where energy expenditure may be 1.3%–41% greater than RMR (133). Meals higher in protein content elicit a higher increase in BMR and may produce greater muscle anabolism during RT. Diets high in protein (relative to CHOs and fat intake) increase satiety (sense of fullness) and energy expenditure (134). Animal and whey proteins induce a greater

thermogenic effect than other proteins (soy) and are thought to increase satiety to a greater extent possibly due to changes in hormones that control hunger (134). High-protein meals are thought to increase thermogenesis by up-regulating uncoupling proteins (134). A meta-analysis showed that diet-induced thermogenesis (after an overnight fast) is higher with high kilocaloric meals compared to low, high protein intake versus lower protein, higher medium-chain TGs versus long-chain TGs, when the individual eats slowly versus rapidly, and may not be affected by meal frequency although some studies show greater diet-induced thermogenesis with a large meal compared to isocaloric meals distributed with higher frequency (133). The BMR increase during exercise is larger when exercise is performed following a meal, showing that exercise can augment diet-induced thermogenesis (1). Light to moderate exercise 1 hour following a meal may be beneficial in individuals trying to lose weight.
- *Environment* — warm environments can produce higher BMRs. Exercise in warm conditions can augment oxygen consumption by ~5% (1). The greater core temperature and physiologic demands of perspiration in the heat poses a stimulus to BMR. Cold temperatures pose a stimulus to BMR. Shivering generates body heat, and BMR can increase to accommodate the cold conditions (1).
- *Other factors* — low kilocalorie diets have the opposite effect. Decreasing kilocalorie intake decreases RMR and leads to weight gain. Stress, and the hormonal response, increases RMR. Catecholamines and thyroid hormones increase BMR. Hormonal control of metabolism is potent and varies based on genetics, nutritional intake, stress levels, and physical activity.

Estimating Resting Energy Expenditure

Estimating resting energy expenditure is important for weight loss/gain programs as direct measurement is impractical. Several population-specific equations have been developed to estimate resting energy expenditure from predictor variables such as body mass or LBM, height, and age that are based on gender. LBM may be the strongest predictor of RMR (135), explaining 53%–88% of the variance in RMR (136). The first equation developed and one still commonly used is the Harris-Benedict equation (137). The Cunningham (138) and Mifflin and St. Jeor (139) equations are commonly used (Table 8.3). These equations were based mostly off of large heterogeneous (*i.e.*, age, bodyweight, body composition components, and fitness levels) cohorts of subjects that may lead to greater variation of prediction when applied to a smaller sample of athletes. In healthy populations, cross-validation studies have shown: (a) the Mifflin and St. Jeor equation to be most reliable within 10% of actual RMR (144) and (b) Harris-Benedict and World Health Organization (WHO; not shown in Table 8.3) equations to be most similar to measured RMR (<10%) while others under predicted (136). Other studies have cross-validated these equations in athletes with most studies showing RMR underestimation

Table 8.3 Resting Metabolic Rate (RMR) Prediction Equations

Equation	Reference
RMR = 66.47 + 6.23 × BW (lb) + 12.67 × Ht (in.) − 6.76 + age (y) in men	Harris and Benedict (140)
RMR = 655.1 + 4.34 × BW (lb) + 4.69 × Ht (in.) − 4.68 + age (y) in women	
RMR = 10 × BM (kg) + 6.25 × Ht (cm) − 5 × age (y) + 5 in men	Mifflin-St Jeor (139)
RMR = 10 × BM (kg) + 6.25 × Ht (cm) − 5 × age (y) − 161 in women	
RMR = 500 + 22 × LBM (kg)	Cunningham (138)
RMR = −857 + 9 × body mass (kg) + 11.7 × height (cm)	*De Lorenzo et al. (141)*
RMR = 88.1 + (2.53 × Ht [cm]) + (8.42 × Mass [kg]) +(19.46 × Age [y]) in female athletes from 11 sports	*Watson et al. (142)*
RMR = 120.81 + (4.88 × Ht [cm]) + (8.24 × FFM [kg]) +(5.71 × Age [y]) in female athletes from 11 sports	
RMR = (24.8 × BM [kg]) + 10 in male and female physique athletes	*Tinsley et al. (143)*
RMR = (25.9 × FFM [kg]) + 284 in male and female physique athletes	

Entries in italics represent studies examining athletes as subjects.

(141,145). The best prediction equations in these studies were Cunningham (135,141,142,145). Jagim et al. (145) reported that the Cunningham equation worked best in women and Harris-Benedict in men; both faring better than the De Lorenzo equation that was developed from a small population of male athletes. Watson et al. (142) developed specific equations for female athletes but also showed the Mifflin/St. Jeor equation a better predictor than other commonly used equations. The lack of consistency in findings indicates that multiple equations can be used depending on the population in question. Table 8.3 also includes equations developed specifically in athletes.

Estimating Energy Expenditure during Exercise

At rest, the average individual requires 0.20–0.35 L of $O_2 \cdot min^{-1}$ or 1.0–1.8 $kcal \cdot min^{-1}$ of energy expenditure (66). A commonly used unit is the MET (metabolic equivalent): 1 MET (resting oxygen consumption) = ~250 $mL \cdot min^{-1}$ for men and ~200 $mL \cdot min^{-1}$ in women (1). 1 MET = a relative VO_2 of 3.5 $mL \cdot kg^{-1} \cdot min^{-1}$. A man with a VO_{2max} of 50 $mL \cdot kg^{-1} \cdot min^{-1}$ exercising at 70% (35 $mL \cdot kg^{-1} \cdot min^{-1}$) is equivalent to 10 METs. Exercise increases energy expenditure with the magnitude dependent on intensity, volume, muscle mass involvement, and

Sidebar Basal Metabolic Rate Estimation in Athletes

Estimation of BMR involves estimation of RMR, diet-induced thermogenesis, and physical activity energy expenditure (PAEE). The following example utilizes the Cunningham (138) equation in a very active 22-year-old athlete who weighs 240 lb and has 11% body fat.

1. The first step is to convert 240 lb to kg (1 lb = 2.2 kg). 240/2.2 = **109.1 kg**.
2. LBM must be calculated. Total mass (109.1 kg) is multiplied by the decimal of body fat percentage (0.11) to calculate fat mass. Fat mass = 109.1 kg × 0.11 = **12 kg**. LBM = total mass − fat mass = 109.1 kg − 12.0 kg = **97.1 kg**. Another method is to multiply total mass (109.1 kg) × 0.89 (1.00 − 0.11 for fat percentage) = **97.1 kg**.
3. Equation (25): RMR = 500 + 22 × LBM (kg): RMR = 500 + 22 × (97.1 kg) = **2,636 kcal**.

4. Diet-induced thermogenesis is calculated. This accounts for ~10% of BMR. TEF = 2,636 kcal × 0.10 = **264 kcal**. Note: a higher percentage (up to 15%) may be used if one consumes a high-protein diet (>1.5 g·kg body mass⁻¹).
5. Determination of PAEE. This could be estimated or the following conversion system can be used: 1.2–1.3 for bedridden individuals, 1.4–1.5 for sedentary occupation without daily movement, 1.5–1.6 for sedentary occupation with daily movement, 1.6–1.7 for occupation with prolonged standing, 1.9–2.1 for strenuous work and physically active. If 1.9 is used for our example, PAEE + RMR = 2,636 kcal × 1.9 = **5,008 kcal**.
6. 5,008 kcal + 264 kcal (TEF) = **5,272 kcal** needed per day to maintain bodyweight.

rest intervals (continuity). Energy cost of sport and exercise is determined via oxygen consumption (Table 8.4). These values are based on a 70-kg man and a 55-kg woman. Larger individuals yield higher values and smaller individuals yield smaller values. Light exercise is considered <5 kcal·min^{-1} in men (<4 METs) and <3.5 kcal·min^{-1} in women (<2.7 METs), moderate exercise is considered 5.0–7.4 kcal·min^{-1} in men (4–6 METs) and 3.5–5.4 kcal·min^{-1} in women (2.8–4.3 METs), and heavy

Table 8.4	Energy Expenditure During Exercise	
Activity	**Men (kcal·min^{-1})**	**Women (kcal·min^{-1})**
Baseball/softball	6.1	4.8
Basketball	8.6	6.8
Boxing (competitive)	14.7	11.6
Hitting bag	7.4	5.8
Cycling		
7.0 mph	5.0	3.9
10.0 mph	7.5	5.9
Football	11.0	8.7
Golf	5.5	4.3
Handball	11.0	8.6
High jump/long jump	7.4	5.8
Judo/jiu jitsu	12.3	9.6
Racquetball	12.3	9.6
Rope jumping	9.8–14.7	7.7–11.2
Rugby	12.3	9.6
Running		
7.5 mph	14.0	11.0
10.0 mph	18.2	14.3
Shot put and discus	4.9	3.9
Soccer	12.2	9.6
Standing	1.8	1.4
Swimming (crawl, 3.0 mph)	20.0	15.7
Tennis	7.1	5.5
Walking		
3.5 mph	5.0	3.9
5.0 mph	9.8	7.7
Weight lifting	8.2	6.4
Wrestling	13.1	10.3

Reprinted with permission from Wilmore JH, Costill DL. *Physiology of Sport and Exercise*. 2nd ed. Champaign (IL): Human Kinetics; 1999; Ainsworth BE, Haskell WL, Whitt MC, et al. Compendium of physical activities: an update of activity codes and MET intensities. *Med Sci Sports Exerc*. 2000;32(Suppl):S498–S516.

exercise is considered >7.5 kcal·min^{-1} in men (>6–7 METs) and >5.5 kcal·min^{-1} in women (4.5–5.5 METs) (1). Most sports exceed the metabolic classifications of heavy exercise, whereas general fitness activities rank light, moderate, or heavy based on intensity. The ACSM has provided several metabolic equations that estimate energy expenditure for walking, running, stepping, and cycling and conversion factors (Table 8.5). Relative VO_2 during exercise is calculated first, converted to absolute VO_2, and converted to kcal·min^{-1} generally by multiplying it by 5. Energy expenditure is higher after exercise cessation as more kilocalories are burned after exercise than would have been if one did not exercise. Estimations of daily energy expenditure are not adequate in factoring the postexercise effects.

Oxygen Consumption and Acute Training Variables

Oxygen consumption increases during exercise in proportion to intensity (Fig. 8.11). There is an exponential rise as exercise approaches steady state (within 1–4 min) termed the *fast component of VO$_2$*. Aerobically trained athletes can reach steady state in a shorter time period than untrained individuals (140). At the onset of exercise, the respiratory and cardiovascular systems do not supply enough oxygen to meet the demands. It takes a few minutes for these systems to catch up, indicating anaerobic systems predominate early in providing energy. The difference between oxygen supply and demand is oxygen deficit and is shown in the shaded area in Figure 8.11. Oxygen deficit is larger during anaerobic (Fig. 8.11B) than aerobic exercise (Fig. 8.11A) and is smaller in aerobically trained athletes than untrained individuals and strength/power athletes (1). Steady state occurs at the VO_2 plateau where oxygen supply meets demand and is where aerobic metabolism predominates. Steady state can occur at various levels of VO_2 depending on intensity. At higher intensities (above the lactate threshold), VO_2 can rise gradually to meet additional energy costs termed the *slow component of VO$_2$* and is attributed to increased core temperature, pulmonary ventilation, and the recruitment of FT muscle fibers (2).

Oxygen consumption remains elevated during recovery following exercise. The magnitude depends on exercise intensity and duration and is proportional to the oxygen deficit accrued at the onset of exercise (1,146). There is little elevated VO_2 after light, short-duration exercise. However, intense aerobic and anaerobic exercise of sufficient duration results in a large rise in VO_2 after exercise. The additional oxygen consumed over baseline levels following exercise is termed excess postexercise oxygen consumption (EPOC), or formerly known as oxygen debt. The EPOC period consists of a rapid initial component followed by a slow component. The rapid component elicits recovery in VO_2 within the first few minutes. The slow component may persist for an hour but may take as long as 24 hours to return to homeostatic VO_2 (1) depending on exercise intensity and duration. Several factors contribute to EPOC. The cardiovascular and respiratory systems remain elevated, which results in greater VO_2 needed to resynthesize ATP and PC, oxidize lactate (and restore pH)

Table 8.5	The ACSM's Metabolic Equations

Activity	Equation
Walking	$VO_2 = 3.5 + 0.1$ (walking speed) $+ 1.8$ (speed) (percent grade)
Running	$VO_2 = 3.5 + 0.2$ (running speed) $+ 0.9$ (speed) (percent grade)
Stepping	$VO_2 = 3.5 + 0.2$ (step rate) $+ 2.4$ (step rate) (step height)
Leg cycling	$VO_2 = 7 + 1.8$ (work rate)/body mass
Arm cycling	$VO_2 = 3.5 + 3$ (work rate)/body mass

Conversion Factors for Metabolic Equations

$$\frac{(\dot{V}O_2 \text{ in } L\cdot min^{-1}) \times 1{,}000}{\text{body mass}} = \dot{V}O_2 \text{ in } mL\cdot min^{-1}\cdot kg^{-1} \qquad \frac{(\dot{V}O_2 \text{ in } mL\cdot min^{-1}\cdot kg^{-1})\,(\text{body mass})}{1{,}000} = \dot{V}O_2 \text{ in } mL\cdot min$$

$$\dot{V}O_2 \text{ in METs} \times 3.5 = \dot{V}O_2 \text{ in } mL\cdot min^{-1}\cdot kg^{-1} \qquad \frac{(\dot{V}O_2 \text{ in } mL\cdot min^{-1}\cdot kg^{-1})}{3.5} = \dot{V}O_2 \text{ in METs}$$

$$\dot{V}O_2 \text{ in } mL\cdot min^{-1} \times 5 = \text{energy exp. in } kcal\cdot min^{-1} \qquad \frac{(\text{energy exp. in } kcal\cdot min^{-1})}{5} = \dot{V}O_2 \text{ in } L\cdot min^{-1}$$

$$(\text{speed in mph}) \times 26.8 = \text{speed in } m\cdot min^{-1} \qquad \frac{\text{speed in } m\cdot min^{-1}}{26.8} = \text{speed in mpho}$$

$$\frac{\text{speed in kph}}{0.06} = \text{speed in } m\cdot min^{-1} \qquad (\text{speed in } m\cdot min^{-1}) \times 0.06 = \text{speed in kph}$$

$$\frac{\text{work rate in } kg\cdot m\cdot min^{-1}}{6} = \text{power in W} \qquad (\text{power in W}) \times 6 = \text{work rate in } kg\cdot m\cdot min^{-1}$$

(*Note:* $kg\cdot m\cdot min^{-1}$ is not technically a unit of power; also conversion with the acceleration of gravity yields a correction factor of 6.12; however, the ACSM uses 6 as a reasonable approximation for exercise prescriptions.)

$$(\text{weight in lb}) \times 2.2 = \text{mass in kg} \qquad \frac{\text{Mass in kg}}{2.2} = \text{Weight in lb}$$

(*Note:* Pounds are not a unit of mass but can be converted with the factor 2.2 when the mass in question is subject to earth's gravity; for greater precision, a factor of 2.2046 can be used.)

$$(\text{height in inches}) \times 0.0254 = \text{height in m} \qquad \frac{\text{height in m}}{0.0254} = \text{height in inches}$$

Units: VO_2 ($mL\cdot min^{-1}\cdot kg^{-1}$); speed ($m\cdot min^{-1}$); work rate ($kg\cdot m\cdot min^{-1}$); body mass (kg); step rate (steps per minute); step height (m).

Reprinted with permission from Swain DP, Leutholtz BC. *Exercise Prescription: A Case Study Approach to the ACSM Guidelines.* 2nd ed. Champaign (IL): Human Kinetics; 2007. p. 49–69.

and resynthesize glycogen from lactate, restore oxygen to myoglobin, and increase oxygen content in the blood and other tissues. Tissue repair, elevated protein synthesis, and redistribution of minerals require energy and higher VO_2. Thermogenesis is enhanced due to lingering effects of the sympathetic nervous system and several hormones (catecholamines, thyroid hormones, glucocorticoids, growth hormone superfamily), and the acute rise in body temperature (1). The elevated EPOC period has also been attributed to increased sodium-potassium pump activity and triglyceride-fatty acid cycling. The EPOC period results in greater energy expenditure and is important for body fat reductions and weight loss.

Resistance Training and Oxygen Consumption

Resistance exercise increases VO_2 during and after a workout. Several factors influence the response. Studies have shown:

- VO_2 is greater during large muscle group exercises than smaller muscle group exercises (147–149). Large muscle mass exercises elicit aerobic energy expenditure values of ~8–11.5 $kcals\cdot min^{-1}$ versus ~5.0–7.3 $kcals\cdot min^{-1}$ seen in smaller mass exercises (150). A lower-body workout may elicit metabolic responses up to ~60% of VO_{2max} (49) showing that traditional RT programs (moderate to high

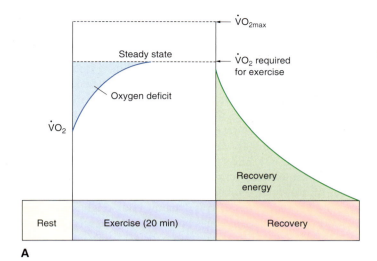

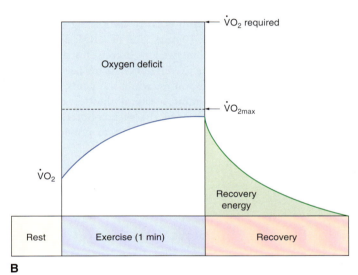

FIGURE 8.11 **A and B.** Oxygen consumption during exercise and excess postexercise oxygen consumption (EPOC). (Adapted with permission from Cramer JT. Bioenergetics of exercise and training. In: Baechle TR, Earle RW, National Strength and Conditioning Association, editors. *Essentials of strength training and conditioning*. 3rd ed. Champaign (IL): Human Kinetics; 2008. 35 p.)

intensity, at least 1–2 min rest intervals) have limited effects on increasing VO_{2max} in fit individuals. Resistance exercises such as squats and deadlifts elicit higher energy expenditure and VO_2 compared to exercises such as the bench press, shoulder press, row, lat pulldown, and curl (148,150,151). The leg extension elicits higher acute VO_2 than the chest press and shoulder press (152). The leg press elicits nearly double the acute VO_2 response than the chest fly (153). Multijoint strength and power exercises (squat, deadlift, bench press, and power clean) performed in sequence produces similar energy expenditure values to performing four strongman exercises (sled drag, farmer's walk, 1-arm dumbbell clean and press, and tire flip) in a row, *e.g.*, median values of 9.1 and 8.9 kcals·min^{-1}, respectively (154). Selection of large muscle mass exercises

is important when designing training programs targeting increased energy expenditure.

- VO_2 may vary based on lifting velocity. The results from studies have been equivocal and may be indicative of an interactive effect of intensity, volume, and repetition velocity. One study showed exercises (matched for rep number) performed with slow to moderate velocities yielded greater VO_2 than fast velocities (155). Another study showed time under tension increases energy expenditure when matched for volume and intensity (156). In contrast, some data indicate higher velocities produce higher energy expenditure especially when more reps are performed (157). Another study showed greater aerobic energy expenditure (7.3 vs. 6.4 kcal·min^{-1}) when explosive squats were performed compared to a 2-second squat (60% of 1 RM) (78), and maximal velocity resulted in greater energy expenditure for other exercises than 2-seconds reps in a follow-up study (151). Lastly, another study showed no difference between 2- and 4-seconds reps in energy expenditure (158).
- VO_2 is greater when exercises are performed with high (80%–90% of 1 RM) > moderate (60%–70% of 1 RM) > low (20%–50% of 1 RM) intensity (72,148,159,160) when similar numbers of reps are performed. If sets are taken to failure, greater rep number and workload seen during light or moderate intensity may lead to greater energy expenditure compared to heavy weight with fewer reps (157). Thus, it appears that the interaction of volume and intensity is critical to energy expenditure when sets are taken to failure or near failure.
- VO_2 and energy expenditure are greater when exercises are performed for high rep number compared to low rep number, or multiple sets compared to single sets (161–163).
- VO_2 is greater when exercises are performed with short versus long rest intervals (74,164,165). The lack of continuity with long rest intervals limits the metabolic response (74,166) and could pose a limitation to increasing VO_{2max} among fit populations. This is also the case when other modalities such as battling rope workouts are performed with short rest intervals (167).
- VO_2 and energy expenditure for a workout is not affected by exercise order (168). However, VO_2 may be lower for an exercise when it was performed first versus last (168). Performing an exercise such as the bench press after the squat can augment the metabolic response compared to if it is performed before the squat when short rest intervals are used (165).
- VO_2, energy expenditure, and blood lactate are greater when reciprocal super set workouts are used compared to traditional set structure, *i.e.*, 34.7 versus 26.3 kJ·min^{-1}, with greater energy expenditure during the immediate EPOC period (169).
- Time-efficient metabolic training programs performed with moderate to high intensities yield large metabolic demands (170) and can increase aerobic fitness, muscle strength, power, and endurance (171–173).
- VO_2 is high during circuit, metabolic RE protocols compared to traditional RE structure (174). For example, a 10-minute circuit of KB swings yielded energy expenditure of ~12.5 kcals·min^{-1} (175). Figure 8.12 depicts relative oxygen consumption data taken from a sandbag RE protocol using Tabata intervals (8 exercises, 20-s exercise, and 10-s

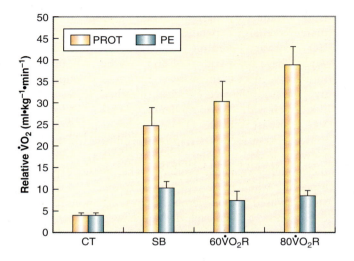

FIGURE 8.12 Oxygen consumption during a sandbag RE workout compared to running at 60% and 80% of $\dot{V}O_{2max}$ reserve. PROT, protocol; PE, post exercise; CT, control (no exercise); SB, sandbag protocol; $60\dot{V}O_2R$, running at 60% of $\dot{V}O_2$ Reserve; $80\dot{V}O_2R$, running at 80% of $\dot{V}O_2$ Reserve. (From Ratamess NA, Kang J, Kuper JD, et al. Acute cardiorespiratory and metabolic effects of a sandbag resistance exercise protocol. *J Strength Cond Res.* 2018;32(6):1491–502.)

rest in continuity repeated for 3 circuits with 2-min rest between circuits) (176). In this study, we compared the sandbag workout to running at 60% and 80% of $\dot{V}O_{2max}$ reserve. $\dot{V}O_2$ during each protocol was higher during both running protocols. On average, the sandbag workout yielded aerobic energy expenditure of ~10.6 kcals·min^{-1} compared to 12.8 and 16.6 kcals·min^{-1}, respectively, for the 60% and 80% running workouts. However, EPOC and energy expenditure following the sandbag workout was 33% and 18% greater than running at 60% and 80%, respectively, during the 30-minutes post exercise period thereby showing metabolic effects of RE play a large role post exercise. Use of Tabata intervals for other modalities such as dynamic bodyweight squat variations (177) and kettlebells has shown high levels of energy expenditure, *e.g.*, 9.5 kcals·min^{-1} for a 12-minute kettlebell workout with peak averages of 12.4 kcals·min^{-1} (178).

- Different modalities of RE elicit different $\dot{V}O_2$ responses. Table 8.6 depicts data from a study comparing traditional resistance exercises (3 × 10 reps, 75% of 1 RM, 2-min rest) to battling rope and bodyweight exercises matched for time (150). Battling rope exercise and the burpee produced the largest metabolic responses, while the plank produced the lowest response. Adding a lateral shuffle or crawl to the push-up greatly increased the metabolic response by 37%–39%. The burpee has been shown to provide a large

Table 8.6 Metabolic Responses to Traditional RE, Battling Rope, and Bodyweight Exercises

	Mean $\dot{V}O_2$ (mL·kg^{-1}·min^{-1})	Peak $\dot{V}O_2$ (mL·kg^{-1}·min^{-1})	EE (kcal·min^{-1})	RER
Baseline	2.5 ± 0.9		1.1 ± 0.4	0.80 ± 0.1
Squat	19.6 ± 1.8	32.5 ± 5.0	8.2 ± 1.1	1.08 ± 0.1
BP	12.5 ± 2.1	19.8 ± 4.0	5.2 ± 0.9	1.11 ± 0.1
Curl	12.3 ± 2.1	20.2 ± 3.0	5.1 ± 0.8	1.05 ± 0.1
BOR	12.2 ± 1.7	22.4 ± 3.6	5.1 ± 0.7	1.10 ± 0.1
HP	14.2 ± 3.2	25.2 ± 5.0	6.0 ± 1.3	1.00 ± 0.1
Lunge	17.3 ± 2.6	28.7 ± 4.6	7.2 ± 1.3	1.03 ± 0.1
DL	18.9 ± 3.0	31.2 ± 5.1	7.8 ± 1.2	1.15 ± 0.1
Burpee	22.9 ± 2.1	35.9 ± 4.1	9.6 ± 1.3	1.00 ± 0.1
Plank	7.9 ± 0.7	12.8 ± 1.6	3.3 ± 0.7	0.90 ± 0.1
BR	24.6 ± 2.6	38.6 ± 4.7	10.3 ± 1.4	1.21 ± 0.1
PU	11.9 ± 1.3	18.9 ± 1.4	4.9 ± 0.6	1.11 ± 0.1
BOSU PU	11.9 ± 1.0	20.3 ± 1.7	5.0 ± 0.7	1.10 ± 0.1
PU-LC	19.5 ± 2.9	31.0 ± 4.9	8.1 ± 1.1	1.05 ± 0.1

All data were significantly different from BL. EE, energy expenditure; RER, respiratory exchange ratio; BP, bench press; BOR, bent-over barbell row; HP, high pull; DL, deadlift; BR, battling rope; PU, push-up; PU-LC, push-up with lateral crawl.

Ratamess NA, Rosenberg JG, Klei S, et al. Comparison of the acute metabolic responses to traditional resistance, body-weight, and battling rope exercises. *J Strength Cond Res.* 2015;29:47–57.

metabolic response (179), and isometric exercises yield a substantially lower metabolic response than traditional dynamic and ballistic exercises (177).

The culmination of these program variables affects the acute metabolic response. Workouts that consist of moderate to high intensity, moderate to high number of repetitions, large muscle mass exercises, with short rest intervals greatly increase VO_2. Circuit weight training (performing exercises continuously from station to station with minimal rest in between) increases acute VO_2 and VO_{2max}. A similar effect is seen with endurance training programs consisting of high reps, low weight, and short rest intervals. Strength and power workouts elicit small VO_2 increases due primarily to long rest intervals and low reps. High metabolic demand is important for body fat reductions and muscle endurance enhancement.

Resistance exercise elicits substantial EPOC in men and women (74,180–183), and the magnitude may be greater than that of aerobic exercise (176,184). When combined, the sequence of aerobic and RT does not appear to affect EPOC (185). Circuit weight training elicits a greater EPOC than AT in women (182). The magnitude for either modality depends on the degree of disturbance to homeostasis. Greater thermogenesis, hormonal response, glycogen depletion, lactate elevations and reductions in pH, and cardiorespiratory demand yields substantial EPOC. EPOC following resistance exercise is biphasic (with a rapid component <1 h and a slow component) and may last up to 48 hours (180,181,186) especially as protein synthesis increases and muscle damage is present. Resting energy expenditure is greater 72 hours after a workout that produces muscle damage (187). Resistance exercise has the advantage of increasing energy expenditure throughout the day following a workout. Binzen et al. (180) showed an 18.6% increase in EPOC and greater fat oxidation over 2 hours after exercise in women. However, the overall net kilocalorie expenditure may be low despite the elevation in EPOC (183).

Body Fat Reductions

Reducing body fat involves proper diet and exercise. Energy expenditure must exceed energy intake so a net kilocalorie deficit is seen. Dietary recommendations include consuming a well-balanced diet from major food groups and high water intake (at least eight glasses per day). Individuals should consume ~55%–60% of kilocalories from CHOs (preferably complex CHOs), at least 15% of kilocalories from protein, and <25% of kilocalories from fats (mostly unsaturated fats). Increasing BMR is important, *i.e.*, maintaining a higher protein intake than the RDA values, early morning workouts, and avoiding simple sugars. The frequency (*i.e.*, high meal frequency or low [1–2] meals per day during an isocaloric diet) and timing of meals (*i.e.*, fasting, skipping breakfast, presleep nutrient intake) have been studied with equivocal findings, so it is difficult to conclude if there is an optimal strategy or if the response is individualized where multiple nutrient patterning strategies could be effectively used depending on the individual's metabolism. Aerobic exercise is highly recommended for its role in increasing fat oxidation during exercise and EPOC. Diet appears to be the key factor with aerobic exercise complimentary. RT is beneficial as the higher LBM increases BMR and energy expenditure throughout the day. Similar to AT, RT increases energy expenditure and yields substantial EPOC. The combination of AT and RT augments each other in comprehensively reducing body fat. Total body workouts (traditional or integrated metabolic HIIT) of moderate to high volume (multiple sets per exercise of at least 10–12 reps), moderate to high intensity, and short rest intervals have profound effects on reducing body fat. Scientific body fat loss (not through crash dieting) is a relatively slow process but one that has a more profound effect on long-lasting fat loss.

Interpreting Research
Oxygen Consumption and Rest Interval Manipulation

Ratamess NA, Falvo MJ, Mangine GT, et al. The effect of rest interval length on metabolic responses to the bench press exercise. *Eur J Appl Physiol*. 2007;100:1–17.

Ratamess et al. (74) studied the metabolic responses to rest interval manipulation during 5 sets of the bench press using either 10 or 5 RM loads with 30-second, 1-minute, 2-minute, 3-minute, or 5-minute rest intervals. Rep number was maintained in each set while weight was reduced when necessary. They found a continuum of effects such that highest VO_2 values were seen with 30-second rest intervals and lowest VO_2 values were seen with 5-minute rest intervals. The acute response pattern was similar between 5 and 10 RM loading protocols; however, the VO_2 response was higher in 10 than 5 RM for most rest intervals demonstrating a volume/intensity effect. EPOC elevations were shown for all protocols. However, the 30-second and 1-minute protocols elicited greater EPOC during 5 RM protocols but had no substantial effect during 10 RM protocols. The highest relative VO_2 obtained was ~16 mL·kg^{-1}·min^{-1} (30 s) and the lowest was ~8 mL·kg^{-1}·min^{-1} (5 min), both of which were below the threshold needed to increase VO_{2max}. Energy expenditure for 30-second protocols was ~6.8–7.3 kcal·min^{-1}, whereas 5-minute protocols elicited values of 4.9–5.3 kcal·min^{-1}. Figure 8.13 depicts the 30-second and 5-minute VO_2 responses. VO_2 was lower during each set (due to the anaerobic nature of lifting and possible Valsalva maneuvers) but increased during the first 30-seconds to 1-minute of recovery and then rapidly decreased (5-min protocol). The 30-second protocol led to the most pronounced and continuous response, but large levels of recovery were seen with 5-minute rest intervals. A quantitative effect was shown where VO_2 increased from set to set peaking by the fourth set. Figure 8.14 shows that VO_2 area under the curve was highest with short rest (30 s and 1 min) and lowest with 5-minute rest intervals.

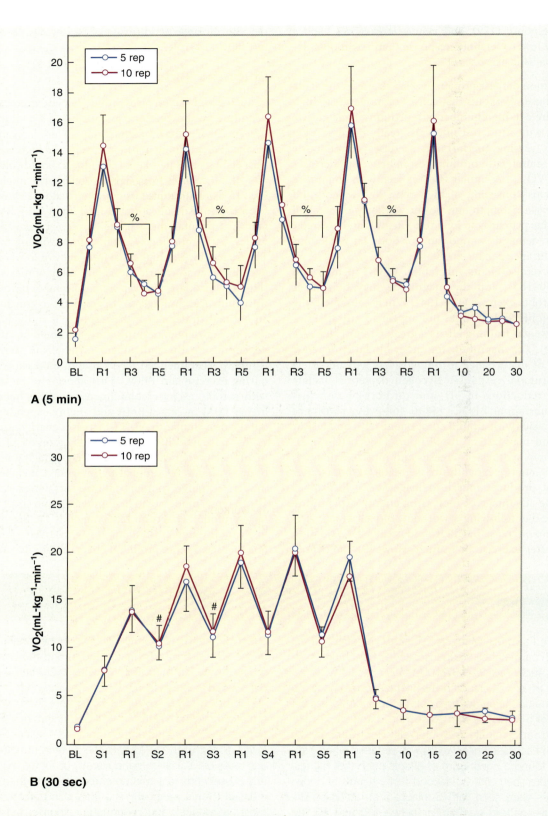

FIGURE 8.13 A and B. Metabolic responses to resistance exercise: 30 seconds vs. 5 minutes. BL, baseline; S1, set 1, R1, rest interval 1 minute, and so on. (Reprinted with permission from Ratamess NA, Falvo MJ, Mangine GT, Hoffman JR, Faigenbaum AD, Kang J. The effect of rest interval length on metabolic responses to the bench press exercise. *Eur J Appl Physiol*. 2007;100:1–17.)

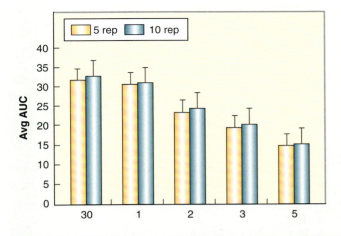

FIGURE 8.14 Total oxygen consumption area under the curve using various rest intervals. (Reprinted with permission from Ratamess NA, Falvo MJ, Mangine GT, Hoffman JR, Faigenbaum AD, Kang J. The effect of rest interval length on metabolic responses to the bench press exercise. *Eur J Appl Physiol.* 2007;100:1–17.)

Myths & Misconceptions
Low-Intensity, Moderate-Duration Exercise Is the Single Best Way to Burn Body Fat and Lose Weight Independent of Diet

Some experts have exclusively recommended low-intensity, moderate-duration exercise (30–60 min of leisure walking) as the best way to burn body fat. Fat is the preferred fuel for energy at rest and during low-intensity exercise when oxygen supply meets demand. However, fat is an energy-dense macronutrient. An 18-C fat molecule can generate a total of 460 ATP, >12 times that of glucose. Although fat oxidation prevails during low-intensity exercise, a molecule of fat goes a long way, so very little will be oxidized and low-intensity exercise is not a potent stimulus to increase aerobic capacity. The critical element to fat loss is to increase VO_{2max}. Fat burning becomes more efficient when VO_{2max} improves. Prescription including high-intensity training (>60%–70% of VO_{2max}) in addition to long, slow-duration AT workouts is the best way to lose body fat. Increasing VO_{2max} is important in building a base by which fat burning becomes easier. So yes, long, slow-duration cardio workouts are beneficial; however, they are more effective when VO_{2max} is improved with moderate- to high-intensity AT.

SUMMARY POINTS

- Bioenergetics is the flow of energy change within the human body. The high-energy compound that provides substantial energy for all of the cell's needs from hydrolysis of chemical bonds is known as adenosine triphosphate (ATP).
- Three major energy systems resynthesize ATP, the ATP-PC, glycolysis, and oxidative systems. ATP-PC system fuels high-intensity exercise up to ~10 seconds in duration. Glycolysis fuels moderate-to-high-intensity exercise lasting up to a few minutes. The oxidative system resynthesizes ATP aerobically when oxygen supply meets demand.
- Anaerobic and AT elicit specific metabolic adaptations that enhance performance via greater substrate storage, altered enzyme activity, or breakdown rates during exercise.
- Metabolic acidosis occurs during exercise that stresses glycolysis. Specific training can increase buffer capacity and allow the athlete to tolerate greater levels of acidity.
- BMR is the minimal level of energy needed to sustain bodily functions. Control of BMR is critical to body fat reductions and weight control. BMR is affected by body mass, exercise, environment, dietary-induced thermogenesis, and hormonal control.
- VO_2 and energy expenditure increase during exercise (and for up to 48–72 h after exercise) with the response in proportion to muscle mass involvement, intensity, volume/duration, and rest interval length.

REVIEW QUESTIONS

1. The majority of energy liberation during a 1 RM set of the deadlift exercise will come from
   a. ATP-PC system (phosphagens)
   b. Fast glycolysis
   c. Slow glycolysis
   d. Aerobic system

2. The elevation of oxygen consumption during recovery from exercise is known as
   a. Excess postexercise oxygen consumption (EPOC)
   b. Oxygen deficit
   c. VO_{2max}
   d. Oxygen requirement

3. An enzyme that catalyzes the reaction that breaks down glycogen to glucose-1-phosphate is
   a. Hexokinase
   b. Phosphorylase
   c. PFK
   d. Pyruvate kinase

4. Capillary and mitochondrial density typically _____ after traditional RT resulting in large muscle hypertrophy
   a. Increase
   b. Decrease
   c. Do not change
   d. None of the above

5. Which of the following does not act as a skeletal muscle/blood buffer?
   a. Creatine phosphate
   b. Bicarbonate
   c. Triglycerides
   d. Carnosine

6. CHO consumption during and immediately following resistance exercise is critical to
   a. Delaying fatigue
   b. Maximizing glycogen repletion during recovery
   c. Sparing muscle glycogen breakdown
   d. All of the above

7. Approximately 65% of PC is replenished within 90 seconds of recovery from exercise.
   a. T
   b. F

8. Creatine supplementation has been shown to increase muscle size, strength, and power in several studies.
   a. T
   b. F

9. Both aerobic and RT decrease resting glycogen stores over time.
   a. T
   b. F

10. The blood lactate response curve to exercise shifts to the right with training at or beyond the lactate threshold.
    a. T
    b. F

11. Aerobic and resistance exercises increase energy expenditure acutely but have very limited effects on postexercise metabolism.
    a. T
    b. F

12. During resistance exercise, small muscle mass exercises increase oxygen consumption to a greater extent than large muscle mass exercises.
    a. T
    b. F

REFERENCES

1. McArdle WD, Katch FI, Katch VL. *Exercise Physiology: Energy, Nutrition, and Human Performance*. 6th ed. Philadelphia (PA): Lippincott Williams & Wilkins; 2007. p. 123–228.
2. Kang J. *Bioenergetics Primer for Exercise Science*. Champaign (IL): Human Kinetics; 2008. p. 3–104.
3. McMahon S, Jenkins D. Factors affecting the rate of phosphocreatine resynthesis following intense exercise. *Sports Med*. 2002;32:761–84.
4. Cramer JT. Bioenergetics of exercise and training. In: Baechle TR, Earle RW, editors. *Essentials of Strength Training and Conditioning*. 3rd ed. Champaign (IL): Human Kinetics; 2008. p. 21–39.
5. Rehunen S, Naveri H, Kuoppasalmi K, Harkonen M. High-energy phosphate compounds during exercise in human slow-twitch and fast-twitch muscle fibres. *Scand J Clin Lab Invest*. 1982;42:499–506.
6. Spencer M, Bishop D, Dawson B, Goodman C. Physiological and metabolic responses of repeated-sprint activities: specific to field-based team sports. *Sports Med*. 2005;35:1025–44.
7. Ratamess NA. *Coaches Guide to Performance-Enhancing Supplements*. Monterey (CA): Coaches Choice Books; 2006.
8. Williams MH. *The Ergogenics Edge*. Champaign (IL): Human Kinetics; 1998.
9. Hirvonen J, Nummela A, Rusko H, Rehunen S, Harkonen M. Fatigue and changes of ATP creatine phosphate and lactate during the 400-m sprint. *Can J Sport Sci*. 1992;17:141–4.
10. Hirvonen J, Rehunen S, Rusko H, Harkonen M. Breakdown of high-energy phosphate compounds and lactate accumulation during short supramaximal exercise. *Eur J Appl Physiol*. 1987;56:253–9.
11. Mendez-Villanueva A, Edge A, Suriano R, Hamer P, Bishop D. The recovery of repeated-sprint exercise is associated with PCr resynthesis, while muscle pH and EMG amplitude remain depressed. *PLoS One*. 2012;7:e51977.
12. Bishop D, Edge J, Thomas C, Mercier J. Effects of high-intensity training on muscle lactate transporters and postexercise recovery of muscle lactate and hydrogen ions in women. *Am J Physiol Regul Integr Comp Physiol*. 2008;295:R1991–8.
13. Edge J, Eynon N, McKenna MJ, et al. Altering the rest interval during high-intensity interval training does not affect muscle or performance adaptations. *Exp Physiol*. 2013;98:481–90.

14. MacDougall JD, Ward GR, Sale DG, Sutton JR. Biochemical adaptation of human skeletal muscle to heavy resistance training and immobilization. *J Appl Physiol.* 1977;43:700–3.

15. Walker PM, Brunotte F, Rouhier-Marcer I, et al. Nuclear magnetic resonance evidence of different muscular adaptations after resistance training. *Arch Phys Med Rehabil.* 1998;79:1391–8.

16. Tesch PA, Thorsson A, Colliander EB. Effects of eccentric and concentric resistance training on skeletal muscle substrates, enzyme activities and capillary supply. *Acta Physiol Scand.* 1990;140:575–80.

17. Dawson B, Fitzsimons M, Green S, Goodman C, Carey M, Cole K. Changes in performance, muscle metabolites, enzymes and fibre types after short sprint training. *Eur J Appl Physiol Occup Physiol.* 1998;78:163–9.

18. Ross A, Leveritt M. Long-term metabolic and skeletal muscle adaptations to short-sprint training: implications for sprint training and tapering. *Sports Med.* 2001;31:1063–82.

19. Johansen L, Quistorff B. 31P-MRS characterization of sprint and endurance trained athletes. *Int J Sports Med.* 2003;24:183–9.

20. Costill DL, Coyle EF, Fink WF, Lesmes GR, Witzmann FA. Adaptations in skeletal muscle following strength training. *J Appl Physiol.* 1979;46:96–9.

21. Thorstensson A, Sjodin B, Tesch P, Karlsson J. Actomyosin ATPase, myokinase, CPK and LDH in human fast and slow twitch muscle fibres. *Acta Physiol Scand.* 1977;99:225–9.

22. Komi PV, Viitasalo JT, Rauramaa R, Vihko V. Effect of isometric strength training on mechanical, electrical, and metabolic aspects of muscle function. *Eur J Appl Physiol.* 1978;40:45–55.

23. Tesch PA, Komi PV, Häkkinen K. Enzymatic adaptations consequent to long-term strength training. *Int J Sports Med.* 1987;8(Suppl):66–9.

24. Thorstensson A, Hulten B, von Dolben W, Karlsson J. Effect of strength training on enzyme activities and fibre characteristics in human skeletal muscles. *Acta Physiol Scand.* 1976;96:392–8.

25. Tesch PA, Thorsson A, Fujitsuka N. Creatine phosphate in fiber types of skeletal muscle before and after exhaustive exercise. *J Appl Physiol.* 1989;66:1756–9.

26. Tesch PA, Thorsson A, Essen-Gustavsson B. Enzyme activities of FT and ST muscle fibers in heavy-resistance trained athletes. *J Appl Physiol.* 1989;67:83–7.

27. Cadefau J, Casademont J, Grau JM, et al. Biochemical and histochemical adaptation to sprint training in young athletes. *Acta Physiol Scand.* 1990;140:341–51.

28. Lehnen AM, Angelis KD, Markowski MM, Schaan BDA. Changes in the GLUT 4 expression by acute exercise, exercise training and detraining in experimental models. *J Diabetes Metab.* 2012;S10:002.

29. Hargreaves M. The metabolic systems: carbohydrate metabolism. In: Tipton CM, editor. *ACSM's Advanced Exercise Physiology.* Philadelphia (PA): Lippincott Williams & Wilkins; 2006. p. 385–95.

30. Hearris MA, Hammond KM, Fell JM, Morton JP. Regulation of muscle glycogen metabolism during exercise: implications for endurance performance and training adaptations. *Nutrients.* 2018;10:E298.

31. Knuiman P, Hopman MTE, Mensink M. Glycogen availability and skeletal muscle adaptations with endurance and resistance exercise. *Nutr Metab.* 2015;12:59.

32. Abernethy PJ, Thayer R, Taylor AW. Acute and chronic responses of skeletal muscle to endurance and sprint exercise. A review. *Sports Med.* 1990;10:365–89.

33. Pascoe DD, Costill DL, Fink WJ, Robergs RA, Zachwieja JJ. Glycogen resynthesis in skeletal muscle following resistive exercise. *Med Sci Sports Exerc.* 1993;25:349–54.

34. Robergs RA, Pearson DR, Costill DL, et al. Muscle glycogenolysis during different intensities of weight-resistance exercise. *J Appl Physiol.* 1991;70:1700–6.

35. Bell DG, Jacobs I. Muscle fiber-specific glycogen utilization in strength-trained males and females. *Med Sci Sports Exerc.* 1989;21:649–54.

36. Tesch PA, Colliander EB, Kaiser P. Muscle metabolism during intense, heavy-resistance exercise. *Eur J Appl Physiol.* 1986;55:362–6.

37. Churchley EG, Coffey VG, Pedersen DJ, et al. Influence of pre-exercise muscle glycogen content on transcriptional activity of metabolic and myogenic genes in well-trained humans. *J Appl Physiol.* 2007;102:1604–11.

38. Alghannam AF, Gonzalez JT, Betts JA. Restoration of muscle glycogen and functional capacity: role of post-exercise carbohydrate and protein co-ingestion. *Nutrients.* 2018;10:E253.

39. American College of Sports Medicine, American Dietetic Association, & Dieticians of Canada. Joint Position Stand. Nutrition and athletic performance. *Med Sci Sports Exerc.* 2009;41:709–31.

40. Andrews JL, Sedlock DA, Flynn MG, et al. Carbohydrate loading and supplementation in endurance-trained women runners. *J Appl Physiol.* 2003;95:584–90.

41. Goforth HW, Arnall DA, Bennett BL, Law PG. Persistence of supercompensated muscle glycogen in trained subjects after carbohydrate loading. *J Appl Physiol.* 1997;82:342–7.

42. Paul DR, Mulroy SM, Horner JA, et al. Carbohydrate-loading during the follicular phase of the menstrual cycle: effects on muscle glycogen and exercise performance. *Int J Sport Nutr Exerc Metab.* 2001;11:430–41.

43. Rauch LH, Rodger I, Wilson GR, et al. The effects of carbohydrate loading on muscle glycogen content and cycling performance. *Int J Sport Nutr.* 1995;5:25–36.

44. Burgomaster KA, Heigenhauser GJ, Gibala MJ. Effect of short-term sprint interval training on human skeletal muscle carbohydrate metabolism during exercise and time-trial performance. *J Appl Physiol.* 2006;100:2041–7.

45. LeBlanc PJ, Howarth KR, Gibala MJ, Heigenhauser GJ. Effects of 7 wk of endurance training on human skeletal muscle metabolism during submaximal exercise. *J Appl Physiol.* 2004;97:2148–53.

46. Perry CG, Heigenhauser GJ, Bonen A, Spriet LL. High-intensity aerobic interval training increases fat and carbohydrate metabolic capacities in human skeletal muscle. *Appl Physiol Nutr Metab.* 2008;33:1112–23.

47. Yeo WK, Paton CD, Garnham AP, Burke LM, Carey AL, Hawley JA. Skeletal muscle adaptation and performance responses to once a day versus twice every second day endurance training regimens. *J Appl Physiol.* 2008;105:1462–70.

48. Holloszy JO, Kohrt WM, Hansen PA. The regulation of carbohydrate and fat metabolism during and after exercise. *Front Biosci.* 1998;3:D1011–27.

49. Tesch PA. Short- and long-term histochemical and biochemical adaptations in muscle. In: *Strength and Power in Sport.* Boston (MA): Blackwell Scientific Publications; 1992. p. 239–48.

50. Burgomaster KA, Moore DR, Schofield LM, Phillips SM, Sale DG, Gibala MJ. Resistance training with vascular occlusion: metabolic adaptations in human muscle. *Med Sci Sports Exerc.* 2003;35:1203–8.

51. Van Proeyen K, Szlufcik K, Nielens H, Ramaekers M, Hespel P. Beneficial metabolic adaptations due to endurance exercise training in the fasted state. *J Appl Physiol*. 2011;110:236–45.

52. Roberts AD, Billeter R, Howald H. Anaerobic muscle enzyme changes after interval training. *Int J Sports Med*. 1982;3:18–21.

53. Chesley A, Heigenhauser GJ, Spriet LL. Regulation of muscle glycogen phosphorylase activity following short-term endurance training. *Am J Physiol*. 1996;270:E328–35.

54. MacDougall JD. Adaptability of muscle to strength training—a cellular approach. In: *Biochemistry of Exercise VI*. Champaign (IL): Human Kinetics; 1986. p. 501–13.

55. Green H, Dahly A, Shoemaker K, Goreham C, Bombardier E, Ball-Burnett M. Serial effects of high-resistance and prolonged endurance training on Na^+-K^+ pump concentration and enzymatic activities in human vastus lateralis. *Acta Physiol Scand*. 1999;165:177–84.

56. Wang N, Hikida RS, Staron RS, Simoneau JA. Muscle fiber types of women after resistance training—quantitative ultrastructure and enzyme activity. *Pflugers Arch*. 1993;424:494–502.

57. Robergs RA, Ghiasvand F, Parker D. Biochemistry of exercise-induced metabolic acidosis. *Am J Physiol Regul Integr Comp Physiol*. 2004;287:R502–16.

58. Favero TG, Zable AC, Colter D, Abramson JJ. Lactate inhibits Ca^{2+}-activated Ca(2+)-channel activity from skeletal muscle sarcoplasmic reticulum. *J Appl Physiol*. 1997;82:447–52.

59. Posterino GS, Dutka TL, Lamb GD. L(+)-lactate does not affect twitch and tetanic responses in mechanically skinned mammalian muscle fibres. *Pflugers Arch*. 2001;442:197–203.

60. Bonen A. The expression of lactate transporters (MCT1 and MCT4) in heart and muscle. *Eur J Appl Physiol*. 2001;86:6–11.

61. Juel C. Current aspects of lactate exchange: lactate/H+ transport in human skeletal muscle. *Eur J Appl Physiol*. 2001;86:12–6.

62. McGinley C, Bishop DJ. Rest interval duration does not influence adaptations in acid/base transport proteins following 10 wk of sprint-interval training in active women. *Am J Physiol Regul Integr Comp Physiol*. 2017;312:R702–17.

63. McGinley C, Bishop DJ. Influence of training intensity on adaptations in acid/base transport proteins, muscle buffer capacity, and repeated-sprint ability in active men. *J Appl Physiol*. 2016;121:1290–305.

64. Mohr M, Krustrup P, Nielsen JJ, Nybo L, Rasmussen MK, Juel C, Bangsbo J. Effect of two different intense training regimens on skeletal muscle ion transport proteins and fatigue development. *Am J Physiol Regul Integr Comp Physiol*. 2007;292:R1594–602.

65. Enoki T, Yoshida Y, Lally J, Hatta H, Bonen A. Testosterone increases lactate transport, monocarboxylate transporter (MCT) 1 and MCT4 in rat skeletal muscle. *J Physiol*. 2006;577:433–43.

66. Wilmore JH, Costill DL. *Physiology of Sport and Exercise*. 2nd ed. Champaign (IL): Human Kinetics; 1999.

67. Edge J, Hill-Haas S, Goodman C, Bishop D. Effects of resistance training on H+ regulation, buffer capacity, and repeated sprints. *Med Sci Sports Exerc*. 2006;38:2004–11.

68. Marcinik EJ, Potts J, Schlabach G, Will S, Dawson P, Hurley BF. Effects of strength training on lactate threshold and endurance performance. *Med Sci Sports Exerc*. 1991;23:739–43.

69. Tomlin DL, Wenger HA. The relationship between aerobic fitness and recovery from high intensity intermittent exercise. *Sports Med*. 2001;31:1–11.

70. Medbo JI, Sejersted OM. Acid-base and electrolyte balance after exhausting exercise in endurance-trained and sprint-trained subjects. *Acta Physiol Scand*. 1985;125:97–109.

71. Parkhouse WS, McKenzie DC. Possible contribution of skeletal muscle buffers to enhanced anaerobic performance: a brief review. *Med Sci Sports Exerc*. 1984;16:328–38.

72. Collins MA, Cureton KJ, Hill DW, Ray CA. Relation of plasma volume change to intensity of weight lifting. *Med Sci Sports Exerc*. 1989;21:178–85.

73. Kraemer WJ, Noble BJ, Clark MJ, Culver BW. Physiologic responses to heavy-resistance exercise with very short rest periods. *Int J Sports Med*. 1987;8:247–52.

74. Ratamess NA, Falvo MJ, Mangine GT, Hoffman JR, Faigenbaum AD, Kang J. The effect of rest interval length on metabolic responses to the bench press exercise. *Eur J Appl Physiol*. 2007;100:1–17.

75. Volek JS, Boetes M, Bush JA, Putukian M, Sebastianelli WJ, Kraemer WJ. Response of testosterone and cortisol concentrations to high-intensity resistance exercise following creatine supplementation. *J Strength Cond Res*. 1997;11:182–7.

76. Ojasto T, Häkkinen K. Effects of different accentuated eccentric loads on acute neuromuscular, growth hormone, and blood lactate responses during a hypertrophic protocol. *J Strength Cond Res*. 2009;23:946–53.

77. Brandenburg J, Docherty D. The effect of training volume on the acute response and adaptations to resistance training. *Int J Sports Physiol Perform*. 2006;1:108–21.

78. Mazzetti S, Douglass M, Yocum A, Harber M. Effect of explosive versus slow contractions and exercise intensity on energy expenditure. *Med Sci Sports Exerc*. 2007;39:1291–301.

79. Yarrow JF, Borsa PA, Borst SE, Sitren HS, Stevens BR, White LJ. Neuroendocrine responses to an acute bout of eccentric-enhanced resistance exercise. *Med Sci Sports Exerc*. 2007;39:941–7.

80. Kang J, Hoffman JR, Im J, et al. Evaluation of physiological responses during recovery following three resistance exercise programs. *J Strength Cond Res*. 2005;19:305–9.

81. Reynolds TH, Frye PA, Sforzo GA. Resistance training and the blood lactate response to resistance exercise in women. *J Strength Cond Res*. 1997;11:77–81.

82. Dudley GA. Metabolic consequences of resistive-type exercise. *Med Sci Sports Exerc*. 1988;20(Suppl):S158–61.

83. Costill DL, Barnett A, Sharp R, Fink WJ, Katz A. Leg muscle pH following sprint running. *Med Sci Sports Exerc*. 1983;15:325–9.

84. Sahlin K, Harris RC, Hultman E. Creatine kinase equilibrium and lactate content compared with muscle pH in tissue samples obtained after isometric exercise. *Biochem J*. 1972;152:173–80.

85. Gordon SE, Kraemer WJ, Pedro JG. Increased acid-base buffering capacity via dietary supplementation: anaerobic exercise implications. *J Appl Nutr*. 1991;43:40–8.

86. Vukovich MD, Sharp RL, Kesl LD, Schaulis DL, King DS. Effects of a low-dose amino acid supplement on adaptations to cycling training in untrained individuals. *Int J Sport Nutr*. 1997;7:298–309.

87. Davey CL. The significance of carnosine and anserine in striated skeletal muscle. *Arch Biochem Biophys*. 1960;89:303–8.

88. Trexler ET, Smith-Ryan AE, Stout JR, et al. International Society of Sports Nutrition Position Stand: Beta-alanine. *J Int Soc Sports Nutr*. 2015;12:30.

89. Parkhouse WS, McKenzie DC, Hochachka PW, et al. The relationship between carnosine levels, buffering capacity, fiber types and anaerobic capacity in elite athletes. In: Knuttgen H, Vogel J, Poortmans J, editors. *Biochemistry of Exercise*. Champaign (IL): Human Kinetics; 1983. p. 275–8.

90. Derave W, Ozdemir MS, Harris RC, et al. Beta-alanine supplementation augments muscle carnosine content and attenuates fatigue during repeated isokinetic contraction bouts in trained sprinters. *J Appl Physiol.* 2007;103:1736–43.

91. Hoffman JR, Ratamess NA, Faigenbaum AD, et al. Short-duration beta-alanine supplementation increases training volume and reduces subjective feelings of fatigue in college football players. *Nutr Res.* 2008;28:31–5.

92. Hoffman JR, Ratamess NA, Ross R, et al. Beta-alanine and the hormonal response to exercise. *Int J Sports Med.* 2008;29:952–8.

93. Kendrick IP, Harris RC, Kim HJ, et al. The effects of 10 weeks of resistance training combined with beta-alanine supplementation on whole body strength, force production, muscular endurance and body composition. *Amino Acids.* 2008;34:547–54.

94. Sahlin K. Intracellular pH and energy metabolism in skeletal muscle of man. *Acta Physiol Scand Suppl.* 1978;455:1–56.

95. Sharp RL, Costill DL, Fink WJ, King DS. Effects of eight weeks of bicycle ergometer sprint training on human muscle buffer capacity. *Int J Sports Med.* 1986;7:13–7.

96. Jacobs I, Esbjornsson M, Sylven C, Holm I, Jansson E. Sprint training effects on muscle myoglobin, enzymes, fiber types, and blood lactate. *Med Sci Sports Exerc.* 1987;19:368–74.

97. Sahlin K, Henriksson J. Buffer capacity and lactate accumulation in skeletal muscle of trained and untrained men. *Acta Physiol Scand.* 1984;122:331–9.

98. Bell GJ, Wenger HA. The effect of one-legged sprint training on intramuscular pH and nonbicarbonate buffering capacity. *Eur J Appl Physiol.* 1988;58:158–64.

99. Nevill ME, Boobis LH, Brooks S, Williams C. Effect of training on muscle metabolism during treadmill sprinting. *J Appl Physiol.* 1989;67:2376–82.

100. Argyropolous G, Harper ME. Uncoupling proteins and thermoregulation. *J Appl Physiol.* 2002;92:2187–98.

101. Steinberg GR. Role of the AMP-activated protein kinase in regulating fatty acid metabolism during exercise. *Appl Physiol Nutr Metab.* 2009;34:315–22.

102. Spriet LL. Regulation of skeletal muscle fat oxidation during exercise in humans. *Med Sci Sports Exerc.* 2002;34:1477–84.

103. Kiens B. Skeletal muscle lipid metabolism in exercise and insulin resistance. *Physiol Rev.* 2006;86:205–43.

104. Watt MJ. Triglyceride lipases alter fuel metabolism and mitochondrial gene expression. *Appl Physiol Nutr Metab.* 2009;34:340–7.

105. Jensen MD. Lipolysis: contributions from regional fat. *Annu Rev Nutr.* 1997;17:127–39.

106. Horowitz JF, Klein S. Lipid metabolism during endurance exercise. *Am J Clin Nutr.* 2000;72(Suppl):558S–63.

107. Hansen D, De Strijcker D, Calders P. Impact of endurance exercise training in the fasted state on muscle biochemistry and metabolism in healthy subjects: can these effects be of particular clinical benefit to type 2 diabetes mellitus and insulin-resistant patients? *Sports Med.* 2017;47:415–28.

108. Romijn JA, Coyle EF, Sidossis LS, et al. Regulation of endogenous fat and carbohydrate metabolism in relation to exercise intensity and duration. *Am J Physiol.* 1993;265:E380–91.

109. Romijn JA, Coyle EF, Sidossis LS, Zhang XJ, Wolfe RR. Relationship between fatty acid delivery and fatty acid oxidation during strenuous exercise. *J Appl Physiol.* 1995;79:1939–45.

110. Fatouros IG, Chatzinikolaou A, Tournis S, et al. Intensity of resistance exercise determines adipokine and resting energy expenditure responses in overweight elderly individuals. *Diabetes Care.* 2009;32:2161–7.

111. Goto K, Ishii N, Sugihara S, Yoshioka T, Takamatsu K. Effects of resistance exercise on lipolysis during subsequent submaximal exercise. *Med Sci Sports Exerc.* 2007;39:308–15.

112. Ormsbee MJ, Thyfault JP, Johnson EA, Kraus RM, Choi MD, Hickner RC. Fat metabolism and acute resistance exercise in trained men. *J Appl Physiol.* 2007;102:1767–72.

113. Ormsbee MJ, Choi MD, Medlin JK, Geyer GH, Trantham LH, Dubis GS, Hickner RC. Regulation of fat metabolism during resistance exercise in sedentary lean and obese men. *J Appl Physiol.* 2009;106:1529–37.

114. Ratamess NA, Bush JA, Kang J, et al. The effects of supplementation with p-synephrine alone and in combination with caffeine on metabolic, lipolytic, and cardiovascular responses during resistance exercise. *J Am Coll Nutr.* 2016;35:657–69.

115. Schenk S, Horowitz JF. Coimmunoprecipitation of FAT/CD36 and CPT I in skeletal muscle increases proportionally with fat oxidation after endurance exercise training. *Am J Physiol Endocrinol Metab.* 2006;291:E254–60.

116. McCall GE, Byrnes WC, Dickinson A, Pattany PM, Fleck SJ. Muscle fiber hypertrophy, hyperplasia, and capillary density in college men after resistance training. *J Appl Physiol.* 1996;81:2004–12.

117. Staron RS, Malicky ES, Leonardi MJ, Falkel JE, Hagerman FC, Dudley GA. Muscle hypertrophy and fast fiber type conversions in heavy resistance-trained women. *Eur J Appl Physiol.* 1989;60:71–9.

118. Holloway TM, Snijders T, Van Kranenburg J, Van Loon LJC, Verdijk LB. Temporal response of angiogenesis and hypertrophy to resistance training in young men. *Med Sci Sports Exerc.* 2018;50:36–45.

119. Holloway TM, Morton RW, Oikawa SY, et al. Microvascular adaptations to resistance training are independent of load in resistance-trained young men. *Am J Physiol Regul Integr Comp Physiol.* 2018;315:R267–73.

120. Bell DG, Jacobs I. Muscle fibre area, fibre type & capillarization in male and female body builders. *Can J Sport Sci.* 1990;15:115–9.

121. Kadi F, Eriksson A, Holmner S, Butler-Browne GS, Thornell LE. Cellular adaptation of the trapezius muscle in strength-trained athletes. *Histochem Cell Biol.* 1999;111:189–95.

122. Hostler D, Schwirian CI, Campos G, et al. Skeletal muscle adaptations in elastic resistance-trained young men and women. *Eur J Appl Physiol.* 2001;86:112–8.

123. Luthi JM, Howald H, Claassen H, Rosler K, Vock P, Hoppeler H. Structural changes in skeletal muscle tissue with heavy-resistance exercise. *Int J Sports Med.* 1986;7:123–7.

124. MacDougall JD, Sale DG, Moroz JR, Elder GCB, Sutton JR, Howald H. Mitochondrial volume density in human skeletal muscle following heavy resistance training. *Med Sci Sports.* 1979;11:164–6.

125. Masuda K, Choi JY, Shimojo H, Katsuta S. Maintenance of myoglobin concentration in human skeletal muscle after heavy resistance training. *Eur J Appl Physiol.* 1999;79:347–52.

126. Schantz PG, Kallman M. NADH shuttle enzymes and cytochrome b5 reductase in human skeletal muscle: effect of strength training. *J Appl Physiol.* 1989;67:123–7.

127. Tang JE, Hartman JW, Phillips SM. Increased muscle oxidative potential following resistance training induced fibre hypertrophy in young men. *Appl Physiol Nutr Metab.* 2006;31:495–501.

128. Thibault MC, Simoneau JA, Cote C, et al. Inheritance of human muscle enzyme adaptation to isokinetic strength training. *Hum Hered.* 1986;36:341–7.

129. MacDougall JD, Hicks AL, MacDonald JR, et al. Muscle performance and enzymatic adaptations to sprint interval training. *J Appl Physiol.* 1998;84:2138–42.

130. Lemmer JT, Ivey FM, Ryan AS, et al. Effect of strength training on resting metabolic rate and physical activity: age and gender comparisons. *Med Sci Sports Exerc.* 2001;33:532–41.

131. Bryner RW, Ullrich IH, Sauers J, et al. Effects of resistance vs. aerobic training combined with an 800 calorie liquid diet on lean body mass and resting metabolic rate. *J Am Coll Nutr.* 1999;18:115–21.

132. Geleibter A, Maher MM, Gerace L, et al. Effects of strength or aerobic training on body composition, resting metabolic rate, and peak oxygen consumption in obese dieting subjects. *Am J Clin Nutr.* 1997;66:557–63.

133. Quatela A, Callister R, Patterson A, MacDonald-Wicks L. The energy content and composition of meals consumed after an overnight fast and their effects on diet induced thermogenesis: a systematic review, meta-analyses and meta-regressions. *Nutrients.* 2016;8:E670.

134. Paddon-Jones D, Westman E, Mattes RD, et al. Protein, weight management, and satiety. *Am J Clin Nutr.* 2008;87(Suppl):1558S–61.

135. Thompson J, Manore MM. Predicted and measured resting metabolic rate of male and female endurance athletes. *J Am Diet Assoc.* 1996;96:30–4.

136. Flack KD, Siders WA, Johnson L, Roemmich JN. Cross-validation of resting metabolic rate prediction equations. *J Acad Nutr Diet.* 2016;116:1413–22.

137. Harris JA, Benedict FG. *A Biometric Study of Basal Metabolism in Man. Publication number 279.* Washington (DC) Carnegie Institution; 1919. p. 1–266.

138. Cunningham JJ. Body composition and resting metabolic rate: the myth of feminine metabolism. *Am J Clin Nutr.* 1982;36:721–6.

139. Mifflin MD, St. Jeor ST, Hill LA, Scott BJ, Daugherty SA, Koh YO. A new predictive equation for resting energy expenditure in healthy individuals. *Am J Clin Nutr.* 1990;51:241–7.

140. Harris C, Adams KJ. Exercise physiology. In: Ehrman JK, editor. *ACSM's Resource Manual for Guidelines for Exercise Testing and Prescription.* 6th ed. Philadelphia (PA): Lippincott Williams & Wilkins; 2010. p. 45–77.

141. De Lorenzo A, Bertini I, Candelaro N, et al. A new predictive equation to calculate resting metabolic rate in athletes. *J Sports Med Phys Fitness.* 1999;39:213–9.

142. Watson AD, Zabriskie HA, Witherbee KE, et al. Determining a resting metabolic rate prediction equation for collegiate female athletes. *J Strength Cond Res.* 2019;33:2426–32.

143. Tinsley GM, Graybeal AJ, Moore ML. Resting metabolic rate in muscular physique athletes: validity of existing methods and development of new prediction equations. *Appl Physiol Nutr Metab.* 2019;44:397–406.

144. Frankenfield D, Roth-Yousey L, Compher C. Comparison of predictive equations for resting metabolic rate in healthy non-obese and obese adults: a systematic review. *J Am Diet Assoc.* 2005;105:775–89.

145. Jagim AR, Camic CL, Kisiolek J, et al. Accuracy of resting metabolic rate prediction equations in athletes. *J Strength Cond Res.* 2018;32:1875–81.

146. Quinn TJ, Vroman NB, Kertzer R. Postexercise oxygen consumption in trained females: effect of exercise duration. *Med Sci Sports Exerc.* 1994;26:908–13.

147. Kalb JS, Hunter GR. Weight training economy as a function of intensity of the squat and overhead press exercise. *J Sports Med Phys Fitness.* 1991;31:154–60.

148. Robergs RA, Gordon T, Reynolds J, Walker TB. Energy expenditure during bench press and squat exercises. *J Strength Cond Res.* 2007;21:123–30.

149. Scala D, McMillan J, Blessing D, Rozenek R, Stone M. Metabolic cost of a preparatory phase of training in weight lifting: a practical observation. *J Appl Sports Sci Res.* 1987;1:48–52.

150. Ratamess NA, Rosenberg JG, Klei S, et al. Comparison of the acute metabolic responses to traditional resistance, body-weight, and battling rope exercises. *J Strength Cond Res.* 2015;29:47–57.

151. Mazzetti S, Wolff C, Yocum A, Reidy P, Douglass MS, Cochran H, Douglass MD. Effect of maximal and slow versus recreational muscle contractions on energy expenditure in trained and untrained men. *J Sports Med Phys Fitness.* 2011;51:381–92.

152. Katch FI, Freedson PS, Jones CA. Evaluation of acute cardio-respiratory responses to hydraulic resistance exercise. *Med Sci Sports Exerc.* 1985;17:168–73.

153. Farinatti PTV, Castinhierans Neto AG. The effect of between-set rest intervals on the oxygen uptake during and after resistance exercise sessions performed with large- and small-mass exercises. *J Strength Cond Res.* 2011;25:3181–90.

154. Harris NK, Woulfe CJ, Wood MR, Dulson DK, Gluchowski AK, Keogh JB. Acute physiological responses to strongman training compared to traditional strength training. *J Strength Cond Res.* 2016;30:1397–408.

155. Ballor DL, Becque MD, Katch VL. Metabolic responses during hydraulic resistance exercise. *Med Sci Sports Exerc.* 1987;19:363–7.

156. Scott CB. The effect of time-under-tension and weight lifting cadence on aerobic, anaerobic, and recovery energy expenditures: 3 submaximal sets. *Appl Physiol Nutr Metab.* 2012;37:252–6.

157. Buitrago S, Wirtz N, Yue Z, Kleinöder H, Mester J. Effects of load and training modes on physiological and metabolic responses in resistance exercise. *Eur J Appl Physiol.* 2012;112:2739–48.

158. Barreto AC, Maior AS, Menezes P, et al. Effect of different resistance exercise repetition velocities on excess post-exercise oxygen consumption and energetic expenditure. *Int Sports Med J.* 2010;11:235–43.

159. Hunter GR, Seelhorst D, Snyder S. Comparison of metabolic and heart rate responses to super slow vs. traditional resistance training. *J Strength Cond Res.* 2003;17:76–81.

160. Willoughby DS, Chilek DR, Schiller DA, Coast JR. The metabolic effects of three different free weight parallel squatting intensities. *J Hum Mov Stud.* 1991;21:53–67.

161. Haddock BL, Wilkin LD. Resistance training volume and post exercise energy expenditure. *Int J Sports Med.* 2006;27:143–8.

162. Mookerjee S, Welikonich MJ, Ratamess NA. Comparison of energy expenditure during single-set vs. multiple-set resistance exercise. *J Strength Cond Res.* 2016;30:1447–52.

163. Scott CB, Croteau A, Ravlo T. Energy expenditure before, during, and after the bench press. *J Strength Cond Res.* 2009;23:611–8.

164. Haltom RW, Kraemer RR, Sloan RA, et al. Circuit weight training and its effects on excess postexercise oxygen consumption. *Med Sci Sports Exerc.* 1999;31:1613–8.

165. Ratamess NA, Rosenberg JG, Kang J, et al. Acute oxygen uptake and resistance exercise performance using different rest interval lengths: the influence of maximal aerobic capacity and exercise sequence. *J Strength Cond Res.* 2014;28:1875–88.

166. Ratamess NA. Adaptations to anaerobic training programs. In: Baechle TR, Earle RW, editors. *Essentials of Strength Training and Conditioning.* 3rd ed. Champaign (IL): Human Kinetics; 2008. p. 93–119.

167. Ratamess NA, Smith CR, Beller NA, Kang J, Faigenbaum AD, Bush JA. Effects of rest interval length on acute battling rope exercise metabolism. *J Strength Cond Res.* 2015;29:2375–87.

168. Farinatti PT, Simao R, Monteiro WD, Fleck SJ. Influence of exercise order on oxygen uptake during strength training in young women. *J Strength Cond Res.* 2009;23:1037–44.

169. Kelleher AR, Hackney KJ, Fairchild TJ, Keslacy S, Ploutz-Snyder LL. The metabolic costs of reciprocal supersets vs. traditional resistance exercise in young recreationally active adults. *J Strength Cond Res.* 2010;24:1043–51.

170. Skidmore BL, Jones MT, Blegen M, Matthews TD. Acute effects of three different circuit weight training protocols on blood lactate, heart rate, and ratings of perceived exertion in recreationally active women. *J Sports Sci Med.* 2012;11:660–8.

171. Buckley S, Knapp K, Lackie A, et al. Multimodal high-intensity interval training increases muscle function and metabolic performance in females. *Appl Physiol Nutr Metab.* 2015;40:1157–62.

172. McRae G, Payne A, Zelt JGE, Scribbans TD, Jung ME, Little JP, Gurd BJ. Extremely low volume, whole-body aerobic-resistance training improves aerobic fitness and muscular endurance in females. *Appl Physiol Nutr Metab.* 2012;37:1124–31.

173. Myers, TR, Schneider, MG, Schmale, MS, Hazell, TJ. Whole-body aerobic resistance training circuit improves aerobic fitness and muscle strength in sedentary young females. *J Strength Cond Res.* 2015;29:1592–600.

174. Elliot DL, Goldberg L, Kuehl KS. Effect of resistance training on excess post-exercise oxygen consumption. *J Appl Sports Sci Res.* 1992;6:77–81.

175. Hulsey CR, Soto DT, Koch AJ, Mayhew JL. Comparison of kettlebell swings and treadmill running at equivalent rating of perceived exertion values. *J Strength Cond Res.* 2012;26:1203–7.

176. Ratamess NA, Kang J, Kuper JD, et al. Acute cardiorespiratory and metabolic effects of a sandbag resistance exercise protocol. *J Strength Cond Res.* 2018;32:1491–502.

177. Scott C, Nelson E, Martin S, Ligotti B. Total energy costs of 3 Tabata-type calisthenic squatting routines: isometric, isotonic and jump. *Eur J Hum Mov.* 2015;35:34–40.

178. Williams BM, Kraemer RR. Comparison of cardiorespiratory and metabolic responses in kettlebell high-intensity interval training versus sprint interval cycling. *J Strength Cond Res.* 2015;29:3317–25.

179. Gist NH, Freese EC, Cureton KJ. Comparison of responses to two high-intensity intermittent exercise protocols. *J Strength Cond Res.* 2014;28:3033–40.

180. Binzen CA, Swan PD, Manore MM. Postexercise oxygen consumption and substrate use after resistance exercise in women. *Med Sci Sports Exerc.* 2001;33:932–8.

181. Borsheim E, Bahr R. Effect of exercise intensity, duration and mode on post-exercise oxygen consumption. *Sports Med.* 2003;33:1037–60.

182. Braun WA, Hawthorne WE, Markofski MM. Acute EPOC response in women to circuit training and treadmill exercise of matched oxygen consumption. *Eur J Appl Physiol.* 2005;94:500–4.

183. Melby CL, Tincknell T, Schmidt WD. Energy expenditure following a bout of non-steady state resistance exercise. *J Sports Med Phys Fitness.* 1992;32:128–35.

184. Burleson MA, O'Bryant HS, Stone MH, Collins MA, Triplett-McBride T. Effect of weight training exercise and treadmill exercise on post-exercise oxygen consumption. *Med Sci Sports Exerc.* 1998;30:518–22.

185. Oliveira NL, Oliveira J. Excess postexercise oxygen consumption is unaffected by the resistance and aerobic exercise order in an exercise session. *J Strength Cond Res.* 2011;25:2843–50.

186. Schuenke MD, Mikat RP, McBride JM. Effect of an acute period of resistance exercise on excess post-exercise oxygen consumption: implications for body mass management. *Eur J Appl Physiol.* 2002;86:411–7.

187. Hackney KJ, Engels HJ, Gretebeck RJ. Resting energy expenditure and delayed-onset muscle soreness after full-body resistance training with an eccentric concentration. *J Strength Cond Res.* 2008;22:1602–9.

CHAPTER 9
Responses and Adaptations of the Cardiorespiratory System

OBJECTIVES

After completing this chapter, you will be able to:

- Discuss the chambers of the heart and blood flow during cardiac muscle contraction
- Discuss intrinsic and extrinsic regulation of the heart
- Discuss oxygen transport, consumption, and blood flow at rest and during exercise
- Discuss the cardiovascular response to exercise
- Discuss cardiovascular responses at rest and during exercise following training
- Discuss the respiratory system and adaptations to training

The cardiovascular (CV) system consists of three major components: the heart ("pump"), the blood vessels ("transport portals"), and the blood ("fluid medium"). All other systems depend on the CV system, including the lungs, which are essential for blood oxygenation and removal of CO_2, which occurs during respiration. The CV system performs a number of critical functions to life including delivery of nutrients, oxygen, and hormones to all tissues; removal of waste products and CO_2; temperature control; pH control; immunity; and hydration. The length of blood vessels within an average-sized man would extend more than 100,000 miles if stretched from end-to-end (1). This chapter discusses the basic anatomy and physiology of the CV system and the acute responses and chronic adaptations to exercise.

Anatomy of the Heart

The heart acts as a pump circulating blood throughout the body. It consists of four chambers (Fig. 9.1) with approximately two-thirds of its mass located on the left side. On average, the heart weighs ~11 oz in men and 9 oz in women, and its weight is proportional to body size (1). Two of the chambers are receivers (*atria*), whereas the other two chambers (*ventricles*) act to pump blood away from the heart. Blood returns to the heart from the rest of the body through the right atrium (via the superior and inferior vena cava) and then passes through the right ventricle. A *tricuspid valve* opens (between the right atrium and ventricle) as the pressure within the atrium builds up to allow passage of blood to the ventricle and closes to prevent backward flow of blood. Contraction of the right ventricle pumps blood to the lungs through the pulmonary *semilunar valve* of the pulmonary artery. Blood becomes oxygenated in the lungs and returns to the heart (left atrium) via the pulmonary vein. Contraction of the left atrium pumps blood through the *bicuspid (mitral) valve* into the left ventricle. The left ventricle is the largest chamber as blood is pumped via the aorta to all parts of the circulatory system. The *chordae tendineae* are chord-like tendons that connect the valves to the papillary muscles. They prevent backward flow of blood by preventing the valves from inversion. The *papillary muscles* contract to tighten and stabilize the chordae tendineae. The atria and ventricles are separated by *septum*, the *interatrial* and *interventricular septum*, respectively.

Cardiac Musculature

Cardiac muscle, or myocardium, is one of three major types of muscle. It contracts on its own and is capable of hypertrophy and adapting to exercise. The thickness of cardiac muscle is affected by stress, and thicker cardiac muscle is stronger. This is particularly true for the left ventricle. The T tubules are fewer in number, larger, broader, and are located along the Z line compared to skeletal muscle. This, in part, allows cardiac muscle to contract forcefully at a lower rate. Cardiac cells, or cardiocytes, have the ability to communicate directly with adjacent cells via connective tissue structures known as *intercalated discs*.

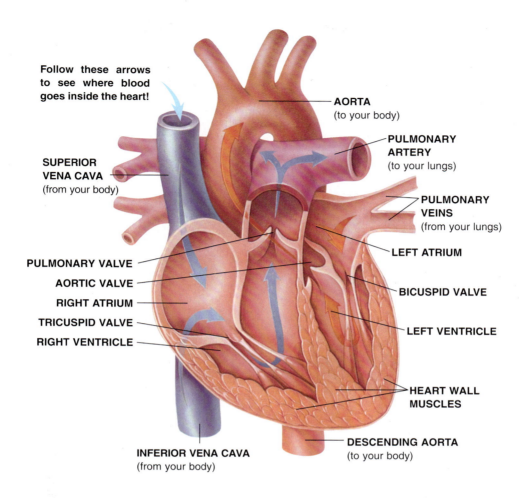

FIGURE 9.1 Anatomy of the heart.

Intercalated discs enable the rapid spread of action potentials and the synchronized contraction of heart musculature. They enable cardiac muscle in all four chambers to act as one large fiber during sequential contraction of the atria and ventricles. Gap junctions are located within the intercalated disks and act as passages between cells. They allow the heart to contract in a network referred to as a *functional syncytium* that occurs in a squeezing-like fashion thereby ejecting the blood in a fluent manner.

 Major Blood Vessels

Blood vessels provide the major routes by which blood is pumped (Fig. 9.2). Because humans have a closed circulatory system, vessels form a large interconnecting network responsible for blood delivery to all tissues, nutrient/waste exchange, and return to the heart. *Arteries* are high-pressure vessels that deliver oxygen-rich blood to tissues. Arteries have walls that contain smooth muscle and elastic fibers. The elastic recoil is large, enabling arteries to forcefully circulate blood. The aorta is the largest artery and has an ascending and descending branch that exits the left ventricle. It acts as a distributor with many branches. Arteries decrease in size and diameter as they approach the tissue level. Smaller arteries form *arterioles*. Arterioles constrict or relax to regulate blood flow at the tissue level. Approximately 17% of the body's total blood supply circulates through arteries at rest (1). Arterioles branch and form smaller vessels called *metarterioles* that end the arterial side of circulation and form a network of capillaries. Capillaries are thin (7–10 μm) vessels that serve as the site for nutrient/oxygen exchange at the tissue level. In skeletal muscle, each metarteriole interfaces with ~8–10 capillaries (1). Approximately 8% of total blood supply circulates through capillary beds at rest, and capillaries in skeletal muscle are densely populated, *e.g.*, 2,000–3,000 capillaries per square millimeter of tissue (1). Capillaries have precapillary sphincters that constrict or dilate to regulate blood flow. The opposite side of the capillary bed forms the venous side of circulation. Small veins (*venules*) continue the circulatory route from capillary beds. Venules form larger veins, and all veins circulate blood into the inferior (from lower body) and superior (from upper body) vena cava. Veins are low-pressure structures with extensible walls. Blood is stored in veins when circulatory demands are low and is compelled into circulation when demand necessitates greater activity. Approximately 68% of total blood supply circulates in veins at rest (1).

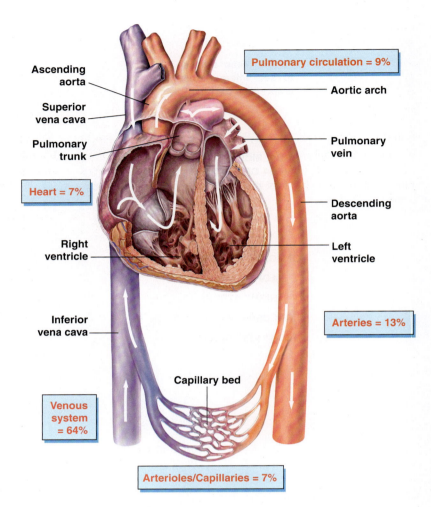

FIGURE 9.2 Circulatory system. Percentages indicate the amount of blood circulating through each region at rest. (Adapted from an asset provided by Anatomical Chart Co.)

 Regulation of the Heart

Cardiac function stems largely from the heart's force of contraction and rate. Although the heart contracts involuntarily, it operates under the control of intrinsic and extrinsic factors. Intrinsic factors relate to the heart's own conduction system as well as the role venous return to the heart plays in cardiac contractility. Extrinsic factors that control CV function relate to stimuli from other major physiological systems including the nervous and endocrine systems. Both intrinsic and extrinsic factors are critical to mediating CV function at rest and during exercise.

Intrinsic Regulation of the Heart

The heart has the ability to regulate its own rhythm (Fig. 9.3). The action potential is spontaneously generated in the *sinoatrial node* (SA node). The SA node is located in the right atrium and is the pacemaker of the heart. The wave of depolarization spreads across the atria to the *atrioventricular node* (AV node). The AV node places a delay (~0.10–0.13 s) to allow the atria more time to contract and allow adequate

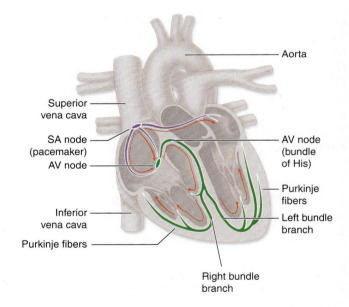

FIGURE 9.3 Conductive system of the heart. (From McArdle WD, Katch FI, Katch VL. *Exercise Physiology: Nutrition, Energy, and Human Performance*. 7th ed. Baltimore (MD): Lippincott Williams & Wilkins; 2010.)

filling time for the ventricles. The AV node gives rise to the *Bundle of His*, which continues the wave of depolarization. Depolarization rapidly spreads through the ventricles via the *left and right bundle branches* and *Purkinje fibers*. The right and left bundle branches send the wave of depolarization toward the heart's apex and then outward. The terminal branches become Purkinje fibers that spread the depolarization throughout the ventricles. Purkinje fibers transmit action potentials at a rate that is approximately six times faster than other cardiac areas (1). The heart's conduction system keeps rate around 60–110 beats per minute depending on one's conditioning level.

Extrinsic Regulation of the Heart

Extrinsic regulation is important to prepare the heart to tolerate stress and exercise. Extrinsic control stems from the nervous and endocrine systems. The medulla oblongata contains a cardiac center that regulates heart rate (HR) and force of contraction, a vasomotor center that controls blood pressure (BP) and vessel diameter, and a respiratory center that controls breathing rate and depth. Feedback from sensory and motor centers in the brain stimulates CV centers to increase HR and force of contraction. The autonomic nervous system plays a substantial role in regulating cardiac function. Sympathetic nervous system stimulation increases cardiac contractility and rate, whereas parasympathetic nervous system (mainly through stimulation of the *vagus nerve*) has the opposite effect and returns CV function back toward homeostasis. Catecholamines (epinephrine and norepinephrine) are secreted, bind to receptors on the surface of the heart, and increase HR and force of contraction. They also lead to an anticipatory rise in CV function prior to exercise. Norepinephrine is most effective when it is released as a neurotransmitter from sympathetic nerves, whereas epinephrine accounts for most of the catecholamines (~80%) secreted by the adrenal medulla.

Blood Components

Blood accounts for ~7% of human body weight and is responsible for transportation of several molecules throughout the human body. Molecules such as oxygen, glucose, fatty acids, amino acids, vitamins, minerals, enzymes, antibodies, and hormones travel through the blood to target tissues. Waste products are removed by blood. Blood volume is dependent on body size and level of aerobic conditioning, but is generally around 5–6 L in men and 4–5 L in women (2). The major components of blood include its liquid portion (plasma) and the segment of formed elements. Plasma comprises 55%–60% of blood volume of which ~90% is water, 7% plasma proteins, and the remaining 3% nutrients and waste (2). Formed elements comprise ~40%–45% of total blood volume. The percent of formed elements

relative to total blood volume is the hematocrit. Hematocrit can change based on hydration levels and is often used to investigate potential blood doping in athletes.

Red blood cells (RBCs, erythrocytes) comprise 99% of the formed elements and up to 1% is composed of white blood cells and *platelets* (2). The body contains >25 trillion RBCs, and RBC production is increased by testosterone (1). RBCs lack a nucleus and organelles. They transport oxygen primarily bound to the iron-containing protein hemoglobin. Although a small percent of oxygen is transported in plasma (~1.5%), most (98.5%) oxygen is transported via hemoglobin. Approximately 65–70 times more oxygen is transported by hemoglobin than plasma dissolution (1). Each RBC contains ~250–280 million hemoglobin molecules; each contains iron and can bind four oxygen molecules. There are ~15 g of hemoglobin per 100 mL of blood in men and ~14 $g \cdot dL^{-1}$ of blood in women (1,2).

Oxygen binding to hemoglobin is cooperative because binding of one oxygen molecule increases the affinity of others. However, oxygen must be dissociated before it is taken up into tissues. Figure 9.4 illustrates the oxygen-hemoglobin dissociation curve at normal pH (7.4) and temperature (37°C) and at pHs of 7.6 and 7.2. Cooperative oxygen binding is a factor leading to the S-shaped curve. The *x*-axis depicts the partial pressure of oxygen (PO_2), and the *y*-axis depicts the percent of hemoglobin saturated with oxygen. The partial pressure is the pressure generated independent of other gases. It is a measure of the quantity of gas present. The air we breathe is composed of 79.04% nitrogen, 20.93% oxygen, and 0.03% CO_2. At sea level, the atmospheric pressure is 760 mm Hg, which creates a PO_2 of 159 mm Hg (760 mm Hg × 0.21). This PO_2 drops to 100–105 mm Hg when air is inhaled as it mixes with water vapor

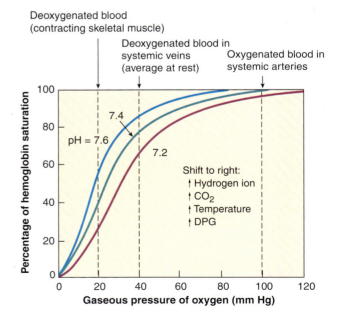

FIGURE 9.4 Oxygen-hemoglobin dissociation curve. (From *Stedman's Medical Dictionary*. 27th ed. Baltimore (MD): Lippincott Williams & Wilkins; 2000.)

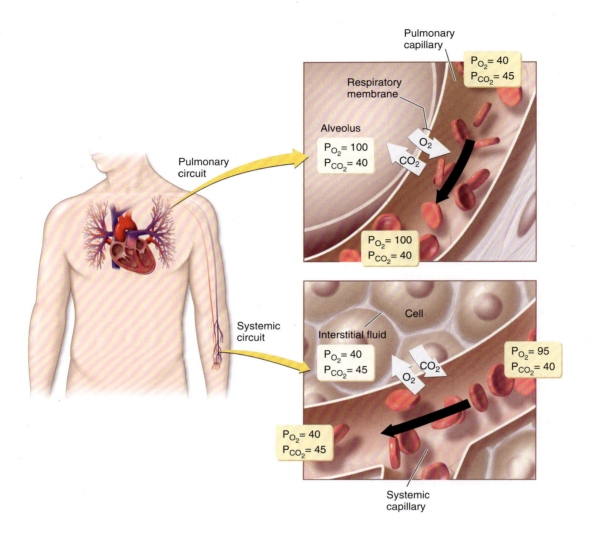

FIGURE 9.5 Partial pressure of oxygen and carbon dioxide. (From Premkumar K. *The Massage Connection Anatomy and Physiology*. Baltimore (MD): Lippincott Williams & Wilkins; 2004.)

and CO_2 in the alveoli. Differences in PO_2 between the lungs (100 mm Hg) and alveolar capillaries (40 mm Hg) and between arterial circulation (100 mm Hg) and the tissues (40 mm Hg) allow diffusion of oxygen (Fig. 9.5). The latter is the arteriovenous oxygen difference (a-VO_2 difference) and is ~4–5 mL of oxygen per dL of blood at rest but may increase up to 15 mL of oxygen per dL of blood during exercise (1). The large PO_2 gradient from the alveoli to the capillaries of 60–65 mm Hg drives oxygen into circulation and is known as the oxygen diffusion capacity. At rest, ~250 mL of oxygen diffuses into pulmonary circulation each minute, and this number is far greater in highly trained endurance athletes (1).

In Figure 9.4, hemoglobin saturation remains high (~75%–80%) at PO_2 above 40 mm Hg. Under resting conditions, about 20%–25% of oxygen is unloaded from hemoglobin into capillary beds. This curve can shift to the right or left. A shift to the right and down indicates greater tissue oxygen unloading, whereas a shift to the left and up has the opposite effect. Four major factors cause a right/down shift in the curve. A reduction in pH (increased H^+), increased temperature, higher levels of CO_2 (increased partial pressure of CO_2 [PCO_2]), and increased *2,3-diphosphoglycerate* (2,3-DPG) can increase oxygen dissociation. Exercise has a similar influence. A right/down shift in the curve resulting from changes in pH and CO_2 is known as the Bohr Effect (named after scientist Christian Bohr). 2,3-DPG is found in RBCs and binds to hemoglobin with higher affinity than oxygen. As a result, 2,3-DPG elevations increase oxygen unloading. 2,3-DPG concentrations are higher in athletes than untrained individuals and higher in women than men (1) reflecting greater potential to unload oxygen with training and, in women, a compensatory mechanism to accommodate lower hemoglobin.

CO_2 must be removed while oxygen is consumed. Like oxygen, CO_2 moves via diffusion from high to low PCO_2 values (Fig. 9.5). Blood PCO_2 is 46 mm Hg versus an alveolar PCO_2 of 40 mm Hg. CO_2 travels in the blood by three routes. In plasma, 5%–10% of CO_2 is transported in a dissolved state. Free CO_2 is important for establishing PCO_2 values. Sixty to eighty percent of CO_2 is transported via bicarbonate. In tissues, the reaction catalyzed by the enzyme *carbonic anhydrase* is

$$CO_2 + H_2O \rightarrow H_2CO_3 \rightarrow H^+ + HCO_3^-.$$

The bicarbonate ion (HCO_3^-) buffers pH while transporting CO_2. In the lungs, the carbonic anhydrase/bicarbonate reaction is reversed where CO_2 (and H_2O) is reformed where it is then expired. Lastly, ~20% of CO_2 is transported with hemoglobin (*carbaminohemoglobin*). Oxygenated hemoglobin has less ability to bind CO_2, whereas deoxygenated hemoglobin has higher affinity for CO_2, a concept known as the Haldane effect. Dissociation occurs in the lungs leading to CO_2 release via expiration.

RBCs have a life span of ~4 months, so they must be replaced adequately. Some RBCs may be destroyed during exercise (*sports anemia*) where mechanical stress via pounding of the feet during running and jarring of kidneys may contribute. Platelets are small molecules required for blood clotting (in addition to several proteins including *fibrin*), whereas white blood cells are critical to immune function. Blood is critical for temperature regulation and pH balance. Blood picks up heat from the body's core and dissipates heat throughout. Skin blood flow increases during exercise, which assists in cooling. Lastly, blood can buffer acids to restore pH.

Blood Flow

Blood flow to working muscles is critical to exercise performance. The body contains ~5 L of blood although the vascular system has the potential to hold four times more than that (1). At rest, skeletal muscle receives ~15%–20% of total blood flow as most blood flows to other organs: 25% to the liver, 20% to the kidneys, 10% to the skin, 14%–15% to the brain, and the remaining ~10%–12% to the heart and other tissues (11). During exercise, blood flow to skeletal muscle may increase to >80% of total flow (via redistribution) to meet the metabolic demands. Blood flow to inspiratory and expiratory muscles during exercise may increase to ~14%–16% of total cardiac output (Q_c) (12). Blood flow is maintained or increased to the brain during exercise. Blood flow to the brain increases as exercise intensity increases to ~60% of VO_2max, where it may plateau or decrease afterward (13). Increased arteriole vasodilation takes place in the brain due to increased PCO_2, decreased PO_2, increased metabolism and activity of muscle mechanoreceptors, and greater mean arterial pressure (13).

Contraction of skeletal muscle is necessary to increase venous blood flow back to the heart. Muscle contraction forces blood against gravity, and venous valves prevent blood from backward flow in healthy veins. Muscle contraction helps create

Sidebar — Blood Doping in Athletes

Blood doping (dates back to the early 1960s) refers to intravenous infusion of blood or blood products to increase athletic performance. Blood may come from a donor (*homologous infusion* or *allotransfusion*) or the athlete (*autologous infusion*) spaced over weeks, frozen in glycerol, and reinfused 3–5 days before the competition. Blood doping increases RBC (and hemoglobin) content up to ~10% (3), and marked improvements take place within 24 hours. Although this technique was banned by the International Olympic Committee in 1984, the drug *erythropoietin* (EPO) became the new method to boost blood in 1988. EPO is a glycoprotein hormone produced by the kidneys and liver, which stimulates the production of RBCs upon binding to receptors on bone marrow. Hypoxia (via expression of hypoxia-inducible factors such as HIF-1α) increases EPO gene expression and hormone production. The actions of EPO are augmented by testosterone, growth hormone, and IGF-1 (4). The synthetic form of EPO (recombinant EPO) is injected to increase RBC count and hemoglobin concentrations. The early form of recombinant EPO had short half-lives of 8–24 hours requiring frequent dosing (5). Since, other preparations with long half-lives (3–6 d) became available. EPO injections (20–50 IU kg body mass^{-1} three times per week) may increase hemoglobin by ~6%–11% and hematocrit by 6%–8.3%, decrease blood lactate during exercise, increase VO_2max by 7%, and run time to exhaustion by 17% (6). A review of the literature has shown that EPO may increase VO_2max by 6%–8% (5). Blood doping or EPO use enhances sea level endurance performance via increased VO_2max, buffer capacity, blood volume, skeletal muscle mitochondrial oxidative phosphorylation capacity, and heat tolerance. Blood doping increases VO_2max by up to 11%, 5-mile treadmill run time, 10-km race time, and running and cycling time to exhaustion by 13%–26% (6–8), and the effects are most notable in athletes with high VO_2max (9). A recent study investigated recombinant EPO administration (50 IU kg body mass^{-1} every 2 d for 4 wk) in native moderate-altitude endurance athletes (Kenyan runners) and found hemoglobin and hematocrit increased in the Kenyan runners to a smaller extent than native sea level runners; however, similar increases in VO_2max and time trial performance were seen showing that EPO administration may still augment physiological performance in athlete's already exposed to erythropoietic hypoxia via altitude exposure (10). It has been estimated that 15%–22% of highly-trained endurance athletes (based on inquiry and testing results) have engaged in some form of blood doping (5). In addition, *HIF stabilizers* (which increase renal production of EPO) have been added to the banned list of blood doping agents used by athletes to enhance performance (5). Negative side effects associated with blood doping include increased blood viscosity, which increases the risk of stroke and myocardial infarction, and potentially an increase in blood pressure (5).

a vibrant circulatory system. Increased muscle blood flow is responsible for the muscle pump associated with resistance training (RT). Muscle blood flow is occluded with contractions >20% of MVC. The mechanical shortening/lengthening of muscle fibers and/or ISOM contraction against a resistance constricts blood vessels and temporarily decreases blood flow. However, greater blood flow circulates to muscle upon relaxation or low-level contractions (reactive hyperemia). One study reported a 38% increase in reactive hyperemia (forearm blood flow) following acute RE (14). Reactive hyperemia may be limited when large muscle mass is involved. That is, a muscle group may receive more blood flow when it is exercising individually than when several muscle groups are exercised simultaneously (15). During resistance exercise, the lifter may feel blood flow increase to the active muscles in between sets rather than during the set. Acutely, RE may produce greater increases in limb blood flow compared to aerobic exercise (14). Ischemia associated with RT is a stimulus for muscle hypertrophy as is blood flow restriction training discussed in other chapters.

Blood flow is tightly regulated. Blood flow follows general principles of hydrodynamics where blood flow is dependent upon the pressure gradient within the vessel (large gradient = greater flow), resistance to flow (lower resistance = greater flow), blood thickness or viscosity (greater viscosity = reduced flow), blood vessel length (greater length = reduced flow), and blood vessel diameter or radius (greater diameter = greater flow) (1). Poiseuille law is defined as:

$$Q = \frac{\pi(P_1 - P_2)r^4}{8\eta L}$$

Exercise presents a potent sympathetic nervous system response where blood vessel vasoconstriction is customary. Vasoconstriction increases BP but reduces flow to that specified region. Blood flow can be redirected from other peripheral tissues to skeletal muscle. Local regulatory factors increase blood flow to skeletal muscle during exercise. The metabolic demands, hypoxia, shear stress of increased flow, and temperature cause the release of several vasoactive substances that increase blood vessel vasodilation. CO_2, reduced pH, adenosine, magnesium, potassium, prostacyclin (prostaglandin I2), and nitric oxide stimulate local vasodilation (1). Figure 9.6 depicts an artery undergoing vasodilation. Endothelial cells release vasodilatory substances (shown is nitric oxide) which reduce sympathetic nervous system vasoconstriction, induce smooth muscle relaxation, and expands the arterial lumen to increase blood flow. Thus, changes in endothelial function are important for mediating improvements in blood flow to skeletal muscle.

Endurance athletes have greater reactive blood flow per min to working muscles during exercise than untrained individuals (15). Swimmers and cyclists have been shown to have superior endothelium-dependent and independent vasodilation, muscle perfusion, and vascular conductance during exercise than untrained individuals (16). A meta-analysis of 42 studies showed that AT significantly improves endothelial function with the largest improvements seen in individuals with clinical disorders (17). Positive relationships were shown between AT intensity and flow-mediated dilation where every 10% increase in relative intensity was accompanied by a 1% improvement in flow-mediated dilation (17). Endurance-trained men may have a greater or similar peak vasodilatory capacity compared to resistance-trained men although both training modalities increase flow-mediated vasodilatation (18,19). Kawano et al. (20) compared reactive blood flow responses following 4 months of high-intensity RT (3 × 10 reps with 80% of 1 RM), moderate-intensity RT (3 × 16 reps with 50% of 1 RM), or combined high-intensity RT with aerobic training (30 min at 60% max heart rate) in previously untrained subjects. They showed that moderate-intensity RT and combined RT and AT increased forearm blood flow response to reactive hyperemia, but not high-intensity RT by itself. A meta-analysis showed that RT improves endothelial function and that frequency of RT is related to the changes in flow-mediated dilation (17). In addition, the combination of AT and RT improves endothelial function (17).

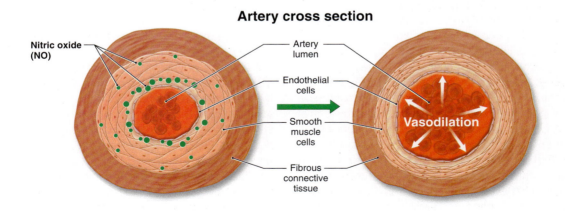

FIGURE 9.6 Arterial vasodilation. From McArdle WD, Katch FI, Katch VL. *Exercise Physiology: Energy, Nutrition, and Human Performance*. 6th ed. Philadelphia (PA): Lippincott Williams & Wilkins; 2007.

Nitric oxide is a gas produced from its precursor L-arginine (with oxygen via the enzyme *nitric oxide synthase*), which is a potent signaling molecule and vasodilatory agent known to produce many functions in the human body. It freely diffuses across cell membranes, is highly reactive, and acts quickly upon arteriole smooth muscle causing relaxation and vasodilation. Nitric oxide regulates skeletal muscle contractility and exercise-induced glucose uptake (21). Training may increase nitric oxide bioavailability, and exercise-induced increases in flow shear stress enhance the synthesis and release of nitric oxide (17).

Arterial Compliance

Arterial compliance is the ability of the walls of the arteries to distend and increase volume with greater pressure. It depends on the elastic properties of the artery, and reduced compliance is accompanied by increased *arterial stiffness*. Arterial stiffness is associated with several pathologies including diabetes and atherosclerosis and may be caused by oxidative stress, inflammation, reduced nitric oxide, smooth muscle proliferation, and increased release of vasoconstriction agents (22). Increased arterial stiffness may lead to increased systolic blood pressure (SBP), left ventricular hypertrophy, and other CV issues (23). Arterial stiffness is measured by examining pulse wave velocity or augmentation index. A meta-analysis showed that AT reduced arterial stiffness (via changes in pulse wave velocity and augmentation index) with greater reductions shown in individuals with stiffer arteries prestudy, when intensity was higher, and when training was longer than 10 weeks (22). Aerobic training produced more changes in peripheral indices than central possibly due to the effects of enhanced nitric oxide release (22). Resistance training had no effect on arterial stiffness, and combined RT and AT had only a small nonsignificant reduction in arterial stiffness (22). Some studies have shown that RT increased arterial stiffness (22). An earlier meta-analysis concluded that high-intensity RT increased arterial stiffness, whereas moderate-intensity RT did not (23). Although the effects of RT on arterial stiffness are unclear and not known if it may occur in response to large acute elevations in mean arterial pressure during lifting, Miyachi (23) concluded that the levels of arterial stiffening seen in the reviewed studies may not have clinically adverse effects in young healthy adults.

Cardiovascular Function

Several CV variables can be measured and used for health/performance evaluations. These variables include HR, HR variability, BP, stroke volume (SV) (and ejection fraction), and Q_c.

- **Heart rate** is the frequency the heart beats per minute. Average resting HR values range from 60–100 beats per minute. Resting HR is affected by age, gender (adult women average 5–10 beats per minute faster than men), posture (standing yields a 10–12 beats per minute greater HR than lying), food intake (digestion increases metabolism and HR), stress/emotion (increases HR), smoking (increases HR), and environmental and body temperature (HR increases when body temperature increases and during hot and humid weather) (11).
- **Heart rate variability** (HRV) represents variation in the time interval between heartbeats (*e.g.*, R-wave to R-wave intervals) and is considered an indirect, noninvasive measure of cardiac autonomic activity, specifically the balance between sympathetic and parasympathetic branches. Following data collection and correction, HRV may be determined in a number of ways including time domain and/or frequency-domain measures. Time-domain has been consistently used and is computed by taking the standard deviation of the R-R intervals (SDRR) and the root mean square (RMSSD) or standard deviation (SD) of successive differences in R-R intervals (24). Decreased parasympathetic nervous system activity is characterized by a decrease in HRV which has been associated with various health risks (25). In athletes, HRV may be used for tracking the time course of training adaptations and recovery.
- **Blood pressure** is the pressure in the arteries following contraction of the left ventricle (systole). SBP is the pressure in the left ventricle during systole and averages ~120 mm Hg. Diastolic blood pressure (DBP) represents peripheral resistance to flow during relaxation (diastole) and averages ~80 mm Hg. Mean arterial pressure averages ~93 mm Hg and is calculated as DBP + (0.333[SBP − DBP]).
- **Stroke volume** is the volume of blood ejected from the left ventricle each beat. SV averages ~60–70 mL of blood per beat and is the difference between the blood volume in the left ventricle after filling (*end diastolic volume*; averages ~100 mL of blood) and the blood volume after systole (*end systolic volume*; averages ~40 mL of blood). The proportion of blood pumped from the left ventricle each beat is the *ejection fraction*. It is calculated by (SV/end diastolic volume) × 100. Ejection fraction averages 60% at rest although strength athletes and endurance athletes have been shown to have values ~67%–73% (26,27).
- **Cardiac output** (Q_c) is the total volume of blood pumped by the heart per minute. It is the product of HR and SV. Q_c averages 5 L·min^{-1} at rest and tends to be higher in a supine position than standing or sitting.

Cardiovascular Responses to Exercise

Aerobic and anaerobic exercise lead to substantial acute CV responses in men and women. Exercise increases oxygen demand, nutrient usage, waste buildup, and body core temperature that all require augmented CV response to meet the additional needs. Recovery from exercise requires augmented CV system response to return to homeostatic levels. Essentially all components of the CV system are modified during exercise.

In this section, HR, HRV, SV, Q_c, BP, plasma volume (PV), and oxygen consumption are discussed.

Heart Rate Response

HR increases during exercise from resting values to rates >195 beats per minute during maximal exercise (1). The upper limits for HR during exercise can be calculated based on the maximum predicted HR (see Chapter 17). The magnitude of HR increase depends on muscle mass use, exercise intensity, and the degree of continuity of exercise. At low to moderate to high intensities of exercise, HR will increase linearly up until maximal. If work rate is held constant, HR plateaus after an initial rise at the onset of exercise. The plateau is the *steady-state HR* and is optimal to meet the current workload. For each increase in intensity beyond this point, a new steady-state value will be reached within 1–2 minutes (2). HR may remain at this point if intensity remains constant. However, during prolonged aerobic exercise, HR may subtly increase at the same intensity when it is >15 minutes in duration. This is known as **cardiovascular drift** where the HR increase compensates for reduced SV caused by fluid loss (1). Interval and RT elicit potent increases in HR. Fluctuations are seen due to the breaks in continuity of the exercise modalities. HR increases following each set at the onset of resistance exercise. HR increases progressively after each set for the first 4 sets (of a 5-set protocol) and plateaus (28). During each repetition, HR responds similarly between ECC and CON phases (29). Circuit protocols and workouts with short rest intervals may yield a potent HR response with less fluctuation than traditional RT with long rest intervals (30,31). Battling rope workouts with 1–2 minutes of rest in between sets can generate high HR values with peaks >180 beats per minute and mean HR range of 140–164 beats per minute in men and women (31), with mean HR response that exceeds traditional RT workouts (32). High, better-sustained HRs are seen during HIIT workouts that utilize Tabata intervals, *e.g.*, with sandbags (mean of ~170 beats per minute) (30) and kettlebells (33). Attempts have been made to maintain higher HRs during resistance exercise (RE) besides using circuits or short rest intervals. For example, performing aerobic exercise in between sets of RE, a concept known as **cardioacceleration training**, is performed to combine AE and RE for concurrent training but also to engage in RT with a higher HR during each set (34). Because HR decreases during rest intervals, adding 30 seconds to 1 minute of aerobic exercise in between sets can help maintain HR.

Heart Rate Variability Response

HRV during exercise has mostly been studied during aerobic exercise. Exercise elicits a curvilinear dose-response reduction in HRV (SDRR, RMSSD) when expressed in the time and frequency domain metrics, and the response is associated with high exercise intensity (24,35). The reduction in HRV appears to reach a threshold point where it stabilizes, and this point corresponds to the lactate threshold (24). Long duration exercise may reduce HRV especially when CV drift occurs (24). Combined aerobic and RT workouts decrease HRV during and through 30 minutes post exercise (36). The reduction represents parasympathetic (vagal) withdrawal and sympathetic nervous system activation during exercise. Resistance exercise may decrease HRV during a workout, and the postexercise response may involve a prolonged decrease in vagal modulation and increase in sympathetic activity in resistance-trained men (37). The reduced HRV seen during RE may be greater than reductions seen during aerobic exercise possibly due to greater FT muscle fiber recruitment, catecholamine release, accumulation of metabolites, and plasma volume shifts (37). When exercise is completed, HRV demonstrates a time-dependent recovery and return to preexercise levels, with a rapid recovery taking place within minutes but full recovery could take as long as 48 hours (24). Recovery may take longer when exercise intensity is high (24). Less of a reduction in HRV may be seen post exercise following 8 weeks of combined AT and RT thereby demonstrating enhanced recovery (36).

Stroke Volume Response

SV increases during exercise and physiological factors such as blood volume returning to the heart, arterial pressure, ventricular contractility, and distensibility contribute to the magnitude of SV increase (2). Remember, the venous system acts as a storage site for blood at rest. Exercise increases blood flow in circulation and causes greater venous return to the heart. Greater venous return increases end-diastolic volume in the left ventricle and the heart's force of contraction. Myocardial fibers stretch via greater *preload*, and the effect is a stronger force of contraction. Greater preload-induced stretch places cardiac muscle fibers in a more conducive length to generate force. This is known as the *Frank-Starling mechanism*. Cardiac contractility increases independent of venous return. Sympathetic nervous system stimulation and catecholamines increase cardiac contractility. Vasodilation decreases total peripheral resistance to flow from the heart, which decreases *afterload*. In combination, these factors contribute to greater SV augmentation during exercise.

SV increases linearly up to ~40%–60% of maximal exercise capacity in untrained and moderately trained individuals (2) where a plateau occurs as exercise progresses. However, SV may increase beyond this intensity in highly trained endurance athletes (2). SV may increase to 100–120 mL in untrained individuals but up to 200 mL in highly trained individuals (2). Critical to SV increases is body position. At rest, SV is higher during supine or recumbent positions due to greater venous return. Upright positions yield lower SV due to gravity causing venous pooling in the lower extremities. During exercise, the SV increase is higher in an upright position than supine due to the lower starting value seen in the supine position. SV increases take place despite increases in HR, which decrease chamber filling times. SV increases during resistance exercise (38). When examining each rep, SV does not increase during the CON phase but may increase during the ECC phase (29). In some cases, SV is lower during CON actions (29). This may be the result of including a Valsalva maneuver (temporary breath-holding) that increases *intrathoracic pressure* (the pressure developed within the chest cavity) and *intra-abdominal pressure*, which increases SBP and DBP. A substantial load (increased BP) is placed on the CV system during lifting (39). The rise in pressure may impede SV temporarily during CON actions. SV rebounds during rest intervals where elevations are seen.

Cardiac Output Response

Q_c is the product of HR and SV. A linear increase in Q_c is seen during aerobic exercise (Fig. 9.7). HR and SV increase during exercise. However, SV may plateau as intensity rises; therefore, an increase in HR is needed at high exercise intensities to reach maximal Q_c. Q_c may increase to 20–40 L·min^{-1} depending on the athlete's aerobic fitness level (2). During resistance exercise, Q_c increases over the course of a workout. Similar to SV, the response is limited during CON actions but higher during ECC actions when analyzing individual reps (29). A compensatory increase in Q_c takes place during rest intervals when SV increases. Cardiac output remains elevated post aerobic exercise but is reduced following RE (40).

Blood Pressure Response

Blood pressure (BP) is controlled in different ways. Sympathetic nervous system activity increases vasoconstriction, which increases BP, and the parasympathetic nervous system has the opposite effect. Central command of the CV system stimulates the vasomotor center of the brainstem to alter BP. Feedback from sensory and motor centers in the brain stimulates CV centers to increase BP. Stretch-sensitive sensory receptors located in the walls of blood vessels (aortic arch and carotid sinuses) known as baroreceptors detect pressure and stimulate the brainstem to modulate BP via negative feedback control. Baroreceptors decrease BP in response to an increase in BP and prevent large elevations in BP during exercise (1). The renin-angiotensin system and the hormone aldosterone (discussed in Chapter 7) regulate BP. Renin leads to the activation of angiotensin II, which causes vasoconstriction. Aldosterone increases sodium retention, which increases BP.

BP increases during exercise. During steady-state aerobic exercise, SBP increases during the first several minutes but plateaus and/or slightly decreases when steady state is reached (1). Vasodilation reduces peripheral resistance so SBP may decline. DBP does not change much. During progressive aerobic exercise, SBP increases linearly as intensity increases, whereas DBP remains constant or decreases (1). SBP values of up to 250 mm Hg are seen in endurance athletes (2). Upper-body exercise increases SBP (by ~18–45 mm Hg) and DBP (by ~20–28 mm Hg) much more than lower-body exercise (1). Smaller muscle mass in the upper body provides greater resistance to blood flow thereby increasing BP to a greater extent. The increase in SBP helps assist in accelerating blood flow and fluid movement through the capillaries (2).

BP increases during RE with the increase proportional to effort. The response is dependent upon the use of the Valsalva maneuver, muscle mass activation, muscle action, and the intensity/duration of the set (29). Blood flow occlusion during muscle contraction increases BP. The increase is needed to overcome greater peripheral resistance. Mean BPs of 320/250 and 345/245 mm Hg may occur during a high-intensity leg press and squat, respectively, with a peak of 480/350 mm Hg shown (41). Mean SBP of 290–307 mm Hg and DBP of 220–238 mm Hg during the leg press (80%, 95%, and 100% of 1 RM) have been shown (42). Other studies showed SBP values of 198–230 mm Hg and DBP values of 160–170 mm Hg (29). Valsalva maneuvers increase BP response to RE and may be unavoidable when lifting weights ≥80% of 1 RM (41,43,44). Breath-holding increases intrathoracic (ITP) and intra-abdominal pressures (IAP), and cerebrovascular transmural pressure, and BP increases proportionally as a result (43,45,46). Some resistance exercises are more likely to raise ITP or IAP more than others. In a systematic review, Blazek et al. (43) showed that (a) the highest IAP was seen during squats (over 200 mm Hg), followed by dead lift, slide row, and leg press (161–176 mm Hg); (b) the lowest IAP was measured during the bench press (79 ± 44 mm Hg); (c) the clean and jerk was associated with high IAP (161–261 mm Hg) but large variation in the response; (d) the highest ITP was seen in the leg press, dead lift, and box lift (105–130 mm Hg) which were higher than the bench press (95 ± 37 mm Hg) and row (88 ± 32 mm Hg); and (e) IAP and ITP increased with loading. Other studies have shown that mean BP during a 1 RM leg press was 311/284 mm Hg with a Valsalva maneuver and 198/175 mm Hg without (47). Higher mean BP for the arm curl (166/112 vs. 148/101 mm Hg) and knee extension (166/108 vs. 151/99 mm Hg) occurred when Valsalva maneuvers were used (48).

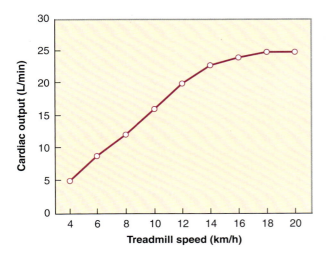

FIGURE 9.7 Cardiac output response to aerobic exercise. (Adapted with permission from Wilmore JH, Costill DL. *Physiology of Sport and Exercise*. 4th ed. Champaign (IL): Human Kinetics; 2008. 230 p.)

Muscle mass activation plays a role in the BP response. Mean BPs are greater during the leg press (320/250 mm Hg) than arm curl (255/190 mm Hg) (41). Higher BP is seen during squats than arm curls (46). The BP response is greater during the CON versus ECC phase of each rep and increases nonlinearly with the magnitude of active muscle mass (29,41). BP increases further during the exercise's sticking point (44). Many times the sticking point is where an exaggerated Valsalva maneuver may be used by the lifter. BP increases as sets progress. Gotshall et al. (49) had subjects perform 3 sets of the leg press for 10 reps and showed a progressive rise in SBP and DBP with each successive rep (Fig. 9.8). Peak SBP were 238, 268, and 293 mm Hg, respectively, for each set. However, it is clear from Figure 9.8 that BP recovers very quickly during the rest intervals when blood flow is restored to working muscles. Prolonged increases are not seen but only during active sets. Peak BP is higher when a set is performed to failure (41,42,50). Sets performed to failure at 70%–85% 1 RM produced a greater BP response than during a 1 RM leg press (51).

Blood pressure drops post exercise, a phenomenon known as **post exercise hypotension** (PEH). A number of factors contribute but appear, in part, as a response to decreased vascular resistance and prolonged vasodilation (due mostly to local factors including histamine release), reduced sympathetic and increased parasympathetic stimulation, and arterial baroreflex resetting following aerobic exercise (40). However, the PEH seen following RE may be due largely to attenuated cardiac output (from reduced stroke volume) as opposed to peripheral vasodilation (40).

SBP and DBP may be reduced by ~4–5 and 3 mm Hg over the subsequent 24-hour period with larger magnitudes of reduction seen during the first few hours post exercise (52). However, great variability in the responses are seen relating to the population (*e.g.*, hypertensive vs. healthy), training status, age, type of workout, time of day, and measurement environment and position (52). PEH occurs following aerobic and RE; however, the effect may be larger following aerobic exercise, *e.g.*, jogging (52). A meta-analysis showed that the PEH response (both SBP and DBP) was larger when exercise intensity and/or duration is higher, in younger individuals, and when more sets of RE are performed versus less (52). Carpio-Rivera et al. (52) reported that SBP dropped by an average of 1.6 mm Hg in athletes, and by 6.2, 3.4, and 7.3 mm Hg, respectively, following aerobic exercise, RE, and concurrent exercise. Intermittent and incremental workouts yielded larger SBP reductions than constant AE (7–11 vs. 4 mm Hg drop). Carpio-Rivera et al. (52) also reported that DBP dropped by an average of 2.7 mm Hg in athletes, and by 3.8, 2.7, and 2.9 mm Hg, respectively, following aerobic exercise, RE, and concurrent exercise. Similar reductions in SBP and DBP were seen between traditional and circuit RE workouts (52). During the first 10–60 minutes post RE, reductions in SBP, DBP, and MAP of 3–12 mm Hg, 6–18 mm Hg, and 7–16 mm Hg, respectively, have been shown with some reductions in DBP and MAP favoring a workout using 1- versus 2-minute rest intervals (53). Many studies have shown PEH following RE with a few studies showing PEH magnitude may depend on the interaction of volume and intensity of the workout (54,55), PEH is greater following total-body versus a split routine (upper or lower body only workout) (56), PEH is greater in higher versus lower-volume workouts (57,58), but may not be affected by the sequence of concurrent RT and AT (59), structure between traditional and super-set–based workouts (60), or the exercise sequence (61).

Plasma Volume

PV is reduced during exercise. PV reductions occur as fluid shifts from the blood to the interstitial spaces and intracellular domains. PV shifts take place as the BP increase forces water into the interstitial space and metabolic waste products build up in muscle (increasing *osmotic pressure*) causing a shift of fluid into muscle (2). Fluid loss from perspiration results in additional PV reductions. When PV decreases, RBCs increase via *hemoconcentration*, and this increases blood viscosity and reduces oxygen transport. PV reductions of up to 20% occur during endurance exercise. Reduced PV can impair endurance performance and VO$_2$max (62). SV is reduced as venous return decreases with fluid loss. Consequently, Q$_c$ and VO$_2$max are reduced. VO$_2$max correlates to PV (63); therefore, reductions in PV during an endurance exercise bout can lead to reduced performance.

A bout of RE decreases PV by 7%–14% (64) and in some cases by >20% immediately postexercise (65,66), with the magnitude dependent on intensity and duration (64). PV may almost fully recover within 30–60 minutes after exercise (65,67), especially when fluid intake accompanies the workout. PV reductions begin during the first set of the first exercise with a concomitant change in fluid regulatory factors such as renin, angiotensin II, and atrial peptide (68) and are affected by the type of program used. Craig et al. (69) showed a 22.6% PV reduction after 10 RM workout (3 sets of nine exercises) versus a 13% reduction after a 5 RM workout. Ploutz-Snyder et al. (65) examined a 6 × 10 squat protocol with 2-minute rest intervals

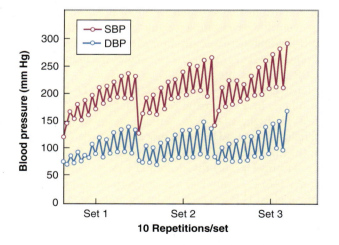

FIGURE 9.8 Blood pressure response to 3 sets of the leg press exercise. SBP, systolic blood pressure; DBP, diastolic blood pressure. (From Gotshall RW, Gootman J, Byrnes WC, Fleck SJ, Valovich TC. Noninvasive characterization of the blood pressure response to the double-leg press exercise. *J Exerc Physiol.* 1999;2:1–6.)

and showed a 22% PV reduction. Muscle CSA of thigh muscles increased by 5%–10% and correlated highly with PV reductions. Fluid shifts correspond to acute muscle size expansion seen during resistance exercise, *e.g.*, a muscle "pump."

Oxygen Consumption

Oxygen consumption, or VO$_2$, increases proportionally during exercise in relation to intensity, muscle mass activation, and degree of continuity (as shown in Chapter 8). Oxygen consumption is represented by the Fick equation, which states that VO$_2$ = Q$_c$ × A-VO$_2$ difference. The structural hierarchy of the circulatory system is as follows:

> large arteries → smaller arteries →
> arterioles → metarterioles → capillary beds →
> venules → small veins → large veins.

Oxygen diffuses through capillary membranes into tissues. The A-VO$_2$ difference is the amount of oxygen in the arterial side versus the venous side and represents tissue oxygen extraction. At rest, arterial oxygen content is ~20 mL of O$_2$ per 100 mL of blood (2). However, this value drops to ~15–16 mL of O$_2$ per 100 mL of blood as blood passes through capillaries into venules (Fig. 9.9). At rest, this value is ~4–5 mL of O$_2$ per 100 mL of blood (2). The A-VO$_2$ difference can increase up to ~15–16 mL of O$_2$ per 100 mL of blood or more during endurance exercise (2). The increase reflects greater oxygen extraction from arterial blood into skeletal muscles. The combination of the increased Q$_c$ and oxygen extraction leads to an increase in VO$_2$ during exercise.

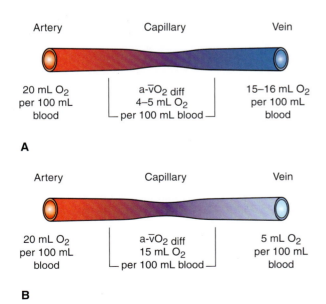

FIGURE 9.9 The A-VO$_2$ difference. **A.** The A-VO$_2$ difference at rest. **B.** The A-VO$_2$ difference during exercise. (Reprinted with permission from Wilmore JH, Costill DL. *Physiology of Sport and Exercise*. 2nd ed. Champaign (IL): Human Kinetics; 1999. 256 p.)

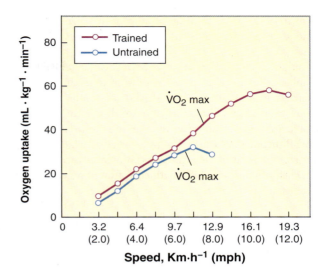

FIGURE 9.10 Relationship between exercise intensity and oxygen consumption. (Reprinted with permission from Wilmore JH, Costill DL. *Physiology of Sport and Exercise*. 2nd ed. Champaign (IL): Human Kinetics; 1999. 140 p.)

VO$_2$ increases during exercise (Fig. 9.10). A linear rise in VO$_2$ is seen with increasing intensity. Increasing the speed of movement, level of inclination (or using a more compliant surface), adding resistance, or increasing the amount of muscular involvement (adding arm exercise to a lower-body exercise modality) during endurance exercise yields proportional increases in oxygen consumption. VO$_2$ increases during anaerobic exercise. However, the lower level of continuity produces abrupt fluctuations. VO$_2$ will rise abruptly during and immediately following a maximal sprint but declines soon thereafter during the rest period. VO$_2$ fluctuates during resistance exercise where short rest intervals yield a greater sustained rise; however, long rest intervals yield an initial abrupt increase but a prolonged period of decline during recovery (28). The limited continuity poses great challenges for increasing VO$_2$max. VO$_2$ during RE increases with higher intensities, short rest intervals, large muscle mass exercises, and slow to moderate repetition velocities. A bodybuilding lower-body workout (multiple sets, squats, leg press and other lower-body exercises, 6–12 reps, with <2 min rest intervals) produces an increase in VO$_2$ to only ~45%–60% of VO$_2$max (70), usually below the threshold needed to increase VO$_2$max in trained to highly trained populations. High-intensity interval training workouts yield large increases in oxygen consumption (30) as does battling rope exercise (31,32).

Chronic Adaptations at Rest and During Exercise

Aerobic and anaerobic training lead to comprehensive changes to the CV system at rest. Dr. Joel Morganroth proposed in the mid-1970s that training produced two general types of overload, pressure, and volume overload. *Pressure overload* results from the rise in BP and intrathoracic pressure that accompany exercise. Pressure overload can alter several CV variables positively over time in addition to leading to changes in cardiac musculature. *Volume overload* results from greater venous return and blood flow to the heart during exercise. Aerobic exercise is superior for volume overload due to the higher level of continuity. Volume overload leads to positive changes in several CV variables and increases cardiac chamber size. These changes not only alter CV function at rest but also acute responses to exercise.

Cardiac Dimensions

Training leads to cardiac muscle alterations. Adaptations are thought to be governed by the *Law of Laplace*, which states that wall tension is proportional to pressure and size of the radius of curvature (39). Greater heart size is characterized by greater left ventricular (LV) cavity (*eccentric hypertrophy*) and thickening of cardiac walls (*concentric hypertrophy*). Myocardial overload and stretch via exercise stimulates higher rates of protein synthesis leading to hypertrophy (1). Cardiac muscle fibers become more sensitive to calcium and contract stronger when stretched leading to greater contractility (1). Volume overload results in an increase in sarcomeres in series (greater chamber size and end-diastolic volumes), whereas pressure overload increases the number of sarcomeres in parallel (greater wall thickness). The LV is the primary chamber studied with respect to exercise although more studies recently have examined the right ventricle. Large changes in LV structure take place with smaller changes affecting the left atrium. A meta-analysis showed that endurance athletes had greater right ventricular (RV) mass, EDV, and stroke volume compared to untrained individuals (71). A study in untrained middle-aged men showed that HIIT and continuous AT increased RV EDV and ESV within 2 weeks of training (72). Another study showed that endurance athletes and strength athletes had similar RV wall thickness with both groups exhibiting greater RV wall thickness than untrained individuals (73). Lastly, cardiac structure is related to body surface area, so changes in cardiac mass may accompany changes in lean tissue mass (71).

Aerobic training leads to comprehensive improvements in cardiac function. In untrained individuals, changes in chamber size occur early with modest changes in wall thickness (76). One study reported increases in LV mass, LV mass index, and LV EDV within the first 6 months of endurance training in previously untrained individuals (77). Cross-sectional comparisons between endurance athletes, strength/power athletes, and nonathletes are difficult because athletes from many sports embark upon endurance, sprint/plyometric, and RT. That concern notwithstanding, cardiac dimensions in athletes are greater than nonathletes having 10% greater chamber size and 15%–20% greater wall thicknesses (76). Naylor et al. (76) reviewed >40 studies and reported that endurance athletes had greater LV mass (25 of 27 studies), posterior wall thickness (25 of 32 studies), interventricular septal wall thickness (19 of 28 studies), and LV cavity dimensions (27 of 32 studies) than control subjects. Another study showed that endurance athletes had greater LV EDV (~149.4 vs. 118.2 mL), greater peak velocity blood flow from LV relaxation in early diastole, but similar ESV values compared to a group of strength athletes (26). Critical

Myths & Misconceptions
Cardiac Muscle Hypertrophy Only Occurs as a Result of Cardiovascular Disease

Heart size and chamber volume increase during training mostly in the LV. These changes are positive; however, at one time, they were viewed as negative. Because hypertrophy of cardiac muscle occurs as a consequence of CV disease, some associated all hypertrophy as negative. However, investigations of the hearts of athletes revealed hypertrophy independent of CV disease. This concept of the *athlete's heart* is associated with positive CV effects (greater SV and Q_c). Changes in resting function can be attributed, in part, to cardiac muscle hypertrophy. The size of the heart increases as body size increases. There has been some difficulty in quantifying changes in cardiac hypertrophy independent of body mass changes during RT. Often, cardiac muscle mass changes will be expressed relative to body surface area or body mass. These concerns notwithstanding, aerobic and anaerobic training positively increase cardiac muscle size. An issue facing cardiologists or team doctors is how to discern exercise-induced cardiac remodeling from *hypertrophic*

cardiomyopathy, which is the leading cause of exercise-related sudden cardiac death in athletes who had an underlying CV disease that was not diagnosed (74). Hypertrophic cardiomyopathy affects around 1:500 individuals, with most cases caused by genetic mutations often in cardiac sarcomere protein genes (75). Some physicians have used advanced imaging and echocardiographic techniques to try to distinguish between the types during examination. Diagnostic tools such as LV wall thickness cut-off values (*i.e.*, >15 mm), nonconcentric LV hypertrophy, small LV cavity size, lateral ECG changes, assessment of low strain and strain rate, and delayed LV diastolic untwisting have been used as criteria for concern (74,75). However, some athletes experience a level of adaptation that overlaps between physiological and pathological adaptation (sometimes referred to as a "gray area" such as LV thickness of 12–13 mm) thereby making it difficult in some cases to discern a potential problem (74,75).

to the increased LV EDV is reduced pericardial restraint and greater compliance seen in trained endurance athletes (78). Training volume positively increases LV mass in endurance athletes (76). Some studies showed greater LV mass increases during AT than RT, whereas others have shown no differences or greater LV mass in resistance-trained athletes (76). One study showed that strength athletes had greater septal (11.3 vs. 9.7 mm) and posterior wall (11.6 vs. 9.2 mm) thickness compared to a group of endurance athletes but both groups of athletes had similar LV mass index, *i.e.*, ~63–65 g·m^{-2} (26). Powerlifters were shown to have greater LV mass, posterior wall thickness, and septal wall thickness than endurance athletes (27). Different techniques have been used to measure cardiac chamber thickness, which may explain some of the noted contrasting findings; a meta-analysis concluded that AT and RT may induce similar changes in LV wall thickness (71). Female long-distance runners have greater LV wall thickness, mass, and interventricular septal thickness than sprinters (79). In addition, some data indicate greater left atrium (LA) diameter and volume index in endurance athletes compared to strength athletes (26,27).

RT leads to changes in cardiac muscularity; however, these changes rarely exceed the upper normal levels of cardiac wall thickness/mass and are less in magnitude than individuals with CV disease (29). Spence et al. (77) showed that no significant increases in LV mass were present in previously untrained men following the first 6 months of RT. In the long-term, resistance-trained individuals have absolute greater LV wall thickness and interventricular septal thickness than untrained individuals (29,38). However, relative changes (to body mass or surface area) are small or nonexistent (29). Elite junior weightlifters have greater absolute and relative LV wall thickness and mass than untrained controls (80,81). However, other studies showed no such relative changes (42). Although the increased BP and ITP during lifting is attributed to concentric hypertrophy, some have argued that the pressure rise is counterbalanced by reduced *transmural pressure* (LV pressure minus ITP) thereby reducing potential training effects (independent of body size changes) (42,45). Nevertheless, absolute increases in cardiac thickness occur during RT. Bodybuilders have high LV mass and wall thickness (29); however, many bodybuilders perform AT to reduce body fat. Anabolic steroid use was not controlled for in some studies and could have contributed to LV mass changes as steroid users may have greater LV posterior and septal wall thickness than drug-free lifters (82). Most cardiac muscle thickness increases are brought about by changes in LBM. The training program determines potential cardiac changes, *i.e.*, the intensity, volume, muscle mass activation, and rest intervals.

Traditional RT elicits very small to no changes in LV cavity size as chamber size increases respond to volume overload. Some studies have shown lifters to have larger chamber size than untrained controls (29,83), whereas others have shown no differences (42,77). Expression of chamber size relative to body surface area or LBM reduces the increases seen in lifters (29). Bodybuilders, but not weightlifters, may have greater LV chamber volume than controls (84) possibly due to integrated training.

Cardiac Output

The CV system adapts by augmenting the Q_c response to exercise. Aerobic training has a profound influence on SV. Resting and exercise-induced SV are enhanced. One study reported resting SV of ~98.4 mL in a group of endurance athletes (26). Untrained individuals possess a SV response of 80–110 mL to exercise; however, trained and highly trained endurance athletes possess a SV response of 130–150 mL and 160 to >220 mL during exercise, respectively (2). Aerobic training leads to greater PV and end-diastolic volume. Coupled with greater cardiac contractility, elastic recoil, and reduced HR (to enhance filling time), SV increases in aerobically trained individuals allowing more blood pumped per beat (2). Ejection fraction during exercise may increase (2). Greater end-diastolic volume with similar end-systolic volume yields a greater SV response. RT may have limited impact on resting SV and ejection fraction during the first 6 months (77).

Aerobic training reduces resting HR. An untrained individual may have a resting HR of 60–80 beats per minute on average. However, AT reduces resting HR to <60 beats per minute, and some elite endurance athletes have a resting HR of <35 beats per minute (2). One study reported a group of endurance athletes at a mean resting HR of 52.1 beats per minute, whereas a group of strength athletes had a resting HR of ~69 beats per minute (26). The reduced resting HR is due to greater parasympathetic or reduced sympathetic nervous system stimulation. Aerobic training leads to a reduced HR response to submaximal exercise (Fig. 9.11) and a quicker recovery of HR immediately after exercise. Because SV is increased, HR does not need to increase much to attain a threshold Q_c. However, the HR response to maximal exercise is constant. Although some endurance athletes have maximal HR lower than age-matched controls, often maximal HR remains similar during AT (2).

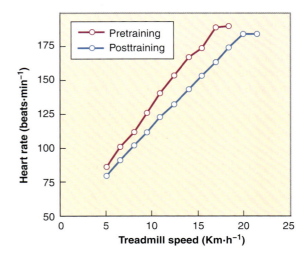

FIGURE 9.11 Heart rate response during exercise before and after training. (Reprinted with permission from Wilmore JH, Costill DL. *Physiology of Sport and Exercise.* 2nd ed. Champaign (IL): Human Kinetics; 1999.)

When coupled together (greater SV and similar maximal HR), Q_c increases with improved fitness. Elite endurance athletes have $Q_c > 30$ L·min^{-1} during maximal exercise (2).

Resting SV may slightly increase or not change (expressed relative to LBM) during RT (29). A group of strength athletes were shown to have normal resting SV of ~69 mL (26). SV is related to body size. Muscle hypertrophy is a stimulus for SV increases, and SV increases during exercise after RT. Strength-trained athletes have greater SV responses and ejection fraction increases during static exercise than controls (38,85). During each rep, SV falls (as ITP increases when a Valsalva maneuver is present) during the CON and ECC phases by nearly 20 mL but returns to baseline during the intraset rest interval (86). However, SV rises higher than resting level during rest intervals between exercises. The response is augmented in strength athletes but far less than that observed in endurance athletes.

Resting HR may not change or slightly decrease during RT. Short-term RT studies have shown reduced resting HR of 4%–13% (29). The largest effects occur in individuals who have below-average aerobic conditioning. The program is critical as more continuous types of programs, *e.g.*, circuit weight training, reduce resting HR (87), and increase VO$_2$max (88,89). Nevertheless, any potential HR reduction from RT is much lower than AT. Junior and senior Olympic weightlifters, powerlifters, and bodybuilders had resting HR ranging from 60 to 78 beats per minute, which was similar to or slightly lower than matched controls (29). Greater reductions in resting HR occur when AT is performed in addition to RT. After RT, the HR response to exercise is decreased for a given submaximal workload (29). The reduction in exercise HR occurs for RT and other exercise modalities such as walking and cycling (29). Bodybuilders have lower HR during submaximal and maximal lifting compared to lesser-trained individuals and controls (51). These data show that RT lessens the stress to the heart during regular physical activity. The culmination of HR and SV data indicate that RT increases the capacity to increase Q_c during exercise but to a lesser extent than AT.

Several studies have shown that AT can increase HRV at rest. The increase in HRV reflects greater cardiac parasympathetic tone at rest (indicative of reduced cardiac stress) and is thought to be an adaptation that may lower CV risks and improve autonomic function at rest and following exercise (36). Levy et al. (90) showed that 6 months of AT increased HRV by 68% in older men and by 17% in young men. Concurrent AT and RT increases resting HRV and poses less of a reduction during the postexercise period indicative of improved recovery ability (36). RT may have minimal effects on resting HRV over time in healthy individuals (37). In athletes, HRV can be used as a training and recovery monitoring tool (25). Athletes of different sports have shown an overall increase in HRV and parasympathetic cardiac modulation compared to untrained individuals (25). This was confirmed in a meta-analysis where athletes were shown to have a small increase in HRV at rest and a moderate increase in postexercise HRV indicating an increase in postexercise parasympathetic HR modulation as a positive training adaptation (91).

VO$_2$ Max

VO$_2$max is the gold standard of aerobic fitness and increases during training due to increases in SV (and Q_c) and a small increase in the A-VO$_2$ difference (up to 20 vol% or 15%) (1,92). Aerobic training is the preferred mode of exercise for increasing VO$_2$max. Aerobic training leads to VO$_2$max increases of 10%–30% during the first 6 months (92). Endurance athletes possess higher VO$_2$max than anaerobic or mixed athletes. Figure 9.12 shows that male endurance athletes (cross-country skiers, distance runners, and cyclists) have higher VO$_2$max values than do mixed athletes (soccer and basketball players) and strength athletes (bodybuilders, powerlifters, and weightlifters). Elite athletes Bjorn Daehlie (retired Olympic champion cross-country skier), Lance Armstrong (multi Tour de France winner), and Greg LeMond (retired multi Tour de France winner) had VO$_2$max values of 96, 84, and 92.5 mL·kg^{-1}·min^{-1}, respectively. Several factors influence VO$_2$max, such as exercise mode (VO$_2$max is higher during treadmill tests than cycling or swimming), gender

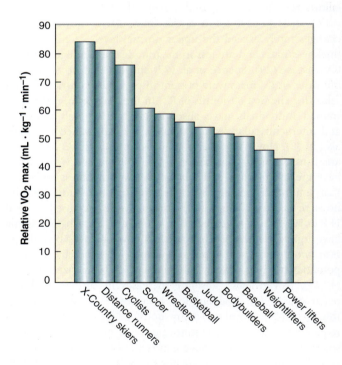

FIGURE 9.12 Comparison of VO$_2$max data from different male athletes. (Data compiled from McArdle WD, Katch FI, Katch VL. *Exercise Physiology: Energy, Nutrition, and Human Performance*. 6th ed. Philadelphia (PA): Lippincott Williams & Wilkins; 2007. p. 314–63; Hoffman JR. *Norms for Fitness, Performance, and Health*. Champaign (IL): Human Kinetics; 2006. p. 67–80; Häkkinen K, Alen M, Komi PV. Neuromuscular, anaerobic, and aerobic performance characteristics of elite power athletes. *Eur J Appl Physiol Occup Physiol*. 1984;53: 97–105; MacFarlane N, Northridge DB, Wright AR, Grant S, Dargie HJ. A comparative study of left ventricular structure and function in elite athletes. *Br J Sports Med*. 1991;25:45–8; Raven PB, Gettman LR, Pollock ML, Cooper KH. A physiological evaluation of professional soccer players. *Br J Sports Med*. 1976;10: 209–16.)

(women have VO₂max values 15%–30% lower than men due to less muscle mass, higher body fat, less testosterone, and lower hemoglobin), age (VO₂max declines with age), body size, and genetics (1). Highest VO₂max values in athletes are seen during the specific mode by which they train. Genetics contribute ~20%–50% to VO₂max (1,92). High-intensity interval training for 3–15 weeks has been shown to increase VO₂max by 4%–26% with the improvements similar, smaller, or larger than continuous AT (93). A meta-analysis has shown a large HIIT effect on VO₂max with largest increases in individuals with lower levels of fitness, and VO₂max increases with HIIT are comparable to continuous AT when longer repetitions are used (93).

Anaerobic training has minimal effects on increasing VO₂max. Weightlifters and powerlifters have VO₂max values similar to or slightly larger than untrained individuals although one study reported a mean VO₂max of ~34 mL·kg⁻¹·min⁻¹ in powerlifters (27). In comparison, bodybuilders have larger VO₂max values than other lifters (94) because bodybuilders train with short rest intervals and often aerobically train. RT with long rest intervals allows HR recovery between sets and rarely reaches a threshold VO₂ level needed to increase VO₂max in trained individuals. RT may increase VO₂max in populations with low levels of aerobic fitness. Olympic weightlifting programs (29,95) and circuit weight training can increase VO₂max by up to 8% (88,89). However, if RT elicits an increased VO₂max, the magnitude is far less than AT. The combination of RT and AT increases VO₂max Performing RT lessens the volume of AT needed to increase VO₂max (96). Programs of moderate to high intensity, high volume, large muscle mass exercises, and short rest intervals may slightly improve VO₂max. Metabolic RT programs (using bodyweight exercises, weight training, or multimodal approaches) 4–6 weeks in duration can increase VO₂max by 7%–11% (97–99). Sprint training can increase VO₂max (100). Concurrent AT and RT increases VO₂max when they are performed separately or when combined into a single workout, *e.g.*, using the cardioacceleration method (34).

Blood Pressure

Aerobic training may lead to reduced SBP and DBP at rest (2). An individual with normal BP may or may not experience a reduction in BP following endurance training, but a hypertensive individual most likely will see reductions. In the American College of Sports Medicine (ACSM) Position Stand on Exercise and Hypertension (106), it was concluded on an abundance of research that BP decreases following AT although the adaptations are quite variable. These studies reported that SBP drops ~3.4–4.7 mm Hg and DBP drops ~2.4–3.1 mm Hg, with the largest drops seen in hypertensive groups. The mechanisms involved are not completely understood. However, alterations in sodium excretion, decreased peripheral resistance, improved vasodilation, and reduced sympathetic nervous system activity and catecholamine release play substantial roles (2,106). The BP

Sidebar	Limitations of VO₂ Max

One topic of debate in the exercise sciences is the question, what factors limit VO₂max? Everyone has an upper limit to VO₂max and debate has centered on factors limiting VO₂max. Central and peripheral factors have been identified and some have argued for central, whereas some have argued for peripheral limitations (101). Central factors entail limitations in oxygen delivery and include Q$_c$ (estimated to account for ~70%–85% of limitation), SV (due to pericardial restraint), oxygen-carrying capacity, and arterial saturation (102). Oxygen delivery can limit VO₂max. Beginning in the lungs, a limitation with alveolar diffusion of oxygen from the atmosphere to hemoglobin in the blood reduces oxygen delivery to mitochondria. Some highly trained endurance athletes experience arterial desaturation during maximal exercise to ~87%, which is 5% lower than expected. This reduction decreased VO₂max by ~5 mL·kg⁻¹·min⁻¹ (103) but only accounts for VO₂max limitations in trained athletes. Mechanical limits to ventilation that are reached in conjunction with attainment of VO₂max occur in endurance athletes; the greater the ventilatory response, the greater the degree of mechanical limitation (104). Expiratory flow limitations can reduce hyperventilation and may limit pulmonary function during maximal exercise (105). Limitations on SV and Q$_c$ limit VO₂max. Comparative studies between one- and two-leg and arm exercise showed that muscle blood flow was limited when large amounts of

muscle mass were activated (showing Q$_c$ could not keep up with the demand). Blood doping increases VO₂max showing oxygen-carrying capacity and blood volumes are limitations.

Peripheral factors entail oxygen transfer from the capillary bed to the mitochondria and include A-VO₂ difference, mitochondrial number and enzyme activity, and capillary density. Oxygen extraction from blood requires dissociation from hemoglobin, diffusion of oxygen from RBCs into muscle fibers, and diffusion and transport of oxygen to the mitochondria. Myoglobin facilitates oxygen dissociation from hemoglobin (in addition to the PO₂ gradient) as myoglobin's affinity for oxygen is approximately five times greater than hemoglobin. Some have argued that in highly trained aerobic athletes, blood flow rate is so great that blood passes by muscle too rapidly to allow for optimal oxygen diffusion. High rates of blood flow may limit saturation as blood moves too quickly through the pulmonary circulation. This effect may be minimal, however, as capillary density increases, which increases surface area for diffusion and controls blood flow velocity. Lastly, the number and size of mitochondria, as well as mitochondrial enzyme activity, play critical roles (2). Because AT increases mitochondrial size, density, and enzyme activity, the athlete's ability to utilize oxygen increases. It seems that no one single factor limits VO₂max, but all contribute.

response to submax and maximal exercise may not change or only be slightly reduced by 6–7 mm Hg during submaximal exercise (106). World-class endurance runners have similar acute SBP responses to untrained individuals (~205–210 mm Hg) during maximal exercise but have lower DBP values (~65 vs. 80 mm Hg) (2). The ACSM recommends at least moderate intensity (40%–60% of VO_2 reserve) continuous or intermittent aerobic exercise for 30 min·day^{-1} to reduce BP (106). HIIT can improve blood pressure with the effects comparable with those resulting from continuous, moderate-intensity AT (107).

RT may not affect or reduce resting BP. Reductions in SBP and MAP have been shown during the first 6 months of RT in untrained individuals (77). Strength-trained athletes have average or below-average resting BP (29). Powerlifters were shown to have resting BP of ~130/82 mm Hg compared to 116/72 mm Hg in endurance athletes (27). A meta-analysis of the RT literature has shown that SBP and DBP may be reduced by 2%–4% (108,109). Another meta-analysis has shown that isometric RT decreases SBP by ~5 mm Hg, DBP by ~1.6 mm Hg, and MAP by ~3 mm Hg (110). The ACSM concludes that RT decreases BP in adults (106) but not quite to the extent of AT. A small 3 mm Hg reduction in BP decreases the risk of CV disease by 5%–9% and stroke by 8%–14% (106). The rate pressure product (HR × SBP) is used to estimate myocardial work and decreases after RT (29). This indicates that the LV performs less work over time and is a positive adaptation (29). After RT, the acute BP response to exercise is lower (29,39). Concurrent AT and RT can decrease SBP and DBP when performed in sequence or combined into a single workout (34).

Blood Volume

Aerobic training increases blood volume, or hypervolemia, mostly from an increase in plasma (2). PV increases 12%–20% within the first few weeks of AT with noticeable increases taking place after the first workout (1). Endurance athletes have blood volumes ~35% greater than untrained individuals (1). The PV increase is attributed to hormonal changes (aldosterone and ADH) and increased protein content in the blood, which increases the osmotic pressure forcing greater fluid

movement (2). RBC content may increase, which contributes to the greater blood volume. PV expands more than the RBC number increases, thereby leading to a decrease in hematocrit (39). The increased blood volume, along with greater capillary density, vasodilation, and more effective blood redistribution, contributes to greater blood flow to working skeletal muscles in endurance-trained athletes (2). Aerobic training reduces blood flow to muscles during submaximal exercise (due to greater oxidative potential and vasodilation of skeletal muscles) and increases blood flow during maximal exercise (due to greater Q_c, redistribution of blood, and increased capillary density and arteriogenesis) (1). The increased blood volume is a critical adaptation that allows SV to increase via the Frank-Starling mechanism. A substantial reduction in PV expansion can be observed within 1 week of detraining (1). Less is known concerning hypervolemia following RT although it is thought that RT may have a limited effect.

Blood Lipids and Lipoproteins

Lipids perform several critical functions including energy storage and liberation, protection, insulation, providing structure to cell membranes, vitamin transport, and cellular signaling. Circulating blood lipids and lipoproteins are major factors for CV health. These include triglycerides (glycerol backbone with three fatty acids), cholesterol, low-density lipoprotein cholesterol (LDL-C), very low-density lipoprotein cholesterol (VLDL-C), high-density lipoprotein cholesterol (HDL-C), and lipoprotein A. Cholesterol plays several critical roles including serving as a precursor in steroid synthesis, cell membrane structure, and bile and vitamin D synthesis. However, elevated cholesterol is a risk factor for CV disease. Lipoproteins provide the major means lipids are transported in the blood. Elevations in LDL-C (carry ~60%–80% of total cholesterol) and VLDL-C (transport triglycerides to muscle and adipose tissue and contain the highest lipid component) pose major risk factors, whereas elevations in HDL-C lower the risk for CV disease. Lipoprotein A is thought to play a role in coagulation but at high levels is atherogenic. Triglyceride levels of <150 mg·dL^{-1}, total cholesterol levels <200 mg·dL^{-1}, LDL-C < 100 mg·dL^{-1}, HDL-C

Myths & Misconceptions
Resistance Training Is Bad for the Heart and Leads to Hypertension

In the past, some have criticized RT as having negative CV effects on the heart. The evidence overwhelming supports RT as having positive benefits for the heart. Because of the pressure overload, changes in cardiac wall thickness enable individuals to tolerate greater stress. The heart becomes stronger and more resistant to stress. Although the adaptations are less comprehensive than AT, concentric hypertrophy poses health and wellness benefits to the individual. Some feared RT due to the myth that it causes chronic elevated BP or hypertension. As eloquently stated in the ACSM's position stand (106),

RT at the very least will cause no change or can decrease resting BP over time. Although an acute rise in BP is observed during a workout (via a rise in ITP and peripheral resistance), the heart adapts to where BP can be reduced following and be lower over time during physical activity. Although BP may increase at rest in individuals who use anabolic steroids or are overtrained, these are exceptions and not the norm. Overwhelming evidence supports RT as safe and beneficial for the CV system and is recommended in some form by the ACSM for essentially all healthy and clinical populations.

> 40 mg·dL^{-1}, and lipoprotein A <14 mg·dL^{-1} are recommended values for minimizing risk factors for CV disease (1).

Several factors influence blood lipid and lipoprotein content including genetics. Diet is the major factor for increasing HDLs and decreasing LDLs and VLDLs. High dietary fiber intake, mono- and polyunsaturated fats, low saturated and *trans* fat intake, and low alcohol consumption positively affect blood lipid and lipoprotein levels. Reducing stress and eliminating cigarette smoking have substantial positive effects. Blood lipid and lipoprotein levels are coupled with changes in body weight, so weight reduction is critical to lowering blood lipids (2). Exercise produces favorable changes and reduces risk factors for CV disease (independent of weight loss). Reductions in total cholesterol, triglycerides, and LDL-C with concomitant increases in HDL-C occur following AT (2), whereas some studies have shown minimal changes. The increases in HDL-C appear more responsive to AT than LDL-C reductions (1). The ratio of LDL-C to total cholesterol/HDL-C (a major CV risk factor) decreases following AT (2). A dose-response relationship is seen where a threshold of exercise volume/duration is needed. Some suggest that the threshold may be ~15–20 miles per week or 1200–2200 kcal of energy expenditure per week (111). This exercise level is associated with 2–3 mg·dL^{-1} increases in HDL-C and 8–20 mg·dL^{-1} reductions in blood triglycerides (111). Higher levels of AT may produce more substantial changes as aerobic athletes (with high Vo$_2$max) have much higher HDL-C and lower blood triglycerides than nonathletes (2,111). Lipoprotein A does not change during training or dietary changes; however, distance runners and bodybuilders have shown elevations (112).

RT may have no or very small effects in improving blood lipid and lipoprotein profiles. RT may increase HDL-C by 10%–15%, decrease LDL-C by 5%–39%, decrease total cholesterol by 3%–16%, or produce no changes or slight increases in LDL-C (29). Strength-trained athletes have normal, lower, or higher HDL-C, LDL-C, and total cholesterol (29). Several confounding variables are thought to influence these results. Some studies did not adequately control for diet or weight loss. Cross-sectional studies cannot eliminate other factors such as AT. Bodybuilders have lower total cholesterol, LDL-C, and VLDL-C compared to weight-matched controls (113), and powerlifters have lower HDL-C and higher LDL-C than bodybuilders and runners (114). However, bodybuilders perform AT, so it is difficult to ascertain how much of a role AT played in these results. Anabolic steroid (alone and in combination with human growth hormone) use increases LDL-C by up to 61%, total cholesterol, decrease HDL-C by up to 55%, increase LDL-C to HDL-C ratio by more than 300% (114–117), and increases coronary artery calcification (115) with the negative effects reversed upon discontinuation in a time frame dependent on the magnitude and duration of steroid use (118,119). Other lipoproteins (lipoprotein-A) and *apolipoprotein* variants (proteins that bind to fats to form lipoproteins) are negatively affected by anabolic steroid use (118). Independent effects of RT do not change or slightly improve blood lipid and lipoprotein profiles. It is thought that RT volume plays a significant role, similar to AT, as reductions have been seen during high-volume phases (29). The best way to improve lipid and lipoprotein profiles is to combine proper diet with AT and RT.

Case Study 9.1

Ben is a high school soccer player who is going to begin an off-season strength and conditioning program. The program consists of total-body RT for 2 days per week and endurance training (running) for 3 days per week. He was told that RT and AT would yield positive benefits to his heart and would increase his stamina on the field. However, Ben is an inquisitive student athlete and was searching for a response that was more specific and physiologically based.

Question for Consideration: How would you describe the CV benefits of strength and endurance training to Ben?

The Respiratory System

The respiratory system is essential for introducing oxygen into the body and removing CO_2. Respiration includes breathing, pulmonary diffusion, oxygen transport, and gas exchange (Fig. 9.13). Breathing brings air into and out of the lungs. The average-size adult's lungs weigh ~1 kg and can hold ~4–6 L of air (1). Air enters the body through the nose or mouth and travels through the pharynx, larynx, trachea, bronchi, bronchioles, and the alveoli. The alveoli are sites of gas exchange. Inspiration is an active event that leads to air entering the lungs. Several muscles contract but inspiration is largely due to contraction of the diaphragm and external intercostal muscles. The diaphragm is a large dome-shaped muscle that provides airtight separation between the thoracic and abdominal cavities. During exercise, several other rib cage and abdominal muscles contract to support forced breathing. Muscle contraction causes the ribs to move up and out thereby expanding the thorax. The diaphragm contracts, flattens, and moves as much as 10 cm (1). The pressure in the lungs decreases (as space increases) causing air from the outside to enter. A pressure gradient is formed where the pressure in the lungs (*intrapulmonary pressure*) is lower than the pressure outside of the body. The pressure gradient allows air to move into the lungs. At the end of inspiration, the pressure in the lungs and outside of the body equilibrates. Expiration is a passive process (at rest) where air exits the lungs and the body. During expiration, inspiratory muscles relax, the diaphragm rises (relaxes), and the thorax is depressed as air exits. The lung pressure is greater than the pressure outside of the body. Air exits and is greatly enhanced by elastic recoil of the lungs. The lungs contain *surfactant*, which reduces surface tension on the alveoli and increases lung compliance. During exercise, other muscles (*e.g.*, abdominal muscles) contract for forced breathing. Air enters the alveoli where gas exchange takes place. Pulmonary diffusion involves the diffusion of

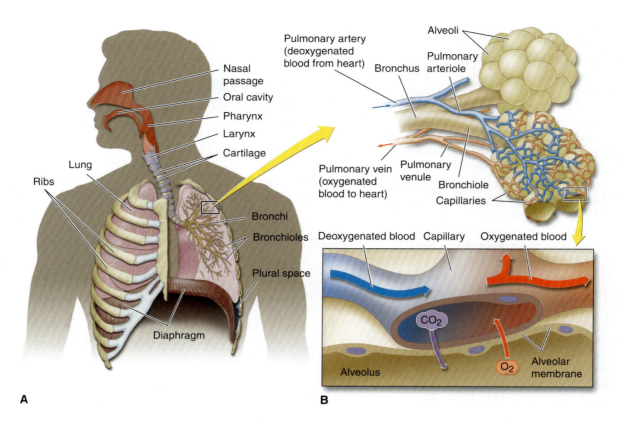

FIGURE 9.13 The human respiratory system. **A.** Major pulmonary structures. **B.** Respiratory passages, alveoli, and gas exchange within the alveoli. (From McArdle WD, Katch FI, Katch VL. *Exercise Physiology: Nutrition, Energy, and Human Performance*. 7th ed. Baltimore (MD): Lippincott Williams & Wilkins; 2010.)

oxygen from the alveoli into the pulmonary capillaries across the thin (0.5–4.0 μm) respiratory membrane. The lungs contain >600 million alveoli with a large blood supply and have thin walls that greatly expand the opportunity for gas exchange (1).

Lung Volumes and Capacities

Several lung volumes and capacities are used to measure lung function. These include the following:

- *Tidal volume*: volume of air inspired or expired every breath (~500 mL in women and ~600 mL in men)
- *Inspiratory reserve volume*: volume of air inspired after normal tidal volume (~1,900 mL in women and ~3,000 mL in men)
- *Expiratory reserve volume*: volume of air expired after normal tidal volume (~800 mL in women and ~1,200 mL in men)
- *Residual volume*: volume of air left in lungs after maximal expiration (~1,000 mL in women and ~1,200 mL in men)
- *Total lung capacity*: volume of air in lungs after maximal inspiration (~4,200 mL in women and ~6,000 mL in men)
- *Forced vital capacity*: maximal volume of air expired after maximal inspiration (~3,200 mL in women and ~4,800 mL in men)
- *Inspiratory capacity*: maximal volume of air after tidal volume expiration (~2,400 mL in women and ~3,600 mL in men)

- *Functional residual capacity*: volume of air in lungs after tidal volume expiration (~1,800 mL in women and ~2,400 mL in men)
- *Forced expiratory volume (FEV_1)*: volume of air maximally expired forcefully in 1 second after maximal inhalation. Often expressed relative to forced vital capacity and is typically ~85%.
- *Maximum voluntary ventilation (MVV)*: maximum volume of air breathed rapidly in 1 minute or number of maximal breaths in 15 seconds extrapolated to 1 minute (~80–120 $L \cdot min^{-1}$ in women and 140–180 $L \cdot min^{-1}$ in men).
- *Minute ventilation (V_E)*: volume of air breathed per minute; is the product of breathing rate and tidal volume. At rest, is typically 6 $L \cdot min^{-1}$ (12 breaths·$min^{-1} \times 0.5$ L). During exercise, breathing rate may increase to 35–45 breaths·min^{-1} to healthy adults but may increase to 60–70 breaths·min^{-1} in elite endurance athletes (1,33). Tidal volume increases during exercise up to 2.0 L or more leading to V_E increases of 100 $L \cdot min^{-1}$ or more (1,33). Peak tidal volumes of ~2.6 L have been shown during HIIT (33). At high exercise intensities, an increase in breathing rate more than tidal volume accounts for the rise in V_E (12). Elite endurance athletes have values of >160–180 $L \cdot min^{-1}$ (1,2). V_E increases linearly as VO_2 rises. However, V_E increases exponentially after the ventilatory threshold (the point at which V_E and CO_2 rise exponentially) is reached (1). During resistance

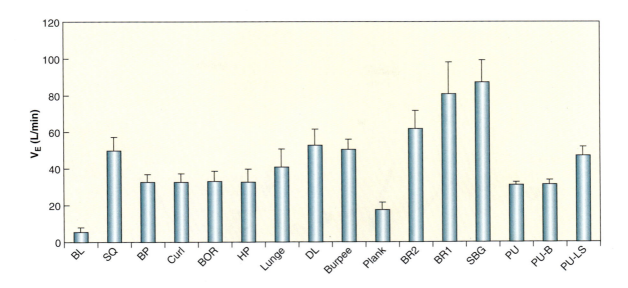

FIGURE 9.14 Ventilation responses to different resistance exercises. BL, baseline; BP, bench press; BOR, bent-over barbell row; HP, high pull; DL, dead lift; BR1, battling rope 1-min rest; BR2, battling rope 2-min rest; SBG, sandbag Tabata interval protocol; PU, push-up; PU-B, push-up on BOSU ball; PU-LC, push-up with lateral crawl. (Data from Ratamess NA, Smith CR, Beller NA, Kang J, Faigenbaum AD, Bush JA. Effects of rest interval length on acute battling rope exercise metabolism. *J Strength Cond Res.* 2015;29:2375–87; Ratamess NA, Rosenberg JG, Klei S, et al. Comparison of the acute metabolic responses to traditional resistance, body-weight, and battling rope exercises. *J Strength Cond Res.* 2015;29:47–7; Ratamess NA, Kang J, Kuper JD, et al. Acute cardiorespiratory and metabolic effects of a sandbag resistance exercise protocol. *J Strength Cond Res.* 2018;32:1491–502.)

exercise, short rest intervals and higher volume produce greater acute increases in V_E (28). Peak value obtained postexercise using 30-second rest intervals for 10 RM sets (5 sets) was 68.2 L·min^{-1} compared to 44.8 L·min^{-1} when 5-minute rest intervals were used for the bench press (28), still considerably lower than values seen during endurance exercise. V_E values of ~45–60 L·min^{-1} have been shown kettlebell workouts using Tabata intervals (33). Figure 9.14 depicts V_E responses from a few studies examining different RE and modalities in men. Most traditional RE yield V_E values of 32–53 L·min^{-1} when performed for 3 sets of 10 reps with 2-minute rest intervals (31). Battling rope workouts using 1 minute of rest in between sets yield higher mean V_E values than when 2-minute rest intervals were used, *e.g.*, 81 versus 61 L·min^{-1} respectively, with peak values >100 L·min^{-1} in men versus 50 and 39 L·min^{-1} in women (32). The largest response was seen during a sandbag protocol (3 rounds of 8 exercises) using Tabata intervals (20 s set, 10-s rest) (30). Not all air that enters the body reaches the alveoli. Some air remains in the nose, mouth, trachea, and other areas (*anatomic dead space*) and ranges between 150 and 200 mL (1). The air that reaches the alveoli is known as alveolar ventilation.

Control of Breathing

Breathing is an involuntary action but can be controlled voluntarily to some extent. Ventilation is controlled by neural and humoral factors (Fig. 9.15). The medulla oblongata and pons of the brainstem contain respiratory centers that control inspiration and expiration. Large networks of respiratory neurons conduct action potentials via the spinal cord to the phrenic nerve (stimulates the diaphragm), intercostal, and abdominal muscle motor nerves (12) to control rate and depth of breathing. Inspiration results in stretching of the lungs that stimulates stretch receptors and inhibits further inspiration and stimulates expiration. The lack of stretch during deflation stimulates the respiratory neurons to increase inspiration. Inspiratory muscles relax and expiration occurs passively. Precise coordination of motor output to respiratory muscles is critical. Inspiratory and expiratory groups of neurons in the brainstem discharge independently and not simultaneously (12). Inspiratory neuronal discharge inhibits expiratory neuronal discharge and vice versa via reciprocal inhibition, which enables full inspiration and expiration to take place, respectively. Proprioceptors located in joints and skeletal muscles stimulate the respiratory centers to alter ventilation during exercise (1). Parallel communication with the motor cortex, cerebellum, and the hypothalamus stimulate the respiratory centers during exercise via a process known as *central command* (12). Rhythmic muscle contraction and frequency of muscular contractions (as seen in AT) provide potent feedback to respiratory centers, whereas increased muscle contraction force poses little effect on increasing V_E during exercise (12).

Circulatory (humoral) factors play substantial roles in ventilation. Changes in arterial PO_2, PCO_2, pH, and temperature provide feedback to the medulla to control ventilation. Reduced PO_2 stimulates increased V_E. Oxygen levels (and PCO_2 and pH) are detected by peripheral *chemoreceptors* located in the medulla, aorta, and carotid bodies, and low PO_2 stimulates

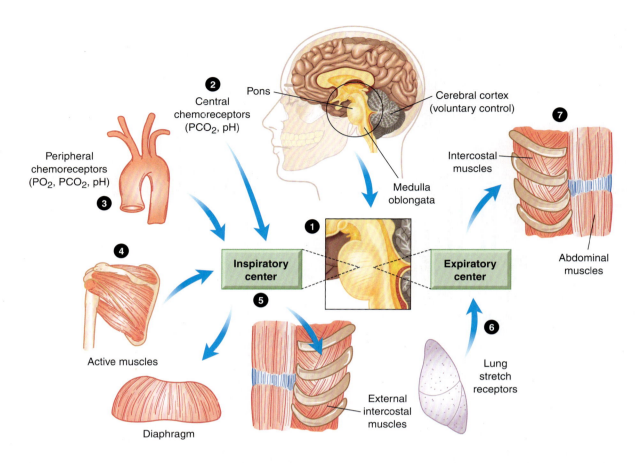

FIGURE 9.15 Overview of respiratory control. (Adapted with permission from Wilmore JH, Costill DL. *Physiology of Sport and Exercise*. 2nd ed. Champaign (IL): Human Kinetics; 1999. 260 p.)

respiratory centers to increase V_E at rest and during exercise. However, V_E changes during exercise are more sensitive to reductions in pH, increased temperature, and increased PCO_2. Higher ventilation rates are especially important during exercise to reduce acidity by removing excess CO_2. Hyperventilation decreases PCO_2 and is important for reducing acidity.

During exercise, there is a rapid increase in V_E followed by a slower rise as exercise progresses (Fig. 9.16). A rise in VO_2 and VCO_2 occur in an intensity-dependent manner with a reduction in respiratory dead space (12). The initial steep rise may be produced by feedback from proprioceptors in joints and muscles and the motor cortex that stimulates contraction of inspiratory muscles (2). The increased V_E is proportional to increases in VCO_2 and oxygen demand. The gradual increase as exercise progresses may be due to peripheral feedback from reduced pH and increased PCO_2 (2). Rapid recovery is seen at the completion of exercise.

Pulmonary Adaptations to Training

There appears to be only little change in lung volumes and capacities with traditional AT in healthy individuals. The lack of direct resistance applied to respiratory muscles during land-based exercise may pose a weak stimulus to direct strengthening of respiratory muscles. No relationship between VO_2max and FVC has been reported (1). Further evidence has been gained where some studies in athletes have shown similar FVC, TLC, and FEV_1 values to untrained control subjects (1). In contrast, one study showed only slightly higher FVC, FEV_1, and

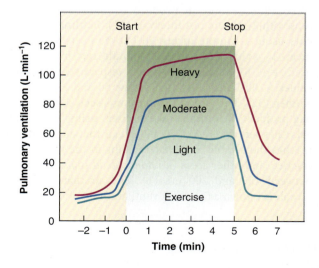

FIGURE 9.16 Pulmonary ventilation during exercise. (Reprinted with permission from Wilmore JH, Costill DL. *Physiology of Sport and Exercise*. 2nd ed. Champaign (IL): Human Kinetics; 1999.)

VC values in hybrid endurance athletes than power athletes and control subjects (120). Given that height and body size correlate to pulmonary function, some groups of taller athletes have shown higher FVC, FEV$_1$, and VC values (121). However, swimmers may have augmented lung volumes given the positive effects being submerged in a pool has on the strength of inspiratory muscles (1). One study reported that bodybuilders and endurance athletes had similar FVC, FEV$_1$, RV, ERV, IC, and TLC; however, bodybuilders had much greater max inspiratory pressure (MIP) and max expiratory pressure (MEP) (tests used to measure respiratory muscle strength) than the endurance athletes (122). Greater strength of respiratory muscles likely due to the high need for development of IAP and subsequent bracing of trunk muscles during lifting did not impact pulmonary capacities (122). The diaphragm is a key muscle playing critical roles in respiration and postural/core stability. Athletes with diaphragms that lack endurance and strength may not breathe properly (and show limited diaphragm excursion), and this could reduce postural stability (123). Ideal diaphragmatic breathing involves lateral expansion of the lower ribs, reduced upper thoracic motion during inhalation, and increased abdominal displacement (123).

Vital capacity may increase slightly or not change, and residual volume may slightly decrease (2). Tidal volume does not change at rest or low-intensity exercise but will increase during maximal exercise especially in endurance-trained athletes (2,12). Respiratory rate decreases at rest and during submaximal exercise but increases during maximal exercise (2). Pulmonary V$_E$ (and alveolar ventilation) does not change or may slightly decrease at rest and during submaximal exercise but increases during maximal exercise to high levels in trained endurance athletes (2,12). Resistance-trained individuals have similar resting V$_E$ values to untrained individuals (28). Pulmonary diffusion does not change at rest or during submaximal exercise but increases during maximal exercise (2). Gender differences exist. Women have pulmonary structural differences than age- and height-matched men that include smaller vital capacity and maximal expiratory flow rates, reduced airway diameter, and a smaller diffusion surface (124). Women have smaller airways and lung volumes, lower resting maximal expiratory flow rates, and higher metabolic costs of breathing relative to men (125). Female athletes develop expiratory flow limitations more often than men and have greater increases in end-expiratory and end-inspiratory lung volume at maximal exercise (125). Female athletes have ~7% and 6% greater end-inspiratory and end-expiratory lung volumes, respectively, compared to men (105). Women have a higher work cost of breathing that is twice that of men at ventilations >90 L·min^{-1} (105).

Respiratory Muscle-Specific Training

Ventilatory, or respiratory muscle-specific training, has increased in popularity greatly over the years in clinical and athletic populations. One reason for use is to offset respiratory muscle fatigue (i.e., decreased MIP or MEP over time), which could limit some sporting activities. Respiratory muscle

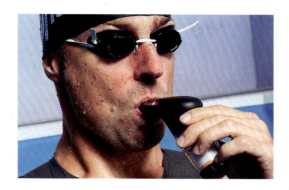

FIGURE 9.17 Photo of an athlete using an RMT device. (Originally published in: https://www.220triathlon.com/training/swim-training/12-swim-tools-to-improve-technique-and-fitness/)

training (RMT) involves direct targeting of the muscles involved in breathing either through *inspiratory muscle training* (IMT), *expiratory muscle training* (EMT), or a combination of both. Resistance is applied during inspiration or expiration; therefore, respiratory muscles are directly stimulated in a manner traditional exercise may not provide (Fig. 9.17). IMT comprises two popular methods of resistive breathing. One method involves breathing forcefully into a mouthpiece attached to a T-piece with a one-way valve on one side and an inspiratory resistance located on the other side. The valve closes during inspiration so the individual breathes against the resistance (a percent of one's *maximal inspiratory mouth pressure*), and expiration is unimpeded. Another modality includes threshold loading. A mouthpiece connected to a valve is used which is attached to a threshold loading device.

Many studies indicate that RMT may improve endurance exercise capacity through a number of potential mechanisms including decreasing the inspiratory muscle motor drive while preserving pressure generation and increasing ventilatory efficiency, increasing diaphragm hypertrophy, inducing favorable fiber-type adaptations in the external intercostal muscles, attenuating the respiratory muscle **metaboreflex** (*i.e.*, a sympathetically mediated vasoconstriction that may redirect blood flow away from limb muscles due to accumulation of metabolites in the respiratory muscles that activates group III and IV nerve afferents), decreasing RPE and breathlessness, improving respiratory muscle economy, reducing respiratory work, and increasing respiratory muscle strength and endurance (126,127).

Several studies have shown that RMT can increase respiratory muscle strength (MIP) by an average of ~30%, MVV, FVC, FEV$_1$, running time to exhaustion, repeated sprint ability, cycling and rowing time trial performance, power output, and improve swimming performance in athletes and healthy populations (126–133), with limited effects on VO$_2$max (129,132–134). In contrast, one meta-analysis reported no effects of RMT with linear workload devices on MVV, FVC, and FEV$_1$ (130). In addition, performing RMT along with traditional exercise may have beneficial performance effects (127). Meta-analyses confirm the findings of enhanced performance from RMT (126,130). One study reported that RMT increased performance 11% more than non-RMT or control conditions, and the responses were greater in less-fit individuals than highly trained athletes, and improvements were greater with long-duration exercise (126). Another meta-analysis reported greater improvements with RMT than training alone (128). These studies have typically used training programs that had 30 breaths per workout performed 1–2 times per day, 2–7 days per week, with 30%–80% of P_{max} or max inspiratory pressure, for 3–12 weeks (127,130). However, some studies have reported no performance effects, but the majority of studies have shown at least some positive effects. IMT is used to improve physical function and reduce painful breathing in clinical populations such as those with chronic obstructive pulmonary disease (COPD) (135–137). The ACSM has recommended IMT for 30 min·day^{-1} or two 15-minute sessions daily, 4–5 days per week with at least 30% of one's maximal inspiratory pressure for those individuals with pulmonary disease (135).

SUMMARY POINTS

◆ The cardiorespiratory system includes the heart, blood vessels, lungs, and associated respiratory muscles. Oxygenated blood from the lungs returns to the heart (left atrium) and is pumped to the rest of the body via the left ventricle. Deoxygenated blood returns to the right atrium and is transported to the lungs in a cyclical process.

◆ Aerobic and anaerobic exercises result in pressure overload (rise in BP and ITP) on the heart, whereas aerobic exercise increases volume overload (greater venous return and blood flow) to the heart. Pressure overload yields adaptations in cardiac wall muscularity, whereas volume overload yields increased cardiac chamber size.

◆ Key CV variables include HR and HR variability, BP, SV (and ejection fraction), and Q_c. AT leads to lower HR, BP, increased SV, and Q_c at rest. RT produces minor changes at rest.

◆ AT and RT can lead to a reduced HR and BP response to submaximal exercise.

◆ VO_2max is most improved via AT, whereas anaerobic training only produces small increases.

◆ Few changes are observed in pulmonary function at rest and during submaximal exercise following aerobic and anaerobic training. However, acute pulmonary response is enhanced during maximal exercise after AT.

◆ RMT use has increased in athletes, and several studies show that it may be useful for increasing respiratory muscle strength and in enhancing some elements of athletic performance.

REVIEW QUESTIONS

1. As an adaptation to RT
   a. Right ventricular wall decreases in thickness and septal wall thickness decreases
   b. BP (systolic and diastolic) increases
   c. Total cholesterol increases
   d. Resting HR and systolic and diastolic BP may decrease slightly

2. The Fick equation states that VO_2max is the product of Q_c and _____
   a. $A\text{-}VO_2$ difference
   b. SV
   c. HR
   d. SBP

3. The part of the heart that pumps blood to the rest of the body is the
   a. Right atrium
   b. Left atrium
   c. Right ventricle
   d. Left ventricle

4. A highly trained endurance athlete may reach a SV of _____ during maximal exercise
   a. 70 mL
   b. 90 mL
   c. 120 mL
   d. 180 mL

5. The volume of air in the lungs after maximal inspiration is known as _____
   a. Residual volume
   b. Tidal volume
   c. Total lung capacity
   d. Minute ventilation

6. Although RT is not the most potent modality to stimulate improvements in VO_2max, which of the following workouts would most likely lead to a higher VO_2max?
   a. 5 exercises for the upper body, 3 sets of 6–8 reps each, 3-minute rest intervals
   b. 8 exercises—total body, 3 sets of 8–10 reps each, 2-minute rest intervals
   c. 5 exercises—lower body, 1 set of 10–12 reps each, 1-minute rest intervals
   d. 10 exercises—total body, 1 set of 10–12 reps performed in a circuit, 3 circuits performed altogether, 15-second rest intervals

7. The rhythm of a healthy heart initiates in the SA node.
   a. T
   b. F

8. An increase in pH and decrease in temperature increase oxygen dissociation from hemoglobin during exercise.
   a. T
   b. F

9. RT can increase left ventricular wall thickness.
   a. T
   b. F

10. A Valsalva maneuver used during weight lifting decreases intra-abdominal pressure and BP and reduces torso rigidity.
    a. T
    b. F

11. The volume of air left in lungs after maximal expiration is minute ventilation.
    a. T
    b. F

REFERENCES

1. McArdle WD, Katch FI, Katch VL. *Exercise Physiology: Energy, Nutrition, and Human Performance*. 6th ed. Philadelphia (PA): Lippincott Williams & Wilkins; 2007. p. 314–63.
2. Wilmore JH, Costill DL. *Physiology of Sport and Exercise*. 2nd ed. Champaign (IL): Human Kinetics; 1999.
3. Leigh-Smith S. Blood boosting. *Br J Sports Med*. 2004;38:99–101.
4. Sgrò P, Sansone M, Sansone A, Romanelli F, Di Luigi L. Effects of erythropoietin abuse on exercise performance. *Phys Sportsmed*. 2018;46:105–15.
5. Atkinson TS, Kahn MJ. Blood doping: then and now. A narrative review of the history, science and efficacy of blood doping in elite sport. *Blood Rev*. 2020;39:100632.
6. American College of Sports Medicine. The use of blood doping as an ergogenic aid. *Med Sci Sports Exerc*. 1996;28:i–viii.
7. Brien AJ, Simon TL. The effects of red blood cell infusion on 10-km race time. *JAMA*. 1987;257:2761–5.
8. Williams MH, Wesseldine S, Somma T, Schuster R. The effect of induced erythrocythemia upon 5-mile treadmill run time. *Med Sci Sports Exerc*. 1981;13:169–75.
9. Sawka MN, Young AJ, Muza SR, Gonzalez RR, Pandolf KB. Erythrocyte reinfusion and maximal aerobic power. An examination of modifying factors. *JAMA*. 1987;257:1496–9.
10. Haile DW, Durussel J, Mekonen W. Effects of EPO on blood parameters and running performance in Kenyan athletes. *Med Sci Sports Exerc*. 2019;51:299–307.
11. Housh TJ, Housh DJ, de Vries HA. *Applied Exercise and Sport Physiology*. 2nd ed. Scottsdale (AZ): Holcomb Hathaway Publishers; 2006. p. 57–80.
12. Dempsey JA, Miller JD, Romer LM. The respiratory system. In: Tipton CM, editor. *ACSM's Advanced Exercise Physiology*. Philadelphia (PA): Lippincott Williams & Wilkins; 2006. p. 246–99.
13. Querido JS, Sheel AW. Regulation of cerebral blood flow during exercise. *Sports Med*. 2007;37:765–82.
14. Collier SR, Diggle MD, Heffernan KS, Kelly EE, Tobin MM, Fernhall B. Changes in arterial distensibility and flow-mediated dilation after acute resistance vs. aerobic exercise. *J Strength Cond Res*. 2010;24:2846–52.
15. Saltin B. Exercise hyperaemia: magnitude and aspects on regulation in humans. *J Physiol*. 2007;583:819–23.
16. Walther G, Nottin S, Karpoff L, Pérez-Martin A, Dauzat M, Obert P. Flow-mediated dilation and exercise-induced hyperaemia in highly trained athletes: comparison of the upper and lower limb vasculature. *Acta Physiol (Oxf)*. 2008;193:139–50.
17. Ashor AW, Lara J, Siervo M, Celis-Morales C, Oggioni C, Jakovljevic DG, Mathers JC. Exercise modalities and endothelial function: a systematic review and dose–response meta-analysis of randomized controlled trials. *Sports Med*. 2015;45:279–96.
18. Baynard T, Jacobs HM, Kessler CM, Kanaley JA, Fernhall B. Fibrinolytic markers and vasodilatory capacity following acute exercise among men of differing training status. *Eur J Appl Physiol*. 2007;101:595–602.
19. Baynard T, Miller WC, Fernhall B. Effects of exercise on vasodilatory capacity in endurance-and resistance-trained men. *Eur J Appl Physiol*. 2003;89:69–73.
20. Kawano H, Fujimoto K, Higuchi M, Miyachi M. Effect of combined resistance and aerobic training on reactive hyperemia in men. *J Physiol Sci*. 2009;59:457–64.
21. Bredt DS. Endogenous nitric oxide synthesis: biological functions and pathophysiology. *Free Radic Res*. 1999;31:577–96.
22. Ashor AW, Lara J, Siervo M, Celis-Morales C, Mathers JC. Effects of exercise modalities on arterial stiffness and wave reflection: a systematic review and meta-analysis of randomized controlled trials. *PLoS One*. 2014;9:e110034.
23. Miyachi M. Effects of resistance training on arterial stiffness: a meta-analysis. *Br J Sports Med*. 2013;47:393–6.
24. Michael S, Graham KS, Davis GM. Cardiac autonomic responses during exercise and post-exercise recovery using heart rate variability and systolic time intervals: a review. *Front Physiol*. 2017;8:301.
25. Dong JG. The role of heart rate variability in sports physiology. *Exp Ther Med*. 2016;11:1531–6.
26. D'Andrea A, Riegler L, Cocchia R, et al. Left atrial volume index in highly trained athletes. *Am Heart J*. 2010;159:1155–61.
27. Silva DV, Waclawovsky G, Kramer AB, et al. Comparison of cardiac and vascular parameters in powerlifters and long-distance runners: comparative cross-sectional study. *Arq Bras Cardiol*. 2018;111:772–81.
28. Ratamess NA, Falvo MJ, Mangine GT, Hoffman JR, Faigenbaum AD, Kang J. The effect of rest interval length on metabolic responses to the bench press exercise. *Eur J Appl Physiol*. 2007;100:1–17.
29. Fleck SJ. Cardiovascular responses to strength training. In: Komi PV, editor. *Strength and Power in Sport*. 2nd ed. Malden (MA): Blackwell Science; 2003. p. 387–406.
30. Ratamess NA, Kang J, Kuper JD, et al. Acute cardiorespiratory and metabolic effects of a sandbag resistance exercise protocol. *J Strength Cond Res*. 2018;32:1491–502.
31. Ratamess NA, Smith CR, Beller NA, Kang J, Faigenbaum AD, Bush JA. Effects of rest interval length on acute battling rope exercise metabolism. *J Strength Cond Res*. 2015;29:2375–87.
32. Ratamess NA, Rosenberg JG, Klei S, et al. Comparison of the acute metabolic responses to traditional resistance, body-weight, and battling rope exercises. *J Strength Cond Res*. 2015;29:47–57.
33. Williams BM, Kraemer RR. Comparison of cardiorespiratory and metabolic responses in kettlebell high-intensity interval training versus sprint interval cycling. *J Strength Cond Res*. 2015;29:3317–25.
34. Davis WJ, Wood DT, Andrews RG, Elkind LM, Davis WB. Concurrent training enhances athletes' cardiovascular and cardiorespiratory measures. *J Strength Cond Res*. 2008;22:1503–14.

35. Gronwald T, Hoos O. Correlation properties of heart rate variability during endurance exercise: a systematic review. *Ann Noninvasive Electrocardiol*. 2020;25:e12697.

36. Figueiredo C, Antunes BM, Giacon TR, et al. Influence of acute and chronic high-intensity intermittent aerobic plus strength exercise on BDNF, lipid and autonomic parameters. *J Sports Sci Med*. 2019;18:359–68.

37. Kingsley JD, Figueroa A. Acute and training effects of resistance exercise on heart rate variability. *Clin Physiol Funct Imaging*. 2016;36:179–87.

38. Adler Y, Fisman EZ, Koren-Morag N, et al. Left ventricular diastolic function in trained male weight lifters at rest and during isometric exercise. *Am J Cardiol*. 2008;102:97–101.

39. Hoffman JR. The cardiorespiratory system. In: Chandler TJ, Brown LE, editors. *Conditioning for Strength and Human Performance*. Philadelphia (PA): Lippincott Williams & Wilkins; 2008. p. 20–39.

40. Romero SA, Minson CT, Halliwill JR. The cardiovascular system after exercise. *J Appl Physiol*. 2017;122:925–32.

41. MacDougall JD, Tuxen D, Sale DG, Moroz JR. Arterial blood pressure response to heavy exercise. *J Appl Physiol*. 1985;58:785–90.

42. Haykowsky M, Taylor D, Teo K, Quinney A, Humen D. Left ventricular wall stress during leg-press exercise performed with a brief Valsalva maneuver. *Chest*. 2001;119:150–4.

43. Blazek Z, Stastny P, Maszczyk A, et al. Systematic review of intra-abdominal and intrathoracic pressures initiated by the Valsalva manoeuvre during high-intensity resistance exercises. *Biol Sport*. 2019;36(4):373–86.

44. MacDougall JD, McKelvie RS, Moroz JR, Sale DG, McCartney N, Buick F. Factors affecting blood pressure during heavy weight lifting and static contractions. *J Appl Physiol*. 1992;73:1590–7.

45. Haykowsky MJ, Dressendorfer R, Taylor D, Mandic S, Humen D. Resistance training and cardiac hypertrophy: unraveling the training effect. *Sports Med*. 2002;32:837–49.

46. Palatini P, Mos L, Munari L, et al. Blood pressure changes during heavy-resistance exercise. *J Hypertens*. 1989;7(suppl):S72–3.

47. Narloch JA, Brandstater ME. Influence of breathing technique on arterial blood pressure during heavy weight lifting. *Arch Phys Med Rehabil*. 1995;76:457–62.

48. Linsenbardt ST, Thomas TR, Madsen RW. Effect of breathing techniques on blood pressure response to resistance exercise. *Br J Sports Med*. 1992;26:97–100.

49. Gotshall RW, Gootman J, Byrnes WC, Fleck SJ, Valovich TC. Noninvasive characterization of the blood pressure response to the double-leg press exercise. *J Exerc Physiol*. 1999;2:1–6.

50. Sale DG, Moroz DE, McKelvie RS, MacDougall JD, McCartney N. Comparison of blood pressure response to isokinetic and weight-lifting exercise. *Eur J Appl Physiol Occup Physiol*. 1993;67:115–20.

51. Fleck SJ, Dean LS. Resistance-training experience and the pressor response during resistance exercise. *J Appl Physiol*. 1987;63:116–20.

52. Carpio-Rivera E, Moncada-Jiminez J, Salazar-Rojas W, Solera-Herrera A. Acute effects of exercise on blood pressure: a meta-analytic investigation. *Arq Bras Cardiol*. 2016;106:422–33.

53. Figueiredo T, Willardson JM, Miranda H, et al. Influence of rest interval length between sets on blood pressure and heart rate variability after a strength training session performed by prehypertensive men. *J Strength Cond Res*. 2016;30:1813–24.

54. Duncan MJ, Birch SL, Oxford SW. The effect of exercise intensity on post resistance exercise hypotension in trained men. *J Strength Cond Res*. 2014;28:1706–13.

55. Figueiredo T, Willardson JM, Miranda H, Bentes CM, Reis VM, Simão R. Influence of load intensity on postexercise hypotension and heart rate variability after a strength training session. *J Strength Cond Res*. 2015;29:2941–8.

56. de Freitas MC, Ricci-Vitor AL, Quizzini GH, de Oliveira JVNS, Vanderlei LCM, Lira FS, Rossi FE. Postexercise hypotension and autonomic modulation response after full versus split body resistance exercise in trained men. *J Exerc Rehabil*. 2018;14:399–406.

57. Figueiredo T, Rhea MR, Peterson M, Miranda H, Bentes CM, dos Reis VM, Simão R. Influence of number of sets on blood pressure and heart rate variability after a strength training session. *J Strength Cond Res*. 2015;29:1556–63.

58. de Freitas Brito A, Brasileiro-Santos MDS, Coutinho de Oliveira CV, da Cruz Santos A. Postexercise hypotension is volume-dependent in hypertensives: autonomic and forearm blood responses. *J Strength Cond Res*. 2019;33:234–41.

59. Stone WJ, Schafer MA, Arnett SW, Lyons TS. Post exercise hypotension following concurrent exercise: does order of exercise modality matter? *Int J Exerc Sci*. 2020;13:36–48.

60. Paz GA, Iglesias-Soler E, Willardson JM, Maia MF, Miranda H. Postexercise hypotension and heart rate variability responses subsequent to traditional, paired set, and superset resistance training methods. *J Strength Cond Res*. 2019;33:2433–42.

61. Tomeleri CM, Nunes JP, Souza MF, et al. Resistance exercise order does not affect the magnitude and duration of postexercise blood pressure in older women. *J Strength Cond Res*. 2020;34:1062–70.

62. Gledhill N, Warburton D, Jamnik V. Haemoglobin, blood volume, cardiac function, and aerobic power. *Can J Appl Physiol*. 1999;24:54–65.

63. Yoshida T, Nagashima K, Nose H, et al. Relationship between aerobic power, blood volume, and thermoregulatory responses to exercise-heat stress. *Med Sci Sports Exerc*. 1997;29:867–73.

64. Collins MA, Cureton KJ, Hill DW, Ray CA. Relation of plasma volume change to intensity of weight lifting. *Med Sci Sports Exerc*. 1989;21:178–85.

65. Ploutz-Snyder LL, Convertino VA, Dudley GA. Resistance exercise-induced fluid shifts: change in active muscle size and plasma volume. *Am J Physiol*. 1995;269:R536–43.

66. Ratamess NA, Kraemer WJ, Volek JS, et al. Androgen receptor content following heavy resistance exercise in men. *J Steroid Biochem Mol Biol*. 2005;93:35–42.

67. Collins MA, Hill DW, Cureton KJ, DeMello JJ. Plasma volume change during heavy-resistance weight lifting. *Eur J Appl Physiol Occup Physiol*. 1986;55:44–8.

68. Kraemer WJ, Fleck SJ, Maresh CM, et al. Acute hormonal responses to a single bout of heavy resistance exercise in trained power lifters and untrained men. *Can J Appl Physiol*. 1999;24:524–37.

69. Craig SK, Byrnes WC, Fleck SJ. Plasma volume during weight lifting. *Int J Sports Med*. 2008;29:89–95.

70. Tesch PA, Komi PV. Short- and long-term histochemical and biochemical adaptations in muscle. In: *Strength and Power in Sport*. Boston (MA): Blackwell Scientific Publications; 1992. p. 239–48.

71. Utomi V, Oxborough D, Whyte GP, et al. Systematic review and meta-analysis of training mode, imaging modality and body size influences on the morphology and function of the male athlete's heart. *Heart*. 2013;99:1727–33.

72. Heiskanen MA, Leskinen T, Heinonen IH, et al. Right ventricular metabolic adaptations to high-intensity interval and moderate-intensity continuous training in healthy middle-aged men. *Am J Physiol Heart Circ Physiol*. 2016;311:H667–75.

73. Utomi V, Oxborough D, Ashley E, et al. The impact of chronic endurance and resistance training upon the right ventricular phenotype in male athletes. *Eur J Appl Physiol*. 2015;115:1673–82.

74. Wasfy MM, Weiner RB. Differentiating the athlete's heart from hypertrophic cardiomyopathy. *Curr Opin Cardiol*. 2015;30:500–5.

75. Augustine DX, Howard L. Left ventricular hypertrophy in athletes: differentiating physiology from pathology. *Curr Treat Options Cardiovasc Med*. 2018;20:96.

76. Naylor LH, George K, O'Driscoll G, Green DJ. The athlete's heart: a contemporary appraisal of the "Morganroth Hypothesis." *Sports Med*. 2008;38:69–90.

77. Spence AL, Naylor LH, Carter HH, et al. A prospective randomised longitudinal MRI study of left ventricular adaptation to endurance and resistance exercise training in humans. *J Physiol*. 2011;589:5443–52.

78. Levine BD. VO₂max: what do we know, and what do we still need to know? *J Physiol*. 2008;586(1):25–34.

79. Venckunas T, Raugaliene R, Mazutaitiene B, Ramoskeviciute S. Endurance rather than sprint running training increases left ventricular wall thickness in female athletes. *Eur J Appl Physiol*. 2008;102:307–11.

80. Fleck SJ, Henke C, Wilson W. Cardiac MRI of elite junior weight lifters. *Int J Sports Med*. 1989;10:329–33.

81. Fleck SJ, Pattany PM, Stone MH, Kraemer WJ, Thrush J, Wong K. Magnetic resonance imaging determination of left ventricular mass: junior Olympic weightlifters. *Med Sci Sports Exerc*. 1993;25:522–7.

82. Dickerman RD, Schaller F, Zachariah NY, McConathy WJ. Left ventricular size and function in elite bodybuilders using anabolic steroids. *Clin J Sports Med*. 1997;7:90–3.

83. Menapace FJ, Hammer WJ, Ritzer TF, et al. Left ventricular size in competitive weight lifters: an echocardiographic study. *Med Sci Sports Exerc*. 1982;14:72–5.

84. Deligiannis A, Zahopoulou E, Mandroukas K. Echocardiographic study of cardiac dimensions and function in weight lifters and body builders. *Int J Sports Cardiol*. 1988;5:24–32.

85. Fisman EZ, Embon P, Pines A, et al. Comparison of left ventricular function using isometric exercise Doppler echocardiography in competitive runners and weightlifters versus sedentary individuals. *Am J Cardiol*. 1997;79:355–9.

86. Lentini AC, McKelvie RS, McCartney N, Tomlinson CW, MacDougall JD. Left ventricular response in healthy young men during heavy-intensity weight-lifting exercise. *J Appl Physiol*. 1993;75:2703–10.

87. Wilmore JH, Parr RB, Girandola RN, et al. Physiological alterations consequent to circuit weight training. *Med Sci Sports*. 1978;10:79–84.

88. Gettman LR, Ward P, Hagan RD. A comparison of combined running and weight training with circuit weight training. *Med Sci Sports Exerc*. 1982;14:229–34.

89. Haennel R, Teo KK, Quinney A, Kappagoda T. Effects of hydraulic circuit training on cardiovascular function. *Med Sci Sports Exerc*. 1989;21:605–12.

90. Levy WC, Cerqueira MD, Harp GD, et al. Effect of endurance exercise training on heart rate variability at rest in healthy young and older men. *Am J Cardiol*. 1998;82:1236–41.

91. Bellenger CR, Fuller JT, Thomson RL, Davison K, Robertson EY, Buckley JD. Monitoring athletic training status through autonomic heart rate regulation: a systematic review and meta-analysis. *Sports Med*. 2016;46:1461–86.

92. Brawner CA, Keteyian SJ, Saval M, Ehrman JK. Adaptations to cardiorespiratory exercise training. In: *ACSM's Resource Manual for Guidelines for Exercise Testing and Prescription*. 6th ed. Philadelphia (PA): Lippincott Williams & Wilkins; 2010. p. 476–88.

93. Milanović Z, Sporiš G, Weston M. Effectiveness of high-intensity interval training (HIT) and continuous endurance training for VO₂max improvements: a systematic review and meta-analysis of controlled trials. *Sports Med*. 2015;45:1469–81.

94. Häkkinen K, Alen M, Komi PV. Neuromuscular, anaerobic, and aerobic performance characteristics of elite power athletes. *Eur J Appl Physiol Occup Physiol*. 1984;53:97–105.

95. Sentija D, Marsic T, Dizdar D. The effects of strength training on some parameters of aerobic and anaerobic endurance. *Coll Anthropol*. 2009;33:111–6.

96. Nakao M, Inoue Y, Murakami H. Longitudinal study of the effect of high intensity weight training on aerobic capacity. *Eur J Appl Physiol Occup Physiol*. 1995;70:20–5.

97. Buckley S, Knapp K, Lackie A, et al. Multimodal high-intensity interval training increases muscle function and metabolic performance in females. *Appl Physiol Nutr Metab*. 2015;40:1157–62.

98. McRae G, Payne A, Zelt JGE, Scribbans TD, Jung ME, Little JP, Gurd BJ. Extremely low volume, whole-body aerobic-resistance training improves aerobic fitness and muscular endurance in females. *Appl Physiol Nutr Metab*. 2012;37:1124–31.

99. Myers TR, Schneider MG, Schmale MS, Hazell TJ. Whole-body aerobic resistance training circuit improves aerobic fitness and muscle strength in sedentary young females. *J Strength Cond Res*. 2015;29:1592–600.

100. MacDougall JD, Hicks AL, MacDonald JR, et al. Muscle performance and enzymatic adaptations to sprint interval training. *J Appl Physiol*. 1998;84:2138–42.

101. Saltin B, Strange S. Maximal oxygen uptake: "old" and "new" arguments for a cardiovascular limitation. *Med Sci Sports Exerc*. 1992;24:30–7.

102. Di Prampero PE. Metabolic and circulatory limitations to VO₂max at the whole animal level. *J Exp Biol*. 1985;115:319–31.

103. Sutton JR. Limitations to maximal oxygen uptake. *Sports Med*. 1992;13:127–33.

104. Johnson BD, Saupe KW, Dempsey JA. Mechanical constraints on exercise hyperpnea in endurance athletes. *J Appl Physiol*. 1992;73:874–86.

105. Guenette JA, Witt JD, McKenzie DC, Road JD, Sheel AW. Respiratory mechanics during exercise in endurance-trained men and women. *J Physiol*. 2007;581:1309–22.

106. American College of Sports Medicine. Position stand: exercise and hypertension. *Med Sci Sports Exerc*. 2004;36:533–53.

107. Campbell WW, Kraus WE, Powell KE, et al.; For the 2018 Physical Activity Guidelines Advisory Committee. High-intensity interval training for cardiometabolic disease prevention. *Med Sci Sports Exerc*. 2019;51:1220–6.

108. Kelley GA. Dynamic resistance exercise and resting blood pressure in adults: a meta-analysis. *J Appl Physiol*. 1997;82:1559–65.

109. Kelley GA, Kelley KS. Progressive resistance exercise and resting blood pressure: a meta-analysis of randomized controlled trials. *Hypertension*. 2000;35:838–43.

110. López-Valenciano A, Ruiz-Pérez I, Ayala F, Sánchez-Meca J, Vera-Garcia FJ. Updated systematic review and meta-analysis on the role of isometric resistance training for resting blood pressure management in adults. *J Hypertens*. 2019;37:1320–33.

111. Durstine JL, Grandjean PW, Davis PG, et al. Blood lipid and lipoprotein adaptations to exercise: a quantitative analysis. *Sports Med*. 2001;31:1033–62.

112. MacKinnon LT, Hubinger LM. Effects of exercise on lipoprotein(a). *Sports Med*. 1999;28:11–24.

113. Yki-Jarvinen H, Koivisto VA, Taskinen MR, Nikkila E. Glucose tolerance, plasma lipoproteins and tissue lipoprotein lipase activities in body builders. *Eur J Appl Physiol Occup Physiol*. 1984;53:253–9.

114. Hurley BF, Seals DR, Hagberg JM, et al. High-density-lipoprotein cholesterol in bodybuilders v powerlifters. Negative effects of androgen use. *JAMA*. 1984;252:507–13.

115. Santora LJ, Marin J, Vangrow J, et al. Coronary calcification in body builders using anabolic steroids. *Prev Cardiol*. 2006;9:198–201.

116. Webb OL, Laskarzewski PM, Glueck CJ. Severe depression of high-density lipoprotein cholesterol levels in weight lifters and body builders by self-administered exogenous testosterone and anabolic-androgenic steroids. *Metabolism*. 1984;33:971–5.

117. Zuliani U, Bernardini B, Catapano A, et al. Effects of anabolic steroids, testosterone, and HGH on blood lipids and echocardiographic parameters in body builders. *Int J Sports Med*. 1989;10:62–6.

118. Hartgens F, Rietjens G, Keiser HA, Kuipers H, Wolffenbuttel BH. Effects of androgenic-anabolic steroids on apolipoproteins and lipoprotein (a). *Br J Sports Med*. 2004;38:253–9.

119. Kuipers H, Wijnen JA, Hartgens F, Willems SM. Influence of anabolic steroids on body composition, blood pressure, lipid profile and liver functions in body builders. *Int J Sports Med*. 1991;12:413–8.

120. Durmic T, Popovic BL, Svenda MZ, et al. The training type influence on male elite athletes' ventilatory function. *BMJ Open Sport Exerc Med*. 2017;3:e000240.

121. Durmic T, Lazovic B, Djelic M, et al. Sport-specific influences on respiratory patterns in elite athletes. *J Bras Pneumol*. 2015;41:516–22.

122. Hackett DA, Johnson N, Chow C. Respiratory muscle adaptations: a comparison between bodybuilders and endurance athletes. *J Sports Med Phys Fitness*. 2013;53:139–45.

123. Nelson N. Diaphragmatic breathing: the foundation of core stability. *NSCA J*. 2012;34:34–40.

124. Harms CA. Does gender affect pulmonary function and exercise capacity? *Respir Physiol Neurobiol*. 2006;151:124–31.

125. Sheel AW, Guenette JA. Mechanics of breathing during exercise in men and women: sex versus body size differences? *Exerc Sport Sci Rev*. 2008;36:128–34.

126. Illi SK, Held U, Frank I, Spengler CM. Effect of respiratory muscle training on exercise performance in healthy individuals a systematic review and meta-analysis. *Sports Med*. 2012;42:707–24.

127. Shei RJ. Recent advancements in our understanding of the ergogenic effect of respiratory muscle training in healthy humans: a systematic review. *J Strength Cond Res*. 2018;32:2665–76.

128. HajGhanbari B, Yamabayashi C, Buna TR, et al. Effects of respiratory muscle training on performance in athletes: a systematic review with meta-analyses. *J Strength Cond Res*. 2013;27:1643–63.

129. Inbar O, Weiner P, Azgad Y, Rotstein A, Weinstein Y. Specific inspiratory muscle training in well-trained endurance athletes. *Med Sci Sports Exerc*. 2000;32:1233–7.

130. Karsten M, Ribeiro GS, Esquivel MS, Matte DL. The effects of inspiratory muscle training with linear workload devices on the sports performance and cardiopulmonary function of athletes: a systematic review and meta-analysis. *Phys Ther Sport*. 2018;34:92–104.

131. Klusiewicz A, Borkowski L, Zdanowicz R, Boros P, Wesolowski S. The inspiratory muscle training in elite rowers. *J Sports Med Phys Fitness*. 2008;48:279–84.

132. Riganas CS, Vrabas IS, Christoulas K, Mandroukas K. Specific inspiratory muscle training does not improve performance or VO$_2$max levels in well trained rowers. *J Sports Med Phys Fitness*. 2008;48:285–92.

133. Williams JS, Wongsathikun J, Boon SM, Acevedo EO. Inspiratory muscle training fails to improve endurance capacity in athletes. *Med Sci Sports Exerc*. 2002;34:1194–8.

134. Sperlich B, Fricke H, de Marees M, Linville JW, Mester J. Does respiratory muscle training increase physical performance? *Mil Med*. 2009;174:977–82.

135. American College of Sports Medicine. *ACSM's Guidelines for Exercise Testing and Prescription*. 8th ed. Philadelphia (PA): Lippincott Williams & Wilkins; 2010. p. 262–3.

136. Geddes EL, O'Brien K, Reid WD, Brooks D, Crowe J. Inspiratory muscle training in adults with chronic obstructive pulmonary disease: an update of a systematic review. *Respir Med*. 2008;102:1715–29.

137. Padula CA, Yeaw E. Inspiratory muscle training: integrative review. *Res Theory Nurs Pract*. 2006;20:291–304.

CHAPTER 10

Principles of Strength Training and Conditioning

OBJECTIVES

After completing this chapter, you will be able to:

◆ Describe the importance of progressive overload in strength training and conditioning and provide examples of how it can be used in program design

◆ Describe the principle of training specificity and discuss the importance of designing a program most specific to the needs of the athlete

◆ Describe how the human body adapts specifically to the muscle actions trained, velocity of movement, range of motion, muscle groups trained, energy systems used, and the movement patterns trained

◆ Describe the importance of variation in program design for continued progression

◆ Describe the impact proper supervision has on training regarding progression in strength gains

Basic strength training and conditioning (S&C) principles underlie program design. These principles can be applied to all training programs in numerous ways. Ultimately, progression is a long-term goal associated with many S&C practitioners. The advantage of S&C is that there are many ways to design effective programs. An examination of the training logs of elite athletes or programs used by coaches and trainers would show great diversity of program design while basic principles are adhered to. Many programs can work effectively provided that guidelines are followed. S&C can be described as a large "toolbox" where each component is a critical "tool" in the development of the individual. Using the "tools" wisely in accordance with established scientific principles is fundamental to progression. This is a critical concept for S&C students to understand as one may become bombarded with a spectrum of training advice. This chapter focuses on the three key principles of progressive overload, specificity, and variation (Fig. 10.1). In addition, the principles of individualization and reversibility (detraining) are discussed.

Progressive Overload

Progressive overload refers to the gradual increase in stress placed on the human body during training (1). The concept of progressive overload is not new, and dates back a few thousand years to the ancient Greek strongman and Olympic wrestling champion *Milo of Crotona* (see Chapter 1). The human body has no need to become larger, stronger, powerful, or more durable unless it is forced to meet higher physical demands. The lack of progressive overload in a program is a leading factor for stagnant progress. The use of progressive overload can overcome accommodation. Accommodation is the staleness resulting from a lack in change in the training program (2). Adaptations to a training program take place within a few weeks. Proper manipulation of acute program variables alters the training stimulus, and if the stimulus exceeds the individual's conditioning threshold, then further improvements in muscular fitness can take place. There are several ways to introduce progressive overload during S&C. The following sections discuss resistance training (RT); flexibility; speed, power, and agility; and aerobic training (AT). Brief examples are given, but more specific training recommendations and examples are given in subsequent chapters.

Resistance Training

Progressive overload can be incorporated into RT programs in many ways. These include the following:

1. The resistance/loading may be increased. The athlete may train with a higher relative percentage of his or her one-repetition maximum (1 RM) or use greater absolute loading within a constant repetition scheme. For example, during

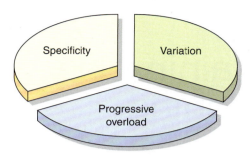

FIGURE 10.1 Critical components of training program design. The key components to programs targeting progression are progressive overload, specificity, and variation.

weeks 1–3, the athlete uses 70% of 1 RM for several structural exercises. During weeks 4 and 5, 75% of 1 RM is used. During weeks 6–8, 80% of 1 RM is used. This example applies when a true 1 RM is known for structural exercises and the loading is calculated by taking the 1 RM and multiplying it by 0.70 (and by 0.75 and 0.80, respectively). For an absolute loading example: during weeks 1 and 2, the athlete lifts 220 lb in the bench press for 8 reps. During weeks 3 and 4, the athlete adds weight and performs the bench press with 225 lb for 8 reps (5 lb is added while repetition number stays the same).

2. Repetitions may be added to current workload. For example (8–12 RM loading zone where the athlete performs a range [8–12] of reps for an exercise), during weeks 1 and 2, the athlete lifts 220 lb in the bench press for 3 sets of 8 reps. During weeks 3 and 4, the athlete maintains loading at 220 lb but performs 3 sets of 10 reps. During weeks 5 and 6, the athlete increases rep number to 12 for 3 sets with 220 lb. Once 3 sets of 12 reps are performed over two successive workouts, the athlete adds weight and performs 8 reps and repeats the cycle.

3. Lifting velocity with submaximal loads may be increased to increase the neural response once technique is mastered. The intent is to lift the weight as fast as possible. Because force = mass × acceleration, increasing rep velocity (while mass remains constant) results in higher peak force and greater strength enhancement.

4. Rest intervals may be lengthened to enable greater loading. In combination with previous strategies, lengthening the rest interval will enable more recovery in between sets to tolerate heavier loading. For endurance and hypertrophy training, the rest interval could be reduced, decreasing recovery in between sets. For high-intensity interval training, exercises can be performed continuously with minimal rest in between to stress conditioning improvements. In addition, rest intervals can be added in between reps or blocks of reps to increase the force, power, and velocity of each rep, a technique known as *rest-pause* or *cluster training*.

5. Training volume may be increased within reasonable limits (2%–5%) or varied to accommodate heavier loads (3). From novice to intermediate training, small increases in volume can enhance RT. However, with further progression, it is the variation of volume and intensity that becomes most important in program design.

6. The source of resistance can be manipulated. Although free weights and machines are popular, the use of implements provides a unique type of resistance. In some cases (*i.e.*, logs, kegs), fluid shifts cause unbalanced resistance. Other implements such as sand bags can provide unstable resistance. The resistance could vary such as through bands or chains. Devices such as kettlebells or thick bars augment gripping to a larger extent making them useful for grip strength training.

7. Other supramaximal-loading training techniques may be introduced. For example, techniques such as forced repetitions, heavy negatives, partial repetitions in the strongest area of the range of motion (ROM), overloads, and variable resistance devices can be used to load either a segment of the ROM or a muscle action with >100% of 1 RM. These techniques should only be used sparingly by experienced individuals.

Flexibility

For flexibility training, the intensity, volume, duration, and frequency can be increased for progressive overload. *Intensity* refers to the ROM of the stretch, as higher-intensity stretching expands joint ROM and poses more discomfort to the individual. Volume (number of reps) and duration (length of each stretch) can be increased with progression. The frequency of stretching can increase with progression. Lastly, progression in exercise selection may take place. For example, single-joint or isolation stretches could be used initially to specifically target a general muscle group. However, progression to multiple-joint or total-body stretches can be used. These stretches target many areas of the body and require a coordinated effort therefore stressing not only major muscle groups but the inner-connecting fascial structures. Some also require greater strength, balance, and postural control elements. Thus, balance, coordination, mobility, and functional performance are all targeted in addition to flexibility enhancement. Multiple- or total-body stretches are common to yoga practice, and research indicates the positive effects on flexibility, balance, muscle strength, and endurance (4,5).

Power, Speed, and Agility

Similar to RT, intensity, volume (and frequency), and rest intervals can be altered for progressive overload. For plyometric, speed, and agility drills, more complex exercises or drills can be introduced, resistance (*i.e.*, weighted vest, bands, sleds, etc.) may be used or increased, and longer or higher jumps or throws (drills that require greater power) may be used to increase intensity. For plyometrics, transitions from bilateral exercises to unilateral exercises can be incorporated. Intensity also increases as athletes increase their speed, jumping ability, power, and agility. Volume may be increased within reasonable limits as conditioning improves. However, caution must be used

Myths & Misconceptions
The Act of Resistance Training Itself Will Build Huge Muscles

Some individuals fear RT because of the misconception that they will develop huge muscles. This is primarily a concern in women who appear to believe in this myth to a greater extent. Part of this concern may commence from viewing female bodybuilders in magazines and making the assumption that RT led entirely to the development of their physiques. However, anabolic steroids and other growth agents are mostly responsible for this extreme level of hypertrophy. Anabolic drug–free women have low concentrations of testosterone, and it is not physiologically possible to gain extreme amounts of muscle mass. Education is important in debunking this myth. One study showed that women who trained under the supervision of a personal trainer were less likely to believe this myth compared to women who trained on their own (6). This fear is unfounded because it takes a great deal of hard work and dedication and not just simply an act of lifting light weights. Lifting weights does not guarantee increases in size and strength. In order for RT to build size and strength, the stimulus must become gradually more difficult. If one lifts below their threshold of adaptation, then very little will be gained. It takes years of hard training so the fear of excessive hypertrophy is unfounded.

as volume and intensity are inversely related so proper recovery in between workouts is mandatory. Rest intervals can be manipulated to target power specifically or high-intensity endurance.

Aerobic Endurance

To progressively overload an AT program, one may increase volume, duration, and intensity and decrease rest intervals. Volume and duration are altered by increasing the distance covered or the length of the exercise bouts. Intensity can be increased modestly by exercising at faster rates, adding resistance, and exercising uphill. It is important to note that intensity cannot increase greatly or the workout can become anaerobic. Aerobic and anaerobic interval training can be used to exercise at higher intensities. Decreasing rest intervals in between bouts increases the continuity of exercise and is effective for increasing aerobic endurance. The modality can be altered as each modality (*i.e.*, running, cycling, swimming, cross-country skiing, rope skipping, rowing, etc.) provides the trainee a unique physical stress regarding muscle mass involvement and tissue recruitment, the level of resistance encountered, and complexity of movement. Using a variety of modalities is an excellent way to improve total body conditioning and add overload to aerobic endurance training.

Case Study 10.1

David is in his second year of RT. For the past 2 months, he has not progressed. Upon examination of his training program, David has performed the same exercises, has performed the same number of reps, and has not added weight to any of his exercises. That is, he has followed the same program without altering any variable. At this point, David has become discouraged and is considering discontinuing RT.

Question for Consideration: What advice would you give David regarding his lack of progress?

Specificity

The principle of specificity entails that all training adaptations are specific to the stimulus applied. Although nonspecific improvements take place, most improvements will take place specific to the stimuli. Training adaptations are specific to the muscle actions involved, velocity of movement and rate of force development (RFD), ROM, muscle groups trained, energy metabolism, movement pattern, and intensity/volume of training (7). Specificity becomes most evident during progression to more advanced RT as many studies have shown a multitude of transfer training effects in untrained and moderately trained individuals. This transfer of training effect applies to

- Strength carryover from unilateral training (to the opposite limb) or to multiple-joint activities
- Strength carryover from the trained muscle action to a nontrained action
- Strength and hypertrophy carryover from limited-ROM training to other areas of the ROM or full ROM
- Strength carryover from one velocity to another velocity
- Motor performance (jumping ability, sprint speed, and sport-specific movements) improvements resulting from other modalities of training
- Possible attenuation of endurance or strength/power performance due to concurrent strength and endurance training (see Chapter 17)

Muscle Action

RT with eccentric (ECC), concentric (CON), and isometric (ISOM) actions increases muscle strength. Much of the strength gains are specific to the type of muscle action trained (7). Training with CON muscle actions yields the greatest increases in CON muscle strength. However, some transferred training effects occur. When comparing ISOM to dynamic RT, ISOM training can increase dynamic strength (especially when multiple joint angles are trained) and dynamic training can increase ISOM muscle strength (8). Dynamic muscle strength increases are greatest when ECC actions are included (9). Because most training programs include CON and ECC muscle actions, strength will increase mostly in these muscle actions. Although ISOM strength may increase (as there are ISOM actions present during dynamic RT), the most effective way to increase ISOM strength is through specific ISOM training at various joint angles.

Velocity of Movement

Velocity specificity indicates that greatest strength increases take place at or near the training velocity. Some carryover effects to nontrained velocities may occur as well as carryover velocity effects between muscle actions (ISOM training can increase ISOM RFD and dynamic movement velocity) (7). Research has focused on isokinetic RT where velocity specificity is seen plus some carryover above and below the training velocity (1). Collectively, these studies show that training at a moderate velocity (180°–240° per second) produces the greatest strength increases across all testing velocities (3). RT with dynamic muscle actions demonstrates specificity and carryover increases to other nontrained lifting velocities. The greatest carryover effects are seen in untrained or moderately trained individuals. Advanced trainees benefit greatly from training at a velocity specific to their needs. Strength/power athletes benefit most from high-velocity movements (or the intent to maximally accelerate the load) (10,11).

Range of Motion

Specificity of ROM is seen during limited-ROM dynamic, isokinetic, or ISOM strength training. Dynamic limited-ROM training can increase strength in the trained ROM, with some carryover increases throughout full ROM (7). ISOM-training strength increases are specific to the joint angles trained (angular specificity) but may carry over to ±20°–30° of the trained angle (12). The magnitude of carryover is greatest at joint angles at greater muscle lengths. These studies show the importance of training in a full ROM for maximal improvements. There are some exceptions to where dynamic partial ROM repetitions may be beneficial. However, RT is most effective when repetitions are performed in a full ROM. Muscle hypertrophy may occur during full and partial ROM RT; thus, the addition of some partial ROM sets to full ROM training may have benefits for athletes (13). For ISOM training, it is recommended that multiple joint angles are trained corresponding to full joint ROM.

Muscle Groups Trained

Adaptations to training take place predominantly in those muscle groups that were trained (14). Ideally, training will target all major muscle groups. Nevertheless, some areas may be untrained or trained submaximally. Adaptations to training can only take place when muscle group–specific exercises are performed. Training all major muscle groups is important for attaining muscle balance, reducing injuries, and optimizing performance.

Energy Metabolism

Adaptations to training are specific to the energy system involvement. Energy systems adapt mostly by increasing enzyme activity or substrate storage/usage (see Chapter 8). The interaction between volume, intensity, movement velocity, and rest-interval length is critical to eliciting acute metabolic responses that target different energy systems. Although all metabolic systems are actively engaged, one may predominate based on the training stimulus. Much of the energy demands of resistance exercise are met by the ATP-PC and glycolytic metabolic pathways. Anaerobic glycolysis becomes increasingly important during intense, long-duration sets and when short rest intervals are used.

Movement Patterns

Although a transfer of training effect may occur and is desired when it comes to performing motor skills, specificity in program design relates to movement patterns. Adaptations are specific to the types of movement patterns used during training.

Interpreting Research
The Intent to Lift Weights Rapidly Is Critical to Strength Development

Behm DG, Sale DG. Intended rather than actual movement velocity determines velocity-specific training response. *J Appl Physiol*. 1993;74:359–68.

A study was conducted by David Behm and Digby Sale in 1993 (10). In this study, men and women trained 3 days per week for 16 weeks using ISOM or dynamic ballistic ankle dorsiflexions against resistance for 5 sets of 10 reps. Training produced similar velocity-specific strength and RFD increases.

Interestingly, the observed training responses previously attributed to high-velocity training also occurred during ISOM ballistic training where the intent was to maximize RFD. The authors concluded that the intent to perform a ballistic, high-velocity action was the key and not the muscle action or resultant velocity per se. The practical application indicates that the major stimulus for strength/power training may be the intent to maximally accelerate the weight.

Examples of the movement patterns examined include free weights versus machines, open- versus closed-chain kinetic exercises, unilateral versus bilateral training, and movement-specific training.

Free Weights versus Machines

Specificity of adaptations is seen during training with free weights and machines (advantages and disadvantages of each modality are discussed in Chapter 13). Although both are effective for increasing muscle strength, it is difficult to state which modality favors greater strength increases. The testing device is critical as free-weight training leads to greater improvements on free-weight tests and machine training results in greater performance on machine tests (15). When a neutral testing device is used, strength improvement from free weights and machines are similar (16). Free-weight training appears more applicable to motor skill enhancement, *e.g.*, vertical jump performance, due to the restricted nature and stabilization effects of machines. A recent study showed that both free-weight and machine RT in older adults produced significant strength increases although free weights added some advantage for leg and triceps strength (17). Carryover effects may be observed. For example, we previously showed that 6 weeks of multiple-joint isokinetic machine RT (chest press, row: 5 sets of 6–10 reps at 75%–85% of peak strength, velocity = 0.15 m·s^{-1} or 3-s CON: 3-s ECC) in women increased 1 RM strength in the bench press (by 10.2%), bent-over barbell row (by 11.2%), and maximal modified push-up endurance performance (by 28.6%) in addition to chest press and row isokinetic strength increases indicating a carryover of training effects to dynamic exercise performance (18). Thus, best results are achieved through modality-specific training; however, carryover or additive effects can provide the trainee with benefits and are often sought in an attempt to maximize performance during comprehensive multimodality training programs.

Open- versus Closed-Chain Kinetic Exercises

A closed-chain kinetic exercise is one where the distal segments are fixed (leg press, squat, deadlift), while an open-chain kinetic exercise (leg extension, leg curl) enables the distal segment to freely move against loading. Many closed-chain exercises stress multiple joints, while many open-chain exercises are single joint. Moderate-to-high relationships between closed-chain exercise and vertical/long jump performance have been shown (19,20) indicating that performance in closed-chain exercises is strongly related to various motor performance skills. Augustsson et al. (21) compared 6 weeks of barbell squat training to knee extension and hip adduction exercises on machines and showed that squat training increased vertical jump by 10%, whereas no difference was found after open-chain exercise training. Closed-chain exercises have been recommended to a greater extent by some exercise professionals compared to open-chain exercises because they are regarded as more functional, provide more proprioceptive feedback, produce less joint shear force, have different torque/ROM curves, and alter the recruitment pattern of muscles (22). This concept was supported as the onset of neuromuscular activity in the lower extremity during closed-chain exercises occurred earlier (22). It was also shown that vastus medialis activity was greater during closed-chain exercise but rectus femoris activity was greater during open-chain exercise (22).. Other studies have shown that closed-chain exercise training led to greater increases in femoral neck bone mineral density (BMD) and balance improvements in postmenopausal women (23), and led to greater strength and muscle size increases and reduced Q angle in patients with patellar chondromalacia (24). In the upper body, closed-chain training produced greater improvements in shoulder power and throwing velocity (by 3.4% vs. 0.5%) in Division 1 softball players (25). Greater shoulder and trunk muscle activation has been shown during closed-chain exercises (26). However, meta-analyses examining anterior cruciate ligament (ACL) patients with reconstructed knees have shown similar efficacy between closed and open-chain exercise training (27,28). Thus, both appear beneficial for a variety of goals but closed-chain exercises appear superior for athletic performance.

Unilateral versus Bilateral Training

Unilaterally or bilaterally (one vs. two arms or legs) performed exercises affect the neuromuscular adaptations to training. *Cross education* refers to strength gained in the nontrained limb during unilateral training. The strength increase in the untrained limb may range as high as 22% (mean increase = ~8%) and is thought to occur predominately via neural adaptations (29,30). *Bilateral deficit* refers to the strength produced by both limbs contracting bilaterally, which is smaller than the sum of the limbs contracting unilaterally. Unilateral training (although it increases bilateral strength) contributes to a greater bilateral deficit, whereas bilateral training reduces the bilateral deficit (31). Specificity is observed as unilateral RT results in better performance of unilateral tasks than bilateral training (32). Athletes involved in sports where unilateral strength and power are important and those with glaring weakness on the opposite side may benefit from unilateral training. This was recently shown in basketball players where unilateral RT (squats, drop jumps, and countermovement jumps) produced better improvements in change of direction performance, unilateral power development, and reduced limb imbalances compared to bilateral RT using the same exercises (33). Optimal training may involve the inclusion of both bilateral and unilateral exercises with the ratio of bilateral to unilateral contractions based on the needs of the sport. The American College of Sports Medicine (ACSM) has recommended the inclusion of both into RT programs targeting progression (34).

Unilateral resistance exercise (RE) requires greater balance, stability, and asymmetric loading. For example, performing a one-arm incline dumbbell press (with only one dumbbell)

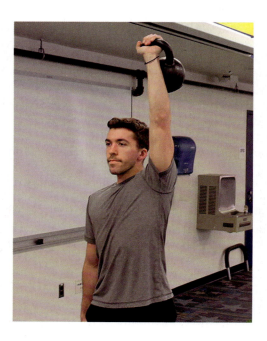

FIGURE 10.2 Overhead single kettlebell walk.

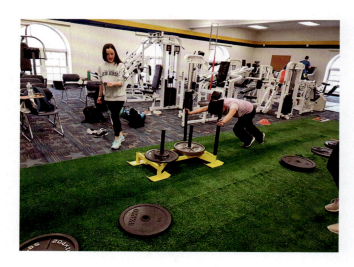

FIGURE 10.3 The sled push exercise.

requires the trunk muscles to contract intensely to offset the torque produced by unilateral loading and enable the athlete to maintain proper posture throughout the exercise. Altered trunk muscle (*i.e.*, external oblique, rectus abdominis) activation strategies have been shown comparing 1- versus 2-arm kettlebell swing (35), rowing (36), and shoulder press (37) exercises resulting from the differences in torques produced. *Unilateral asymmetric loading* can be implemented as training tool in a number of ways from using a single free weight or resistance implements (*i.e.*, dumbbell, kettlebell, bar, medicine ball, etc.) during RE or various implements can be added to locomotor movements such as walking (for carries; Fig. 10.2), jogging, jumping, and other biomotor skills to increase core muscle activation to a greater extent than unloaded or bilaterally loaded conditions.

Movement-Specific Training

Traditional RT involved selecting exercises that targeted specific muscle groups. For example, the quadriceps muscles could be trained by selecting exercises such as squats, lunges, and leg press. However, *movement-specific training* entails the use of loaded exercises that train or target specific movements (Fig. 10.3) rather than targeting specific muscle groups. The intent is to improve motor performance through RT and to provide a link between muscular strength gained through traditional RT and movement-specific strength. Many exercises involve the entire body. Training consists of multiplanar movements stressing multiple loading vectors, sometimes performed in unstable environments to enhance stabilizer muscle function with various pieces of equipment such as bands, medicine balls, dumbbells, stability balls, kettlebells, ropes, and other devices.

Overweight/Underweight Implements

A common training tool among athletes is to perform sport-specific exercises against a resistance, *e.g.*, overweight implements. Overweight implements allow the athlete to overload a sport-specific motion, thereby eliciting a resisted motor pattern similar to the motion itself as a method of strength training. It is thought that the overload enhances the neural response possibly via potentiation and that the enhanced neural responses lead to greater strength and power development with subsequent training. Training with overweight implements targets the force component of the force-velocity relationship. Underweight implements have been used primarily by throwing athletes. Underweight implements target the velocity component of the force-velocity relationship where athletes mimic the motor skill by throwing an object lighter than the ball used for the sport. For throwing athletes, studies have supported the use of over- and underweight implement training to enhance throwing velocity, and it has been suggested that the implement used be 5%–20% of normal load for throwing athletes (38). Overweight implements are used for any motor skill but have mostly been studied during overarm throwing in baseball and handball players. A biomechanical study in high school and college pitchers showed reduced pelvis, trunk, shoulder, and elbow angular velocities, and reduced shoulder and elbow joint torques and forces as pitching with a progressive increase in ball mass was performed (from 5 to 32 oz) (39). Van den Tillaar (40) reported that overweight implements increased throwing velocity by 5%–11%, underweight implements (20%–25% less than ball weight) increased velocity by 2%–7% (with best results found when combined with regulation balls during training), and the combination of over- and underweight implements increased throwing velocity by 3%–6%. A recent review of the literature showed that 7 out of 10 studies demonstrated increases in baseball pitching velocity (from 2 to >11 mph) resulting from training with overweight, underweight, or a combination of balls (41). Other examples include using a

| Sidebar | Use of Overweight/Underweight Implements for Increasing Bat Swinging Velocity |

Szymanski DJ, DeRenne C, Spaniol FJ. Contributing factors for increased bat swing velocity. *J Strength Cond Res.* 2009;23:1338–52.

Several studies investigated various training or warm-up potentiation effects for increasing bat swing velocity either acutely or over time as a function of training with overweight and underweight implements. Szymanski et al. (42) reviewed the literature and reported the following:

- Acute studies examining swinging either lighter bats or heavier bats (*i.e.*, with donuts, sleeves, or larger weighted bats) as a potentiation warm-up prior to hitting increased bat velocity as long as the weight differential was within 12% of the weight of the game bat. Very heavy or very light bats had adverse effects on bat velocity.
- Chronic studies examining training with heavier (8%–100% heavier than normal bat weight) or combined heavy or lighter implements (within 12% of bat weight) showed that: (a) heavy implement training — two studies showed increased bat velocity (by ~8% in one of the studies), whereas one study did not. (b) Overweight and underweight training — two out of two studies showed increased bat velocity (by 6%–10%) as a function of training. These studies ranged in training protocols from 240 to 600 swings per week for 6–12 weeks.
- Most general RT studies showed increases in bat swing velocity and that muscle strength, power, and lean body mass (LBM) have correlated to bat swing velocity in most studies.

chute, sled, or weighted vest during sprinting and jumping, swinging weighted bats, and using bands during a motor skill. Overweight and underweight implements should be used in conjunction with normal training as the velocity used with heavier implements may be slower.

Variation

Training variation requires alterations in one or more program variables over time to keep the stimulus optimal. Because the human body adapts rapidly to stress, variation is critical for subsequent adaptations to take place. Studies show that the systematic variation of volume and intensity is most effective for long-term progression as compared to programs that did not alter any program variable (43). Workouts can be varied in infinite ways. The S&C practitioner should think of each design characteristic as a tool in the proverbial toolbox, which provides a wide array of strategies for progression. Many ways exist to increase health- and skill-related fitness components, so the trainer benefits by including several methods of variation into program design. Training philosophies that support minimal variation will have limited effectiveness.

Progression and Program Design

Training Status and Progression

Training status dictates the pattern of progression for a fitness component. Training status reflects a continuum of adaptations such that fitness level, training experience, and genetic endowment each make a contribution. For example, the largest rates of strength improvement occur in untrained individuals as the window of adaptation is greatest during this time. Resistance-trained individuals show a slower rate of progression. In a position stand published by the ACSM in 2002 (44), >150 studies at that time were reviewed and showed strength increases of

- ~40% in untrained individuals
- ~20% in moderately trained individuals
- ~16% in trained individuals
- ~10% in advanced individuals
- ~2% in elite athletes

These studies ranged from 4 weeks to over 2 years in duration, and the training programs and testing procedures varied greatly. It is very difficult if not impossible to accurately classify an individual as trained or moderately trained because each classification comprises an interaction between fitness level and years of experience, *e.g.*, some individuals with many years of experience possess less strength than some with limited experience and vice versa. However, one can see that progression becomes more difficult as one's conditioning improves. Similar results were shown where untrained individuals responded most favorably while less increases were seen in trained individuals (45). Although these studies have focused on muscle strength, the same can be said about any fitness variable. The difficulty in strength progression occurs within as little as several months of training. Each improvement brings the individual closer to his or her genetic limit. Short-term studies (<16 weeks) show that the majority of strength increases take place within the first 4–8 weeks (46). The rate and magnitude of progression decrease with higher levels of conditioning. Plateaus occur as individuals get closer to their genetic ceiling and it becomes more difficult to improve (*principle of diminishing returns*). Training programs need to incorporate progressive overload, specificity, and variation to progress to a higher level.

General-to-Specific Model of Progression

When learning a new skill or participating in a new activity, a progression pattern from basic to more complex applications can be made. Whether one is learning to play a musical instrument, dance, play a new sport, or begin martial arts training, basic skills are first learned and practiced and then progression to a higher level ensues. Strength and conditioning practices follow similar principles. Because untrained individuals respond favorably to any training program, less-specific or general program design is all that is needed initially. There is no need for complexity at this stage as most programs will work. This initial phase is characterized by learning proper technique and building a conditioning base for progressive training. The ACSM has recommended general program structures to start (44). However, trained individuals show a slower rate of progression and demonstrate a cyclical pattern to their training (47). Training cycles provide greater opportunities for variation, and variation is needed in program design. Training progression occurs in an orderly manner from a general, or less-specific, program design initially to a more specific design with higher levels of training (Fig. 10.4). Advanced training targeting progression is more complex and requires great variation specific to training goals. Figure 10.4 is a simplified schematic representing a theoretical continuum of the amount of variation needed, known as a *general-to-specific model* for training progression. The narrow segment of the triangle (novice) suggests that limited variation is suitable in this population as it is important to begin gradually. However, the triangle widens as the individual progresses suggesting that more variation (specific training cycles) is necessary.

Individualization

All individuals respond differently to training. Figure 10.5 depicts individualized data from a study in our laboratory (48). Subjects engaged in 10 weeks of combined RT and sprint/plyometric training and individual 1 RM squat and 60-m sprint time improvements are presented. Everyone improved differently despite following the same training program. Genetics, training status, nutritional intake, and the program itself play substantial roles in the level of adaptation. One needs to be aware of individual response patterns and the need for variation if the response is minimal. The most effective programs are those designed to meet individual needs. This can oftentimes be difficult especially if one is training several athletes at once. When practical, program individualization is beneficial for progression.

Detraining (Principle of Reversibility)

Detraining is the complete cessation of training or substantial reduction in frequency, volume, or intensity that results in performance reductions and a loss of some of the beneficial physiological adaptations associated with training. The length of the detraining period and the training status of the individual dictate the magnitude of performance loss. Performance reductions may occur in as little as 2 weeks, and possibly sooner in trained athletes. In recreationally trained men, muscle strength may be reduced within 4 weeks of detraining (49), whereas other research shows very little change in strength during the first 6 weeks detraining (50). In trained individuals, detraining may result in greater losses in muscle power than strength (51). Strength reductions are related to neural mechanisms initially with atrophy of skeletal muscle predominating as the detraining period extends. Detraining leads to other physiological changes such as muscle fiber (IIa to IIx) transitions (49), reduced anaerobic substrate concentrations, and enzyme activity (52). Interestingly, the level of muscle strength, even after detraining, is rarely lower than pretraining levels showing that training has a residual effect when it is discontinued. However, when the individual returns to training, the rate of strength acquisition is high (53).

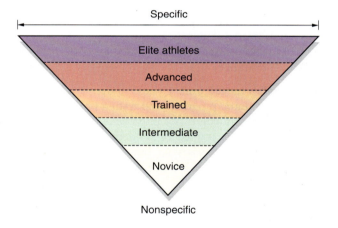

FIGURE 10.4 General-to-specific model of training and progression. The narrow part of the triangle refers to the magnitude of variation needed for beginning trainees. Because beginners progress easily, there is no need for complexity or great variation here. General or less-specific programs are recommended during this phase. However, with progression, gains take place more slowly. Greater variation is needed in program design (represented by the wide walls of the triangle). Advanced and elite athletes benefit greatly from cycling training. (This theoretical model is proposed based on current literature by the ACSM American College of Sports Medicine. Position Stand: Progression models in resistance training for healthy adults. *Med Sci Sports Exerc.* 2002;34:364–80; Kraemer WJ, Ratamess NA. Fundamentals of resistance training: progression and exercise prescription. *Med Sci Sports Exerc.* 2004;36:674–8.)

Importance of Supervision

Supervision by a certified professional is a critical component to any training program. Not only does supervised training result in less injuries and better technique, but performance

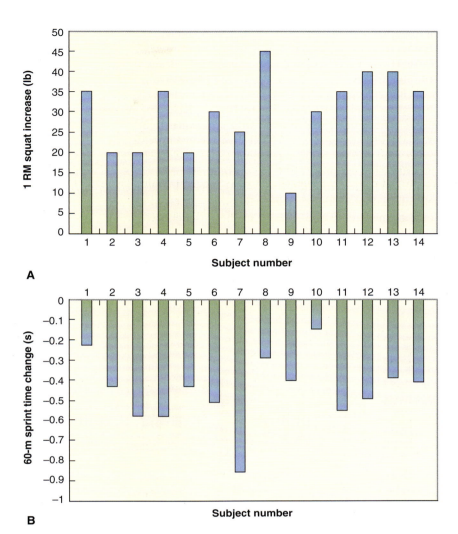

FIGURE 10.5 Individual responses to training. Individual responses to 10 weeks of combined sprint/plyometric and RT. **A.** Increases in 1 RM squat. **B.** Reductions in 60-m sprint times. Both panels show variable magnitudes of improvements for each subject. (Adapted with permission from Ratamess NA, Kraemer WJ, Volek JS, et al. The effects of ten weeks of resistance and combined plyometric/sprint training with the Meridian Elyte athletic shoe on muscular performance in women. *J Strength Cond Res*. 2007;21:882–7.)

is enhanced to a greater extent. Athletes who are supervised progress at a higher rate than those training on their own. This was shown by Mazzetti et al. (54) who compared 12 weeks of supervised versus unsupervised RT and found the supervised group increased maximal strength to a greater extent (>10%). Supervised training (in the form of a coach, trainer, or at least a partner) poses several advantages to the athlete targeting progression.

Supervision positively affects the intensities individuals self-select in unsupervised RT. Men and women tend to self-select training loads that are in the range of 40%–57% of their 1 RM per respective exercise (55–57). By many standards, these loads can be considered suboptimal or too low for muscle strength and hypertrophy increases in trained populations especially if the repetition number is low to moderate (*i.e.*, far below the point of muscular exhaustion). We compared

Myths & Misconceptions
Detraining Will Turn Muscle into Fat

Detraining leads to strength, power, and endurance reductions with the magnitude dependent upon training status and the detraining period duration. Although neural adaptations are mostly responsible for strength reductions initially, detraining periods of at least a few weeks or more result in a loss of muscle mass. The muscle mass lost is, in fact, lost and not directly converted to fat. Muscle mass is critical to enhancing the athlete's metabolism and kilocalorie expenditure on a daily basis. With muscle loss, a reduction in basal metabolic rate may ensue. This, coupled with other factors such as dietary kilocalorie intake and lower activity level, increases the likelihood of one increasing his or her body fat. Therefore, an increase in body fat can take place with detraining but not from direct conversion of lost muscle.

self-selected RT intensities of women who trained with and without a personal trainer (6). The women were carefully instructed to select a weight they would perform for 10 repetitions in their own workouts and were subsequently tested for 1 RM strength on four exercises: leg press, leg extension, chest press, and seated row. Figure 10.6 depicts some of the results. The women who trained with a personal trainer had greater 1 RM strength. For self-selected relative intensity, the group who trained with a personal trainer selected higher intensities for leg press (50% vs. 41%), chest press (57% vs. 48%), and seated row (56% vs. 42%). Overall, the average self-selected intensity for all exercises was ~51.4% in the personal trainer group and ~42.3% in the unsupervised group, showing positive benefits of supervision and an important role for a personal trainer in RT. A follow-up study showed similar results in men and women where self-selected training loads were higher for those who had a personal trainer by 12%–27% for the leg press, bench press, leg extension, and arm curl exercises (58). In comparison, self-selected intensity for RT was below recommended levels (44%–60% of 1 RM) in recreationally trained men and women; however, the same trainees self-selected higher and more appropriate intensities (~84% of peak heart rate) for AT thereby showing a greater likelihood of self-selecting lower intensities during RT (59).

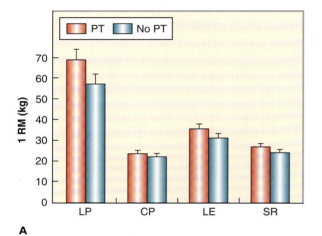

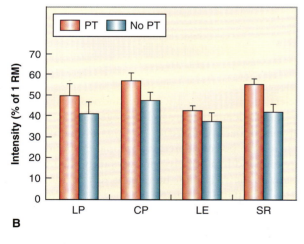

FIGURE 10.6 The effects of a personal trainer on self-selected RT intensities in healthy women. **A.** 1 RM strength data in the group who trained with (PT) and without (No PT) a personal trainer. **B.** Self-selected training intensities in the PT and No PT groups. LP, leg press; CP, chest press; LE, leg extension; SR, seated row. Women in the PT group had higher 1 RM strength values and self-selected higher relative loads than women who resistance trained without a personal trainer. (Reprinted with permission from Ratamess NA, Faigenbaum AD, Hoffman JR, Kang J. Self-selected resistance training intensity in healthy women: the influence of a personal trainer. *J Strength Cond Res.* 2008;22:103–11).

SUMMARY POINTS

- The three most important principles in program design are progressive overload, specificity, and variation. A program is effective when these principles are addressed.
- Supervised training programs are most effective when they are designed based on individual needs.
- Untrained individuals respond favorably to training, provided a threshold volume and intensity are prescribed. It is recommended that general program design be used initially while trainees learn proper technique and build a conditioning base. With training progression, greater specificity is needed to optimally target various training goals.
- The effects of training can be lost upon cessation, or detraining, when the stimulus is removed or the volume and intensity are drastically reduced.

REVIEW QUESTIONS

1. Which of the following is not an example of progressive overload?
    a. Increasing the amount of weight for an exercise while keeping the repetition number the same
    b. Maintaining the same amount of weight for an exercise while increasing the repetition number
    c. Decreasing the amount of weight for an exercise while decreasing the number of repetitions performed at the same velocity
    d. Increasing the amount of weight for an exercise while slightly decreasing the number of repetitions

2. Which of the following exercises is an example of a closed-chain kinetic exercise?
    a. Arm curl
    b. Leg press
    c. Triceps pushdown
    d. Lateral raise

3. The strength gained in a nontrained limb resulting from unilateral training is
   a. Cross education
   b. Bilateral deficit
   c. Detraining
   d. Accommodation

4. An athlete begins an 8-week weight training program. His weights increased substantially during training; however, he was tested using an ISOM device, and his scores only improved minimally. This testing tool appears to have been a violation of the principle of
   a. Specificity
   b. Variation
   c. Progressive overload
   d. Supervision

5. A general-to-specific model of training progression implies that
   a. Novice lifters require great variation in program design
   b. General programs work best in advanced to elite athletes
   c. Advanced to elite athletes require greater specificity in program design for progression
   d. None of the above

6. The staleness resulting from a lack in change in the training program is known as
   a. Specificity
   b. Variation
   c. Accommodation
   d. Progressive overload

7. The principle of diminishing returns entails progression, and it becomes more difficult as an athlete gets closer to his or her genetic ceiling.
   a. T
   b. F

8. The window of adaptation for strength gains is greatest in an elite strength athlete and least in an untrained individual.
   a. T
   b. F

9. Supervised training results in a greater rate of performance improvement.
   a. T
   b. F

10. ISOM training at one joint angle will not induce a strength carryover to adjacent nontrained areas of the ROM.
    a. T
    b. F

11. Detraining can lead to Type IIa to IIx fiber transitions.
    a. T
    b. F

REFERENCES

1. Hoffman JR, Ratamess NA. *A Practical Guide to Developing Resistance-Training Programs*. 2nd ed. Monterey (CA): Coaches Choice; 2008.
2. Zatsiorsky V, Kraemer WJ. *Science and Practice of Strength Training*. 2nd ed. Champaign (IL): Human Kinetics; 2006.
3. Fleck SJ, Kraemer WJ. *Designing Resistance Training Programs*. 3rd ed. Champaign (IL): Human Kinetics; 2004.
4. Polsgrove MJ, Eggleston BM, Lockyer RJ. Impact of 10-weeks of yoga practice on flexibility and balance of college athletes. *Int J Yoga*. 2016;9:27–34.
5. Tran MD, Holly RG, Lashbrook J, Amsterdam EA. Effects of hatha yoga practice on the health-related aspects of physical fitness. *Prev Cardiol*. 2001;4:165–70.
6. Ratamess NA, Faigenbaum AD, Hoffman JR, Kang J. Self-selected resistance training intensity in healthy women: the influence of a personal trainer. *J Strength Cond Res*. 2008;22:103–11.
7. Kraemer WJ, Ratamess NA. Fundamentals of resistance training: progression and exercise prescription. *Med Sci Sports Exerc*. 2004;36:674–8.
8. Morrissey MC, Harman EC, Johnson MJ. Resistance training modes: specificity and effectiveness. *Med Sci Sports Exerc*. 1995;27:648–60.
9. Dudley GA, Tesch PA, Miller BJ, Buchanan MD. Importance of eccentric actions in performance adaptations to resistance training. *Aviat Space Environ Med*. 1991;62:543–50.
10. Behm DG, Sale DG. Intended rather than actual movement velocity determines velocity-specific training response. *J Appl Physiol*. 1993;74:359–68.
11. Behm DG, Sale DG. Velocity specificity of resistance training. *Sports Med*. 1993;15:374–88.
12. Knapik JJ, Mawdsley RH, Ramos MU. Angular specificity and test mode specificity of isometric and isokinetic strength training. *J Orthop Sports Phys Ther*. 1983;5:58–65.
13. Newmire DE, Willoughby DS. Partial compared with full range of motion resistance training for muscle hypertrophy: a brief review and an identification of potential mechanisms. *J Strength Cond Res*. 2018;32:2652–64.
14. Kraemer WJ, Nindl BC, Ratamess NA, et al. Changes in muscle hypertrophy in women with periodized resistance training. *Med Sci Sports Exerc*. 2004;36:697–708.
15. Boyer BT. A comparison of the effects of three strength training programs on women. *J Appl Sports Sci Res*. 1990;4:88–94.
16. Willoughby DS, Gillespie JW. A comparison of isotonic free weights and omnikinetic exercise machines on strength. *J Hum Mov Stud*. 1990;19:93–100.
17. Schott N, Johnen B, Holfelder B. Effects of free weights and machine training on muscular strength in high-functioning older adults. *Exp Gerontol*. 2019;122:15–24.
18. Ratamess NA, Beller NA, Gonzalez AM, et al. The effects of multiple-joint isokinetic resistance training on maximal isokinetic and dynamic muscle strength and local muscular endurance. *J Sports Sci Med*. 2016;15:34–40.
19. Augustsson J, Thomee R. Ability of closed and open kinetic chain tests of muscular strength to assess functional performance. *Scand J Med Sci Sports*. 1998;10:164–8.
20. Blackburn JR, Morrissey MC. The relationship between open and closed kinetic chain strength of the lower limb and jumping performance. *J Orthop Sports Phys Ther*. 1998;27:430–5.
21. Augustsson J, Esko A, Thomee R, Svantesson U. Weight training of the thigh muscles using closed vs. open kinetic chain exercises:

a comparison of performance enhancement. *J Orthop Sports Phys Ther*. 1998;27:3–8.

22. Stensdotter AK, Hodges PW, Mellor R, Sundelin G, Hager-Ross C. Quadriceps activation in closed and in open kinetic chain exercises. *Med Sci Sports Exerc*. 2003;35:2043–7.

23. Thabet AAE, Alshehri MA, Helal OF, Refaat B. The impact of closed versus open kinetic chain exercises on osteoporotic femur neck and risk of fall in postmenopausal women. *J Phys Ther Sci*. 2017;29:1612–6.

24. Bakhtiari AH, Fatemi E. Open versus closed kinetic chain exercises for patellar chondromalacia. *Br J Sports Med*. 2008;42:99–102.

25. Prokopy MP, Ingersoll CD, Nordenschild E, et al. Closed-kinetic chain upper-body training improves throwing performance of NCAA Division I softball players. *J Strength Cond Res*. 2008;22:1790–8.

26. Pozzi F, Plummer HA, Sanchez N, Lee Y, Michener LA. Electro-myography activation of shoulder and trunk muscles is greater during closed chain compared to open chain exercises. *J Electromyogr Kinesiol*. 2019;102306. doi: 10.1016/j.jelekin.2019.05.007.

27. Glass R, Waddell J, Hoogenboom B. The effects of open versus closed kinetic chain exercises on patients with ACL deficient or reconstructed knees: a systematic review. *N Am J Sports Phys Ther*. 2010;5:74–84.

28. Jewiss D, Ostman C, Smart N. Open versus closed kinetic chain exercises following an anterior cruciate ligament reconstruction: a systematic review and meta-analysis. *J Sports Med (Hindawi Publ Corp)*. 2017;2017:4721548.

29. Munn J, Herbert RD, Gandevia SC. Contralateral effects of unilateral resistance training: a meta-analysis. *J Appl Physiol*. 2004;96:1861–6.

30. Shima SN, Ishida K, Katayama K, Morotome Y, Sato Y, Miyamura M. Cross education of muscular strength during unilateral resistance training and detraining. *Eur J Appl Physiol*. 2002;86:287–94.

31. Kuruganti U, Parker P, Rickards J, Tingley M, Sexsmith J. Bilateral isokinetic training reduces the bilateral leg strength deficit for both old and young adults. *Eur J Appl Physiol*. 2005;94:175–9.

32. McCurdy KW, Langford GA, Doscher MW, Wiley LP, Mallard KG. The effects of short-term unilateral and bilateral lower-body resistance training on measures of strength and power. *J Strength Cond Res*. 2005;19:9–15.

33. Gonzalo-Skok O, Tous-Fajardo J, Suarez-Arrones L, et al. Single-leg power output and between-limbs imbalances in team-sport players: unilateral versus bilateral combined resistance training. *Int J Sports Physiol Perform*. 2017;12:106–14.

34. American College of Sports Medicine. Position Stand: Progression models in resistance training for healthy adults. *Med Sci Sports Exerc*. 2009;41:687–708.

35. Andersen V, Fimland FS, Gunnarskog A, et al. Core muscle activation in one-armed and two-armed kettlebell swing. *J Strength Cond Res*. 2016;30:1196–204.

36. Saeterbakken A, Andersen V, Brudeseth A, Lund H, Fimland MS. The effect of performing bi- and unilateral row exercises on core muscle activation. *Int J Sports Med*. 2015;36:900–5.

37. Saeterbakken A, Fimland MS. Muscle activity of the core during bilateral, unilateral, seated and standing resistance exercise. *Eur J Appl Physiol*. 2012;112:1671–8.

38. Escamilla RF, Speer KP, Fleisig GS, Barrentine SW, Andrews JR. Effects of throwing overweight and underweight baseballs on throwing velocity and accuracy. *Sports Med*. 2000;29:259–72.

39. Fleisig GS, Diffendaffer AZ, Aune KT, Ivey B, Laughlin WA. Biomechanical analysis of weighted-ball exercises for baseball pitchers. *Sports Health*. 2017;9:210–5.

40. Van den Tillaar R. Effect of different training programs on the velocity of overarm throwing: a brief review. *J Strength Cond Res*. 2004;18:388–96.

41. Caldwell JME, Alexander FJ, Ahmad CS. Weighted-ball velocity enhancement programs for baseball pitchers: a systematic review. *Orthop J Sports Med*. 2019;7:1–14.

42. Szymanski DJ, DeRenne C, Spaniol FJ. Contributing factors for increased bat swing velocity. *J Strength Cond Res*. 2009;23:1338–52.

43. Fleck SJ. Periodized strength training: a critical review. *J Strength Cond Res*. 1999;13:82–9.

44. American College of Sports Medicine. Position Stand: Progression models in resistance training for healthy adults. *Med Sci Sports Exerc*. 2002;34:364–80.

45. Rhea MR, Alvar BA, Burkett LN, Ball SD. A meta-analysis to determine the dose-response for strength development. *Med Sci Sports Exerc*. 2003;35:456–64.

46. Hickson RC, Hidaka K, Foster C. Skeletal muscle fiber type, resistance training, and strength-related performance. *Med Sci Sports Exerc*. 1994;26:593–8.

47. Häkkinen K, Pakarinen A, Alen M, Kauhanen H, Komi PV. Neuromuscular and hormonal adaptations in athletes to strength training in two years. *J Appl Physiol*. 1988;65:2406–12.

48. Ratamess NA, Kraemer WJ, Volek JS, et al. The effects of ten weeks of resistance and combined plyometric/sprint training with the Meridian Elyte athletic shoe on muscular performance in women. *J Strength Cond Res*. 2007;21:882–7.

49. Terzis G, Stratakos G, Manta P, Georgladis G. Throwing performance after resistance training and detraining. *J Strength Cond Res*. 2008;22:1198–204.

50. Kraemer WJ, Koziris LP, Ratamess NA, et al. Detraining produces minimal changes in physical performance and hormonal variables in recreationally strength-trained men. *J Strength Cond Res*. 2002;16:373–82.

51. Izquierdo M, Ibanez J, Gonzalez-Badillo JJ, et al. Detraining and tapering effects on hormonal responses and strength performance. *J Strength Cond Res*. 2007;21:768–75.

52. MacDougall JD, Ward GR, Sale DG, Sutton JR. Biochemical adaptation of human skeletal muscle to heavy resistance training and immobilization. *J Appl Physiol*. 1977;43:700–3.

53. Staron RS, Leonardi MJ, Karapondo DL, et al. Strength and skeletal muscle adaptations in heavy-resistance-trained women after detraining and retraining. *J Appl Physiol*. 1991;70:631–40.

54. Mazzetti SA, Kraemer WJ, Volek JS, et al. The influence of direct supervision of resistance training on strength performance. *Med Sci Sports Exerc*. 2000;32:1175–84.

55. Cotter JA, Garver MJ, Dinyer TK, Fairman CM, Focht BC. Ratings of perceived exertion during acute resistance exercise performed at imposed and self-selected loads in recreationally trained women. *J Strength Cond Res*. 2017;31:2313–8.

56. Focht BC. Perceived exertion and training load during self-selected and imposed-intensity resistance exercise in untrained women. *J Strength Cond Res*. 2007;21:183–7.

57. Glass S, Stanton D. Self-selected resistance training intensity in novice weightlifters. *J Strength Cond Res*. 2004;18:324–7.

58. Dias MRC, Simao RF, Saavedra FJF, Ratamess NA. Influence of a personal trainer on self-selected loading during resistance exercise. *J Strength Cond Res*. 2017;31:1925–30.

59. Dias MRC, Simao RF, Saavedra FJF, Buzzachera CF, Fleck S. Self-selected training load and RPE during resistance and aerobic training among recreational exercisers. *Percept Mot Skills*. 2018;125:769–87.

PART III

Strength Training and Conditioning Program Design

CHAPTER 11

Warm-Up, Flexibility, and Myofascial Release

OBJECTIVES

After completing this chapter, you will be able to:

◆ Discuss the physiological effects of a warm-up and the importance of warming up for injury prevention and performance enhancement

◆ Design general and specific warm-ups

◆ Discuss factors that affect flexibility

◆ Describe different modalities of stretching

◆ Discuss flexibility training guidelines and design a flexibility training program

◆ Discuss myofascial release and the benefits of foam rolling

◆ Discuss the importance of including a cooldown following a workout

---

An athlete can only attain peak performance when he or she has been properly prepared. Preparation can be viewed in terms of chronic and acute. Chronic preparation consists of the athlete's training program, diet, and recovery strategies used over a period of time. Acute preparation focuses on the athlete's strategic plan before a workout or competition. Included in acute preparation are dietary intake and fluid consumption, mental focus and visualization, competition strategy, and the warm-up. The warm-up is used to prepare the body for high-intensity and/or high-volume exercise and reduce the potential risk of injury. A warm-up generally includes some aerobic exercises and/or exercises that increase joint range of motion (ROM) such as very light stretching, dynamic calisthenics, and sport-specific drills. Joint ROM impacts the athlete's flexibility. Flexibility is a health-related fitness component known to affect performance and health. In this chapter, the physiological and performance benefits of a proper warm-up, myofascial release, and flexibility training are discussed.

Warm-Up

A warm-up consists of performing lower-intensity exercise to prepare the body for more intense physical activity, and it is widely accepted that warming-up prior to exercise is vital for performance, although reduction of injury risk has not been established (1). The warm-up begins very light and should increase in intensity progressively until the athlete is prepared for the intensity of the workout. A warm-up can be passive (where muscle temperature is increased without exercise via a sauna, hot shower or water immersion, or heat application) or active (via movement and exercise). Both types of warm-ups increase muscle temperature effectively and augment performance compared to no warm-up (2,3). Active warm-ups tend to result in better short-term performance than passive warm-ups and enhance moderate- and longer-duration exercise, provided the active warm-up is not fatiguing (2,3). There are two types of active warm-ups: general and specific. A *general warm-up* consists of low-intensity exercise such as slow jogging and/or stationary cycling that lasts for 5–10 minutes. A *specific warm-up* consists of dynamic or very light static movements similar to the sport/activity and may last between 5 and 15 minutes. Specific warm-ups vary greatly depending on the sport. Often, a general warm-up precedes a specific warm-up. The specific warm-up segment provides the athlete with a good opportunity to incorporate corrective exercises or exercises that facilitate core stability in preparation for intense workouts or practices. Figure 11.1 depicts a general warm-up followed by two specific warm-ups: one for a sprint workout and the other for a lower-body weight training workout where the first exercise in sequence is the barbell back squat (exercises are described in other chapters).

The optimal warm up is still up for debate, though it likely varies by sport or activity. The main goal of the warm up is to improve muscle temperature, $\dot{V}O_2$, neuromuscular

251

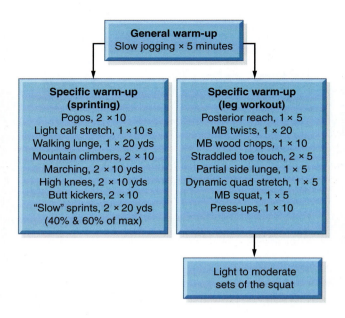

FIGURE 11.1 Examples of general and specific warm-ups.

athlete first selects an activity for the general warm-up, perhaps cycling or light jogging for 5–10 minutes. The intensity should be low and should not fatigue the athlete. A specific warm-up follows. Exercises selected for the specific warm-up vary greatly and may consist of calisthenics, technique drills, resistance exercises, medicine ball exercises, dynamic flexibility exercises (see Sidebar: Dynamic Flexibility Exercises), and low-to-moderate-intensity plyometric, sprint, and agility preparatory exercises. Several of these exercises are described in other chapters. These are low-to-moderate intensity initially but progress to moderately high intensity if the athlete is preparing for explosive exercise. Some high-intensity exercises may be used for the potentiation of the athletic skills. Five to ten drills can be selected and performed for 1–3 sets totaling 5–15 minutes. For aerobic training, the general warm-up can progress into the main workout or can precede a specific warm-up. Alternatively, a warm-up consisting of light stretches, calisthenics, or corrective exercises may precede the aerobic warm-up. The goal is to have the athlete prepare the body for exercise prior to beginning an aerobic segment; then they can immediately progress from the low-intensity aerobic segment to the workload segment. For resistance exercise, the specific warm-up may consist of calisthenics, corrective exercises, and dynamic flexibility exercises and progress into light weight training sets. Inclusion of low-intensity plyometric drills may help facilitate performance especially if the workout begins

control, and flexibility and minimize fatigue prior to exercise (4). Many coaches and athletes experiment with different warm-ups and eventually design one individualized to meet their needs. Designing a warm-up is relatively simple. The

Sidebar: Some Dynamic Flexibility Exercises Used in Specific Warm-ups

- Arm circles (front and back)
- Neck rotations
- Hip circles (standing or kneeling)
- Overhead medicine ball (MB) lassos
- Toe touches
- Medicine ball front raises
- Medicine ball figure eights
- Arm cross-face circles
- Quadruped
- Crab kicks
- Jumping jacks
- Burpee
- Front/back kicks
- Trunk circles from a straddled position
- Wrist "praying" flexion/extension
- Ankle rolls
- Torso rotations/side bends/bent-over T-rotations
- 3-point thoracic rotation
- Knee circles
- Standing/walking knee hugs
- Cross-body kicks
- Side leg swings
- Shoulder crossovers (horizontal adduction/abduction)
- Straddled medicine ball rollouts/circles
- Lunge/lateral lunge with or without rotation
- Groiner/groiner with rotational reach
- Catcher-squat to hamstring stretch
- Supine or standing hip medial/lateral rotation
- Fire hydrant
- High-knee crossovers
- Windshield wipers
- Body weight squats
- Mountain climbers
- Glute bridge
- Triceps extensions with MB (with posterior reach)
- Stability ball (SB) arm circles (from kneeling, flexed position)
- Press-ups
- SB supine slides (into bridge)
- Overhead claps
- Diagonal reaches
- Rockers (with knees/hips flexed)
- Woodchops

with heavy multiple-joint exercises or explosive exercises such as the Olympic lifts. For sprint, plyometric, and agility training, the specific warm-up may consist of low-intensity drills and progress to high-intensity drills. For sport-specific warm-ups, general drills can be incorporated, which culminate into sport-specific activities, *e.g.*, throwing/hitting for baseball, shooting/layup drills for basketball.

Physiology of Warming Up

A proper warm-up prepares the body for exercise and is thought to reduce the risk of injury. Although very little scientific research supports the contention that a warm-up reduces the incidence of muscular/connective tissue (CT) injury, at the very least a proper warm-up can enhance performance and may reduce injury potential (1,5). Several physiological responses occur during an active warm-up. These include (2,6,7).

- Increased muscle and core temperature
- Increased blood flow
- Increased speed of metabolic reactions, phosphocreatine use, and ATP turnover
- Increased muscle cross-bridge cycling rate
- Increased release of oxygen from hemoglobin and myoglobin (Bohr effect)
- Increased heart rate and cardiac output
- Increased nerve conduction velocity and neural activation
- Increased oxygen consumption
- Decreased joint/CT and skeletal muscle viscosity and resistance
- Increased compliance of ligaments and tendons
- Increased muscle glycogen breakdown and glycolysis
- Increased mental preparedness and psychological functioning

These acute responses are thought to elicit greater strength, power, ROM, speed, agility, and endurance following a warm-up.

Performance Effects

Most studies show an acute warm-up enhances performance more than not performing a warm-up (5,8). Vertical jump, swimming time, running time, and cycling power are enhanced after 3–5 minutes of low- to moderate-intensity warm-up (3). Much of the enhancement is attributed to increased muscle temperature (2). However, some studies have not shown enhancement, and a few studies have shown reduced performance, suggesting the warm-up was too intense or did not include enough recovery time before assessment (2,3). Warm-ups enhance performance of intermediate-duration activities. It is thought that, in addition to higher muscle temperatures, performing a warm-up before an intermediate- or long-duration activity increases the initial $\dot{V}O_2$ level, thereby reducing oxygen deficit and increasing the contribution of aerobic metabolism throughout the event (3). The longer the duration of the event, the less likely a warm-up will affect performance. *It is recommended that a general warm-up consisting of aerobic exercise at 40%–60% of $\dot{V}O_{2max}$ for 5–10 minutes (with ~5 min of recovery before the event begins) be used to enhance athletic performance* (3,9,10). The ACSM recommends a dynamic warm-up involving large muscle groups of no longer than 15 minutes (9). An endurance-trained athlete may require a higher intensity (70% of $\dot{V}O_{2max}$) to adequately increase muscle temperature (10,11). The key elements to the warm-up are to (a) increase muscle temperature, (b) increase $\dot{V}O_2$, and (c) minimize fatigue (ATP-PC and glycogen depletion, blood lactate).

High-Intensity Warm-Up: Postactivation Potentiation (PAP) and Postactivation Performance Enhancement (PAPE)

One concept of interest is a warm-up consisting of high-intensity exercise. Although some strength and conditioning (S&C) professionals view a warm-up as a low-to-moderate-intensity activity used to prepare the body for more challenging exercises, others view potentiation (*e.g.*, PAP and the more recently termed PAPE) protocols as high-intensity warm-ups (12) (Fig. 11.2). PAP and PAPE are most commonly used for high-intensity exercises and consists of a gradual progression in intensity (while minimizing fatigue). During PAP, activated motor units stay facilitated for a short period of time following maximal or near-maximal muscle contractions as evidenced by enhanced evoked muscle twitch force. However, performance of subsequent exercise may be enhanced for a period of time following a traditional PAP period thereby indicating multiple mechanisms are contributing to the performance enhancement; hence the concept of PAPE (12). Mechanisms suggested to enhance performance include increased neural drive and reflex activity, increased muscle temperature, increased phosphorylation of myosin regulatory light chains, increased calcium sensitivity and mobilization, and increased muscle–tendon stiffness; and the response may be augmented to a larger extent in athletes with larger percentages of fast-twitch fibers and higher levels of strength (7,12). During this time of facilitation, muscle strength, power, and endurance can be enhanced (12–14). Studies have shown that performing back or front squats with 30%–90% of 1-RM enhanced 40-m sprint speed (15,16); performing heavy squats (5 sets of 1 rep with 90% of 1-RM) increased jump power

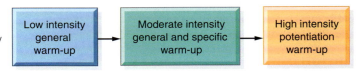

FIGURE 11.2 The warm-up continuum. Warm-ups exist on an intensity continuum and occur from general to specific. (LI, low intensity; MI, moderate intensity; HI, high intensity.)

in trained athletes but not recreationally trained individuals (17); performing half squats (20%–90% of 1-RM) increased jump peak force and height and greater improvements were seen in those athletes with higher levels of strength (18,19); performing the bench press (6 reps with 65% of 1-RM) increased bench press peak power (20); and performing a 1-RM back squat protocol increased max vertical jump height by 3% (21). Performing drop jumps or weighted jumps may augment power performance by 2%–5% (7). A meta-analysis has shown that exercises of moderate intensity (60%–84% 1-RM) produced a greater response compared to high-intensity (85% 1-RM) contractions, multiple sets were better than single sets, rest intervals of 7–10 minutes following PAP were better than 3–7 minutes and >10 minutes, and the effects were more prevalent in athletes compared to untrained individuals (22). Thus, several studies have shown enhanced performance following high-intensity exercise or PAP/PAPE warm-up protocols. However, some studies have not shown acute potentiation (19).

Dynamic versus Static Warm-Ups

Most studies show that dynamic warm-ups enhance performance (3). The mean performance improvement following dynamic flexibility exercises is ~1.3% but could exceed 7% when the set duration >90 seconds (23). However, a major topic of debate is the decision to include intense static stretching into the warm-up. For many years, static stretching was widely accepted for use in warm-ups with the intent to increase muscle temperature and ROM, and to reduce injury risk. This was particularly evident for athletes whose sports required high levels of flexibility (gymnastics). However, the last 30 years of research has yielded some interesting findings regarding intense (not light) static stretching prior to strength and power events thereby leaving its use in question. Many researchers, coaches, and practitioners have opted to include dynamic warm-up protocols in lieu of intense static stretching.

Warm-ups that include static stretching have been shown to impair performance (muscle strength and power performance, *e.g.*, vertical jump height, power, agility, and sprinting speed) in multiple studies (24–31). The reduction in muscle strength has been termed the *stretching-induced force deficit* (32). Performance reductions were shown, with prolonged static stretching having the most profound effects (33). The reduced performance effects linger for up to 2 hours, and the strength/power reductions occur while joint ROM is increased following stretching (34). In direct comparison (10 min of static, ballistic, or proprioceptive neuromuscular facilitation [PNF] stretching), acute vertical jump performance was reduced by 4%, 2.7%, and 5.1%, respectively, but fully recovered after 15 minutes (35). Other studies have shown greater strength performance reductions following PNF stretching than static stretching (36). A few reviews and meta-analyses have attempted to quantify the performance changes seen following acute static stretching. Kay and Blazevich (33) reported acute static stretching durations of <30 seconds and 30–45 seconds have no significant del-

eterious performance effects; however, a dose-response effect is seen where significant reductions take place with durations ≥60 seconds. Behm et al. (37) reported an overall mean reduction in performance of 3.7% following static stretching with a 4.6% reduction seen in stretching duration ≥60 seconds and a trivial reduction of 1.1% with short duration stretching. The reductions were larger in strength-based activities than power. PNF stretching produced a mean performance reduction of 4.4%. Critical to these findings are that many studies post-test subjects within minutes (mean of ~3–5 min) of stretching and did not include dynamic exercises (37). Intense static stretching for long durations (60 s) as part of a warm-up can potentially reduce acute strength and power performance; thus, dynamic stretching during the warm-up is recommended (9).

The two major mechanism proposed to reduce force performance have been reduced neural drive and reduced musculotendinous stiffness. Reduced electromyographic (EMG) activity of muscles accompanies strength and power deficits following stretching, thereby indicating reduced neural drive (32,38). Behm et al. (37) tested subjects following 20 minutes of static stretching of the quadriceps and showed a 12% reduction in maximal voluntary contractile force and reduced neural activation ranging from 2% to 20%. It is thought that high-intensity stretching reduces musculotendinous stiffness thereby lessening the ergogenic effects of the stretch-shortening cycle. Musculotendinous stiffness is related to maximal concentric (CON) and isometric (ISOM) force production (39) and decreases following static stretching (40). Dynamic stretching may not produce much of a performance deficit and may be a favorable alternative. Interestingly, upper-body static stretching may not be a limiting factor for upper-body strength and power (41). Although performance of dynamic warm-up exercise after static stretching may reduce some of the deficit (29), some studies have shown reductions linger even if dynamic exercise is performed (29,42). The critical element is the intensity and duration/volume of the static stretching protocol. Minimal effects are seen with light stretching only for a few sets (43,44). The use of light stretching coupled with dynamic warm-up protocols is effective for optimizing performance (45). Acute stretching may increase running economy but a stretching program may not affect running economy in the long term (46). For those strength/power athletes who require high levels of flexibility (gymnasts, martial artists), some static stretching may be necessary but caution must be used to not overstretch and reduce performance. For example, rhythmic gymnasts generally warm up for ~45 minutes, a slow jog initially followed by sport-specific warm-up exercises and static stretching (47) to achieve the high level of ROM needed for the sport. The need for high flexibility trumps the undesirable effects of prolonged static stretching. However, intense stretching is recommended following the workout as part of a cooldown for strength/power athletes.

Notwithstanding the acute deficits of strength and power following high-intensity static stretching, some data indicate that long-term performance could be impacted. Performing

> **Interpreting Research**
> **Acute Static or Ballistic Stretching on Maximal Strength Performance**
>
> Bacurau RF, Monteiro GA, Ugrinowitsch C, et al. Acute effect of a ballistic and a static stretching exercise bout on flexibility and maximal strength. *J Strength Cond Res*. 2009;23: 304–308.
>
> Bacurau et al. (48) studied three conditions: (a) 20 minutes of static stretching, (b) 20 minutes of ballistic stretching, and (c) control condition. Immediately following each session was the determination of the 1-RM leg press. 1-RM was lower following static stretching (a reduction of ~28 kg) but 1-RM did not decrease after ballistic stretching. These results demonstrate that maximal strength performance can be negatively affected by intense prestatic stretching.

flexibility training prior to resistance training (RT) may reduce total RE (muscle endurance) volume by 9%–24% (49). Barroso et al. (50) reported that only PNF stretching before RT decreased leg press 1-RM by 5.5%; however, PNF, static, and ballistic decreased number of reps of the leg press at 80% of 1-RM by 18%–23%. A recent study showed that 10 weeks of RT following flexibility training produced inferior increases in muscle CSA and total lifting volume throughout compared to RT only; however, flexibility training before RT did not negatively affect 1-RM strength increases despite the volume differences (51). These studies show that flexibility training should follow RT when performed during the same workout. See Interpreting Research: Acute Static or Ballistic Stretching on Maximal Strength Performance.

Stretching and Flexibility

Flexibility is a measure of joint ROM without injury and is an important health-related component of fitness. *Static flexibility* describes ROM about a joint during active (unassisted) or passive (assisted) movement (where the final position is held), whereas *dynamic flexibility* (*functional flexibility*) describes ROM during movement. Another type of dynamic flexibility, *ballistic flexibility*, has been defined as ROM attained during explosive- or bouncing-type movements. Stretching is generally thought to improve flexibility.

Having adequate flexibility has many health and performance benefits. Flexibility training helps maintain appropriate muscle lengths and increase joint flexibility (52) where side-to-side symmetry should be the goal. In some cases, muscle shortening or tightness can take place over time (53), and flexibility training may help improve muscle length and balance. Flexibility training helps improve muscular weaknesses by increasing muscle strength and is thought to reduce the risk of certain types of injury although direct links to reduced injury have been inconsistent (54). Flexibility training can improve posture and the ability to move, relieve stress, and reduce the risk of low-back pain. From an athletic standpoint, improved flexibility may increase performance for several athletic skills. For example:

- Increased flexibility of the shoulders helps the Olympic weightlifter attain the proper overhead position in the snatch
- Increased flexibility of the hips helps the gymnast attain proper position during a split
- Increased flexibility of the hips and shoulders is crucial to the ice hockey goalie who needs to block the puck at many difficult angles
- Increased flexibility of the shoulder is crucial to the tennis player for maximizing the velocity and the accuracy of the serve
- Increased flexibility of the shoulders can help the volleyball player block a shot and spike the ball
- Increased flexibility of the hips and hamstrings is essential for the hurdler who must elevate over the hurdle without much deviation from his or her normal stride

Positive relationships exist between ankle flexibility and flutter kicking speed in female swimmers (55) although flexibility may not correlate to sprint performance (56). A 12-week static stretching program (resulting in an 18.1% increase in flexibility) increased long and vertical jump performance by 2.3% and 6.7%, respectively, 20-m sprint speed by 1.3%, maximal strength by 15%–32%, and endurance by 28%–32% (57). Overall, flexibility may enhance certain types of athletic performance, while poor flexibility may limit performance of some skills.

Flexibility and Injury Prevention

It is generally thought that greater joint flexibility decreases the risk of pain and injury, though there has not been consistent scientific evidence in support of this claim (1). Stretching, and the increase in flexibility, is thought to increase compliance of the tendon unit, thereby increasing the tendons' ability to absorb energy (58). Acute static stretching and static stretching programs reduce acute tendon stiffness, decrease hysteresis (the amount of energy lost as heat during the elastic recoil), and increase tendon compliance (59,60). These changes enhance joint ROM. However, studies examining the effects of stretching and injury incidence produced conflicting results (58). Some studies connect static stretching with reduced injury where reduced ankle dorsiflexion ROM was associated with greater incidence of patellar tendinopathy in volleyball players

(61), lower incidence rates of low-back pain were shown in military recruits who included static stretching compared to those who did not stretch (62), and an ~12.4% lower injury rate was shown in military basic trainees who stretched the hamstrings regularly than those trainees who did not stretch (63). In contrast, research has shown no benefits of stretching on reducing the incidence of lower-body injuries (64). Hip abduction flexibility was not associated with reducing the risk of groin injuries in National Hockey League (NHL) hockey players (65), and flexibility was not related to injury prevention in soccer players (66). The benefits of greater flexibility in injury prevention are up for debate, but increased flexibility is advantageous for fitness and performance.

Factors Affecting Flexibility

An individual's joint flexibility is determined by many factors. These factors include the following (6,67).

- Joint structure—the type of joint will dictate how many planes of motion are possible. Ball-and-socket joints enable motion in three planes, whereas hinge joints predominately allow motion in one plane. The size of the bones at the articulation site plays a critical role. Large bones with convex surfaces that articulate with a deep fossa or concave surface provide more stability and less mobility than smaller bones/fossa.
- Muscular imbalance—muscle strength and length imbalances reduce flexibility. Unequal pull by antagonist muscles or *hypertonic* (shortened) muscles reduce flexibility.
- Muscular control—for some movements (hip abduction from a lying position), a certain degree of strength and balance is needed to reach a certain level of the ROM. A lack of strength and balance can decrease flexibility.
- Age—flexibility decreases with age. Older, sedentary individuals lose motor units and muscle fibers while fibrous CT expands. The higher collagen content reduces compliance and flexibility.
- Gender—women tend to be more flexible than men in some areas, especially in the hips. Anatomical, structural, and hormonal (estrogen, progesterone) differences between genders account for flexibility differences. Women have larger pelvic girdles and broader and shallower hips than men, which enhances flexibility in the pelvic/hip region. Joint *hypermobility* syndrome is three times more likely in women, is highly genetic, and may increase risk of certain injuries while causing pain and discomfort.
- Connective tissue (CT)—tendons, ligaments, fascia, joint capsules, and skin affect flexibility. Collagen and elastin content affects CT elasticity and plasticity. Training alters CT plasticity.
- Bulk—an increase in muscle bulk or percent body fat can limit joint ROM and decrease flexibility scores. The additional tissue mass acts as an obstruction to joint motion limiting bony segment movement with a high degree of ROM. Elite bodybuilders may have less elbow flexion ROM mostly due to large upper-arm mass rather than poor flexibility of the elbow extensors. Similar restrictions are seen with obesity. An overweight or obese person may have difficulty scoring well on the *sit-and-reach flexibility test* (a test of hamstring, gluteal, and lower-back flexibility) partially due to abdominal bulk rather than neuromuscular factors affecting joint ROM. Thus, ROM and flexibility are not exactly equitable as joint flexibility is limited by CT restrictions, whereas ROM can be negatively affected by factors (bulk) independent of joint flexibility. In addition, body segment lengths can affect flexibility scores (68,69).
- Training in a limited ROM—training (especially RT) in a limited ROM can reduce flexibility over time. Training in a full exercise–prescribed ROM is recommended.
- Activity level—active individuals tend to be more flexible than sedentary adults.

See Myths & Misconceptions: Flexibility Is Mostly Genetic and Very Limited Improvements Can Be Expected with Training.

Types of Stretching

Stretching requires positioning a body segment to at least a mild level of resistance or discomfort within the joint's ROM. A force is needed to stretch each joint. An *active stretch* is produced when the athlete provides the force, whereas a

---

Myths & Misconceptions
Flexibility Is Mostly Genetic and Very Limited Improvements Can Be Expected with Training

Some have argued that genetics is the primary factor affecting one's flexibility. Although genetics contributes to flexibility to some extent, other trainable factors contribute and can be enhanced with regular flexibility training. Consistent flexibility training consisting of dynamic movements and static stretching can increase flexibility.

Studies have shown that 6–20 weeks of static stretching or Yoga training increases joint ROM by more than 10° or more than 18% (5,70–72). Improvements may take place within the first few weeks (54). Although genetics may pose some limitation, everyone can increase flexibility with training.

passive stretch is produced when a partner or device provides the force. Some research indicates that active stretching is superior to increasing hamstring flexibility than passive stretching over short-term periods (4–6 weeks) of training (73,74), but passive stretching is superior over longer periods (>8 weeks) (73). Four types of stretching are used in training programs: static, dynamic, ballistic, and PNF.

Static Stretching

Static stretching involves holding a joint position (statically) with some level of discomfort for at least 15–20 seconds. The athlete maintains complete control over the movement and static holding of the joint position. Static stretching is very effective for increasing joint ROM but is most productive post exercise when the goal is to increase flexibility. Some static stretches isolate a muscle group. The advantage is that the stretch in isolation can thoroughly stretch the muscle group leading to increased flexibility. Other stretches target several muscle groups. The advantage is that the muscle/tendon complex is stretched but so are the myofascial slings that connect muscles to other muscles. This may add an additional mobility component to the muscle flexibility component. Both examples of static stretches are presented later in this chapter.

Dynamic Stretching

Dynamic stretching involves actively moving a joint through its full ROM without any relaxation or holding of joint positions. These stretches are functional in nature and often replicate sport-specific movements. Specific movements are emphasized rather than individual muscle groups. Some examples include forward and backward arm circles, trunk circles (from a straddled position), and walking knee lifts. Dynamic stretching offers clear advantages to static stretching when included as part of a warm-up (23,45). Dynamic stretches offer similar physiological responses that assist in preparing the body for exercise yet do not result in the same level of reduced musculotendinous stiffness characteristic of static stretching (which yields reductions in strength and power). Dynamic stretching offers the advantage of warming up several muscle groups simultaneously, which could potentially increase the efficiency of the warm-up. These stretches may be performed as repetitions in place or in series covering a specific distance. In either case, the progression should take place from light, gradual movements to more intense, quicker movements when preparing for strength/power activities (67).

An explosive type of dynamic stretching is ballistic stretching. The movement is ballistic, resulting in a bouncing type of motion where the final position is not held. The utility of ballistic stretching has been controversial. Opponents argue that it may increase the risk of injury and result in greater muscle/CT damage and soreness. Ballistic stretching activates the muscle spindles to initiate the stretch reflex, which facilitates agonist contraction and not relaxation. This may defeat the purpose of stretching for increased flexibility (6). Although ballistic stretching can increase flexibility (6,75), it is believed that the stimulus applied may be too short to optimize increases in flexibility compared to the prolonged lower force application of static stretching (6). Proponents of ballistic stretching argue that it can be effective and safe when performed properly and may help prepare the body for ballistic exercise more effectively (76). Nevertheless, most S&C coaches and athletes prefer dynamic stretching (without ballistic movements) for warming up. Research shows that acute ballistic stretching results in less vertical jump performance decrement than static and PNF stretching (35), enhances acute vertical jump height (75), and does not affect acute 1-RM strength while static stretching acutely decreases 1-RM (48).

Proprioceptive Neuromuscular Facilitation Stretching

PNF stretching was developed in the late 1940s by Herman Kabat as part of rehabilitation for polio patients (6,77). Different from other forms of stretching, PNF stretching incorporates combinations of CON, eccentric (ECC), and ISOM muscle actions, and passive stretching. The physiological rationale is to cause relaxation via muscle inhibition of the agonist muscle group to facilitate greater ROM. PNF has been shown to increase flexibility (up to 33% (6,77) or acutely by 3°–9°(77)), alter sprint biomechanics and increase stride length by 9% (78) and enhance muscle strength, endurance, and joint stability (6). Acute PNF stretching may increase joint ROM with effects lasting up to 90 minutes or more (79). It is thought that PNF stretching enhances an athlete's stretch tolerance or perception thereby enabling greater acute ROM increases and flexibility improvements (77). However, PNF stretching performed as a warm-up before intense strength and power activity has similar negative effects as static stretching but may improve performance of submaximal exercise (35,79).

Some neuromuscular mechanisms are thought to play critical roles in muscle relaxation and include *autogenic inhibition,* which involves reflex relaxation that occurs in an agonist muscle group following fatiguing contraction via Golgi tendon organ activation (6), *reciprocal inhibition*, which involves antagonist muscle relaxation resulting from contracting the agonist muscle group where ISOM muscle action may slightly alter muscle spindle function to favor relaxation (6), and *stress relaxation* of the musculotendinous unit, which may occur when the muscle/tendon complex is under constant stress that reduces the viscoelastic force and allows enhanced ROM (79). The combination of pain and pressure during PNF stretching is thought to simultaneously activate GTOs and pain receptors (nociceptors) thereby reducing pain perception in the CNS, a phenomenon known as *Gate Control Theory* (79).

Several variations of PNF stretching may be performed. These variations typically require the help of a partner but an athlete may self-apply PNF techniques manually as well. Four commonly used PNF techniques include (a) hold-relax, (b) contract-relax, (c) hold-relax with agonist contraction, and (d) contract-relax with agonist contraction. The term *hold* refers to an ISOM action and *contract* refers to CON contraction of the agonist or antagonist muscle group. *Relax* refers to passive static stretching. There are numerous ways to use PNF stretching to attempt to increase flexibility. The American College of Sports Medicine recommends that individuals hold a light-moderate contraction for 3 to 6 second (at 20%–75% of maximal voluntary contraction [MVC]) followed by a 10- to 30-second assisted stretch (9,54). Comparisons of the contraction intensity, *e.g.*, 20% to 100% of MVC force, have shown similar acute increases in joint ROM (80). It is recommended that PNF stretching be performed at least 1–2 days per week (77).

Hold-Relax
- Technique begins with a passive stretch held at the point of mild discomfort for ~10 seconds.
- Partner applies force to resist the agonist muscles and instructs athlete to hold the position.
- The athlete ISOM contracts and resists the partner's force for ~6 seconds.
- Athlete relaxes and partner passively stretches athlete deeper in the ROM for ~20–30 seconds.
- Cycle may be repeated until final segment of ROM is reached (Fig. 11.3).

Contract-Relax
- Technique begins with a passive stretch held at the point of mild discomfort for ~10 seconds
- Partner applies force to resist the agonist muscle group, while the athlete CON contracts the agonist group through the joint ROM
- Athlete relaxes and partner applies passive stretch in deeper area of ROM for ~20–30 seconds.
- Cycle may be repeated until final segment of ROM is reached.

Hold-Relax with Antagonist Contraction
- Technique begins with a passive stretch held at the point of mild discomfort for ~10 seconds.
- Partner applies force to resist the antagonist muscle group and instructs athlete to hold the position.
- Passive stretch is applied to athlete and is held for ~20–30 seconds.
- Cycle may be repeated until final segment of ROM is reached.

Contract-Relax with Antagonist Contraction
- Technique begins with a passive stretch held at the point of mild discomfort for ~10 seconds.
- Partner applies force to resist the antagonist muscle group while the athlete CON contracts through the joint ROM.
- Athlete relaxes and partner applies passive stretch in a deeper area of ROM for ~20–30 seconds, while the athlete CON contracts.
- Cycle may be repeated until final segment of ROM is reached.

Myofascial Release and Foam Rolling

Myofascia is the connective tissue that covers various layers of skeletal muscle (see Chapter 5 for review). Fascia connects muscles of the body together, so motion (and force transmission) results in a coordinated contractile effort of multiple muscles ("sling-like") (81). It has been suggested that myofascial disruption may pose limitations to flexibility, postural alignment, and mobility, in addition to muscle strength, endurance, and coordination (82). Myofascial limitations in one region of the body could alter the load placed on other

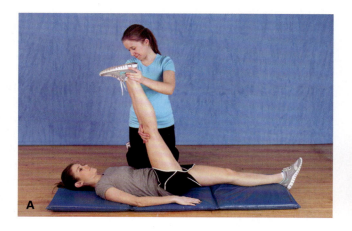
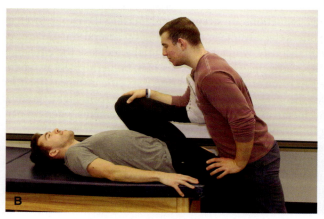

FIGURE 11.3 Hold-relax PNF stretching of the hamstrings **(A)** and hip flexors/extensors **(B)** muscle groups.

Myths & Misconceptions
Resistance Training Will Decrease Flexibility

Some have had great concern that RT (muscle hypertrophy) will make one "muscle-bound" and decrease flexibility. This could potentially occur if the athlete does not include any flexibility exercises. Although some athletes with large levels of muscle mass may have poor flexibility, this is most likely the result of initial flexibility deficits or a lack of stretching. It is possible for an athlete who does not resistance train or train for flexibility to lose flexibility regardless of the magnitude of muscle mass. The lack of stretching is the key. RT alone may improve flexibility in some joints especially in sedentary and elderly populations with initial low levels of flexibility (11,83). Although some studies have shown RT may not increase flexibility (51), RT did not inhibit flexibility increases when a stretching program was used concomitantly with RT (84). Olympic weightlifters have superior shoulder flexibility

(from performing the snatch and related lifts) compared to bodybuilders, power lifters, and football players. The combination of RT and stretching is the most effective method to increase flexibility with concomitant muscle hypertrophy. To enhance flexibility during RT solely, exercises need to be performed in a fully prescribed ROM and the ECC phase of each rep can be emphasized. Several exercises, by design, can increase joint ROM, including the squat, snatch, power clean and front squat, stiff-leg deadlift, and lunge, to name a few. The squat may increase ankle and hip flexibility. The snatch can increase shoulder, spine, and hip flexibility. The power clean and front squat can also increase wrist flexibility due to the nature of the catch position. The stiff-leg deadlift can increase hamstring flexibility. The lunge (and lateral lunge) can increase hip and ankle flexibility.

parts of the body. Various causes of myofascial limitations have been suggested and include injury, overuse, inflammation, scar tissue, ischemia-induced spasms, and fascial adhesions (85). Myofascial restrictions or stiffness is attributed to muscle changes such as hypertrophy and hypertonicity, direct muscle fiber insertion into fascia, contraction of myofibroblasts, changes in the hydration state of myofascia, and the formation of fascial adhesions and subsequent "trigger points" (*i.e.*, sensitive areas within a muscle that may cause pain or dysfunction) (85). In addition to reduced joint motion and mobility, myofascial adhesions could lead to pain and discomfort. *Myofascial release* is the technique used to remedy myofascial limitations by reducing fascial adhesions, lengthening fascia, altering fluid content, reducing scar tissue and trigger points, and restoring extensibility to the myofascial unit. However, other possible mechanisms contributing to acute ROM and performance enhancement seen with myofascial release include increased muscle blood flow and reduced arterial stiffness, augmented mechanoreceptor-induced relaxation, increased pain tolerance, and tissue thixotropy from rolling friction-induced heat (85,86).

Various modes are used including massage therapy. Massage therapy involves manual soft tissue manipulation in order to treat pain, stress, dysfunction, and promote health, recovery, and well-being. Many types or techniques may be used during massage therapy including Swedish massage, acupressure, deep tissue, trigger point, shiatsu, clinical and sports massage, and many others. Single applications of massage therapy have been shown to reduce blood pressure, heart rate, and anxiety while multiple applications can reduce pain (87). One meta-analysis showed that postexercise massage had limited effects on recovery (88). A recent meta-analysis showed that sports

massage posed some benefits by eliciting small improvements in flexibility (by 7%) and measures of delayed onset muscle soreness (by 13%) but had no effect on muscle strength, power, speed, or endurance (89). Thus, some health benefits may be gained, but further research is needed to examine athletic performance.

Self-myofascial release has grown in popularity significantly in S&C where the athlete may self-induce deep fiber stimulation using a variety of equipment such as foam rollers (of various sizes, shape, and densities), baseballs/softballs, tennis balls, massage sticks, PVC pipes, medicine balls, or devices such as the "Peanut" (Fig. 11.4). The athlete is able to roll over the desired area, find the "trigger point," and continue to roll for a number of reps or duration to relieve the area. The athlete may control the pressure or intensity by altering body position or control the percent of their body weight compressed during loading, which is guided by pain. One strategy used in myofascial release is to start with a pliable foam roller while one becomes accustomed to the pressure, and then progress to a denser device as tolerance and conditioning improve.

Foam rolling has several benefits that may enhance performance or decrease injury risk, though these connections have only been suggested and more research is needed for confirmation. Foam rolling for 30–60 seconds (but in as little as 10 s) acutely increases joint ROM by 3%–23% for up to 20–30 minutes post exercise and reduces stiffness by up to 24% (85,86,90). Foam rolling one area of the body may increase ROM in remote areas (85). Foam rolling may enhance recovery and reduce acute muscle soreness and pain (90). Unlike static stretching or PNF, rolling acutely increases ROM without compromising muscle strength, power, or speed (85,86). Some studies have

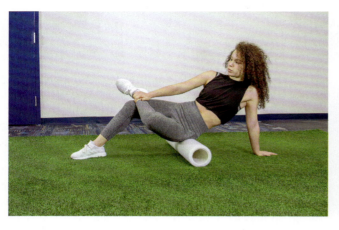 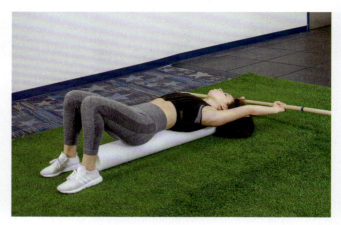
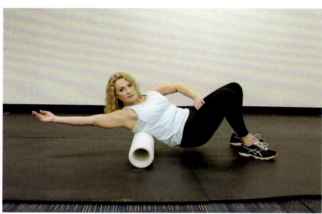 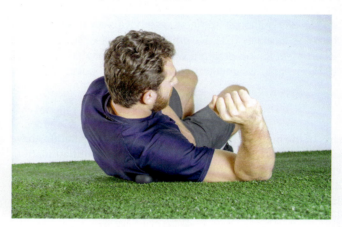

FIGURE 11.4 Shown here is self-myofascial release for the hip rotators, latissimus dorsi, overhead mobility, and scapular/rotator cuff muscle release (using the Peanut). Please visit thePoint to view the other exercises.

shown augmented strength and power (*e.g.*, vertical and long jump, sprint speed, 1-RM strength, agility) performance following rolling (85,91) although others have shown no augmented effects over other types of warm-ups (92,93).

Optimal foam rolling regiments have not been established and likely vary by type body region, symptoms, and goal of the sessions. As with other modalities, it is expected that the intensity, frequency, volume, and duration of myofascial release per muscle group will affect the response. Phillips et al. (94) showed that 5 minutes of foam rolling (compared to 1 min) produced better performance of a kneeling lunge (16% vs. 12.5%) but had negative effects on vertical jump and pro-agility performance. Interestingly, Monteiro et al. (95) examined the effects of 60 and 120 seconds of foam rolling of the antagonist muscles (hamstrings) in between sets of 10-rep leg extension protocol and showed foam rolling reduced the number of reps performed in a dose-response manner. Passive recovery led to best performance, whereas foam rolling for 120 seconds yielded the fewest reps. Thus, it appears 30–60 seconds per set of rolling appears effective when used as a warm-up. Studies 1–3 weeks in duration using myofascial release have shown increased flexibility, whereas one study 8 weeks in duration showed no change (86). Hodgson et al. (96) compared 4 weeks of foam rolling the quadriceps and hamstrings (4×30 s) for either 3 or 6 days per week and showed that rolling did not affect ROM and strength. The use of myofascial release in conjunction with static stretching appears to be most effective for augmenting the effects of myofascial release especially in athletes accustomed to foam rolling (97). It has been recommended that myofascial release be used in conjunction with stretching, strengthening, and mobility exercises to correct postural issues and improve performance (82).

Exercises

Static Stretches

The following section illustrates and describes several popular static stretches. See the exercise boxes to see the proper positioning and movement, step-by-step instructions, as well as variations and cautions of performing the static stretches.

Visit thePoint to view more exercises and variations in the online appendix.

Neck Rotation

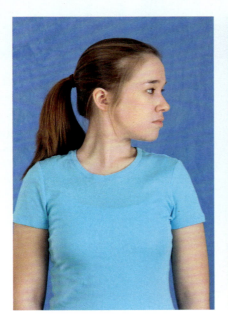
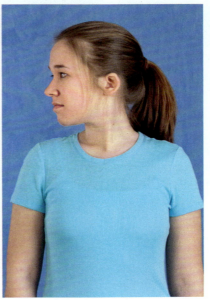

FIGURE 11.5 Neck rotation.

- Athlete maintains a standing or seated position with the head and neck upright and turns head left and holds the position (Fig. 11.5).
- Head returns to the starting position and turns to the right and is statically held.
- Muscles stretched: *neck rotators*

> **CAUTION!** A slow and controlled velocity should be used during rotation.

Neck Flexion/Extension/Lateral Flexion

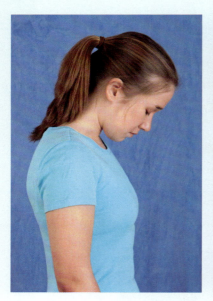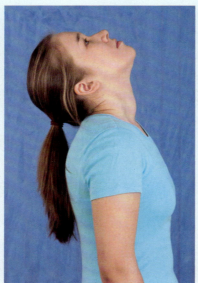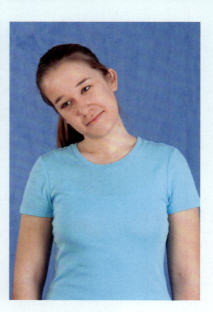

FIGURE 11.6 Neck flexion/extension/lateral flexion.

- Athlete stands, sits, or lies supine on a bench with head and neck upright and flexes neck by tucking chin toward chest. The position is held (Fig. 11.6).
- Head returns to starting position and extends and hyperextends back. Position is held.
- Head returns to anatomical position and athlete laterally flexes neck to the right, holds the position, and laterally flexes neck to the left (and holds the position).
- Muscles stretched: *neck extensors*, *flexors*, and *lateral flexors*

Pectoral Wall Stretch

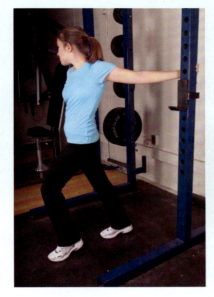
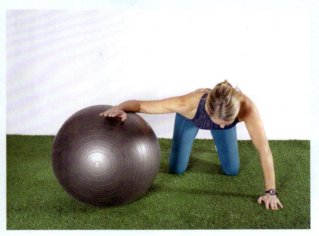
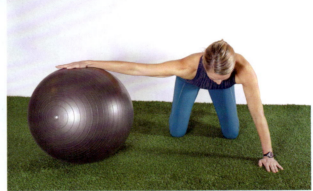

FIGURE 11.7 Pectoral wall stretch.

- Athlete stands against an object (open doorway or weight machine) with arms bent at 90° angles with elbows positioned at shoulder level.
- Athlete leans body forward until stretch is felt in upper chest.
- Stretch can be performed with one arm against the wall or weight machine (shown in Fig. 11.7). In this variation, torso rotation helps expand the ROM of the stretch. This stretch can be performed between two benches, chairs, or SBs. A static variation may be performed on a SB where the athlete assumes a position on their knees and leans forward or uses the floor for leverage as in the arm/shoulder pigeon. A dynamic variation could be used where the athlete places the palm of the hand on the SB and rotates the SB clockwise or counterclockwise while maintaining the bent-over body position (shown in Figure 11.7).
- Another variation is to assume a supine position on a bench with light dumbbells (DB) in hand. Similar to performing a negative fly, the athlete lowers the DBs in an arc fashion until the final position is attained. This position is held.
- Muscles stretched: *pectoralis major*, *shoulder girdle protractors*, and *anterior deltoid*

Bent-Over Shoulder/Pectoral Stretch

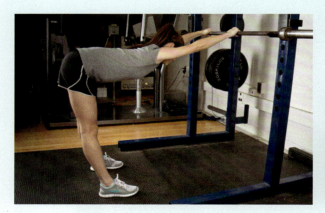
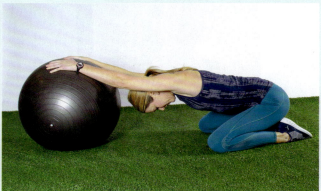
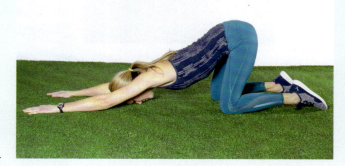

FIGURE 11.8 Bent-over shoulder/pectoral stretch.

- Athlete assumes a shoulder-width grip with shoulders flexed (elbows may be bent as a variation), grasps a bar or bench or power rack, bends over at the waist, and assumes a position where the upper body is parallel to the ground (Fig. 11.8).
- Athlete relaxes the shoulders and continues to bend as far as possible to where the head will be level or lower than the arms.
- This stretch may be performed on the knees with the athlete's hands facing down on the mat or floor. A variation shown is to perform the exercise using a SB, wall, or the floor (shown above).
- Muscles stretched: *shoulder flexors and scapular protractors*

Posterior Shoulder Hyperextension

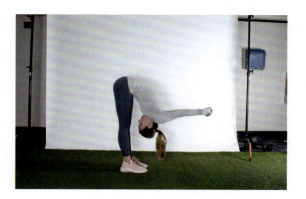

- Athlete stands with arms behind back, the elbows are extended, and fingers interlocked with palms facing each other. The neck is relaxed and head is upright (Fig. 11.9).
- A variation is to use a broomstick or light bar instead of clasping the fingers together.
- Elbows are fully extended while arms are slowly raised, or shoulders hyperextended. A variation is to perform the stretch from a bent-over straddled position or from a seated position.
- Muscles stretched: *shoulder flexors*

FIGURE 11.9 Posterior shoulder hyperextension.

Seated Posterior Lean

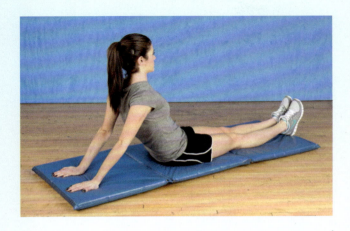

- Athlete sits with legs straight and arms extended with palms on the floor (pointing away from the body) behind the hips (Fig. 11.10).
- As the hands slide backward, the body leans back.
- Muscles stretched: *shoulder flexors*

FIGURE 11.10 Seated posterior lean.

Anterior Cross-Arm Stretch

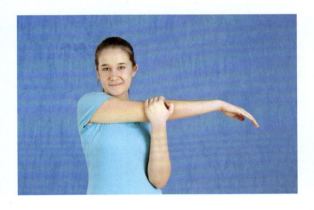
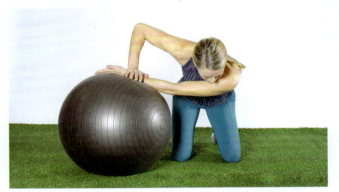

FIGURE 11.11 Anterior cross-arm stretch.

- Athlete stands or sits with left elbow slightly flexed, arm horizontally adducted across the body, and the right hand pulls the left arm across chest (Fig. 11.11).
- Position is held and repeated for opposite limb. A variation shown is performing the stretch on a SB or on the floor.
- Muscles stretched: *upper-back muscles* and *posterior deltoid*

Flexed Arms Above Head Stretch

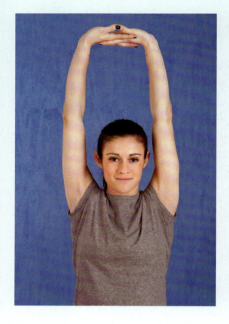
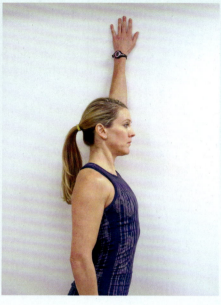

FIGURE 11.12 Flexed arms above head stretch.

- Athlete stands with arms stretched in front of the torso, fingers interlocked, and palms facing out (Fig. 11.12).
- Arms straighten (shoulder flexion) above head (palms now face up) and athlete reaches upward and back to expand ROM. This position is held.
- A variation is to lean in and use a pull-up bar for leverage. A single-arm version is shown where the athlete flexes one arm and leans into a wall.
- Muscles stretched: *upper-back and shoulder muscles*

Single-Arm Lat Stretch

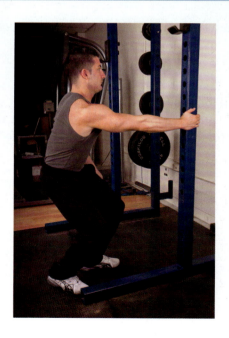

- Athlete grasps the uprights of a power rack with arms at or near shoulder level (Fig. 11.13).
- Athlete flexes hips/knees, leans back, and stretches upper-back muscles. Position is held.
- Muscles stretched: *upper-back muscles* and *shoulder girdle retractors*

FIGURE 11.13 Single-arm lat stretch.

Internal/External Shoulder Rotation Stretch

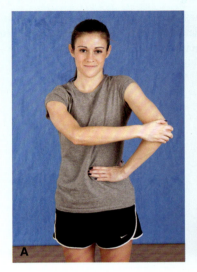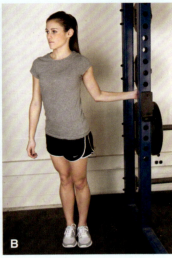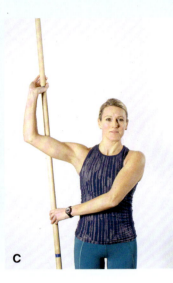

FIGURE 11.14 Internal/external shoulder rotation stretch.

- Athlete stands/sits with elbow flexed and hand on hip or behind the back (Fig. 11.14A). Opposite arm applies force to elbow to facilitate internal rotation. Position is held, and stretch is repeated for opposite arm.
- Athlete stands with elbow flexed at 90° against the side of a wall or power rack (Fig. 11.14B). Force is applied by rotating the body to facilitate external rotation. Position is held and stretch is repeated for opposite arm. A variation is shown where a stick, towel, or band can be used to facilitate greater rotation, while the opposite arm applies pressure (Figure 11.14C).
- Muscles stretched: *shoulder internal* and *external rotators*
- Another stretch for the rotator cuff is the **sleeper stretch** where the athlete lies on their side with the bottom arm flexed to 90° and elbow flexed to 90°. The athlete presses down and forward on the hand/wrist as ROM permits thereby stretching the external rotators and posterior shoulder.

Behind-the-Neck Triceps Stretch

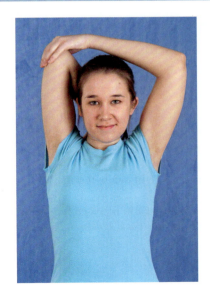

- Athlete stands or sits with right shoulder abducted and elbow flexed (Fig. 11.15).
- Left hand grasps right elbow, pulls the elbow behind the head, position is held, and repeated for opposite arm.
- Muscles stretched: *triceps brachii*

> **CAUTION!** Do not push neck forward during the stretch.

FIGURE 11.15 Behind-the-neck triceps stretch.

Forward Triceps Stretch

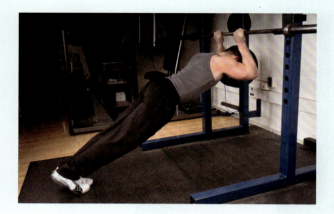

- Athlete assumes narrow grip on a bar located in front of the body. Athlete leans the body forward while flexing the elbows, and final position is held (Fig. 11.16).
- Muscles stretched: *triceps brachii*

FIGURE 11.16 Forward triceps stretch.

Biceps Stretch

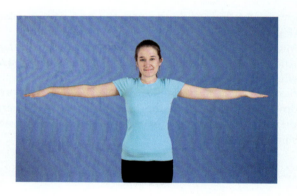

- Athlete abducts the shoulders and keeps the elbows extended. The forearm is pronated to stretch the elbow flexors and supinator further. A wall or power rack may be used for support (Fig. 11.17).
- Muscles stretched: *elbow flexors* and *supinator*

FIGURE 11.17 Biceps stretch.

Pretzel

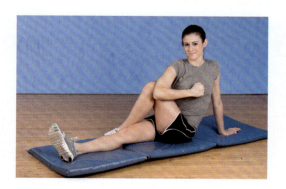

- Athlete assumes a seated position, left foot is placed to the side of right knee, and knee is bent. The back part of the right elbow pushes against the left side of knee. Left arm is used for support (Fig. 11.18).
- Left knee is pushed right, while the chest is opened and athlete faces posterior.
- Position is maintained and repeated for opposite side.
- Muscles stretched: *low back*, *abdominals*, and *obliques*

FIGURE 11.18 Pretzel.

Supine Hip Flexion

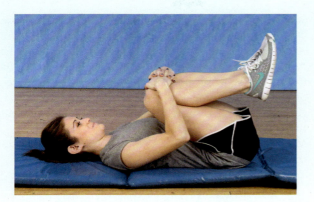

FIGURE 11.19 Supine hip flexion.

- Athlete lies on back with legs straight. Both legs are pulled inward to chest (with hands above knees). Final position is held (Fig. 11.19).
- Muscles stretched: *low back, hip extensors*

> **VARIATIONS** A variation is to stretch one side at a time. Another variation is to roll back onto shoulders (with upper arms assisting in support) while releasing hands from knees. Hands support torso as gravity pulls legs downward to head.

Semi-Leg Straddle

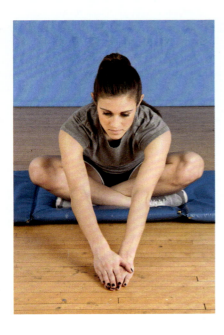

FIGURE 11.20 Semi-leg straddle.

- Athlete's knees and hips are flexed with toes pointed outward. Another variation is to sit on a chair rather than the floor (Fig. 11.20).
- Athlete leans forward from the waist as the arms extend forward.
- Muscles stretched: *low back* and *hip extensors*

> **VARIATIONS** A variation is to keep the body upright but to bend the knee to 90° and pull the leg upward at the ankle/lower leg.

Lying Torso Stretch

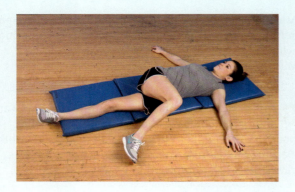

FIGURE 11.21 Lying torso stretch.

- Athlete lies on the mat with shoulders abducted to close to 90° and elbows extended. Hips and knees are flexed.
- Athlete rotates hips all the way to right and position is held. Athlete rotates to the left and position is held. The elbow flexors and shoulder horizontal adductors can be stretched on the ipsilateral side during torso rotation.
- An alternative is to have one leg to rotate while the other remains straight (Fig. 11.21).
- Muscles stretched: *low back*, *hip extensors/abductors*, and *trunk rotators*

> **VARIATIONS** A variation is to keep the knees extended while rotating. Another is to rotate the hip of the bottom leg (a stretch known as the "brettzel").

Forward Lunge Stretch

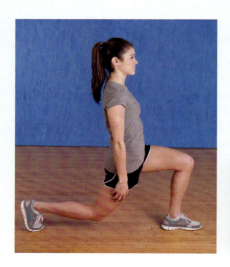 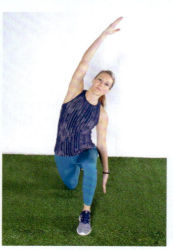

FIGURE 11.22 Forward lunge stretch.

- From standing position, athlete takes stride forward with left leg and flexes left knee until it is directly over left foot (Fig. 11.22).
- Left foot is flat on the floor with toes pointed in the same direction and back knee is slightly bent.
- Hips move forward and downward. Position is held and opposite side is stretched.
- Muscles stretched: *hip flexors and opposite side hip extensors*

> **VARIATIONS** A variation is to perform this stretch from a kneeling position. A torso rotation, flexed arm overhead, or other upper-body stretch can be added.

Press-Up Stretch

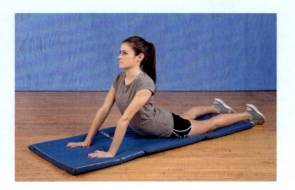

- Athlete lies prone on the mat in a push-up position. Athlete pushes upper body upward while keeping hips and lower extremities static. Final position is held (Fig. 11.23).
- Muscles stretched: *hip flexors* and *abdominals*

> **CAUTION!** Hips should remain in contact with the ground.

FIGURE 11.23 Press-up stretch.

Side Bend Stretch (Straight or Flexed Arms)

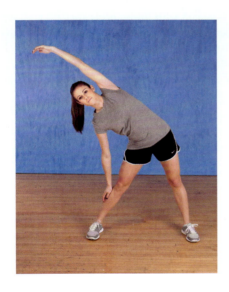

- Athlete stands with feet greater than shoulder width apart, left arm overhead, and right arm down by side (Fig. 11.24).
- Athlete reaches and laterally flexes the trunk to the right side. Position is held and other side is stretched.
- Muscles stretched: *obliques* and *latissimus dorsi*

> **VARIATIONS** An alternative is to have the athlete stand with feet hip-width apart, and fingers interlaced with palms facing outward and away from torso, or the athlete can perform the stretch from a seated, straddled position.

FIGURE 11.24 Side bend stretch, straight or flexed arms.

Partner Hip Flexor Stretch

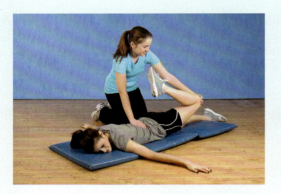

FIGURE 11.25 Partner hip flexor stretch.

- Athlete lies prone on a bench, floor, or table. A partner is positioned at the side (Fig. 11.25).
- Partner applies pressure to low back and lifts up the flexed leg (under the knee) while athlete contracts the gluteal muscles.
- Position is held and opposite side is stretched. Pressure can be applied to the foot by the partner to assist in stretching the quadriceps simultaneously. A variation was shown earlier in this chapter for PNF stretching where a partner applies force to the leg while the athlete is lying on a table.
- Muscles stretched: *hip flexors*

Seated Toe Touch Stretch

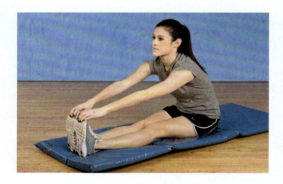

FIGURE 11.26 Seated toe touch stretch.

- Athlete is seated with upper body vertical with legs straight. Body leans forward using hip flexors and arms to reach toward toes or ankles (depending on flexibility) (Fig. 11.26).
- Legs remain straight and position is held.
- Muscles stretched: *erector spinae*, *hamstrings*, and *plantar flexors*

Semistraddle Stretch

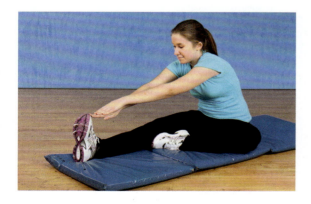

FIGURE 11.27 Semistraddle stretch.

- Athlete is seated with upper body nearly vertical and right leg straight. Sole of left foot is placed on the inner side of right knee (Fig. 11.27).
- Athlete leans forward using hip flexors and arms to reach toward toes. Position is held and opposite side is stretched.
- Muscles stretched: *erector spinae*, *hamstrings*, and *plantar flexors*

> **CAUTION!** The nonstretched leg should rotate inward and not outward, which places undue stress on the knees (a variation known as the hurdler's stretch).

Straddle Stretch

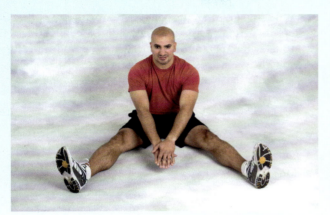
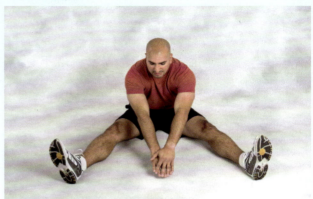
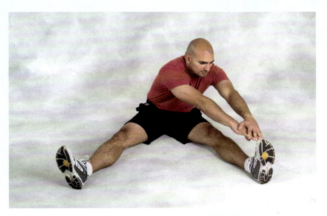

FIGURE 11.28 Straddle stretch.

- Athlete assumes a seated position with legs abducted in a wide stance or foot position (Fig. 11.28).
- The athlete bends forward and grasps the ankles or toes while keeping the knees extended. The final position is held.
- Muscles stretched: *erector spinae, hamstrings, hip adductors,* and *plantar flexors*

> **VARIATIONS** A variation is to perform the stretch supine against a wall where the hips are abducted (with knees extended) while touching the wall. A partner could apply pressure to deepen the stretch. This variation targets mostly the hip adductors.

Butterfly Stretch

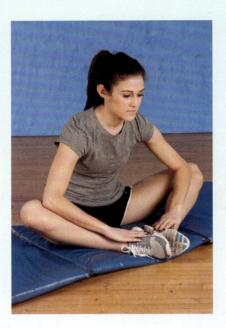

- Athlete assumes an upright position with knees flexed and hips rotated outward with soles of feet touching (Fig. 11.29).
- Athlete attempts to touch knees to floor and leans forward from the waist causing hip abduction.
- Muscles stretched: *hip adductors/internal rotators*

FIGURE 11.29 Butterfly stretch.

Kneeling Hip Adductor Stretch

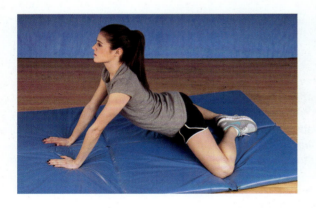

- Athlete assumes a kneeling position on the mat and gradually abducts the hips (widens the base) until the position is attained (Fig. 11.30). Feet can be touching in the rear. This stretch can be performed with the knees extended from a standing position.
- Athlete relaxes and drops body weight downward to stretch the hips.
- Muscles stretched: *hip adductors/internal rotators*

FIGURE 11.30 Kneeling hip adductor stretch.

Standing Quadriceps Stretch

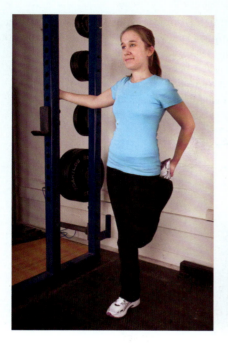
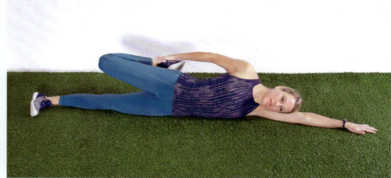

FIGURE 11.31 Standing quadriceps stretch.

- Athlete stands and supports body weight by holding on to a wall or power rack. This stretch may be performed lying with the legs straight. Front of ankle is grasped with left hand and pulled toward glutes, flexing left knee. Position is held and opposite side is stretched. A variation shown is to perform the exercise lying on the side (Fig. 11.31).
- Muscles stretched: *quadriceps*

> **VARIATIONS** A variation is to position the foot of the stretched leg against a wall and lean backward or by performing the stretch while lying on one's side.

Squat Stretch

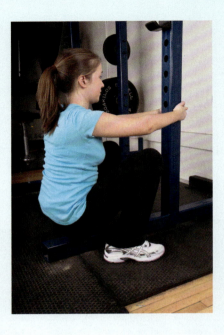

FIGURE 11.32 Squat stretch.

- Athlete assumes a standing position with shoulder width stance and squats as low as possible and maintains the final position (Fig. 11.32).
- The athlete may use a power rack for support or may rotate hips forward to deepen the stretch.
- Muscles stretched: *quadriceps* and *hip extensors*

Partner Quadriceps Stretch

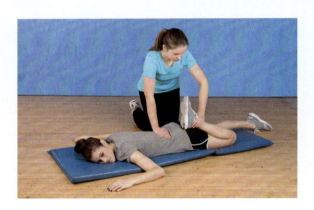

FIGURE 11.33 Partner quadriceps stretch.

- Athlete assumes prone position on bench or floor and flexes one or both knees (Fig. 11.33).
- Partner supplies force to athlete's ankles to enhance ROM. A partner may not be needed for this as the athlete can self-stretch but does benefit the efficacy of the stretch.
- Muscles stretched: *quadriceps*

Piriformis Stretch

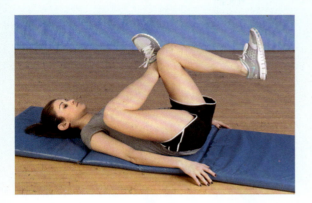

FIGURE 11.34 Piriformis stretch.

- Athlete assumes a standing, seated, or lying position (Fig. 11.34). The left hip and knee are flexed and right leg is crossed over the left leg.
- Pressure is applied to the right knee to stretch the hip rotators. Left hip flexes to assist in expanding ROM. Athlete can semisquat if in the standing position. Final position is maintained and opposite side is stretched.
- Muscles stretched: *hip rotators*
- A variation is the 90/90 hip stretch. The athlete may add torso rotation (left) or lean forward (right) to deepen the stretch.

Lying Hip External Rotation Stretch

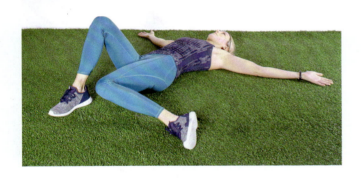

FIGURE 11.35 Lying hip external rotation stretch.

- Athlete assumes a standing, seated, or lying position (Fig. 11.35). The left hip is medially rotated as far as possible while the opposite knee is flexed or straight.
- Final position is maintained and opposite side is stretched.
- Muscles stretched: *hip external rotators*

Standing Hamstring Stretch

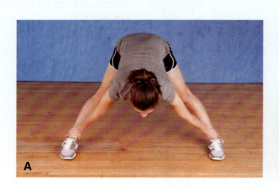
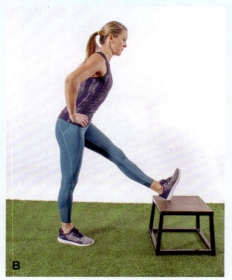

FIGURE 11.36 Standing hamstring stretch.

- Athlete assumes a wide, straddled stance with upright torso and bends at waist (keeping knees extended) and touches right or left toes (if possible) or flexes toward the center (Fig. 11.36).
- Final position is held and opposite side is stretched.
- Muscles stretched: *hamstrings*, *lower back*, and *glutes*

> **VARIATIONS** A variation is to narrow the stance and cross one leg over the other where the rear leg is actively stretched. Another variation is to flex one leg forward and elevate it off of the floor onto an object (step, bench) (Figure 11.36B). While keeping the toes pointed up, the athlete bends forward (with knee extended) stretching the hamstrings in the process.

Standing Adductor Stretch

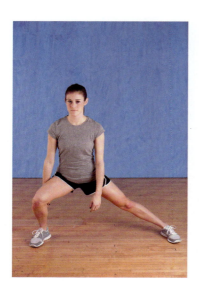

- Athlete stands in a straddle stance with feet wider than shoulder width and performs a side lunge until stretch is felt in the athlete's adductors (groin) (Fig. 11.37).
- Final position is maintained and opposite side is stretched.
- Muscles stretched: *hip adductors* and *hamstrings*

> **CAUTION!** Athlete should try to maintain a vertical trunk posture as much as possible.

FIGURE 11.37 Standing adductor stretch.

Supine Hamstrings Stretch

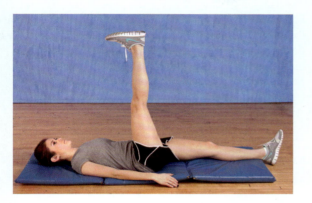

- Athlete lies flat on back with legs extended and flexes right hip with knee flexed and extends knee. Final position is held and opposite side is stretched (Fig. 11.38).
- Muscles stretched: *hamstrings*

> **VARIATIONS** A variation is to perform this stretch standing (with hip flexed) or seated in a chair.

FIGURE 11.38 Supine hamstrings stretch.

Wall Calf Stretch

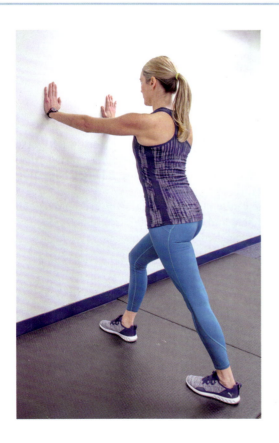

- Athlete faces the wall with feet shoulder width apart and leans forward with hands on the wall (Fig. 11.39).
- One leg steps back while front leg flexes at knee. Athlete extends back leg trying to lower heel to the floor. Final position is held and opposite side is stretched.
- Muscles stretched: *plantar flexors*
- Using a bent knee position can target the soleus.

FIGURE 11.39 Wall calf stretch.

Step Stretch

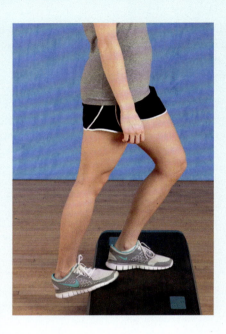

FIGURE 11.40 Step stretch.

- Ball of one foot is at the edge of a step with other foot flat on the step. Heel of foot on edge of the step is lowered toward the floor with a straight leg (Fig. 11.40).
- Final position is held and opposite side is stretched.
- Muscles stretched: *plantar flexors*
- Using a bent knee position can target the soleus.

Prone Hip Abductor Stretch

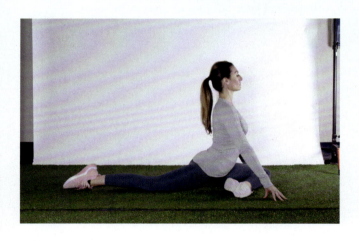

FIGURE 11.41 Prone hip abductor stretch.

- Athlete begins in a prone push-up position. Right leg moves forward and inward by hip flexion, internal rotation, and adduction to where it is crosses the body beneath the trunk (Fig. 11.41).
- Athlete gently places weight downward onto leg. Final position is held and opposite side is stretched.
- Muscle stretched: *hip abductors*

Stretches Involving Several Muscle Groups

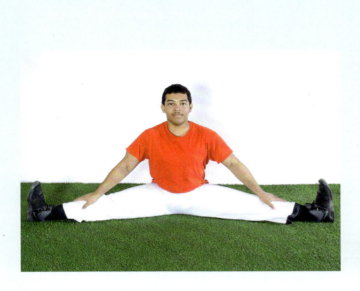
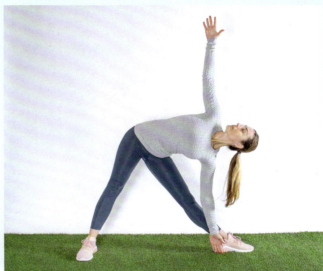
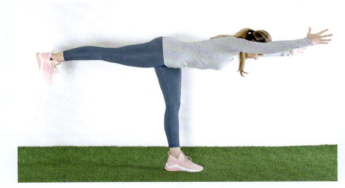
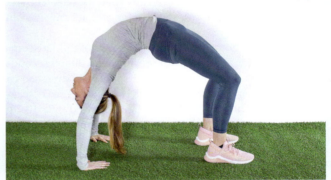

FIGURE 11.42 Stretches involving several muscle groups.

Several stretches simultaneously stress multiple muscle groups. The advantage is that not only the targeted muscles are stretched but the interconnecting myofascia is also lengthened. The resultant stimulus appears advantageous for improving mobility and functional performance. Figure 11.42 depicts several stretches plus some advanced stretches including various splits. Additional exercises are shown on thePoint.

Flexibility Training Guidelines

Although dynamic exercise may increase joint flexibility, stretching is the key component of a flexibility training program. Stretching to improve flexibility should be performed following a workout or following a general warm-up (where flexibility or corrective exercises are the sole modality) as muscles can be safely stretched to a greater ROM when they are warm. Stretching early or after a workout produces similar increases in flexibility (98) so the latter is preferred if anaerobic exercise is performed during the same workout (to avoid the potential detrimental performance effects of static stretching).

An optimal stretching regiment has not been established with studies indicating that increased frequency per week (99), but not per day is beneficial and that the duration of each bout of stretching of 30–60 seconds is likely mort beneficial (100–102).

The ACSM (9,54) has recommended the following flexibility training guidelines:

- Selection of stretches that work each major muscle group.
- The program should be of at least 10-minute duration and should include at least 2–4 repetitions per muscle group for at least 2–3 days per week. Greater gains in flexibility may be gained with higher frequency.

Table 11.1 A Novice, Progressive 10-Week Flexibility Training Program[a]

Stretch/Exercise	Weeks 1–3	Weeks 4–7	Weeks 8–10
General Warm-up — jogging	5 min	5 min	5 min
Foam rolling — 1 set — calves, hamstrings, hips, quads, back, lats/shoulders	30 s	30 s	30 s
Dynamic stretching — 1 × 10 reps: 3 exercises: choose from arm circles, lunges, MB rotations, toe touches, press-ups, etc.	1 × 10 reps	1 × 10 reps	1 × 10 reps
Standing Quadriceps Stretch	3 × 30 s	3 × 40 s	4 × 40 s
Butterfly Stretch	3 × 30 s	3 × 40 s	4 × 40 s
Semistraddle Stretch	3 × 30 s	3 × 40 s	4 × 40 s
Pretzel Stretch	3 × 30 s	3 × 40 s	4 × 40 s
Bent-Over Shoulder/Pectoral Stretch	3 × 30 s	3 × 40 s	4 × 40 s
Anterior Cross-Arm Stretch	3 × 30 s	3 × 40 s	4 × 40 s
Behind-the-Neck Triceps Stretch	3 × 30 s	3 × 40 s	4 × 40 s

[a]Each stretch is taken to the point of mild discomfort and held for the designated period of time; the program is performed 3 days per week.

- Dynamic, static, and PNF stretches may be selected, and ballistic stretching may be suitable for athletes involved in explosive sports.
- Static stretches should be taken to the point of mild discomfort and held for at least 10–30 seconds, and 30–60 seconds in older adults. Each muscle group should be stretched in total for at least 60 seconds. For PNF stretches, a 3- to 6-second contraction at 20%–75% MVC followed by a 10- to 30-second assisted stretch is recommended.

Table 11.1 depicts a sample progressive 10-week novice flexibility training program. Designing a flexibility training program begins with the selection of exercises and a training frequency. Unlike other modalities, stretching can be performed every day or multiple times per day (although there may be no additional benefit with performing the stretch multiple times per day). Advanced flexibility training may involve higher frequencies. Flexibility training should be performed after the exercise session to maximize joint ROM and minimize performance decrements from overstretching during a warm-up. All major muscle groups should be stretched (or at least those trained during the workout). Two to four repetitions (or more can be performed depending on the needs of the athlete) of static stretches are common and each should be held at the point of slight discomfort. This position may vary especially as one's flexibility increases. The intensity can increase based on the level of stretch or discomfort. Lastly, stretches should be held for at least 15–30 seconds, for a total of 60 seconds per body region stretched. Progression for flexibility training involves increasing stretch ROM, duration, and repetition number gradually. This sample program begins with a general warm-up followed by foam rolling for 1 set of 30 seconds per muscle group. The next component consists of dynamic stretches with exercises rotated (exercises from Sidebar: Dynamic Flexibility Exercises). The main progressive component consists of static stretching. The stretches included here are basic isolation stretches that are easily performed by a novice. Exercises may be varied from week to week. The individual may progress to more complex stretches over time and partner-assisted or PNF stretching.

Case Study 11.1

Dwight is a wrestler who is beginning an off-season training program. Last season Dwight tested well in several assessments. He was at the top or near the top in all strength and power assessments, and he scored well in muscle endurance tests. However, Dwight scored poorly in flexibility. As a result, Dwight has committed himself to increasing his flexibility during the off-season. He would like to increase flexibility for all major muscle groups; however, his emphasis is on increasing his shoulder and hip flexibility. Dwight will be lifting weights 3 days per week and plans on incorporating a stretching program at the conclusion of his weight lifting workouts.

Questions for Consideration: Based on Dwight's goals, what flexibility training advice would you give him?

 ## The Cooldown

The cooldown is a postworkout light exercise activity, which provides an adjustment period between exercise and rest. It helps return the body to homeostasis in a controlled manner. Waste removal is facilitated, cardiovascular responses are reduced appropriately, and a greater sense of well-being is instituted following a cooldown. The cooldown period provides an excellent opportunity for postexercise stretching to increase flexibility. The athlete may perform a light activity such as walking/cycling for 5–10 minutes and include static stretching.

SUMMARY POINTS

- A warm-up consists of a general and specific component. Warm-ups yield several acute physiological changes that help prepare the body for more intense exercise. A high-intensity warm-up may elicit post-activation potentiation, which can augment strength and power performance.
- Dynamic warm-ups are preferred as prolonged high-intensity static stretching can reduce strength and power performance. If stretching is to be performed, it should only be of light-to-moderate intensity. It is acceptable for athletes who require high levels of flexibility to perform prolonged static stretching during the warm-up.
- Flexibility is increased by stretching. Factors that influence or limit flexibility include joint structure, muscular imbalance and control, age, genetics, gender, connective tissue, bulk, performing exercises in a limited ROM, and physical activity level.
- Stretching may be active or passive. The types of stretching include static, dynamic, ballistic, and PNF stretching.
- Myofascial release, such as foam rolling, can acutely increase ROM without sacrificing strength and power performance. Myofascial release coupled with stretching is recommended for chronic flexibility training.
- Recommendations for flexibility training include selection of stretches that work all major muscle groups, 2–3 days per week, at an intensity of mild discomfort, at least 2–4 repetitions per muscle group, and held for 10–30 seconds or longer for advanced stretching.

REVIEW QUESTIONS

1. Which of the following is true concerning flexibility?
   a. Males tend to be more flexible than females in the hips.
   b. Active individuals are more flexible than sedentary individuals.
   c. Training in a limited ROM maximizes flexibility.
   d. Tendons and other CT structures play a limited role in joint flexibility.

2. The "pretzel" stretch works which major muscle group?
   a. Obliques
   b. Soleus
   c. Gastrocnemius
   d. Pectoralis major

3. Reflex relaxation that occurs in an agonist muscle group following fatiguing contraction via Golgi tendon organ activation is known as
   a. Autogenic inhibition
   b. Proprioceptive neuromuscular facilitation
   c. Reciprocal inhibition
   d. Hysteresis

4. A stretch that involves bouncing near the end of the ROM is known as
   a. PNF stretching
   b. Static stretching
   c. Passive stretching
   d. Ballistic stretching

5. A warm-up may
   a. Increase tissue resistance
   b. Reduce muscle blood flow
   c. Increase muscle temperature
   d. Decrease cardiac output

6. The semistraddle stretch works primarily the _____ muscle group
   a. Triceps brachii
   b. Pectoralis major
   c. Hamstrings
   d. Quadriceps

7. Performing a light 5-minute jog is an example of a specific warm-up.
   a. T
   b. F

8. High-intensity stretching performed as a part of a specific warm-up can maximize vertical jump and sprint performance.
   a. T
   b. F

9. A potentiation protocol consisting of 3 sets of squats for 1–2 reps with 85% of 1-RM can augment maximal vertical jump performance.
   a. T
   b. F

10. An athlete who concurrently is involved in an RT and flexibility program will most likely lose flexibility due to muscle hypertrophy.
    a. T
    b. F

11. The press-up stretch is used to stretch the abdominal and hip flexor muscles.

a. T
b. F

12. The cooldown is a critical segment of the workout because it helps return the body to homeostasis in a controlled manner.

a. T
b. F

REFERENCES

1. Fradkin AJ, Gabbe BJ, Cameron PA. Does warming up prevent injury in sport? The evidence from randomised controlled trials? *J Sci Med Sport*. 2006;9(3):214–220.
2. Bishop D. Warm up I: potential mechanisms and the effects of passive warm up on exercise performance. *Sports Med*. 2003;33:439–54.
3. Bishop D. Warm up II: performance changes following active warm up and how to structure the warm up. *Sports Med*. 2003;33:483–98.
4. Silva LM, Neiva HP, Marques MC, Izquierdo M, Marinho DA. Effects of warm-up, post-warm-up, and re-warm-up strategies on explosive efforts in team sports: a systematic review. *Sports Med*. 2018;48:2285–2299.
5. Fradkin AJ, Zazryn TR, Smoliga JM. Effects of warming-up on physical performance: a systematic review with meta-analysis. *J Strength Cond Res*. 2010;24:140–148.
6. Alter MJ. *Science of Flexibility*. 2nd ed. Champaign (IL): Human Kinetics; 1996. p. 32–142.
7. McGowan CJ, Pyne DB, Thompson KG, Rattray B. Warm-up strategies for sport and exercise: mechanisms and explanations. *Sports Med*. 2015;45:1523–46.
8. McCrary JM, Ackermann BJ, Halaki M. A systematic review of the effects of upper body warm-up on performance and injury. *Br J Sports Med*. 2015;49:935–942.
9. American College of Sports Medicine. *ACSM's Guidelines for Exercise Testing and Prescription*. 11th ed. Philadelphia (PA): Lippincott Williams & Wilkins; 2020.
10. Woods K, Bishop P, Jones E. Warm-up and stretching in the prevention of muscular injury. *Sports Med*. 2007;37:1089–99.
11. Barbosa AR, Santarem JM, Filho WJ, Marucci MDFN. Effects of resistance training on the sit-and-reach test in elderly women. *J Strength Cond Res*. 2002;16:14–8.
12. Blazevich AJ, Babault N. Post-activation potentiation versus post-activation performance enhancement in humans: historical perspective, underlying mechanisms, and current issues. *Front Physiol*. 2019;10:1359.
13. Boullosa D, Del Rosso S, Behm DG, Foster C. Post-activation potentiation (PAP) in endurance sports: a review. *Eur J Sport Sci*. 2018;18:595–610.
14. Seitz LB, Haff GG. Factors modulating post-activation potentiation of jump, sprint, throw, and upper-body ballistic performances: a systematic review with meta-analysis. *Sports Med*. 2016;46:231–240.
15. McBride JM, Nimphius S, Erickson TM. The acute effects of heavy-load squats and loaded countermovement jumps on sprint performance. *J Strength Cond Res*. 2005;19:893–7.
16. Yetter M, Moir GL. The acute effects of heavy back and front squats on speed during forty-meter sprint trials. *J Strength Cond Res*. 2008;22:159–65.
17. Chiu LZ, Fry AC, Weiss LW, et al. Postactivation potentiation response in athletic and recreationally trained individuals. *J Strength Cond Res*. 2003;17:671–7.
18. Gourgoulis V, Aggeloussis N, Kasimatis P, Mavromatis G, Garas A. Effect of a submaximal half-squats warm-up program on vertical jumping ability. *J Strength Cond Res*. 2003;17:342–4.
19. Hodgson M, Docherty D, Robbins D. Post-activation potentiation: underlying physiology and implications for motor performance. *Sports Med*. 2005;35:585–95.
20. Baker D. The effect of alternating heavy and light resistances on power output during upper-body complex power training. *J Strength Cond Res*. 2003;17:493–7.
21. Hoffman JR, Ratamess NA, Faigenbaum AD, Mangine GT, Kang J. Effects of maximal squat exercise testing on vertical jump performance in American college football players. *J Sports Sci Med*. 2007;6:149–50.
22. Wilson JM, Duncan NM, Marin PJ, et al. Meta-analysis of postactivation potentiation and power: effects of conditioning activity, volume, gender, rest periods, and training status. *J Strength Cond Res*. 2013;27:854–9.
23. Behm DG, Blazevich AJ, Kay AD, McHugh M. Acute effects of muscle stretching on physical performance, range of motion, and injury incidence in healthy active individuals: a systematic review. *Appl Physiol Nutr Metab*. 2016;41:1–11.
24. Fletcher IM, Anness R. The acute effects of combined static and dynamic stretch protocols on fifty-meter sprint performance in track-and-field athletes. *J Strength Cond Res*. 2007;21:784–7.
25. Holt BW, Lambourne K. The impact of different warm-up protocols on vertical jump performance in male collegiate athletes. *J Strength Cond Res*. 2008;22:226–9.
26. McMillian DJ, Moore JH, Hatler BS, Taylor DC. Dynamic vs. static-stretching warm up: the effect on power and agility performance. *J Strength Cond Res*. 2006;20:492–9.
27. Nelson AG, Driscoll NM, Landin DK, Young MA, Schexnayder IC. Acute effects of passive muscle stretching on sprint performance. *J Sports Sci*. 2005;23:449–54.
28. Samuel MN, Holcomb WR, Guadagnoli MA, Rubley MD, Wallmann H. Acute effects of static and ballistic stretching on measures of strength and power. *J Strength Cond Res*. 2008;22:1422–8.
29. Taylor KL, Sheppard JM, Lee H, Plummer N. Negative effect of static stretching restored when combined with a sport specific warm-up component. *J Sci Med Sport*. 2009;12:657–61.
30. Vetter RE. Effects of six warm-up protocols on sprint and jump performance. *J Strength Cond Res*. 2007;21:819–23.
31. Young WB, Behm DG. Effects of running, static stretching and practice jumps on explosive force production and jumping performance. *J Sports Med Phys Fitness*. 2003;43:21–7.
32. Cengiz A. EMG and peak force responses to PNF stretching and the relationship between stretching-induced force deficits and bilateral deficits. *J Phys Ther Sci*. 2017;27:631–4.
33. Kay AD, Blazevich AJ. Effect of acute static stretch on maximal muscle performance: a systematic review. *Med Sci Sports Exerc*. 2012;44:154–64.
34. Power K, Behm D, Cahill F, Carroll M, Young W. An acute bout of static stretching: effects on force and jumping performance. *Med Sci Sports Exerc*. 2004;36:1389–96.
35. Bradley PS, Olsen PD, Portas MD. The effect of static, ballistic, and proprioceptive neuromuscular facilitation stretching on vertical jump performance. *J Strength Cond Res*. 2007;21:223–6.

36. Sa MA, Matta TT, Carneiro SP, et al. Acute effects of different methods of stretching and specific warm-ups on muscle architecture and strength performance. *J Strength Cond Res.* 2016;30:2324–9.

37. Behm DG, Button DC, Butt JC. Factors affecting force loss with prolonged stretching. *Can J Appl Physiol.* 2001;26:261–72.

38. Marek SM, Cramer JT, Fincher AL, et al. Acute effects of static and proprioceptive neuromuscular facilitation stretching on muscle strength and power output. *J Athl Train.* 2005;40:94–103.

39. Wilson GJ, Murphy AJ, Pryor JF. Musculotendinous stiffness: its relationship to eccentric, isometric, and concentric performance. *J Appl Physiol.* 1994;76:2714–9.

40. Ryan ED, Herda TJ, Costa PB, et al. Determining the minimum number of passive stretches necessary to alter musculotendinous stiffness. *J Sports Sci.* 2009;27:957–61.

41. Torres EM, Kraemer WJ, Vingren JL, et al. Effects of stretching on upper-body muscular performance. *J Strength Cond Res.* 2008;22:1279–85.

42. Pearce AJ, Kidgell DJ, Zois J, Carlson JS. Effects of secondary warm up following stretching. *Eur J Appl Physiol.* 2009;105:175–83.

43. Robbins JW, Scheuermann BW. Varying amounts of acute static stretching and its effect on vertical jump performance. *J Strength Cond Res.* 2008;22:781–6.

44. Young W, Elias G, Power J. Effects of static stretching volume and intensity on plantar flexor explosive force production and range of motion. *J Sports Med Phys Fitness.* 2006;46:403–11.

45. Faigenbaum AD, McFarland JE, Schwerdtman JA, Ratamess NA, Kang J, Hoffman JR. Dynamic warm-up protocols, with and without a weighted vest, and fitness performance in high school female athletes. *J Athl Train.* 2006;41:357–63.

46. Barnes KR, Kilding AE. Strategies to improve running economy. *Sports Med.* 2015;45:37–56.

47. Giudetti L, DiCagno A, Gallotta MC, et al. Precompetition warm-up in elite and subelite rhythmic gymnastics. *J Strength Cond Res.* 2009;23:1877–82.

48. Bacurau RF, Monteiro GA, Ugrinowitsch C, et al. Acute effect of a ballistic and a static stretching exercise bout on flexibility and maximal strength. *J Strength Cond Res.* 2009;23:304–8.

49. Nelson AG, Kokkonen J, Arnall DA. Acute muscle stretching inhibits muscle strength endurance performance. *J Strength Cond Res.* 2005;19:338–43.

50. Barroso R, Tricoli V, Santos Gil SD, Ugrinowitsch C, Roschel H. Maximal strength, number of repetitions, and total volume are differently affected by static-, ballistic-, and proprioceptive neuromuscular facilitation stretching. *J Strength Cond Res.* 2012;26:2432–7.

51. Junior RM, Berton R, Frota de Souza TM, et al. Effect of the flexibility training performed immediately before resistance training on muscle hypertrophy, maximum strength and flexibility. *Eur J Appl Physiol.* 2017;117:767–74.

52. Medeiros DM, Cini A, Sbruzzi G, Lima CS. Influence of static stretching on hamstring flexibility in healthy young adults: systematic review and meta-analysis. *Physiother Theory Pract.* 2016;32:438–445.

53. Ekstrand J, Gillquist J. The frequency of muscle tightness and injuries in soccer players. *Am J Sports Med.* 1982;10:75–78.

54. American College of Sports Medicine. Quantity and quality of exercise for developing and maintaining cardiorespiratory, musculoskeletal, and neuromotor fitness in apparently healthy adults: guidance for prescribing exercise. *Med Sci Sports Exerc.* 2011;43:1334–59.

55. McCullough AS, Kraemer WJ, Volek JS, et al. Factors affecting flutter kicking speed in women who are competitive and recreational swimmers. *J Strength Cond Res.* 2009;23:2130–6.

56. Meckel Y, Atterbom H, Grodjinovsky A, Ben-Sira D, Rotstein A. Physiological characteristics of female 100 metre sprinters of different performance levels. *J Sports Med Phys Fitness.* 1995;35:169–75.

57. Kokkonen J, Nelson AG, Eldredge C, Winchester JB. Chronic static stretching improves exercise performance. *Med Sci Sports Exerc.* 2007;39:1825–31.

58. Witvrouw E, Mahieu N, Danneels L, McNair P. Stretching and injury prevention: an obscure relationship. *Sports Med.* 2004;34:443–9.

59. Kubo K, Kanehisa H, Fukunaga T. Effect of stretching training on the viscoelastic properties of human tendon structures in vivo. *J Appl Physiol.* 2002;92:595–601.

60. Kubo K, Kanehisa H, Kawakami Y, Fukunaga T. Influence of static stretching on viscoelastic properties of human tendon structures in vivo. *J Appl Physiol.* 2001;90:520–7.

61. Malliaris P, Cook JL, Kent P. Reduced ankle dorsiflexion range may increase the risk of patellar tendon injury among volleyball players. *J Sci Med Sport.* 2006;9:304–9.

62. Amako M, Oda T, Masuoka K, Yokoi H, Campisi P. Effect of static stretching on prevention of injuries for military recruits. *Mil Med.* 2003;168:442–6.

63. Hartig DE, Henderson JM. Increasing hamstring flexibility decreases lower extremity overuse injuries in military basic trainees. *Am J Sports Med.* 1999;27:173–6.

64. Thacker SB, Gilchrist J, Stroup DF, Kimsey CD. Effect of stretching on sport injury risk: a review. *Med Sci Sports Exerc.* 2004;36:371–8.

65. Emery CA, Meeuwisse WH. Risk factors for groin injuries in hockey. *Med Sci Sports Exerc.* 2001;33:1423–33.

66. Watson AW. Sports injuries related to flexibility, posture, acceleration, clinical defects, and previous injury, in high-level players of body contact sports. *Int J Sports Med.* 2001;22:222–5.

67. Jeffreys I. Warm-up and stretching. In: Baechle TR, Earle RW, editors. *Essentials of Strength Training and Conditioning.* 3rd ed. Champaign (IL): Human Kinetics; 2008. p. 295–324.

68. Hoeger WW, Hopkins DR. A comparison of the sit and reach and the modified sit and reach in the measurement of flexibility in women. *Res Q Exerc Sport.* 1992;63:191–5.

69. Hopkins DR, Hoeger WWK. A comparison of the sit-and-reach test and the modified sit-and-reach test in the measurement of flexibility for males. *J Appl Sport Sci Res.* 1992;6:7–10.

70. Ferreira GN, Teixeira-Salmela LF, Guimaraes CQ. Gains in flexibility related to measures of muscular performance: impact of flexibility on muscular performance. *Clin J Sport Med.* 2007;17:276–81.

71. Grabara M, Szopa J. Effects of hatha yoga exercises on spine flexibility in women over 50 years old. *J Phys Ther Sci.* 2015;27:361–5.

72. Sainz de Baranda P, Ayala F. Chronic flexibility improvement after a 12-week stretching program utilizing the ACSM recommendations: hamstring flexibility. *Int J Sports Med.* 2010;31:389–96.

73. Fasen JM, O'Connor AM, Schwartz SL, et al. A randomized controlled trial of hamstring stretching: comparison of four techniques. *J Strength Cond Res.* 2009;23:660–7.

74. Meroni R, Cerri CG, Lanzarini C, et al. Comparison of active stretching technique and static stretching technique on hamstring flexibility. *Clin J Sport Med.* 2010;20:8–14.

75. Woolstenhulme MT, Griffiths CM, Woolstenhulme EM, Parcell AC. Ballistic stretching increases flexibility and acute vertical jump height when combined with basketball activity. *J Strength Cond Res*. 2006;20:799–803.

76. Oliveira LP, Vieira LHP, Aquino R, Manechini JPV, Santiago PRP, Puggina EF. Acute effects of active, ballistic, passive, and proprioceptive neuromuscular facilitation stretching on sprint and vertical jump performance in trained young soccer players. *J Strength Cond Res*. 2018;32:2199–2208.

77. Sharman MJ, Cresswell AG, Riek S. Proprioceptive neuromuscular facilitation stretching: mechanisms and clinical implications. *Sports Med*. 2006;36:929–39.

78. Caplan N, Rogers R, Parr MK, Hayes PR. The effect of proprioceptive neuromuscular facilitation and static stretch training on running mechanics. *J Strength Cond Res*. 2009;23:1175–80.

79. Hindle KB, Whitcomb TJ, Briggs WO, Hong J. Proprioceptive neuromuscular facilitation (PNF): its mechanisms and effects on range of motion and muscular function. *J Hum Kinet*. 2012;31:105–13.

80. Feland JB, Marin HN. Effect of submaximal contraction intensity in contract-relax proprioceptive neuromuscular facilitation stretching. *Br J Sports Med*. 2004;38:e18.

81. Ajimsha MS, Al-Mudahka NR, Al-Madhar JA. Effectiveness of myofascial release: systematic review of randomized controlled trials. *J Bodyw Mov Ther*. 2015;19:102–12.

82. Clark MA, Lucett SC. *NASM Essentials of Corrective Exercise Training*. Philadelphia (PA): Lippincott Williams & Wilkins—Wolters Kluwer; 2011. p. 197–209.

83. Thrash K, Kelly B. Flexibility and strength training. *J Appl Sport Sci Res*. 1987;1:74–5.

84. Nobrega ACL, Paula KC, Carvalho ACG. Interaction between resistance training and flexibility training in healthy young adults. *J Strength Cond Res*. 2005;19:842–6.

85. Behm DG, Wilkie J. Do self-myofascial release devices release myofascial? Rolling mechanisms: a narrative review. *Sports Med*. 2019;49:1173–81.

86. Beardsley C, Skarabot J. Effects of self-myofascial release: a systematic review. *J Bodyw Mov Ther*. 2015;19:747–58.

87. Moyer CA, Rounds J, Hannum JW. A meta-analysis of massage therapy research. *Psychol Bull*. 2004;130:3–18.

88. Poppendieck W, Wegmann M, Ferrauti A, Kellmann M, Pfeiffer M, Meyer T. Massage and performance recovery: a meta-analytical review. *Sports Med*. 2016;46:183–204.

89. Davis HL, Alabed S, Chico TJA. Effect of sports massage on performance and recovery: a systematic review and meta-analysis. *BMJ Open Sport Exerc Med*. 2020;6:e000614.

90. Cheatham SW, Kolber MJ, Cain M, Lee M. The effects of self-myofascial release using a foam roller or roller massage on joint range of motion, muscle recovery, and performance: a systematic review. *Int J Sports Phys Ther*. 2015;10:827–38.

91. Peacock CA, Krein DD, Silver TA, et al. An acute bout of self-myofascial release in the form of foam rolling improves performance testing. *Int J Exerc Sci*. 2014;7:202–11.

92. Behara B, Jacobson BH. Acute effects of deep tissue foam rolling and dynamic stretching on muscular strength, power, and flexibility in Division I linemen. *J Strength Cond Res*. 2015;31:888–92.

93. Healey KC, Hatfield DL, Blanpied P, Dorfman LR, Riebe D. The effects of myofascial release with foam rolling on performance. *J Strength Cond Res*. 2013;28:61–8.

94. Phillips J, Diggin D, King DL, Sforzo GA. Effect of varying self-myofascial release duration on subsequent athletic performance. *J Strength Cond Res*. 2018.

95. Monteiro ER, Skarabot J, Vigotsky AD, et al. Maximum repetition performance after different antagonist foam rolling volumes in the inter-set rest period. *Int J Sports Phys Ther*. 2017;12:76–84.

96. Hodgson DD, Lima CD, Low JL, Behm DG. Four weeks of roller massage training did not impact range of motion, pain pressure threshold, voluntary contractile properties or jump performance. *Int J Sports Phys Ther*. 2018;13:835–45.

97. Skarabot J, Beardsley C, Stirn I. Comparing the effects of self-myofascial release with static stretching on ankle range-of-motion in adolescent athletes. *Int J Sports Phys Ther*. 2015;10:203–12.

98. Beedle BB, Leydig SN, Carnucci JM. No differences in pre- and postexercise stretching on flexibility. *J Strength Cond Res*. 2007;21:780–3.

99. Marques AP, Vasconcelos AA, Cabral CM, Sacco IC. Effect of frequency of static stretching on flexibility, hamstring tightness, and electromyographic activity. *Braz J Med Biol Res*. 2009;42:949–53.

100. Ayala F, de Baranda Andujar PS. Effect of 3 different active stretch durations on hip flexion range of motion. *J Strength Cond Res*. 2010;24:430–6.

101. Bandy WD, Irion JM. The effect of time on static stretch on the flexibility of the hamstring muscles. *Phys Ther*. 1994;74:845–50.

102. Bandy WD, Irion JM, Briggler M. The effect of time and frequency of static stretching on flexibility of the hamstring muscles. *Phys Ther*. 1997;77:1090–6.

CHAPTER 12
Resistance Training Program Design

OBJECTIVES

After completing this chapter, you will be able to:

- Discuss the importance of designing individualized resistance training programs for obtaining maximal benefits
- Define each acute program variable and identify ways in which to manipulate each one to target specific training goals
- Discuss the ACSM's recommendations for progression during resistance training
- Discuss various advanced resistance training techniques and their potential usage
- Design a phase of a resistance training program from beginning to end

Resistance training (RT) is well known for improving athletic performance. The critical component to optimal RT is the design of the program in addition to the motivation and dedication of the athlete to follow the program consistently. A RT program is a composite of several variables (Fig. 12.1) that interact with each other to provide a stimulus for adaptation (1). Program design emphasizes the manipulation of these variables to target specific goals (strength, power, hypertrophy, and muscular endurance) and minimize boredom that could accompany training with little variation. Because there are infinite ways to vary programs, many programs can be successful provided that they adhere to general training guidelines. Basic RT guidelines were initially established by the American College of Sports Medicine (ACSM) in 1990 and 1998 (2). Since then, the ACSM (3,4) has expanded these initial guidelines by providing general progression recommendations to maximize strength, power, hypertrophy, and endurance training in healthy young and older individuals. These guidelines and the finer points of program design are discussed in a way to allow the coach/athlete a framework to build a template.

Individualization of Resistance Training Programs

The most effective RT programs are individualized to the athlete's needs and goals. Training goals (see Chapter 1) serve the basis of the program, and most athletes' programs are based on multiple goals. Following medical clearance or completion of health history information, goals, in addition to needs of the sport, are obtained by performing a needs analysis. A needs analysis consists of answering questions based upon goals and desired outcomes, assessments, access to equipment, health, and the demands of the sport. A sample needs analysis is shown in Table 12.1. Individualized RT programs are most effective because they target the goals and needs of the athlete. The questions a needs analysis may address are (5–7)

1. *Are there health/injury concerns that may limit the exercises performed or the exercise intensity?* An injury or health concern may limit some exercises and training intensity until sufficient recovery has ensued. Exercises can be selected to work around an injury.
2. *What type of equipment is available?* Equipment availability is paramount to exercise selection. Although effective programs can be developed with minimal equipment, knowledge of what is available allows one to select appropriate exercises and variations.
3. *What is the training frequency and are there any time constraints that may affect workout duration?* The total number of training sessions per week needs to be derived initially because this will affect all other training variables such as exercise selection, volume, and intensity. Some athletes may be scheduled at specific blocks of time. If this block of time is 1.5 hours, then the program needs to be developed within that time frame. The exercises selected, the number of exercises and total sets performed, and rest intervals between sets and exercises will be affected.

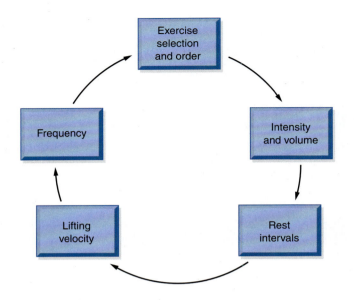

FIGURE 12.1 The acute program variables.

5. *What are the targeted energy systems?* RT programs mostly target the ATP-PC and glycolysis systems. Specific attention can be given to both if they match the metabolic demands of the sport. Although the oxidative system is active during resistance exercise (RE), it is trained more specifically through aerobic training.
6. *What types of muscle actions (CON, ECC, ISOM) are needed?* These are included in all training programs. Some athletes may benefit from targeting one when necessary.
7. *If training for a sport, what are the most common sites of injury?* Special attention can be given to susceptible areas often injured. For example, female athletes are four to eight times more likely to sustain a tear of their anterior cruciate ligament (ACL) than their male counterparts. Special attention can be given to strengthen the kinetic chain to prevent ACL injuries. See Sidebar: Anterior Cruciate Ligament Injuries and Female Athletes.

The Importance of Training Status

Program design differs based on one's level of training. Training status ranges on a continuum from beginner to elite strength/power athlete. Factors to consider include the athlete's history of lifting weights (months and years of experience), level of conditioning (magnitude of strength, power, endurance, and hypertrophy), and sports participation (RT is encountered in several sports and can pose an adaptive stimulus to an athlete independent of weight lifting). Training

4. *What muscle groups require special attention?* All major muscle groups need to be trained but some may require prioritization based upon strengths/weaknesses or the demands of the sport. It is important to maintain muscle balance especially among those muscles with agonist-antagonist relationships, primary stabilizer roles for large muscle mass exercises, and small muscles often weak in comparison to larger muscle groups.

Table 12.1 Sample Needs Analysis

College Baseball Player — Right Fielder Off-Season Strength and Conditioning Program

Sport needs	Throwing, hitting, base running, defensive play, sliding, sprinting, occasional diving, and jumping
Muscle groups	All major muscle groups are emphasized — special attention for core strength/power, shoulder (rotator cuff), grip strength, and hip/quadriceps strength/power
Common injury sites	Shoulder, knee, hamstrings, elbow, low back
Energy demands	ATP-PC system predominately
Fitness needs	Muscle strength, power, endurance, speed, agility, reaction time and coordination, reduced body fat
Equipment restraints	None
Testing results	Scored well in speed and agility tests; scored fairly well in power assessments; scored fairly well in muscle strength
Desired frequency	3 days per week
Training background	5 yr of resistance training experience. Has good form and technique especially for Olympic lifts. Has built a modest-to-good strength base. Based on examination of training history is considered to be an advanced trainee
Workout structure	Periodized, total-body workout. Each workout structured in sequence from Olympic/powerlifts → basic strength → sport-specific needs

Note: This off-season program will strengthen all major muscle groups in a periodized manner to peak strength and power for preseason testing. Plyometric, speed, and agility training will occur separately.

Sidebar — Anterior Cruciate Ligament Injuries and Female Athletes

An ACL tear is a severe injury that is costly in rehabilitation time. More than 100,000 ACL injuries occur each year, and an ACL injury increases the risk of osteoarthritis as early as 10 years following the injury (8). For noncontact ACL injury, the most common mechanism is deceleration with twisting, pivoting, and/or change of direction (9). ACL injuries are up to 8–10 times more likely to occur in female than male athletes (8,10). During cutting tasks, ~60% of female demonstrate a biomechanical deficit that could put them at a higher risk of injury (11). The greater risk is associated with postpubertal females as young females have much lower injury risks similar to that of young males (8). Females have several anatomical and physiological attributes that make them more susceptible to noncontact ACL injuries occurring ~30–100 ms following foot contact with the ground (8). Females have wider pelvic girdles, a larger angle of pull of the quadriceps muscles (*e.g.*, *Q angle*), greater femoral anteversion, less-developed quadriceps muscle size and strength, increased joint laxity and flexibility (leading to more tibial displacement), more tibial torsion, narrower femoral notch (less space to house the ACL), lower hamstring-to-quadriceps muscle strength ratio, higher estrogen concentrations (and subsequent increases during the menstrual cycle), generate force more slowly, exhibit greater impact forces and impact rates of loading, altered hip muscle recruitment patterns for controlling landing (*i.e.*, increased hip torque, lower gluteus maximus and higher rectus femoris activity) and proprioception, and have smaller ACLs in comparison to men (9,10,12). These are factors that decrease knee stability. Other factors such as height and tibia/thigh length, body mass, foot pronation and navicular drop, foot/surface interaction, and prior ACL injury history contribute to the injury risk (12). In fact, rapid changes at puberty have been implicated as the female body size increases without the concomitant increases in muscle strength, size, coordination, and power seen in males undergoing puberty (8). Women have greater *valgus stress* placed on the knee. A valgus stress is one where abduction (outward angulation) of the joint is seen in a joint where abduction is not a prescribed movement. Valgus stresses increase susceptibility to knee injury and result from some of the aforementioned anatomical factors. The research group of Myer, Hewett, and colleagues (8,11,13–15) have identified leading factors contributing to the increased valgus stress. They report that *ligament dominance* (imbalance between muscular and ligamentous control of knee during landing and pivoting; less knee flexion during cutting and landing forcing the quadriceps to pull tibia forward stressing the ACL), *quadriceps dominance* (greater quadriceps activation and coordination relative to the hamstrings), *leg dominance* (one side of body much stronger and powerful than other side by more than 20%), and *trunk dominance* (where lateral

trunk displacement increases with the body shifted over one leg with little knee flexion while the foot is planted flat on the surface; due to core dysfunction) are strong predictors of ACL injuries in female athletes. Many ACL injuries involve a valgus collapse mechanism or "position of no return" where multiplanar loading of the knee is encountered, as well as greater hip adduction and internal rotation, external tibial rotation, and knee with little flexion to hyperextension. Myer et al. (13–15) have shown knee valgus motion (cm) and knee flexion range of motion (ROM; degrees) during landing from a jump, body mass (kg), tibia length (cm), and quadriceps-to-hamstrings strength ratio are strong predictors of ACL injury and developed an algorithm to identify athletes at risk using these variables that contribute to high valgus stress (Fig. 12.2). They showed that these five factors accounted for 78% of the variance seen in knee abductor moments during landing. Each of the five factors are measured and scored by drawing a line from the score to the "points" line. All points are totaled and a line is drawn connecting the point total to the probability line indicating the probability the athlete will attain a knee abductor moment >21.74 Nm during landing. Such data can be useful to the coach and athletes to identify early athletes who are at risk. Panel B depicts mild valgus collapse seen during landing yielding a knee abductor moment placing them at higher risk for injury.

The needs analysis for a female athlete may demonstrate that knee injuries are of concern and special training modifications are needed to strengthen that area. It is recommended that integrated training methods (*i.e.*, referred to as *integrative neuromuscular training* or *neuromuscular training [NMT]*) begin in the female adolescent athlete as strength, power, and coordination improvements in this population may help offset postpubertal issues increasing the risk of ACL injury (8,15,16). NMT involves the integration of resistance, corrective exercise, balance, speed and agility, and plyometric training modes targeting specific deficits in the female body. Prevention of ACL injuries encompasses several concepts that extend beyond focusing on the knee. Rather, strengthening the entire kinetic chain (hip, ankle, and core in addition to the knee) is paramount because the knee may be the weak link. Wilk et al. (9) have defined eight areas of concern for female athletes and have proposed exercises to address each area to reduce ACL injuries. These include exercises that target (a) increased hip strength in three planes (lateral step-over, lunge); (b) strengthened hamstrings to provide greater control of the knee (lateral lunge, slide board); (c) controlled valgus stresses (step-up with band, single-leg squat); (d) controlled knee hyperextension (plyometrics); (e) increased neuromuscular reaction (movement-specific exercises on unstable surfaces); (f) increased thigh musculature (squats, leg press); (g) increased endurance (aerobic training); and (h) increased

(Continued)

speed (sprint drills, backward running). Some recent meta-analyses have examined the efficacy of NMT on ACL injury risk. Myer et al. (15) showed female athletes undergoing NMT had a 72% knee injury reduction (especially for girls 18 yr of age and younger) compared to controls. The rate of injury reduction was 16% for females over 18 years of age (15). Sugimoto et al. (17) reported a 46% reduction in injury risk for those undergoing a NMT program compared to those who were not. They also reported a dose-response effect with NMT where ACL injury prevention was greatest with longer workouts (>20–30 min), multiple workout frequencies (compared to 1 day per week), and with higher volume programs compared to moderate and low volumes. The longer duration workouts decreased ACL injury risk by ~70% (17). Thus, RT programs targeting these biomechanical/physiological deficits are critical to training female athletes.

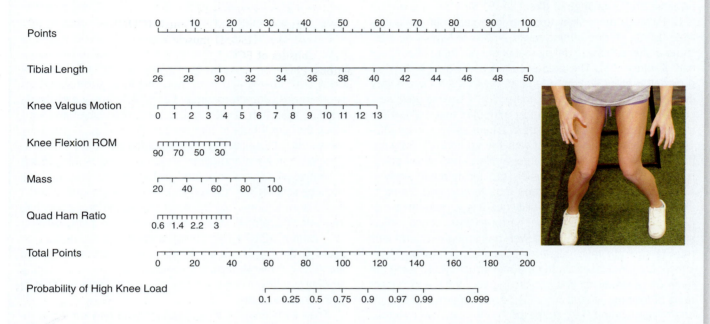

FIGURE 12.2 Knee valgus stress during landing in a female athlete. (Adapted from Figures 2 and 9, Myer GD, Ford KR, Khoury J, Succop P, Hewett TE. Development and validation of a clinic-based prediction tool to identify female athletes at high risk for anterior cruciate ligament injury. *Am J Sports Med*. 2010;38:2025–33.)

status (and responder vs. nonresponder) is a culmination of these factors and can pose difficulty for the coach to determine in some cases. For example, some individuals have lifted weight for several months to years and only experienced small improvements, whereas some individuals with little experience have adapted quickly due to genetics or prior sports participation. Therefore, some difficulty can be encountered in classifying athletes on this continuum. Notwithstanding, a beginner is one who has no or very little experience lifting weights and has a large potential window of adaptation. An intermediate (moderately trained) individual is one who has at least 4–6 months of progressive RT experience and has attained notable improvements. The key is progressive RT experience and not merely working out below one's threshold level of adaptation. A trained individual is one with at least 1 year of consistent progressive RT and has experienced a substantial level of adaptation. Those who truly excel in RT may attain advanced or elite status in which they rank highly in one or more components of fitness. Skill level increases as one progresses from beginner to intermediate to advanced.

Training status identification helps determine the rate and magnitude of progression. Untrained individuals respond favorably to any program, thereby making it difficult to evaluate the effects of different RT programs at this stage. Resistance-trained individuals have a slower rate of progression than untrained or moderately trained individuals (6). In the ACSM's 2002 position stand (3), several studies were reviewed and it was estimated that strength increases the most in untrained individuals followed by moderately trained, trained, advanced, and elite athletes over training periods ranging from 4 weeks to 2 years on a continuum where progression becomes reduced with advancing status. Progression in any fitness component becomes more difficult with training. Because of these trends, it was proposed that RT program design be prescribed in an orderly manner from a *general-to-specific progression* (3). This model is illustrated in Figure 12.3. The narrow segment of the pyramid representing novice individuals illustrates that little variation is needed here. Because many programs yield positive results initially, it is recommended that program design be general to begin (keep it simple!). This general phase is

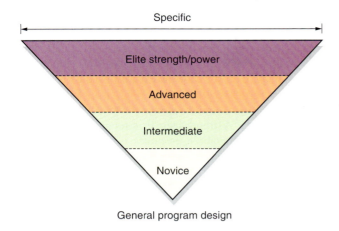

FIGURE 12.3 General-to-specific model of progression. (Data from American College of Sports Medicine. American College of Sports Medicine: Position stand: progression models in resistance training for healthy adults. *Med Sci Sports Exerc*. 2002;34:364–80.)

characterized by low to moderate intensity/volume training where enhancing technique and establishing a conditioning base are primary goals. However, as the window of adaption narrows per conditioning variable with experience, more variation is needed as illustrated by the wider sides of the pyramid. Greater specificity is needed to target each component in a periodized approach. A general RT program may improve several components of fitness simultaneously in an untrained individual. However, this same program may only improve one or two components in a trained individual. Advanced training is characterized by greater specificity and this requires greater variation in the program. Training cycles are common and each cycle may target a few components of fitness. Training plateaus are encountered at higher levels of training, thereby demonstrating the need for variation.

 ## Resistance Training Program Design

The RT program is a composite of several variables that include (a) muscle actions used, (b) intensity, (c) volume, (d) exercises selected and workout structure, (e) the sequence of exercise performance, (f) rest intervals between sets, (g) repetition velocity, and (h) training frequency. Altering one or several of these variables will affect the training stimuli and increase motivation.

Exercise Selection

Exercise selection refers to the exercises included in the RT program. The exercises selected play a significant role in the transfer of muscle strength, power, and endurance from training to athletic performance. Exercises selection is affected by a number of factors including the targeted muscle actions, the size and number of muscle groups targeted, goals of the program and of each exercise, equipment availability and source of the resistance, posture and body positioning, grip/stance widths, uni- versus bilateral exercises, and the intent to isolate muscle groups or target specific movements with resistance (4,6). Each exercise variation should be treated as a separate exercise as any change in position, equipment, hand/foot position or spacing, posture, etc. will result in muscle activation or leverage differences and subsequently affect the amount of weight lifted and/or number of reps performed.

All exercises consist of concentric (CON), eccentric (ECC), and/or isometric (ISOM) muscle actions. Each dynamic repetition consists of ECC, CON, and may include ISOM muscle actions. Physiologically, ECC actions provide greater force per unit of muscle cross-sectional area (CSA), involve less motor unit activation per unit of force, require less energy expenditure per level of tension, result in higher levels of muscle damage, and are more conducive to muscle growth than CON or ISOM muscle actions (4,6). They are important to mediating neuromuscular adaptations to training. Dynamic strength improvements are greatest when ECC actions are emphasized (18). Because dynamic repetitions consist of CON and ECC phases, very little manipulation of these muscle actions occurs. However, each CON or ECC phase can be altered by manipulating the loading, volume, velocity, and rest interval length. Some advanced forms of training involve prioritizing the ECC phase. Another example is *triphasic training* (by strength coach Cal Dietz) where, given the load per exercise, the ECC phase is emphasized (for 5–8 s reps) for a short phase (*e.g.*, 2 wk), the ISOM phase between ECC and CON phases is emphasized (3–5 s) the next 2-week phase, and the CON phase is emphasized the next 2-week phase using fast rep velocities. With traditional RT, most of the effort is applied at the CON sticking region of exercise. The sticking region is the point where bar velocity is minimal. Mechanically, the lifter is in a disadvantageous position when heavy loading is used or fatigue ensues. Weight selection targets the CON sticking region because any more will result in failure, so this limiting factor is present when full ROM repetitions are used. As a consequence, the ECC phase may not receive optimal loading. Accentuated ECC training can provide some additional benefits to the lifter. Acutely, CON strength may be enhanced and it is thought that accentuated ECC training may reduce neural inhibitions leading to greater CON strength. For the bench press, lowering a heavier weight than one's CON 1 RM (105% of 1 RM) yields a greater 1 RM bench press than lowering the CON 1 RM load (19). This was studied by using hooks that became unloaded at the end of the ECC phase. CON 1 RM performance was enhanced by up to ~7 kg (20). Techniques to enhance ECC training include heavy negatives, forced negatives (with partner assistance), and unilateral negatives (*i.e.*, performing the CON phase of a machine exercise with two arms or legs but performing the ECC phase with one).

ISOM muscle actions exist in many forms during RE. Stabilizer muscles contract quasi-isometrically to maintain posture and stability during an exercise. ISOM actions occur in between ECC and CON actions for the agonist muscles. The action may be prolonged if a pause is instituted. Gripping tasks require ISOM muscle actions. ISOM contraction of finger, thumb, and wrist muscles is paramount to gripping the weights, especially during pulling exercises. Grip strength training greatly depends upon ISOM muscle actions. ISOM muscle actions can serve as the primary mode of exercise in a specific area of the ROM. Exercises such as a leg lift and plank are predominantly ISOM. Strong contraction of the trunk muscles is needed to offset the effects of gravity. Another example is the overhead squat. The upper body and trunk muscles mostly isometrically contract to maintain the overhead bar position. The top position of the pull-up exercise can be held for a specific length of time. This involves ISOM contraction of back and arm musculature and may be used to enhance ROM-specific strength and endurance. Position-hold ISOM exercises can be used for strength and endurance improvements. For a number of exercises (loaded or bodyweight), a position within the dynamic ROM may be held for several seconds. Some examples include the ISOM push-up and wall squat where the athlete descends to the mid-range (push-up) or parallel position (squat) and holds that position for a period of time. Lastly, functional ISOM training can be used (discussed later in this chapter). The ACSM recommends ISOM muscle actions be targeted in RT programs (4).

Exercises are generally classified as single or multiple joint. Single-joint exercises target one joint or major muscle group. Although multiple joints may be involved in stability roles, the objective is to target a specific area or muscle group. Multiple-joint exercises target more than one joint or major muscle group with the potential to stress several major muscle groups. Distribution of loading is made to multiple muscle groups involved in the exercise. This was shown by Soares et al. (21) who reported greater reductions in elbow flexor peak torque (27% vs. 15%, which remained reduced at 24 h post-RE) and muscle soreness following 8 sets of 10 reps of a single-joint exercise of the elbow flexors (preacher curl) versus a multiple-joint exercise (seated row). Single- and multiple-joint exercises are effective for increasing muscle strength, endurance, and hypertrophy. Single-joint exercises, *e.g.*, triceps pushdown, lying leg curl, are used to target specific muscle groups and reduce the level of skill and technique involved. Multiple-joint exercises, *e.g.*, bench press, shoulder press, and squat, are more neurally complex and are regarded as most effective for increasing strength because of the lifting of a larger amount of weight (5). Some studies reported limited benefits of adding single-joint exercises to multi-joint RT programs (22); however, the total number of exercises was low in subjects with limited RT experience making it difficult to extrapolate these findings to higher volume athletic programs. Some exercises are closed-chain kinetic exercises where the distal segments are fixed while some exercises are open-chain kinetic exercises where the distal segment freely moves against loading. In comparison, moderate-to-high relationships exist between closed-chain multiple-joint exercises and jump performance (23) indicating a greater potential role for multiple-joint exercises in improving performance (24).

Multiple-joint exercises may be subclassified as basic strength, total-body, or combination exercises. *Basic strength exercises* (squat, bench press) involve at least two to three major muscle groups, whereas *total-body exercises* (Olympic lifts and variations) involve most major muscle groups and are the most complex exercises. These exercises are effective for increasing power because they require rapid force production and fast bodily movements. A trend seen in strength and conditioning to increase the metabolic response is the use of combination exercises. *Combination exercises* involve combining two or more exercises into one sequential movement pattern for a series of repetitions. These may be performed by combining Olympic lifts and variations (a clean from the floor, a front squat, and a push press to finish) or non-Olympic lifts (lunge with torso rotation, squat rotational press, push-up and renegade row, lunge and press, and thruster). Combination exercises are primarily used for increasing muscular endurance and hypertrophy while strength training effects are secondary. The weight lifted for a combination exercise often will be less than the weight lifted if each exercise was performed separately. Thus, maximal strength training is secondary while metabolic conditioning is prioritized. Exercises that stress large muscle groups increase the metabolic demands and provide a potent stimulus for conditioning programs.

Performing exercises unilaterally or bilaterally adds another caveat to RT (25). Neural activity to skeletal muscles varies when exercises are performed unilaterally, bilaterally, alternating, or when exercises involve limb movements that work in opposition (*i.e.*, walking) or cross the midline of the body. Training unilaterally increases muscle strength in both trained and untrained limbs (26). Training bilaterally may increase the ability to produce maximal force simultaneously on both sides, thereby reducing the bilateral deficit. Unilateral exercises require greater balance and stability. Performing a unilateral dumbbell exercise (with one dumbbell using asymmetric loading) requires the trunk muscles to contract intensely to maintain proper posture in order to offset the torque produced by unilateral loading. Asymmetric loading can be utilized bilaterally in multiple ways via specialized implements and through exercises such as partner carries.

Muscle mass involvement is important when selecting exercises. Exercises stressing multiple or large muscle groups produce the greatest acute metabolic responses (27). Large muscle mass, multiple-joint exercises such as deadlifts, jump squats, and Olympic lifts augment the acute testosterone and growth hormone response to RE more than the bench press and shoulder press (28). Single- and multiple-joint exercises may be performed with free weight and machine exercises, both are recommended by the ACSM (4) and loading and performance vary between free weights and a Smith machine for a given exercise (29). Free weight training leads to greater improvements in free weight test performance, and machine training results in greater performance on machine tests (30,31) although free weight training increases machine-based maximal strength and vice versa. When a neutral testing device is

Table 12.2	Sample Workouts Depicting Exercise Selection for Various Training Goals		
Weightlifter	**Strength/Power Athlete**	**Bodybuilder**	**Powerlifter**
Full snatch 5 × 1–3	Hang clean 4 × 3–5	Back squat 5 × 8–10	Bench press 6 × 3–6
Snatch pull 5 × 1–3	Back squat 4 × 5–8	Leg press 3 × 8–10	Bench press (with pause) 3 × 5
Overhead squat 4 × 5	Bench press 4 × 5–8	Leg extension 3 × 10–12	Wide-grip bench press 3 × 5
Good mornings 3 × 5	Barbell step-up 3 × 8	Stiff-leg deadlift 4 × 10–12	Dumbbell shoulder press 3 × 6
Bench press 3 × 5	Bent-over row 3 × 8	Lying leg curl 3 × 10–12	Front raise 3 × 8
	Standing calf raise 3 × 10		Lying triceps extension 3 × 8
	Internal/external rotation 3 × 10		
	Plyo leg raise 3 × 20		

used, strength improvements from free weights and machines appear similar (31,32). The ACSM recommends unilateral and bilateral single- and multiple-joint exercises be included, with emphasis on multiple-joint exercises for maximizing muscle strength, size, and endurance in novice, intermediate, and advanced individuals (4). However, the ACSM recommends the use of predominately multiple-joint exercises for novice, intermediate, and advanced power training (4). Many variations or progressions of single- and multiple-joint exercises can be performed. Table 12.2 illustrates example workouts characteristic of the training of athletes, powerlifters, bodybuilders, and Olympic weightlifters.

Some single- and multiple-joint exercises may be considered "corrective." *Corrective exercises* generally target muscle groups that are prone to strength or length imbalances via adaptation or dysfunction. Imbalances could lead to joint dysfunction and altered movement patterns, thereby increasing the likelihood of overuse injuries and pain. The physiotherapist Vladimir Janda characterized postural distortions linked to pain and dysfunction. Some muscles such as the pectoralis minor and major, psoas group, hamstrings, and anterior neck flexor muscles are more prone to shortening, whereas the gluteus maximus and medius, rhomboids, mid-to-lower trapezius, and multifidus are more prone to lengthening. The resulting effects have been termed *upper cross* and *lower cross syndromes* (Fig. 12.4) leading to postural imbalances such rounded shoulders/forward head and anterior pelvic tilt/hip flexion (33,34). *Pronation distortion syndrome* is characterized by excessive foot pronation, knee flexion, internal rotation, and knee valgus torque (33). In addition, weak core, hip abductors and external rotators, and gluteus maximus muscles have been related to higher incidences of ankle and knee injuries, hamstring strains, and low back pain (33,34). Corrective exercises (plus myofascial release and flexibility exercises) can be used to correct postural deficits and restore neuromuscular function. Corrective exercises can easily be included in programs as part of warm-ups, cool-downs, and during the main lifting segment of the workout.

Exercise Order and Workout Structure

The number of muscle groups trained per workout needs to be considered. There are three basic workout structures to choose from: (a) total-body workouts; (b) upper/lower-body split workouts; and (c) muscle group split routines. Total-body workouts involve performance of exercises that work all major muscle groups (1–2 exercises for each major muscle group or several exercises that stress most major muscle groups). They are common among athletes and Olympic weightlifters. With weightlifting, the Olympic lifts and variations are total-body exercises. The first few exercises in sequence are Olympic lifts (plus variations) and the remainder of the workout may be dedicated to basic strength exercises. Upper/lower-body split workouts involve performance of upper-body exercises only during one workout and lower-body exercises only during the next workout. These are common among athletes, powerlifters, and bodybuilders. Muscle group split routines involve performance of exercises for specific muscle groups during a workout (*e.g.*, a "back/biceps" workout where all exercises for the back are performed then all exercises for the biceps are performed). These are characteristic of bodybuilding programs. Compound split routines involve training more than one muscle per group workout. Isolated split routines involve training only one muscle group per workout. Many times these are used within *double splits* where the lifter may train twice per day. For compound split routines, lifters use different strategies for muscle group organization. Agonist-antagonist (chest/back), synergist (chest, triceps), and unrelated muscle group (shoulders, calves) structures may be used. All of these structures can improve performance. Goals, time/frequency, and personal preferences will determine which structure(s) is selected by the coach or athlete. The major differences between structures are the magnitude of specialization present during each workout (related to the number of exercises performed per muscle group) and the amount of recovery in between workouts. One study reported similar improvements in untrained women between total-body and upper/lower-body split workouts (35).

Upper Crossed Syndrome

**Rounded shoulders
Forward head**

Short Muscles

Upper trapezius
Levator scapulae
Sternocleidomastoid
Scalenes
Latissimus dorsi
Teres major
Subscapularis
Pectoralis major/minor

Lengthened Muscles

Deep cervical flexors
Serratus anterior
Rhomboids
Mid-trapezius
Lower trapezius
Teres minor
Infraspinatus

Possible Injuries

Headaches
Biceps tendonitis
Rotator cuff impingement
Thoracic outlet syndrome

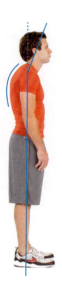

Lower Crossed Syndrome

**Increased lumbar lordosis
Anterior pelvic tilt**

Short Muscles

Gastrocnemius
Soleus
Hip flexor complex
Adductors
Latissimus dorsi
Erector spinae

Lengthened Muscles

Anterior tibialis
Posterior tibialis
Gluteus maximus
Gluteus medius
Transversus abdominis
Internal oblique

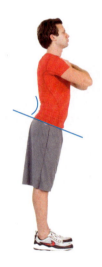

Pronation Distortion Syndrome

**Foot pronation
Knee flexion, internal rotation, adduction**

Short Muscles

Soleus
Peroneals
Adductors
Iliotibial band
Hip flexor complex
Bicep femoris
(short head)

Lengthened Muscles

Posterior tibialis
Vastus medialis
Gluteus medius/maximus
Hip external rotators

Possible Injuries

Posterior tibialis
tendonitis (shin splints)
Patellar tendonitis
Low back pain

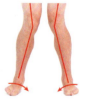

FIGURE 12.4 Upper cross, lower cross, and pronation distortion syndromes. (Reprinted from Clark MA, Lucett SC. *NASM Essentials of Corrective Exercise Training*. Philadelphia (PA): Lippincott Williams & Wilkins–Wolters Kluwer; 2011. p. 197–209.)

Table 12.3 Sample Workouts of Different Training Structures

Total-Body Workout	Upper-Body Workout	Split Routine (Chest/Triceps)
Squat 3 × 10	Bench press 3 × 6–8	Bench press 3 × 6–8
Bench press 3 × 10	Bent-over row 3 × 6–8	Incline bench press 3 × 8
Lat pull-down 3 × 10	Incline dumbbell press 3 × 8	Dumbbell flys 3 × 10
Leg press 3 × 10	Seated row 3 × 10	Cable cross-over 3 × 12
Shoulder press 3 × 10	Lateral raise 3 × 10	Standing triceps extension 3 × 10
Back extension 3 × 15	Lying triceps extension 3 × 10	Reverse pushdowns 3 × 10
Triceps pushdown 3 × 10	Preacher curl 3 × 10	Reverse dips 3 × 20
Standing curl 3 × 10		
Standing calf raise 3 × 15		
Torso rotations 3 × 25		

In the elderly, similar improvements in lower-body strength between total-body and lower-body workouts (of equal volume and intensity) were shown (36). Table 12.3 illustrates example workouts.

Exercise order affects acute lifting performance and the rate of strength increases during RT (37). Exercises performed early in the workout generate higher rep number and weights lifted because less fatigue is present. This is true for low-, moderate-, and high-intensity RT. Single- and multiple-joint exercise performances decline when these exercises are performed later in a workout rather than early (37–41). Critical to strength training is the potential decline in multiple-joint exercise performance. Sforzo and Touey (39) investigated bench press and squat performance. Sequence 1 consisted of the squat, leg extension, leg curl, bench press, shoulder press, and triceps pushdown (4 sets × 8 RM, 2–3-min rest intervals), and sequence 2 was the reverse. There were 75% and 22% declines in bench press and squat performance, respectively, when the reverse order was used. Simao et al. (40,41) compared two sequences: bench press, lat pull-down, shoulder press, biceps curl, triceps extension (3 sets of 10 reps); and the reverse order. When the bench press and lat pull-down were performed at the end, there was a 28% and 8% reduction in the number of reps performed, respectively (Fig. 12.5). Spreuwenberg et al. (42) examined the squat when it was performed first or last in sequence and reported higher number of reps when it was performed first. Interestingly, average power output of the squat was higher when performed after hang pulls, thereby showing an explosive exercise can potentiate performance of a basic strength exercise. Several studies since have consistently shown reduced performance as exercises are performed later in sequence (37,43,44). This is why priority is given to those exercises deemed most critical to RT goals as they are performed early in sequence. Although many of these studies show multiple-joint exercise performance is reduced following single-joint exercises stressing similar muscle groups, the same is true when multiple-joint exercises for similar muscle groups are performed in sequence. We examined a sequence of all multiple-joint exercises (e.g., bench press, incline press, shoulder press, and bent-over row) where we manipulated the rest interval of the bench press but used standard rest intervals for the remaining three exercises. Bench press performance was best with 3-minute rest intervals. However, performance of the incline press and shoulder press were reduced regardless of bench press performance (45). Fatigue from the bench press reduced performance of the incline press and shoulder press

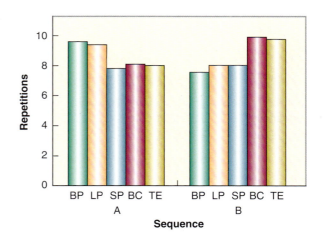

FIGURE 12.5 Resistance exercise performance using two sequences (A and B). BP, bench press; LP, leg press; SP, shoulder press; BC, biceps curl; TE, triceps extension. (Adapted with permission from Simao R, Farinatti PTV, Polito MD, Maior AS, Fleck SJ. Influence of exercise order on the number of repetitions performed and perceived exertion during resistive exercises. *J Strength Cond Res*. 2005;19:152–6.)

but did not affect the bent-over row. Other studies show performance of an exercise may be augmented if the antagonist muscles are stressed in a preceding set (46), thereby providing a basis for agonist-antagonist exercise sequencing. These data show that rotating exercises of varying muscle groups could help maintain repetition performance. Athlete and coaches should expect declines in performance when several exercises are performed stressing similar muscle groups in sequence. Loading modifications are needed to accommodate the fatigued state or the trainees may choose to cycle their training where they will place exercises earlier in sequence to target progression for those specific exercises.

Exercise order affects the neuromuscular responses to some exercises within a RE workout (37,47). For a few exercises in these studies, neural activity was greater for some muscle groups (but not all) earlier in sequence and lower later in sequence. The sequence of REs may affect oxygen consumption for a specific exercise but may not affect oxygen consumption of the entire workout (48–50). We showed that oxygen consumption for the bench press performed with short rest intervals was higher when it followed the squat in sequence compared to when it was performed first in sequence (50). Performance of the squat first or second did not affect oxygen consumption. It is possible performing the smaller mass exercise after the large mass exercise posed a metabolic advantage in viewing the bench press. Large muscle mass exercises performed in a workout with small-mass exercises can augment ISOM strength gains compared to small-mass exercise training alone (51). These data collectively indicate that the sequence of RE may have some effects on neural drive for few muscle groups and an exercise-specific effect on oxygen consumption.

The primary concern for proper exercise sequencing is derived upon the goals of maximal strength and power training. Maximal strength and power are best trained in a nonfatigued state, thereby rendering the sequencing of exercises critically important especially for highly trained athletes. In a review of the literature, Simao et al. (37) showed several augmented strength increases and effect sizes for exercises performed early in sequence compared to later for 8–12 weeks of RT. Considering that multiple-joint exercises are effective for increasing strength and power, the ACSM recommends giving priority to these exercises early in a workout (4). The Olympic lifts require explosive force production, and fatigue antagonizes the neuromuscular response. They are technically demanding and the quality of each rep needs to be maximal. These exercises need to be performed early in the workout. However, exceptions to these principles are acceptable given varying RT goals. Training for muscle endurance and hypertrophy may be accomplished or maximized using a variety of sequencing schemes. Multi-joint to single-joint exercise sequencing and the reverse have led to similar gains in muscle hypertrophy (52). Fatigue is a necessary component of muscle endurance training and to some extent hypertrophy training as well. Several exceptions exist when training to maximize muscle growth and endurance. Sequencing strategies for strength and power training are recommended by the ACSM (4,6) and examples are illustrated in Table 12.4. They can apply to endurance/hypertrophy training as well although exceptions are common. The recommendations/guidelines include

Total-body workout

1. Large muscle exercises should be performed before smaller muscle exercises.
2. Multiple-joint exercises should be performed before single-joint exercises.
3. For power training: total-body exercises (from most to least complex) should be performed before basic strength exercises, *e.g.*, most complex is the snatch (because the bar must

Table 12.4 Sample Workouts Illustrating Various Exercise Orders

Total-Body Workout Sequencing — Muscle Mass	Upper-Body Workout Sequencing — MJ, SJ	Split Workout Sequencing — Muscle Mass	Olympic Lifter/ Athlete Sequencing — OL-BS	Back Workout Sequencing — Intensity
Squat	Decline bench press	Bench press	Barbell snatch	Deadlift 4 × 3–5
Stiff-legged deadlift	Close-grip pull-down	Dumbbell incline press	Hang power clean	Bent-over barbell row 3 × 6–8
Lat pull-down	Incline dumbbell press	Decline fly	Clean pull	Reverse lat pull-down 3 × 8–10
Bench press	Upright row	Lying triceps extension	Front squat	Low pulley row 3 × 10
Barbell shrugs	Triceps pushdown	Rope pushdown	Hyperextension	Straight-arm cable pull-down 3 × 12
Triceps extension	Preacher curl			
Seated curl				

MJ, multiple-joint; SJ, single-joint; OL, Olympic lifts; BS, basic strength exercises.

be moved the greatest distance) and related lifts, followed by cleans, and presses.

4. Rotation of upper- and lower-body exercises or opposing (agonist-antagonist relationship) exercises can be employed (see Sidebar: Sample Push-Pull Exercise Pairings). The rationale is to allow muscles to rest while the opposing muscles are trained. This strategy is beneficial for maintaining high training intensities and targeted repetition numbers.

5. Some exercises targeting different muscle groups can be staggered in between sets of other exercises to increase workout efficiency.

Upper/lower-body split

1. Large muscle exercises should be performed before small muscle group exercises.
2. Multiple-joint exercises should be performed before single-joint exercises.
3. Rotation of opposing exercises may be performed.

Split routines

1. Multiple-joint exercises should be performed before single-joint exercises.
2. Large before smaller muscle mass exercises (when applicable).
3. Higher-intensity exercises should be performed before lower-intensity exercises. The sequence can proceed from heaviest to lightest exercises.

Some exceptions exist to the preceding guidelines for hypertrophy and muscular endurance training. Training to maximize hypertrophy should include strength training so the exercise sequencing recommendations apply. However, muscle hypertrophy is predicated upon mechanical and metabolic stress/hypoxic factors. Strength training maximizes the mechanical factors, whereas training in a fatigued state may potentiate metabolic stress factors that induce muscle growth. The exercise order may vary considerably. Some bodybuilders use a technique known as preexhaustion. *Preexhaustion* is a technique that requires the lifter to perform a single-joint exercise first to fatigue a muscle group. A multiple-joint exercise is performed after. One example is the sequence of dumbbell flys and bench press. When one examines the bench press, often the triceps brachii may be the primary site of fatigue. With preexhaustion, the pectoral group is prefatigued that way when the lifter performs the bench press, it is more likely that the targeted muscle, the pectoral muscles, will fatigue earlier. Less weight is used so this technique targets hypertrophy and endurance mostly, with limited strength training effects. A few studies show the targeted muscles are not activated to a greater extent with preexhaustion (38,53,54). Likewise, preexhaustion results in fewer reps performed during the multiple-joint exercise by 18%–35% (55). Multiple-joint exercise technique may be altered when performed after the single-joint exercise (56). Fatigue needs to be present for adaptations to take place when training to maximize muscle endurance, thereby leaving numerous sequencing strategies available. Warm-up exercises are another exception as some perform a single-joint exercise before a multiple-joint exercise. The key element is the single-joint exercise is performed with light weights and does not cause fatigue.

Intensity

Intensity describes the amount of weight lifted during RT and is dependent upon exercise order, volume, frequency, repetition velocity, and rest interval length. Intensity has been used to describe the level of exertion during RE. For clarity, intensity will be used to describe loading, whereas *exertion* is the preferred term used to describe the level of difficulty of performing RE. Intensities range from low to high (Table 12.5) and intensity prescription depends upon the athlete's training status and goals.

Strength Training

Intensities of 45%–50% of 1 RM or less increase strength in untrained individuals (57). It is important to stress proper form and technique to beginners, and the intensity prescription must accommodate this. Because light to moderate intensity is effective initially, it is recommended that beginners start light and progress gradually over time. Light weights (*i.e.*, 0%–30% of 1 RM) can be effective for increasing strength when they are used during ballistic training at maximal velocity but the maximal strength increases, if seen, are inferior to traditional heavy RT, *e.g.*, 6 RM (58,59). Analysis of the literature has shown that 60% of 1 RM produces the largest strength effects in untrained individuals (60). Strength increases may take place if moderate intensity is accompanied by lifting the weight as rapidly as

---

Sidebar — Sample Push-Pull Exercise Pairings

- Bench press and bent-over barbell row
- Shoulder press and lat pull-down/pull-up
- Triceps pushdown/extension and curls (and variations)
- Upright row and dips
- Back extension and sit-up
- Leg extension and leg curl
- Squat/leg press and hip flexion
- Hip adduction and hip abduction
- Wrist curl and reverse wrist curl
- Flys and reverse flys
- Lateral raise and cable crossover
- Front raise and pullover

Table 12.5 Intensity Classification

Intensity Classification	Percent of 1 RM	Utility
Supramaximal	100–↑	Max strength, partial-ROM, ISOM, and ECC strength, overloads (used cautiously)
Very heavy	95–100	Max strength, hypertrophy, motor unit recruitment
Heavy	90–95	Max strength, hypertrophy, motor unit recruitment
Moderately heavy	80–90	Max strength, power, hypertrophy
Moderate	70–80	Strength, power, hypertrophy, strength endurance
Light	60–70	Power, muscle endurance, hypertrophy
Very light	60–↓	Warm-up, unloading, high endurance, hypertrophy

possible (61). However, high (moderate to very heavy) intensities (≥80%–85% of 1 RM) are needed to increase maximal strength as one progresses to advanced training (62,63). Research supports the concept that at least 80%–85% of 1 RM is needed to maximize strength in trained athletes (Fig. 12.6) (60,64). Recent studies have shown greater strength increases with RT in the 2–5 rep zone than the 8–12 rep zone in RT men (65–67). Heavy lifting produces a neural pattern that is distinct from light to moderate loading, and training the nervous system is critical to strength enhancement since neural adaptations tend to take place before muscle hypertrophy occurs. Maximizing strength, power, and hypertrophy may only occur when the maximal numbers of motor units are recruited. High intensity is necessary at times but the periodization of intensity is most critical to strength training. Zatsiorsky (68) reported that ~8% of training encompassed loads of 60% of competition best or less, 24% was dedicated to 60%–70%, 35% was dedicated to 70%–80%, 26% was dedicated to 80%–90%, and only 7% was dedicated to maximal weights (for competition lifts) in elite weightlifters. Low to moderate intensities for some exercises (corrective) may be preferred especially when training scapular, rotator cuff, spinal, and some muscles of the core. Closed kinetic-chain exercises performed on one leg or arm is more intense as a greater percent of bodyweight must be sustained by limited muscle mass. Light-to-moderate loads may be appropriate and preferred for these types of exercises. With heavier weights comes lower repetition number and vice versa. The number of repetitions performed relative to the 1 RM is variable depending on the exercise and the level of muscle mass involvement. Intensity and volume prescription is most effective when a periodized approach is used (5). Each exercise should be treated as a specific entity as each exercise will have a specific goal and intensity should match that goal. A workout may consist of varying intensities even if the goal is peak strength or power. The commitment to strength training entails heavy weight lifting for some, but not all, exercises.

An inverse relationship exists between the amount of weight lifted and the number of reps that can be successfully performed (69,70). Figure 12.7A and B illustrates the relationship between intensity, velocity, and rep number. Low numbers of reps are performed at high intensities and vice versa. There is a continuum where high intensity and low reps are most conducive to maximal strength development. Strength becomes less targeted and endurance becomes the predominant goal as the curve shifts to the right (with an increase in rep number and decrease in intensity). High-intensity lifting is more conducive to strength increases (61) and a continuum is seen where decreasing the intensity and increasing the volume per set results in a slower rate of strength gains. The number of reps performed relative to the athlete's 1 RM is variable depending on the exercise and the level of muscle mass involvement, as large muscle mass exercises yield higher reps.

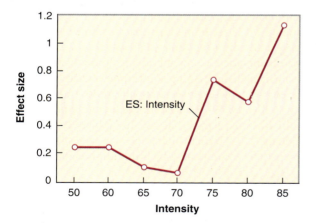

FIGURE 12.6 Dose-response for resistance training intensity. Examination of literature showed than training at ~85% of 1 RM produced greatest effect size (ES) for strength enhancement. Training with 50%–70% of 1 RM produced the least magnitude of strength gains. (Adapted with permission from Peterson MD, Rhea MR, Alvar BA. Maximizing strength development in athletes: a meta-analysis to determine the dose-response relationship. *J Strength Cond Res.* 2004;18:377–82.)

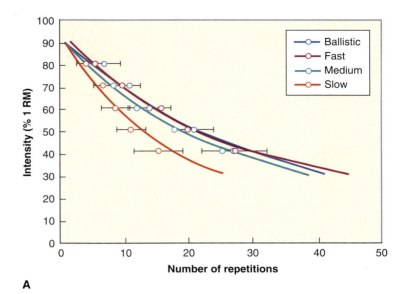

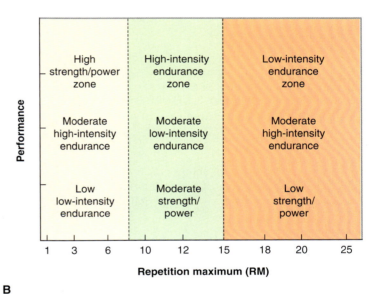

FIGURE 12.7 Relationship between intensity and reps **(A)** and theoretical repetition maximum (RM) continuum **(B)**. (**A** reprinted with permission from Sakamoto A, Sinclair PJ. Effect of movement velocity on the relationship between training load and the number of repetitions of bench press. *J Strength Cond Res.* 2006;20:532–27. **B** adapted with permission from Fleck SJ, Kraemer WJ. *Designing Resistance Training Programs.* 2nd ed. Champaign (IL): Human Kinetics; 1997.)

Table 12.6 provides a general frame of reference for the relationship between intensity and rep number. However, as shown in Table 12.7, this relationship is not so simple and depends on factors such as muscle mass involvement, training status, and gender (70,78). These values are based on performance of one set. Fatigue reduces rep number per intensity zone when multiple sets are performed. Training with loads corresponding to 1–6 RM (>85% of 1 RM) is most effective for increasing maximal strength (6) (Fig. 12.8). Although strength increases will occur using 6–12 RM loads (65%–85% of 1 RM), it is believed this range may not be entirely specific to increasing maximal strength in advanced athletes compared to higher intensities. However, this range is ideal for novice to intermediate-trained athletes (4,6). Intensities lighter than this (≤12–15 RM) have small effects on maximal strength. The higher the RM, the greater the level of muscle twitch contractile fatigue (80), thereby showing high repetitions poses a potent stimulus for endurance enhancement.

Although each training zone on this continuum has its advantages, an athlete should not devote 100% of training time to one general zone (6). Rather, training cycles should be used that employ each range depending on the training goals. For strength training, the ACSM recommends that novice to intermediate athletes train with loads corresponding to 60%–70% of 1 RM for 8–12 reps and advanced individuals cycle training loads of 80%–100% of 1 RM to maximize muscular strength (4). For strength training progression in those athletes training at a specific RM load, it is recommended that a 2%–10% (lower percent for small mass exercises, higher percent for large mass exercises) increase in load be applied when the athlete can perform that workload for 1–2 reps over the desired number on two consecutive sessions. Intensity prescription is exercise dependent. Some exercises, *e.g.*, multiple-joint structural exercises, benefit greatly from high-intensity strength cycles within the periodized training plan. However, other exercises may have other goals associated with them. The intensity may vary in these cases.

Table 12.6	The General Relationship between Intensity and Repetitions Performed
Percent of 1 RM	**Repetitions Performed**
100	1
95	2
93	3
90	4
87	5
85	6
83	7
80	8
77	9
75	10
70	11
67	12
65	15

Source: Baechle TR, Earle RW, Wathen D. Resistance training. In: Baechle TR, Earle RW, editors. *Essentials of Strength Training and Conditioning*. 3rd ed. Champaign (IL): Human Kinetics; 2008. p. 381–412. Ref. (71).

The commitment to strength training entails heavy weight lifting but this does not mean every exercise is high in intensity. Rather, those selected as structural exercises are targeted.

Power Training

Training for maximal power requires a mixed strategy. Power is the product of force and velocity so both components must be trained. This requires a spectrum of intensities. Figure 12.9 depicts changes in the force-velocity curve as a result of power training. A shift to the right is seen where for a given level of force, velocity is higher. This shift indicates improvement in the athlete's rate of force development (RFD). Moderate to heavy loads are required to increase maximal strength. A second training strategy is to incorporate low to moderate intensities performed at explosive lifting velocities to target RFD. Lifting velocity is higher at low intensities and decreases in proportion to loading (81). Maximizing velocity is critical to power training. The intensity may vary depending on the exercise in question and training status of the individual. Peak power is greater for the shoulder throw than shoulder press at both 30% and 40% of 1 RM (82). Most studies show peak power is attained in a range from 15% to 60% of 1 RM for ballistic exercises such as the jump squat and bench press throw (4,81,83–86). Less resistance (bodyweight) may maximize power output during jumps (19,87). McBride et al. (88) showed that jump squat training

Table 12.7	Number of Repetitions Performed at Various Intensities Relative to 1 RM							
Exercise	**40%**	**60%**	**70%**	**75%**	**80%**	**85%**	**90%**	**95%**
Leg press								
UT	80.1	33.9	***	***	15.2–20.3	***	***	***
TR	77.6	45.5	***	***	19.4–21.0	***	***	***
Lat pull-down								
UT	41.5	19.7	***	***	9.8	***	***	***
TR	42.9	23.5	***	***	12.2	***	***	***
Bench press								
UT	34.9	19.7–21.6	***	10.9–10.6	9.1–9.8	***	6.0	***
TR	38.8	21.7–22.6	13.4–14.0	10.0–14.1	9.2–12.2	6.0	4.0	2.2
Leg extension								
UT	23.4	15.4	***	***	9.3	***	***	***
TR	32.9	18.3	***	***	11.6	***	***	***
Sit-up								
UT	21.1	15.0	***	***	8.3	***	***	***
TR	27.1	18.9	***	***	12.2	***	***	***
Arm curl								
UT	24.3	15.3–17.2	***	***	7.6–8.9	***	3.9	***
TR	35.3	19–21.3	***	***	9.1–11.4	***	4.4	***

Table 12.7	Number of Repetitions Performed at Various Intensities Relative to 1 RM (*Continued*)							
Exercise	40%	60%	70%	75%	80%	85%	90%	95%
Leg curl								
UT	18.6	11.2	***	***	6.3	***	***	***
TR	24.3	15.4	***	***	7.2	***	***	***
Squat								
UT	***	35.9	***	***	11.8	***	6.5	***
TR	***	25–29.9	13.5	10.6	8.4–12.3	6.5	4.6–5.8	2.4
Power clean								
UT	***	***	***	***	***	***	***	***
TR	***	***	13.6–17.0	11.5	9.3	7.0	4.6	2.6
Shoulder press								
UT	***	***	***	***	***	***	***	***
TR	***	14.0	***	***	6.0	***	***	***

***Limited data.

UT, untrained; TR, trained.

Data obtained from Hoeger WK, Barette SL, Hale DF, Hopkins DR. Relationship between repetitions and selected percentages of one repetition maximum. *J Appl Sport Sci Res*. 1990;1:11–3; Morales J, Sobonya S. Use of submaximal repetition tests for predicting 1-RM strength in class athletes. *J Strength Cond Res*. 1996;10:186–9 Ref. (72); Mayhew JL, Ball TE, Arnold MD, Bowen JC. Relative muscular endurance performance as a predictor of bench press strength in college men and women. *J Appl Sport Sci Res*. 1992;6:200–6 Ref. (73); Mayhew JL, Ware JS, Bemben MG, et al. The NFL-225 test as a measure of bench press strength in college football players. *J Strength Cond Res*. 1999;13:130–4 Ref. (74); Kraemer WJ, Fleck SJ, Maresh CM, et al. Acute hormonal responses to a single bout of heavy resistance exercise in trained power lifters and untrained men. *Can J Appl Physiol*. 1999;24:524–37 Ref. (75); Ware JS, Clemens CT, Mayhew JL, Johnston TJ. Muscular endurance repetitions to predict bench press and squat strength in college football players. *J Strength Cond Res*. 1995;9:99–103 Ref. (76); Kraemer WJ. A series of studies-the physiological basis for strength training in American football: fact over philosophy. *J Strength Cond Res*. 1997;11:131–42; Kraemer WJ, Fry AC, Ratamess NA, French DN. Strength testing: development and evaluation of methodology. In: Maud PJ, Foster C, editors. *Physiological Assessments of Human Performance*. 2nd ed. Champaign (IL): Human Kinetics; 2006. p. 119–50 Ref. (77); Ratamess (unpublished); Shimano T, Kraemer WJ, Spiering BA, et al. Relationship between the number of repetitions and selected percentages of one repetition maximum in free weight exercises in trained and untrained men. *J Strength Cond Res*. 2006;20:819–23; Hatfield DL, Kraemer WJ, Spiering BA, et al. The impact of velocity of movement on performance factors in resistance exercise. *J Strength Cond Res*. 2006;20:760–6.)

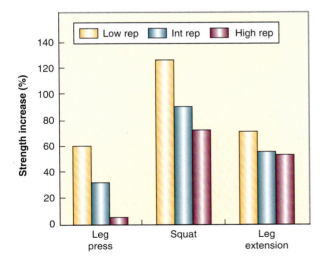

FIGURE 12.8 Strength changes with low reps (4 sets × 3–5 RM, 3-min RI); intermediate reps (3 sets × 9–11 RM, 2-min RI); and high reps (2 sets × 20–28 RM, 1-min RI) for the leg press, squat, and leg extension exercises. (Adapted with permission from Campos GER, Luecke TJ, Wendeln HK, et al. Muscular adaptations in response to three different resistance-training regimens: specificity of repetition maximum training zones. *Eur J Appl Physiol*. 2002;88:50–60. Ref. 79).

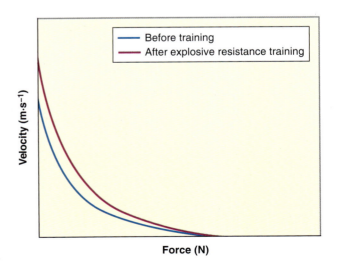

FIGURE 12.9 Shift in the force-velocity curve following training. (Reprinted with permission from Kawamori N, Haff GG. The optimal training load for the development of muscular power. *J Strength Cond Res*. 2004;18:675–84.)

with 30% of 1 RM was more effective for increasing peak power than jump squat training with 80% of 1 RM. Ballistic RE is differentiated from traditional RE because the deceleration phase is eliminated by maximally accelerating the load by jumping or releasing the weight. Traditional reps result in a substantial deceleration phase that limits power development throughout the complete ROM (Fig. 12.10). The length of the deceleration phase depends on the load and average velocity because the load is decelerated for a considerable proportion (24%–40%) of the CON phase (89,90). This percentage increases to 52% when performing the lift with a lower percentage (81%) of 1 RM lifted (89) or when attempting to move the bar rapidly in an effort to train more specifically near the movement speed of the target activity (90). Ballistic RT increases maximal strength and augments upper-body strength gains when added to traditional RT (59,91).

The intensities at which peak power is attained during traditional reps are higher than ballistic exercises due to the variance in deceleration, e.g., 40%–60% of 1 RM for the bench press, 40%–70% for the squat (92,93). Peak power for the Olympic lifts typically occurs ~70%–80% of 1 RM (94). Although any intensity can enhance muscle power, specificity is needed such that training includes a range of intensities but emphasizes the intensity that closely matches the demands of the sport. The ACSM recommends that a power component consisting of 1–3 sets per exercise using light to moderate loading (30%–60% of 1 RM for upper-body exercises, 0%–60% of 1 RM for lower-body exercises) for 3–6 reps is added concurrently to strength training (4). Progression requires various loading strategies in a periodized manner (for 1–6 reps) where heavy loading (85%–100% of 1 RM) is necessary for increasing the force component and light to moderate loading (30%–60% of 1 RM for upper-body exercises, 0%–60% of 1 RM for lower-body exercises) performed at an explosive velocity is necessary for increasing fast force production. The addition of Olympic lifts and variations are recommended using periodized intensities of 30%–85% of 1 RM (or heavier). The selection of loading for ballistic exercises could correspond to the intensities where peak power is produced; however, intensities higher or lower can benefit the athlete depending on the nature of the sport.

Hypertrophy Training

Heavy loads in combination with moderate and light loads are effective for increasing muscle hypertrophy. It is important to note that hypertrophy training needs to be viewed within context of the interaction effects of intensity, volume, rest interval length, and velocity/duration. Heavy loads stress mechanical growth factors while light-to-moderately heavy loads target metabolic stress factors. The 6–12 RM loading zone (65%–85% of 1 RM) has generally been regarded as a "hypertrophy" zone when viewed alone because this loading range has been suggested to elicit a sufficient combination of mechanical and metabolic stress growth-inducing responses (6) compared to other zones. For example, heavy weights for 1–3 repetitions optimize the mechanical components but provide little metabolic stress unless performed for a very large number of sets, which could be counterproductive. Light weights performed for 20–30 repetitions or more maximize the metabolic stress component but limit the level of motor unit recruitment seen

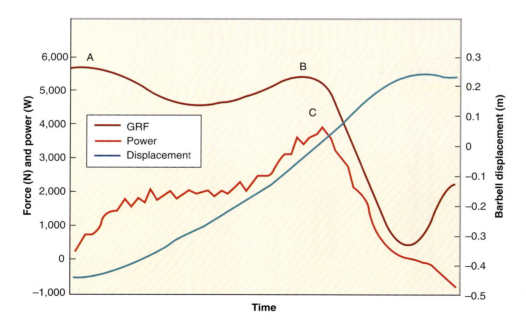

FIGURE 12.10 Force and power during the squat. It is shown that peak ground reaction force (GRF) (*points A and B*) and power (*point C*) occur well before the repetition is completed. The remaining decline is characteristic of the deceleration phase. (Reprinted with permission from Zink AJ, Perry AC, Robertson BL, Roach KE, Signorile JF. Peak power, ground reaction forces, and velocity during the squat exercise performed at different loads. *J Strength Cond Res.* 2006;20:658–64.)

during heavy lifting. The 6–12 repetition zone is frequently targeted by bodybuilders and athletes striving to increase muscle size during hypertrophy-driven training phases. However, short-term studies have shown similar muscle hypertrophy gains between this range and heavy weight training (66,67) with larger effect sizes seen with the moderate-intensity rep range (67) while some support heavier training for maximizing hypertrophy (65). Thus, moderate and heavy loading appear effective for increasing muscle size. Lower intensities yielding 12–15 reps or more can increase muscle hypertrophy presumably mostly through metabolic stress (6) and lighter weights coupled with blood flow restriction. High reps (11–24) coupled with short rest intervals produces muscle hypertrophy more so than 8 RM loading with long rest intervals (95). A meta-analysis showed that hypertrophy gains may be made comparably above and below 60% of 1 RM provided sets are concluded at muscular failure (96). Thus, hypertrophy training is complex and may be viewed as a blend of strength and endurance training to maximize the mechanical and metabolic stresses leading to tissue growth.

The concept of long-term training for muscle hypertrophy has been inadequately addressed in the scientific literature. Long-term maximal hypertrophy training requires a multidimensional periodized approach where a systematic alteration of the training stimulus and a wide spectrum of training loads are recommended. Of concern is that most studies examining muscle hypertrophy use untrained or recreationally trained subjects for short periods of time, which provides limited insight into long-term training effects. In addition, many studies do not address the novelty of changing the training stimulus in subjects with some RT experience, which is a critical element in program design. That is, one training group may perform a RT program they are accustomed to (*e.g.,* 10–rep sets) while another training group performs a RT program that is novel or unaccustomed. Thus, the results of the study may be more reflective of the novelty (or periodization) of the stimulus rather than the program loading per se. Long-term studies need to address the cumulative effects of periodized phases within a hypertrophy-driven training program rather than isolating specific variables over a short period of time. These concerns notwithstanding, the ACSM recommends a loading range of 70%–100% of 1 RM be used for 1–12 reps per set in a periodized manner such that the majority of training is devoted to 6–12 RM and less training devoted to 1–6 RM loading (4) to target the mechanical and metabolic stress factors directly to maximize muscle hypertrophy for advanced hypertrophy training. Higher reps than noted with light-to-moderate loading may also be used in conjunction with moderate-to-heavy loading. Given the variety of intensities that contribute to muscle hypertrophy, it appears the variation of loading as well as the interaction of loading with other acute program variables is critical to maximizing muscle hypertrophy.

Muscle Endurance Training

Basic strategies of endurance training for traditional RT involve performing sets to and beyond exhaustion, progressively increasing rep number with a given load, utilizing high rep sets, and reducing rest intervals in between sets. For novice and intermediate muscle endurance training, it is recommended that light-to-moderate loads be used (10–15 reps or more). For advanced endurance training, it is recommended that various loading strategies be used (10–25 reps or more) in periodized manner (4). Performing 25–35 reps with light weight has been shown to increase submaximal muscle endurance more so than 8–12 reps in RT men (97). Set duration may be the prescription tool for some exercises (ISOM exercises like the plank and flexed arm hang, or implement drill such

Interpreting Research
Training Practices of Strength Competitors

Winwood PW, Keogh JWL, Harris NK. The strength and conditioning practices of strongman competitors. *J Strength Cond Res.* 2011;25:3118–28.

Winwood et al. (98) examined 167 strongman competitors via the use of an extensive online survey. The results showed

◆ 73.7% included specific hypertrophy training in their programs; 82% of these performed sets to failure or near failure; 80% of these performed 8–12 reps for hypertrophy training (with 10 reps the most common); 85% of these performed 3–5 sets per exercise; and 59% used rest intervals <2 minutes.

◆ 97% included maximal strength training; 97% of these performed 4–6 reps per set (3 most common); 71% of these performed 3–5 sets per exercise; and 87% used rest intervals >2 minutes.

◆ 90.4% included specific power training; 88% of these performed 1–6 reps per set (3 most common); 70% of these performed 3–5 sets per exercise; and 58% used rest intervals >2 minutes.

◆ 50.6% reported performing traditional exercises as fast as possible and 41% used a mix of fast and moderate velocities.

◆ 88% reported using Olympic lifts; 30%–40% reported using upper and lower body plyometrics; and 38%–56% reported using chains and bands in training.

◆ 50% reported training only with implements, whereas 50% mixed gym work with implements while most reported using tire flips, log clean and press, stone lifting, farmers walk, and truck pull in training.

Sidebar: Ballistic Training and Maximal Strength

Interest has grown in the potential utility of ballistic RT to enhance maximal strength. In fact, it was shown that loaded sprint training by itself can increase 1 RM squat (99). Ballistic RT alone (not in conjunction with traditional RT) has been shown to

- Not increase 1 RM squat (despite increases in power) in recreationally resistance-trained individuals after 8 weeks of jump squat training with 26%–48% of 1 RM (100)
- Not increase 1 RM squat following 10 weeks of jump squat training with 0%–30% of 1 RM (58)
- Increase 1 RM squat in athletes by 15% and 10.5%, respectively, after 7 weeks of machine jump squat training with either 80% or 20%–43% of 1 RM (101)
- Increase leg press, leg extension, and leg curl strength in untrained individuals after 12 weeks of plyometric training (102)
- Increase leg press, bench press, and half squat strength by 21%, 12%, and 19%, respectively, following ballistic training of these exercises at 30% of 1 RM (59)

The addition of ballistic RT to traditional RT may augment maximal strength. Mangine et al. (91) compared ballistic plus traditional RT to traditional RT only and showed that the combination group increased bench press 1 RM (but not squat 1 RM) to a greater extent than the traditional-only group. The neuromuscular demand of ballistic RT may have potential transfer effects to increasing 1 RM strength given the neuromuscular recruitment patterns of ballistic RT.

---

as sledgehammer swings). In this case, the total set duration can be increased or intensity can be increased while a constant set duration is used for muscle endurance training. Modern muscle endurance conditioning programs have utilized various "metabolic training" strategies where multiple modalities are integrated within each workout, intensity and volume will be moderate to high, rest intervals are short (circuit training manner), and each circuit may progressively decrease time to completion. See Interpreting Research: Training Practices of Strength Competitors and Sidebar: Ballistic Training and Maximal Strength.

Methods of Increasing Resistance Exercise Intensity

There are four general methods (Fig. 12.11) to increase loading during progressive RT: (a) increase relative percents; (b) increase weight within a RM zone; (c) increase absolute amounts of weight to an exercise; and (d) use of velocity-based training (VBT) intensity (discussed later in this chapter). Increasing relative percents is common in periodized programs, especially for structural exercises such as the Olympic lifts and variations, squats, and bench press. Percents can be used to vary intensity from set to set or can be used to quantify a training cycle, e.g., hypertrophy cycle may be characteristic of intensities of 65%–75% of 1 RM versus a strength cycle that may be characteristic of intensities >85% of 1 RM. Over a long training cycle, a relative percent can exceed 100% of 1 RM if the coach is factoring in potential strength gains. Relative percents are useful during unloading weeks and may vary as a result of strength testing. Training within a RM zone requires an increase in repetitions with a workload until a target number is reached. In an 8- to 12 RM zone, the athlete selects an 8 RM load and performs 8 reps. Within a few workouts, the athlete increases reps with that load until 12 reps are performed on consecutive workouts.

Loading is increased and the athlete returns to performing 8 reps. The most practical way to increase loading is by increasing the weight in absolute amounts. For example, an athlete completes 6 reps with 100 kg in the bench press. Subsequently, the athlete continues with 6 reps, however, with a greater load (102.5 kg). When the athlete is stronger, an absolute amount of

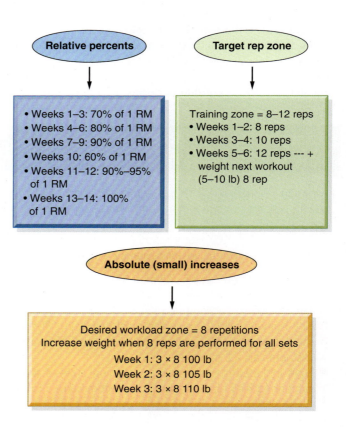

FIGURE 12.11 Examples of ways to increase intensity.

mass or weight is added. The absolute increase depends on the exercise because a large muscle mass exercise (leg press) can tolerate a 5- to 10-kg increase, whereas a small mass exercise may only tolerate 1- to 2-kg increase. All of these methods are effective and it is the preference of the coach/athlete as to which one or combination is used. These methods apply mostly to the external loading provided by free weights and machines. Other types of equipment (discussed in the next chapter) provide unique elements to challenge the athlete to a greater extent. For example, increasing intensity with elastic bands can be accomplished with stretching them further or using thicker, stronger bands. For bodyweight training, progressions take place with variations where a larger percent of bodyweight is overcome, progressing from double-leg/arm exercises to single, or increasing the moment arm of resistance to provide greater loading during the exercise. The continued challenge of overload is needed for RT progression.

Training Volume

Training volume is a measure of the total workload and is the summation of the number of sets and repetitions performed during a workout. Another term used to describe volume is volume load. *Volume load* is calculated by multiplying the load lifted (in kilograms) by the number of sets and repetitions (103). This has greater applicability because it takes into consideration the amount of weight lifted. If two athletes are performing the squat for 4 sets of 8 reps and one lifts 150 kg whereas the second athlete lifts 200 kg, the second athlete would have a greater volume load due to the heavier load (6,400 vs. 4,800 kg, respectively) despite similar volume. Volume load is an effective means of quantifying total work in the weight room and is commonly used to quantify training cycles. See Myths and Misconceptions: Every Set during Resistance Training Needs to Be Performed to Failure.

Myths & Misconceptions
Every Set during Resistance Training Needs to Be Performed to Failure

A concept relating to intensity is when to terminate a set. Should a set conclude when the lifter reaches momentary muscular exhaustion (failure) where another repetition can no longer be performed without assistance at that load using good technique or should a set conclude prior to the lifter reaching failure? Training programs follow a continuum where some athletes conclude many of their sets by reaching failure (bodybuilders), whereas some athletes rarely intentionally encounter muscular failure (Olympic weightlifters) although a missed lift may be viewed as a technical breakdown rather than muscular failure. The rationale for training to failure is to try to maximize motor unit activity and muscular adaptations (104). It is thought to maximize muscle strength, hypertrophy, and endurance. However, sets performed to failure cause a higher level of fatigue and can limit set performance after (105). Benson et al. (105) compared volume of performing elbow flexion for 3 sets to failure at 10 RM loading versus 90% of 10 RM loading first the two sets and going to failure on the third set and reported that volume was 14% lower when going to failure with RM loading primarily for the 2nd and 3rd sets. The reduced volume occurred despite no differences in EMG and MVC reductions between protocols. Thus, the impact of the reduced volume (or load reduction) is unclear as is how many sets in a workout should be performed to failure if any. Analysis of the literature shows that training to failure does not offer any distinct advantages to training to near failure for strength increases (106). A meta-analysis of the literature base concluded that RT not to failure increased muscle strength by 23%–24% while RT to failure increased strength by ~23% (104). A subset analysis revealed that in studies that controlled training volume strength increased by ~30% going to failure versus 25%–26% nonfailure (104), whereas studies that did not control for volume reported 16%

increase in strength going to failure versus 22% increase non-failure. Training to failure may be appropriate under several conditions. Effect size analysis revealed a small advantage to nonfailure training for strength increases. However, the challenge is to designate the proper proportion of the total sets performed to failure while still minimizing overuse. There is evidence showing fatigue related to training to failure or near exhaustion may enhance strength (107). Drinkwater et al. (108) compared training to failure (4 × 6 reps) or not to failure (8 × 3 reps) with similar loading and found training to failure resulted in a greater increase in 6 RM bench press (9.5%) compared to nonfailure (5%). However, Izquierdo et al. (109) showed similar increases in 1 RM squat (23%) and bench press (22%–23%) strength, and power output (26%–29%) following 16 weeks, although training to failure produced greater improvements in muscle endurance. Although it is unclear how to augment the inclusion of sets to failure, evidence supports both philosophies and the goal of the exercise selected may be critical to the decision. Maximal strength and power training may not necessitate inclusion of failure sets, although few sets may provide small benefits. Complex exercises that require high force, velocity, power production (high quality of effort), and proper technique, *i.e.*, Olympic lifts, variations, and ballistic exercises, are best performed with minimal fatigue. Consequently, training to failure may be counterproductive. However, strength training with multiple-joint, basic strength, and single-joint exercises to failure, at least part of the time, may be beneficial. Not every set is performed to failure, but it does appear that at least a few sets can be performed to failure to maximally increase muscle strength at various points in training. Concluding sets at failure may have more impact for muscle endurance and hypertrophy than strength and power training.

Several systems including the nervous, metabolic, hormonal, and muscular systems are sensitive to training volume (6). Manipulating training volume can be accomplished by changing the number of exercises performed per session, the number of reps performed per set, or the number of sets per exercise, and the loading (when referring to volume load). The progression of volume load is related to strength increases in men and women and muscle hypertrophy in women (110). There is an inverse relationship between the number of sets per exercise and the number of exercises performed in a workout. There is an inverse relationship between volume and intensity such that volume should be reduced if major increases in intensity are prescribed. Heavy RE elicits higher neuromuscular fatigue than moderate-intensity RE (111) and, coupled with high volume, could increase the risk of overtraining. Strength training is synonymous with low to moderate training volume as a low to moderate number of reps are performed per set for structural exercises. The set number may be moderate to high but fewer reps are performed per set. Hypertrophy and muscle endurance training are synonymous with low to moderate to high intensity and moderate to high volume. These programs are high in total work and stimulate a potent endocrine and metabolic response (112). Interestingly, the addition of a high-volume single set to multiple sets of heavy loads (3–5 RM) for the same exercises enhance muscle hypertrophy to a greater extent than strength training alone (112). Training volumes of athletes vary considerably and depend on other factors besides intensity, e.g., training status, number of muscle groups trained per workout, nutrition practices, practice/competition schedule, goals, etc. Current volume recommendations for strength training are isolated to the number of sets per exercise and include 1–3 sets per exercise in novice athletes. Multiple sets should be used with systematic variation of volume and intensity for progression into intermediate and advanced training. A dramatic increase in volume is not recommended. This was shown in Olympic weightlifters where a moderate training volume was more effective than low or high volumes for increasing strength (113). However, not all exercises need to be performed with the same number of sets, and that emphasis of higher or lower volume is related to the program priorities (4). Although some data indicate a relationship between total volume (or volume load) and strength and hypertrophy increases, at some point a ceiling may be reached where the variation of the volume along with intensity could be the most critical factor to long-term progression.

Of interest is the number of sets performed per exercise, muscle group, and/or workout. There are few data directly comparing RT programs of varying total sets, thus leaving numerous possibilities for the strength training and conditioning (S&C) professional when designing programs. The results of a meta-analysis showed that high weekly set numbers (≥10) produced greater strength gains in single- and multiple-joint exercises than low weekly set volumes (≤5) (114). Another meta-analysis showed a dose-response effect in the relationship between weekly RT volume and gains in muscle hypertrophy (115). Most volume studies compared single- and multiple-set training programs, or rather one set per exercise performed

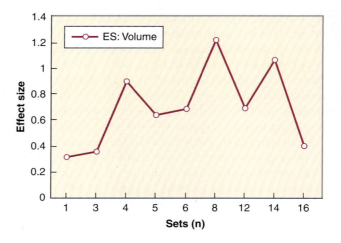

FIGURE 12.12 Number of sets per workout. (Adapted with permission from Peterson MD, Rhea MR, Alvar BA. Maximizing strength development in athletes: a meta-analysis to determine the dose-response relationship. *J Strength Cond Res.* 2004;18:377–82.)

for 8–12 reps at an intentionally slow lifting velocity has been compared to both periodized and nonperiodized multiple-set programs. These studies shown untrained individuals respond well to single and multiple sets. However, multiple sets are needed for higher rates of progression in advancing training status. Regarding total sets per workout, one meta-analysis suggested ~4–8 sets per muscle group yielded the most substantial effects in trained individuals (106) (Fig. 12.12), whereas 4 sets produced the highest effects in untrained individuals (106). Most studies used 2–6 sets per exercise and found substantial strength increases in trained and untrained individuals (6). Typically, 3–6 sets per exercise are common but more and less can be used successfully.

There are no specific recommendations for the total number of sets performed per workout as these values vary greatly and depend on numerous other factors. In addition to loaded free weight, implement, or machine exercises, the use of corrective exercises or low to moderate intensity resisted or bodyweight exercises could result in higher set numbers but are generally well tolerated by the human body. The following guide (comprising examples from total-body, upper/lower-body split, and muscle group split routine workouts) may be useful in selecting set number per workout:

- Total-body workouts: 10–40 sets/workout (3–6 sets or 1–2 exercises per muscle group or use of multiple total-body exercises)
- Upper-body workouts: 10–30 sets/workout (6–9 sets or 1–3 exercises per muscle group)
- Lower-body workouts: 10–30 sets/workout (6–9 sets or 1–3 exercises per muscle group)
- Chest workouts: 6–20 sets per workout (3–6 exercises per workout)
- Back workouts: 6–20 sets per workout (3–6 exercises per workout)

- Quadriceps/hamstrings workouts: 8–25 sets per workout (3–7 exercises per workout)
- Calf workouts: 6–15 sets per workout (2–5 exercises per workout)
- Shoulder/trapezius workouts: 6–18 sets per workout (3–6 exercises per workout)
- Biceps workouts: 5–12 sets per workout (2–5 exercises per workout)
- Triceps workouts: 6–15 sets per workout (2–5 exercises per workout)
- Forearm workouts: 6–12 sets per workout (2–4 exercises per workout)
- Core workouts: 6–20 sets per workout (3–6 exercises per workout)

These workouts provide a range of sets commonly used in various RT programs. Athletes have successfully completed workouts outside of these ranges as well, once again demonstrating great variability here and leaving numerous possibilities to the S&C coach for prescription. Ranges are dependent upon training experience, frequency, intensity, nutrition, and recovery factors. Individuals with more training experience can perform more sets in a given workout. Set number depends on intensity because more sets can be performed at low to moderate intensities than high. Frequency is critical. If a muscle group is only trained once per week, then a high number of sets can be performed. However, if a muscle group is trained two to three times per week (within a total-body or upper/lower-body split workout), then fewer sets are performed per workout. Nutrition plays a critical role. Protein and carbohydrate (as well as vitamin and mineral) intake must be sufficient to allow athletes to train hard and recover in between workouts. Occasions where athlete's kilocalorie intake is low may require a reduction in the number of sets to prevent overtraining. A factor such as drug usage plays a role. It is not uncommon to read a magazine and view training programs of elite athletes that use higher set numbers than the ranges provided. Anabolic drugs increase recovery ability and enable athletes to train at higher volumes. A drug-free athlete must be aware of this when examining various RT programs. Lastly, the number of sets per workout depends on other modalities of training. If RT is integrated with sprint/plyometric/agility training or aerobic training, modification of volume may be needed. This is the case for in-season RT programs of athletes where the total number of sets per workout will be lower due to the practice/competition demands of the sport.

Although most exercises are performed for 3–6 sets per exercise, there have been some exceptions. For example, some lifters have used high set numbers for 1–2 exercises per workout as a way to promote muscle hypertrophy. One such program, *German Volume Training* (*e.g.*, 10-Set Method), involves performing 10 sets for usually a multi-joint or total-body exercise with ~60% of 1 RM for usually 1–2 exercises per workout with ~1 minute rest interval in between sets. The workout becomes increasingly difficult with each successive set. A few studies have examined German Volume Training or variations and showed it is effective for increasing muscle strength and hypertrophy; however, less effective or similar to performing 5 sets per exercise instead of 10 (116,117). See Myths and Misconceptions: Single Sets of Resistance Training Are Equally as Effective for Maximizing Strength as Multiple Sets.

Myths & Misconceptions
Single Sets of Resistance Training Are Equally as Effective for Maximizing Strength as Multiple Sets

Historically, one issue in S&C has been the use of single versus multiple sets per exercise. The issue itself may be the fact that this topic has been an issue in RT when one examines the literature. Nevertheless, the debate began in the 1970s when the company Nautilus popularized single-set training using their RT equipment. Claims were made stating its efficacy that prompted some investigators to test this program. A common criticism of some studies (as well as some current studies) is that the number of sets per exercise was not separated from other variables. Rather, some of these studies intended to compare programs: one popular single-set program versus various multiple-set programs. That is, one single-set program was compared to other programs where the number of sets was not isolated from other variables. Proponents of single-set training argue these programs are most time efficient, have high exercise adherence rates, are less injurious (slow repetition velocities coupled with machine-based exercises are suggested), and can be as effective as higher volumes of training for all training goals. In their view, much of the improvements in muscle strength take place within the first set; therefore, performing additional sets does not constitute a high benefit:cost ratio. Another way of looking at it is via the *Principle of Diminishing Returns* that entails a reduction in performance improvement (output) despite added time (input) of training. Proponents of single-set training argue that increasing the volume yet experiencing less improvement over time is not necessary.

Those who support multiple-set training contend that single-set programs are adequate for beginners or those individuals involved in short-term maintenance training but long-term progression requires more periodized volume and time dedicated to training. For the athlete, this is critical as strength training is incorporated into training for the sport. Examination of training logs of strength athletes or advanced to elite

(Continued)

lifters show that nearly all train with multiple sets. A survey study concluded that 97% of Division I S&C coaches use multiple-set programs (118). It may be argued that single-set programs limit variation, which is needed during progression. Although more exercises can be performed per workout, variation within each exercise (intensity, volume, rest interval selection) may be limited with performance of only one set. Heavy lifting can be difficult with only one set because many lifters require warm-ups to progress to heavy weights. The feasibility of requiring lifters to perform sets with heavy weights may be limited without proper preparation. Lastly, other aspects of single-set training such as slow lifting velocities, mostly training in an 8–12 RM zone, and utilizing machine-based exercises do not appeal to all training goals. Although the "less-is-best" argument is attractive philosophically, rarely is it seen that maximal benefit is gained using a minimalistic approach. Both sides of the debate have valid points so the ACSM has recommended single or multiple sets for beginners but periodized multiple-set programs for progression (4).

As a result of this debate, many studies and literature reviews have been published. Some studies showed similar results in novice individuals (119), whereas several studies have shown multiple sets superior in this population (120–125). However, periodized, multiple-set programs are superior during progression to intermediate and advanced stages of training in all studies (60,126–132) but one (133). One study (using a crossover design) in resistance-trained postmenopausal women showed that multiple-set training resulted in a 3.5%–5.5% strength increase, whereas single-set training resulted in a 1.1%–2.0% reduction in strength (134). Several reviews and meta-analyses were published examining this topic (131,135–139). Collectively, these reviews have shown the following:

◆ Prior to 1998, 13 studies were published; 6 showed similar strength improvements between single and multiple sets and 7 showed multiple sets provided additional benefits. Of the studies showing similar strength increases, 4 used untrained subjects and 2 used trained subjects. Of the studies showing multiple-set superiority, 1 used UT subjects and 6 used trained subjects.
◆ From 1998 to 2003, 8 studies were published of which 1 (trained subjects) showed similar strength increases whereas the other 7 showed multiple-set superiority (5 studies used UT subjects, 2 studies used trained subjects).

◆ From 2003 to the present, several studies examined UT subjects or individuals not currently weight training. Most of these studies demonstrated multiple-set superiority and one showed multiple-set superiority for only one exercise tested out of three using various conditions (140). Munn et al. (141) showed superior increases in strength (48% vs. 25%) using multiple sets versus one set. McBride et al. (142) reported a greater increase in curl 1 RM (22.8% vs. 8.5%) and a trend for greater increase in leg press 1 RM (52.6% vs. 41.2%) following 12 weeks of multiple-set training than single-set. Ronnestad et al. (143) reported greater increases in lower-body strength and hypertrophy with multiple-set RT but similar increases in upper-body strength following 11 weeks of multiple- or single-set training. Kelly et al. (144) compared 1 versus 3 sets of isokinetic leg extensions ($60°\cdot s^{-1}$) for 8 weeks and showed multiple-set training led to increases in peak torque (mostly during the first 4 weeks), whereas single-set training did not increase peak torque. Sooneste et al. (125) showed 3 sets superior for increasing strength (32% vs. 20%) and CSA (13% vs. 8%) of the elbow flexors compared to 1 set in UT men over 12 weeks of RT. Radaelli et al. (123) showed 3 and 5 sets superior to 1 set for increasing 5 and 20 RM strength and muscle size of the elbow flexors and extensors in previously UT men over 6 months of RT. Muscle thickness did not change following 1 set RT, only with 3 (for flexors) and 5 sets (123). One study in trained men showed greater squat increases with 8 sets (but not 4 sets) compared to 1 set (129) and another study showed similar 1 RM bench press and squat increases between 1, 3, and 5 sets; however, multiple sets produced superior muscle hypertrophy (145).
◆ Studies longer than 14 weeks in duration showed multiple sets superior to single sets for long-term performance enhancement (123,136,139).
◆ 2–3 sets per exercise produce ~46% greater gains in strength than single-set training in UT and trained individuals (137)
◆ No study has shown single-set training to be superior to multiple-set training in either trained or UT individuals.
◆ Multiple-set RT produces 40% larger effect sizes for muscle hypertrophy compared to single sets (138); 2–3 sets per exercise yielded similar effects to 4–6 sets per exercise.

Set Structures for Multiple-Set Programs

When multiple sets are used per exercise, the next decision is to determine the structure, *e.g.*, the pattern of loading and volume prescription from one set to the next. The intensity and volume during each set can increase, decrease, or stay the same. Three basic structures (as well as many integrated systems) can be used (Fig. 12.13). Advantages and disadvantages exist for each one. Because all are effective, use of these may be up to the personal preference of the athlete or coach. The first is a constant load/repetition system. The loading and rep number remain constant across all sets (assuming that fatigue does not affect rep number). A *fixed* system can be used where all exercises are performed for the same number of reps (while the loading for each exercise remains constant) or a *variable* system can be used where each exercise can be performed for varying amounts of reps (with constant loading). This system is very effective for increasing strength, power, hypertrophy, and muscle endurance. A second system is to work from light to heavy system. Weight is increased each set while repetitions remain

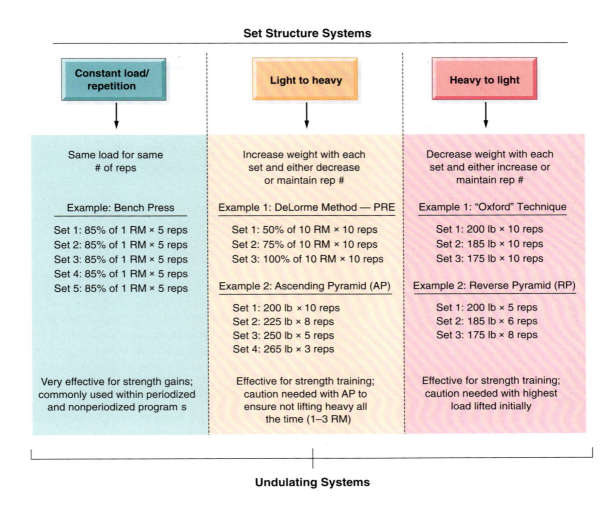

FIGURE 12.13 Set structure systems. (Reprinted with permission from McGuigan M, Ratamess NA. Strength. In: Ackland TR, Elliott BC, Bloomfield J, editors. *Applied Anatomy and Biomechanics in Sport*. 2nd ed. Champaign (IL): Human Kinetics; 2009. p. 119–54.)

the same or decrease. One of the first known light-to-heavy systems was the DeLorme method of *Progressive Resistance Exercise*. Ten reps are performed per set. However, 50%, 75%, and 100% of the athlete's 10 RM weight is used for each of the three sets, respectively (146). The first two sets are ramping sets and the third set is the workload set.

Another popular example of a light to heavy system is the *ascending pyramid* where weight is added and repetitions are reduced each set. Ascending pyramids can be used to target any fitness component by manipulating the intensity and volume (Table 12.8) although a classic ascending pyramid is one which targets maximal strength as the athlete progresses toward a 1 RM. This is advantageous in the sense that there is progression prior to lifting the heaviest weight. Classic ascending pyramids have been criticized because there is a wide range of intensity used (70%–100% of 1 RM) and the athletes typically approach a 1 RM, which could lead to overtraining if used too frequently (68). However, ascending pyramids can be modified to target specific intensities with narrower ranges, *i.e.*, a lower peak intensity based on the goals (75%–80% of 1 RM). Some practitioners suggest ascending pyramids are most effective when a narrow range of intensity is used (10%–20%) (147)

as too wide a range (with a corresponding higher rep number) could result in greater fatigue. Ascending pyramids can be used for any exercise; however, they are more commonly used for multiple-joint basic strength exercises because these exercises typically require at least 3 sets be performed. Not every

Table 12.8 Examples of Ascending Pyramids

"Classic" Ascending Strength Pyramid		Hypertrophy/Endurance Ascending Pyramid	
Set	Weight × Reps	Set	Weight × Reps
1	225 lb × 12 reps	1	135 lb × 20 reps
2	335 lb × 10 reps	2	155 lb × 15 reps
3	415 lb × 8 reps	3	175 lb × 12 reps
4	435 lb × 6 reps	4	185 lb × 10 reps
5	450 lb × 5 reps	5	195 lb × 8 reps
6	485 lb × 1–2 reps		

exercise in a workout may use an ascending pyramid. Rather, a few structural exercises early in the workout may be targeted while the remaining exercises may use a different set structure system. One study showed that it produced similar strength and hypertrophy increases to traditional loading schemes (148).

The third basic system structure is to work from heavy to light. This may be accomplished by decreasing weight with each set and either maintaining or increasing repetition number. Some early studies examined a structure known as the *Oxford technique* (149). The Oxford technique requires the lifter to maintain the same number of reps for all sets of an exercise but decrease the weight with each set in succession. It is effective for increasing strength and produces similar increases in strength as the DeLorme system following 9 weeks of training (150). This system may be effective when short rest intervals are used as loading needs to be reduced to maintain rep number. Another popular example is the *descending pyramid*. The weight is decreased each set while reps increase. The advantage is that the heaviest set is performed first where fatigue may be minimal. Theoretically, this could provide an optimal strength training stimulus. However, critics of this system point out the potential of not being properly warmed up for the heaviest set especially if it is the first exercise in sequence and requires near 1 RM loading. Caution needs to be used. Not every exercise in a workout may be performed using descending pyramids. Rather, the first few exercises may, while others use a different structuring system.

Integrated and/or undulating models (that are based upon constant load/repetition, heavy to light, and light to heavy systems) are used. Integrated models combine two or more of these systems. A true pyramid system combines ascending and descending pyramids. The lifter increases loading and decreases reps on the way up and then decreases loading and increases reps on the way down. Proponents suggest that some potentiation may take place on the way down as loading is reduced. Ultimately, many sets need to be performed per exercise. Another integrated model is a *skewed pyramid*. The progression is similar to an ascending period. However, a *down set* (decreased load, higher rep number) is included at the end rather than the descending portion of a pyramid. Performance of the down set may be enhanced because of the ascending segment of the pyramid via postactivation potentiation (103). Models exist where loading may increase and reps decrease (or vice versa) over multiple sets rather than one. Table 12.9 depicts an integrated model for the squat. Intensity is increased and volume is decreased over a span of two sets rather than one so the ascending pyramid was expanded to increase set number at a specific intensity. This model applies to descending pyramids, and other variations can be applied. Lastly, *undulating models* include heavy and moderate loads alternated across all sets. They are used for multiple-joint exercises comprising several sets (>5 sets). One example is *wave loading*. Although there are many ways to use this system, one requires the athlete perform 3, 2, and 1 repetition, respectively, with 90%, 95%, and 100% of 1 RM in the first wave (ascending pyramid). A second wave is performed for 3, 2, and 1 repetition with 2.5 lb added to each set. The athlete continues until the wave cannot be completed (147). Another undulating example is the double stimulation

Table 12.9	An Integrated Model of Set Structuring: Barbell Squat	
Set	Weight × Reps	Percent of 1 RM
1	400 lb × 8 reps	80
2	400 lb × 8 reps	80
3	450 lb × 5 reps	90
4	450 lb × 5 reps	90
5	475 lb × 2 reps	95
6	475 lb × 2 reps	95

Note: Based on a 500-lb 1 RM; excludes warm-up sets.

model. The athlete alternates between single and moderate reps with an intensity differential of 10%–15% (103). For example, the athlete may perform 1 rep × 90% for set 1, 5 reps × 80% for set 2, 1 rep × 90% for set 3, 5 reps × 80% for set 4, and this pattern repeats until the sets are completed. Undulating models attempt to maximize potentiation that occurs from performing a lower-intensity set following a higher-intensity set.

Rest Intervals

Rest interval length between sets and exercises is dependent upon training intensity, goals, fitness level, and targeted energy system utilization. Rest intervals between exercises are affected by the muscle groups trained, equipment availability, and the time needed to change weights and relocate to another bench, machine, platform, etc. The amount of rest between sets and exercises affects the metabolic, hormonal, and cardiovascular responses to an acute bout of RE, as well as performance of subsequent sets and training adaptations (4,6). Acute strength and power production is compromised with short rest intervals as minimal recovery is allowed to take place, *e.g.*, ATP-PC resynthesis, lactate removal, muscle buffering, and repayment of the oxygen debt (4,126,151), although these short rest intervals are beneficial for hypertrophy and muscle endurance training. Kraemer (126) showed that 10 reps with 10 RM loads were performed for 3 sets when 3-minute rest periods were used for the leg press and bench press but only 10, 8, and 7 reps were performed, respectively, when rest intervals were reduced to 1 minute. Using 4 sets of the squat and bench press, Willardson and Burkett (152) showed that the highest volume attained was with 5-minute rest intervals, followed by 2 and 1 minute, respectively. Miranda et al. (153) compared two sequences of 6 exercises performed for 3 sets of 8 RM loading with 1- or 3-minute rest intervals and showed 3-minute rest intervals yielded a range of 4–6 more reps performed over 3 sets than 1-minute rest intervals. In this study, exercises that worked similar muscle groups were performed in sequence (wide-grip lat pull-down, close-grip lat pull-down, machine row, barbell row). Interestingly, subjects were not able to perform 8 reps on the first set of any exercise after the first, and this effect was exacerbated with 1-minute rest intervals showing exercise performance stressing similar muscle groups may be reduced from prior fatigue.

Figure 12.14 depicts acute lifting performance with various rest intervals. A continuum was shown where greatest reductions in performance were seen with 30-second rest intervals and performance was maintained the best with 5-minute rest intervals (154). Other studies have shown higher rep numbers performed during the squat and bench press with longer rest intervals, e.g., 5 minutes > 3 minutes > 2 minutes > 1 minute or less (45,155–158). The reductions in performance with short rest intervals appear similar between multi- and single-joint exercises (159). Short rest intervals compromise performance, whereas long rest intervals help maintain intensity/volume load, and the reductions seen during short rest intervals are inversely related to maximum strength where stronger athletes show a larger reduction.

The reductions seen with short rest intervals are related to multiple factors. We conducted a series of studies investigating performance effects with different rest interval lengths. We initially showed that children and adolescents were more capable of maintaining volume over 3 sets of up to 10 reps of the bench press with short, moderate, and longer rest intervals (1, 2, and 3 min) than young adult men using similar relative loading (160). In a follow-up study, we used a similar protocol comparing young men and women and showed that women were better able to maintain volume over 3 sets of the bench press using 1-, 2-, and 3-minute rest intervals with differences more notable with 1- and 2-minute rest intervals (155). The common finding was that subjects with lower levels of maximal strength in both studies were better able to maintain training volume regardless of rest interval length. We then examined a cohort of young men and divided them into two groups based on 1 RM bench press strength, a higher group (mean = 141 kg) versus a lower group (mean = 80 kg). The lower group was better able to maintain volume over 3 sets with 1- and 2-minute rest intervals compared to the higher group. Significant negative correlations were observed between 1 RM bench press and total number of reps completed for 1- and 2-minute RIs (155). We also showed that manipulation of rest interval length for the first exercise in sequence (1, 2, or 3 min) did not affect performance of subsequent RE exercises stressing similar muscle groups (45). Although short rest intervals resulted in reduced volume load compared to long, all rest intervals led to similar levels of fatigue when sets were concluded at muscular failure. We concluded that factors that enable an individual to lift a larger amount of weight may not translate into muscle endurance or recovery ability in between sets. Rest interval length may vary depending on strength levels of the athletes where some may benefit from short rest without sacrificing volume load. We then examined the influence of maximal aerobic capacity on rest interval length during performance of 5 sets of up to 10 reps of the squat and bench press in random order. VO_2 max was negatively correlated to 1 RM bench press and squat and was significantly correlated to squat reps but did not correlate to bench press performance especially with short rest intervals (50). Thus, aerobically fit individuals (mostly runners) were better able to maintain volume load with short rest intervals for lower body RE.

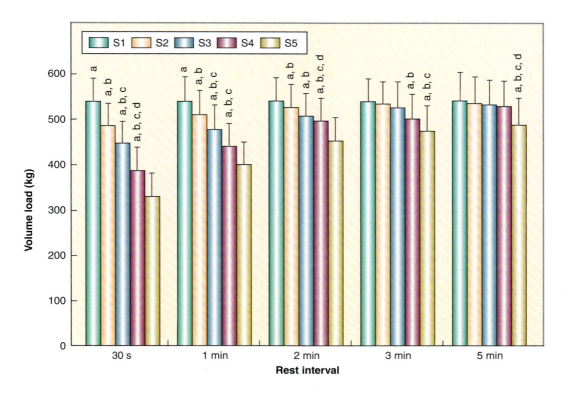

FIGURE 12.14 Lifting performance during 10 repetition sets of the bench press with 30-second, 1-, 2-, 3-, and 5-minute rest intervals. (*a*) Significantly less ($P < 0.05$) than set 1. (*b*) Less than set 2. (*c*) Less than set 3. (*d*) Less than set 4. (Reprinted with permission from Ratamess NA, Falvo MJ, Mangine GT, Hoffman JR, Faigenbaum AD, Kang J. The effect of rest interval length on metabolic responses to the bench press exercise. *Eur J Appl Physiol*. 2007;100:1–17.)

Long-term studies show greater strength increases with long versus short rest intervals between sets, *e.g.*, 2–5 minutes versus 30–60 seconds (4,151,161,162). Several studies have collectively shown 2%–8% greater strength increases with longer rest intervals (>2 min) versus short rest intervals (≥1 min) (163–165). De Salles et al. (151) showed a continuum of bench press and leg press strength increases where largest increases were seen with 5-minute rest intervals, followed by 3 minutes, and 1 minute in resistance-trained men. No strength increases were seen in the bench press using 1-minute rest intervals (161). Total training volume load followed similar pattern where 5 minutes > 3 minutes > 1 minute (161). However, some studies have shown statistically similar strength increases between rest intervals, *e.g.*, 1 versus 2.5 minutes, 2 versus 4 minutes, and 2 versus 5 minutes (166–168). These studies collectively show that strength differentiation mostly occurs when the rest intervals are <2 minutes. Rest interval length will vary based on the goals of that particular exercise (not every exercise will use the same rest interval). For novice, intermediate, and advanced strength and power training, the ACSM recommends that rest intervals of at least 2–3 minutes be used for structural exercises using heavier loads and 1–2 minutes of rest for assistance exercises (4).

These recommendations extend to training for hypertrophy although shorter rest intervals can be effectively used to target both mechanical and metabolic stress factors associated with muscle growth (169,170). Although some data indicate augmented muscle hypertrophy with longer rest intervals (162), hypertrophy can occur with a multitude of rest intervals so it is recommended the rest interval length match the objective of the set (*e.g.*, longer for strength or short to moderate for endurance). Strength and power performance is highly dependent upon the ATP-PC system and it generally takes at least 3 minutes for the majority of repletion to take place. Muscle strength may be increased using short rest intervals but at a slower rate and magnitude. Rest interval selection has a great impact when training for muscular endurance. Training to increase muscular endurance implies the athlete (a) performs high reps (long-duration sets) to enhance submaximal muscle endurance and/or (b) minimizes recovery between sets to enhance high-intensity (or strength) endurance. It is recommended that short rest intervals be used for muscular endurance training, *e.g.*, 1–2 minutes for high-rep sets (>15–20 reps), and <1 minute for moderate (10–15 reps) sets (4). See Sidebar: Kinetics and Kinematics of Lifting Performance during Multiple Sets and Figure 12.15.

Sidebar: Kinetics and Kinematics of Lifting Performance during Multiple Sets

Rest interval length affects performance. Reductions in loading and reps occur with short rest intervals. However, less noticeable changes can take place with fatigue. Peak muscle force and bar velocity can decrease despite no change in rep number. Figure 12.15 depicts data collected from our laboratory during a squat protocol consisting of 6 sets of 10 reps with 75% of 1 RM using 2-minute rest intervals. Loading was maintained for the first 3 sets but was reduced to allow performance of 10 reps for the last 3 sets. Although loading was maintained for the first 3 sets, ground reaction force was reduced with each successive set. Reps can be performed in a fatigued state; however, they are performed more slowly with less force output. Bar velocity can decrease with each set independent of rep number. These data have important ramifications for those athletes training for maximal strength and power that requires a high quality of repetition performance and form a basis for velocity-based RT. Rest interval length needs to be long enough to allow the lifter to maximally perform each rep for strength and power training.

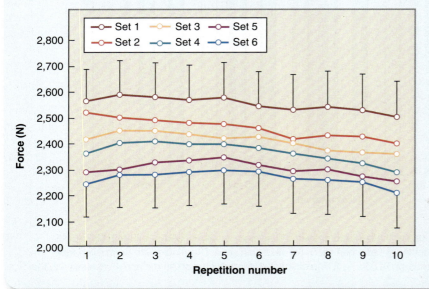

FIGURE 12.15 Kinetic profile of a squat protocol. (Reprinted with permission from McGuigan M, Ratamess NA. Strength. In: Ackland TR, Elliott BC, Bloomfield J, editors. *Applied Anatomy and Biomechanics in Sport*. 2nd ed. Champaign (IL): Human Kinetics; 2009. p. 119–54.)

Repetition Velocity

Repetition velocity affects the neural, hypertrophic, and metabolic responses to training and is dependent upon loading and fatigue (6). A large number of studies have examined isokinetic RE. Isokinetic devices allow for acceleration, deceleration, and a sustained programmed velocity, and the ultimate relative contribution of each component depends on the exercise ROM. Isokinetic devices possess a dynamometer that maintains the lever arm at a sustained constant angular velocity where slow ($\sim 30° \cdot s^{-1}$), moderate ($\sim 180° \cdot s^{-1}$), and fast ($\sim 300° \cdot s^{-1}$ or more) velocities can be selected. The athlete applies maximal muscle force to the dynamometer; however, the velocity is predetermined and torque or force is displayed. Isokinetic devices account for velocity that is uncontrolled with free weights and machines, act as an accommodating resistance device, and can provide greater ECC loading in a safe environment. However, the cost of an isokinetic dynamometer is prohibitive so isokinetic training is not as common as free weight/machine RT. Strength increases specific to the velocity trained with some carryover above and below the training velocity ($30° \cdot s^{-1}$) although all velocities result in strength increases (6). Training at moderate velocity ($180-240° \cdot s^{-1}$) produces the greatest strength increases across all testing velocities (171).

Most athletes train in an environment that is not velocity controlled. Rather, *dynamic constant external RT* predominates where the athlete has control over the velocity of the weight to a large extent. For nonmaximal lifts, the intent to control velocity is critical. Since force = mass × acceleration, reductions in force are observed when the intent is to perform the rep slowly (172). However, there are two types of slow-velocity contractions: unintentional and intentional. Unintentional slow velocities are used during high-intensity reps in which either the loading and/or fatigue are responsible for the slower velocity. The athlete exerts maximal force (and attempts to move the weight rapidly) but due to the heavy loading or fatigue, the resultant velocity is slow. These are seen during heavy sets and present a potent stimulus for strength increases. Repetition velocity may decrease during the last few reps of a set during the onset of fatigue. During a 5 RM bench press, the CON phase for the first 3 reps is ~1.2–1.6 seconds in duration whereas the last two reps may be ~2.5 and 3.3 seconds, respectively (173). Fatigue plays a critical role in lifting velocity especially near set completion.

Intentional slow-velocity reps are used with submaximal weights where the athlete has direct control over the velocity of the weight. These velocities have been used, in part, to increase muscular time under tension. Increasing the time under tension via intentionally slow velocities results in high levels of fatigue (174) that could present a potent stimulus for endurance enhancement. Force production is lower for an intentionally slow velocity (5- to 10-s CON, 5- to 10-s ECC) compared to a traditional (moderate) or explosive velocity with a corresponding lower level of muscle fiber activation (175,176). Intentionally lifting a weight slower forces the athlete to reduce the weight and results in fewer reps performed per load (Fig. 12.16) (175,177,178) and results in lower force and

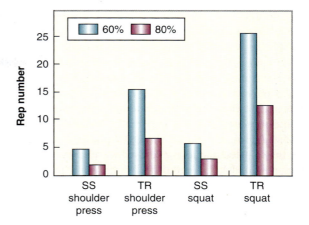

FIGURE 12.16 Comparison of super slow and traditional repetition velocities. Data show significantly more reps performed for 60% and 80% of 1 RM for the traditional (TR) than super slow (SS) velocities for the shoulder press and squat. (Adapted with permission from Hatfield DL, Kraemer WJ, Spiering BA, et al. The impact of velocity of movement on performance factors in resistance exercise. *J Strength Cond Res*. 2006;20:760–6.)

power output (175). Performing a set of 10 reps using a very slow velocity (10-s CON, 5-s ECC) compared to a slow velocity (2-s CON, 4-s ECC) may result in a 30% reduction in load, and this limits strength gains following 10 weeks of training (179). Intentionally slow velocities may be useful for muscular endurance training but appear counterproductive for intermediate and advanced strength and power training. In untrained individuals, Munn et al. (141) showed an 11% greater strength increase with a faster (1-s CON, 1-s ECC) velocity than a slower one (3-s CON, 3-s ECC). In athletes, training with fast velocities (<0.85-s CON, 1.7-s ECC) produced greater increases in bench press (7.9%) and bench pull (5.5%) strength than a slow velocity (1.7-s CON, 1.7-s ECC) (133). Other studies showed 6 weeks of maximal velocity training produced greater increases in squat and bench press strength than slower velocity RT (180,181). Rana et al. (182) showed slower rate of strength increases with super slow training velocity in UT women. However, Neils et al. (183) showed similar strength increases for one of two exercises in UT individuals. A meta-analysis showed that fast and moderate RT velocities produced the highest strength increases (21%–22%) primarily with loads ranging from 60% to 79% of 1 RM (184). Compared to slow velocities, moderate (1- to 2-s CON, 1- to 2-s ECC) and fast (<1-s CON, 1-s ECC) velocities are more effective for enhanced muscular performance, *e.g.*, number of reps performed, work and power output, volume (69,185), and for increasing the rate of strength gains (186). Sakamoto and Sinclair (69) showed that for a slow velocity lifted for 60%–80% of 1 RM, 3–9 reps were performed; however, for fast or ballistic velocities at the same intensity, 5–15 reps were performed for the Smith machine bench press.

The magnitude velocity has on rep performance becomes more substantial at low and moderate intensities (69). A positive linear relationship exists between the velocity of the first rep in a set and the total number of reps performed during that set (187). For strength training, the intent to move the weight as quickly as possible (to optimize the neural response) and the RFD appear to be critical elements (188). The final lifting velocity seen may be viewed as the outcome but the maximal intent to move the bar quickly is critical. This technique has been termed *compensatory acceleration* (189) that requires the athlete to accelerate the load maximally throughout as much of the ROM as possible during the CON phase. A major advantage is that this technique can be used with heavy loads (as well as moderate loads), it is quite effective for multi-joint exercises, and it was shown to be more beneficial for strength training than slower velocities (61,190). The ACSM recommends slow and moderate velocities for UT individuals and moderate velocities for intermediate-trained individuals during strength and hypertrophy training (4). For advanced strength and hypertrophy training, the inclusion of a continuum of velocities from unintentionally slow (for heavy loads) to fast velocities is recommended (4). The velocity selected should correspond to the intensity, and the intent should be to maximize the velocity of the CON muscle action if maximal strength is desired. Power training entails increasing maximal RFD, muscular strength at slow and fast velocities, SSC performance, and coordination or technique (6). Fast velocities (<1-s CON, <1-s ECC) should be used for power training (4).

Training for muscle endurance, and in some respects hypertrophy, requires a spectrum of velocities with various loading strategies. The critical component to muscle endurance training is to prolong the duration of the set. Two recommended strategies used to prolong set duration are (a) moderate reps using a slow velocity and (b) high reps using moderate to fast velocities. Intentionally slow velocity training with light loads (5-s CON, 5-s ECC and slower) places continued tension on the muscles for an extended period of time. However, it is difficult to perform a large number of reps using intentionally slow velocities. When high reps are desired, moderate to fast velocities are preferred. Both slow velocity, moderate reps and moderate to fast velocity, high-repetition training strategies increase the glycolytic and oxidative demands of the stimulus, thereby serving as an effective means of increasing muscle endurance. The ACSM recommends intentionally slow velocities be employed for moderate reps (10–15) and moderate to fast velocities when performing a large number of reps (15–25 or more) (4). See Sidebar: Velocity-Based Training.

Frequency

The number of training sessions performed during a specific period of time may affect training adaptations. Frequency includes the number of times certain exercises or muscle groups

---

Sidebar   Velocity-Based Training

Although many RT programs are governed by intensity prescription via relative percents, RM zones, and absolute loading amounts, *velocity-based training* (VBT) as an intensity prescription option has increased in popularity. VBT uses repetition velocity as a guide rather than relative intensity for multiple-joint exercises (191). It is thought to provide a stable measure of the quality of the rep and could be used to predict 1 RM strength data. VBT entails measuring the average velocity of the concentric (ACV) phase of a rep and terminating a set when a threshold velocity reduction has occurred (as opposed to terminating a set at or near failure). Mean set velocity is maintained whereas performing additional reps would result in reductions (192). Technology such as a Tendo analyzer, GymAware, Bar Sensei, Beast sensor, etc. is needed to measure ACV and provide feedback to the trainee. The rationale is to maximize performance of each rep without performing reps in a fatigued state that are thought to negatively affect the quality of subsequent reps. Repetition velocity decreases with fatigue and an inverse relationship exists between ACV and loading (193). Terminating a set prior to fatiguing reps leaves the trainee with *repetitions in reserve*, and it has been suggested that VBT may limit mechanical and metabolic stress while providing a sufficient strength and power training stimulus. For maximal strength training, it has been recommended that barbell velocities range from 0.15 to

0.35 $m \cdot s^{-1}$, whereas for speed strength, the ACV is 0.45–0.75 $m \cdot s^{-1}$ (193,194). Although ACV provides a stable measure of basic strength exercise performance, peak concentric velocity is more appropriate for the Olympic lifts (191). The ACV of the 1 RM squat may range from 0.22 to 0.43 $m \cdot s^{-1}$ depending on the training status of the athletes, *i.e.*, higher in novices (193), and ~0.10–0.18 $m \cdot s^{-1}$ for bench press, ~0.24 $m \cdot s^{-1}$ for overhead press, and 0.14–0.22 $m \cdot s^{-1}$ for deadlift (194). The ACV may range from 0.84 to 1.19 $m \cdot s^{-1}$ for the squat, bench press, deadlift, and overhead press with loads as light as 35% of 1 RM (194). Studies have shown VBT leads to comparable or in some cases superior increases in muscle strength and jump power (195). Pareja-Blanco et al. (196) compared RT using VBT for the squat (based off of first rep performance) with 20% versus 40% loss of ACV each set for 8 weeks and reported that 40% loss resulted in higher numbers of reps performed per set (4–9) versus 20% loss (2–5); the 20% group trained at a higher ACV; subjects in the 40% group reached failure during 56% of sets; strength increased in 20% and 40% groups by 18% and 13%; VJ only increased in 20% group by 9.5%; the 40% group led to a larger reduction in MHCIIX fiber percents with no change in 20%; and both groups similarly increased muscle CSA. These data show that maintaining set ACV produces significant increases in muscle strength.

are trained per week and is dependent upon several factors such as volume and intensity, exercise selection, level of conditioning and/or training status, recovery ability, nutritional intake, and training goals. Heavy training increases the recovery time needed prior to subsequent training sessions. It has been shown that untrained women only recovered ~94% of their strength 2 days following a lower-body workout consisting of 5 sets of 10 reps with 10 RM loads (197). Numerous studies used frequencies of 2–3 alternating days per week in UT individuals. In comparison, 2- and 3-day frequencies have produced similar results in UT individuals when volume is similar (198). This is an effective initial frequency and recommended for beginning lifters (4). In a few studies, 4–5 days per week were superior to 3 days; 3 days per week superior to 1 and 2 days; and 2 days per week superior to 1 day for increasing maximal strength (199,200). Meta-analysis data show 3 days per week produces the highest effect size in UT individuals and 2 days per week produces the highest effect size in trained individuals (60). An increase in training experience does not necessitate a change in frequency for training each muscle group but may be more dependent upon alterations in other acute variables such as exercise selection, volume, and intensity. Increasing frequency may enable greater exercise selection and volume per muscle group.

Frequency for advanced training varies considerably. One study showed football players training 4–5 days per week achieved better results than those who trained either 3 or 6 days per week (201). Advanced weightlifters and bodybuilders use high-frequency training, *e.g.*, 4–6 sessions per week. The frequency for elite weightlifters and bodybuilders may be even greater. Double-split routines (two training sessions per day with emphasis on different muscle groups) are common, which may result in 8–12 training sessions per week. Frequencies as high as 18 sessions per week have been shown in Olympic weightlifters (68). The rationale is frequent short sessions followed by periods of recovery, supplementation, and food intake allow for a better training stimulus. One study showed greater increases in muscle CSA and strength when training volume was divided into two sessions per day rather than one (202). High or low frequency may result in similar strength and hypertrophy increases if volume is equated (203). Results from meta-analyses support higher training frequency and volume for increasing muscle hypertrophy (204,205). Elite powerlifters typically train 4–6 days per week with each major lift (bench press, squat, deadlift) trained 1–2 times per week (206). Not all muscle groups are trained specifically per workout using a high frequency. Rather, each major muscle group may be trained 2–3 times per week despite the large number of workouts. Strongman competitors were shown to train ~3–5 days per week (207).

Training frequency affects workout structure. The following guide can be used when matching workout structures to different frequencies:

- 1 day per week: total-body workout
- 2 days per week: total-body or upper/lower-body split workouts
- 3 days per week: total-body, upper/lower-body split, or compound split routine workouts
- 4 days per week: total-body (with or without split designations), upper/lower-body split, or compound split routine workouts
- 5 days per week: total-body (with or without split designations) or compound/isolated split routine workouts
- 6–7 days per week and higher: compound/isolated split routine workouts — total body (with or without split designations)

Total-body workouts with split designations refer to Olympic lifting, high-intensity interval training (metabolic), or strength competition type of programs. Because the Olympic lifts are total-body lifts, the workout is considered a total-body workout. However, the split designation refers to the exercises performed after the Olympic lifts. These can be divided into upper- and lower-body exercises.

Case Study 12.1

Lance is a collegiate Division II football player who is ready to begin off-season training. He is a 6′2″ 225-lb linebacker whose goals are to increase maximal strength and power, while gaining some muscle hypertrophy. He has lifted weights for 6 years and is proficient with the Olympic lifts. The athlete's weight room is well equipped with lifting platforms, racks, benches, and free weight equipment but is limited to only a few machines, *i.e.*, lat pull-down, low pulley row, leg press, and cable/pulley system. He has a history of using total-body workouts and is well balanced in strength through his major muscle groups (he has no glaring weaknesses). Lance asks you to design a 10-week training program.

Question for Consideration: What program would you give Lance?

Corrective Exercise Programming

Corrective exercises consist mostly of bodyweight exercises or RE with low levels of loading that target primarily trunk/spine, hip, and shoulder musculature. Corrective exercises (plus myofascial release and flexibility exercises) can be used to correct postural deficits and restore neuromuscular function. Several exercises are depicted in Chapter 14. Corrective exercises comprise single- and multiple-joint exercises using CON, ECC, and ISOM muscle actions that target problem or weakened areas. Corrective exercises can easily be included in programs as part of warm-ups, cooldowns, and integrated into the main lifting segment of the workout. Similar to myofascial release and flexibility exercises, some low-intensity corrective exercises may be performed daily if need be. Although specific guidelines should be individualized, some practical guidelines have recommended that corrective exercises be performed at least 3–5 days per week for at least 1–2 sets per exercise for 10–15 reps, or at least 4-second contractions for positional ISOM exercises (33). Minimal rest is needed between sets or repetitions for many corrective exercises; however, more rest may be given for challenging exercises. Progression may occur from simple to more challenging exercises (*i.e.*, beginning with a double-leg glute bridge → single-leg glute bridge → single-leg glute bridge with limb movement), increasing the time of ISOM contraction duration or repetition number, or by adding light weight to the exercise. Table 12.10 is a sample total-body workout targeting corrective exercises. See Sidebar: Training the Pelvic Floor and Figure 12.17.

Metabolic Training Programming

Metabolic circuit training has been a staple of tactical strength and conditioning for many years and has become popular in general fitness and in the training of athletes especially with the rise of popularity in sports/programs such as high-intensity interval training, which are based on metabolic circuit training. Circuit programs increase training efficiency, yield substantial metabolic and cardiovascular responses, and are effective for increasing anaerobic capacity/endurance. The continuity (or very short rest intervals) is a stimulus for increasing aerobic

Table 12.10	General Warm-Up + Myofascial Release and Light Stretching
Exercise	**Sets × Reps**
Supine knee raises (with core bracing)	2 × 10 reps
Side plank	2 × 20 s each side
ISOM single-leg glute bridge	2 × 20 s each leg
Supine medial hip rotation	2 × 20 s each leg
Quadruped	2 × 10 reps with 2-s ISOM at top
Superman	2 × 20 s position hold
Lying hip abduction (with hip medial rotation)	2 × 10 reps each leg with 2-s ISOM at top
Groiner with trunk rotation	2 × 20 s each side
Scapular circuit (Y, T, L, I, reverse I)	1 × 15 s each position
4-point thoracic rotation	2 × 10 reps
Wall slide	2 × 10 reps

Sidebar   Training the Pelvic Floor

—By Tamara Rial-Rebullido, PhD

The pelvic floor is located at bottom of the pelvis and is a structure composed of several layers of muscles including the ischiococcygeus, internal obturator, and the levator ani as well as connective tissue supporting structures. The pelvic floor muscles (PFMs) are able to increase urethral closure pressure, lift the pelvic floor, and provide structural support to the pelvic organs (*e.g.*, urinary bladder, uterus, vagina, rectum). Of interest, the PFMs not only play an important role in sexuality and parturition but they aid in stabilization of the sacroiliac articulation and breathing mechanics (208). Weakness and loss of functionality of the PFMs can lead to a variety of conditions known as pelvic floor disorders (PFDs). The high prevalence of PFDs in women represents a major public health burden (209). The most common PFDs are urinary incontinence, fecal incontinence, pelvic organ prolapse, pelvic pain, and sexual dysfunction. About 25% of adult women suffer from at least one PFD (209). In addition to high BMI, women who participate in strenuous exercise activities or sports that involve high-impact landing, running, or jumping are at an increased risk (208,209). High impact loading is linked to PFD due to prolonged exposure to increased IAP and ground reaction forces, which can stress the pelvic floor structures and reduce PFM functionality (208). Health care providers, sport coaches, and fitness professionals play an important role in managing modifiable risk factors for PFD such as a high BMI or weak PFM. Professionals involved in the design of exercise programs for females are in a privileged position to raise awareness about PFD and the benefits of PFM training.

PFM training should be considered an essential component of RT programs for women. The concept of progressive RT for the PFM was introduced ~1950s by Arnold Kegel and consequently PFM exercises are commonly called Kegels. The goal of PFM training is to increase the muscular strength, endurance, and neuromuscular facilitation. High-quality evidence supports the use of PFM training for the treatment and prevention of PFD such as urinary incontinence and pelvic organ prolapse (210,211). Qualified supervision and instruction are needed to perform PFM training properly. Over 30% of healthy women and 70% of women with PFD are unable to perform a PFM contraction correctly (212,213). Common errors known as COMMOV (**C**ontraction of **O**ther **M**uscle groups and other **MOV**ements) are likely to occur during PFM training. Effective coaching cues and constructive feedback can reduce COMMOV and increase the efficacy of a PFM program (214). Since PFM training is a learned skill, the type of instruction used to teach proper activation of the PFM can influence the efficacy of PFM contractions. Significant

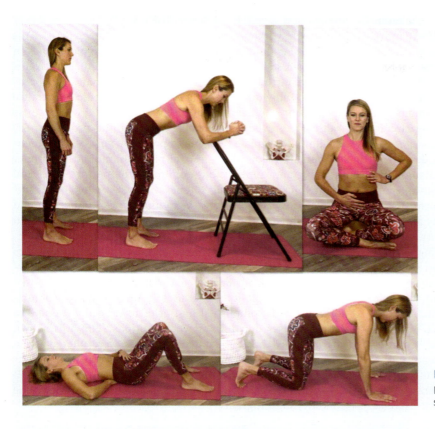

FIGURE 12.17 Examples of body positions to perform pelvic floor muscle contractions: standing, hip-hinging, sitting, quadruped, and supine.

variations of PFM recruitment and displacement are found depending on the verbal instruction used (215). Examples of simple and effective coaching cues to activate the PFM are "stop the flow of urine" and "squeeze the anus."

PFM training consists of a cycle of repetitive PFM contractions and relaxations. The first step is to localize, visualize, and feel the contraction and relaxation of the PFM. A proper cycle consists of the ability to contract and lift the PFM for a few seconds while exhaling and then relax the PFM while inhaling. Once this is achieved for a few reps, the program can progress from gentle contractions of 6–10 seconds in the supine or seated position to more intense contractions for 3–6 seconds in different body positions (*e.g.*, standing, quadruped, hip hinging). Figure 12.17 shows different body positions for PFM training. A general protocol for PFM training can include 1–3 different exercises performed for 1–3 sets of 6–10 reps with proper breathing and adequate rest intervals between reps and sets.

capacity. Often, circuits consist of ~3–12 exercises, low to moderate intensity, for at least 10–15 repetitions with <10–15 seconds between exercises. The number of circuits (or rounds) depends on the number of exercises used, volume, and intensity, as well as the conditioning level of the trainees. Large muscle mass resistance and bodyweight exercises increase the metabolic response and difficulty of the circuit. For example, we have previously shown that exercises such as burpees, battling rope movements, and push-ups with lateral shuffles (bear crawls) increase acute oxygen consumption more so than many traditional REs performed for 3 sets of 10 reps with 2-minute rest intervals (216). We also reported significant acute metabolic responses to performing a sandbag and bodyweight RE protocol using Tabata intervals (3 circuits of 8 multiple-joint exercises performed for as many reps as possible for 20 s followed by a 10-s rest interval before beginning the next exercise with 2 min of rest between circuits) (217). The large acute elevations in oxygen consumption and cardiorespiratory responses make metabolic training not only an established mode of anaerobic training but an attractive alternative to aerobic training.

Muscle strength and power can improve with circuit training as circuits can be designed to target each fitness component. The intensity needs to be higher, exercises should be sequenced to allow partial rest for major muscle groups in between exercise performance, and rep number is lower. It has become popular to include other modalities of training (*e.g.*, sprint, agility, tactical, aerobic, and plyometric drills) within metabolic circuits. Circuit progression can take place by increasing the load, reps, duration or length of drill, and reducing the total time needed to complete the entire circuit, *e.g.*, *timed circuits*. A high-intensity interval training approach used in addition to the aforementioned methods is to use a standard circuit of exercises and reps/durations but to gradually increase the number of rounds completed within a time frame (*i.e.*, 10–15 min). Timed circuits can target speed, quickness, and agility in addition to muscle strength/power endurance. The athlete can perform the entire circuit, rest ~1–2 minutes, and repeat the circuit for the desired number of sets. Circuits are dependent upon equipment availability, spacing, and can be varied a number of ways by altering the exercise selection and number per circuit, loading, and volume.

Several metabolic training programs can be developed given the large number of potential exercises. Structural and compound (large muscle mass) bodyweight, resistance, aerobic, plyometric, sprint, or agility exercises are performed with minimal rest between exercises. The high continuity and large muscle mass involvement (along with the intensity interaction) provide a strong metabolic stimulus targeting cardiovascular and muscle endurance improvements and body fat reductions. These workouts can be very challenging so a gradual progression is needed, perhaps starting with a couple of drills for moderate duration. Volume can increase and rest can decrease progressively over time as the trainee becomes more conditioned. Increasing the workload too quickly or predisposing a novice, deconditioned individual to an advanced, competitive program could result in a greater risk of overuse type injuries such as muscle strains, torn ligaments, stress fractures, and *exertional rhabdomyolysis* so prudent exercise

prescription should be implemented as well as proper recovery in between workouts, nutritional, and fluid intake (218). This has been the topic of discussion as the ACSM recommends in a consensus statement regarding military personnel that trainees (a) are introduced gradually to metabolic training; (b) programs be individualized to needs; (c) seek medical clearance especially if one has a medical issue that could compromise health when exposed to challenging training programs; (d) are allowed adequate rest with appropriate volume and intensity initially followed by gradual progression; and (e) proper nutrition and supervision/monitoring of performance and health, injury, and fatigue/soreness be used to avoid overtraining (218). As is the case with traditional RT, trainees should first be taught proper technique of the exercises and begin with a simple design building a strength and endurance foundation. This is especially true when Olympic lifts, gymnastics variations, tactical drills, plyometrics, or other complex exercises are used. Considering that metabolic programs consist of largely multiple-joint exercises, a solid technical foundation must be accomplished first prior to exposing trainees to these exercises during fatigued conditions. This was shown where barbell back squat biomechanics were altered when performed in a fatigued state (219). Progression with experience will entail the transition to building tolerance to reduced rest within the workouts. See Sidebar: Examples of Metabolic Conditioning Programs.

Sidebar   Examples of Metabolic Conditioning Programs

Sample workout no. 1: A high-intensity interval training workout of the day. The workout is performed for as many rounds as possible in 10 minutes. Rounds are counted — progression entails gradually increasing number of rounds within 10 minutes. Rest may be taken within as needed but less rest is used with progression and improved conditioning.

Pull-ups	5 reps
Push-ups	10 reps
Front squats	15 reps (performed with light loading)

Sample workout no. 2: A sandbag workout using only 11, 20, and 44 kg sandbags (217). The workout is based on Tabata intervals; 20 seconds as many reps as possible followed by 10-second rest for all eight exercises performed in sequence with 2-minute rest intervals in between sets (circuits). Table 12.11 depicts the mean (± standard deviation) of the rep numbers performed by subjects in the study. This workout yielded high blood lactates and heart rates ~160–180+ bpm.

Sample workout no. 3: A multimodal workout performed for three circuits with 2 minutes of rest in between circuits. Light to moderate weights used for barbell and kettlebell exercises.

Barbell squat	10 reps
Battling rope single-arm waves	30 seconds
Box jumps	10 reps
Push-ups	15 reps
Kettlebell swings	15 reps
Medicine ball torso rotations	15 reps
Jumping jacks	50 reps

Sample workout no. 4: A workout focused on adding a sport-specific element performed for five circuits with 1 minute of rest in between circuits.

Landmine barbell unilateral rotational press	10 reps each arm
Boxing heavy bag round (targeting jabs, crosses, hooks, upper cuts, or combinations in different forms for hand speed and power) or speed bag round	1 minute
Push-ups on fists	10 reps
Jump rope	50 reps

Table 12.11	Repetition Performance during the Sandbag Resistance Exercise Protocol			
	Set 1	Set 2	Set 3	Total
Front squat	12.8 ± 1.8	11.3 ± 2.1[a]	8.5 ± 3.4[a,b]	32.5 ± 6.0
Clean	9.4 ± 2.2	9.3 ± 2.0	7.8 ± 2.6	26.4 ± 6.0
Bear hug squat	12.4 ± 2.3	9.8 ± 1.9[a]	7.6 ± 2.8[a]	29.8 ± 5.2
Rotational DL	10.5 ± 2.9	8.5 ± 1.9[a]	7.0 ± 2.9[a,b]	26.0 ± 6.7
Lunge with rotation	8.8 ± 2.6	8.0 ± 1.9	7.8 ± 1.3	24.5 ± 4.3
Lateral drag	11.9 ± 1.6	11.6 ± 1.5	9.9 ± 1.6[a,b]	33.4 ± 4.0
Overhead press	15.3 ± 2.6	12.3 ± 4.1	11.9 ± 5.4	39.9 ± 8.2
Shouldering	8.9 ± 1.1	7.4 ± 2.0[a]	8.8 ± 1.7	25.0 ± 3.2

[a]$P \leq 0.05$ compared with set 1.

[b]$P \leq 0.05$ compared with set 2. DL, deadlift.

Reprinted from Table 2, Ratamess NA, Kang J, Kuper JD, et al. Acute cardiorespiratory and metabolic effects of a sandbag resistance exercise protocol. *J Strength Cond Res.* 2018;32:1491–502.

Advanced Resistance Training Techniques

Some RT techniques better serve trained to advanced individuals. They provide a high degree of overload and can be useful for assisting athletes in overcoming training plateaus. It is not that intermediated-trained individuals cannot benefit from a few of these techniques. Rather, because novice to intermediate individuals progress rapidly with basic programs many suggest incorporating the techniques once a solid strength base has been built. Some of these techniques have been acutely compared to traditional set schemes and shown to produce similar or lower volume loads and similar or higher levels of fatigue for up to 48 hours post-RE. Given the stimulatory nature of some of these fatigue-driven techniques, it appears the best strategy in using these is a periodized approach to compliment traditional RT especially for the athlete striving to maximize muscle hypertrophy. Other techniques targeting maximal strength and power strive to lower the fatigue response and maximize the quality of each repetition. Nevertheless, long-term studies have not addressed the most effective ways to incorporate some of these techniques into advanced RT programs. Advanced techniques are based upon most program variables as well as ROM and a few are used to train past the point of momentary muscular failure. The techniques covered are

- Muscle actions: heavy negatives, forced negatives, functional ISOMs
- Range of motion: partial repetitions, variable resistance
- Intensity (supramaximal: >100% of CON 1 RM to stimulate nervous system): heavy negatives, forced negatives, overloads, forced repetitions, partial repetitions (strongest ROM)

- Rest intervals and volume: breakdown sets, combining exercises, noncontinuous sets, quality training, spectrum repetition/contrast loading combinations

Heavy and Forced Negatives

Heavy negatives involve loading the bar/machine with >100% of 1 RM (usually by 20%–50%) and only performing the ECC phase with a slow cadence (>3–4 s) in the presence of capable spotters or a power rack with the pins set appropriately. CON phases are performed with spotter assistance. Another form of heavy ECC training involves performing a bilateral machine exercise with low to moderate weight and then lowering it with only one limb. The athlete can perform a two-legged knee extension but lower the weight with only one leg and then rotate with each repetition or set. Some machines have been developed with multiple loading capacities that enable greater ECC loading. Additional loading is provided to the ECC phase while the CON phase is performed with less weight, known *accentuated ECC loading*. Repetitions during conventional sets can be enhanced with force applied to ECC phase via a spotter (*forced negatives*). Some have suggested that supramaximal ECC loading leads to greater muscle hypertrophy and strength gains. Brandenburg and Docherty (220) compared 9 weeks of traditional (4 × 10 reps, 75% of 1 RM) to accentuated ECC training (3 × 10 reps, 75% of 1 RM for CON phase, 110%–120% of 1 RM for ECC phase) using the preacher curl and triceps extension exercises and found similar strength increases for the preacher curl. However, ECC-accentuated training led to greater strength improvements in the elbow extensors (24% vs. 15%). Heavy ECC training should be used with caution (4–6-week training cycles for only a few sets per workout) to reduce muscle damage and the risk of overtraining and/or injury.

Functional Isometrics

Functional isometrics were first promoted by Bob Hoffman and involve lifting a barbell in a power rack a few inches until it is pressing or pulling up against the rack's pins. The lifter continues to push/pull as hard and as rapidly as possible for the ISOM action for ~2-6 seconds. The pins are set in two places (when not initiating the reps from the floor), at the starting position that allows the barbell to rest and at the targeted area of the ROM. Because ISOM strength is greater than CON strength, the rationale is to provide greater force at specific areas of the ROM to increase dynamic strength to a greater extent. Functional ISOMs provide a potent metabolic stimulus when compared to traditional RE sets (177). Functional ISOMs can be performed in any area of the ROM but are effective when performed near the sticking region of the exercise. This is an effective strength and power training technique that targets the exercise's weak point. Some exercises commonly targeted with functional ISOM are the bench press, deadlift, squat, and clean pull. A variation of functional ISOM, the mid-thigh ISOM clean pull assessment, is discussed in the Chapter 19. Jackson et al. (221) found 6-second functional ISOM added to dynamic training increased strength by 19.4%, whereas the dynamic-only group increased strength 11.9%. O'Shea and O'Shea (222) compared 6 weeks of functional ISOM to dynamic squat training and showed a greater increase in 1 RM squat strength with functional ISOM than dynamic training (31.8 vs. 13.2 kg, respectively). Giorgi et al. (223) compared dynamic bench press and squat training to dynamic training plus functional ISOM (2-3 s for each rep) and found similar strength increases (functional ISOM = 13%-25%; dynamic = 11%-16%). However, when the six strongest subjects were analyzed, 5%-10% greater strength increases were seen with functional ISOM. Therefore, functional ISOM training may have potential to enhance dynamic strength in athletes who have already developed a strength base.

Partial Repetitions

Partial reps are those performed in a limited ROM. They are useful for those with clinical problems or limited joint ROM in rehabilitation settings. Graves et al. (224) had subjects train using the knee extension for a partial ROM of 120°-60°, 60°-0°, and for full ROM and showed ROM-specific strength gains. In another study, Graves et al. (225) had subjects exercise from 72°-36°, 36°-0°, and full ROM (72°-0°) lumbar extension for 8-12 reps. Strength increased in each respective ROM and training through 36° was effective for increasing strength throughout the full ROM. It was concluded that full ROM strength can be enhanced by training in a partial ROM. Partial reps increase strength in a segment of the ROM, and if these changes translate into full ROM strength gains, then they may provide useful for athletes during strength training.

Most often the reps are performed in the area of maximal strength. Partial reps can be used in different ways. Some athletes have used them to extend sets beyond failure (sometimes known as "burns"). Partial reps allow more reps when the lifter can no longer complete a full CON phase without assistance. This utility of partial reps is mostly seen for those training for maximal hypertrophy or endurance (body builders) where training beyond failure may provide additional benefits. A review of the literature proposed partial reps has a hypertrophic effect on skeletal muscle and may provide some advantages to full ROM training only when training to maximize hypertrophy (226). Another utility is to integrate partial reps into dynamic sets with full ROM reps. Bodybuilders have used these techniques in their training. A technique known as "21s" has been used. The lifter selects an exercise and performs 7 reps in the first half of the ROM, 7 reps in the other half of the ROM, and then finishes with 7 full ROM reps. Another example is the 1½ system. The lifter follows a full ROM rep with a partial ROM rep until the set is completed.

Often partial reps are performed in the area of maximal strength with larger-than-normal loading. The rationale is to reduce neural inhibitions by applying a supramaximal load and train a ROM that is submaximally trained with conventional loading in a full ROM. Bypassing the weak point and overloading the strongest area of the ROM can be used to stimulate the nervous system for strength gains. Training in a partial ROM where sports performance may be specific (a half squat performed to enhance vertical jump performance) has been performed in athletes and termed by some *accentuation* (68). Ascending strength curves are observed for pushing exercises, whereas descending curves are seen with pulling exercises. Maximal force production for the bench press occurs near the lockout phase (68). Supramaximal loads may be lifted in this ROM as the sticking region is bypassed. Partial ROM bench press strength may be ~11%-18% greater than full ROM lifts (173), and the partial ROM bench presses yield higher integrated EMG (IEMG) data than full ROM lifts (Fig. 12.18). Those unfamiliar with partial reps respond favorably by increasing their 1 RM by ~4.5% within a few workouts (173). Clark et al. (227) showed that loads lifted and force production increased as ROM decreased

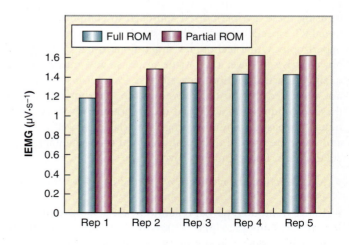

FIGURE 12.18 IEMG during a set of full ROM and partial ROM bench press.

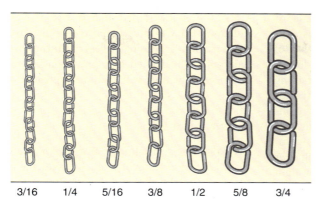

FIGURE 12.19 Chain size information. Note that chain link sizes and their corresponding rates are displayed per linear foot and can be used to calculate additional weights on the bar.

for the bench press, e.g., full versus ¾ versus ½ versus ¼ ROM. Massey et al. (228,229) compared 10 weeks of training consisting of either full ROM bench press, partial ROM bench press, or a combination and showed that all three produced similar 1 RM full ROM bench press increases in UT men. Interestingly, partial ROM training increased full ROM 1 RM bench press but the combination of both did not augment full ROM strength more than full ROM training alone. Strength athletes such as powerlifters may benefit from enhanced strength in this area as many compete with bench press shirts, and bench press shirts provide greatest support near the lowest and midsegments of the ROM. Partial ROM lifts can be incorporated into strength peaking mesocycles (perhaps sequenced following the full ROM structural exercise but before assistance exercises).

Variable Resistance Training

Variable resistance machines modify the loading throughout joint ROM based on ascending/descending human strength curves. These machines have a cam that varies in length so that loading is modified via altering the distance between the load and pivot point. The technology became popularized in the early 1970s when it was used by Nautilus in their machines. An advantage to variable RT is loading is reduced through the sticking region and greater in areas of the ROM that are stronger. By reducing the load in this region, variable RT allows other areas of the ROM to be trained to a greater extent.

Variable RT may not be considered an advanced RT technique. However, there are some variations that have become popular among powerlifters and other athletes. Many athletes have used bands and/or chains to create variable resistance during free-weight training. A survey study showed that 39% and 57% of British powerlifters use bands and chains, respectively, in their training programs (230), and another study reported 38%–56% of strength competitors reported using chains and bands in training (98). Both can be used by themselves as forms of variable resistance. Bands and chains come in many sizes and offer various levels of resistance to the user. For the squat, chains applied to both ends of the bar will be suspended in the air (or at least more than half of the chain will be suspended) during lockout (the athlete supports the majority of chain weight in this strong ROM area). As the athlete descends, more links of the chain are supported by the floor, thereby reducing weight as the athlete descends to the parallel position. Upon ascent, progressively more weight is applied as the chain links are lifted from the floor. The resistance used depends on the weight and size of the chain and the distance of the bar from the floor (more weight is applied when the bar is higher). A 5- to 7-ft chain can accommodate most athletes. Chains oscillate, which increases the stabilization requirement during the exercise. Figure 12.19 depicts chain sizes. Applying one 5/8 chain to each side of the bar would yield ~40 lb added to the upper segment of the exercise. One 5/8 chain and one ½ chain to each side yields ~60 lb. Chains can provide substantial loading.

A similar effect is gained through stretchable bands attached to the floor and bar. The farther the band is stretched, the more resistance applied to the bar. The ergogenic effects of bands and chains are not well understood from a research perspective although these training tools are used successfully by competitive athletes and elite powerlifters (231). Cronin et al. (232) compared 10 weeks of jump squat training with or without bungy cords and found similar improvements in strength between the two (although greater EMG activity was seen during the ECC phase when bungy cords were used). Wallace et al. (233) showed that the use of elastic bands added to the back squat increased force and power output. Bands provide greater neuromuscular loading to barbell exercises but long-term training effects remain to be seen. Ebben and Jensen (234) compared traditional squatting with squatting with either a chain or band (each of which comprised ~10% of 1 RM) and found that all three produced similar muscle activation and mean/peak ground reaction forces. Coker, Berning, and Briggs (235,236) examined chain use during the snatch and power clean in weightlifters (80% and 85% of 1 RM with 5% in chains) and showed no differences in technique or kinetics between conditions. However, all of the lifters perceived working harder with the addition of chains and felt that the oscillations of the chains required greater shoulder, abdominal, and back muscle activity to stabilize the bar. Few studies examined training with chains over time. One study examined band and chain use for speed reps in the bench press over 7 weeks (chains/bands were only used 1 day per week) and showed no augmentation of strength or power in football players (237). However, Anderson et al. (238) examined 7 weeks of bench press and squat training with free weights only or free weights plus elastic bands (bands provided 20% of load) in athletes and showed greater gains in bench press (8% vs. 4%), squat (16% vs. 6%) strength, and jumping power with band usage. McCurdy et al. (239) compared chain-only versus free weight bench press training over 9 weeks and reported chain-only training increased free weight and chain 1 RM bench press strength and vice versa similar to free weight training. Although further research is needed, there are data showing ergogenic effects of band/chain RT.

Overloads

Overloads entail holding a supramaximal load in order to make subsequent sets feel lighter or to engage potential neural inhibiting mechanisms. An athlete preparing to attempt a 1 RM of 375 lb in training/competition may precede this attempt by first loading the bar to ~400 lb and holding the weight in the locked-out position. The intent is to potentiate the neural response to the 375-lb attempt. Powerlifters use this technique for the squat as they will walk out with a supramaximal load (after lifting it off of the rack) and stand (without actually performing the squat) to train the neuromuscular system to accommodate the load. The goal is to use postactivation potentiation to enhance subsequent squat sets.

Forced Repetitions

Forced repetitions are those completed with the assistance of a spotter (although the lifters can spot some exercises themselves like the leg press) beyond failure in an attempt to increase strength, endurance, and hypertrophy. Minimal assistance is applied to allow movement of the weight for ~1–4 reps. Forced repetitions can be used exclusively as a specific set or can be used to extend a set when muscular failure occurs. For the former, a supramaximal load can be used for a few repetitions in which a spotter assists in all repetitions. For the latter, a spotter can assist the lifter in performing a few additional repetitions beyond fatigue. Forced reps produce a greater anabolic hormone response and stress the neuromuscular system to a higher degree. Ahtiainen et al. (240) compared training to failure with a 12 RM versus 12 reps performed with forced repetitions (8 RM load + 4 forced reps) for 8 sets and found both protocols resulted in elevated testosterone, cortisol, and GH. However, the forced repetition workout resulted in greater elevations in cortisol and GH. ISOM strength was reduced by 38.3% following the traditional workout, whereas a 56.5% reduction was seen following the forced rep workout 3 days after, indicating that forced reps provide greater overload to the neuromuscular system and increase the recovery time in between workouts. Training status plays a role in the acute response. Workouts including forced reps lead to greater acute elevations in total testosterone (but not free T or GH) in strength-trained athletes compared to untrained individuals (241). One study reported similar strength gains among three training groups regardless of the number of forced reps per workout (242). Forced reps provide a potent training stimulus and need to be used with caution as greater fatigue may ensue.

Breakdown Sets

Breakdown sets, also known as *descending sets*, *drop sets*, or *multipoundage system*, involve quickly reducing the load with minimal rest, thereby allowing the lifter to perform additional reps. The rationale is when failure occurs, there is still potential to perform more reps with less weight. Breakdown sets are another method used to train beyond failure. Single (for one set) or multiple breakdowns (for multiple sets) may be used. Breakdown sets are most effective when a spotter(s) is present to remove weights or change pins on machine weight stacks. Historically, breakdown sets were used to enhance muscle hypertrophy and endurance and predominately used by bodybuilders. However, breakdown sets can be used to target muscle strength as a near maximal weight can be lifted for 1–2 reps, 5%–10% of the load can be reduced, 1–2 additional reps are performed, etc., until the targeted number of reps are completed. Breakdown sets result in additional fatigue (243,244). Chronic studies show increased muscle strength (when the first set is of equal intensity to heavy loading), endurance, and hypertrophy and in some cases similar to high-load RT (148,245,246). One study showed it could augment muscle hypertrophy (247). Thus, the utility appears mostly hypertrophy or muscular endurance related with less potential to augment strength unless the initial set (prior to the drop sets) is of high intensity.

Combining Exercises

Combining exercises involve performing two or more exercises consecutively with minimal to no rest. Multiple exercises can be combined into one exercise (combination lifts). This is common when using Olympic lifts. A combination lift may involve a clean from the floor, a front squat, and a push press to finish. This sequence is performed for a series of reps. Combination exercises have become more common for non-Olympic lifts as well. Another strategy is to perform all repetitions for one exercise followed by consecutive performance of one or more exercises with minimal rest in between exercises. The following terminology describes three different exercise stacking methods:

- *Supersets* — involve consecutive performance of two different exercises (either for the same muscle group or different muscle groups, *i.e.*, agonist-antagonistic, unrelated). Many times the term *compound set* is used to describe supersets of different exercises involving the same muscle groups.
- *Example*: 10 reps of the incline bench press are immediately followed by 10 reps of the low pulley row. Following a rest interval, the sequence is repeated until the targeted numbers of sets have been completed.

- *Tri-Sets* — involve consecutive performance of three different exercises.
- *Example*: 10 reps of the bench press are immediately followed by 10 reps of bodyweight dips, which are immediately followed by 10 reps of dumbbell flys. Following a rest interval, the sequence is repeated until the targeted numbers of sets have been completed.
- *Giant Sets* — involve consecutive performance of four or more different exercises.
- *Example*: 10 reps of the squat are immediately followed by 10 reps of leg extensions, which are immediately followed by 10 reps of leg curls, which are immediately followed by 10 reps of barbell setups. Following a rest interval, the sequence is repeated until the targeted numbers of sets have been completed.

Combining exercises are primarily used for increasing muscular endurance and hypertrophy, especially if the athlete is trying to minimize workout duration. Although strength can increase with these combinations, most strength enhancement is seen in lesser-trained individuals. In trained men, supersetting the flat and incline bench press (5 sets × 10 RM loading to start) results in less volume load and muscle activation compared to standard sets (248). Combination lifts are used to increase muscular endurance and increase the metabolic demands of a workout as the weight lifted for each exercise is less than what would typically be used if the exercise was performed alone (and dependent on the weakest of the exercises). In our previous example (clean, front squat, press), the weight selected would have to be light enough to accommodate the weakest exercise in sequence (the press) in a fatigued state. Metabolic/endurance goals predominate when using this technique. Many bodybuilders use supersets, tri-sets, and giant sets for increasing muscle hypertrophy and the metabolic demands of the workout to aid in body fat reductions. It is common for these athletes to combine exercises stressing the same muscle groups as many bodybuilders use split routines. The largest benefit is enhanced muscle endurance and size due to the large fatigue effect. Some strength athletes may use super sets to increase muscle strength. Many times the super sets involve opposing or unrelated (upper to lower body) muscle groups so adequate recovery is given and greater loading can be used. This method may be most suitable for strength training out of the methods discussed in this section.

Noncontinuous Sets

Noncontinuous sets involve including an intraset rest interval or a pause in between reps or groups of reps in a set. The rationale is to maximize force and power output of each rep by minimizing fatigue. Figures 12.20 and 12.21 depict data obtained from our laboratory on 10-rep sets of the squat and bench press. These data show that the quality of each rep varies as sets progress. For the squat, peak force occurs in reps 2 through 5 and progressively declines afterward. For the bench press, highest power values were obtained during performance of the first three reps. In both cases, the quality of reps declined after reps 6 and 3, respectively. This is one reason why some S&C practitioners recommend low reps for strength and power training. High quality of repetition performance is critical to several sports including Olympic lifting and powerlifting. Inserting a rest interval in between reps is thought to minimize fatigue effects so that each rep is performed at maximal velocity.

Pause between Repetitions

Inserting a rest interval in between reps or groups of reps can result in more reps performed and higher force/power output (249). It has been suggested that this may be advantageous as each rep may be performed in a less-fatigued state. Workouts stressing glycolysis stimulate hypertrophy. Light loads (coupled with restricted blood flow and increased metabolites) produce similar hypertrophy gains to heavier loads (250). However, the role of metabolites in RT is less clear. Rooney et al. (107) trained subjects for 6 weeks and performed reps either continuously for 6–10 reps or completed each set with a 30-second rest interval in between reps and found strength increased 56.3% when reps were performed continuously (vs. a 41.2% increase when rest intervals were used). Lawton et al. (251) compared bench press training with either 4 × 6 reps or 8 × 3 reps (with a 6 RM load) and showed strength increased 9.7% in the continuous (4 × 6) group versus 4.9% in the noncontinuous (8 × 3) group

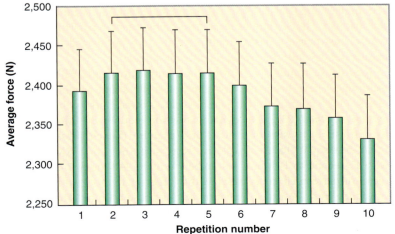

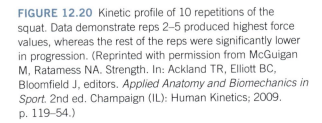

FIGURE 12.20 Kinetic profile of 10 repetitions of the squat. Data demonstrate reps 2–5 produced highest force values, whereas the rest of the reps were significantly lower in progression. (Reprinted with permission from McGuigan M, Ratamess NA. Strength. In: Ackland TR, Elliott BC, Bloomfield J, editors. *Applied Anatomy and Biomechanics in Sport*. 2nd ed. Champaign (IL): Human Kinetics; 2009. p. 119–54.)

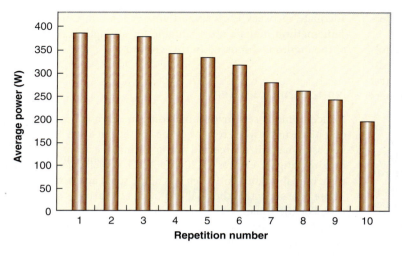

FIGURE 12.21 Power profile of 10 repetitions of the bench press.

indicating that performing reps continuously (inducing more fatigue) was a better strength training stimulus than including intraset rest intervals. However, Folland et al. (252) had UT subjects train 3 days per week for 9 weeks using either 4 × 10 continuous reps (75% of 1 RM) with a 30-second rest between sets versus performing the same volume with 1 rep every 30 seconds and showed similar increases in strength. It is unclear as to the ultimate role fatigue has on strength development as training in fatigued and less-fatigued states increase muscle strength.

Rest-Pause Training and Failure/Nonfailure Variations

Rest-pause training methods allow more reps to be performed especially with maximal or near-maximal weights via short intraset rest periods. The rationale is to increase volume per set with moderately heavy to heavy loading. The short rest intervals enable partial recovery and allow extra reps to be performed with moderately to heavy weights. For example, an athlete may desire to perform 6 reps with a 3 RM load in the bench press. The lifter performs 3 reps without assistance to failure or near-failure, racks the weight, and rests for 15–30 seconds. The lifter then proceeds to perform 1–2 additional reps with the same load, rests for 15–30 seconds, and 1–2 additional reps are performed, etc. until the targeted number of reps are performed. Other rest-pause variations exist. The length of the rest interval can be altered, the loading can range from moderate to very high (using near 100% of 1 RM for single repetitions), and the loads can be slightly reduced with subsequent reps. This type of rest-pause training (high-intensity reps performed to failure and beyond) may cause significant fatigue.

Rest-pause training variations (in combination with VBT techniques) have been used by elite powerlifters and weightlifters. One training system used by elite powerlifters is the *dynamic method* (231). The dynamic method requires the lifter to perform 8–10 sets of a structural exercise (bench press, squat, box squat) for 2–3 explosive reps with ~60% of 1 RM with 45-second to 1-minute rest in between sets. Although 2–3 reps are performed consecutively, the large set number with substantial rest illustrate a variation of rest-pause training. The use of multiple reps is advantageous because some lifters do not attain peak force or power on the first rep.

Cluster training is a method used successfully in the training of Olympic weightlifters and other athletes (189). It involves inserting intraset rest intervals in between reps, inserting interset rest intervals in between smaller groups of reps, or reducing rest intervals in between sets and including a rest interval in the middle of a set (*rest redistribution*). Generally, 5- to 45-second rest intervals are used in between reps or groups of reps depending on the goals (103,253,254). Haff et al. (255) studied cluster training in Olympic weightlifters and track and field athletes. They compared it to traditional methods and showed that clusters (with 30-s rest in between reps) led to greater bar velocity and displacement during 1 × 5 reps of clean pulls especially during the last 3 reps. Hansen et al. (256) compared traditional sets (4 × 6 reps, 3-min rest between sets) of jump squats to different cluster configurations: (a) 4 × 6 singles with 12 seconds of rest between reps; (b) 4 × 3 doubles with 30 seconds of rest between pairs; and (c) 4 × 2 × triples with 60 seconds of rest between triples and showed that each cluster produced higher peak power and velocity than traditional sets especially during the latter reps (reps 4–6). Hardee et al. (257) showed that rest intervals of at least 20 seconds between reps enabled maintenance of technique during the power clean. Other studies have shown advantages of maintaining set quality (power, velocity) with cluster sets (258–264) and lower blood lactates (258,260) and cortisol and GH responses (260) compared to traditional sets. Meta-analytic data provide support for the use of clusters to maximize rep quality (253). The response appears similar between trained and untrained individuals (253,260). Oliver et al. (259) showed that 12 weeks of RT using clusters resulted in greater strength and power improvements, vertical jump power, but led to similar increases in lean mass and MHC IIx to IIa transitions. Cluster sets can be structured in different ways. The load can be kept constant for all reps or can be increased, decreased, or undulated. Clusters can be particularly useful during the Olympic lifts as many times the weight is cautiously dropped to the platform in between reps and the intraset rest interval allows for regripping the bar, possibly changing weight, and reestablishing proper body positioning. Rest intervals of 5–45 seconds are used in between reps or groups of reps can be performed in clusters, *e.g.*, instead of 3 × 10 reps with 70% of 1 RM (totaling 30 reps) 6 × 5 reps or 10 × 3 reps can be performed with the same loading.

Quality Training

Quality training is a technique used to increase muscle endurance and hypertrophy for the most part, with strength increases secondary. Quality training involves reducing rest interval lengths as training progresses. For example, a lifter is currently training the dead lift for 4 sets of 10 reps with 275 lb using 2.5 minutes in between sets. This lifter would then reduce rest interval length to 2 minutes as training progresses and as he improves his conditioning. Perhaps, the goal may be to be able to perform 4 sets of 10 reps with 275 lb using only 1-minute rest intervals. At that point, training becomes more efficient and the lifter then needs to add weight, increase rest interval length, and begin the process once again. One study showed that 8 weeks of RT (along with creatine supplementation) using a constant 2-minute rest interval versus reduced rest intervals of 15 seconds per week (*i.e.*, starting at 2 min and finishing with 30 s) with other program variables similar produced similar increases in muscle strength and CSA (265).

Spectrum Repetition/Contrast Loading Combinations

Many different rep patterns have been used over the years. *Spectrum repetitions* refer to targeting low, moderate, and high reps within a workout. Accordingly, contrast loading takes places where heavy weights are lifted first followed by light/moderate weights, or are alternated. The rep variation can occur within an exercise or between exercises. Multiple fitness components are stressed per workout. For example, one system used by some is the 6–20 system. The athlete performs 6 sets of an exercise such as the squat. The first 3 sets are performed with heavy weights for 6 reps. The last 3 sets are performed with light weights for 20 reps. The goal of this contrast loading system is to recruit as many muscle fibers as possible with heavy weights and then stimulate metabolic stress with low weight and high reps. Another example is the 5-10-20 system. This system involves selecting three exercises that work the same muscle groups. The first exercise is performed with heavy weights for multiple sets of 5 reps; the second with moderate weights for multiple sets of 10 reps; and the third with light weights for multiple sets of 20 reps. A similar rationale is applied here where the lifter begins heavy and proceeds to light to work all areas of the spectrum. Many other variations to these exist. These techniques tend to be used more by bodybuilders where increasing muscle hypertrophy is the primary goal.

 Keeping a Training Log

A training log is a record or diary of all prescribed workouts. It includes every exercise performed, the weights, and numbers of repetitions, rest intervals, and room for general comments.

For example, if an athlete is feeling fatigued or ill, a comment could be left indicating that a poor workout may have been due to confounding variables. Keeping a detailed training log allows the coach and/or athlete to accurately monitor progress and evaluate the efficacy of the RT program. There is little room for error when each workout is accurately recorded. It provides a valuable assessment tool in addition to regularly scheduled assessments. A training log can be used as a motivational tool for the athlete. Viewing past workouts and drawing comparisons to current workouts can motivate the athlete to train harder.

SUMMARY POINTS

- Manipulation of the acute RT variables is critical to program design as programs must continually be altered to avoid training plateaus.
- Individualized training programs are most effective for progression. Performing a needs analysis reveals pertinent information taken into consideration during program design.
- Follow these steps for designing RT programs:
- Make sure athlete has been medically cleared and any known ailments/injuries have been disclosed.
- Determine training goals, needs of the sport, and strengths/weaknesses of the athlete.
- Plan out the yearly training schedule, *e.g.*, off-season, preseason, and in-season periods of time, and the training goals associated with each.
  - Determine the training frequency for RT. Also, decide on what other modalities will be trained simultaneously, *e.g.*, sprints, plyometrics, flexibility, aerobic training. The frequency must coincide with other forms of exercise as well as the demands of the sport (practices, games, and competitions).
  - Determine the workout structure based on the frequency, *i.e.*, total-body, upper/lower-body split, or split routine.
  - Determine the exercises to be used in the program and the sequence. These will be the structural and assistance exercises. Many exercises can be selected and a plan can be used to vary or cycle exercises throughout the training year.
  - Determine the intensity and volume for each exercise per training phase. The intensity could be based on a percent of 1 RM if a 1 RM is known via testing or can be used via a trial-and-error approach. The volume will correspond with the phase and accommodate intensity prescription. When multiple sets are used, set structure needs to be determined.
  - Determine the anticipated or intended repetition velocity for each exercise.
  - Determine the rest intervals in between sets and exercises.
  - Decide if any advanced techniques will be used.
  - Keep a training log. Tables 12.12 and 12.13 are examples of RT programs used by athletes.

Table 12.12 — 15-Week Wrestling Program

Monday	Sets × Reps (Week Numbers)
Power clean	3 × 6 (1–4); 5 (5–8); 4 × 5 (9–12); 5 × 3 (13–15)
Bench press	3 × 10–12 (1–4); 8–10 (5–8); 6–8 (9–12); 3–5 (13–15)
Close-grip bench press	3 × 10–12 (1–4); 8–10 (5–8); 6–8 (9–12); 3–5 (13–15)
Shoulder press	3 × 10–12 (1–4); 8–10 (5–12); 6–8 (13–15)
Pull-up progressions	
Wide-grip pull-ups	3 × 10–25 (1–5)
Towel pull-ups	3 × 10–15 (6–10)
Weighted pull-ups or	3 × 8–10 (11–15)
Unilateral pull-ups	
Internal/external rotations	3 × 10
MB Russian twist	3 × 25–50
Stability ball crunches	3 × 25–50
Manual resistance — neck	2 × 10
Wednesday	**Sets × Reps (Week Numbers)**
Back squat	3 × 10–12 (1–4); 8–10 (5–8); 4 × 6–8 (9–12); 5 × 3–5 (13–15)
Overhead squat	3 × 6–8 (1–7)
Front squat	3 × 6–8 (8–15)
Unilateral leg press	3 × 8–10 (1–7)
Split squat/lunge	3 × 8–10 (8–15)
Stiff-leg deadlift	3 × 10–12 (1–6); 8–10 (7–12); 6–8 (13–15)
Back extensions	3 × 15–20
Calf raise	3 × 15–20
Thick bar deadlift	3 × 10
Plyometric leg raise	3 × 15–25
Trunk stabilization ("plank")	3 × 1 min
Friday	**Sets × Reps (Week Numbers)**
Power snatch	3 × 6 (1–4); 5 (5–8); 4 × 5 (9–12); 5 × 3 (13–15)
Bent-over Barbell row	3 × 10–12 (1–4); 8–10 (5–8); 6–8 (9–12); 3–5 (13–15)
Close-grip lat pull-down	3 × 10–12 (1–5); 8–10 (6–10); 6–8 (11–15)
Weighted dips	3 × 12–15 (1–4); 10–12 (5–8); 8–10 (9–15)
Pullovers	3 × 8–10
Push-up progressions	
Basic	3 × 25–50 (1–5)
Stability ball	3 × 15–30 (6–10)
MB plyo push-ups	3 × 10 (11–15)
Partner plate pass	3 × 25
Weighted curl-ups	3 × 25
Wrist and reverse wrist curls	3 × 10

Intensity: 60%–85% of 1 RM periodized. Rest intervals: 2–3 minutes for structural exercises; 1–2 minutes for assistance exercises; 30 seconds for abs.

Adapted with permission from Hoffman JR, Ratamess NA. *A Practical Guide to Developing Resistance Training Programs*. 2nd ed. Monterey (CA): Coaches Choice Books; 2008. Ref. (266).

Chapter 12 Resistance Training Program Design   **327**

Table 12.13	15-Week 3-Day/Week Tennis Program
Monday	**Sets × Reps (Week Numbers)**
Hang clean	3 × 6 (1–5); 4 × 5 (6–10); 5 × 3 (11–15)
Back squat	3 × 10–12 (1–4); 8–10 (5–8); 4 × 6–8 (9–12); 5 × 3–5 (13–15)
DB bench press	3 × 10–12 (1–5); 8–10 (6–10); 6–8 (11–15)
Lunge	3 × 8–10
DB lateral raise	3 × 10–12
Pullovers	3 × 10–12
Trunk rotations	3 × 25
Internal/external rotations	3 × 10
Wednesday	**Sets × Reps (Week Numbers)**
Leg press	4 × 8–10 (1–5); 6–8 (6–10); 5–6 (11–15)
Stiff-leg deadlift	3 × 10–12 (1–8); 8–10 (9–15)
Front lat pull-downs	3 × 10–12 (1–5); 8–10 (6–10); 6–8 (11–15)
Calf raise	3 × 15–20
Reverse fly	3 × 10
Russian twist	3 × 25–50
Ulnar/radial deviation	2 × 10
Scapula stabilizer circuit	2 × 10
Friday	**Sets × Reps (Week Numbers)**
Hang snatch	3 × 6 (1–5); 4 × 5 (6–10); 5 × 3 (11–15)
Front squat	3 × 10–12 (1–5); 8–10 (6–10); 6–8 (11–15)
Unilateral DB row	3 × 10–12 (1–8); 8–10 (9–15)
Incline DB fly	3 × 10–12
Pullovers	3 × 10–12
Wrist/reverse curls	3 × 10
Internal/external rotations	3 × 10
Stability ball crunches	3 × 25–50

Note: Intensity: 60%–85% of 1 RM periodized. Rest intervals: 2–3 minutes for structural exercises; 1–2 minutes for assistance exercises; 30 seconds for abs.

Modified from Hoffman JR, Ratamess NA. *A Practical Guide to Developing Resistance Training Programs*. 2nd ed. Monterey (CA): Coaches Choice Books; 2008.

REVIEW QUESTIONS

1. A general to specific model of RT progression implies that
   a. Novice lifters require great variation in program design
   b. General programs work best in advanced to elite athletes
   c. Advanced to elite athletes require greater specificity in program design for progression
   d. None of the above

2. The program squat 3 × 6, bent-over row 3 × 10, leg press 3 × 8, bench press 3 × 8, reverse lunge 3 × 6, upright row 3 × 10 is an example of a(n)
   a. "Push/pull" workout
   b. Lower/upper-body exercise sequence
   c. Intensity-based sequence
   d. Muscle group split routine

3. The number of sets performed per workout will be affected by the
   a. Training frequency
   b. Muscle groups trained
   c. Training intensity
   d. All of the above

4. An athlete performs 4 sets of the deadlift exercise in the following manner: 225 × 10; 245 × 8; 265 × 6; 275 × 5. This is an example of
   a. A reverse pyramid
   b. An ascending pyramid
   c. A constant load/repetition system
   d. Progressive resistance exercise (DeLorme technique)

5. Training with an intentionally slow repetition speed is
   a. Most conducive to increasing muscle power
   b. Most effective for increasing maximal muscle strength
   c. Effective for increasing local muscle endurance
   d. None of the above

6. An athlete is following a program designed to peak muscle strength. Which of the following loading patterns would be most appropriate for his or her structural exercises?
   a. Weeks 1–12: 80% of 1 RM
   b. Weeks 1–3: 95%–100% of 1 RM, weeks 4–6: 95% of 1 RM, weeks 7–9: 90% of 1 RM, weeks 10–12: 80% of 1 RM
   c. Weeks 1–3: 80% of 1 RM, weeks 4–6: 90% of 1 RM, weeks 7–9: 95% of 1 RM, weeks 10–12: 95%–100% of 1 RM
   d. Weeks 1–4: 70% of 1 RM, weeks 5–8: 75% of 1 RM, weeks 9–12: 80% of 1 RM

7. A needs analysis consists of answering questions based upon goals and desired outcomes, assessments, access to equipment, health, and the demands of the sport.
   a. T
   b. F

8. Olympic lifts are examples of basic strength exercises.
   a. T
   b. F

9. Performing an exercise such as the barbell squat at the end of a lower-body workout versus first in a workout will not affect the number of repetitions performed or the amount of weight lifted.
   a. T
   b. F

10. Volume load is calculated by multiplying the load lifted (in kilograms) by the number of sets and repetitions.
    a. T
    b. F

11. Forced repetitions are those completed with assistance of a spotter beyond failure to increase strength, endurance, and hypertrophy.
    a. T
    b. F

12. Bands and chains can be added to multiple-joint exercises to be used for variable RT.
    a. T
    b. F

REFERENCES

1. Ratamess NA. Adaptations to anaerobic training programs. In: Baechle TR, Earle RW, editors. *Essentials of Strength Training and Conditioning*. 3rd ed. Champaign (IL): Human Kinetics; 2008. p. 93–119.
2. American College of Sports Medicine. Position stand: the recommended quantity and quality of exercise for developing and maintaining cardiorespiratory and muscular fitness, and flexibility in healthy adults. *Med Sci Sports Exerc*. 1998;30:975–91.
3. American College of Sports Medicine. Position stand: progression models in resistance training for healthy adults. *Med Sci Sports Exerc*. 2002;34:364–80.
4. American College of Sports Medicine. Position stand: progression models in resistance training for healthy adults. *Med Sci Sports Exerc*. 2009;41:687–708.
5. Fleck SJ, Kraemer WJ. *Designing Resistance Training Programs*. 2nd ed. Champaign (IL): Human Kinetics; 1997.
6. Kraemer WJ, Ratamess NA. Fundamentals of resistance training: progression and exercise prescription. *Med Sci Sports Exerc*. 2004;36:674–8.
7. McGuigan M, Ratamess NA. Strength. In: Ackland TR, Elliott BC, Bloomfield J, editors. *Applied Anatomy and Biomechanics in Sport*. 2nd ed. Champaign (IL): Human Kinetics; 2009. p. 119–54.
8. Hewett TE, Myer GD, Ford KR, Paterno MV, Quatman CE. Mechanisms, prediction, and prevention of ACL injuries: cut risk with three sharpened and validated tools. *J Orthop Res*. 2016;34:1843–55.
9. Wilk KE, Arrigo C, Andrews JR, Clancy WG. Rehabilitation after anterior cruciate ligament reconstruction in the female athlete. *J Athl Train*. 1999;34:177–93.
10. Childs SG. Pathogenesis of anterior cruciate ligament injury. *Orthop Nurs*. 2002;21:35–40.
11. Pappas E, Shiyko MP, Ford KR, Myer GD, Hewett TE. Biomechanical deficit profiles associated with ACL injury risk in female athletes. *Med Sci Sports Exerc*. 2016;48:107–13.
12. Hewett TE, Myer GD, Ford KR. Anterior cruciate ligament injuries in female athletes. Part 1: mechanisms and risk factors. *Am J Sports Med*. 2006;34:299–311.
13. Myer GD, Ford KR, Khoury J, Succop P, Hewett TE. Development and validation of a clinic-based prediction tool to identify female athletes at high risk for anterior cruciate ligament injury. *Am J Sports Med*. 2010;38:2025–33.
14. Myer GD, Ford KR, Khoury J, Succop P, Hewett TE. Biomechanics laboratory-based prediction algorithm to identify female athletes with high knee loads that increase risk of ACL injury. *Br J Sports Med*. 2011;45:245–52.

15. Myer GD, Sugimoto D, Thomas S, Hewett YE. The influence of age on the effectiveness of neuromuscular training to reduce anterior cruciate ligament injury in female athletes. *Am J Sports Med.* 2013;41:203–15.

16. Faigenbaum AD, Myer GD, Farrell A, et al. Integrative neuromuscular training and sex-specific fitness performance in 7-year-old children: an exploratory investigation. *J Athl Train.* 2014;49: 145–53.

17. Sugimoto D, Myer GD, Foss KDB, Hewett TE. Dosage effects of neuromuscular training intervention to reduce anterior cruciate ligament injuries in female athletes: meta- and sub-group analyses. *Sports Med.* 2014;44:551–62.

18. Dudley GA, Tesch PA, Miller BJ, Buchanan MD. Importance of eccentric actions in performance adaptations to resistance training. *Aviat Space Environ Med.* 1991;62:543–50.

19. Cormie, P, McBride JM, McCaulley GO. Validation of power measurement techniques in dynamic lower body resistance exercises. *J Appl Biomech.* 2007;23:103–18.

20. Doan BK, Newton RU, Marsit JL, et al. Effects of increased eccentric loading on bench press 1RM. *J Strength Cond Res.* 2002;16: 9–13.

21. Soares S, Ferreira-Junior JB, Pereira MC, et al. Dissociated time course of muscle damage recovery between single-and multi-joint exercises in highly resistance-trained men. *J Strength Cond Res.* 2015;29:2954–9.

22. Gentil P, Soares SRS, Fereira MC, et al. Effect of adding single-joint exercises to a multi-joint exercise resistance-training program on strength and hypertrophy in untrained subjects. *Appl Physiol Nutr Metab.* 2013;38:341–4.

23. Blackburn JR, Morrissey MC. The relationship between open and closed kinetic chain strength of the lower limb and jumping performance. *J Orthop Sports Phys Ther.* 1998;27:430–5.

24. Augustsson J, Esko A, Thomee R, Svantesson U. Weight training of the thigh muscles using closed vs. open kinetic chain exercises: a comparison of performance enhancement. *J Orthop Sports Phys Ther.* 1998;27:3–8.

25. McCurdy KW, Langford GA, Doscher MW, Wiley LP, Mallard KG. The effects of short-term unilateral and bilateral lower-body resistance training on measures of strength and power. *J Strength Cond Res.* 2005;19:9–15.

26. Munn J, Herbert RD, Gandevia SC. Contralateral effects of unilateral resistance training: a meta-analysis. *J Appl Physiol.* 2004;96:1861–6.

27. Ballor DL, Becque MD, Katch VL. Metabolic responses during hydraulic resistance exercise. *Med Sci Sports Exerc.* 1987;19: 363–7.

28. Kraemer WJ, Ratamess NA. Endocrine responses and adaptations to strength and power training. In: Komi PV, editor. *Strength and Power in Sport.* 2nd ed. Malden (MA): Blackwell Science; 2003. p. 361–86.

29. Cotterman ML, Darby LA, Skelly WA. Comparison of muscle force production using the Smith machine and free weights for bench press and squat exercises. *J Strength Cond Res.* 2005;19:169–76.

30. Boyer BT. A comparison of the effects of three strength training programs on women. *J Appl Sports Sci Res.* 1990;4:88–94.

31. Langford GA, McCurdy KW, Ernest JM, Doscher MW, Walters SD. Specificity of machine, barbell, and water-filled log bench press resistance training on measures of strength. *J Strength Cond Res.* 2007;21:1061–6.

32. Willoughby DS, Gillespie JW. A comparison of isotonic free weights and omnikinetic exercise machines on strength. *J Hum Mov Stud.* 1990;19:93–100.

33. Clark MA, Lucett SC. *NASM Essentials of Corrective Exercise Training.* Philadelphia (PA): Lippincott Williams & Wilkins–Wolters Kluwer; 2011. p. 197–209.

34. Page P, Frank CC, Lardner R. *Assessment and Treatment of Muscle Imbalance: The Janda Approach.* Champaign (IL): Human Kinetics; 2010. p. 5–245.

35. Calder AW, Chilibeck PD, Webber CE, Sale DG. Comparison of whole and split weight training routines in young women. *Can J Appl Physiol.* 1994;19:185–99.

36. Campbell WW, Trappe TA, Jozsi AC, et al. Dietary protein adequacy and lower body versus whole body resistive training in older humans. *J Physiol.* 2002;542:631–42.

37. Simao R, de Salles BF, Figueiredo T, Dias I, Willardson JW. Exercise order in resistance training. *Sports Med.* 2012;42:251–65.

38. Gentil P, Oliveira E, Junior VAR, Carmo J, Bottaro M. Effects of exercise order on upper-body muscle activation and exercise performance. *J Strength Cond Res.* 2007;21:1082–6.

39. Sforzo GA, Touey PR. Manipulating exercise order affects muscular performance during a resistance exercise training session. *J Strength Cond Res.* 1996;10:20–4.

40. Simao R, Farinatti PTV, Polito MD, Maior AS, Fleck SJ. Influence of exercise order on the number of repetitions performed and perceived exertion during resistive exercises. *J Strength Cond Res.* 2005;19:152–6.

41. Simao R, Farinatti PTV, Polito MD, Viveiros L, Fleck SJ. Influence of exercise order on the number of repetitions performed and perceived exertion during resistance exercise in women. *J Strength Cond Res.* 2007;21:23–8.

42. Spreuwenberg LPB, Kraemer WJ, Spiering BA, et al. Influence of exercise order in a resistance-training exercise session. *J Strength Cond Res.* 2006;20:141–4.

43. Miranda H, Simao R, Vigario PS, et al. Exercise order interacts with rest interval during upper-body resistance exercise. *J Strength Cond Res.* 2010;24:1573–7.

44. Miranda H, Figueiredo T, Rodrigues B, Paz GA, Simao R. Influence of exercise order on repetition performance among all possible combinations on resistance training. *Res Sports Med.* 2013;21:355–66.

45. Ratamess NA, Chiarello CM, Sacco AJ, et al. The effects of rest interval length manipulation of the first upper-body resistance exercise in sequence on acute performance of subsequent exercises in men and women. *J Strength Cond Res.* 2012;26:2929–38.

46. Baker D, Newton RU. Acute effect on power output of alternating an agonist and antagonist muscle exercise during complex training. *J Strength Cond Res.* 2005;19:202–5.

47. Soncin R, Pennone J, Guimaraes TM, et al. Influence of exercise order on electromyographic activity during upper body resistance training. *J Hum Kinet.* 2014;44:203–9.

48. Farinatti PTV, Simao R, Monteiro WD, Fleck SJ. Influence of exercise order on oxygen uptake during strength training in young women. *J Strength Cond Res.* 2009;23:1037–44.

49. Farinatti PTV, da Silva NSL, Monteiro WD. Influence of exercise order on the number of repetitions, oxygen uptake, and rate of perceived exertion during strength training in younger and older women. *J Strength Cond Res.* 2013;27:776–85.

50. Ratamess NA, Rosenberg JG, Kang J, et al. Acute oxygen uptake and resistance exercise performance using different rest interval lengths: the influence of maximal aerobic capacity and exercise sequence. *J Strength Cond Res.* 2014;28:1875–88.

51. Hansen S, Kvorning T, Kjaer M, Szogaard G. The effect of short-term strength training on human skeletal muscle: the importance

of physiologically elevated hormone levels. *Scand J Med Sci Sports.* 2001;11:347–54.

52. Avelar A, Ribeiro AS, Nunes JP, et al. Effects of order of resistance training exercises on muscle hypertrophy in young adult men. *Appl Physiol Nutr Metab.* 2019;44:420–4.

53. Augustsson J, Thomee R, Hornstedt P, et al. Effect of pre-exhaustion exercise on lower-extremity muscle activation during a leg press exercise. *J Strength Cond Res.* 2003;17:411–6.

54. Soares EG, Brown LE, Gomes WA, et al. Comparison between pre-exhaustion and traditional exercise order on muscle activation and performance in trained men. *J Sports Sci Med.* 2016;15:111–7.

55. Vilaca-Alves J, Geraldes L, Fernandes HM, et al. Effects of pre-exhausting the biceps brachii muscle on the performance of the front lat pull-down exercise using different handgrip positions. *J Hum Kinet.* 2014;42:157–63.

56. Brennecke A, Guimaraes TM, Leone R, et al. Neuromuscular activity during bench press exercise performed with and without the preexhaustion method. *J Strength Cond Res.* 2009;23:1933–40.

57. Anderson T, Kearney JT. Effects of three resistance training programs on muscular strength and absolute and relative endurance. *Res Q Exerc Sport.* 1982;53:1–7.

58. Cormie P, McGuigan MR, Newton RU. Adaptations in athletic performance after ballistic power versus strength training. *Med Sci Sports Exerc.* 2010;42:1582–98.

59. Zaras N, Spengos K, Methenitis S, et al. Effects of strength vs. ballistic-power training on throwing performance. *J Sports Sci Med.* 2013;12:130–7.

60. Rhea MR, Alvar BA, Burkett LN, Ball SD. A meta-analysis to determine the dose response for strength development. *Med Sci Sports Exerc.* 2003;35:456–64.

61. Jones K, Bishop P, Hunter G, Fleisig G. The effects of varying resistance-training loads on intermediate- and high-velocity-specific adaptations. *J Strength Cond Res.* 2001;15:349–56.

62. Häkkinen K, Alen M, Komi PV. Changes in isometric force-and relaxation-time, electromyographic and muscle fibre characteristics of human skeletal muscle during strength training and detraining. *Acta Physiol Scand.* 1985;125:573–85.

63. Hoffman JR, Kang J. Strength changes during an in-season resistance-training program for football. *J Strength Cond Res.* 2003;17:109–14.

64. Peterson MD, Rhea MR, Alvar BA. Maximizing strength development in athletes: a meta-analysis to determine the dose-response relationship. *J Strength Cond Res.* 2004;18:377–82.

65. Mangine GT, Hoffman JR, Gonzalez AM, et al. The effect of training volume and intensity on improvements in muscular strength and size in resistance-trained men. *Physiol Rep.* 2015;3:e12472.

66. Schoenfeld BJ, Ratamess NA, Peterson MD, Contreras B, Tiryaki-Sonmez G, Alvar BA. Effects of different volume-equated resistance training loading strategies on muscular adaptations in well-trained men. *J Strength Cond Res.* 2014;28:2909–18.

67. Schoenfeld BJ, Contreras B, Vigotsky AD, Peterson M. Differential effects of heavy versus moderate loads on measures of strength and hypertrophy in resistance-trained men. *J Sports Sci Med.* 2016;15:715–22.

68. Zatsiorsky V. *Science and Practice of Strength Training.* Champaign (IL): Human Kinetics; 1995.

69. Sakamoto A, Sinclair PJ. Effect of movement velocity on the relationship between training load and the number of repetitions of bench press. *J Strength Cond Res.* 2006;20:523–7.

70. Shimano T, Kraemer WJ, Spiering BA, et al. Relationship between the number of repetitions and selected percentages of one repetition maximum in free weight exercises in trained and untrained men. *J Strength Cond Res.* 2006;20:819–23.

71. Baechle TR, Earle RW, Wathen D. Resistance training. In: Baechle TR, Earle RW, editors. *Essentials of Strength Training and Conditioning.* 3rd ed. Champaign (IL): Human Kinetics; 2008. p. 381–412.

72. Morales J, Sobonya S. Use of submaximal repetition tests for predicting 1-RM strength in class athletes. *J Strength Cond Res.* 1996;10:186–9.

73. Mayhew JL, Ball TE, Arnold MD, Bowen JC. Relative muscular endurance performance as a predictor of bench press strength in college men and women. *J Appl Sport Sci Res.* 1992;6:200–6.

74. Mayhew JL, Ware JS, Bemben MG, et al. The NFL-225 test as a measure of bench press strength in college football players. *J Strength Cond Res.* 1999;13:130–4.

75. Kraemer WJ, Fleck SJ, Maresh CM, et al. Acute hormonal responses to a single bout of heavy resistance exercise in trained power lifters and untrained men. *Can J Appl Physiol.* 1999;24:524–37.

76. Ware JS, Clemens CT, Mayhew JL, Johnston TJ. Muscular endurance repetitions to predict bench press and squat strength in college football players. *J Strength Cond Res.* 1995;9:99–103.

77. Kraemer WJ, Fry AC, Ratamess NA, French DN. Strength testing: development and evaluation of methodology. In: Maud PJ, Foster C, editors. *Physiological Assessments of Human Performance.* 2nd ed. Champaign (IL): Human Kinetics; 2006. p. 119–50.

78. Hoeger WK, Barette SL, Hale DF, Hopkins DR. Relationship between repetitions and selected percentages of one repetition maximum. *J Appl Sport Sci Res.* 1990;1:11–3.

79. Campos GER, Luecke TJ, Wendeln HK, et al. Muscular adaptations in response to three different resistance-training regimens: specificity of repetition maximum training zones. *Eur J Appl Physiol.* 2002;88:50–60.

80. Behm DG, Reardon G, Fitzgerald J, Drinkwater E. The effect of 5, 10, and 20 repetition maximums on the recovery of voluntary and evoked contractile properties. *J Strength Cond Res.* 2002;16:209–18.

81. Cronin J, McNair PJ, Marshall RN. Force-velocity analysis of strength-training techniques and load: implications for training strategy and research. *J Strength Cond Res.* 2003;17:148–55.

82. Dalziel WM, Neal RJ, Watts MC. A comparison of peak power in the shoulder press and shoulder throw. *J Sci Med Sport.* 2002;5:229–35.

83. Baker D, Nance S, Moore M. The load that maximizes the average mechanical power output during explosive bench press throws in highly trained athletes. *J Strength Cond Res.* 2001;15:20–4.

84. Baker D, Nance S, Moore M. The load that maximizes the average mechanical power output during jump squats in power-trained athletes. *J Strength Cond Res.* 2001;15:92–7.

85. Kawamori N, Haff GG. The optimal training load for the development of muscular power. *J Strength Cond Res.* 2004;18:675–84.

86. Wilson GJ, Newton RU, Murphy AJ, Humphries BJ. The optimal training load for the development of dynamic athletic performance. *Med Sci Sports Exerc.* 1993;25:1279–86.

87. Cormie P, McCaulley GO, McBride JM. Power versus strength-power jump squat training: influence on the load-power relationship. *Med Sci Sports Exerc.* 2007;39:996–1003.

88. McBride JM, Triplett-McBride T, Davie A, Newton RU. The effect of heavy- vs. light-load jump squats on the development of strength, power, and speed. *J Strength Cond Res.* 2002;16:75–82.

89. Elliott BC, Wilson GJ, Kerr GK. A biomechanical analysis of the sticking region in the bench press. *Med Sci Sports Exerc.* 1989;21:450–62.

90. Newton RU, Kraemer WJ, Häkkinen K, Humphries BJ, Murphy AJ. Kinematics, kinetics, and muscle activation during explosive upper body movements. *J Appl Biomech*. 1996;12:31–43.

91. Mangine GT, Ratamess NA, Hoffman JR, Faigenbaum AD, Kang J, Chilakos A. The effects of combined ballistic and heavy resistance training on maximal lower- and upper-body strength in recreationally-trained men. *J Strength Cond Res*. 2008;22:132–9.

92. Siegel JA, Gilders RM, Staron RS, Hagerman FC. Human muscle power output during upper- and lower-body exercises. *J Strength Cond Res*. 2002;16:173–8.

93. Zink AJ, Perry AC, Robertson BL, Roach KE, Signorile JF. Peak power, ground reaction forces, and velocity during the squat exercise performed at different loads. *J Strength Cond Res*. 2006;20:658–64.

94. Kawamori N, Crum AJ, Blumert PA, et al. Influence of different relative intensities on power output during the hang power clean: identification of the optimal load. *J Strength Cond Res*. 2005;19:698–708.

95. Fink J, Kikuchi N, Nakazato K. Effects of rest intervals and training loads on metabolic stress and muscle hypertrophy. *Clin Physiol Funct Imaging*. 2018;38:261–8.

96. Schoenfeld BJ, Grgic J, Ogborn D, Krieger JW. Strength and hypertrophy adaptations between low- vs. high-load resistance training: a systematic review and meta-analysis. *J Strength Cond Res*. 2017;31:3508–23.

97. Schoenfeld BJ, Peterson MD, Ogborn D, Contreras B, Sonmez GT. Effects of low- vs. high-load resistance training on muscle strength and hypertrophy in well-trained men. *J Strength Cond Res*. 2015;29:2954–63.

98. Winwood PW, Keogh JWL, Harris NK. The strength and conditioning practices of strongman competitors. *J Strength Cond Res*. 2011;25:3118–28.

99. Ross RE, Ratamess NA, Hoffman JR, Faigenbaum AD, Kang J, Chilakos A. The effects of treadmill sprint training and resistance training on maximal running velocity and power. *J Strength Cond Res*. 2009;23:385–94.

100. Winchester JB, McBride JM, Maher MA, et al. Eight weeks of ballistic exercise improves power independently of changes in strength and muscle fiber type expression. *J Strength Cond Res*. 2008;22:1728–34.

101. Harris NK, Cronin JB, Hopkins WG, Hansen KT. Squat jump training at maximal power loads vs. heavy loads: effect on sprint ability. *J Strength Cond Res*. 2008;22:1742–9.

102. Vissing K, Brink M, Lonbro S, et al. Muscle adaptations to plyometric vs. resistance training in untrained young men. *J Strength Cond Res*. 2008;22:1799–810.

103. Bompa TO, Haff GG. *Periodization: Theory and Methodology of Training*. 5th ed. Champaign (IL): Human Kinetics; 2009.

104. Davies T, Orr R, Halaki M, Hackett D. Effect of training leading to repetition failure on muscular strength: a systematic review and meta-analysis. *Sports Med*. 2016;46:487–502.

105. Benson C, Docherty D, Brandenburg J. Acute neuromuscular responses to resistance training performed at different loads. *J Sci Med Sport*. 2006;9:135–42.

106. Peterson MD, Rhea MR, Alvar BA. Applications of the dose-response for muscular strength development: a review of meta-analytic efficacy and reliability for designing training prescription. *J Strength Cond Res*. 2005;19:950–8.

107. Rooney KJ, Herbert RD, Balnave RJ. Fatigue contributes to the strength training stimulus. *Med Sci Sports Exerc*. 1994;26:1160–4.

108. Drinkwater EJ, Lawton TW, Lindsell RP, et al. Training leading to repetition failure enhances bench press strength gains in elite junior athletes. *J Strength Cond Res*. 2005;19:382–8.

109. Izquierdo M, Ibanez J, Gonzalez-Badillo JJ, et al. Differential effects of strength training leading to failure versus not to failure on hormonal responses, strength, and muscle power gains. *J Appl Physiol*. 2006;100:1647–56.

110. Peterson MD, Pistilli E, Haff GG, Hoffman EP, Gordon PM. Progression of volume load and muscular adaptation during resistance exercise. *Eur J Appl Physiol*. 2011;111:1063–71.

111. Linnamo V, Pakarinen A, Komi PV, Kraemer WJ, Häkkinen K. Acute hormonal responses to submaximal and maximal heavy resistance and explosive exercises in men and women. *J Strength Cond Res*. 2005;19:566–71.

112. Goto K, Nagasawa M, Yanagisawa O, et al. Muscular adaptations to combinations of high- and low-intensity resistance exercises. *J Strength Cond Res*. 2004;18:730–7.

113. Gonzalez-Badillo JJ, Gorostiaga EM, Arellano R, Izquierdo M. Moderate resistance training volume produces more favorable strength gains than high or low volumes during a short-term training cycle. *J Strength Cond Res*. 2005;19:689–97.

114. Ralston GW, Kilgore L, Wyatt FB, Baker JS. The effect of weekly set volume on strength gain: a meta-analysis. *Sports Med*. 2017;47:2585–601.

115. Schoenfeld BJ, Ogborn D, Krieger JW. Dose-response relationship between weekly resistance training volume and increases in muscle mass: a systematic review and meta-analysis. *J Sports Sci*. 2017;35:1073–82.

116. Amirthalingham T, Mavros Y, Wilson GC, et al. Effects of a modified German Volume Training program on muscular hypertrophy and strength. *J Strength Cond Res*. 2017;31:3109–19.

117. Hackett DA, Amirthalingham T, Mitchell L, et al. Effects of a 12-week modified German Volume Training program on muscle strength and hypertrophy — a pilot study. *Sports*. 2018;6:E7.

118. Durell DL, Pujol TJ, Barnes JT. A survey of the scientific data and training methods utilized by collegiate strength and conditioning coaches. *J Strength Cond Res*. 2003;17:368–73.

119. Schlumberger A, Stec J, Schmidtbleicher D. Single- vs. multiple-set strength training in women. *J Strength Cond Res*. 2001;15:284–9.

120. Berger RA. Comparison of the effect of various weight training loads on strength. *Res Q Exerc Sport*. 1963;36:141–6.

121. Borst SE, Dehoyos DV, Garzarella L, et al. Effects of resistance training on insulin-like growth factor-1 and IGF binding proteins. *Med Sci Sports Exerc*. 2001;33:648–53.

122. Messier SP, Dill ME. Alterations in strength and maximal oxygen uptake consequent to Nautilus circuit weight training. *Res Q Exerc Sport*. 1985;56:345–51.

123. Radaelli R, Fleck SJ, Leite T, et al. Dose-response of 1,3, and 5 sets of resistance exercise on strength, local muscular endurance, and hypertrophy. *J Strength Cond Res*. 2015;29:1349–58.

124. Sanborn K, Boros R, Hruby J, et al. Short-term performance effects of weight training with multiple sets not to failure vs. a single set to failure in women. *J Strength Cond Res*. 2000;14:328–31.

125. Sooneste H, Tanimoto M, Kakigi R, Saga N, Katamoto S. Effects of training volume on strength and hypertrophy in young men. *J Strength Cond Res*. 2013;27:8–13.

126. Kraemer WJ. A series of studies-the physiological basis for strength training in American football: fact over philosophy. *J Strength Cond Res*. 1997;11:131–42.

127. Kraemer WJ, Ratamess N, Fry AC, et al. Influence of resistance training volume and periodization on physiological and performance adaptations in college women tennis players. *Am J Sports Med.* 2000;28:626–33.

128. Kramer JB, Stone MH, O'Bryant HS, et al. Effects of single vs. multiple sets of weight training: impact of volume, intensity, and variation. *J Strength Cond Res.* 1997;11:143–7.

129. Marshall PWM, McEwen M, Robbins DW. Strength and neuromuscular adaptation following one, four, and eight sets of high intensity resistance exercise in trained males. *Eur J Appl Physiol.* 2011;111:3007–16.

130. Marx JO, Ratamess NA, Nindl BC, et al. The effects of single-set vs. periodized multiple-set resistance training on muscular performance and hormonal concentrations in women. *Med Sci Sports Exerc.* 2001;33:635–43.

131. Paulsen G, Myklestad D, Raastad T. The influence of volume of exercise on early adaptations to strength training. *J Strength Cond Res.* 2003;17:113–8.

132. Rhea MR, Alvar BA, Ball SD, Burkett LN. Three sets of weight training superior to 1 set with equal intensity for eliciting strength. *J Strength Cond Res.* 2002;16:525–9.

133. Hass CJ, Garzarella L, Dehoyos D, Pollock ML. Single versus multiple sets and long-term recreational weightlifters. *Med Sci Sports Exerc.* 2000;32:235–42.

134. Kemmler WK, Lauber D, Engelke K, Weineck J. Effects of single- vs. multiple-set resistance training on maximum strength and body composition in trained postmenopausal women. *J Strength Cond Res.* 2004;18:689–94.

135. Frohlich M, Emrich E, Schmidtbleicher D. Outcome effects of single-set versus multiple-set training—an advanced replication study. *Res Sports Med.* 2010;18:157–75.

136. Galvao DA, Taaffe DR. Single- vs. multiple-set resistance training: recent developments in the controversy. *J Strength Cond Res.* 2004;18:660–7.

137. Krieger JW. Single versus multiple sets of resistance exercise: a meta-regression. *J Strength Cond Res.* 2009;23:1890–901.

138. Krieger JW. Single vs. multiple sets of resistance exercise for muscle hypertrophy: a meta-analysis. *J Strength Cond Res.* 2010;24:1150–9.

139. Wolfe BL, LeMura LM, Cole PJ. Quantitative analysis of single- vs. multiple-set programs in resistance training. *J Strength Cond Res.* 2004;18:35–47.

140. Landin D, Nelson AG. Early phase strength development: a four-week training comparison of different programs. *J Strength Cond Res.* 2007;21:1113–6.

141. Munn J, Herbert RD, Hancock MJ, Gandevia SC. Resistance training for strength: effect of number of sets and contraction speed. *Med Sci Sports Exerc.* 2005;37:1622–6.

142. McBride JM, Blaak JB, Triplett-McBride T. Effect of resistance exercise volume and complexity on EMG strength and regional body composition. *Eur J Appl Physiol.* 2003;90:626–32.

143. Ronnestad BR, Egeland W, Kvamme NH, et al. Dissimilar effects of one- and three-set strength training on strength and muscle mass gains in upper and lower body in untrained subjects. *J Strength Cond Res.* 2007;21:157–63.

144. Kelly SB, Brown LE, Coburn JW, et al. The effect of single versus multiple sets on strength. *J Strength Cond Res.* 2007;21:1003–6.

145. Schoenfeld BJ, Contreras B, Krieger J, et al. Resistance training volume enhances muscle hypertrophy but not strength in trained men. *Med Sci Sports Exerc.* 2019;51:94–103.

146. DeLorme TL, Watkins AL. Technics of progressive resistance exercise. *Arch Phys Med Rehabil.* 1948;29:263–73.

147. Poliquin C. *Modern Trends in Strength Training. Volume 1: Reps and Sets.* 2nd ed. Canada: CharlesPoliquin.net; 2001.

148. Angieri V, Ugrinowitsch C, Libardi CA. Crescent pyramid and drop-set systems do not promote greater strength gains, muscle hypertrophy, and changes on muscle architecture compared with traditional resistance training in well-trained men. *Eur J Appl Physiol.* 2017;117:359–69.

149. Zinovieff AN. Heavy-resistance exercises the "Oxford technique". *Br J Phys Med.* 1951;14:129–32.

150. Fish DE, Krabak BJ, Johnson-Greene D, DeLateur BJ. Optimal resistance training: comparison of DeLorme with Oxford techniques. *Arch Phys Med Rehabil.* 2003;82:903–9.

151. De Salles BF, Simao R, Miranda H, et al. Strength increases in upper and lower body are larger with longer inter-set rest intervals in trained men. *J Sci Med Sport.* 2010;13:429–33.

152. Willardson JM, Burkett LN. A comparison of 3 different rest intervals on the exercise volume completed during a workout. *J Strength Cond Res.* 2005;19:23–6.

153. Miranda H, Fleck SJ, Simao R, et al. Effect of two different rest period lengths on the number of repetitions performed during resistance training. *J Strength Cond Res.* 2007;21:1032–6.

154. Ratamess NA, Falvo MJ, Mangine GT, Hoffman JR, Faigenbaum AD, Kang J. The effect of rest interval length on metabolic responses to the bench press exercise. *Eur J Appl Physiol.* 2007;100:1–17.

155. Ratamess NA, Chiarello CM, Sacco AJ, et al. The effects of rest interval length on acute bench press performance: the influence of gender and muscle strength. *J Strength Cond Res.* 2012;26:1817–26.

156. Richmond SR, Godard MP. The effects of varied rest periods between sets to failure using the bench press in recreationally trained men. *J Strength Cond Res.* 2004;18:846–9.

157. Willardson JM, Burkett LN. The effect of rest interval length on bench press performance with heavy vs. light loads. *J Strength Cond Res.* 2006;20:396–9.

158. Willardson JM, Burkett LN. The effect of rest interval length on the sustainability of squat and bench press repetitions. *J Strength Cond Res.* 2006;20:400–3.

159. Senna G, Willardson JM, de Salles BF, et al. The effect of rest interval length on multi and single-joint exercise performance and perceived exertion. *J Strength Cond Res.* 2011;25:3157–62.

160. Faigenbaum AD, Ratamess NA, McFarland J, et al. Effect of rest interval length on bench press performance in boys, teens, and men. *Pediatr Exerc Sci.* 2008;20:457–69.

161. De Salles BF, Simao R, Miranda F, et al. Rest interval between sets in strength training. *Sports Med.* 2009;39:765–77.

162. Schoenfeld BJ, Pope ZK, Benik FM, et al. Longer interset rest periods enhance muscle strength and hypertrophy in resistance-trained men. *J Strength Cond Res.* 2016;30:1805–12.

163. Pincivero DM, Campy RM. The effects of rest interval length and training on quadriceps femoris muscle. Part I: knee extensor torque and muscle fatigue. *J Sports Med Phys Fitness.* 2004;44:111–8.

164. Pincivero DM, Lephart SM, Karunakara RG. Effects of rest interval on isokinetic strength and functional performance after short-term high intensity training. *Br J Sports Med.* 1997;31:229–34.

165. Robinson JM, Stone MH, Johnson RL, Penland CM, Warren BJ, Lewis RD. Effects of different weight training exercise/rest intervals on strength, power, and high intensity exercise endurance. *J Strength Cond Res.* 1995;9:216–21.

166. Ahtiainen JP, Pakarinen A, Alen M, Kraemer WJ, Häkkinen K. Short vs. long rest period between the sets in hypertrophic resistance training: influence on muscle strength, size, and hormonal adaptations in trained men. *J Strength Cond Res*. 2005;19:572–82.

167. Buresh R, Berg K, French J. The effect of resistive exercise rest interval on hormonal response, strength, and hypertrophy with training. *J Strength Cond Res*. 2009;23:62–71.

168. Willardson JM, Burkett LN. The effect of different rest intervals between sets on volume components and strength gains. *J Strength Cond Res*. 2008;22:146–52.

169. Grgic J, Lazinica B, Mikulic P, Krieger JW, Schoenfeld BJ. The effects of short versus long inter-set rest intervals in resistance training on measures of muscle hypertrophy: a systematic review. *Eur J Sport Sci*. 2017;17:983–93.

170. Henselmans M, Schoenfeld BJ. The effect of inter-set rest intervals on resistance exercise-induced muscle hypertrophy. *Sports Med*. 2014;44:1635–43.

171. Kanehisa H, Miyashita M. Specificity of velocity in strength training. *Eur J Appl Physiol*. 1983;52:104–6.

172. Schilling BK, Falvo MJ, Chiu LZF. Force-velocity, impulse-momentum relationships: implications for efficacy of purposely slow resistance training. *J Sports Sci Med*. 2008;7:299–304.

173. Mookerjee S, Ratamess NA. Comparison of strength differences and joint action durations between full and partial range-of-motion bench press exercise. *J Strength Cond Res*. 1999;13:76–81.

174. Tran QT, Docherty D, Behm D. The effects of varying time under tension and volume load on acute neuromuscular responses. *Eur J Appl Physiol*. 2006;98:402–10.

175. Hatfield DL, Kraemer WJ, Spiering BA, et al. The impact of velocity of movement on performance factors in resistance exercise. *J Strength Cond Res*. 2006;20:760–6.

176. Keogh JWL, Wilson GJ, Weatherby RP. A cross-sectional comparison of different resistance training techniques in the bench press. *J Strength Cond Res*. 1999;13:247–58.

177. Gentil P, Oliveira E, Bottaro M. Time under tension and blood lactate response during four different resistance training methods. *J Physiol Anthropol*. 2006;25:339–44.

178. Wickwire PJ, McLester JR, Green JM, Crews TR. Acute heart rate, blood pressure, and RPE responses during super slow vs. traditional machine resistance training protocols using small muscle group exercises. *J Strength Cond Res*. 2009;23:72–9.

179. Keeler LK, Finkelstein LH, Miller W, Fernhall B. Early-phase adaptations of traditional-speed vs. superslow resistance training on strength and aerobic capacity in sedentary individuals. *J Strength Cond Res*. 2001;15:309–14.

180. Gonzalez-Badillo JJ, Rodriguez-Rosell D, Sanchez-Medina L, Gorostiaga EM, Pareja-Bianco F. Maximal intended velocity training induces greater gains in bench press performance than deliberately slower half-velocity training. *Eur J Sport Sci*. 2014;14:772–81.

181. Pareja-Blanco F, Rodriguez-Rosell D, Sanchez-Medina L, Gorostiaga EM, Gonzalez-Badillo JJ. Effect of movement velocity during resistance training on neuromuscular performance. *Int J Sports Med*. 2014;35:916–24.

182. Rana SR, Chleboun GS, Gilders RM, et al. Comparison of early phase adaptations for traditional strength and endurance, and low velocity resistance training programs in college-aged women. *J Strength Cond Res*. 2008;22:119–27.

183. Neils CM, Udermann BE, Brice GA, Winchester JB, McGuigan MR. Influence of contraction velocity in untrained individuals over the initial early phase of resistance training. *J Strength Cond Res*. 2005;19:883–7.

184. Davies TB, Kuang K, Orr R, Halaki M, Hackett D. Effect of movement velocity during resistance training on dynamic muscular strength: a systematic review and meta-analysis. *Sports Med*. 2017;47:1603–17.

185. Morrissey MC, Harman EA, Frykman PN, Han KH. Early phase differential effects of slow and fast barbell squat training. *Am J Sports Med*. 1998;26:221–30.

186. Hay JG, Andrews JG, Vaughan CL. Effects of lifting rate on elbow torques exerted during arm curl exercises. *Med Sci Sports Exerc*. 1983;15:63–71.

187. Beckham GK, Olmeda JJ, Flores AJ, et al. Relationship between maximum pull-up repetitions and first repetition mean concentric velocity. *J Strength Cond Res*. 2018;32:1831–7.

188. Behm DG, Sale DG. Intended rather than actual movement velocity determines the velocity-specific training response. *J Appl Physiol*. 1993;74:359–68.

189. Verkhoshansky Y, Siff M. *Supertraining*. 6th ed. Ultimate Athlete Concepts; 2009. p. 393–400.

190. Jones K, Hunter G, Fleisig G, Escamilla R, Lemak L. The effects of compensatory acceleration on upper-body strength and power in collegiate football players. *J Strength Cond Res*. 1999;13:99–105.

191. Mann JB, Ivey PA, Sayers SP. Velocity-based training in football. *Strength Cond J*. 2015;37:52–7.

192. Weakley J, Ramirez-Lopez C, McLaren S, et al. The effects of 10%, 20%, and 30% velocity loss thresholds on kinetic, kinematic, and repetition characteristics during the barbell back squat. *Int J Sports Physiol Perform*. 2019;16:1–23.

193. Fahs CA, Rossow LM, Zourdos MC. Analysis of factors relate to back squat concentric velocity. *J Strength Cond Res*. 2017;32:2435–41.

194. Fahs CA, Blumkaitis JC, Rossow LM. Factors related to average concentric velocity of four barbell exercises at various loads. *J Strength Cond Res*. 2019;33:597–605.

195. Dorrell HF, Smith MF, Gee TI. Comparison of velocity-based and traditional percentage-based loading methods on maximal strength and power adaptations. *J Strength Cond Res*. 2019;34(1):46–53.

196. Pareja-Blanco F, Rodriguez-Rosell D, Sanchez-Medina L, et al. Effects of velocity loss during resistance training on athletic performance, strength gains and muscle adaptations. *Scand J Med Sci Sports*. 2017;27:724–35.

197. Häkkinen K. Neuromuscular fatigue and recovery in women at different ages during heavy resistance loading. *Electromyogr Clin Neurophysiol*. 1995;35:403–13.

198. Candow DG, Burke DG. Effect of short-term equal-volume resistance training with different workout frequency on muscle mass and strength in untrained men and women. *J Strength Cond Res*. 2007;21:204–7.

199. Graves JE, Pollock ML, Leggett SH, et al. Effect of reduced training frequency on muscular strength. *Int J Sports Med*. 1988;9:316–9.

200. Hunter GR. Changes in body composition, body build, and performance associated with different weight training frequencies in males and females. *J Strength Cond Res*. 1985;7:26–8.

201. Hoffman JR, Kraemer WJ, Fry AC, Deschenes M, Kemp DM. The effect of self-selection for frequency of training in a winter conditioning program for football. *J Appl Sport Sci Res*. 1990;3:76–82.

202. Häkkinen K, Kallinen M. Distribution of strength training volume into one or two daily sessions and neuromuscular

203. Thomas MH, Burns SP. Increasing lean mass and strength: a comparison of high frequency strength training to lower frequency strength training. *Int J Exerc Sci*. 2016;9:159–67.

204. Schoenfeld BJ, Ogborn D, Krieger JW. Effects of resistance training frequency on measures of muscle hypertrophy: a systematic review and meta-analysis. *Sports Med*. 2016;46:1689–97.

205. Wernbom M, Augustsson J, Thomee R. The influence of frequency, intensity, volume and mode of strength training on whole muscle cross-sectional area in humans. *Sports Med*. 2007;37:225–64.

206. Gadomski SJ, Ratamess NA, Cutrufello PT. Range of motion adaptations in powerlifters. *J Strength Cond Res*. 2018;32:3020–8.

207. Winwood PW, Dudson MK, Wilson D, et al. Tapering practices of strongman athletes. *J Strength Cond Res*. 2018;32:1181–96.

208. Rebullido Rial T, Chulvi-Medrano I, Faigenbaum AD, Stracciolini A. Pelvic floor dysfunction in female athletes. *Strength Cond J*. 2020;42(4):82–92.

209. Wu JM, Vaughan CP, Goode PS, Redden DT, Burgio KL, Richter HE, Markland AD. Prevalence and trends of symptomatic pelvic floor disorders in U.S. women. *Obstet Gynecol*. 2014;123:141–8.

210. Cacciari LP, Dumoulin C, Hay-Smith EJ. Pelvic floor muscle training versus no treatment, or inactive control treatments, for urinary incontinence in women: a Cochrane systematic review abridged republication. *Braz J Phys Ther*. 2019;23:93–107.

211. Li C, Gong Y, Wang B. The efficacy of pelvic floor muscle training for pelvic organ prolapse: a systematic review and meta-analysis. *Int Urogynecol J*. 2016;27:981–92.

212. Talasz H, Himmer-Perschak G, Marth E, Fischer-Colbrie J, Hoefner E, Lechleitner M. Evaluation of pelvic floor muscle function in a random group of adult women in Austria. *Int Urogynecol J Pelvic Floor Dysfunct*. 2008;19:131–5.

213. Tibaek S, Dehlendorff C. Pelvic floor muscle function in women with pelvic floor dysfunction: a retrospective chart review, 1992-2008. *Int Urogynecol J*. 2014;25:663–9.

214. Neels H, De Wachter S, Wyndaele JJ, Van Aggelpoel T, Vermandel A. Common errors made in attempt to contract the pelvic floor muscles in women early after delivery: a prospective observational study. *Eur J Obstet Gynecol Reprod Biol*. 2018;220:113–7.

215. Ben Ami N, Dar G. What is the most effective verbal instruction for correctly contracting the pelvic floor muscles? *Neurourol Urodyn*. 2018;37:2904–10.

216. Ratamess NA, Rosenberg JG, Klei S, et al. Comparison of the acute metabolic responses to traditional resistance, body-weight, and battling rope exercises. *J Strength Cond Res*. 2015;29:47–57.

217. Ratamess NA, Kang J, Kuper JD, et al. Acute cardiorespiratory and metabolic effects of a sandbag resistance exercise protocol. *J Strength Cond Res*. 2018;32:1491–502.

218. Bergeron MF, Nindl BC, Deuster PA, et al. Consortium for Health and Military Performance and American College of Sports Medicine consensus paper on extreme conditioning programs in military personnel. *Curr Sports Med Rep*. 2011;10:383–9.

219. Hooper DR, Szivak TK, Comstock BA, et al. Effects of fatigue from resistance training on barbell back squat biomechanics. *J Strength Cond Res*. 2014;28:1127–34.

220. Brandenburg JP, Docherty D. The effects of accentuated eccentric loading on strength, muscle hypertrophy, and neural adaptations in trained individuals. *J Strength Cond Res*. 2002;16:25–32.

221. Jackson A, Jackson T, Hnatek J, West J. Strength development: using functional isometrics in an isotonic strength training program. *Res Q Exerc Sport*. 1985;56:234–7.

222. O'Shea KL, O'Shea JP. Functional isometric weight training: its effects on static and dynamic strength. *J Appl Sport Sci Res*. 1989;3:30–3.

223. Giorgi A, Wilson GJ, Weatherby RP, Murphy AJ. Functional isometric weight training: its effects on the development of muscular function and the endocrine system over an 8-week training period. *J Strength Cond Res*. 1998;12:18–25.

224. Graves JE, Pollock ML, Jones AE, Colvin AB, Leggett SH. Specificity of limited range of motion variable resistance training. *Med Sci Sports Exerc*. 1989;21:84–9.

225. Graves JE, Pollock ML, Leggett SH, Carpenter DM, Fix CK, Fulton MN. Limited range-of-motion lumbar extension strength training. *Med Sci Sports Exerc*. 1992;24:128–33.

226. Newmire DE, Willoughby DS. Partial compared with full range of motion resistance training for muscle hypertrophy: a brief review and an identification of potential mechanisms. *J Strength Cond Res*. 2018;32:2652–64.

227. Clark RA, Bryant AL, Humphries B. An examination of strength and concentric work ratios during variable range of motion training. *J Strength Cond Res*. 2008;22:1716–9.

228. Massey CD, Vincent J, Maneval M, Moore M, Johnson JT. An analysis of full range of motion vs. partial range of motion training in the development of strength in untrained men. *J Strength Cond Res*. 2004;18:518–21.

229. Massey CD, Vincent J, Maneval M, Johnson JT. Influence of range of motion in resistance training in women: early phase adaptations. *J Strength Cond Res*. 2005;19:409–11.

230. Swinton PA, Lloyd R, Aqouris I, Stewart A. Contemporary training practices in elite British powerlifters: survey results from an international competition. *J Strength Cond Res*. 2009;23:380–4.

231. Simmons L. What if? *MILO*. 1996;4:25–9.

232. Cronin J, McNair PJ, Marshall RN. The effects of bungy weight training on muscle function and functional performance. *J Sports Sci*. 2003;21:59–71.

233. Wallace BJ, Winchester JB, McGuigan MR. Effects of elastic bands on force and power characteristics during the back squat exercise. *J Strength Cond Res*. 2006;20:268–72.

234. Ebben WP, Jensen RL. Electromyographic and kinetic analysis of traditional, chain, and elastic band squats. *J Strength Cond Res*. 2002;16:547–50.

235. Berning JM, Coker CA, Briggs DL. The biomechanical and perceptual influence of chain resistance on the performance of the Olympic clean. *J Strength Cond Res*. 2008;22:390–5.

236. Coker CA, Berning JM, Briggs DL. A preliminary investigation of the biomechanical and perceptual influence of chain resistance on the performance of the snatch. *J Strength Cond Res*. 2006;20:887–91.

237. Ghigiarelli JJ, Nagle EF, Gross FL, Robertson RJ, Irrgang JJ, Myslinski T. The effects of a 7-week heavy elastic band and weight chain program on upper-body strength and upper-body power in a sample of Division 1-AA football players. *J Strength Cond Res*. 2009;23:756–64.

238. Anderson CE, Sforzo GA, Sigg JA. The effects of combining elastic and free weight resistance on strength and power in athletes. *J Strength Cond Res*. 2008;22:567–74.

239. McCurdy K, Langford G, Ernest J, Jenkerson D, Doscher M. Comparison of chain- and plate-loaded bench press training on strength, joint pain, and muscle soreness in Division II baseball players. *J Strength Cond Res*. 2009;23:187–95.

240. Ahtiainen JP, Pakarinen A, Kraemer WJ, Häkkinen K. Acute hormonal and neuromuscular responses and recovery to forced

240. vs maximum repetitions multiple resistance exercises. *Int J Sports Med.* 2003;24:410–8.

241. Ahtiainen JP, Pakarinen A, Kraemer WJ, Häkkinen K. Acute hormonal responses to heavy resistance exercise in strength athletes versus nonathletes. *Can J Appl Physiol.* 2004;29:527–43.

242. Drinkwater EJ, Lawton TW, McKenna MJ, et al. Increased number of forced repetitions does not enhance strength development with resistance training. *J Strength Cond Res.* 2007;21:841–7.

243. Costa BDV, Ferreira MEC, Gantois P, et al. Acute effect of drop-set, traditional, and pyramidal systems in resistance training on neuromuscular performance in trained adults. *J Strength Cond Res.* 2019; Online ahead of print. doi: 10.1519/JSC.0000000000003150.

244. Raeder C, Wiewelhove T, Westphal-Martinez MP, et al. Neuromuscular fatigue and physiological responses after five dynamic squat exercise protocols. *J Strength Cond Res.* 2016;30:953–65.

245. Johannsmeyer S, Candow DG, Brahms CM, Michel D, Zello GA. Effect of creatine supplementation and drop-set resistance training in untrained aging adults. *Exp Gerontol.* 2016;83:112–9.

246. Ozaki H, Kubota A, Natsume T, et al. Effects of drop sets with resistance training on increases in muscle CSA, strength, and endurance: a pilot study. *J Sports Sci.* 2018;36:691–6.

247. Fink J, Schoenfeld BJ, Kikuchi N, Nakazato K. Effects of drop set resistance training on acute stress indicators and long-term muscle hypertrophy and strength. *J Sports Med Phys Fitness.* 2018;58:597–605.

248. Wallace W, Ugrinowitsch C, Stefan M, et al. Repeated bouts of advanced strength training techniques: effects on volume load, metabolic responses, and muscle activation in trained individuals. *Sports (Basel).* 2019;7:E14.

249. Denton J, Cronin JB. Kinematic, kinetic, and blood lactate profiles of continuous and intraset rest loading schemes. *J Strength Cond Res.* 2006;20:528–34.

250. Shinohara M, Kouzaki M, Yoshihisa T, Fukunaga T. Efficacy of tourniquet ischemia for strength training with low resistance. *Eur J Appl Physiol Occup Physiol.* 1998;77:189–91.

251. Lawton T, Cronin J, Drinkwater E, Lindsell R, Pyne D. The effect of continuous repetition training and intra-set rest training on bench press strength and power. *J Sports Med Phys Fitness.* 2004;44:361–7.

252. Folland JP, Irish CS, Roberts JC, Tarr JE, Jones DA. Fatigue is not a necessary stimulus for strength gains during resistance training. *Br J Sports Med.* 2002;36:370–4.

253. Latella C, Teo WP, Drinkwater EJ, Kendall K, Haff GG. The acute neuromuscular responses to cluster set resistance training: a systematic review and meta-analysis. *Sports Med.* 2019;49(12):1861–77.

254. Stone MH, Stone M, Sands WA. *Principles and Practice of Resistance Training.* Champaign (IL): Human Kinetics; 2007.

255. Haff GG, Whitley A, McCoy LB, et al. Effects of different set configurations on barbell velocity and displacement during a clean pull. *J Strength Cond Res.* 2003;17:95–103.

256. Hansen KT, Cronin JB, Newton MJ. The effect of cluster loading on force, velocity, and power during ballistic jump squat training. *Int J Sports Physiol Perform.* 2011;6:455–68.

257. Hardee JP, Lawrence MM, Zwetsloot KA, et al. Effect of cluster set configurations on power clean technique. *J Sports Sci.* 2013;31:488–96.

258. Garcia-Ramos A, Gonzalez-Hernandez JM, Banos-Pelegrin E, et al. Mechanical and metabolic responses to traditional and cluster set configurations in the bench press exercise. *J Strength Cond Res.* 2020;34(3):663–70.

259. Oliver JM, Jagim AR, Sanchez AC, et al. Greater gains in strength and power with intraset rest intervals in hypertrophic training. *J Strength Cond Res.* 2013;27:3116–31.

260. Oliver JM, Kreutzer A, Jenke SC, et al. Acute response to cluster sets in trained and untrained men. *Eur J Appl Physiol.* 2015;115:2383–93.

261. Oliver JM, Jenke SC, Mata JD, Kreutzer A, Jones MT. Acute effect of cluster and traditional set configurations on myokines associated with hypertrophy. *Int J Sports Med.* 2016;37:1019–24.

262. Tufano JJ, Brown LE, Haff GG. Theoretical and practical aspects of different cluster set structures: a systematic review. *J Strength Cond Res.* 2017;31:848–67.

263. Wagle JP, Taber CB, Carroll KM, et al. Repetition-to-repetition differences using cluster and accentuated eccentric loading in the back squat. *Sports (Basel).* 2018;6:E59.

264. Wetmore AB, Wagle JP, Sams ML, et al. Cluster set loading in the back squat: kinetic and kinematic implications. *J Strength Cond Res.* 2019;33(Suppl):S19–25.

265. Souza-Junior TP, Willardson JM, Bloomer R, et al. Strength and hypertrophy responses to constant and decreasing rest intervals in trained men using creatine supplementation. *J Int Soc Sports Nutr.* 2011;8:17.

266. Hoffman JR, Ratamess NA. *A Practical Guide to Developing Resistance Training Programs.* 2nd ed. Monterey (CA): Coaches Choice Books; 2008.

CHAPTER 13

Resistance Training Equipment and Safety

OBJECTIVES

After completing this chapter, you will be able to:

- Discuss different modalities and equipment used in resistance training
- Discuss advantages and disadvantages of free weights and machines
- Review general safety procedures for effective resistance training
- Discuss ways in which resistance training can reduce the risk of injury

Theoretically, any piece of equipment that supplies some degree of resistance can be used for training. In the past 30 years, numerous pieces of resistance training (RT) equipment have been developed. Some equipment is new and innovative, and some manufacturers have expanded upon other pieces used throughout the history of RT. One can design quality RT programs with inexpensive equipment, so the cost should not preclude one from training effectively.

 ## Resistance Training Modalities

Bodyweight

The human body is the most basic form of resistance in existence. Exercises such as bodyweight squats, push-ups, and pull-ups all require the athlete to overcome his or her bodyweight to perform a series of repetitions. Other modalities such as calisthenics, balance, sprint, plyometric, endurance, flexibility, and agility training all require the athlete to overcome bodyweight. In the absence of adding external weight, bodyweight exercises can be made more difficult by changing grip/stance width, changing posture or body position, leverage (moment arm of resistance), cadence, adding additional movements (*e.g.*, combination exercises), or by using uni- and bilateral contractions (one vs. two arms or legs). The magnitude of the athlete's bodyweight will contribute to the difficulty or intensity of the exercise. It is important to note that the basic principles of RT for acute program variable exercise prescription must still be followed even when the resistance is supplied by bodyweight, *i.e.*, adequate relative intensity must be maintained if strength adaptations are the goal of the training. Although a number of bodyweight exercises can be performed, some general classifications of bodyweight exercises include

- Push-ups
- Pull-ups
- Dips
- Squats
- Lunges
- Hyperextensions
- Climbing/crawling/obstacle
- Abdominal/core
- Burpees
- Gymnastics
- Dance
- Corrective/mobility
- Suspension
- Sport specific

The push-up is a prime example (Fig. 13.1). The push-up can be made easier by performing it on the knees (*modified push-up*), which reduces the resistance arm and allows the ground to support some of the bodyweight. Studies have shown that 64%–75% of bodyweight (depending on posture and range of motion [ROM]) is supported (with more force in the bottom than top positions) during a regular traditional push-up, and 49%–62% of bodyweight is supported during a modified push-up (1–3). The difficulty of the push-up can increase when strength and endurance improves. An athlete may widen, narrow, or stagger his or her hand spacing or

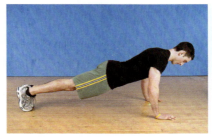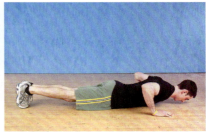

FIGURE 13.1 Push-up.

place hands further in front of the body (head level); elevate the feet on a bench or upper body between chairs, ball, or platform; maintain contact with the floor with only one foot (or cross feet); add a twist to exercise (rotation at the top position), pause, or forward walk with the hands; alter the cadence; and eventually progress to a single-arm push-up. For example, performing the push-up with upper body elevated on a bench reduces loading (*e.g.*, 41% of bodyweight) whereas elevating the feet on the bench increases the loading more so than the traditional push-up (1). Push-ups can be performed on the fingertips or backs of hands, which increase difficulty as well as require greater hand and wrist strength. The prone push-up position is a potent core exercise so manipulation of limbs while maintaining this position stresses core musculature (one- vs. two-arm plank) (1). All of these variations alter muscle activation and complexity to some degree without adding external resistance to increase difficulty and intensity. Metabolically, similar responses were shown between traditional push-ups on the floor versus a BOSU ball. However, adding a lateral crawl (or shuffle) to the push-up increased oxygen consumption and energy expenditure by 39% (4).

Bodyweight training has been a primary modality for several groups of individuals including dancers, gymnasts, and tactical athletes. Athletes such as gymnasts who train against bodyweight possess high levels of muscle strength and power owing to the efficacy of understanding biomechanics and how to use bodyweight as a training tool. Bodyweight is a form of resistance that anyone can use for RT at no cost and exercises can be performed in most places (4). Bodyweight exercises are commonly included in metabolic or high-intensity interval training programs. For example, it was previously shown that oxygen consumption and energy expenditure during the bodyweight burpee exercises was greater than several traditional resistance exercises performed for 3 sets of 10 reps at 75% of 1RM (4) (Table 13.1). It is important for the strength and conditioning (S&C) professional to realize that, due to either a lack of sufficient strength or large amount of weight, some bodyweight exercises may be impractical for certain populations. For example, some individuals may not be able to complete one dip or pull-up. In these cases, other strengthening exercises (machine dip, lat pull-down) may be used initially until the individual develops the ability to perform a bodyweight exercise without assistance. Lastly, some pieces of equipment can be useful for performing some bodyweight exercises. For example, dip bars can assist in performing dips, bars can be useful for pull-ups, and benches can be used for reverse dips, crunches, sit-ups, and leg raises. See Myths & Misconceptions: The Best Resistance Training Workouts Involve Costly Equipment.

Suspension training is popular where the athlete performs a bodyweight exercise suspended where all or a segment of bodyweight serves as resistance. *Gymnastic rings* form a parallel strap system with dual anchor points where the athlete' entire weight is supported during various exercises, *e.g.*, pull-ups, dips, iron cross, or other gymnastics movements (6). The difficulty is greater because rings are often suspended high off of the ground forcing the athlete to perform the exercise against all of their bodyweight. In addition, the instability of the straps makes the exercise more challenging. However, other devices are used to partition bodyweight at multiple angles and positions. A popular piece of bodyweight equipment is the TRX Suspension Trainer (Fig. 13.2). The TRX is one type of suspension training device common to fitness facilities, *e.g.*, one versus two anchor points. The TRX consists of two straps with adjustable handles and foot attachments that can be suspended or anchored from the ceiling, a door, beams, or from a multipurpose resistance exercise device like a cable unit or power rack that forms a "V"-shaped suspension system. The adjustable straps enable the performance of hundreds of movement-specific bodyweight exercises. The straps are freely moveable yet supportive, which creates a desirable training stimulus. It is based on a pendulum system where manipulation of the athlete's body position (distance from anchor, strap length, body angle relative to floor, height of the starting position and center of gravity [COG], and size of base support) dictates the percent of bodyweight that needs to be overcome. For example, the more upright the body (feet back), the easier the exercise is (less weight to support) for some upper body exercises. The closer to the ground (feet closer to anchor), the more difficult the exercise is as a larger percent of bodyweight must be overcome. Giancotti et al. (7) examined the TRX push-up at seven body positions with different strap lengths from near vertical to near horizontal at flexed and extended elbow positions. They found that trainees had to support 19.1% (near vertical position) to 43.5% (near horizontal position) of their bodyweight with the elbows extended and 41.5%–58.2% of bodyweight with the elbows flexed. Gulmez (8) also reported greater loading with near horizontal position compared to more vertical positions and during flexed versus extended elbow positions at each angle. Muscle activation of the triceps brachii, rectus abdominis, erector spinae, pectoralis major, and upper trapezius per repetition is greater when push-ups are performed on a suspension device compared to the floor (9,10) with the results

Table 13.1	Metabolic Responses to the Resistance Exercise Protocols[a]			
	Mean $\dot{V}O_2$ (mL·kg^{-1}·min^{-1})	Peak $\dot{V}O_2$ (mL·kg^{-1}·min^{-1})	EE (kcal·min^{-1})	RER
Baseline	2.5 ± 0.9		1.1 ± 0.4	0.80 ± 0.1
Squat	19.6 ± 1.8[b]	32.5 ± 5.0[b]	8.2 ± 1.1[b]	1.08 ± 0.1
BP	12.5 ± 2.1[c]	19.8 ± 4.0[c]	5.2 ± 0.9[c]	1.11 ± 0.1
Curl	12.3 ± 2.1[d]	20.2 ± 3.0[e]	5.1 ± 0.8[d]	1.05 ± 0.1
BOR	12.2 ± 1.7[f]	22.4 ± 3.6[g]	5.1 ± 0.7[f]	1.10 ± 0.1
HP	14.2 ± 3.2[h]	25.2 ± 5.0[i]	6.0 ± 1.3[h]	1.00 ± 0.1
Lunge	17.3 ± 2.6[j]	28.7 ± 4.6[b]	7.2 ± 1.3[j]	1.03 ± 0.1
DL	18.9 ± 3.0[k]	31.2 ± 5.1[k]	7.8 ± 1.2[k]	1.15 ± 0.1
Burpee	22.9 ± 2.1[l]	35.9 ± 4.1[m]	9.6 ± 1.3[l]	1.00 ± 0.1
Plank	7.9 ± 0.7[l]	12.8 ± 1.6[l]	3.3 ± 0.7[l]	0.90 ± 0.1
BR	24.6 ± 2.6[l]	38.6 ± 4.7[n]	10.3 ± 1.4[l]	1.21 ± 0.1
PU	11.9 ± 1.3[o]	18.9 ± 1.4[p]	4.9 ± 0.6[o]	1.11 ± 0.1
BOSU PU	11.9 ± 1.0[q]	20.3 ± 1.7[q]	5.0 ± 0.7[q]	1.10 ± 0.1
PU-LC	19.5 ± 2.9[r]	31.0 ± 4.9[s]	8.1 ± 1.1[r]	1.05 ± 0.1

[a]All data were significantly different from BL. EE, energy expenditure; RER, respiratory exchange ratio; BP, bench press; BOR, bent-over barbell row; HP, high pull; DL, deadlift; BR, battling rope; PU, push-up; BOSU, both sides up; PU-LC, push-up with lateral crawl.

[b]$P \leq 0.05$ compared with all exercises except DL and PU-LC.

[c]$P \leq 0.05$ compared with all exercises except CU, BOR, PU, BOSU PU.

[d]$P \leq 0.05$ compared with all exercises except BP, BOR, PU, and BOSU PU.

[e]$P \leq 0.05$ compared with all exercises except BP, PU, and BOSU PU.

[f]$P \leq 0.05$ compared with all exercises except BP, CU, HP, PU, and BOSU PU.

[g]$P \leq 0.05$ compared with all exercises except BP, HP, PU, and BOSU PU.

[h]$P \leq 0.05$ compared with all exercises except BOR and BOSU PU.

[i]$P \leq 0.05$ compared with all exercises except BOR.

[j]$P \leq 0.05$ compared with all exercises except DL.

[k]$P \leq 0.05$ compared with all exercises except SQ, LN, PU-LC.

[l]$P \leq 0.05$ compared with all exercises.

[m]$P \leq 0.05$ compared with all exercises except BR.

[n]$P \leq 0.05$ compared with all exercises except burpee.

[o]$P \leq 0.05$ compared with all exercises except BP, CU, BOR, and BOSU PU.

[p]$P \leq 0.05$ compared with all exercises except BP, CU, and BOSU PU.

[q]$P \leq 0.05$ compared with all exercises except BP, CU, BOR, HP, and PU.

[r]$P \leq 0.05$ compared with all exercises except SQ and DL.

[s]$P \leq 0.05$ compared with all exercises except SQ, LN, and DL.

Reprinted from Ratamess NA, Rosenberg JG, Klei S, et al. Comparison of the acute metabolic responses to traditional resistance exercise, bodyweight, and battling rope exercises. *J Strength Cond Res.* 2015;29:47–57.

Myths & Misconceptions
The Best Resistance Training Workouts Involve Costly Equipment

Albeit some popular and effective pieces of RT equipment are expensive, quality RT programs can be developed for free and/or at very low cost (5). This has large ramifications for training at home, on the road, or training groups of athletes with limited resources. The most basic source of resistance is one's bodyweight. Bodyweight exercises can be made more difficult (or easy) by altering biomechanics, intensity, repetition number, exercises selected, and rest intervals. Bodyweight workouts can be effective for athletes at all fitness levels. Manual RT (self-imposed or partner resistance) is free and can be performed anywhere. Other sources of resistance can be purchased at low cost. Bands, tubing, medicine balls (MBs), dumbbells, and kettlebells (KBs) can be purchased at low cost and are easily transportable. Implements or some items around the home/yard (sledgehammer, cinder blocks, wheelbarrow, couch, etc.) can be used. Larger pieces of free-weight equipment, machines, and gym memberships are more costly and/or prohibitive for home purchase. They also require more space. For example, barbell sets (depending on the amount of plates and weights) are sold per pound and can range in price from $100 to several hundreds of dollars. Free-weight benches can be low in cost but better-quality equipment (equipment designed for more extensive use) can cost hundreds of dollars. Lifting platforms and power racks cost several hundred to a couple of thousand dollars. Machines are quite costly and limit the number of exercises performed. Gym memberships usually cost a few hundred to >$1,000 per year. Cost may preclude some equipment use. However, it is a myth that it is costly to improve physical conditioning.

differing between suspension devices (9). Greater muscle activity of the rectus abdominis, external oblique, and erector spinae muscles has been shown during the TRX plank versus the floor (11). Similar kinetic results were shown for the TRX row where 37%, 53%, 68%, and 79% of bodyweight were supported from vertical to horizontal positions (30°, 45°, 60°, and 75° from vertical) (12). Thus, suspension training devices can augment muscle activation during bodyweight exercise under certain conditions and provide a unique stimulus supplementing traditional bodyweight training.

The bodyweight of other individuals or partners can be a beneficial RT tool. A multitude of exercises such as the squat, bench press, push-up, shoulder press, abdominal crunch/back extension, clean, deadlift, rows, bear hug lifts, stand-up, suplex arch, and various carries can be performed with the bodyweight of a partner. A partner's weight determines how many repetitions can be performed. It is unique that bodyweight distribution is not balanced, so performing an exercise with a 150-lb partner will be more difficult than performing the exercise with a 150-lb barbell. Other partner exercises such as wheelbarrow walks, hops, or push-ups require the partner to support part of the trainee's bodyweight to maintain a specific position. A partner may also be used as a guide for different drills. For example, the partner jump over and crawl under involves a trainee jumping over the body of partner (while they maintain a 4-point position on their hands and knees) and then immediately

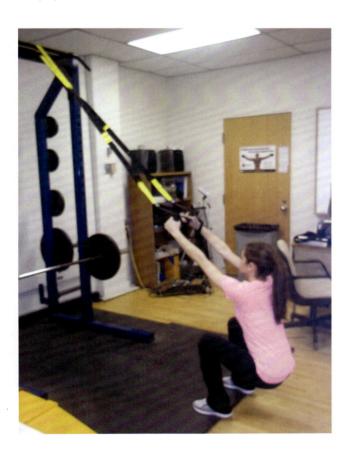

FIGURE 13.2 A TRX squat.

Case Study 13.1

The push-up exercise was discussed in the previous section. Using the same logic, apply biomechanical principles to the basic bodyweight squat.

Question for Consideration: Discuss ways an athlete can make the exercise more difficult without adding external weight.

dropping to the floor and crawling under the partner. Thus, partner exercises can add a unique element to an S&C program.

Visit thePoint to view more exercises in the online appendix.

Manual or Partner Resistance

An athlete or partner may provide self-resistance for relatively slow repetitions (Fig. 13.3). The advantages of manual or partner dynamic or isometric (ISOM) RT exercises are they can be performed anywhere at very little to no cost, risk of injury is low, high resistance can be applied throughout the ROM, many individuals can be trained at once, resistance can be adjusted based on fatigue, and they can add variety to a traditional RT program (13,14). These exercises can be effective for complete strength development, provided intensity is sufficient. Some examples of manual resistance exercises include unilateral elbow flexion/extension, towel leg press, ISOM chest squeeze and wall push, front raise (held with opposite arm), supine row (with legs) and chest press (on legs), upright row (held with opposite arm), shrug, hip adduction/abduction with arms, ISOM knee extension, knee raise (against arms), and four-way neck manual resistance exercises. These exercises work best when an exercise is opposed by a muscle group stronger than the agonists (which is not always the case). A partner can supply the resistance directly or with the use of a towel. A partner may be useful for some exercises difficult for one to perform manually, *e.g.*, leg curl, rowing, shoulder press, lateral raise, push-up, and so on. A partner has an advantage of using two arms or his or her whole body for resistance. Thus, loading can be greater than self-resistance. Disadvantages with manual/partner RT include the difficulty in consistently quantifying how much resistance is being used, relatively low exercise selection, and using a partner with a sufficient level of size and strength. Partners (or spotters) must fully communicate with the athlete, watch and monitor technique, and adjust tension when necessary to accommodate fatigue or stronger areas of the ROM.

Free Weights

Free weights are named because the athlete must control and can move the weight freely in any direction. Free weights include barbells, dumbbells, plates, collars/clamps, PlateMates (1.25-lb magnetic weights that stick to weights; can be used when 2.5-lb weights are too heavy), and various accessories and specialty bars that enable greater free-weight exercise selection. Free weights have many advantages compared to other RT modalities, especially when it comes to ease of loading and the ability to perform a large number of exercises with them.

Barbells

Barbells are bars of various lengths that can be loaded with weights or plates. Typically, barbells are between 5 and 7 ft in length and may vary in thickness. An Olympic barbell is most commonly used (Fig. 13.4). This is the type used with Olympic weights or plates (those with a larger 2-in. central hole to accommodate an Olympic bar) commonly seen in health clubs, gyms, and weight rooms. They are ~7 ft in length and weigh ~45 lb, although some may be slightly lighter or heavier. They have knurling to increase friction between the hands and bar for better gripping. The bar tends to be ~1 in. in diameter. The bearings, *e.g.*, roller, ball, and needle, allow the weights to freely rotate. Barbells may be used in a multitude of ways for traditional exercises but are popularly used for anchored RT exercises where one end of the bar is lifted while the opposite end is anchored to a ground-based apparatus and may be suspended from a power rack to create pendulum barbell exercises. Light weight (15-lb) aluminum bars are nice for beginners or young athletes just learning proper technique. A cambered Olympic bar allows the athlete to have more ROM during the bench press or be able to perform shrugs while seated on a bench. Another type of barbell is the *thick bar* (15,16). Thick bars come in various diameters, *e.g.*, 2, 2¾, and 3 in., and typically weigh between 20 and 50 lb. Because of the thicker diameter, thick bars are mostly used for grip strength training. Thick bars have minimal effects on pushing exercises such as the bench press and shoulder press (16). However, pulling exercises such as the deadlift, bent-over row, arm curl, and upright row are affected in proportion to the thickness of the bar. For the deadlift and bent-over row, 1RM lifts are ~28% and 55% lower for the 2- and 3-in. bars, respectively, and ~9% and 37% for the bent-over row. Interestingly, reductions in loading correlate to hand size and maximal ISOM grip strength (16). Grip adapters (*i.e.*, Fat Gripz) can be cost effective and placed on barbells and dumbbells to increase diameter for thick bar training.

Other specialty bars have been developed in recent years. The *Tsunami barbell* is flexible (made of composite and thermoplastic material) and bends and oscillates as the lifter performs repetitions. It creates a form of vibration training where

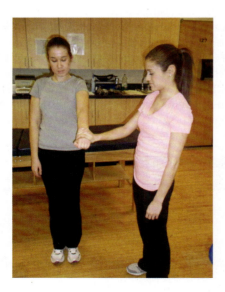

FIGURE 13.3 Manual resistance front raise (with partner assistance).

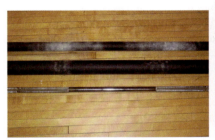 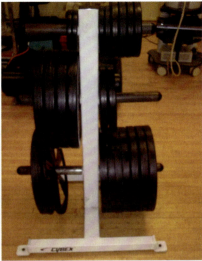

FIGURE 13.4 Olympic bar and thick bars plus plates.

the lifter is required to increase muscle activation to stabilize the bar throughout the ROM despite using lighter weights than a standard barbell. It is ~3 in. in diameter, is 78–90 in. in length, and weighs 13–17 lbs depending on which bar is used. The *Bandbell Earthquake Bar* contains wooden grooves on both sides to allow the trainee to hang kettle bells from bands to create oscillations. The *Freak bar* (Westside Barbell in Columbus, OH) allows the lifter to slide the hands in and out during performance of an exercise such as the bench press. It allows for pushing and pulling the barbell on the horizontal axis with resistance provided by springs within the bar. This added effect encountered during each repetition is thought to increase muscle activation and provide a novel strength training effect. Ghigiarelli et al. (17) examined 6 weeks of bench press training with the Freak bar versus a regular bar and reported significant strength increases in both training groups with no difference between groups. They also concluded that training with the Freak bar trains the lifter to apply lateral and medial forces and may have an advantage for increasing muscular strength at multiple areas of the ROM during the bench press.

Standard barbells have smaller ends than Olympic bars and are used to accommodate standard plates. They weigh less and may accommodate up to ~400 lb. Some gyms have fixed barbells. These are preloaded barbells with a specific weight. Like dumbbells, a range of fixed barbells may be seen, *e.g.*, 10–100 lb or more. These are advantageous because they do not require any loading or unloading so they are nice when performing sets with short rest intervals. Specialty bars may be seen in many gyms. Curl bars (E-Z bars) are bent in the middle to allow more pronation when gripping. This removes some stress from the wrists when performing exercises such as curls or triceps extensions. These are nearly 4-ft long and weigh 15–25 lb. Triceps bars are narrow but allow the individual to use a midrange hand position for arm curl or extensions exercises. Trap bars, or *hex bars*, have a diamond-shaped middle section that is used for performing shrugs, deadlifts, jump squat, and farmer's walk. The hex bar deadlift allows for a more upright posture reducing torque at the hip joint. This alters muscle activation and enables a higher 1RM (18). Using a hex bar for a loaded jump squat enables high power output without having a barbell on the shoulders. Safety squat bars have two padded bars extending at 90° angles from the bar base. These can be used as grips but they allow the bar to rest comfortably on the shoulders without support. Some athletes will use their arms to grasp a power rack during the squat for support or assistance during the ascent and descent.

Weights, or plates, are added to bars for loading. Plates typically come in weight sizes of 1.25, 2.5, 5, 10, 25, 35, 45, and 100 lb, or in kg measures. Standard plates are used for standard bars, and Olympic plates are used for Olympic bars. Many Olympic plates are solid. However, some newer models have grips within that make it easier for loading and, in some cases, to perform an exercise with them. Rubberized plates are common. Because they are rubberized, they can easily be dropped or thrown without causing damage. Some rubberized plates are actually cast iron plates coated in rubber. These plates can potentially damage bars and platforms. However, bumper plates are completely rubberized and are specifically designed to be dropped without damaging platforms and floors and to withstand punishment from explosive lifting. This is important when performing the Olympic lifts/variations because one is taught to drop the weight during an unsuccessful attempt and to drop the weight once the lift is complete. Plates are held in place by various collars and clamps including twist/lock (Muscle Clamp), spin/lock, screw-on, or squeeze/lock (spring). They typically weigh <1 lb although some may weigh nearly 6 lb.

Dumbbells

Dumbbells are small versions of barbells designed mostly for single-arm use (although a single dumbbell can be used for several exercises). Many types of dumbbells exist from solid, fixed, one-piece units to adjustable (a bar that can be loaded with different weights and supported by clamps/collars) and nonadjustable weight-loaded units. Some dumbbells have rotating handles. Selectorized dumbbells (PowerBlocks) are dumbbells with blocks that support several stacks of small plates. Poundage is selected and the dumbbell is lifted up off of the block with the targeted weight. As with plates, some dumbbells are rubberized, which assist in dropping them with little to no damage. Dumbbells come in many sizes and are stacked in pairs in order on a tiered rack from the smallest (5 lb) to the largest (125 lb or more) usually in 5-lb increments. Their greatest utility is the large movement potential and ROM they provide. Weight magnets may be attached to dumbbells to add 1.25- or 2.5-lb increments.

Free-Weight Equipment

Many other pieces of equipment are available that enable free weight use. These are commonly found in most weight rooms, gyms, and clubs. They are advantageous for allowing the athlete to alter body posture or position when performing free-weight exercises. The following list outlines many of these key pieces of equipment.

- Olympic benches: flat, incline, and decline
- Portable benches (some which are adjustable)
- Shoulder press benches
- Sit-up benches
- Dip/leg raise benches
- Glute-ham raise or hyperextension benches
- Reverse hyperextension bench and Nordic leg curl bench
- Lifting platforms: essential for performing Olympic lifts
- Power racks (with adjustable pins) and rigs — for multiple exercises
- Multiple rack units — with benches, dipping, and chinning bars
- Squat racks
- Preacher curl benches (standing and seated)
- Plyo boxes — for stepping up, box squats, or other ballistic exercises
- Wrist rollers
- Belts — for performing loaded dips or pull-ups
- Head/neck harness
- T-bar
- Landmine — for anchored barbell exercises
- Suspension Straps (*e.g.*, Henny) — for creating barbell pendulum exercises

Machines

Several types of RT machines may be found in clubs and gyms. Some machines offer the athlete a constant level of tension throughout the ROM. Linear motion is produced as is the case with some types of leg press machines. Another example found in many gyms is the *Smith machine*. The Smith machine (named after Rudy Smith, who improved upon the initial design by fitness legend Jack La Lanne in the 1950s) consists of a barbell that can only move vertically upward and downward on steel runners, although some models allow for angled movement. The Smith machine is versatile and allows performance of many exercises such as bench press (and variations), shoulder press, squats, rows, and several others. It enhances safety as catches can be used to stop the bar if fatigue sets in and prevents any side-to-side or front-to-back movements of the bar. A series of slots run behind each runner in which the bar can be hooked or secured at various locations.

Cable pulley machines consist of a cable that runs through one or more pulleys connected to a weight stack (Fig. 13.5). Many times the weight is selected by placing a pin at the desired location (as most machine plates range from 5 to 20 lb). The individual applies a force to the cable, the force is redirected by the pulley, and the plates (at the level of the pin and all of those plates above) are lifted to provide tension. Weight stacks (and pulley arrangements) vary when going from one machine to another. An athlete must adjust load or repetition number accordingly because performing an exercise on one machine may be easy but difficult on another using similar loading. Many cable machines are adjustable so that a multitude of unilateral and/or bilateral exercises can be performed. The pulley can be placed low, high, and at many sites in between. Although cable pulley machines are machines (free-form) per se, they do not provide as much stabilization as other types of machines so the athlete can benefit from stabilizer muscle cocontraction. Multipurpose cable pulley units are common in gyms and health clubs as many exercises can be performed. Many different types of bars/handles/ropes can be used to vary exercises. Some cable pulley machines are nonadjustable, more specific, and only enable performance of a few exercises, *e.g.*, low pulley row, lat pull-down.

Plate-loaded machines (Fig. 13.6) require the athlete to load weights for resistance. As opposed to a weight stack, plates

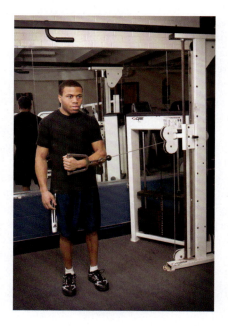

FIGURE 13.5 Cable pulley machine.

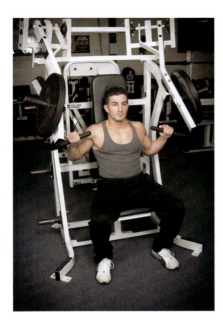

FIGURE 13.6 A plate-loaded (Hammer Strength) chest press machine.

are loaded to the machine, which offers a few advantages: (a) athletes are provided with a wider range of loading, *i.e.*, 2.5-lb weights can be used to target those desired resistances that may be difficult with weight stacks and (b) greater loading may be used as many weight-stack machines plateau at a resistance that may be insufficient for strong athletes. Some plate-loaded machines, *e.g.*, Hammer Strength, use convergent and divergent arcs of motion and use counterbalanced lever arms to vary the resistance throughout the ROM (a variable resistance machine). At the starting position, the lever is rotated out so the athlete does not have to bear the entire load. However, the lever arm moves toward the horizontal as the weight is lifted, therefore, increasing the loading on the individual (19).

Older variable resistance machines used a sliding lever to change the point of application of the resistance on the weight stack. Newer variable resistance machines use a cam to alter the loading throughout the ROM. The cam is an ellipse connected to the machine arm by which the cable or belt is located (20). The shape of the cam dictates the variable resistance to mimic human strength curves. Muscle torque production varies throughout the full joint ROM. Some machines attempt to accommodate these tension variations by altering the shape of the cam to make it more difficult in that segment of the ROM where greater torque is produced and to make it easier in the ROM where less torque is produced. For example, an inverted U-shaped cam can be used for ascending-descending strength curves (single-joint exercises), an oblong-shaped cam with the largest radius at the distal end can be used for ascending strength curves (multiple-joint pushing exercises), and an oblong-shaped cam with the largest radius at the proximal end can be used for descending strength curves (multiple-joint pulling exercises) (21). Other nonmachine equipment, *e.g.*, elastic bands, springs, tubing, and chains, can provide variable resistance.

Hydraulic resistance machines have a lever arm connected to a hydraulic piston that provides resistance against the oil-filled chamber it is set in (21). Some machines have a flow control, which changes the fluid velocity and the resistance. The resistance matches the effort of the athlete (the faster the individual moves the more resistance). Some machines use a pressure-release valve to allow fluid flow once a force greater than the valve resistance is applied to open the valve (19). This type provides more constant resistance (19). Hydraulic resistance machines utilize a concentric (CON)/CON movement minimizing loaded eccentric (ECC) muscle actions. The machine has a dual-exercise component stressing antagonist muscles.

Pneumatic resistance machines (such as Keiser) were first designed in the late 1980s and use air pressure for resistance. A ram or piston (similar to a syringe) is preloaded using compressed air. During the lifting phase, the ram compresses the air further providing resistance for CON and ECC phases (19). The athlete can adjust the resistance by letting air out during a set, which can be advantageous. Proponents of pneumatic machines cite smooth, fluid movements and ease of changing resistance as advantages of pneumatic machines compared to those using weight stacks. A pneumatic machine has no inertial effects due to the lack of a weight stack; thus, the resistance is consistent over the entire ROM regardless of the lifting velocity.

We are living in the computer age and computerized resistance machines have been developed. These machines provide variable resistance through gears and belts connected to a motor. A touch screen, button, or foot pedal allows the manipulation of resistance, and some can load the ECC component more than CON.

Isokinetic machines possess a dynamometer that maintains the lever arm at a constant angular velocity for most of the ROM. The utility is that repetition velocity is controlled and acts passively as an accommodating resistance device (22,23). A velocity is selected rather than a resistance. The cost of an isokinetic machine can be prohibitive as isokinetic machines are mostly found in research laboratories, training rooms, and clinical facilities. Isokinetic machines are computerized devices where the velocity is predetermined. They are useful for strength assessment because there are many measures that can be monitored, including peak and mean torque, angle-specific peak torque, total work, time to peak torque, and torque at various time intervals. The variables available depend on the brand and model of dynamometer used, as well as the software package accompanying it.

Free Weights versus Machines

Several advantages and disadvantages exist when examining RT with free weight and machines. Free-weight exercises (especially multiple-joint exercises) may pose a greater risk of injury under certain conditions because they require the individual to completely control the exercise (maintain body stability and displacement of the resistance), whereas machines may reduce the risk of acute injury because they assist in stabilizing the body and movement of the resistance. However, the risk of developing chronic inflammation in tendons may be greater with machines that limit motion flexibility. One study examined RT-related injuries in 12 athletes and reported that 9 of the injuries occurred using free weights and 3 injuries occurred during machine exercises (24). In either case, the risk of injury during RT is very low. Hamill (25) reported 0.012 and 0.0013 injuries per 100 hours of activity, respectively, for weight training and weightlifting. Although both modalities may cause injury, proper program design and supervision are mandatory.

Free weights and machines offer other advantages/disadvantages (22). The athlete must control repetition velocity, and free-weight training movements are more similar to those found in athletics. Free weights require greater coordination and muscle stabilizer activity than machines (26) because free weights must be controlled through all spatial dimensions, whereas machines generally involve uniplanar control. Thus, stabilization muscles may be more effectively trained with free weights. This can be an advantage or disadvantage depending on the individual's skill level. Some individuals with poor balance and impaired motor function may benefit from machine-based RT initially. Another practical reason for using free weights is their low cost and availability. Both free weights and machines are effective for increasing strength (27). Research shows that free-weight training leads to greater improvements in strength assessed with free weights and machine training results in greater performance on machine tests (28). When a neutral testing device is used, strength improvement from free weights and machines are similar (29). The choice to use free weights or machines is based on the level of training status and familiarity with specific exercise movements, as well as the primary training objective. Both are recommended by the American College of Sports Medicine (ACSM) for progression during RT.

Olympic lifts and variations are performed with free weights as these require large muscle mass recruitment, which cannot be adequately performed within the constructs of machines. Some exercises are difficult to perform optimally with free weights (lying leg curl, leg extension) so machines are a more favorable alternative. Free weights involve CON and ECC muscle activities. Eccentric muscle activity is limited on some hydraulic machines or with some isokinetic dynamometers. Free weights allow the desired ROM, whereas some machines can be restrictive if it is not possible to get a proper fit between the individual and the machine configuration. Similar to free weights, machines must be closely maintained. This includes checking for lose screws; worn parts; frayed cables, chains, or pulleys; and torn upholstery and grip supports. It is imperative that machines are adjusted properly to the individual and that they are operating smoothly; improper lubrication or a misalignment of the device may add unknown resistance to the machine. This includes making sure that the machine plates do not stick together.

Medicine Balls, Stability Balls, BOSU Balls, and Other Balance Devices

Medicine balls are weighted rubber or leather balls that vary in size (Fig. 13.7). They can be used for general RT, calisthenics, and plyometric exercises. Historically, the first so-called MBs (which were merely sand-filled bladders) were used by wrestlers nearly 3,000 years ago. In the 19th and early 20th centuries, they were commonly used in physical education classes and for gymnastics training. Later they became extensively used for the core training of boxers, *e.g.*, to simulate a body punch. Most MBs today are made of rubber. Rubber MBs are useful because they bounce and can be thrown safely with no damage. An athlete using an MB for an explosive overhead throw could throw the ball against a wall and have the ball rebound back to him or her for multiple reps. MBs come in sizes of 1–30 lb (~5–11 in.) and have developed over the years beyond their initial design. For example, core balls are MBs with handles to facilitate better gripping. These balls can be used similar to dumbbells or thrown explosively for plyometric exercises. Slam balls are MBs with ropes attached. The athlete can grip the rope and throw or slam the ball on the floor or wall for several power exercises. These are beneficial for rotational core exercises. Some MBs (NRG ball) have handles on one or both sides to vary exercise selection. Some MBs are less elastic, which makes them useful for exercises where they can be slammed on the floor or wall without large amplitudes of rebound. Lastly, rebounding units (that resemble trampolines) have facilitated MB training. These allow the athlete to throw the ball against the unit and a rebound ensues. The athlete may catch the ball in rebound to facilitate the stretch-shortening cycle and enhance plyometric training. See Sidebar: Comparison of Free Weights and Machines.

Stability balls (SBs), also known as *Exercise Balls, Physio Balls,* or *Swiss Balls*, are inflatable balls (Fig. 13.8) that come in many sizes (~30–85 cm). First used for clinical purposes prior to World War II, SBs are currently used to train in an unstable environment. They create postural disequilibrium by increasing postural sway and through surface distortion, thereby attempting to increase the activity of some core and limb muscles compared to performing the same exercise at the same relative

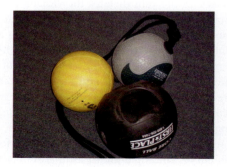

FIGURE 13.7 Medicine ball, core ball, and slam ball.

Sidebar — Comparison of Free Weights and Machines

Machines

Advantages

- Safe to use and easy to learn. Familiarization is easier and technique is simplified. Higher stability for beginners and special populations.
- Changing resistance is simple by either moving the pin (for weight stack machines) or modifying resistance on other machines (hydraulic, pneumatic). Plate-loaded machines require weight change similar to free weights.
- Some machines provide variable resistance in an attempt to accommodate strength curves. Although strength curves cannot be completely replicated, variable resistance machines provide altered loading, which can be somewhat similar to normal joint mechanics.
- Isokinetic machines control velocity and allow the individual to produce maximal effort and slow, moderate, and fast velocities of muscle action.
- RT can be performed unilaterally or bilaterally.
- Easy to evaluate progress. Monitoring resistance and rep number is easy. Some machines are computerized and can store training information.
- Allow performance of some exercises that may be difficult with free weights.
- Usually does not require the use of a spotter although spotters can be beneficial with machine-based exercises (especially a Smith machine).
- Hydraulic and pneumatic machines reduce momentum and provide smooth rep cadence.
- Some machines are multiunit and allow performance of several exercises.
- Can be a major attraction for a facility selling memberships.
- Effective for increasing all health- and skill-related components of fitness to some degree, provided the training program is progressive.
- Some machines were designed for functional or sport-specific purposes, *e.g.*, ground-based jammer (for football), tire flipping, and rope climbing.

Disadvantages

- Are much more costly and require more maintenance than free weights. Machines are large and heavy, making them difficult to move.
- May hinder the development of optimal neuromuscular coordination, and the additional stability lessens the body's need to stabilize itself. Antagonist and stabilizer muscle activities are lower. The machine does some of the work for the individual.
- On some machines, only one or a few exercises may be performed. Some limitations can restrict grip or foot angles/widths.
- Hydraulic/pneumatic machines produce less of an increase in strength and power when compared to free-weight training. Since hydraulic/pneumatic apparatus furnish no preload at the beginning of a movement, they limit strength increases early in the ROM (30,31).
- Some machines do not provide enough resistance for strong individuals. Loading varies greatly when going from one machine to another when performing the same exercise.
- Can be difficult to thoroughly accommodate individuals of different height, weight, and limb length based on machine setting restrictions.

Free Weights

Advantages

- Less expensive and require less maintenance than machines.
- Require greater antagonist and stabilizer muscle activity to support the body in all planes of motion. Allows multidirectional movement that must be controlled. A better stimulus for balance and coordination is present.
- Allow more variation for hand/foot spacing, etc., to alter the stimulus.
- Can perform a multitude of exercises with little equipment. Exercise selection is greater. Some pieces of equipment can be easily moved.
- Resistance training can be performed unilaterally or bilaterally.
- Can target CON, ECC, and ISOM muscle actions.
- Easy to evaluate progress. Monitoring resistance and repetition number is easy.
- Allow performance of Olympic lifts. Optimize acceleration for power training. Free weights are more conducive for explosive training and better for developing power and speed.
- Very easy to replicate motions seen in athletics or activities of daily living.
- Effective for increasing all health- and skill-related components of fitness.

Disadvantages

- May potentially pose a greater risk of injury due to the greater stabilization requirements.
- Takes longer to change weights and put them away in between sets and exercises.
- May require more time to learn a proper technique, especially for the Olympic lifts.
- May require a spotter on some exercises (bench press, shoulder press, and squat).
- Line of resistance is vertically downward, thus some exercises performed in a transverse plane (relative to the anatomical position) may not receive maximal resistance unless a pendulum barbell setup with suspension straps are used to anchor the barbell to a large unit such as a power rack.

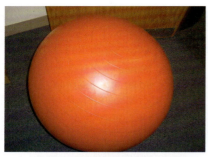
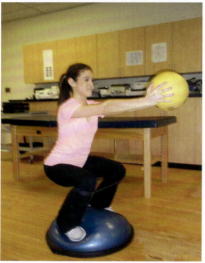

FIGURE 13.8 Stability ball **(top)** and BOSU ball **(bottom)**.

intensity on a stable surface (32). SBs are used mostly to target core musculature as stabilizer muscles must contract to a greater extent to keep the athlete from rolling off the ball. SBs can be used with free-weight and bodyweight exercises and are selected by having the athlete sit on the ball and the hips should flex to ~90°. Because force production is greatest under the most stable bodily conditions, loading for exercises performed on a SB will be lower than the same exercise performed on a bench or floor as ISOM and dynamic 1RM strength, power, and velocity have been shown to be lower on a SB compared to a bench (for the bench press) (33). It was proposed that an increase in joint stiffness, *e.g.*, a "stiffening strategy," may be employed during the threat of instability, which could contribute to the decrement in force and power output (32). Smaller balls pose advantageous for some exercises because they can be used for exercises requiring the athlete to support the ball between the feet/legs, or because a smaller ball is closer to the ground, it can make a basic exercise more challenging, *e.g.*, SB rollout. For some exercises (push-up), an SB that is somewhat deflated may be more beneficial (less stability); however, a ball highly inflated is more prone to roll and is more challenging for some exercises (curl-up).

BOSU balls (Balance Trainer) resemble SBs with the exception that the bottom is flat with a stable base (measuring ~21–25 in. in diameter and 12 in. in height when fully inflated). Several exercises are performed on it, and it has been popular since its invention in 1999. The top portion allows for instability, whereas the ball will not roll due to the flat base. BOSU stands for either "both sides utilized" or "both sides up" as the ball can be used either way. Dome side down enables the BOSU ball to be used like a wobble board. Similar to a SB, muscle force and activity may vary depending on the exercise compared to performing an exercise on a stable surface. Saeterbakken and Fimland (34) examined ISOM squat strength on a BOSU ball versus a stable platform and showed force was 19% lower on a BOSU ball. Lower body and core muscle activity were similar with the exception of the rectus femoris, which was higher on the stable surface. See Sidebar: Stability Ball Exercise and Training Research.

Other balance devices have been used in RT. Collectively, these devices provide an unstable environment for training. Balance steps are small vinyl balls filled with air or water that can be used flat side down or up. They can be stepped on during movement or stood upon during exercise to improve balance. Balance discs are small versions of instability equipment that are 14–24 in. in diameter. Likewise, a multitude of exercises can be performed on these. Squatting on a balance disc increases activation of the soleus, erector spinae, and abdominal muscles to maintain stability (48). Balance pads (Airex) (Fig. 13.9) function similarly as they provide instability when stood upon. Balance and wobble boards (Fig. 13.9) possess a circular center with a wooden platform located on top. The platform can move side to side and front to back (or wobble) and requires the individual to balance during exercise. These stress the ankle inversion and eversion muscles nicely in addition to plantar- and dorsiflexors. See Interpreting Research: Comparison of Various Balance Devices.

Elastic Bands, Cords, Tubing, Chains, and Springs

Elastic bands, cords, and tubing provide *variable resistance* to the athlete. Resistance increases as the band or tubing is stretched further matching an ascending strength curve. Remember from Chapter 2 that elastic force = stiffness × stretch length. Thus, stiffer bands and greater lengths of band displacement yield higher levels of resistance. The range of resistance can be from minimal to more than 45 kg depending on the length and type of band used (49). Some band companies provide a chart depicting how many pounds of force are provided at various band lengths. This information is pertinent to the athlete as one can control the tension by positioning the body at a point corresponding to the desired band length/tension. There a number of types of bands on the market (*i.e.*, therapy, compact resistance, lateral, figure 8, heavy-duty, etc.) often color coded to denote the level of resistance. Bands have multiple uses. They can be used to

- Perform traditional RT or bodyweight exercises like presses, squats, lunges, and rows.

Sidebar: Stability Ball Exercise and Training Research

SB exercise has been a topic of research interest (35). Electromyography (EMG) studies show conflicting results regarding the chest press exercise where the SB chest press produced similar rectus abdominis muscle activation to a chest press on a bench (36). However, other studies show higher abdominal and lower-back muscle activation when the exercise is performed on an SB (37–39). Bench press muscle activation (pectoralis major, triceps brachii, anterior deltoid) is similar when performing the bench press on the ball versus a bench (40), whereas deltoid activity was higher during an SB chest press in one study (38).

SB exercises may result in greater selected trunk muscle activation during core exercises (41). Core exercises performed on SBs increase abdominal muscle activation by 28% compared to a stable surface (37). SB crunches result in greater abdominal muscle activation than crunches performed on a floor primarily when the ball is located under the lower back (as opposed to when the ball is located under the upper-back region) (42). SB curl-ups resulted in 14% and 5% greater activation of the rectus abdominis and external oblique muscles, respectively, compared to a stable surface (43). In contrast, squats and deadlifts with at least 50%–70% of 1RM yielded higher lumbar muscle activity than unloaded exercises (bridge, back extension, quadruped) (44). Most research indicates performing trunk exercises on an SB provides a novel training stimulus.

Of great importance to RT is the effect performing exercises on SBs has on loading. Reduced loading is used when exercises are performed on an SB. Anderson and Behm (36) showed that maximum ISOM chest press force was ~60% lower on an SB compared to a flat bench. McBride et al. (45) showed that maximum ISOM squat force and rate of force development (and agonist muscle activation) was 40%–46% lower on an unstable surface then on a floor. Work capacity during chest press training on an SB (compared to bench) was 12% lower (46). However, Goodman et al. (40) showed similar 1RM bench press strength performances between SB and bench. The majority of research supports the concept that loading (and rep number with a specific load) must be reduced when performing nonbodyweight exercises on SBs.

Cowley et al. (46) showed that 3 weeks of chest press training on an SB or bench in untrained women produced similar increases in strength (assessed both on a bench and SB). Training specificity appears to be preserved where bench press training on a SB produces the greatest strength increases (when tested on a SB) but does have a smaller transfer effect to bench pressing with dumbbells or on a Smith machine (47).

- Train multi-joint, total-body movements in all three motion planes.
- Provide variable resistance to free-weight exercises.
- Load exercises for corrective or kinesthetic strategies, *i.e.*, placing bands around ankles during side-shuffling, lateral movements, hip flexion, or any foot movement drill to strengthen hip ab/adductors, flexors, extensors, rotators; placed around knees to strength hips in order to reduce valgus collapse.
- Provide support (self-spotting) for exercises such as pull-ups or negative hamstring curls.
- Provide multiple angles and directions to change the loading vectors for many exercises.
- Augment ECC loading the greater they are stretched.
- Load power exercises such as vertical jumping and sprinting to increase jump performance and acceleration ability.
- Load sport-specific exercises or movements to provide resistance to motor skills such as throwing, hitting, striking, kicking, body throwing, etc.
- Support plates or KBs when attached to a bar to provide oscillations that make the exercise more difficult to perform. The *oscillation bench press* (Fig. 13.10) loads the shoulder flexors/adductors and elbow extensors but increases the stabilization muscle activity to control bar path during the lowering and raising of the bar.

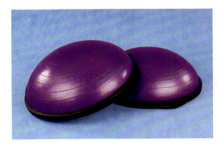 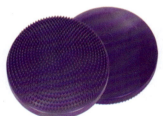 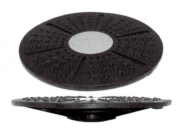

FIGURE 13.9 BOSU balls and balance discs.

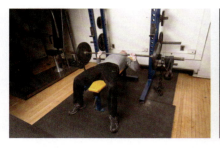 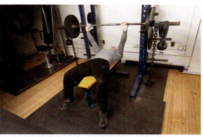

FIGURE 13.10 The oscillation bench press with chains and kettlebells attached to bar with bands.

Bands and tubing are light and portable. They can be transported anywhere and used for home training or for RT while traveling. Many companies make different styles of bands. Usually, they are color coded based on the amount of resistance they supply and may be labeled anywhere from extra light to super heavy. Bands can be placed under the feet or other bodily region and grasped for tension, or placed around a stable object (mounted to wall or post) and grasped for tension. Some short bands can be placed around both legs to resist frontal plane lower-body movements, *e.g.*, side steps, shuffling, lateral movements, or to increase gluteus medius/minimus activity during squats and jumps. The latter is used as a training tool for ACL injury prevention in female athletes to reduce knee valgus stress by increasing hip strength. Elastic band RT is beneficial for increasing muscular strength, power, endurance, and functional performance (20,50–52). Progression in intensity is accomplished via stretching the band further or switching to thicker bands. A disadvantage is that the level of resistance is unknown. A recent study examined the benefit of interfacing a load cell with elastic bands (to provide force feedback to the trainee) during training and showed that it could be valuable during band training although it did not augment the strengthening effect more so than band training without feedback (53).

Another utility of bands (and chains) is to provide variable resistance to a barbell exercise. Bands can be added to barbells especially for exercises such as the bench press and squat. Several elite powerlifters use them quite effectively since their inception of use at the Westside Barbell Club in Columbus, Ohio. Because the squat and bench press are multiple-joint exercises that exemplify ascending strength curves, bands provide greater resistance as the lift progresses (where the athlete is in a stronger area of the ROM). Bands are used for the deadlift exercise. A study by Wallace et al. (54) compared a free-weight squat (85% of 1RM) to squats using bands, one condition where bands accounted for 20% of the resistance and a second condition where bands accounted for 35% of the resistance. They showed that peak force and power were greater with bands compared to the free-weight squat. The lower resistance observed early in the exercise ROM may allow for greater velocity and the extra resistance added toward the end of the ROM may help reduce the deceleration phase common to traditional resistance exercises, thereby increasing average bar velocity and power throughout the rep (55). During the deadlift, highest forces were recorded with free weights only; however, rep velocity and power increased more so as band resistance increased (15% and 35% of total resistance) to replace part of the free-weight resistance (56). Bands used to supply ~15% of 1RM resistance added to the deadlift and box squat (totaling 85% of 1RM) have been shown to induce greater postactivation potentiation during a standing broad jump then with free weights alone (57). When combined with barbell training (*i.e.*, 15%–20% of average loading for band resistance plus 80%–85% from free weights), the addition of elastic bands to barbells was shown to be 4%–10% more effective than barbell training alone for increasing 1RM bench press and squat strength (58–60). However, some studies did not report significant 1RM strength augmentation of bands added to barbells during periodized training in novice individuals (61) suggesting its efficacy may be greater in trained individuals.

Chains are used in a similar manner for performing the squat, bench press, and variations. Chains are typically 6–7 ft in length, 12 lb and heavier, and attach easily to a clamp on the barbell. Multiple chains can be attached at each side to provide greater resistance. A segment of the chain rests on the floor at the low end of the ROM so the athlete only has to support and lift a fraction of the chain's weight. Less chain weight is supported by the floor during bar ascent (as more links leave the floor), which forces the athlete to produce more tension. The chains oscillate, which increases the stability requirement. Small chains (3/16–5/16 in. links) provide 1 lb or less weight per foot of length, whereas larger chains (5/8–3/4 in. links) provide 3–5 lb of weight per foot of length. A few studies examined acute lifting performance using chains. Ebben et al. (62) showed no effects of chains (with chains replacing 10% of the load) on ground reaction force and muscle activation. Coker et al. (63) and Berning et al. (64) showed no difference in ground reaction force and bar velocity of the snatch and clean with chains (replacing 5% of the load) although subjects reported feeling they worked harder with chains. Nijem et al. (65) showed lower ground reaction force and gluteus maximus muscle activation and no difference in rate of force development with chain use (20% of load) during the deadlift. McCurdy et al. (66) examined bench press training in baseball players with chains providing nearly the entire weight versus traditional loading and showed similar increase in strength in both groups. Chains are used as the sole source of resistance during many exercises (Fig. 13.11).

Visit thePoint to view more exercises in the online appendix.

Springs provide variable resistance. As springs are pulled apart, greater tension is encountered. The use of spring RT was

Chapter 13 Resistance Training Equipment and Safety   349

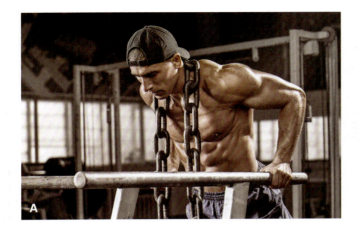 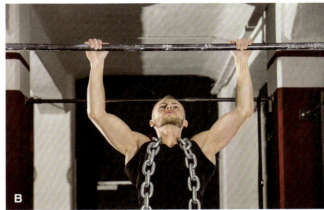

FIGURE 13.11 **A and B.** The dip and pull-up performed with chains.

popular in the 1950s and for decades after when strength training entrepreneurs were searching for alternative methods of training to free weights. Some spring devices are still used but they are not as popular.

Movement-Specific Resistance Devices

Movement-specific resistance devices are those that enable loading to a specific motor skill. For example, power chutes and harnesses are used to resist sprinting. Harnesses may be useful for other acceleration skills for other sports, *e.g.*, resisted takedowns in wrestling or mixed martial arts. Weighted vests are used to resist sprinting, jumping, and numerous other motor skills. Sleds are used to resist sprinting and plyometric drills (Fig. 13.12). Elastic bands have many uses including resisting sport-specific movements. Treadmills have been developed to resist sprinting without additional loading to the skeletal system. For example, the Woodway Force 3.0 treadmill provides loading within the belt via an electromagnetic braking system of up to 150 lb of resistance. Training on this treadmill has been shown to be effective for increasing land-based speed (68). Many devices are used to resist movements with the intent to increase muscle strength, power, and acceleration ability.

Ropes and Battling Ropes

Ropes are used in a number of capacities. Historically, they were mostly used for climbing, pulling, and suspension training (Fig. 13.13) and used extensively in various settings including physical education classes, gymnastics training, and the training of tactical and combat athletes. Figure 13.13 also depicts the evolution of rope climbing and pulling machines (Marpo Kinetics) that evolved over the years to increase the efficiency of rope exercise especially if space is an issue in the facility or if the trainee has difficulty climbing ropes yet wants to participate in rope training. Given the efficacy of ropes in strength and conditioning, ropes (*i.e.*, *battling ropes* popularized by John Brookfield) have recently been

Interpreting Research
Comparison of Various Balance Devices

Wahl MJ, Behm DG. Not all instability training devices enhance muscle activation in highly resistance-trained individuals. *J Strength Cond Res.* 2008;22:1360–1370.

A study by Wahl and Behm (67) examined muscle activation to standing and squatting on Dyna Discs, BOSU ball, wobble board, an SB, and the floor. The results showed:

- During standing, soleus muscle activity was highest on the wobble board compared to other modalities, and lower abdominal muscle activity was highest using the wobble board, and second on an SB.
- During standing, the SB increased rectus femoris muscle activity the most, the wobble board increased biceps femoris activity the highest, and the SB and wobble board increased erector spinae muscle activity the most.
- During squatting, soleus activity was highest on the wobble board, and lower abdominal activity was highest on the wobble board and SB.
- Dyna Discs and BOSU balls provided a minimal muscle stimulus in resistance-trained subjects.

The authors concluded that modalities that provided greater instability (SB and wobble board) were more effective for increasing muscle activation than those that provide mild instability (Dyna Discs, BOSU).

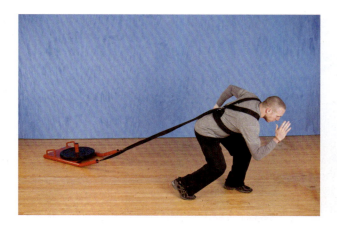

FIGURE 13.12 Illustration of resisted running with a sled.

Sleds and Automobiles

The use of sleds in training has increased greatly in popularity in S&C. Historically, most studies examined the use of towing sleds as a method of speed and acceleration training and showed that resisted speed training with sleds (light to moderate loading, i.e., <50% of bodyweight) can increase speed, power, and acceleration. Heavy sled pushing is commonly used by athletes to increase muscle strength along a horizontal force vector. This is especially important to athletes who have to overcome the force of an opponent such as football players or wrestlers. The use of automobiles is used in a similar manner for heavy pushing and pulling exercises. Berning et al. (73) examined the metabolic responses to all-out pushing and pulling a 1,960-kg automobile for 400 m and showed that $\dot{V}O_2$ and heart rate reached 65% and 96% of max (with no differences between pushing and pulling), respectively, and led to substantial fatigue, dizziness, and nausea, thereby showing the great physical challenge posed by this training implement. Sled pushing (and pulling) is commonly included in high-intensity interval (i.e., metabolic) training programs because they elicit potent metabolic and cardiovascular responses over long distances or when short rest intervals are used. A number of exercises are performed with sleds (Fig. 13.15) such as pushing and pulling, sprints, bear crawls, lunges, pull-through, low pulley rows, plank rope pulls, and side lateral shuffles. Sled can be loaded with heavy weights but the magnitude will depend on the surface as the coefficient of friction will vary. A smooth surface will make the exercise easier and a rougher surface (turf) will reduce sled motion and force the athlete to exert more force throughout the entirety of the rep.

used for undulations, or wave training, to increase strength, endurance, and provide potent metabolic and cardiovascular responses (Fig. 13.14). Waves are generated via multiple movement patterns as the ropes are anchored at a fixed point. Many exercises can be performed, e.g., single- and double-arm waves, and several others can be performed when using different postures (standing, seated, kneeling, prone, lunge, squat) and integrated with other modalities such as plyometric drills, calisthenics, and footwork agility (lateral shuffles, hops, etc.). The length and diameter of the ropes, as well as the velocity and amplitude of the waves, govern exercise intensity to a certain extent (69). Ropes are typically 10–100 ft in length, 1–2 in. in diameter, and weigh ~0.46–0.98 lbs per foot of rope depending on the diameter and type of rope used. Studies show battling rope exercises and training (e.g., single- and double-arm waves, double-arm slams) produce substantial metabolic responses (Table 13.1) comparable to or exceeding other modalities of anaerobic exercise (4,70,71). The metabolic responses are greater with short rest intervals (72).

Strength Implements

The use of strength implements in RT has increased in popularity in recent times. However, some of these implements were

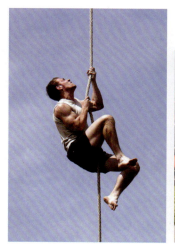
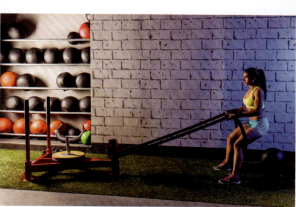
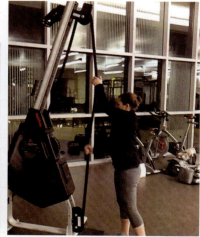

FIGURE 13.13 The use of ropes for climbing, pulling, and the Marpo Kinetics Rope Climbing Machine. (From Shutterstock and Marpo Fitness, https://marpofitness.com/products)

events (Strongest Man in the World competition), strength athletes incorporated these implements into their own programs. In fact, it was shown that the majority of strength competitors include implements and perform the tire flip (82%), log clean and press (95%), stone lifting (94%), farmer's walk (96%), truck pull (49%), axle (80%), yoke (>75%), kegs (60%), sleds (60%), and sandbags (45%) routinely in training (74). The efficacy and popularity have carried over to other goals as many strength/power athletes now frequently integrate implements into a general RT program. Strength training with implements has been shown to produce increases in maximal strength, speed, agility, and power comparable to traditional RT in rugby players (75). Implements provide a different stress to the athlete than free weights as many implements provide unbalanced resistance and the gripping may be more difficult. Some exercises with implements cannot be replicated with free weights. The following section discusses some popular implements. It is important to note that other implements not discussed have been used, *e.g.*, trucks for pulling/towing and other heavy objects.

Kegs

Kegs are fluid-filled drums used in RT. Kegs can weigh as little as 20–30 lb or more than 300 lb. Keg weight is determined by the training status of the athlete, goals of the program, and the targeted exercises. Some facilities have kegs of various weights for training variation. Because kegs are filled with fluids (and sand), there is a greater balance requirement especially if fluid is used over sand. Fluid moves as the kegs are lifted, thereby requiring the athlete to alter force production and muscle activation for stabilization. As a result, athletes who perform exercises with kegs similar to free-weight exercises need to select lighter kegs to accommodate the stabilization effect. Gripping is important. Although kegs have grip supports, athletes will

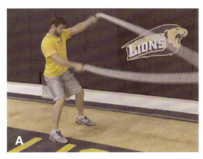
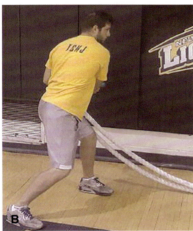

FIGURE 13.14 Battling rope alternate waves **(A)** and grappler rotation exercises **(B)**. (Reprinted from photos 4 & 6, Stanforth D, Brumitt J, Ratamess NA, Atkins W, Keteyian SJ. Toys and training … bells, ropes, and balls—oh my! *ACSM's Health Fit J*. 2015;19:5–11.)

used for many years in RT. The idea to use these implements stemmed from strength competitions in which various implements were used. As training specificity increased for these

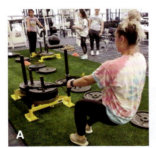
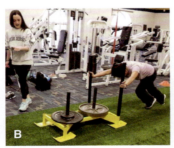
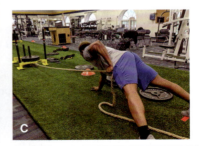
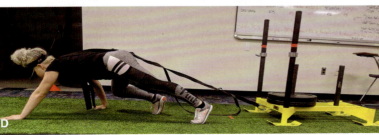
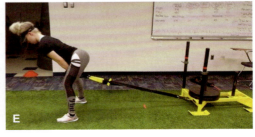

FIGURE 13.15 A–E. The sled pull, push, plank pull, bear crawl, and pull through exercises.

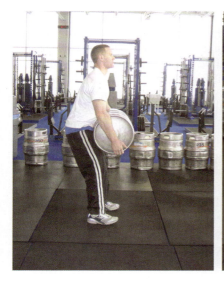
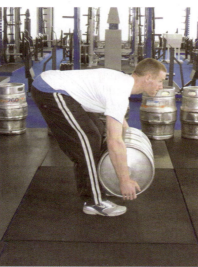

FIGURE 13.16 Illustration of a deadlift with a keg. (Reprinted with permission from Chandler J, Brown L. *Conditioning for Strength and Human Performance*. Baltimore (MD): Lippincott Williams & Wilkins; 2008.)

not have the same strong grip with kegs as they would with a barbell. Many traditional exercises can be performed with kegs including squats, lunges, deadlifts, bench press, and rows (Fig. 13.16). Strength/power-specific exercises such as keg toss, chops, swings, cleans, shouldering, bearhug variations, slams, carries, and throws can be performed.

Kettlebells

Kettlebells (KBs) were used for weighing crops in the 1700s in Russia but ultimately were used in strength festivals and became a training tool for Soviet army. They became a popular piece of training equipment in Europe and Russia since the 1940s and were introduced in America in the 1990s (76). Competitive KB lifting is known as *Girevoy* sport, which began in Russia in the 1960s. It consists of 3 lifts: snatch (with 1 KB), jerk (with 2 KBs), and the long jerk (with 2 KBs cleaned) with a standard KB size (e.g., 16–32 kg). Competition format includes a biathlon (number of jerks in 10 min followed by the number of snatches in 10 min) and the long cycle (number of long jerks in 10 min). It is a rigorous sport that contests muscle strength, power, and endurance. A recent study examining simulated Girevoy KB snatches with a 16-kg KB showed a cardiorespiratory response capable of eliciting increased aerobic capacity (77).

KBs are circular weights with handles attached (Fig. 13.17). They come in sizes similar to dumbbells. KBs provide unique challenges to the athlete separate from the effects of dumbbells. KBs are beneficial for enhancing grip strength because the grips are thicker. The handle is designed to allow the KB to swing freely. Leverage changes as it is lifted, placing greater strength on hand/forearm musculature and requiring greater activation of stabilizer muscles to support the added movement of the KB. As opposed to a dumbbell (which is grasped near the COG as the handle is located between the weights), KBs are grasped off of the COG (for several gripping styles) with the handle located on top of the weight. More rotation occurs during some KB exercises forcing the athlete to adapt by greater grip support.

KBs can be grasped in a number of ways to vary exercises and create a grip strength training challenge. Common gripping styles include

- Bottom's up
- 2-hand
- Press
- Horn
- Crush
- Side
- Waiter
- Push-up
- Palm

Visit thePoint to view these gripping styles and more exercises in the online appendix..

KB training can be implemented in many ways. One critical element in learning several KB exercises initially is to learn the proper rack position. This position is important for overhead lifts, carries, and for support during squats and lunges. Exercises performed with dumbbells can be performed with KBs. However, popular KB exercises and related variations

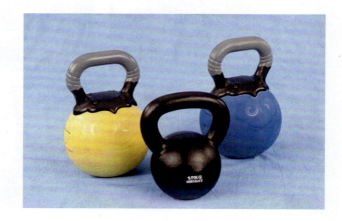

FIGURE 13.17 Illustration of kettlebells.

include swings, presses and jerks, rows, cleans, snatch, windmills, squats, lunges, and Turkish get-ups. Exercises can be performed with 1 or 2 KBs but some are more effective with 1 KB (*i.e.*, Turkish get-up) and use of 1 KB for several exercises provides asymmetrical loading to stress core/trunk musculature. A number of studies have examined muscle activation and metabolic responses to KB exercises, as well as chronic effects of KB training on muscle strength, power, endurance, and aerobic capacity, and shown KB training elicits significant metabolic responses (when the program is targeting endurance) as well as significant chronic training effects showing KBs to be a useful RT modality (78–80).

Logs

Tree logs and log bars have been used in training. Smaller tree logs may be used for carries and larger logs used for deadlifts and related exercises. The military has used large logs for team carry drills. Log bars allow weights to be added to each side. However, they have a midrange grip support, which allows athletes to use them with a pronated forearm position. Some logs are filled with water to add resistance and, similar to kegs, forces the individual to increase stabilizer muscle activity. Many exercises can be performed including cleans, presses, jerks, rows, squats, deadlifts, and lunges.

Farmer's Walk Bars

Farmer's walk bars are implements that allow the athlete to grasp a heavy weight and walk/run with it for a specified distance. Farmer's walk is a popular contested strength competition event. These bars enable training for this event plus have a carryover effect for improving general strength, power, and fitness. These bars are effective for enhancing grip strength. Because of their design, limited exercise selection is seen compared to some other implements. Various models of Farmer's walk bars have been developed. Nylon webbing (for grasping) can be used in conjunction with dumbbells to replicate the Farmer's walk. Some will also use dumbbells, single weight plates, or hex bars to perform the farmer's walk.

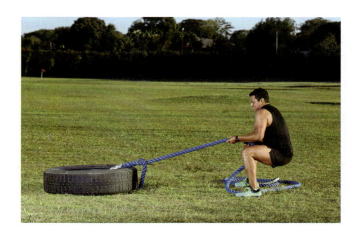

FIGURE 13.18 Use of tires for pulling exercises. (Image from Shutterstock.)

Tires and Sledgehammers

The use of tires for a number of exercises is common to the S&C of athletes. Historically, tires were used for agility drills in sports such as football. Tires are used for dragging (or towed) and pulling exercises in a manner similar to sleds (Fig. 13.18). Tires are used for resisted carry drills. In addition, tires are used for grappling drills where two athletes come together and try to wrestle the tire away and/or drag their opponent in the process of reaching a finish line (see thePoint online). Tires from trucks and heavy equipment provide a great deal of resistance for athletes, primarily for end-to-end flipping. Tire flipping involves a triple extension of the hips, knees, and ankles that is beneficial for increasing strength and power (Fig. 13.19). The tire is lifted off the ground by pushing the body into it; hands are adjusted and extended to flip the tire. The tire flip is described in 4 phases. Keogh et al. (81) showed mean tire flip time took ~2.9 seconds (range = ~1.9–3.72 s) and that the 1st pull, 2nd pull, transition, and push phases took ~0.74 second (range = 0.71–0.77 s), 1.12 (range = 0.38–1.7 s), 0.15 (range = 0.15–0.17 s), and 0.95 second (range = 0.66–1.14 s), respectively. Tire flipping (2 sets of 6 flips) elicits potent cardiometabolic demands, *e.g.*, mean heart rate of 180 bpm, blood lactate ~10.4 mmol·L^{-1} (81). Experienced athletes select a tire that is about twice their

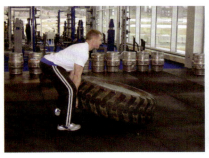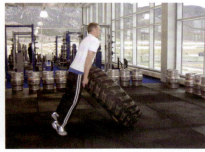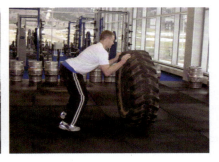

FIGURE 13.19 Illustration of tire flipping. (Reprinted with permission from Chandler J, Brown L. *Conditioning for Strength and Human Performance.* Baltimore (MD): Lippincott Williams & Wilkins; 2008.)

bodyweight to start, and with the tire lying flat, that comes to around knee level. A disadvantage is that a facility may need several tires of different sizes and weights to accommodate many athletes. Larger tires are used for strength and metabolic training, whereas smaller or moderate-sized tires may be used for speed, power, metabolic, and endurance training. Muscle endurance is enhanced by performing more reps, flipping for greater distance, or using timed intervals. Other devices (*i.e.,* Flip'T Trainer and The Tread) and machines (*e.g.,* Tire Flip 180) have been developed to replicate tire flipping in more practical terms. Devices such as the Flip'T Trainer and The Tread have handles/straps to help with gripping and allow it to be used for carries or the farmer's walk.

Tires serve as a target for *sledgehammer training.* Swinging sledgehammers is an excellent exercise that stresses core and grip musculature. Sledgehammers come in various sizes ranging from 8 to 20 lb and are used for vertical, horizontal, and diagonal swings. The athlete explosively strikes the tire with the sledgehammer in a repetitive manner. The athlete must control the rebound of the hammer from the tire. The exercise can be made more difficult by increasing the resistance arm by grasping the hammer closer to the end of the handle or more explosive by grasping the hammer closer to the head for speed and power. Timed intervals or high-rep sets are common for sledgehammer training. Sledge hammers are used for strengthening exercises involving ISOM actions or grip/forearm strength training.

Visit thePoint to view more exercises in the online appendix.

Sandbags and Heavy Bags

Sandbags have plastic bags filled with sand enclosed within a larger bag. They range in size, shape, and weight from being light to over 100 lbs and many styles have handles enabling easier gripping. Sandbags provide the athlete with unbalanced resistance, which forces the athlete to increase stabilizer muscle activation for proper technique. They are effective for increasing grip strength because they must be grasped with very little support especially for those styles that do not have handles. It is thought that sandbag training may provide the athlete with a larger transfer of training effects to performance of occupational tasks, which is why they are commonly used by tactical athletes. Many exercises can be performed with sandbags including squats, drags, lunges, Turkish get-ups, presses, deadlifts, pulls, cleans, rows, bear hug throws, burpees, carries, twists, etc. We examined a sandbag protocol consisting of 8 exercises performed in 3 rounds using Tabata intervals (*e.g.,* 20 s of exercise with 10 s of rest) and reported energy expenditure values similar to those obtained during running at 60% of $\dot{V}O_{2max}$ (82). The sandbag protocol produced a large cardiometabolic response. Thus, sandbags can effectively be used for strength, power, and endurance training depending on program structure.

Like sandbags, heavy bags (punching bags) have multiple uses in S&C. Heavy bags are commonly used in striking sports such as boxing, martial arts, and mixed martial arts to build strength, power, and speed for various types of strikes with the hands, feet, elbows, and knees when hanging suspended from a support. They are used on the ground for improving "ground and pound" skills of mixed martial arts fighters. Heavy bags are used for RT. They can be used for exercises such as squats, front squats, drags, carries, runs, and bear hug throws. These are beneficial for grappling athletes as they mimic an opponent and can be thrown or lifted in multiple directions.

Visit thePoint to view more exercises in the online appendix.

Stones

Stone lifting dates back thousands of years possibly to the beginning of time and is regarded by some as one of the ultimate forms of strength as it greatly challenges all major muscle groups throughout the phases of lifting (83). Organized stone lifting for training and competition has been a staple of training especially in countries such as Scotland, Wales, Iceland, Denmark, Norway, Sweden, and Finland for the last several hundreds of years. Many types of unique and aptly named stones have originated in these countries and have been used weighing from 30 to 50 lbs to more than 500 lbs. For example, the Husafell stone in Iceland weighs ~409–420 lbs, the Inver stone in Scotland weighs ~265–268 lbs, and the Barevan stone in Scotland weighs ~231 lbs. The Dinnie stones are a pair (~317 and 414 lbs) with ring handles that are either lifted from a straddle position or from a farmer's walk position. The McGlashen, or Atlas, stones (which range in size from ~220 lbs to more than 350 lbs in the World's Strongest Man competition) are popular and have been used especially in strength competitions. The technique used to lift stones is unique and depends on the stone's size, shape, texture, weight, and balance (83). The trainee straddles the stone, cradles the stone between the elbows and forearms with hands as low as possible, deadlifts the stone, sits back and loads the stone into the lap, readjusts arm positioning, and squats to the standing position rolling the stone up to the chest where it can be hoisted over the shoulder, pressed overhead, carried, or placed on a loading platform (Fig. 13.20). Other than lifting real stones, equipment such as stone molds, stone trainers, heavy sandbags, and medicine balls have been developed to mimic and aid in stone lift training.

Super Yoke

The Super Yoke stems from strength competitions. It requires the athlete to walk or partial squat a heavy weight on the shoulder in the yoke apparatus. The super yoke walk poses a large physical challenge to the athlete requiring strength and balance to keep the yoke from swaying. Given the level of loading, the yoke walk can be used for progressive distances or timed intervals.

Water and the Environment

Water and the environment are other sources of resistance. Certain properties of water enable it to create resistance to motion. The buoyancy of water is defined as the upward force

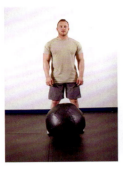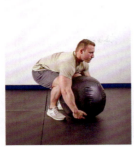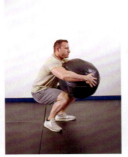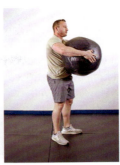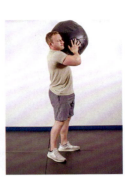

FIGURE 13.20 The proper technique of stone lifting.

acting in the opposite direction of gravity and is related to the specific gravity of the athlete immersed in the water (84). Specific gravity is the ratio of the mass of an object to its mass of water displacement. The specific gravity of the human body is less than the specific gravity of water (1.0); therefore, humans float. Greater resistance to motion is supplied when athletes move downward against the force of buoyancy. Upward motion encounters less resistance because the buoyancy force supports the movement. Buoyancy forces allow the athlete's limbs to remain parallel to the pool with little effort, *e.g.*, during horizontal abduction (84). Hydrostatic pressure provides resistance to motion in water as depth increases. Resistance in the water is encountered due to the water's viscosity. Human movement through water causes adjacent water molecules to collide, which increases fluid resistance and resists motion. The resistance encountered is increased when the athlete moves at faster rates or uses equipment to increase the amount of surface area exposed to water molecular flow (84).

In addition to swimming, aquatic RT programs are popular. They involve performing exercises in the water against natural water resistance or using aquatic resistance devices, *e.g.*, aqua dumbbells, belts, fan paddles and gloves, wrist and ankle cuffs, and training shoes. Aquatic resistance exercise reduces stress on the joints and skeletal system, which make it attractive for special populations and athletes rehabilitating injuries or general all-purpose training. There is less cardiovascular and thermoregulatory demand. However, there is less of an ECC component with aquatic resistance exercise. Aquatic RT is effective for increasing muscle strength, grip strength, hypertrophy, flexibility, endurance, and functional performance in various populations (43,85,86). Plyometric training in the water is effective for increasing vertical jump performance (87). See Interpreting Research: Mechanical Analysis of Strongmen Events.

Environmental factors such as hills (downhill and uphill) and terrain provide added resistance. Running uphill provides a greater neuromuscular and metabolic challenge to the athlete than running on a flat surface. This is evident in athletes who frequently run up (and down) stadium steps. Downhill running has a substantial ECC component and is more likely to result in muscle damage and delayed onset muscle soreness. Rougher surfaces are more challenging physiologically and place more strain on the joints then smooth, even surfaces. For example, walking in sand or snow increases metabolic energy expenditure two to three times (89). Terrain can be used to enhance training, especially walking, jogging, and sprinting.

Interpreting Research
Mechanical Analysis of Strongmen Events

McGill SM, McDermott A, Fenwick CMJ. Comparison of different strongman events: trunk muscle activation and lumbar spine motion, load, and stiffness. *J Strength Cond Res.* 2009;23:1148–1161.

McGill et al. (88) analyzed muscle activation and spinal loading characteristics of several strongmen events: farmer's walk, suitcase carry, super yoke walk, tire flip, log lift, Atlas stone lift, and the keg walk. They found

- Greatest spinal compression was seen during the super yoke walk.
- Greatest L4/L5 vertebrae moments were seen in the tire flip followed by the keg walk and log lift.
- The tire flip and Atlas stone lift produced the greatest activation of rectus abdominis, internal and external obliques, latissimus dorsi, gluteus medius and maximus, biceps femoris, erector spinae, and rectus femoris muscles. The log lift also produced high erector spinae activity.
- All events produced great challenges to the core and hip musculature to stabilize the spine. Carrying events produced differential activation patterns than lifting events.

Case Study 13.2

Lisa is a high school student who is considering trying out for the school's basketball team. Although Lisa has been playing some pick-up basketball games with her friends to get in shape, she very much wants to begin RT to increase her chances of making the team. Rather than join a gym or lift weights in the high school weight room, Lisa wants to train in the privacy of her own home. She has limited space in the garage and her father has agreed to purchase some inexpensive equipment for her.

Questions for Consideration: Based on her situation, what RT modalities would you recommend for Lisa? What type of equipment is reasonably priced and may be of great benefit to her? How would you advise Lisa to begin her RT program?

Vibration Devices and Training

Vibrations are mechanical oscillations that are defined by their frequency (number of cycles per second) and amplitude (half difference between minimum and maximum oscillatory values) (90). The magnitude of vibration can be represented by the acceleration (g or $m \cdot s^{-2}$) in addition to amplitude (91). Vibrations using different waveforms can be added to the exercise, *i.e., vibration training,* by (a) applied directly to an exercising muscle via a handheld vibrating unit or (b) via a vibrating platform (known as *whole-body vibration training*). Although vibration training dates back to the 1960s, the latter has become more popular in recent times not only in athletes but also in elderly and special populations. Adding vibrations to an exercise is a common feature to the oscillation bench press or other exercise using a tsunami barbell or chains and elastic bands with kettlebells (discussed previously in this text), the *Bodyblade*, and the *Shake Weight*. The Bodyblade can be used for a large number of exercises as oscillations are supplied by the vibrating blade during contraction. The Shake Weight is dumbbell-like, which vibrates while it is being lifted during an exercise. For total body vibration training, whole-body vibration plates have reciprocal vertical displacement (on left and right) or whole-plate uniform up and down oscillations. Most vibration units provide a frequency in the range of 15–60 Hz, displacements of <1–10 mm, and up to 15-g acceleration (92).

Vibrations elicit responses to several physiological systems. The proposed performance improvement effects are thought to occur via enhanced neural responses. Vibrations are thought to stimulate the primary endings of muscle spindles (Ia afferents), which potentiates motoneuron discharge to agonist muscles, called a *tonic vibration reflex* (91). More efficient motor patterns, recruitment, and synchronization result and dynamic muscle force and power production are thought to be enhanced. It has been suggested that vibrations compensate for fatigue by increasing motor unit output (91). It has been suggested that vibration training may also augment energy expenditure and increase weight loss (93), and prior bodyweight exercise combined with WBV can augment energy expenditure during subsequent aerobic exercise than with no vibration (94). WBV provides a stimulus capable of increasing muscle hypertrophy in a variety of populations (95). Of concern are potential hazards associated with vibrations. In animal and workplace studies, vibrations were associated with cardiovascular stress, lung damage, bone/joint damage, low-back problems, and neurological disorders (91). However, the magnitude of vibrations exposed to athletes appears lower, provided caution is used. Vibration devices have the potential to expose athletes to high levels of vibration that could be injurious; however, training studies have been short term using moderate stimuli.

Whole-body vibration devices have been studied during acute exercise and training (Fig. 13.21). The stimulus is defined

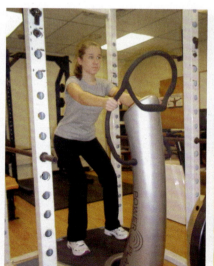
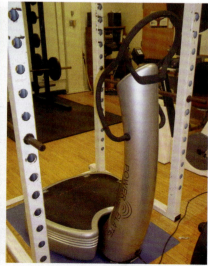

FIGURE 13.21 Illustration of the Power Plate vibration training system.

by the interaction of its frequency (number of stimuli per second), amplitude (oscillation displacement), acceleration (angular frequency^2 × amplitude), and duration in addition to the type of exercise performed on the plate. A large number of dynamic and isometric exercises can be performed on a vibration plate where the feet, knees, hands, arms, trunk, or buttocks are in contact with the plate. Some units have attachments for elastic bands and other modalities such as free weights, medicine balls, and kettlebells can be used during the exercise performed on the vibration plate. Upper-body studies have typically used elbow flexion, whereas whole-body vibration studies have mostly used squatting and lunging movements (91). It is important to note that erect standing positions can cause greater vibratory transmission to the head; thus, greater flexion of the knee can alleviate the stress to the head. Most studies examined vibration training at frequencies of 30–40 Hz (up to 50 Hz) with amplitudes ranging from 2 to 6 mm (up to 12 mm) and accelerations of 2–14 g (up to 18 g) for sets of 30–60 seconds (96). Foot position does not affect amplitude for vertical vibration plates; however, foot position does play a role in side-to-side vibration plates.

Vibration training was shown to augment strength and power, whereas some studies reported no ergogenic effects compared to an identical protocol performed without vibration exposure. Acute studies using vibrations of 26–44 Hz, 3–10 mm, and 30–170 m·s^{-2} have shown vibrations enhanced lower body muscle power by 5%–12%, jump height by 1%–9%, strength by 3%–10%, and produced elevated testosterone and growth hormone and reduced cortisol (90,92,96–100). Some studies showed acute upper body power enhancement of 8%–14% (96). Quadriceps muscle activity was higher during uni- and bilateral ISOM squats on a vibrating platform than with no vibration (85,101). Hazell et al. (102) showed vibration exercise resulted in 1%–7% greater lower-body muscle activation and only greater triceps brachii activation in the upper body. However, higher frequencies (>35 Hz) and amplitudes (4 vs. 2 mm) of vibration produced the highest increases in muscle activation. Whole-body vibration increases muscle temperature, which may augment the acute performance enhancement seen in some vibration studies (96). In contrast, some studies did not show any ergogenic potential of vibration training (90–92,96). Chronic vibration training of 1–8 weeks may increase muscle strength (by 4%–50%), power (by 8%–18%), and flexibility (91,96,100). Longer-term (>8 weeks) studies have shown beneficial effects of vibration training on power, velocity, strength, and flexibility (103–107). However, some studies have shown no effects on strength, power, speed, vertical jump, or agility in athletes (90,108,109). Two meta-analyses (110,111) were performed examining vibration training effects on muscle strength and power and showed (a) acute changes in strength and power were negligible; (b) chronic RT with vibration may have positive impact on strength and power especially with vertical vibration platforms; (c) untrained individuals experienced much larger strength effect sizes than athletes; (d) dose-responses were mostly noted for frequency, amplitude, and volume for strength and power effects; (e) larger strength and power effects were seen when dynamic and ISOM exercises were used compared to ISOM only and the lower-body strength effects were larger when squats and lunges were used compared to squats only; and (f) the power effects were larger in older than younger individuals.

Injury Prevention

Resistance training is thought to play an important role in reducing the risk of injury — not only injuries encountered in the weight room (which are very low) but also injuries encountered in athletics, recreation, or during performance of activities of daily living. Greater muscular strength increases joint stability, which enables the athlete to offset high levels of force encountered during ballistic activities. Tendons, ligaments, and bone adapt to RT by increasing stiffness (tendons), cross-sectional area, and bone mineral density, which provide greater support to the skeletal system and increase force transmission efficiency. Proper RT, *e.g.*, training all muscle groups and improving weaknesses, increases muscle balance. Increasing muscle balance is thought to reduce injury risk; however, more research is needed to show a definitive link between muscle balance and injury prevention. Muscle balance should be maintained between muscles of both sides of the body and those that have antagonistic relationships. Muscle balance entails ensuring that muscle strength and length are at comparable levels. Muscle balance training may be important for reducing the risk of overuse injuries (knee ligament sprains/strains, hamstring tears, shoulder injuries, and low-back pain/injury). For example, gender differences (hormonal, anatomical, strength imbalances) make female athletes more susceptible to ACL injuries (112). Strength balance between the internal and external shoulder rotators is important for reducing shoulder injuries in athletes (113). It is suggested that the ratio of hamstring-to-quadriceps strength be at least 60%, and <10% strength difference be between dominant and nondominant legs. This may be higher in athletes as collegiate female athletes were shown to be at higher risk for leg injury if there was >15% difference in knee flexion strength between right and left legs and hamstrings-quadriceps ratio <75% (114). Lastly, strengthening of the abdominal, hamstrings, hip extensors, and spinal muscles is critical to prevention of low-back injuries. See Box Myths & Misconceptions: Resistance Training Poses a High Risk of Joint Injury and Damage.

Myths & Misconceptions
Resistance Training Poses a High Risk of Joint Injury and Damage

Some have stated that RT is highly injurious. However, studies show that RT poses less of a risk of injury compared to other competitive sports when it is performed properly (25,115). For general RT, the most common site of injury is the lower back and the type of injury mostly encountered is a muscle strain (115). The major causes of RT-related injuries are (a) improper lifting technique or poor form; (b) improper loading (increasing load too fast); (c) lack of supervision; (d) overtraining; (e) muscular imbalances; (f) improper warm-up; and (g) weight room accidents. Many of these injury mechanisms stem from inexperience or lack of supervision. A novice individual with poor technique and limited knowledge of program design, and who does not have supervision or an individual (trainer, coach) present for assistance (or spotting), may be at a slightly higher risk. Weight room accidents can occur regardless of experience level, but novice individuals tend to be more susceptible. Experienced athletes are more susceptible to overtraining-related injuries as these individuals train intensively for extended periods of time. Another factor implicated in increasing the injury risk is the use of anabolic steroids (116). Primarily based on some animal data, anabolic steroids increase collagen degeneration (primarily through aromatizing estrogenic effects of anabolic steroid metabolism), thereby placing tendons at greater risk of injury (116). Tendons adapt to loading more slowly than skeletal muscles so an athlete using anabolic steroids who experiences rapid gains in muscular strength and hypertrophy may not have optimal tendinous support at that point in time. As a result, force transmission to bone is compromised and anabolic steroids can be viewed as indirectly increasing the risk of myotendinous injury. However, with proper supervision and exercise prescription, there is a very low risk of injury resulting from drug-free RT.

There is a higher incidence of injury with advanced RT or competitive lifting. These individuals take themselves to their physical limits regularly, thus exposing themselves to a higher risk of injury. This is inherent to training at a high level. Many studies examined injury rates and types in competitive lifting sports of weightlifting, bodybuilding, powerlifting, strength competitions, CrossFit, and the *Highland Games* (*e.g.*, the Highland Games involve contested events such as the caber toss, stone put, Scottish hammer throw, weight throws for distance and height, and the sheaf toss). A few examples are discussed in this section. Keogh et al. (117) examined 101 competitive powerlifters and reported an average of 1.2 injuries per year or 4.4 injuries per 1,000 hours of training. In this sample, 36% reported shoulder injuries, 24% reported low-back injuries, and 11% reported elbow injuries. Goertzen et al. (118) examined 358 bodybuilders and 60 powerlifters and reported that 84% reported some type of injury (pulls, sprains, and tendonitis). Shoulder and elbow injuries were most common (>40%) and low-back and knee injuries were common. Powerlifters showed twice the injury rate as bodybuilders. Raske and Norlin (119) reported that weightlifters exhibited higher frequency of low-back and knee injuries, whereas shoulder injuries were more prominent in powerlifters. In a review of the literature, Keogh and Winwood (120) reported injury rates of 0.12–0.7 injuries per lifter per year and 0.24–1 injury per 1,000 hours in bodybuilders, 0.3–0.4 injuries per lifter per year and 1.0–1.1 injuries per 1,000 hours in powerlifters, 2.0 injuries per lifter per year and 5.5 injuries per 1,000 hours of training in strongman competitors, 2.4–3.3 injuries per 1,000 hours in weightlifters, 3.1 injuries per 1,000 hours in CrossFit, and 7.5 injuries per 1,000 hours of training and competition in Highland Games competitors. Across the lifting sports, the five most commonly injured sites were the shoulder, lower back, knee, elbow, and wrist/hand.

Safe and Effective Resistance Training

For RT to be safe and effective, general procedures should be followed not only to ensure the safe and effective participation of the athlete, but other athletes working out in the facility. In addition to following general safety (and common sense) procedures, proper gym etiquette should be followed to ensure a productive lifting environment for everyone. The safety/etiquette checklist in the Safety Checklist Sidebar can be used to ensure an optimal RT environment. See the later sidebar for tips on becoming an effective spotter.

Sidebar — Safety Checklist

- Obtain medical clearance before initiating RT. Although an individual may appear healthy and the risk of serious illness or death via a cardiovascular event during exercise is very low (<6 individuals per 100,000), it is recommended that screening take place. The ACSM, American Heart Association (AHA), and National Strength and Conditioning Association (NSCA) have published guidelines addressing the procedures used for obtaining medical clearance (121,122). The ACSM and AHA recommend all exercise facilities screen individuals prior to participation with a medical history questionnaire or health appraisal document. All exercise professionals should adhere to the recommendations of these organizations when screening individuals for RT.
- Proper athletic screening. Athletic screening (see Chapter 19) can determine athletes' strengths and weaknesses. Separate from medical clearance, athletic screening can point out glaring motor weaknesses the athlete may have prior to training. Such weaknesses may encompass strength, endurance, flexibility, balance, coordination, and technique deficits that need to be addressed. For example, an athlete with limited flexibility of the hips and ankles who cannot perform a proper squat (posture and depth) with no weight should not begin loaded squat training until motor performance improves. Loading improper motor patterns can be problematic and increase injury risk. Technical (and perhaps flexibility) training will prepare the athlete for greater loading. Although weaknesses may not preclude the athlete from initiating RT, program design should stress weaknesses prior to more advanced RT.
- Proper, nonoffensive clothing should be worn. Nonrestrictive, comfortable clothing (shorts, sweatpants, T-shirts, tank tops, compression shorts, workout pants, leggings, sweat-shirts, yoga pants, etc.) should be worn to allow optimal joint ROM during resistance exercise. Clothing should reflect ambient temperatures as clothing should be worn to keep the individual cool in hot, humid conditions or warm in cool conditions. Proper athletic shoes should be worn to allow comfort, stability, and ease of movement to the athlete.
- Know how each piece of equipment functions and its proper usage. Prior to RT, each athlete should understand how each exercise is performed and how each piece of equipment works prior to use. Lack of knowledge in this area could lead to injury.
- Practice proper form and technique with each exercise, especially with free weights. Although injury risk is low, improper technique, especially with free weights, can increase the risk of injury. A trainer, supervisor, or coach should be consulted if an individual is unclear as to the correct performance of an exercise.
- Before using machines, check for frayed pulleys, loose screws, loose pads, and proper movement. Damage or wear and tear to machines can be injurious. If damage is present, a staff member should be consulted immediately, and the machine should not be used until it is fixed. An "out of order" sign should be placed on the machine subsequently.
- Make sure seat adjustments are correct and pins are all the way through their holes. Each machine will have a proper adjustment point based on the target musculature. For example, in performing a leg extension exercise, the knees should be aligned with the machine's axis of rotation and the seat or back pad should be adjusted accordingly. On a chest press machine, the seat can be adjusted so the grips are positioned at the lower (sternal) chest level. However, positioning the seat above or below this point can shift muscle activation to the upper or lower pectoral muscles, respectively. For machines requiring a pin to change resistance, the pin should be placed all the way through the hole in the weight stack. A partially placed pin may not secure loading appropriately.
- Do not bounce the weight stacks and never put fingers near the stack when someone is using it. Bouncing the weight stack reflects a lack of control, especially during the ECC phase. Weights should be lifted in control and this would negate any loud, clanging bouncing of the weight stack. One should never place fingers or hands near a weight stack while in use. A finger caught in a stack could be very painful or even result in a loss of the finger. Some athletes perform breakdown sets in which a spotter may be located at the weight stack to quickly pull the pin in between sets for an individual to lower the weight. This technique is acceptable; however, spotters must communicate clearly with the individual as to when a set ends and the next set begins. Spotters should keep their hands away from the weight stack except when changing the weight in between sets.
- Never bother anyone while they are in the middle of a set. Common courtesy. Individuals are focused on the task at hand during a set and do not need to be distracted by others in the facility (unless an emergency exists, or the individual is placed at great risk for injury where intervention is necessary). Distraction can place the individual at a higher risk for injury or result in poor performance of the exercise. When communicating with someone in the weight room, it is appropriate to do so upon completion of the exercise or in between sets.
- No horseplay in the facility. Common sense but may occur in younger populations. Poor behavior can result in injury or being asked to leave the gym or club.

(Continued)

- Caution with use of cell phones in the gym. Although they may be positively used as a source of music for the trainee, a watch or timer for set durations, or a source for training information, they can also be a major source of distraction that could leave a trainee temporarily unaware of their surroundings.
- Never attempt to lift ultra-heavy weights without a spotter or safety rack. For certain exercises such as the squat, bench press and variations, and shoulder press, a spotter is recommended when heavy weights are lifted. Because of the position of the body at the lower point of each exercise, the athlete could be trapped under the bar if unable to complete the repetition. Spotters assist in lifting the weight until completion where the bar can be safely racked. If lifting in a power rack, the weight can be safely placed on the pins. For the squat, multiple spotters can be used depending on the amount of weight.
- Make sure dumbbells are tightened. For dumbbells that are not solid (one-piece) but have plates placed on either side that are fastened in place, it is important that these dumbbells remain tightened. Loose dumbbells can result in plates sliding off of one or both sides, perhaps striking the athlete and causing injury.
- Make sure bars are loaded properly and evenly. When loading barbells, it is important to make sure the same amount of weight is placed on both sides. Improper loading can result in one side being heavier than the other, causing disproportionate lifting technique. Caution must be used when unloading bars or plate-loaded machines. One should not take off weight entirely on one side. This could cause the bar to tip and hit someone or cause a small machine to tip. It is important to remove plates from bars equally on both sides.
- Use clamps with barbells to prevent slipping of the weights. Clamps or collars keep plates in place on bars, preventing them from slipping off. Although clamps are not used for various reasons, they do increase safety by keeping plates fixed on barbells.
- Make sure there is enough room between you and other people. Space is an important safety consideration. Lifting too close to someone could result in bodily injury via contact with a bar, dumbbell, kettlebell, battling rope, medicine ball, tire, or any other piece of equipment. The athlete should be aware of extended bars on racks (and other moving parts) to prevent walking into them. Colliding into someone while lifting can disrupt that person's set as well as put him or her at greater risk of injury. Athletes should be aware of the surroundings and always look before moving from one area to the next. This is especially true for lifting platforms where individuals are performing the Olympic lifts. These are explosive lifts and can be dangerous if one gets too close to the bar when another is in the middle of a set. From a weight room perspective, standards have been set by various profes-

sional organizations (122) detailing adequate spacing between pieces of equipment. Gym and club owners should be aware of these guidelines and design facilities accordingly.
- Store equipment properly. One should not leave equipment on the floor in another's walkway. This is a safety issue and a measure of etiquette. Leaving free-weight equipment or MBs could result in tripping, loss of balance, and falling, causing injury. It is important for an individual to replace weights when finished. Individuals must share the gym with others and leaving bars loaded and dumbbells at specific stations (away from racks) requires others to house clean in order to use the equipment. Proper gym etiquette mandates individuals return equipment when they have finished using it.
- Exercise using a fully prescribed ROM. Excellent results are obtained when individuals perform exercises in a fully prescribed ROM. Although some advanced techniques require athletes to perform partial ROM exercises, under many conditions, it is imperative for athletes to perform each exercise in a full ROM.
- Properly warm-up prior to RT. The benefits of a warm-up were discussed previously in this text. It is imperative that athletes properly warm-up before lifting weights to reduce the risk of injury and enhance performance.
- Always make sure the athlete is in a stable position when beginning an exercise. It is important to make sure the athlete is focused, prepared, and ready to begin a set when performing an exercise with a heavy weight. This entails being in the proper body position when initiating an exercise. In some cases, a spotter may be used to help the athlete lift the weight to a starting position (a "lift-off"). This is customary when performing a bench press, behind-the-neck press, and when heavy dumbbells are handed to the athlete for various exercises. Spotters need to make sure the athletes are ready to receive the load, so communication is paramount. Handing or lifting off a weight to an athlete unprepared could cause injury.
- Use proper control when lifting weights and placing them down. Athletes should control the weights; the weights should not control the athlete. Proper loading is essential to assisting in controlling weights especially during the ECC phase. A common mistake by beginners is to let gravity control the weight during the ECC phase. Accentuating the ECC phase is critical to maximal strength and hypertrophy development. Not controlling the ECC phase increases the risk of injury and limits performance improvement. In some cases, athletes drop or throw free weights upon completion of a set if they are in a compromised position. For example, some athletes drop dumbbells to the floor after completion of a set of dumbbell bench presses. This is because the athlete must rise off of the bench and it is difficult to do

(Continued)

so with heavy dumbbells in hand. Athletes drop weights upon completion of an Olympic lift on a platform using bumper plates. Several examples can be mentioned but the key is to use caution and control in these situations.

♦ When lifting weights from the floor, use the lower body and proper posture as much as possible. Proper lifting technique is important for reducing the risk of low-back injuries. Low-back injuries stem from different factors (poor extensor muscle endurance and strength, length/strength imbalances, spinal muscle atrophy, reduced neural/muscle activation or coactivation), but improper lifting technique places great stress on lumbar vertebrae, potentially causing injury. Repeated trunk flexion places large amounts of stress on lumbar discs, in some cases enough to cause bulging or herniation. Proper technique involves increasing spinal stability while minimizing spinal loading. This is accomplished in a few ways. First, the athlete must increase spinal stability by increasing IAP. A technique known as abdominal bracing is used. Abdominal bracing involves contraction of all layers of abdominal muscles in unison (123). Lumbar extensor muscles cocontract to increase spine rigidity. This maintains the lordotic arch (flat-back position), which reduces spinal shear stress. It is important to teach athletes the correct posture, hip hinge, and bracing technique early in training. It could be described as retracting the shoulder girdle, sticking the chest out, and bracing the core. This position should be maintained for all exercises and not solely for lifting weights off of the ground. A rounded (flexed) spine places the athlete at greater risk of injury. IAP increases in response to a Valsalva maneuver, or temporary breath holding, which compounds the stabilizing effects of bracing. Second, the athlete should lift with the legs as much as possible. This involves strong contraction of the hip extensor muscles especially the gluteus maximus. Contracting the hip musculature reduces spinal loading forcing the hips to do most of the work. Abdominal bracing and correct lifting technique are the best ways to prevent acute low-back injuries.

♦ Make sure spotters are capable. It is important to select spotters who have experience and know how to spot for a given exercise. Communication with spotters is critical to the type of spot needed by the athlete. Some individuals prefer the spotter to provide no assistance until failure and some individuals prefer to have a spotter assist before failure. Some individuals prefer minimal assistance from the spotter (just enough force to keep the bar moving) while some prefer more assistance. The spotter needs to have sufficient strength. For strong athletes performing a heavy exercise, it is mandatory that the spotter be strong enough to assist if failure occurs. Although spotters many times only need to provide low levels of force, if greater force is needed, the spotter has to be strong enough to accommodate. In rare cases, a poor spotter can increase the risk of injury.

♦ When perspiring, make sure to carry a towel or clean equipment after use. For proper gym etiquette, it is a good idea to have a towel to prevent excessive perspiration on the equipment. If not, then wiping down the equipment with cleanser after use is recommended. Although perspiration is desired, leaving a pool of sweat on the equipment is not desirable and inconsiderate to other athletes in the facility. Individuals should make sure to wash their hands or use a hand sanitizer upon completion of a workout. This is important for reducing the risk of catching a cold, flu, or other infection. Although many individuals clean equipment upholstery after perspiration, bars, dumbbells, machine handles, MBs, etc. (pieces of equipment that are gripped with the hands) are rarely cleaned and are the first line by which infections may be passed. Gripping equipment that hundreds of other individuals gripped and placing one's hands on the facial region are easy ways to contaminate oneself.

♦ Always practice proper breathing. Proper breathing entails exhaling on the positive phase (more difficult segment) and inhaling on the negative (easier phase because muscles are stronger during ECC muscle actions) for many exercises. Some repetitive exercises require rhythmical breathing, *e.g.*, bear crawl or various types of carries. Some exercises (*e.g.*, Turkish get-up, various Olympic lifts) have more than the usual three phases of lifting and require cyclical breathing patterns depending on the level of exertion within each phase. Under many conditions (low- to moderate-intensity exercise), proper breathing should be performed during resistance exercise to maximize performance and reduce cardiovascular stress. However, there are exceptions. Holding one's breath (Valsalva maneuver) increases IAP, intrathoracic pressure, and torso rigidity. For example, a powerlifter during a maximal squat may inhale during the decent to the area of the sticking region, temporarily hold his or her breath at the bottom of the descent through early ascent past the sticking region, and then exhale for the completion of the lift. The sticking region is the most difficult part of the exercise and an area that increases vulnerability to a low-back injury. Postural stability is crucial here to develop the force necessary to ascend with a heavy weight while protecting the spine. A temporary Valsalva maneuver can increase IAP and protect the spine at this critical position. Valsalva maneuvers are seen during other explosive activities as well such as the delivery phase of pitching in baseball or during a maximal vertical jump. Postural stability trumps the undesirable effects of the Valsalva maneuver under explosive or heavy-loaded conditions. It is important to note that this is an exception to the breathing principle, and proper breathing should be used under most circumstances.

♦ If you feel any pain or discomfort while training, stop immediately. It may not be in the best interest of the

(Continued)

athlete to attempt to ascertain the cause or nature of the pain at that point; thus, it is wise to stop lifting and prevent further injury from taking place.

◆ Use proper gym etiquette. Proper gym etiquette should be followed at all times. This includes communicating with others when using equipment. When approaching a piece of equipment, make sure no one else is currently using it. If another athlete is using the equipment, then communicating by asking, "can I work in?" or "how many sets do you have left?" is common courtesy. It is not proper to occupy equipment when not using it because other athletes may be waiting to use it. If an athlete needs a spot, the individual should ask politely and the athlete will oblige or decline courteously. It is important to be courteous to others and this includes not using profanity or rude language, cleaning up after oneself and putting equipment away, and not acting like one owns the gym and aggressively trains without concern for others.

Distracting others is discouraged. The gym is not a social place per se as many are there to train and not socialize. Sometimes it becomes more difficult to lift when gyms are crowded. Individuals have to wait for equipment and may feel rushed as others are waiting for them to finish an exercise. These can be challenging times for maintaining proper etiquette, but it is critical for individuals to identify the congested environment and act accordingly. Communication and courteous behavior is helpful in dealing with crowded gyms. Having a backup plan (other exercises, rest intervals) can help in these situations. Lastly, following the facility's rules is important. Most facilities will have rules posted or provide lifters with a list of rules. Facilities may have policies on dress or attire, music, noise, cell phones, use of lifting chalk, cleaning equipment, dropping weights or leaning plates on equipment, and how some pieces of equipment are to be used, so it is important to respect and follow the rules.

Sidebar	Becoming an Effective Spotter

Many athletes (and training partners) provide spots during RT. A spotter is defined as a person who applies assistance to an individual in need. Spotting ability becomes better with repeated exposure. The following is a checklist of items that make one an effective spotter:

◆ Be familiar with the exercise for which you are spotting.
◆ Effectively communicate with the athlete about the type of spot preferred, the amount of assistance to apply, when to intervene and assist, if a lift-off is needed, where the athlete prefers to be spotted (around the waist or shoulders for the squat, under the elbows or stabilizing the wrists for presses), how many reps the athlete is targeting, the potential for forced reps, and if the athlete needs assistance racking the weight upon completion.
◆ Do not crowd the athlete when spotting and give the athlete adequate space to complete the exercise. For example, when spotting the bench press, do not stand too close to the athlete's head to avoid contact during the exercise.
◆ Make sure you are strong enough to provide assistance for strong athletes.
◆ When spotting for squats (with only one spotter located behind the athlete), follow the athlete down each repetition to maintain proper position and should avoid accidentally pushing the athlete forward when assisting.
◆ Make sure you provide just enough force to keep the bar moving. This ensures the athlete is working maximally. Do not take the weight away from the athlete unless it is an emergency situation or a 1RM test.

◆ Know when to intervene if the athlete needs assistance. This will occur after a 1–3 seconds period where the bar is stagnant.
◆ Be sure to check and clear the area of obtrusive objects before the athlete begins the lift.
◆ Double-check the bar and make sure the bar is evenly loaded with collars secured. When transferring dumbbells to the athlete, make sure the grips are exposed and easily grasped and hand the weights to the athlete in the starting position of the exercise.
◆ Maintain proper spotting posture and body position throughout the exercise. Stay focused and do not become distracted by others in the gym.
◆ Spotting for machine exercises may occur. If so, provide assistance to the athlete's limbs or machine's grip support and use caution if applying pressure to cables.
◆ Spotting for Olympic lifts is not common and not recommended as athletes are coached to safely release the bar during failed attempts.
◆ For some exercises, multiple spotters may be needed if heavy weights are used or one spotter alone may be needed in a compromised position to assist.
◆ For some exercises (leg press, unilateral arm curls or triceps extensions, seated calf raises), an athlete may be able to self-spot himself or herself upon failure.
◆ In some cases, a spotter may apply resistance for forced negatives or manual resistance exercise. The amount of resistance depends on the strength and goals of the athlete. This must be communicated prior to beginning the exercise.

SUMMARY POINTS

◆ Several different modalities are used for RT. Free weights and machines are recommended because they enable great exercise selection and are easily quantifiable.

◆ Bodyweight, manual or partner resistance, and the environment can be used for RT. These are essentially free and can be used independent of one's budget.

◆ Free weights and machines have advantages and disadvantages in direct comparison, and the ACSM has recommended the inclusion of both in an RT program.

◆ MBs come in various sizes and are used for a multitude of exercises. They can be thrown for plyometric training.

◆ Instability equipment increases balance and stabilizer muscle activation. SBs, BOSU balls, wobble boards, pads, and balance discs are commonly used in RT.

◆ Elastic bands, tubing, cables, and chains have increased in popularity because they are portable and can be used for variable RT.

◆ As strength competitions have increased in popularity, so have the training methods used. Strength implements have been successfully incorporated into many RT programs.

◆ RT is very safe provided that general rules and guidelines are followed.

REVIEW QUESTIONS

1. Free weights include
   a. Barbells
   b. Dumbbells
   c. Plates
   d. All of the above

2. Resistance exercise machines that use air pressure for resistance are known as
   a. Hydraulic machines
   b. Pneumatic machines
   c. Smith machines
   d. Plate-loaded machines

3. Free weights are advantageous because
   a. They are more costly than machines
   b. Require greater antagonist and stabilizer muscle activity to support the body in all planes of motion
   c. They limit exercise selection
   d. They do not require the use of spotters

4. Variable resistance can be provided solely by
   a. Medicine balls
   b. Stability balls
   c. Elastic bands
   d. Kettlebells

5. Which of the following is not characteristic of an effective spotter?
   a. Is familiar with the exercise being spotted
   b. Is strong enough to provide adequate assistance if the individual fails during the set
   c. Does not communicate with the individual regarding the set
   d. Checks to make sure area is clear before initiating the exercise

6. Abdominal bracing involves contracting trunk muscles to increase IAP and spinal stability.
   a. T
   b. F

7. The risk of injury during a supervised resistance training program is much lower than the injury risk from playing competitive sports.
   a. T
   b. F

8. Performing a 1RM bench press on an SB will yield a higher value than performing the 1RM on a stable bench.
   a. T
   b. F

9. Performing exercises on an SB, a BOSU ball, or a wobble board increases stabilizer muscle activation due to the unstable environment.
   a. T
   b. F

10. The use of strength implements is advantageous because some provide unbalanced resistance and some exercises are difficult to replicate with free weights.
    a. T
    b. F

11. Chains may be advantageous because they apply variable resistance to a free-weight exercise.
    a. T
    b. F

12. Proper breathing during resistance exercise entails exhaling on the negative phase and inhaling on the positive phase.
    a. T
    b. F

REFERENCES

1. Contreras B, Schoenfeld B, Jonathan M, Tiryaki-Somnez G, Cronin J, Elsbeth V. The biomechanics of the push-up: implications for resistance training programs. *Strength Cond J*. 2012;34:41–6.

2. Ebben WP, Wurm B, VanderZanden TL, et al. Kinetic analysis of several variations of push-ups. *J Strength Cond Res*. 2011;25:2891–4.

3. Suprak DN, Dawes J, Stephenson MD. The effect of position on the percentage of body mass supported during traditional and modified push-up variants. *J Strength Cond Res*. 2011;25:497–503.

4. Ratamess NA, Rosenberg JG, Klei S, et al. Comparison of the acute metabolic responses to traditional resistance exercise, body-weight, and battling rope exercises. *J Strength Cond Res.* 2015;29:47–57.

5. Hoffman JR, Ratamess NA. *A Practical Guide to Developing Resistance-Training Programs.* 2nd ed. Monterey (CA): Coaches Choice; 2008.

6. Kochanowicz A, Niespodziński B, Mieszkowski J, Marina M, Kochanowicz K, Zasada M. Changes in the muscle activity of gymnasts during a handstand on various apparatus. *J Strength Cond Res.* 2019;33(6):1609–18.

7. Giancotti GF, Fusco A, Varalda C, Capranica L, Cortis C. Biomechanical of suspension training push-up. *J Strength Cond Res.* 2018;32:602–9.

8. Gulmez I. Effects of angle variations in suspension push-up exercise. *J Strength Cond Res.* 2017;31:1017–23.

9. Calatayud J, Borreani S, Colado JC, et al. Muscle activation during push-ups with different suspension training systems. *J Sports Sci Med.* 2014;13:502–10.

10. Snarr RL, Esco MR. Electromyographic comparison of traditional and suspension push-ups. *J Hum Kinet.* 2013;39:75–83.

11. Snarr RL, Esco MR. Electromyographical comparison of plank variations performed with an without instability devices. *J Strength Cond Res.* 2014;28:3298–305.

12. Melrose D, Dawes J. Resistance characteristics of the TRX™ suspension training system at different angles and distances from the hanging position. *J Athl Enhance.* 2015;4:1.

13. Dorgo S, King GA, Rice CA. The effects of manual resistance training on improving muscular strength and endurance. *J Strength Cond Res.* 2009;23(1):293–303.

14. Hedrick A. Manual resistance training for football athletes at the U.S. Air Force Academy. *Strength Cond J.* 1999;21:6–10.

15. Kubik B. *Dinosaur Training: Lost Secrets of Strength & Development.* 5th ed. Louisville (KY): Brooks Kubik Enterprises, Inc.; August 1, 2006.

16. Ratamess NA, Faigenbaum AD, Mangine GT, Hoffman JR, Kang J. Acute muscular strength assessment using free weight bars of different thickness. *J Strength Cond Res.* 2007;21:240–4.

17. Ghigiarelli JJ, Pelton LM, Gonzalez AM, et al. Effects of a 6-week bench press program using the freak bar in a sample of collegiate club powerlifters. *J Strength Cond Res.* 2018;32:938–49.

18. Andersen V, Fimland MS, Mo DA, et al. Electromyographic comparison of barbell deadlift, hex bar deadlift, and hip thrust exercises: a cross-over study. *J Strength Cond Res.* 2018;32:587–93.

19. Newton R. Biomechanics of conditioning exercises. In: Chandler TJ, Brown LE, editors. *Conditioning for Strength and Human Performance.* Philadelphia (PA): Wolters Kluwer, Lippincott Williams & Wilkins; 2008. p. 77–93.

20. Kraemer WJ, Keuning M, Ratamess NA, et al. Resistance training combined with bench-step aerobics enhances women's health profile. *Med Sci Sports Exerc.* 2001;33:259–69.

21. Stoppani J. *Encyclopedia of Muscle and Strength.* Champaign (IL): Human Kinetics; 2006. p. 23–37.

22. Kraemer WJ, Fry AC, Ratamess NA, French DN. Strength testing: development and evaluation of methodology. In: Maud PJ, Foster C, editors. *Physiological Assessments of Human Performance.* 2nd ed. Champaign (IL): Human Kinetics; 2006. p. 119–50.

23. Kraemer WJ, Mazzetti SA, Ratamess NA, Fleck SJ. Specificity of training modes. In: Brown LE, editor. *Isokinetics in Human Performance.* Champaign (IL): Human Kinetics; 2000. p. 25–41.

24. Van der Wall H, Mc Laughlin A, Bruce W, et al. Scintigraphic patterns of injury in amateur weight lifters. *Clin Nucl Med.* 1999;24:915–20.

25. Hamill BP. Relative safety of weightlifting and weight training. *J Strength Cond Res.* 1994;8:53–7.

26. Nosse LJ, Hunter GR. Free weights: a review supporting their use in training and rehabilitation. *Athl Train.* 1985;20:206–9.

27. Schwanbeck SR, Cornish SM, Barss T, Chilibeck PD. Effects of training with free weights versus machines on muscle mass, strength, free testosterone, and free cortisol levels. *J Strength Cond Res.* 2020;34(7):1851–9.

28. Boyer BT. A comparison of the effects of three strength training programs on women. *J Appl Sports Sci Res.* 1990;4:88–94.

29. Willoughby DS, Gillespie JW. A comparison of isotonic free weights and omnikinetic exercise machines on strength. *J Hum Mov Stud.* 1990;19:93–100.

30. Hunter G, Culpepper M. Knee extension torque joint position relationships following isotonic fixed resistance and hydraulic resistance training. *Athl Train.* 1988;23:16–20.

31. Hunter G, Culpepper M. Joint angle specificity of fixed masses hydraulic resistance knee flexion training. *J Strength Cond Res.* 1995;9:13–6.

32. Behm DG, Drinkwater EJ, Willardson JM, Cowley PM. The use of instability to train the core musculature. *Appl Physiol Nutr Metab.* 2010;35:91–108.

33. Koshida S, Urabe Y, Miyashita K, Iwai K, Kagimori A. Muscular outputs during dynamic bench press under stable and unstable conditions. *J Strength Cond Res.* 2008;22:1584–8.

34. Saeterbakken AH, Fimland MS. Muscle force output and electromyographic activity in squats with various unstable surfaces. *J Strength Cond Res.* 2013;27:130–6.

35. Vera-Garcia FJ, Grenier SG, McGill SM. Abdominal muscle response during curl-ups on both stable and labile surfaces. *Phys Ther.* 2000;80:564–9.

36. Anderson KG, Behm DG. Maintenance of EMG activity and loss of force output with instability. *J Strength Cond Res.* 2004;18:637–40.

37. Behm DG, Leonard AM, Young WB, Bonsey WA, MacKinnon SN. Trunk muscle electromyographic activity with unstable and unilateral exercises. *J Strength Cond Res.* 2005;19:193–201.

38. Marshall PW, Murphy BA. Increased deltoid and abdominal muscle activity during Swiss ball bench press. *J Strength Cond Res.* 2006;20:745–50.

39. Norwood JT, Anderson GS, Gaetz MB, Twist PW. Electromyographic activity of the trunk stabilizers during stable and unstable bench press. *J Strength Cond Res.* 2007;21:343–7.

40. Goodman CA, Pearce AJ, Nicholes CJ, Gatt BM, Fairweather IH. No difference in 1RM strength and muscle activation during the barbell chest press on a stable and unstable surface. *J Strength Cond Res.* 2008;22:88–94.

41. Mori A. Electromyographic activity of selected trunk muscles during stabilization exercises using a gym ball. *Electromyogr Clin Neurophysiol.* 2004;44:57–64.

42. Sternlicht E, Rugg S, Fujii LL, Tomomitsu KF, Seki MM. Electromyographic comparison of a stability ball crunch with a traditional crunch. *J Strength Cond Res.* 2007;21:506–9.

43. Tsourlou T, Benik A, Dipla K, Zafeiridis A, Kellis S. The effects of a twenty-four-week aquatic training program on muscular strength performance in healthy elderly women. *J Strength Cond Res.* 2006;20:811–8.

44. Nuzzo JL, McCaulley GO, Cormie P, Cavil MJ, McBride JM. Trunk muscle activity during stability ball and free weight exercises. *J Strength Cond Res.* 2008;22:95–102.

45. McBride JM, Cormie P, Deane R. Isometric squat force output and muscle activity in stable and unstable conditions. *J Strength Cond Res.* 2006;20:915–8.

46. Cowley PM, Swensen T, Sforzo GA. Efficacy of instability resistance training. *Int J Sports Med.* 2007;28:829–35.

47. Saeterbakken AH, Andersen V, Behm DG, et al. Resistance-training exercises with different stability requirements: time course of task specificity. *Eur J Appl Physiol.* 2016;116:2247–56.

48. Anderson KG, Behm DG. Trunk muscle activity increases with unstable squat movements. *Can J Appl Physiol.* 2005;30:33–45.

49. Shoepe TC, Ramirez DA, Almstedt HC. Elastic band prediction equations for combined free-weight and elastic band bench presses and squats. *J Strength Cond Res.* 2010;24:195–200.

50. Andersen V, Fimland MS, Cumming KT, Vraalsen O, Saeterbakken AH. Explosive resistance training using elastic bands in young female team handball players. *Sports Med Int Open.* 2018;2:E171–8.

51. Hostler D, Schwirian CI, Campos G, et al. Skeletal muscle adaptations in elastic resistance-trained young men and women. *Eur J Appl Physiol.* 2001;86:112–8.

52. Rogers ME, Sherwood HS, Rogers NL, Bohlken RM. Effects of dumbbell and elastic band training on physical function in older inner-city African-American women. *Women Health.* 2002;36:33–41.

53. Picha KJ, Almaddah MR, Barker J, et al. Elastic resistance effectiveness on increasing strength of shoulders and hips. *J Strength Cond Res.* 2019;33:931–43.

54. Wallace BJ, Winchester JB, McGuigan MR. Effects of elastic bands on force and power characteristics during the back squat exercise. *J Strength Cond Res.* 2006;20:268–72.

55. Garcia-Lopez D, Hernandez-Sanchez S, Martin E, et al. Free-weight augmentation with elastic bands improves bench press kinematics in professional rugby players. *J Strength Cond Res.* 2016;30:2493–9.

56. Galpin AJ, Malyszek KK, Davis KA, et al. Acute effects of elastic bands on kinetic characteristics during the deadlift at moderate and heavy loads. *J Strength Cond Res.* 2015;29:3271–8.

57. Strokosch A, Louit L, Seitz L, Clarke R, Hughes JD. Impact of accommodating resistance in potentiating horizontal-jump performance in professional rugby league players. *Int J Sports Physiol Perform.* 2018;13:1223–9.

58. Anderson CE, Sforzo GA, Sigg JA. The effects of combining elastic and free weight resistance on strength and power in athletes. *J Strength Cond Res.* 2008;22:567–74.

59. Bellar DM, Muller MD, Barkley JE, et al. The effects of combined elastic-and free-weight tension vs. free-weight tension on one-repetition maximum strength in the bench press. *J Strength Cond Res.* 2011;25:459–63.

60. Riviere M, Louit L, Strokosch A, Seitz LB. Variable resistance training promotes greater strength and power adaptations than traditional resistance training in elite youth rugby league players. *J Strength Cond Res.* 2017;31:947–55.

61. Shoepe TC, Ramirez DA, Rovetti RJ, Kohler DR, Almstedt HC. The effects of 24 weeks of resistance training with simultaneous elastic and free weight loading on muscular performance of novice lifters. *J Hum Kinet.* 2011;29:93–106.

62. Ebben WP, Jensen RL. Electromyographic and kinetic analysis of traditional, chain, and elastic band squats. *J Strength Cond Res.* 2002;16:547–50.

63. Coker CA, Berning JM, Briggs DL. A preliminary investigation of the biomechanical and perceptual influence of chain resistance on the performance of the snatch. *J Strength Cond Res.* 2006;20:887–91.

64. Berning JM, Coker CA, Briggs D. The biomechanical and perceptual influence of chain resistance on the performance of the Olympic clean. *J Strength Cond Res.* 2008;22:390–5.

65. Nijem RM, Coburn JW, Brown LE, Lynn SK, Ciccone AB. Electromyographic and force plate analysis of the deadlift performed with and without chains. *J Strength Cond Res.* 2016;30:1177–82.

66. McCurdy K, Langford G, Ernest J, Jenkerson D, Doscher M. Comparison of chain-and plate-loaded bench press training on strength, joint pain, and muscle soreness in Division II baseball players. *J Strength Cond Res.* 2009;23:187–95.

67. Wahl MJ, Behm DG. Not all instability training devices enhance muscle activation in highly resistance-trained individuals. *J Strength Cond Res.* 2008;22:1360–70.

68. Ross RE, Ratamess NA, Hoffman JR, Faigenbaum AD, Kang J, Chilakos A. The effects of treadmill sprint training and resistance training on maximal running velocity and power. *J Strength Cond Res.* 2009;23:385–94.

69. Stanforth D, Brumitt J, Ratamess NA, Atkins W, Keteyian SJ. Toys and training … bells, ropes, and balls—oh my! *ACSM's Health Fit J.* 2015;19:5–11.

70. Faigenbaum AD, Kang J, Ratamess NA, et al. Acute cardiometabolic responses to a novel training rope protocol in children. *J Strength Cond Res.* 2018;32:1197–206.

71. Fountaine CJ, Schmidt BJ. Metabolic cost of rope training. *J Strength Cond Res.* 2015;29:889–93.

72. Ratamess NA, Smith CR, Beller NA, Kang J, Faigenbaum AD, Bush JA. Effects of rest interval length on acute battling rope exercise metabolism. *J Strength Cond Res.* 2015;29:2375–87.

73. Berning JM, Adams KJ, Climstein M, Stamford BA. Metabolic demands of "junkyard" training: pushing and pulling a motor vehicle. *J Strength Cond Res.* 2007;21:853–6.

74. Winwood PW, Keogh JWL, Harris NK. The strength and conditioning practices of strongman competitors. *J Strength Cond Res.* 2011;25:3118–28.

75. Winwood PW, Cronin JB, Posthumus LR, Finlayson SJ, Gill ND, Keogh JWL. Strongman vs. traditional resistance training effects on muscular function and performance. *J Strength Cond Res.* 2015;29:429–39.

76. Tsatsouline P. *The Russian Kettlebell Challenge: Xtreme Fitness for Hard Living Comrades.* St. Paul (MN): Dragon Door Publications; 2001.

77. Chan M, MacInnis MJ, Koch S, et al. Cardiopulmonary demand of 16-kg kettlebell snatches in simulated Girevoy sport. *J Strength Cond Res.* 2020;34:1625–33.

78. Falatic JA, Plato PA, Holder C, et al. Effects of kettlebell training on aerobic capacity. *J Strength Cond Res.* 2015;29:1943–7.

79. Manocchia P, Spierer DK, Lufkin AK, Minichiello J, Castro J. Transference of kettlebell training to strength, power, and endurance. *J Strength Cond Res.* 2013;27:477–84.

80. Williams BM, Kraemer RR. Comparison of cardiorespiratory and metabolic responses in kettlebell high-intensity interval training versus sprint interval cycling. *J Strength Cond Res.* 2015;29:3317–25.

81. Keogh JWL, Payne AL, Anderson BB, Atkins PJ. A brief description of the biomechanics and physiology of a strongman event: the tire flip. *J Strength Cond Res.* 2010;24:1223–8.

82. Ratamess NA, Kang J, Kuper JD, et al. Acute cardiorespiratory and metabolic effects of a sandbag resistance exercise protocol. *J Strength Cond Res.* 2018;32:1491–502.

83. Jancsis M, Crawford B. *Stonelifting: An Ancient Test of Strength Revived.* Middletown (DE); 2018. p. 7–117.

84. Thein JM, Brody LT. Aquatic-based rehabilitation and training for the shoulder. *J Athl Train.* 2000;35:382–9.

85. Poyhonen T, Sipila S, Keskinen KL, Hautala A, Savolainen J, Malkia E. Effects of aquatic resistance training on neuromuscular performance in healthy women. *Med Sci Sports Exerc.* 2002;34:2103–9.

86. Volaklis KA, Spassis AT, Tokmakidis SP. Land versus water exercise in patients with coronary artery disease: effects on body composition, blood lipids, and physical fitness. *Am Heart J.* 2007;154:560.e1–6.

87. Stemm JD, Jacobson BH. Comparison of land- and aquatic-based plyometric training on vertical jump performance. *J Strength Cond Res.* 2007;21:568–71.

88. McGill SM, McDermott A, Fenwick CMJ. Comparison of different strongman events: trunk muscle activation and lumbar spine motion, load, and stiffness. *J Strength Cond Res.* 2009;23:1148–61.

89. McArdle WD, Katch FI, Katch VL. *Essentials of Exercise Physiology.* 3rd ed. Philadelphia (PA): Lippincott Williams & Wilkins; 2005. p. 279–80.

90. Luo J, McNamara B, Moran K. The use of vibration training to enhance muscle strength and power. *Sports Med.* 2005;35:23–41.

91. Jordan MJ, Norris SR, Smith DJ, Herzog W. Vibration training: an overview of the area, training consequences, and future considerations. *J Strength Cond Res.* 2005;19:459–66.

92. Cardinale M, Wakeling J. Whole body vibration exercise: are vibrations good for you? *Br J Sports Med.* 2005;39:585–9.

93. Cristi-Montero C, Cuevas MJ, Collado PS. Whole-body vibration training as complement to programs aimed at weight loss. *Nutr Hosp.* 2013;28:1365–71.

94. Kang J, Bush JA, Ratamess NA, et al. Acute effects of whole-body vibration on energy metabolism during aerobic exercise. *J Sports Med Phys Fitness.* 2016;56:834–42.

95. Chen H, Ma J, Lu B, Ma XL. The effect of whole-body vibration training on lean mass: a PRISMA-compliant meta-analysis. *Medicine.* 2017;96:e8390.

96. Cochrane DJ. Vibration exercise: the potential benefits. *Int J Sports Med.* 2011;32:75–99.

97. Bosco C, Cardinale M, Tsarpela O. Influence of vibration on mechanical power and electromyogram activity in human arm flexor muscles. *Eur J Appl Physiol Occup Physiol.* 1999;79:306–11.

98. Bosco C, Colli R, Introini E, et al. Adaptive responses of human skeletal muscle to vibration exposure. *Clin Physiol.* 1999;19:183–7.

99. Bosco C, Iacovelli M, Tsarpela O, et al. Hormonal responses to whole-body vibration in men. *Eur J Appl Physiol.* 2000;81:449–54.

100. Issurin VB, Tenenbaum G. Acute and residual effects of vibratory stimulation on explosive strength in elite and amateur athletes. *J Sports Sci.* 1999;17:177–82.

101. Roelants M, Verschueren SM, Delecluse C, Levin O, Stijnen V. Whole-body-vibration-induced increase in leg muscle activity during different squat exercises. *J Strength Cond Res.* 2006;20:124–9.

102. Hazell TJ, Jakobi JM, Kenno KA. The effects of whole-body vibration on upper-and lower-body EMG during static and dynamic contractions. *Appl Physiol Nutr Metab.* 2007;32:1156–63.

103. Annino G, Padua E, Castagna C, et al. Effect of whole body vibration training on lower limb performance in selected high-level ballet students. *J Strength Cond Res.* 2007;21:1072–6.

104. Fagnani F, Giombini A, Di Cesare A, Pigozzi F, Di Salvo V. The effects of a whole-body vibration program on muscle performance and flexibility in female athletes. *Am J Phys Med Rehabil.* 2006;85:956–62.

105. Issurin VB, Liebermann DG, Tenenbaum G. Effect of vibratory stimulation training on maximal force and flexibility. *J Sports Sci.* 1994;12:561–6.

106. Mahieu NN, Witvrouw E, Van de Voorde D, Michilsens D, Arbyn V, Van den Broecke W. Improving strength and postural control in young skiers: whole-body vibration versus equivalent resistance training. *J Athl Train.* 2006;41:286–93.

107. Mester J, Kleinoder H, Yue Z. Vibration training: benefits and risks. *J Biomech.* 2006;39:1056–65.

108. Cochrane DJ, Legg SJ, Hooker MJ. The short-term effect of whole-body vibration training on vertical jump, sprint, and agility performance. *J Strength Cond Res.* 2004;18:828–32.

109. Delecluse C, Roelants M, Diels R, Koninckx E, Verschueren S. Effects of whole body vibration training on muscle strength and sprint performance in sprint-trained athletes. *Int J Sports Med.* 2005;26:662–8.

110. Marin PJ, Rhea MR. Effects of vibration training on muscle strength: a meta-analysis. *J Strength Cond Res.* 2010;24:548–56.

111. Marin PJ, Rhea MR. Effects of vibration training on muscle power: a meta-analysis. *J Strength Cond Res.* 2010;24:871–8.

112. Henry JC, Kaeding C. Neuromuscular differences between male and female athletes. *Curr Womens Health Rep.* 2001;1:241–4.

113. Chandler TJ, Kibler WB, Stracener EC, Ziegler AK, Pace B. Shoulder strength, power, and endurance in college tennis players. *Am J Sports Med.* 1992;20:455–8.

114. Knapik JJ, Bauman CT, Jones DH, Harris JM, Vaughan L. Preseason strength and flexibility imbalances associated with athletic injuries in female collegiate athletes. *Am J Sports Med.* 1991;19:76–81.

115. Mazur LJ, Yetman RJ, Risser WL. Weight-training injuries. Common injuries and preventative methods. *Sports Med.* 1993;16:57–63.

116. Hoffman JR, Ratamess NA. Medical issues associated with anabolic steroid use: are they exaggerated? *J Sports Sci Med.* 2006;5:182–93.

117. Keogh J, Hume PA, Pearson S. Retrospective injury epidemiology of one hundred one competitive Oceania power lifters: the effects of age, body mass, competitive standard, and gender. *J Strength Cond Res.* 2006;20:672–81.

118. Goertzen M, Schoppe K, Lange G, Schulitz KP. Injuries and damage caused by excess stress in body building and power lifting. *Sportverletz Sportschaden.* 1989;3:32–6.

119. Raske A, Norlin R. Injury incidence and prevalence among elite weight and power lifters. *Am J Sports Med.* 2002;30:248–56.

120. Keogh JWL, Winwood PW. The epidemiology of injuries across the weight-training sports. *Sports Med.* 2017;47:479–501.

121. American College of Sports Medicine & American Heart Association. Joint position stand: recommendations for cardiovascular screening, staffing, and emergency policies at health/fitness facilities. *Med Sci Sports Exerc.* 1998;30:1009–18.

122. National Strength and Conditioning Association. *Strength and Conditioning Professional Standards and Guidelines.* Colorado Springs (CO): NSCA; May 2001.

123. McGill S. *Ultimate Back Fitness and Performance.* 4th ed. Waterloo, Canada: Backfitpro Inc.; 2009. p. 112–23.

CHAPTER 14

Resistance Training Exercises

OBJECTIVES

After completing this chapter, you will be able to:

- Demonstrate proper breathing during resistance exercise
- Describe the proper performance of several barbell, dumbbell, and machine resistance exercises for lower body, upper body, and core musculature
- Describe how exercises can be combined into a single exercise to increase complexity
- Describe methods of grip strength training
- Describe the proper performance of the Olympic lifts and their variations
- Describe the performance of exercises with different modalities including medicine balls, stability balls, BOSU balls, sand bags, kettlebells, ropes, and other implements

There are a multitude of exercises that can be performed and incorporated into a resistance training (RT) program. Historically, many traditional resistance exercises were chosen to target specific muscle groups. This approach is still very common and effective. Another approach is to select exercises that target specific movements rather than muscle groups. This "functional" or *movement-specific* approach is popular and effective as well[23]. Most S&C programs will consist of both types of exercises. Considering that many devices/pieces of equipment have been developed, the numbers of possible exercises are numerous. Selecting the proper exercises is an important task for the coach and athlete. Exercises need to be selected such that they target specific goals and are similar in movement to motor skills found in the sport. Beginners should focus on a few basic exercises initially and expand to more complex exercises with experience. Technique mastery is important and should be used as a guide to select proper loading and as a prerequisite to advancing to more complex and challenging exercises. This chapter discusses proper performance of more than 70 exercises and lists more than 600 variations with many of them shown on thePoint. Alteration of an athlete's body position or posture, hand/foot width, and hand/foot position changes muscle activation slightly so each variation must be regarded independently regarding loading and the number of repetitions performed. Several exercises can be performed unilaterally (one arm or leg) as well as bilaterally (two arms or legs). Performing an exercise on one leg, *e.g.*, can be used to enhance muscular strength and balance. Performing an exercise with one arm provides asymmetric loading requiring greater muscle coactivation to maintain balance. The use of a stable or unstable surface affects exercise performance and subsequent adaptation. This chapter describes exercises based on whether they primarily stress upper-body limb muscles, lower-body muscles, the core, or total-body musculature. Exercises performed with free weights (barbells [BBs], dumbbells [DBs], and plates), body weight (BW), stability balls (SBs) and BOSU, medicine balls (MBs), elastic bands/tubing, kettlebells (KBs), sand bags, and other implements (kegs, chains, and strength competition equipment) are described.

Visit thePoint to view more exercises in the online appendix.

Exercise Kinesiology

Human motion is described relative to the anatomical position (standing erect with joints extended, palms facing forward, and feet parallel) and occurs in three planes of motion (Fig. 14.1). A sagittal plane divides the body into right and left segments (Fig. 14.2). Movements occur in a sagittal plane about a transverse (or mediolateral) axis of rotation and take place in a front-to-back manner (flexion, extension from the anatomical position) and vice versa. A frontal plane divides the body into anterior and posterior regions (Fig. 14.3). Movements occur in

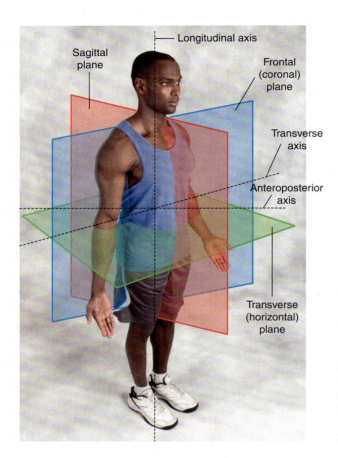

FIGURE 14.1 Planes of motion and axes of rotation of the human body. Sagittal, frontal, and transverse planes are shown as well as their corresponding axes of rotation (which are perpendicular to the plane). (Reprinted with permission from Thompson W, editor. *ACSM's Resources for the Personal Trainer*. 3rd ed. Baltimore (MD): Lippincott Williams & Wilkins; 2010.)

a frontal plane about an anteroposterior axis of rotation and take place in a side-to-side manner (adduction, abduction) from anatomical position. Transverse planes divide the body into upper (superior) and lower (inferior) regions (Fig. 14.4). Movements occur in a transverse plane about a longitudinal axis of rotation and take place in a horizontal manner (rotation, supination, and pronation) from anatomical position.

Many human movements are multiplanar and take place in two or three planes of motion. Motion planes can vary when a movement is initiated from other postures different than the anatomical position, *e.g.*, elbow flexion can occur in any plane depending on the starting position of the shoulder and could occur in two or three planes simultaneously depending on the starting position and motion of other joints.

Myths & Misconceptions
An Athlete Should Never Hold His or Her Breath When Lifting

Proper breathing is critical to RT. Breathing patterns may vary depending on the complexity and intensity of exercise. Under many circumstances, it is recommended that the athlete exhale during the more difficult part (the concentric [CON] or positive phase) and inhale during the easier segment (the eccentric [ECC] or negative phase) for several exercises. Breathing patterns for complex lifts may vary corresponding to the difficulty of the phase. However, there are exceptions to this general rule. During the lifting of heavy loads for exercises that require high levels of intra-abdominal pressure (IAP) and lumbar spine support (deadlift, squat, bent-over row, Olympic lifts), many athletes temporarily hold their breath during the most difficult part. During a heavy squat, an athlete may inhale during the decent, temporarily hold his or her breath at the bottom position and during the initial ascent (until the sticking region is surpassed), and then exhale during the upper segment of the ascent. Breath holding helps increase torso rigidity and enables better exercise performance. Valsalva maneuvers are unavoidable during intense resistance exercise (>80% of 1 RM) or when sets approach muscular failure (1). An incremental rise in IAP is seen as intensity and effort increase (1). The greater postural stability enables better strength and power performance from the individual. Valsalva maneuvers are avoided under many circumstances, but there are occasions where holding one's breath is advantageous.

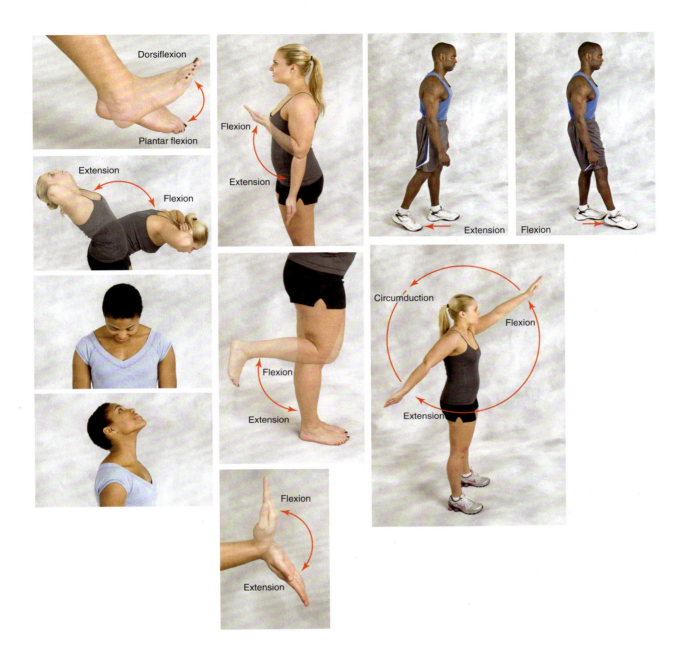

FIGURE 14.2 Movements in a sagittal plane. The movements flexion, extension, hyperextension, plantarflexion, and dorsiflexion are shown. (Reprinted with permission from Thompson W, editor. *ACSM's Resources for the Personal Trainer*. 3rd ed. Baltimore (MD): Lippincott Williams & Wilkins; 2010.)

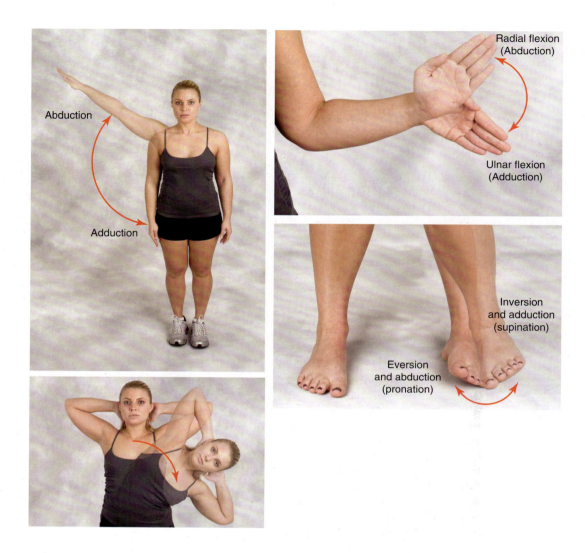

FIGURE 14.3 Movements in a frontal plane. The movements abduction, adduction, lateral flexion, radial/ulnar deviation, inversion, and eversion are shown. (Reprinted with permission from Thompson W, editor. *ACSM's Resources for the Personal Trainer*. 3rd ed. Baltimore (MD): Lippincott Williams & Wilkins; 2010.)

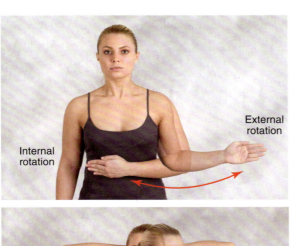
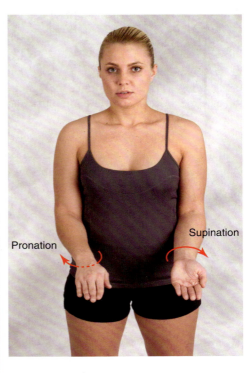
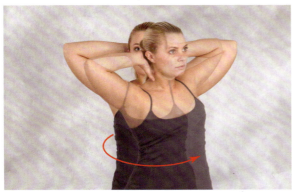

FIGURE 14.4 Movements in a transverse plane. The movements rotation, pronation, and supination are shown. (Reprinted with permission from Thompson W, editor. *ACSM's Resources for the Personal Trainer*. 3rd ed. Baltimore (MD): Lippincott Williams & Wilkins; 2010.)

Exercise

Resistance Exercises

The following sections discuss many exercises commonly performed in RT. Different modalities may be used. BW, BB, DB, SB, BOSU ball, MB, thick bar (TB), KB, bands/tubing, kegs, sand bags, tires, logs, and other implements are discussed. Each exercise is given a complexity rating allowing the reader to differentiate between simple and challenging exercises to learn. The rating system consists of three classifications: An "A" rating indicates the exercise is simple to perform and has a short learning period. Most exercises with an "A" rating are single joint with limited balance requirements. Some machine-based multiple-joint exercises are given an "A" rating. A "B" rating indicates the exercise is somewhat challenging to perform and has a longer learning period than an A-rated exercise. These exercises are multiple joint with sufficient balance requirements. A "C" rating indicates the exercise is very challenging and has either a long learning period or a strong core strength requirement. These exercises are multiple joint with large balance and coordination requirements.

Lower-Body Exercises

Lower-body exercises encompass motion in three planes (sagittal, transverse, and frontal) about the hip, knee, and ankle joints. Several major muscle groups (Fig. 14.5) produce these motions and must contract isometrically to stabilize the joints when they are not considered to be prime movers. Some are multiarticular or produce motion at multiple joints (Table 14.1).

Table 14.1 Kinesiology of Lower-Body Motion

Joint	Type of Joint	Joint Movement	Muscle Involvement
Hip	Ball and socket	Flexion	Psoas major and minor, iliacus, pectineus, rectus femoris, sartorius, tensor fasciae latae, adductor brevis and longus, gracilis
		Extension/hyperextension	Hamstrings (biceps femoris, semimembranosus, semitendinosus), gluteus maximus, adductor magnus
		Abduction	Gluteus medius, minimus, and maximus, sartorius, tensor fasciae latae, piriformis, and hip external rotators
		Adduction	Pectineus, adductors brevis, longus, and magnus, gracilis, gluteus maximus
		Internal and external rotation	IR: gluteus medius, maximus, and minimus, tensor fascia latae, adductors ER: sartorius, piriformis, superior/inferior gamelli, obturator externus/internus, quadratus femoris
Knee[a]	Modified hinge	Flexion	Hamstrings (biceps femoris, semimembranosus, semitendinosus), gracilis, popliteus, sartorius, gastrocnemius
		Extension	Quadriceps (rectus femoris, vastus intermedius, lateralis, and medialis)
Ankle	Hinge	Dorsiflexion	Tibialis anterior, extensor hallucis longus, extensor digitorum longus, peroneus tertius
		Plantar flexion	Peroneus brevis, peroneus longus, gastrocnemius, soleus, tibialis posterior, flexor digitorum longus, flexor hallucis longus
Subtalar	Plane/gliding	Inversion	Tibialis anterior, extensor hallucis longus, tibialis posterior, gastrocnemius, soleus, flexor digitorum longus, flexor hallucis longus
		Eversion	Peroneus brevis, peroneus longus, extensor digitorum longus, peroneus tertius

[a]Internal and external rotation of the knee is possible when the hip is flexed.

Chapter 14 Resistance Training Exercises 373

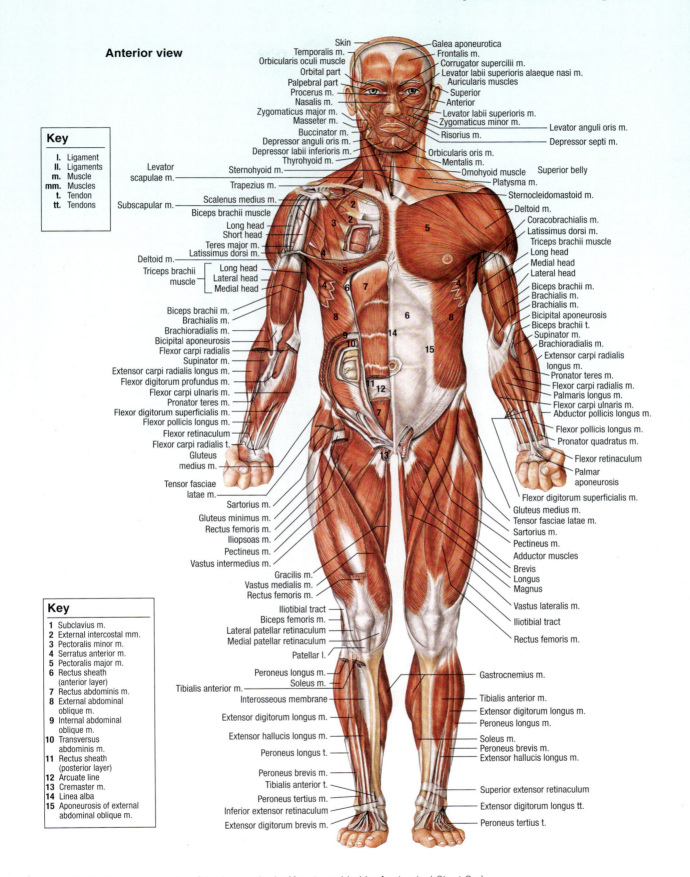

FIGURE 14.5 Major muscles of the human body. (Asset provided by Anatomical Chart Co.)

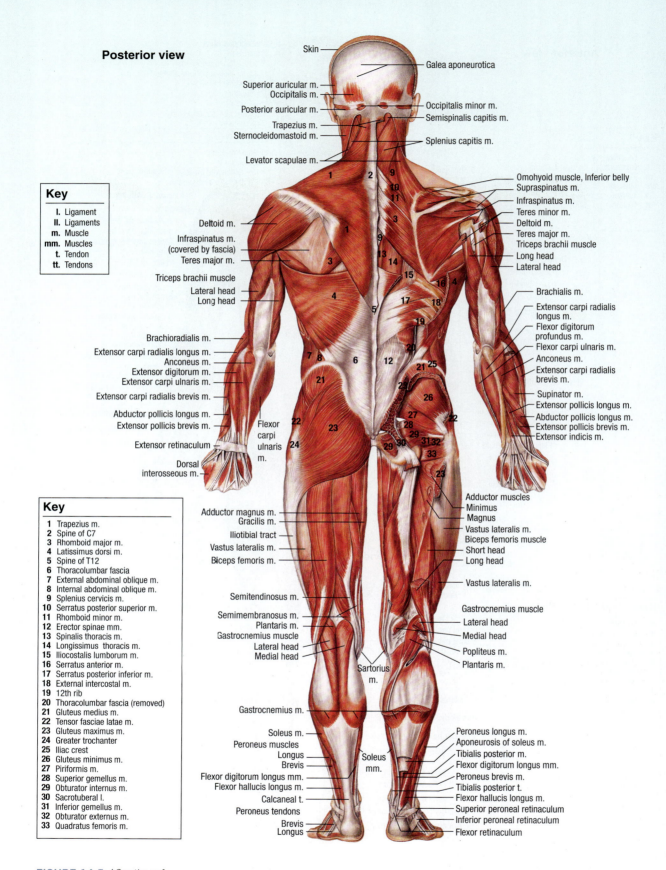

FIGURE 14.5 (*Continued*)

Squat

Rating: B

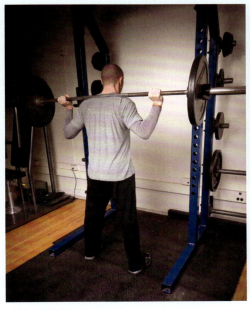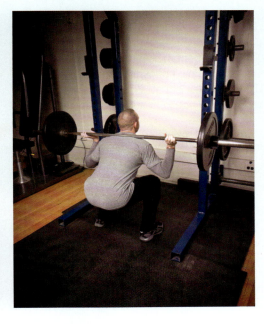

FIGURE 14.6 Squat.

- The bar rests on shoulders in a low bar (across the posterior deltoids and in the middle of the trapezius) or high bar (above the posterior deltoid at the base of the neck) position with shoulders abducted upward and scapula retracted to create a shelf for the bar (Fig. 14.6).
- Bar is grasped with a closed, pronated grip slightly wider than shoulder width.
- Feet are parallel and shoulder width apart or wider with toes pointing slightly outward.
- Head is tilted upward with the eyes focused directly ahead at or above eye level.
- Hips and knees are flexed during descent and bar is lowered in a curvilinear pattern with control while keeping an erect and braced torso (chest out, shoulders back).
- Descent continues until the top of the thighs are parallel to the ground.
- Ascent occurs via extension of the hips, knees, and ankles.
- May have one spotter on each side of bar or one spotter behind the athlete. It is important to follow the athlete downward during descent. When needed, force may be applied around the athlete's chest/upper torso or to the bar. It is important not to push the athlete forward when applying assistance.
- *Coaching tip:* Teaching the bottom position of the exercise is a good place to start for a beginner. Some new lifters have difficulty reaching this position and lack the confidence to squat down and back. Teaching this position first makes it easier for the athlete to descend with proper technique.

Using a box or bench as a low-point location marker can be beneficial as the athlete must descend until gluteal contact with the box or bench.

Single-leg versions of squats are common in training and athletic assessment. Because many sports require movements where one leg is pushing off to accelerate the body, single-leg squats force hip, knee, and ankle stabilizers to forcefully contract for stability and assist in sport-specific strength development. They require bodily control over the planted leg, thus reflective of hip/knee strength and postural control. Gender differences are seen in the ability to perform single-leg squats where women display greater motion in the frontal plane and greater valgus forces on the knee (2).

CAUTION! Knees too far ahead relative to toes, excessive forward lean, not performing exercise in a fully prescribed range of motion (ROM), and head facing downward are common mistakes. The athlete should be instructed to contract the gluteal, hamstring, and quadriceps muscles as forcefully as possible to reduce lower-back strain. Some advocate using a board to elevate the heels in athletes with poor ROM. A board is not needed. Rather, the coach should work on improving the athlete's ROM. A good pair of lifting shoes, by design, slightly elevates the heels.

> **OTHER VARIATIONS AND SIMILAR EXERCISES** Front squat (arms over bar), hack squat, DB/KB/sand bag squat, DB squat (with shoulders flexed parallel to ground), Smith machine squat, split squat (many variations similar to lunges), box (or bench) squat, squat with chains or bands, pause squat, lateral squat, staggered (stance) squat, single-leg squat (floor, BOSU), single-leg squat (rear leg supported by SB or bench), single-leg squat (elevated on bench to allow opposite leg to relax downward), TRX single-leg squat, Zercher squat, rack squats, belt squat, sissy squat, machine squat, safety squat, SB wall squats, SB single-leg lateral squat (outer or inner leg), single-leg SB squat, ISOM wall squats, squats with bands around ankles (to increase hip abductor strength), BW squats, BW squats with TRX, deck squat, MB squat (with shoulders flexed), knee squats, buddy squat, keg squat, sand bag squats, landmine squat, BOSU or balance board squats, single-DB sumo squat, BW/DB duck walks, balance squat (one-leg support, one-leg hip flexion from BB squat position), KB swing squat, partner stand-up, fireman pickup, and jump squats (DB, MB, KB, Smith machine, sand bag, weighted vest).

Interpreting Research
Biomechanical Analysis of Foot Position during the Squat

Escamilla RF, Fleisig GS, Lowry TM, Barrentine SW, Andrews JR. A three-dimensional biomechanical analysis of the squat during varying stance widths. *Med Sci Sports Exerc.* 2001;33:984–98.

Escamilla et al. (3) analyzed the BB squat with a narrow (~107% of shoulder width), medium (~142% of shoulder width), and wide (~169% of shoulder width) stance width and found that in comparison to a narrow stance, the wider stance produced:

◆ 7°–12° greater horizontal thigh position
◆ 6°–11° greater hip flexion
◆ 6° greater hip external rotation
◆ 5°–9° greater vertical shank (lower-leg) position

These results show that varying stance width affects squat kinematics. Some athletes perform the squat with varying stance widths to alter muscle activation, strengthen muscles in a different way, and add variety to a workout.

Leg Press

Rating: A

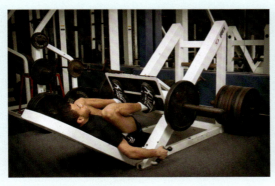 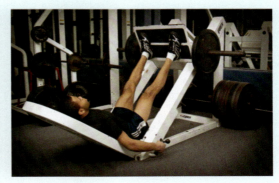

FIGURE 14.7 Leg press.

- Body is positioned according to machine type (seated, angled, or lying supine) (Fig. 14.7).
- Feet are placed on the sled approximately shoulder width apart with knees and hips aligned about 90° when starting from the bottom position.
- The hands grasp the supports firmly at sides or by shoulders (depending on where they are located) while the torso remains straight and flat against the support pads.
- Legs push forward on the sled to extend the knees and hips (without locking out knees).
- It is important to complete a full ROM while maintaining proper foot position.
- Once the repetition is completed, the carriage is returned under control to the starting position.
- One can self-spot by pushing on the legs when assistance is needed or have a spotter located laterally applying pressure to the carriage when assistance is needed.

> **OTHER VARIATIONS** Supine leg press, vertical leg press, side leg press, and unilateral leg press. An athlete can alter foot spacing and position. The athlete may perform a BB (bilateral or unilateral) leg press or ballistic leg press using a pendulum strap in a power rack while seated on an angled or L-shaped bench.

Deadlift

Rating: B

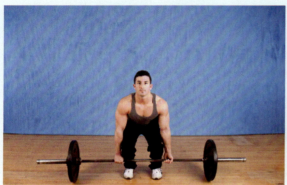
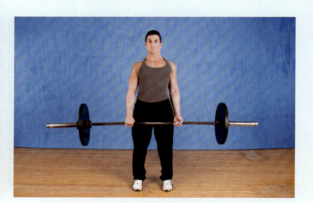

FIGURE 14.8 Deadlift.

- Feet are positioned shoulder width apart and flat on the floor with knees inside of arms (for conventional-style deadlift) or arms inside of legs with a wider stance (for sumo-style deadlift). Research has shown that (a) sumo style yields a more parallel thigh position, greater vertical posture, wider stance with greater hip external rotation, greater muscle activation of the quadriceps and tibialis anterior, and 8%–10% less load shear force at L4/L5 vertebrae position compared to conventional style and (b) conventional deadlift yields 25%–40% greater bar distance moved, work, and energy expenditure compared to sumo style (4–6) (Fig. 14.8).
- Grasp bar with a closed grip (pronated or alternated) slightly wider than or close to shoulder width and extend arms fully. The alternated grip allows the athlete more support when grasping the bar and may result in greater weights being lifted.
- Lower body by flexing the knees and hips.
- Position the bar over the feet close to shins with shoulders slightly ahead of bar vertically.
- The back should be maintained flat by hyperextension while holding the chest up and out and pulling the shoulder blades toward each other. Core is braced.
- The bar is pulled upward by extending the knees and moving the hips forward while raising the shoulders. The first third of the movement is predominantly knee extension; the second third is a combination of knee and hip extension; the final segment is predominantly hip extension. Athlete should forcefully contract hip extensors to lower strain on the lumbar spine.
- With elbows extended, the bar is lifted upward while maintaining close position to the body.
- Upon complete hip and knee extension, the body assumes an erect standing position.
- With control, bar is then lowered to starting position by flexion of hips and knees.
- Although presented in this section, the deadlift stresses several upper-body pulling muscles and is an excellent total-body mass/strength-building exercise.

> **CAUTION!** Raising the hips prior to moving the bar (without knee extension) place additional stress on the lower back. The bar should be lifted off of the ground by extension of the knees.

> **OTHER VARIATIONS AND SIMILAR EXERCISES** Deadlift (with bands), stiff-legged deadlift, DB/KB (one or two) deadlift, T-bar stiff-legged deadlift, deadlift pulls (in rack), deadlift with a DL bar or thick bar (predominantly a forearm exercise), deadlift from a small elevation (deficit), deadlift with keg or sand bag, partner (BW) deadlift, sand bag/heavy bag deadlift with a bear hug (could finish with a throw), sandbag rotational deadlift, DB/KB (one or two) single-leg deadlift (with contralateral leg extended), cable pull-through, stone DL, hex-bar DL, partner DL, partner suplex arch, and landmine DL.

Barbell Lunge

Rating: B

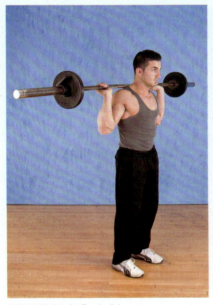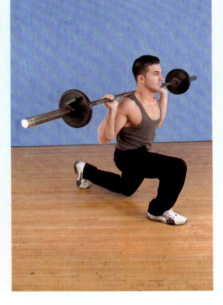

FIGURE 14.9 Barbell lunge.

- Bar is grasped with a closed, pronated grip slightly wider than shoulder width and is placed on shoulders in a high bar position (above the posterior deltoids at the base of neck) similar to the back squat.
- Feet are placed close to or slightly wider than shoulder width.
- A step forward is taken with a larger than normal step and knees are aligned with toes with the toes pointing straight ahead or slightly inward (Fig. 14.9).
- During the step, the lead knee is flexed under control directly above the lead foot while the training knee is lowered to the floor but no contact is made.
- The torso remains erect throughout and core is braced.
- Athlete pushes off with lead leg and returns to starting position in one large (or two small) step(s).
- The same movement is performed with the opposite leg.
- Lunges involve a step with each repetition whereas a similar exercise, the split squat (and variations), involves maintaining the split position without stepping each repetition.

> **OTHER VARIATIONS (SINGLE OR ALTERNATE LEGS) AND SIMILAR EXERCISES** DB/KB/MB/BW/sand bag lunge, reverse lunge (DB,KB, and BB), side lunge, Smith machine lunge, Cossack lunge, box lunge, walking lunge, lunge or reverse lunge with keg or sand bag, buddy lunge, lunge onto BOSU, power lunge, star lunge, lunge/reverse lunge with torso rotation (MB), lunge from an overhead squat BB position, DB/KB (one or two) overhead lunge, DB/MB reaching lunge (front, side), DB lunge with shoulder press or lateral raise, curtsy, landmine lunge/reverse lunge, mountain climbers (BW), SB circles, and elastic bands at various angles and loading positions and lunges or forward/backward walks using pendulum straps and a belt in a power rack.

Step-Up

Rating: B

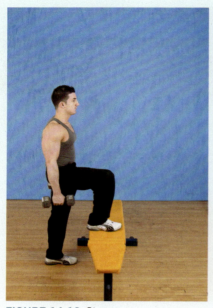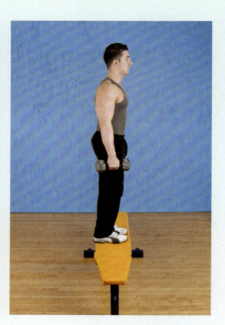

FIGURE 14.10 Step-up.

- Athlete stands erect 30–45 cm from a box or bench that is 30–45 cm high (or a height that will create a 90° angle at the knee joint when foot is on box) with a DB in each hand (or BB placed on shoulders) (Fig. 14.10).
- Athlete steps up with the lead leg onto the top of the bench, placing the foot in the center.
- Without leaning forward, BW is shifted to the lead leg and the body ascends unilaterally into a standing position on the top of the bench.
- The trailing leg is not used to push off but just follows to the top of the bench.
- Athlete steps off the bench with trailing leg to starting position (or if a cycle is used, the lead leg steps off first). As trailing foot is placed on the floor, BW shifts to trailing leg.
- Athlete steps off bench with lead leg and returns to starting position and repeats.

> **OTHER VARIATIONS (SINGLE OR ALTERNATE LEGS)** BB/KB/MB/BW step-ups, step-ups with keg or sand bag, side step-up (with or without crossover), step-ups with knee lift, partner step-ups, overhead step-ups, step-ups with a curl and press, and plyometric step-ups.

Several other single-joint hip exercises can be performed with machines, cable devices, bands/tubing, or ankle weights. These include machine and cable hip abduction/adduction, machine and cable hip flexion and extension, cable straight-leg hip extension, lying hip extension, hip extension with partner resistance, flexion, abduction/adduction, prone kneeling bent-leg hip extension, supine bent-leg hip extension (on the floor with contralateral hip flexion), lying hip abduction with straight leg and hip medial rotation, glute adductor squeeze, glute squeeze, and "clamshell."

Leg Curl

Rating: A

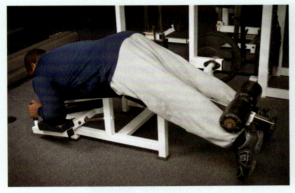 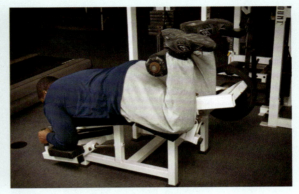

FIGURE 14.11 Leg curl.

- Athlete lies face down on a bench or machine with hips and chest flat against pads (Fig. 14.11).
- Knees are positioned below the bottom edge of the thigh pad and are aligned with the axis of rotation of the machine and ankles under heel pads while hands grasp the grips.
- Hips remain in contact with bench as knees flex (heels curl close to buttocks).
- Ankle position is important. Knee flexion torque generated is higher when the ankle is dorsiflexed than plantar flexed (7). The gastrocnemius is a multiarticular muscle, which assists in flexing the knee. Performing a leg curl with the ankles dorsiflexed puts the gastrocnemius at a length more conducive to producing force.
- Legs are slowly lowered with control to starting position.
- A spotter could apply pressure to the ankles during knee flexion if assistance is needed.
- The reverse leg curl (*i.e.*, Russian leg curl, Nordic leg curl) is a variation common among athletes and shown to reduce risk of hamstring injuries in some groups of athletes.

> **OTHER VARIATIONS AND SIMILAR EXERCISES** Standing unilateral curl, stated machine leg curl, DB/KB/MB leg curl, cable leg curls, reverse leg curl (with legs supported), reverse leg curl (with bands), leg curl with bands/tubing or partner, razor leg curl, SB (one or two legs) leg curls, and TRX leg curl (one or two legs).

Leg Extension

Rating: A

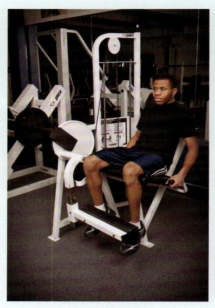 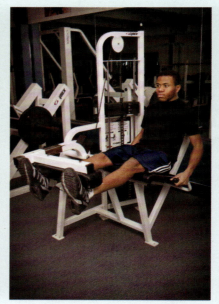

FIGURE 14.12 Leg extension.

- Athlete sits with back flat against the back support, knees aligned with the machine's axis of rotation, ankles in contact with the roller pads, and hands firmly grasping the handles (to keep hips on the seat when heavy loading is used) (Fig. 14.12).
- Buttocks and back should maintain their position on the machine while fully extending knees.
- The athlete slowly lowers the resistance arm to starting position.

- Mistakes include performing the exercise in a limited ROM and not firmly grasping the hand supports. Greater torque and power can be produced when the body is stabilized.

> **OTHER VARIATIONS** Unilateral leg extension, DB/KB/band leg extension, ISOM leg extension, SB leg extension, and performing the exercise with varied seat angles.

Calf (Toe) Raise

Rating: A

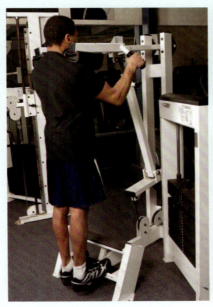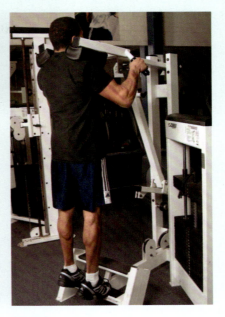

FIGURE 14.13 Calf (toe) raise.

- Grip bar with a closed, pronated grip slightly wider than shoulder width or place shoulders under pad if using a machine (Fig. 14.13).
- Stance is hip-to-shoulder width and knees are fully extended.
- To increase ROM and extend fully, the balls of the feet are near the edge of a raised surface. Pointing the toes inward, outward, or maintaining a neutral position shifts emphasis to different regions of the muscle.
- The athlete ascends (plantar flexion) onto toes as high as possible while maintaining fully extended knees, and toes are kept in a plantarflexed position for a brief time.
- The weight is lowered until heels are below the level of the toes at the starting position.
- Performing the exercise in a limited ROM is a common mistake.
- Training the ankle dorsiflexors, inverters, and everters is important for balance. Dorsiflexion exercises can be performed with bands, a plate placed over the feet, or a device known as the DARD (dynamic axial resistance device). Balance equipment (wobble board, BOSU) and single-leg exercises train these muscles as well.

> **OTHER VARIATIONS AND SIMILAR EXERCISES** Calf raise on leg press (angled, horizontal, or vertical), smith machine (or BB) calf raise, DB/KB/keg/sand bag calf raise, DB/BW unilateral calf raise, donkey calf raise, calf squats, partner calf raise, seated calf raises (machine, BB, or DB), and ankle dorsiflexion.

Upper-Body Exercises

Upper-body exercises encompass motion in three planes (sagittal, transverse, and frontal) about the shoulder, shoulder girdle, elbow, radioulnar, and wrist joints. Several major muscle groups produce these motions and must contract isometrically to stabilize the joints when they are not considered to be prime movers. Some are multiarticular or produce motion at multiple joints (Table 14.2).

Table 14.2	Kinesiology of Upper-Body Motion		
Joint	**Type of Joint**	**Joint Movement**	**Muscles**
Sternoclavicular	Saddle	Elevation	Serratus anterior, levator scapulae, rhomboid major/minor, trapezius
		Depression	Pectoralis minor, subclavius, lower trapezius
		Protraction	Serratus anterior, pectoralis minor
		Retraction	Levator scapulae, rhomboid major/minor, trapezius
		Upward rotation	Serratus anterior, trapezius
		Downward rotation	Levator scapulae, rhomboid major/minor
Acromioclavicular	Gliding	—	—
Glenohumeral	Ball and socket	Flexion	Pectoralis major, coracobrachialis, anterior/medial deltoid, biceps brachii
		Extension/hyperextension	Subscapularis, posterior deltoid, latissimus dorsi, teres major, long head of triceps brachii
		Adduction	Pectoralis major, coracobrachialis, biceps brachii, latissimus dorsi, teres major/minor, long head of triceps brachii
		Abduction	Supraspinatus, medial deltoid, infraspinatus
		Medial rotation	Pectoralis major, subscapularis
		Lateral rotation	Infraspinatus, teres minor
Elbow (humeroulnar)	Hinge	Flexion	Biceps brachii, brachialis, brachioradialis, pronator teres
		Extension	Triceps brachii, anconeus
		Pronation	Pronator teres, pronator quadratus
Radioulnar	Pivot	Supination	Biceps brachii, supinator
Radiocarpal (wrist)	Condyloid	Extension	Extensor carpi radialis brevis/longus, extensor carpi ulnaris, extensor digitorum, extensor digiti minimi, extensor pollicis brevis/longus, extensor indicis
		Flexion	Flexor carpi radialis, flexor carpi ulnaris, palmaris longus, flexor digitorum superficialis and profundus, flexor/abductor pollicis longus
		Ulnar deviation	Flexor carpi ulnaris, extensor carpi ulnaris
		Radial deviation	Flexor carpi radialis, flexor digitorum superficialis, extensor carpi radialis brevis/longus

Bench Press

Rating: B

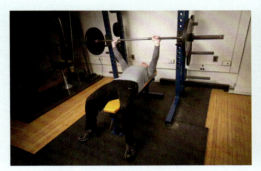
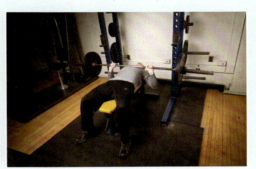

FIGURE 14.14 Bench press.

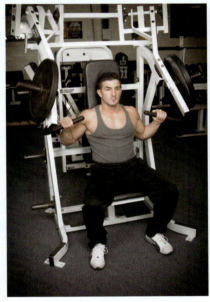
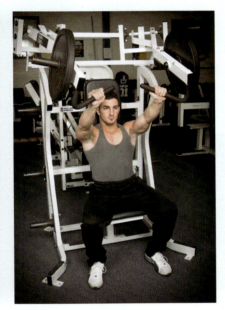

FIGURE 14.15 Chest press machine.

- The athlete lies supine on a bench with feet flat on the floor. The scapulae are retracted and the chest is forced out (Fig. 14.14).
- Bar is grasped with a closed, pronated grip slightly wider than shoulder width. Starting with the palms on the rear of the bar and rotating the hands help place the palms under the bar when lifting off and help lock the shoulders into the bench.
- Bar is removed from the rack and positioned directly over the chest with elbows fully extended.
- With control, the bar is lowered until it touches the lower chest near the nipples.
- Bar is lifted upward in a curvilinear manner until elbows are fully extended. The body remains flat on the bench.
- Bar is returned to the rack after completion of set.
- A spotter is located at the head of the bench and can apply enough force to keep the bar moving slowly when assistance is needed.
- This exercise can be performed on a chest press machine (Fig. 14.15) in an upright position. Similar technique applies to this variation. There are several machines that can be used that alter the grip position (midrange and pronated) and width (narrow, medium, wide). Seats may be adjusted to target different areas of the chest, *e.g.*, adjusting the seat high (with grips near the lower chest) to target lower chest musculature and vice versa.

> **CAUTION!** Bouncing the bar off of the chest and excessive arching of the back off of the bench are common mistakes. A mild-to-moderate arch with buttocks still in contact with the bench is a technique commonly used by powerlifters to increase performance by improving leverage. Some lifters like to place their feet on the bench during the bench press. This reduces stability and alters the technique. It is not recommended when lifting heavy weights.

> **OTHER VARIATIONS AND SIMILAR EXERCISES** DB bench press (unilateral or bilateral), close-grip bench press (especially effective for triceps development), decline bench press, reverse-grip bench press, wide-grip bench press, Smith machine bench press, ballistic bench press, keg, mastiff bar, or sand bag bench press, floor press, use of specialty bars, board press, bench press with pause, SB DB/KB bench press (with body parallel to ground, incline, decline), bench press in rack (functional isometrics, partial ROM, negatives), bench press with chains/bands, bench press to neck, oscillation bench press (with bands, KBs, and/or plates), and machine chest press. Standing elastic band presses are shown. Progression may occur from parallel stance to staggered stance to one leg, and from bilateral to alternating to unilateral pressing. Standing presses increase the trunk muscle recruitment to maintain stability and bands provide variable resistance. Vertical BB ballistic or traditional bench presses can be performed using an L bench with pendulum straps in a power rack.

Incline Bench Press

Rating: B

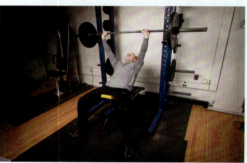

FIGURE 14.16 Incline bench press.

- Athlete lays ~45° (angle can vary) on an incline bench with feet flat on the floor similar to the bench press (Fig. 14.16).
- The bar is grasped with a closed, pronated grip slightly wider than shoulder width.
- Bar is removed from the rack and positioned directly over the upper chest with elbows fully extended.
- With control, bar is lowered until it touches the upper chest near the clavicles.
- Bar is lifted upward in a curvilinear manner until arms are fully extended. Body remains on the bench without excessive back arching or bouncing of weight off the chest.
- Bar is returned to the rack after completion of set.
- A spotter is located at the head of the bench and can apply enough force to keep the bar moving slowly when assistance is needed.

> **OTHER VARIATIONS** Similar to many of those listed for the flat bench press. Variations can be performed on a decline bench (Fig. 14.17).

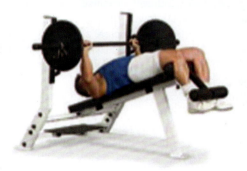

FIGURE 14.17 Decline bench press.

Interpreting Research
Muscle Activation during Variations of the Bench and Shoulder Press

Barnett C, Kippers V, Turner P. Effects of variations of the bench press exercise on the EMG activity of five shoulder muscles. *J Strength Cond Res.* 1995;9:222–7.

Barnett et al. (8) studied muscle activity and strength during the decline, flat, incline, and shoulder press with wide and narrow grips (Fig. 14.18). Body position affected maximum strength as the shoulder press yielded the lowest 1 RM and the decline bench press the highest. The middle (sternocostal) portion of the pectoralis major was most active during the flat bench press whereas similar activity was seen between flat and incline bench presses for the upper (clavicular) pectoralis major. Anterior deltoid activity increased in proportion from the decline press to the shoulder press. Triceps brachii activity was highest during the decline and flat bench presses. Latissimus dorsi activity was greatest during the decline press.

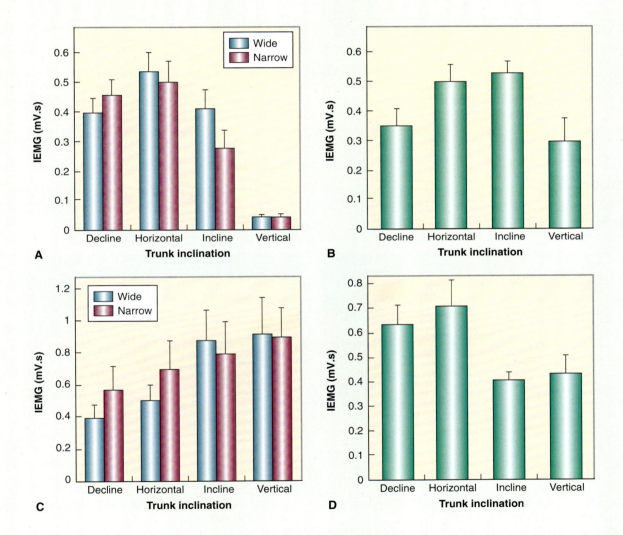

FIGURE 14.18 Muscle activation during the bench press. These figures show that trunk inclination and grip width affect muscle activity during the bench press. **A.** Shows the mid-sternal segment off the pectoralis major activity is highest during the flat bench press. **B.** Shows the clavicular (upper) part of the pectoralis major is most active during the incline and flat bench presses. **C.** Shows the anterior deltoid is most active during the shoulder press (and incline bench press). **D.** Shows triceps brachii activity is highest during the flat bench press (followed by the decline press).

(Continued)

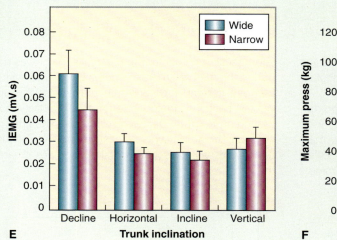
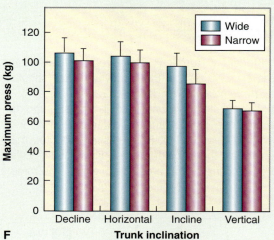

FIGURE 14.18 (*Continued*) **E.** Shows latissimus dorsi activity is highest during the decline press. **F.** Shows the largest amount of weight is lifted during the decline press, followed by the flat bench press, and shoulder press. (Reprinted with permission from Barnett C, Kipper V, Turner P. Effects of variations of the press exercise of the EMG activity of five shoulder muscles. *J Strength Cond Res.* 1995;9:222–7.)

Dumbbell Fly

Rating: A

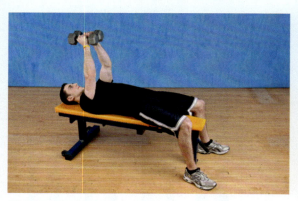

FIGURE 14.19 Dumbbell fly.

- Athlete lies flat on a bench (or can be inclined or declined) with feet flat on the floor (Fig. 14.19).
- DBs are grasped with a closed, pronated grip above the chest with arms fully extended and are rotated so that the palms of the hands face each other and the elbows point out (elbows are slightly flexed).
- DBs are lowered with control in a wide arc with elbows slightly flexed.
- Arms horizontally adduct a wide arc until they return to the starting arm position above the chest. (Performance note: flexing the elbow during the up phase decreases the moment arm of resistance and makes the exercise easier. Thus, elbow position should be maintained as best as possible throughout the ROM).
- One can spot by applying pressure medially to the wrist/forearms.

> **OTHER VARIATIONS AND SIMILAR EXERCISES** Incline DB/KB fly, machine (pec-deck) fly, cable fly, rotation fly, SB DB fly, SB cable fly, MB fly, TRX fly, standing cable crossover (with multiple postures and arm positions), and supine DB/KB arm bar (with trunk rotation).

Parallel Bar Dips

Rating: B

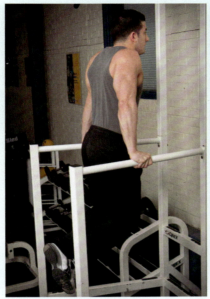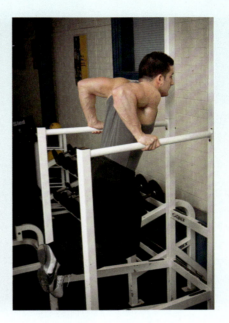

FIGURE 14.20 Parallel bar dips.

- Body is positioned and supported on the bars with the arms fully extended and knees flexed. Arms are shoulder width apart; torso is erect with a slight forward lean (to increase chest muscle activity) (Fig. 14.20).
- In control, the body is lowered until the upper arms are parallel to the ground and then lifted back to the starting position.

> **OTHER VARIATIONS AND SIMILAR EXERCISES** Reverse dips (primarily for the triceps), SB reverse dips, ring (gymnastic rings) dips and stabilization, and machine dips (with support). The exercise can be performed in a power rack with use of two Olympic bars.

Push-Up

Rating: B

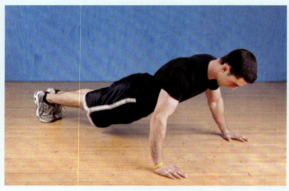 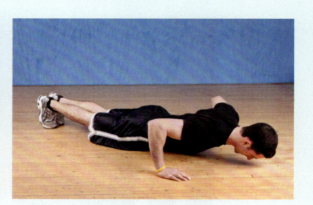

FIGURE 14.21 Push-up

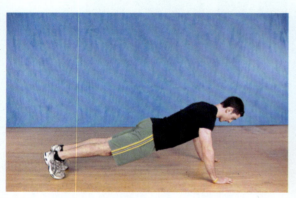 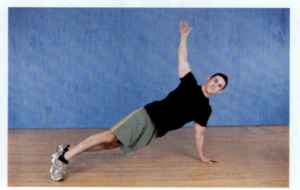

FIGURE 14.22 T-rotation.

- Athlete begins in prone position with wrists below shoulders, weight supported by arms vertical to the floor, legs extended, toes tucked under, and core contracted (Fig. 14.21).
- With control, the athlete flexes elbows (~90°) and horizontally abducts shoulders to where chest is located just above the floor.
- Athlete extends elbows and horizontally adducts shoulders to elevate body back up to the starting position.

OTHER VARIATIONS, SIMILAR EXERCISES, AND CRAWLING Modified push-up (on knees), push-ups with various grip widths and hand positions (wide, narrow), push-ups with staggered hand positions, push-ups on finger tips/wrists/fists, push-ups with feet elevated (decline, incline), pike push-up, one-arm push-ups, push-ups on MB (two hands, one hand on ball), MB push-up with shuffle or cross-over, plyo push-up on SB (arms on ball, feet on ball [shins, toes, one leg on SB]), core board, and BOSU (both sides), push-ups with walkout, push-up with T rotation (Fig. 14.22), Spiderman push-up, swivel push-up, corkscrew push-up, blast-off push-up, side-to-side push-up, archer push-up, birddog push-up, renegade on DB/KB, dive bomb/yoga push-up, push-up jack, TRX push-up, push-up with unilateral shoulder flexion at top (single-arm support works core) or anterior reach, ISOM half push-up, scapular push-ups, SB stabilization, walkouts, upper body step-up, partner push-up variations, elbow push-up, army crawls bear crawls, side crawls wheelbarrows, wheelbarrow drags (dragging plate on floor with feet), push-up walks, push-ups with various stances (feet together, apart, on top of one another, one leg with other extended), wall push-up, push-ups on DB/KB/bars, and handstand/handstand push-ups.

Bent-Over Barbell Row

Rating: B

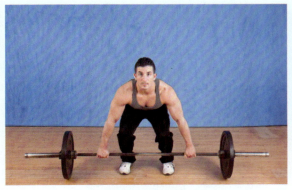
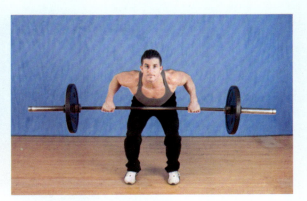

FIGURE 14.23 Bent-over barbell row.

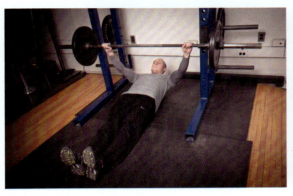
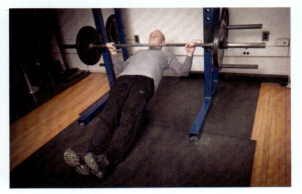

FIGURE 14.24 Inverted row.

- Athlete stands with feet shoulder width apart and knees flexed (Figs. 14.23).
- Bar is grasped from the floor with a closed, pronated grip wider than shoulder width while the back is flat, chest out, shoulders retracted, head is tilted forward, elbows are fully extended, and torso is flexed forward 10°–30° above horizontal.
- Athlete should remain flexed forward throughout the exercise.
- Bar is pulled upward (using back muscles mostly and not the elbow flexors) touching the upper abdomen.
- The elbows are pointed up with a rigid torso and the back should remain hyperextended (straight) throughout the movement.
- Bar is lowered with control until elbows are fully extended.

CAUTION! Standing too upright greatly limits ROM and muscle development. A common mistake is to see this exercise performed with the athlete maintaining nearly an upright posture.

OTHER VARIATIONS AND SIMILAR EXERCISES Reverse-grip bent-over row, bent-over DB row (with various grip positions), BB bench row, T-bar row, Smith machine row, machine rows, rows with keg, or sand bag, one-arm DB/core ball/band/tubing row, one-arm cable row, thick bar, DB/KB row (single leg for balance), landmine rows, partner rows, renegade row with DB or KB, one-arm bench row, and inverted row (BW with bar or TRX and feet elevated on bench/SB or placed on the floor, pronated or supinated grip) (Fig 14.24), and elastic band rowing. Progression may occur from parallel stance to staggered stance to one leg, to bent-over position, and from bilateral to alternating to unilateral rowing.

Lat Pull-Down

Rating: A

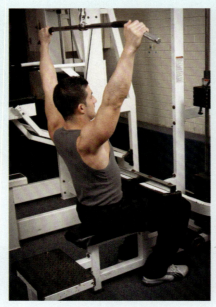
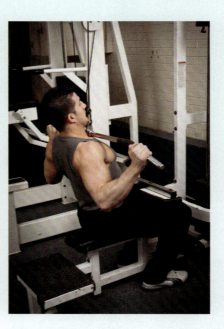

FIGURE 14.25 Lat pull-down.

- The bar (several lat bars to choose from) is grasped with a closed, pronated grip wider than shoulder width (but may vary depending on the variation performed) (Fig. 14.25).
- Athlete is seated on the bench with arms fully extended, back hyperextended slightly, chest out, shoulders retracted, and thighs secured under the properly adjusted thigh/hip pad.
- The bar is pulled downward in control to touch the upper chest or below chin level and then the bar is returned to the starting position. Athlete should avoid using momentum generated by the core to complete the lift.
- A spotter may apply downward pressure to the bar if assistance is needed.

OTHER VARIATIONS AND SIMILAR EXERCISES Wide-grip lat pull-down parallel grip lat pull-down, close-grip lat pull-down, reverse lat pull-down, machine pull-down (with various machines), rear lat pull-down, straight-arm pull-down, and cable double pull-down.

Pull-Up

Rating: B

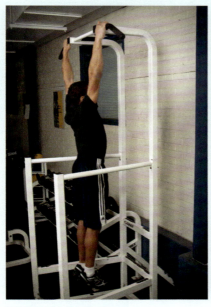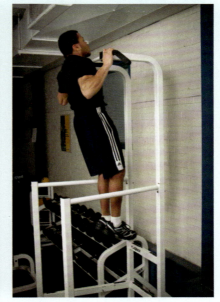

FIGURE 14.26 Pull-up.

- Using a chinning bar about 6 in. higher than an extended arm overhead position, the bar is held with an overhand grip with hands wider than shoulder width as the body hangs (chest out, back hyperextended) motionless (with knee flexed or straight). The straight-leg position increases the difficulty. Flexing the hips reduces the resistance arm and may allow for additional reps to be performed (Fig. 14.26).
- The body is pulled upward to where the chin surpasses the bar and returns in control to the starting position. The athlete should minimize sway as much as possible. A machine or elastic bands may be used if the athlete cannot lift his or her BW for the desired number of repetitions.
- A spotter may apply pressure to the hips or under the feet for assistance.

> **OTHER VARIATIONS, SIMILAR EXERCISES, AND ROPE CLIMBING** Chin-up (supinated grip), sternum chin-ups, weighted pull-ups (with different grips and grip widths), towel chin-ups, single-arm pull-up, rear pull-up, pull-up and press (muscle up), kipping pull-ups, commando pull-ups, negative pull-ups, ring pull-ups, flexed arm hang, machine assisted, monkey bar pull-ups or obstacles, rope pulls or climbs, climb pulls, and rope pulls on a Marpo Kinetics device.

Interpreting Research
Muscle Activation during Variations of the Lat Pull-down

Signorile JF, Zink AJ, Szwed SP. A comparative electromyographical investigation of muscle utilization patterns using various hand positions during the lat pull-down. *J Strength Cond Res*. 2002;16:539–46.

Signorile et al. (9) examined muscle activation during the wide-grip lat pull-down (front and rear), reverse grip pull-down, and narrow grip (parallel bar) pull-down and showed that the wide-grip lat pull-down to the front increased latissimus dorsi and teres major activity the most. Posterior deltoid activity was greatest during the close-grip lat pull-down (Fig. 14.27).

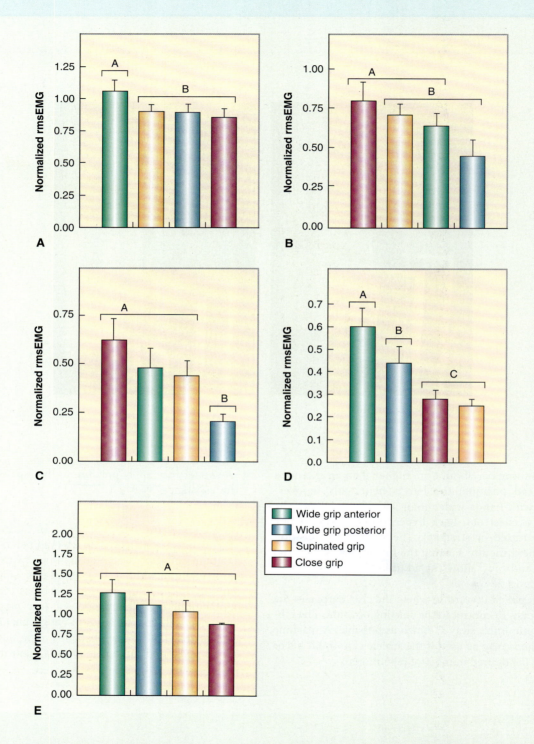

FIGURE 14.27 Muscle activation during variations of the lat pull-down. **A, D, and E.** Show latissimus dorsi, triceps brachii, and teres major activity were highest during the wide-grip front lat pull-down. **B and C.** Show pectoralis major and posterior deltoid muscle activity were highest during the close-grip lat pull-down. (Data from Signorile JF, Zink AJ, Szwed SP. A comparative electromyographical investigation of muscle utilization patterns using various hand positions during the lat pull-down. *J Strength Cond Res*. 2002;16:539–46.)

Low-Pulley Row

Rating: A

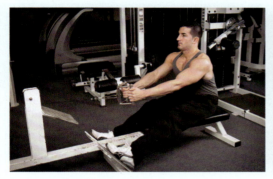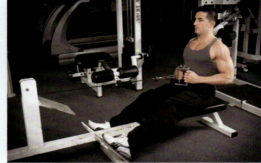

FIGURE 14.28 Low-pulley row.

- Athlete sits facing the machine with torso perpendicular to the floor, chest out, shoulders retracted, and knees slightly flexed with feet against foot support (Fig. 14.28).
- The handles are grasped with a closed grip and elbows fully extended.
- With an erect torso, the bar is pulled toward the upper abdomen with control and then returned to the starting position.

> **OTHER VARIATIONS AND SIMILAR EXERCISES** Machine rows (with various types of machines) and cable rows with various grips and bars (reverse, wide, narrow grip, pronated and supinated grips).

Pullover

Rating: A

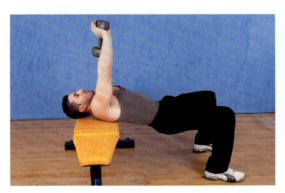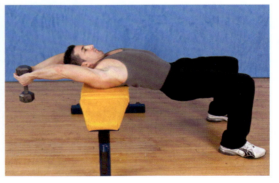

FIGURE 14.29 Pullover.

- Athlete lies on the side of a flat bench (cross bench) with the shoulders aligned over the bench and the rest of the body off. The hips should be descended lower than the level of the bench with flexed knees and feet flat on the floor (Fig. 14.29).
- The chest is out, neck is straight, and arms are extended straight over the chest with a DB in between.
- The shoulders are flexed until the upper arm is at the level of the head and then the shoulders extend back to the starting position in control.

> **OTHER VARIATIONS AND SIMILAR EXERCISES** BB pullover, machine pullover, MB pullover, DB/KB/MB/band/bag pullover (one or two arms) on SB, and pullover and press.

Standing Shoulder Press (Military Press)

Rating: B

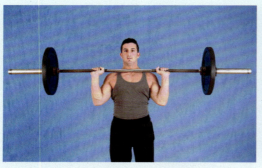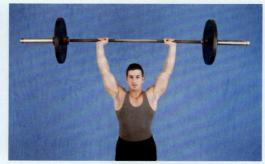

FIGURE 14.30 Standing shoulder press (military press).

- Bar is grasped with a closed, pronated grip slightly wider than or at shoulder width at shoulder height (Fig. 14.30).
- The elbows are kept under the bar with the wrists hyperextended. Feet should be slightly wider than shoulder width and knees are slightly flexed.
- The bar is lifted upward until elbows are fully extended and then lowered to shoulder level with control.
- The body is kept upright throughout the movement. Standing press increases core muscle activity more so than seated versions.

> **OTHER VARIATIONS AND SIMILAR EXERCISES** Standing DB/KB shoulder press (with pronated or midrange grip; one or two arms), MB/core ball press, Neider press, Sots press, keg or sand bag press, mastiff bar press, press with bands/tubing, standing DB Arnold press (with rotation), standing DB/KB rotation press, MB/DB "Y" press, shoulder press on BOSU or wobble board, plate/MB squat rotation press, shoulder-to-shoulder press, landmine rotational press/throw, landmine clean and press, landmine single-arm press, KB side press, wall slides, forearm wall slides, wall circles, band presses (multiple loading vectors) horizontal/angled prone press out, steering wheel, and angled BB presses using pendulum straps in a power rack.

Seated Shoulder Press

Rating: A

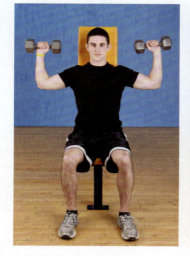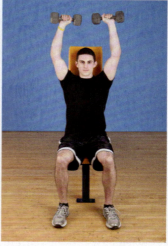

FIGURE 14.31 Seated shoulder press.

- Athlete sits on a bench with back support (head faces forward and back supported by the bench), chest out, back hyperextended, and feet are flat on the floor.
- The bar is grasped with a closed, pronated grip wider than shoulder width.
- The bar is lifted from the rack to an extended elbow position above the head.
- With control, the bar is lowered to below chin level and pressed overhead until elbows are fully extended.
- When DBs are used (Fig. 14.31), the athlete begins with a pronated grip at or near shoulder level, presses the DBs upward, and returns to the starting position. The exercise can be adapted to target balance by performing it on one leg (see the sidebar below).

> **OTHER VARIATIONS AND SIMILAR EXERCISES** Seated behind-the-neck BB shoulder press, seated KB shoulder press (using pronated or midrange hand positions), SB shoulder press, seated DB Arnold press, Smith machine shoulder press, seated shoulder press rack work (partial ROM, negatives, functional isometrics), and machine shoulder press (various types of machines).

Sidebar: Altering a Basic Exercise to Improve Balance

Muscle force production is greater when the body is in a most stable position. For example, athletes can lift large amounts of weight in the shoulder press when performing seated on a stable bench or when standing with proper posture and a large base support. However, when an athlete performs an exercise in a less stable bodily position, other stabilizer muscles are recruited to keep the body still and less weight is lifted. The goal becomes improving balance (and stabilizer muscle activity) rather than improving maximal strength. In our previous example, if one trained specifically for balance when performing the shoulder press, then some variations can be used. The athlete can perform the exercise while sitting on an SB; standing on a BOSU ball, wobble board, or Airex pads; or standing on one leg (one- or two-arm presses), which narrows the base support (Fig. 14.32); the athlete can close his or her eyes and/or add a reaction component to the exercise. Balance exercises have increased in popularity over the past several years. These exercises should be used specifically to enhance balance and stabilize muscle activity; the great weight reductions needed to create an inferior stimulus for maximal strength training.

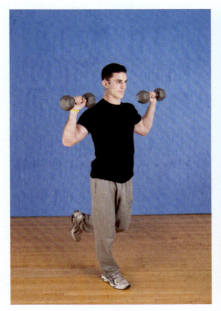 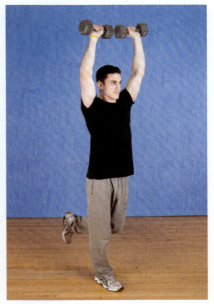

FIGURE 14.32 One-leg DB standing shoulder press.

Shrug

Rating: A

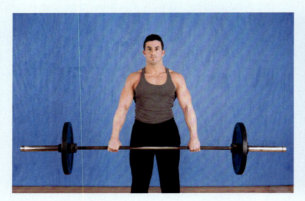 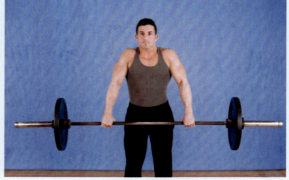

FIGURE 14.33 Shrug.

- The bar (Fig. 14.33) or DBs are grasped with a closed, pronated grip resting at arm's length at side of thighs (for DBs) or in front of the upper thighs (for BB).
- Feet are slightly wider than shoulder width and knees are slightly flexed.
- The weight is lifted by elevating shoulders while maintaining the body in an upright position with elbows fully extended. Shoulders are shrugged or elevated as high as possible and returned to the starting position (depressed) in control.

> **OTHER VARIATIONS AND SIMILAR EXERCISES** Power shrugs, machine shrugs, cable shrugs, keg/sand bag shrugs, seated DB/KB shrugs, seated trap bar shrugs, DB overhead shrug, thick bar, and behind-the-back BB shrugs.

Upright Row

Rating: A

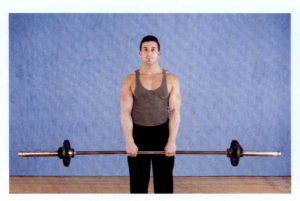 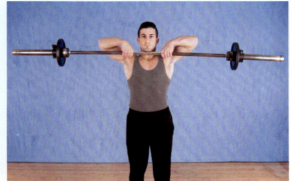

FIGURE 14.34 Upright row.

- Bar is grasped with a closed, pronated grip with hands about 20–30 cm apart (Fig. 14.34).
- The feet are kept slightly wider than shoulder width, knees are slightly flexed, and the bar rests with elbows fully extended on the thighs.
- The bar is lifted upward close to the body toward the chin (the elbows should be higher than the wrist and above the shoulders). A common mistake is to use the lower body or back to generate momentum to lift the weight. The weight should be lifted with an isolated effort from the upper-body musculature.
- With control, the bar is lowered to the starting position.

> **OTHER VARIATIONS AND SIMILAR EXERCISES** DB/KB/MB upright row, wide-grip upright row, cable upright row, partner manual resistance towel upright row, one-arm upright row, upright row on BOSU or wobble board, DB step-up with upright row, and upright row with bands/tubing.

Dumbbell Lateral Raise

Rating: A

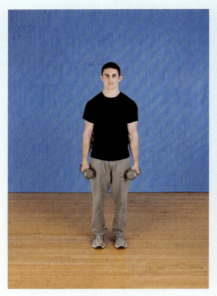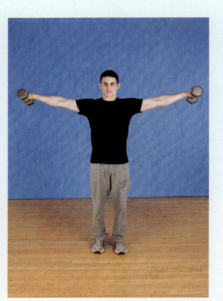

FIGURE 14.35 Dumbbell lateral raise.

- DBs are grasped with a closed, pronated grip in front of the hips with the elbows slightly flexed and are rotated so that the palms face each other with the elbows pointed outward (Fig. 14.35).
- Feet are kept slightly wider than shoulder width, knees are slightly flexed, and back is straight with eyes focused straight ahead.
- DBs are raised laterally until the elbows and wrists are parallel to the floor and in line with the shoulders. A common mistake is to use momentum to swing DBs.
- With control, DBs are lowered to the starting position. This exercise can be added to other exercises (lunge, squat, side plank, push-up) to form a combo exercise.

> **OTHER VARIATIONS, SIMILAR EXERCISES, AND SCAPULAR CORRECTIVE EXERCISES** Seated lateral raise, ISOM lateral hold/front raise, cable side laterals, machine lateral raise, rear lateral raise (DB or cable), bent-over lateral raise, kneeling lateral raise on SB, machine reverse fly, cable reverse fly, SB reverse fly, cross-cable laterals, BB front raise, lateral/front raise with core ball, DB/KB/MB front raise, alternate arm front raise, 45° front raise (with arm internally rotated), angled front raise, standing plate front raise (with a twist steering wheel), standing lateral/front raise on BOSU, standing horizontal abduction/adduction, scaption (empty, full can), DB punches (jabs, upper cuts, with rotation), DB arm swings, prone/seated/standing shoulder extensions, and scapular Y, T, W, L, I, reverse I, 3-point rotation (knees, toes).

Internal/External Shoulder Rotations

Rating: A

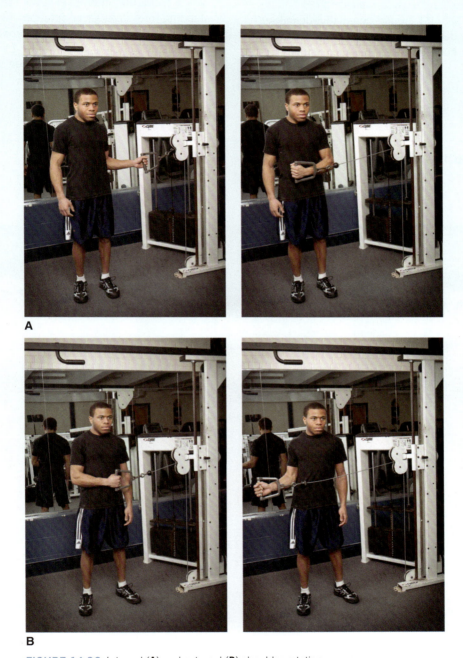

FIGURE 14.36 Internal (**A**) and external (**B**) shoulder rotation.

- Athlete stands with feet shoulder width apart near a cable pulley system or bands/tubing. The pulley is aligned with the elbow as the arms are relaxed at the sides (Fig. 14.36).

- Arm is flexed ~90° and externally rotated ~60°–80° to the starting position.

- The arm is rotated medially through complete ROM (while maintaining proper body position) while the upper arm remains at the side and then returns to the starting position.
- Weight is changed (internal shoulder rotators are stronger than external rotators) and body is rotated 180°.
- Elbow is flexed to ~90° and shoulder medially rotated ~90°.
- The arm is rotated externally through complete ROM (while maintaining proper body position) and then returns to the starting position.

> **OTHER VARIATIONS AND SIMILAR EXERCISES** Machine internal/external rotations, standing DB internal/external rotations, lying cross-bench T crucifix, internal/external rotations with bands, standing internal/external rotations (with upper arm parallel to the floor) with bands, prone external rotations on bench or SB, and lying internal/external rotations (on side midrange between supine and prone).

Scapula Retraction/Protraction

Rating: A

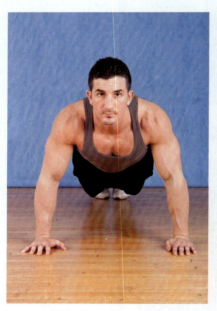 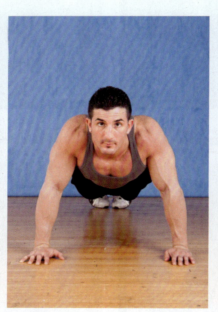 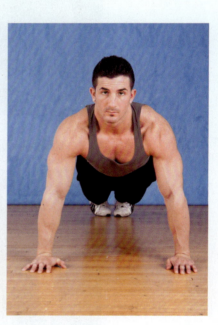

FIGURE 14.37 Scapula retraction/protraction.

- Athlete lies prone in a push-up position with a slightly wider than shoulder width hand position (Fig. 14.37).
- The shoulder blades (scapulae) are retracted or pulled back while keeping arms extended in a push-up position, and then returned to the starting position.
- From here, scapulae are protracted or pulled forward while keeping arms extended in a push-up position and then returned to the starting position.

> **OTHER VARIATIONS AND SIMILAR EXERCISES** Serratus punch. Same exercise can be performed from a bench press position, on SB/BOSU, with DB, or leaning against a wall.

Stability Ball Slaps

Rating: A

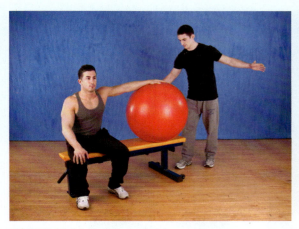 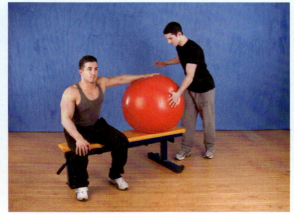

FIGURE 14.38 Stability ball slaps.

- An SB is held in place at the side of the athlete (or in front) supported on a bench. The ball is maintained in a stable position by the athlete isometrically contracting shoulder musculature to hold the ball still (Fig. 14.38).
- A partner slaps the ball at different locations with different intensities with altered timing. This forces the individual to react to the slaps by strongly contracting shoulder muscles.
- Athlete switches arms and supports the SB with the opposite arm while reacting to the partner's slaps.

> **OTHER VARIATIONS** Exercise can be performed while standing, lying prone or supine, or kneeling.

Triceps Pushdown

Rating: A

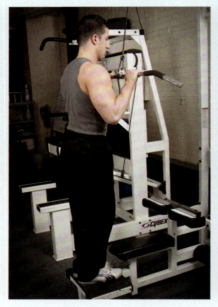
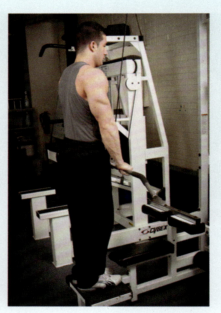

FIGURE 14.39 Triceps pushdown.

- The bar on a cable unit is grasped with a closed, pronated grip 10–15 cm apart with thumbs over the top of the bar and feet placed shoulder width apart with knees slightly flexed (Fig. 14.39).
- Body is kept upright throughout movement with elbows positioned next to torso.
- The bar is pushed down until the elbows reach full extension and then, with control, the bar is lowered to the starting position. A common mistake is to use the trunk to generate momentum to lift the weight or to perform the exercise in a limited ROM.

OTHER VARIATIONS AND SIMILAR EXERCISES Rope pushdowns, V-bar pushdowns, power pushdown, cross-body pushdown (one arm), reverse pushdown (with various bars), and incline bench pushdown (with various bars).

Seated Triceps Extension

Rating: A

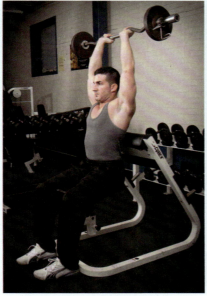
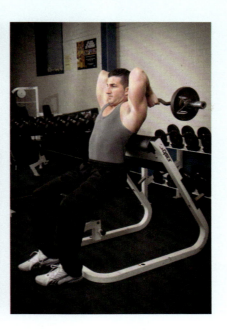

FIGURE 14.40 Seated triceps extension.

- Athlete is seated on a bench with feet flat on the floor and back supported (Fig. 14.40).
- Bar or DB(s) is grasped with a closed, pronated grip and lifted to a position above the head with the elbows fully flexed and pointed outward.
- The weight is extended upward until elbows are fully extended (while proper posture is maintained) and returned to the starting position under control.

> **OTHER VARIATIONS AND SIMILAR EXERCISES** Bilateral or unilateral triceps extension (with on DB) and seated BB triceps extension (with straight or EZ curl bar). Incline BB or DB triceps extension. Several variations can be performed standing. Machine triceps extension, seated reverse-grip BB triceps extension, DB extensions (with hand rotation), seated (or incline) cable triceps extension (with various bars or rope), bent-over prone cable triceps extension, BB, cable, or DB kickbacks (bent-over or lying).

Lying Triceps Extension (Skull Crushers)

Rating: A

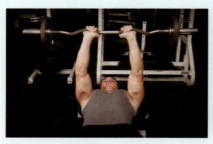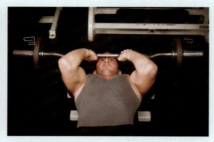

FIGURE 14.41 Lying triceps extension (skull crushers).

- Athlete lies supine on the bench with feet flat on the floor (Fig. 14.41).
- The bar is grasped with a closed, pronated grip with hands 15–25 cm apart and elbows are extended above the upper chest.
- With control, the bar is lowered to the forehead, and upper arms remain perpendicular to the floor.
- The bar is pushed upward until elbows return to the fully extended position.

> **OTHER VARIATIONS AND SIMILAR EXERCISES** Lying reverse-grip BB extension, lying DB triceps extension (midrange hand position), cross-face DB extensions, cable triceps extension (with various bars or rope), decline, lying BB, cable, or DB extensions with upper arm at 45° angle to the floor, and fixed-bar body extension.

Standing Biceps Curl (Olympic/EZ Curl Bar)

Rating: A

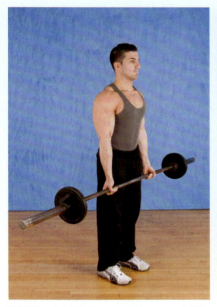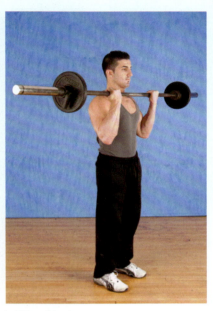

FIGURE 14.42 Standing biceps curl (Olympic/EZ curl bar).

- The bar is grasped shoulder width or slightly wider with a closed, supinated (palms facing forward) grip with elbows extended (Fig. 14.42).
- Feet are shoulder width apart, knees are slightly flexed, back is straight, eyes are focused straight ahead, and upper arms are positioned against trunk perpendicular to the floor.
- Bar is lifted in an arc toward the anterior deltoids by flexing the elbows and then lowered in control to the starting position. DB variations can be added to exercises (lunge, squat) to form combo exercises.
- Common mistake includes using momentum to lift the weight up or not using a full ROM.

> **OTHER VARIATIONS AND SIMILAR EXERCISES** Wide-grip curl, cheat curls, slide (drag) curl, DB curls, alternate DB curls, cable curls, standing concentration curl, high cable curls, curls (one leg), Zottman curls, and DB rotation curls.

Seated Dumbbell Biceps Curl

Rating: A

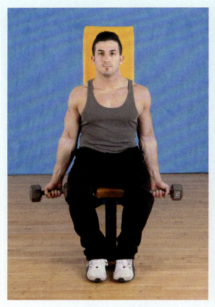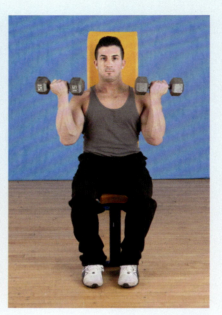

FIGURE 14.43 Seated dumbbell biceps curl.

- Athlete sits on the bench with feet flat on the floor and the back supported by pad (Fig. 14.43).
- DBs are grasped with the elbows extended at the sides with a closed, supinated grip.
- DBs are lifted in an arc toward the anterior deltoid by flexing the elbows and then lowered in control to the starting position.
- May be performed by alternating each arm unilaterally or simultaneously bilaterally.

OTHER VARIATIONS AND SIMILAR EXERCISES Seated cable curls, incline DB curls, incline cable curls, DB concentration curl, prone bench curl (DB, cables, or BB), machine curls, supine cable curls, supine DB curl, and landmine curl.

Hammer Curl

Rating: A

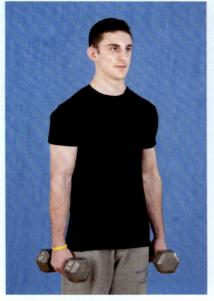
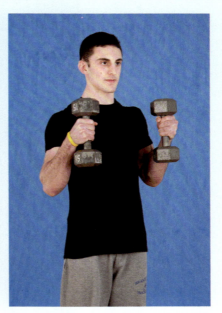

FIGURE 14.44 Hammer curl.

- DBs are grasped with elbows extended at the sides in closed, supinated midrange grip (palms of the hands are facing the body) with feet shoulder width apart and knees slightly flexed. Back is straight and eyes are focused straight ahead (Fig. 14.44).
- DBs are raised in an arc toward the anterior deltoid by flexing the elbows and then lowered with control to the starting position.
- Exercise can be performed by alternating each arm unilaterally or bilaterally.

> **OTHER VARIATIONS** Cross-body hammer curls and cable hammer curls.

Preacher Curl (Olympic/EZ Curl Bar)

Rating: A

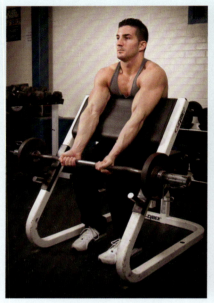 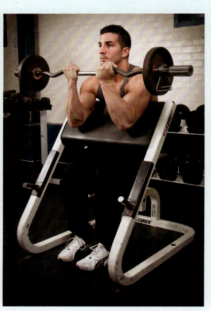

FIGURE 14.45 Preacher curl (Olympic/EZ curl bar).

- A preacher bench is used. The bar is grasped with a narrow, closed, supinated grip while athlete is seated (Fig. 14.45).
- Back is straight, eyes are focused straight ahead, and upper arms rest against support pad.
- Bar is lifted in an arc toward the anterior deltoids by flexing the elbows and lowered in control to the starting position.
- A spotter can apply force to the bar during the upward movement if necessary.

OTHER VARIATIONS DB preacher curl, one-arm DB preacher curl, cable preacher curl, Scott curls, and machine preacher curls.

Wrist Curl

Rating: A

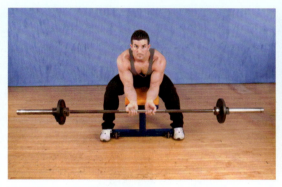 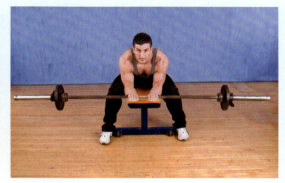

FIGURE 14.46 Wrist curl.

- Athlete sits on the end of a bench and grasps the bar (straight or EZ curl bar) with an open, supinated grip with hands 20–30 cm apart. Wrists are hyperextended (Fig. 14.46).
- Feet are flat on the floor with the torso leaning forward and elbows and forearms resting on the thighs (or bench) throughout the movement.
- The bar is lifted by flexing fingers and wrist and then returning to the starting position.

OTHER VARIATIONS AND SIMILAR EXERCISES DB wrist curl, cable wrist curls, behind-the-back BB wrist curls (standing or seated), behind-the-back DB or cable wrist curls, machine wrist curls, wrist curls on a preacher bench, wrist rolls (with a roller or similar device such as a Gripedo), and wrist circles (radial/ulnar deviation).

Reverse Wrist Curl

Rating: A

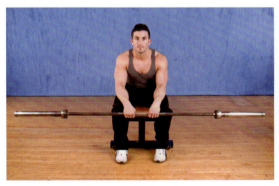 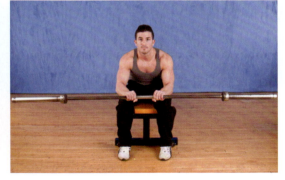

FIGURE 14.47 Reverse wrist curl.

- Athlete sits on the end of a bench and grasps the bar with a closed, pronated grip, wrists flexed, and hands held 20–30 cm apart (Fig. 14.47).
- Feet are flat with the torso leaning forward and elbows and forearms resting on the thighs (or bench) throughout the movement.
- The bar is raised by extending and hyperextending the wrists.

OTHER VARIATIONS AND SIMILAR EXERCISES DB or cable reverse wrist curl, machine reverse wrist curl, wrist rows, and reverse wrist rolls (with a roller or similar device such as a Gripedo), KB ISOM hold.

Reverse Curl

Rating: A

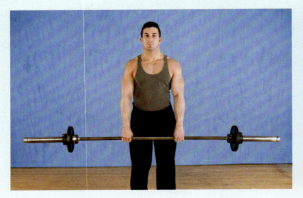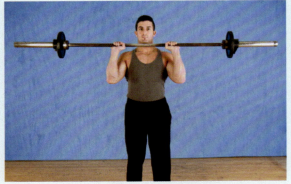

FIGURE 14.48 Reverse curl.

- Bar is grasped shoulder width or slightly wider with a closed, pronated grip with elbows extended (Fig. 14.48).
- Feet are shoulder width apart, knees are slightly flexed, back is straight, eyes are focused straight ahead, and upper arms are positioned against trunk perpendicular to the floor.
- Bar is lifted in an arc toward the anterior deltoids by flexing the elbows (and extending wrists) and then lowered in control to the starting position.

> **OTHER VARIATIONS** Standing reverse curl (DB, cables) and machine reverse curl.

Core Exercises

Core exercises encompass motion in three planes about the spinal column and pelvic girdle. Several major muscle groups produce these motions and must ISOM contract to stabilize the joints when they are not considered to be prime movers (Table 14.3). Flexion occurs when anterior muscles contract bilaterally (both sides of vertebral column). Extension occurs when posterior muscles contract bilaterally. Lateral flexion and/or rotation occur when muscles contract unilaterally. Stability when the athlete is standing (while externally loaded), bridged supine on ground with shoulders and feet (knees bent), and prone on all fours (plank) is trained. There are a large number of exercises and variations that develop a strong, durable core.

Table 14.3	Kinesiology of Core Motion		
Joint	**Type of Joint**	**Joint Movement**	**Muscles**
Cervical	Hinge, pivot (C1-C2)	Lateral flexion rotation	Rectus capitis (lateralis, anterior), longus capitis and colli, sternocleidomastoid, splenius capitis and cervicis, suboccipital group, levator scapulae, semispinalis capitis and cervicis, multifidus, longissimus capitis, trapezius, rotatores cervicis
		Flexion	Rectus capitis (lateralis, anterior), longus capitis and colli, hyoid muscles, sternocleidomastoid, scalenes
		Extension/ hyperextension	Splenius capitis and cervicis, suboccipital group, semispinalis capitis and cervicis, erector spinae, multifidus, levator scapulae, longissimus capitis, trapezius, scalenes, sternocleidomastoid, rotatores cervicis
Thoracic lumbar		Flexion	Rectus abdominis, external/internal oblique, quadratus lumborum
		Extension	Spinalis, iliocostalis, and longissimus thoracis, semispinalis thoracis, multifidus, iliocostalis lumborum, rotatores thoracis
		Rotation and lateral flexion	Semispinalis thoracis, erector spinae, multifidus, external/internal oblique, rectus abdominis, psoas major/minor, iliocostalis lumborum, quadratus lumborum
		Abdominal hollowing	Transversus abdominis
Rib cage[a]		Elevation, inspiration	Diaphragm, serratus posterior superior, internal intercostals, levator costarum, transversus thoracis
		Depression, expiration	Serratus posterior inferior, external intercostals

[a]Primary respiration muscles.

Proper Position for Core Exercises

Contraction of abdominal and spinal muscles is essential to maintaining spine stability. One muscle, the transversus abdominis, resembles an internal girdle. Its major function is hollowing (or compression) where the abdominal wall is drawn in toward the spine (10) and is activated before other muscles during movement. Special attention has been given to this muscle because of its role in low-back pain. Many therapists, coaches, and trainers teach athletes to draw in the abs by contracting the transversus abdominis. It is assessed by having the athlete lie supine and contract the transversus abdominis with the trainer's hand under the lumbar spine to measure pressure. The exercise is practiced from other positions, *e.g.*, prone, seated, and standing (11). A complex variation is the dead bug (Fig. 14.49) where the arms and legs are elevated off of the floor. Other core muscles need to contract to generate high IAP via bracing (12). Bracing involves ISOM contraction of the transversus abdominis as well as the internal and external obliques, rectus abdominis, quadratus lumborum, and lumbar muscles and increases lumbar stability (12). Strengthening the top (diaphragm) and bottom (pelvic floor) of the abdomen is important for core stability. The Sidebar below discusses some ways in which core exercises can be made more difficult once proper position is attained.

Sidebar: Making Core Exercises More Difficult

Several core exercises can be made more difficult by altering the position of the limbs, thereby increasing the moment arm of resistance. For example, a curl-up is more difficult when the arms are extended over-head rather than crossed across the chest. For some SB exercises, less BW can be supported by the ball or one leg can be used instead of two. Bending the knees during the leg raise makes it easier than with extended knees. Several progressions can be developed to increase the difficulty of an exercise without adding additional loading.

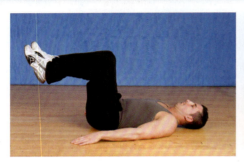
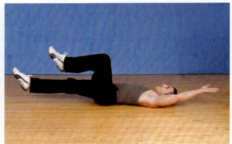

FIGURE 14.49 "Dead bug."

Core Exercises

Crunch (Curl-Up)

Rating: A

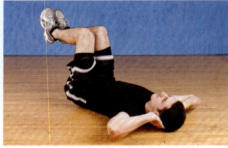
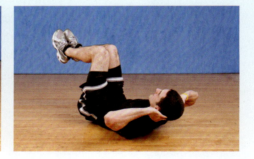

FIGURE 14.50 Crunch (curl-up).

- Athlete lies supine on a mat or floor with hips and knees elevated to form a 90° angle (Fig. 14.50).
- Hands are placed at the sides of the head or folded across the chest with chin tucked into the chest.
- Torso is flexed (curled) toward the thighs until shoulders are off the floor and returned in control to the starting position.

> **OTHER VARIATIONS (WITH PLATES, DB MACHINES, MB, KB, SAND BAG) AND SIMILAR EXERCISES** Ab crunches (with feet straight, bent knees, pike position), decline crunches, machine crunches, cable crunches (standing or kneeling), reverse crunch (with SB or MB), ISOM crunch, side (oblique) crunches, SB oblique crunch, cable side crunches, partner (base, bottom man down) crunches, SB crunches, BOSU crunches, crunches with arms overhead (DB/MB), and hanging side crunches.

Bent-Knee Sit-Up

Rating: A

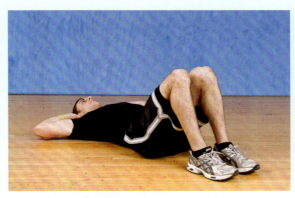 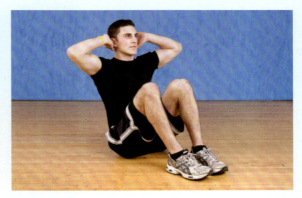

FIGURE 14.51 Bent-knee sit-up.

- Athlete lies supine on the floor with knees flexed and heels close to buttocks (Fig. 14.51).
- Hands are placed at the sides of the head or folded across the chest with chin tucked into the chest.
- Trunk and hips are flexed toward thighs until trunk is off the floor and returned in control to the starting position.

> **OTHER VARIATIONS (WITH PLATES, DB, MACHINES, MB, KB SAND BAG) AND SIMILAR EXERCISES** Sit-ups on decline bench, glute-ham sit-up, Roman chair sit-ups, sit-ups with MB toss, straight-leg sit-ups, sit-ups with straight arms, suspended sit-ups, and sit-ups with BB, DB, plate, or MB press, Janda sit-ups, and landmine sit-up.

Bent-Knee Twists

Rating: A

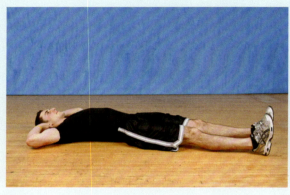 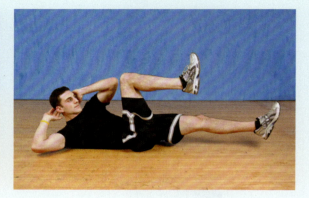

FIGURE 14.52 Bent-knee twists.

- Athlete lies supine on the floor with knees flexed, heels close to buttocks, and hands placed on the side of the head with elbows pointed forward (Fig. 14.52).
- Torso is flexed and rotated during ascent off of the floor as the elbow approaches the opposite knee (right elbow to left knee) and then returns in control to the starting position.
- Next repetition is performed using the opposite elbow to knee.

> **OTHER VARIATIONS, SIMILAR EXERCISES, AND WINDMILLS** Roman chair twisting sit-ups, decline twisting sit-ups, twisting crunches (flat, decline, Roman chair, with knee raise), cable twisting crunches, reverse trunk twists, SB reverse trunk twist (windshield wiper), SB trunk rotations, machine trunk rotations, Russian twists (flat, sit-up bench, decline with DB, plate, MB, landmine), SB/BOSU twisting knee-ups, SB/BOSU twisting crunches (with bands), partner plate pass, MB side throws, standing/seated twists (with BB, DB, or MB), bent-over trunk rotations (with stick, BB, DB, or MB), and KB high/low windmill.

Side Bends

Rating: A

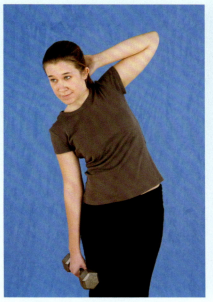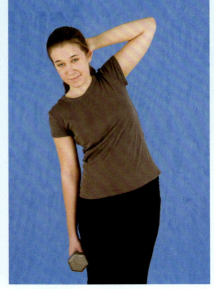

FIGURE 14.53 Side bends.

- Athlete stands with shoulder width stance grasping a DB in one hand and opposite arm positioned on the side of the head (Fig. 14.53).
- Athlete laterally flexes (bends) to the side grasping the DB and returns in control to the starting position.
- After the required number of repetitions is performed, individual grasps DB with opposite hand and repeats the exercise. A common mistake is to use two DBs for this exercise. The second DB acts as a counterbalance and reduces loading on the core.

> **OTHER VARIATIONS AND SIMILAR EXERCISES** Cable, BB, SB, or stick side bends, lateral flexion (on hyperextension bench or glute-ham), arms overhead, and lying side bends.

Plank

Rating: A

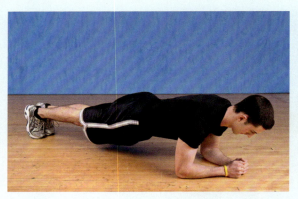

FIGURE 14.54 Plank.

- Athlete begins in a push-up postural position with BW supported by the feet and hands or elbows (which are in contact with the floor) (Fig. 14.54).
- Torso remains in a straight line with the hip level for the duration of the exercise.
- Athlete maintains this ISOM hold position with proper body alignment and requires trunk musculature to contract strongly against the force of gravity. A common mistake is to allow the hips to drop too low or rise too high during fatigue.

> **OTHER VARIATIONS AND SIMILAR EXERCISES** SB plank (hands on ball — push-up position; SB under feet — push-up position), MB plank, plank with one leg elevated, one-arm plank, one-arm plank with contralateral arm movement, ISOM side plank (on elbows or hands), side plank with hip abduction (star plank) or contralateral shoulder lateral raise, KB/DB, angled plank (with BB or bench), TRX plank, TRX side plank, TRX plank with leg scissors, plank-up, plank jack, plank side hop, plank walk, side glide (against wall), dynamic side bridge, prone twist, plank band pull, plank hip dip (rotation), reverse plank, side plank trunk rotation, plank/side plank band row, and plank lateral drag.

Stability Ball Roll-Out

Rating: B

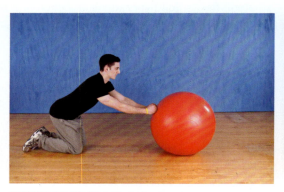 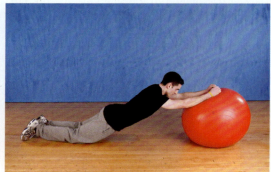

FIGURE 14.55 Stability ball roll-out.

- Athlete begins on knees in an upright position (with slight forward lean) with forearms/wrists near the side of SB (Fig. 14.55).
- Athlete leans forward as ball rolls. Forearms stay in contact with ball (and roll over the ball to elbow level) as the shoulders flex.
- Core muscles contract to maintain posture. Athlete continues to roll the ball until trunk, arms, and shoulders are aligned. With control, the ball is rolled back to starting position via shoulder extension with core muscles contracting to maintain proper position.
- Exercise is more difficult with the body closest to the ground (with a BB, DB, or Ab Roller) or when it is performed from a standing or elevated body position.
- Because of upper-body involvement, shoulder extensors are worked.

> **OTHER VARIATIONS** Ab Roller, standing SB roll-out, elevated SB roll-out, BB/DB roll-out, MB roll-out, and landmine roll-out.

Lying Leg Raise

Rating: A

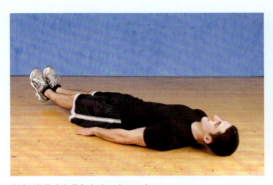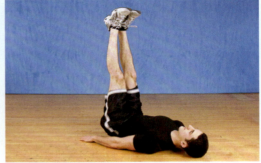

FIGURE 14.56 Lying leg raise.

- Athlete lies supine on the floor with hips and knees extended in front (Fig. 14.56).
- Trunk is kept tight, legs are raised with knees slightly bent until they are perpendicular to the floor, and returned in control to the starting position.
- May use BW, SB, or MB for resistance.

> **OTHER VARIATIONS AND SIMILAR EXERCISES** Plyometric leg raise (with partner), vertical (dip) bench straight- or bent-leg raise, hanging straight- or bent-leg raise (BW or MB), circular (360°) straight leg raise, bent knee-ups (floor, bench, seated, and decline), cable/band knee-ups, alternate leg knee-ups, knee-ups + abdominal crunch, lying V-ups, SB side leg lift, lying flutter kicks, lying scissors, ISOM leg raise holds (6 in.), lying side knee-ups, side flutter kicks, side jackknife, SB prone knee-ups (ball under shins, toes, or one leg), SB twisting knee-ups, SB prone pike knee-up, TRX knee-up and twisting knee-up, TRX pike knee-up, TRX windshield wiper, KB/MB/DB L-sit, Rocky leg lift, partner knee tucks, and kips.

Stability Ball Exchange

Rating: B

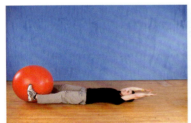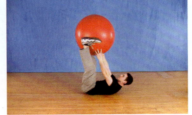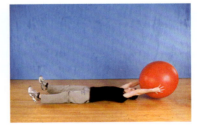

FIGURE 14.57 Stability ball exchange.

- Athlete begins in a supine position with legs and arms extended in opposite directions. An SB is placed between hands and held in an overhead position (Fig. 14.57).
- Shoulders extend, trunk flexes, and hips flex bringing arms and legs toward the center of the body.
- At the top of the movement, the SB is exchanged from hands to feet (ball is held between the legs near the ankles) and arms and legs are returned in control to the starting position.

> **OTHER VARIATIONS** MB exchange.

Medicine Ball Woodchop

Rating: A

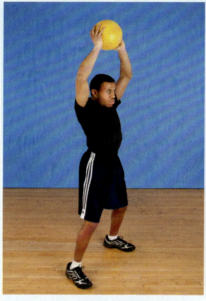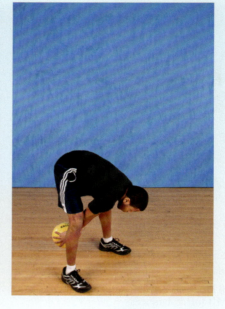

FIGURE 14.58 Medicine ball woodchop.

- Feet are placed wider than shoulder width. MB is held with both hands above the head (Fig. 14.58).
- MB is swung forcefully downward between the legs flexing the trunk, hips, and extending the shoulders.
- The movement is reversed back to the starting position.

OTHER VARIATIONS DB woodchop, rotational woodchop, diagonal woodchop, cable woodchop, chop and lift, reverse woodchop, and MB slam.

Cable Rotations

Rating: A

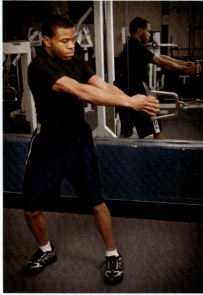
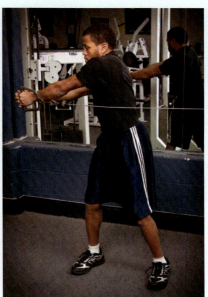

FIGURE 14.59 Cable rotations.

- Athlete adjusts a cable pulley system to shoulder height and assumes a position facing away from the machine at a 90° angle a few feet away (Fig. 14.59).
- A shoulder width stance is used. With feet planted securely, the athlete rotates the trunk to grasp the handle with both hands.
- Keeping the lower body still, the athlete rotates 180° with arms in an extended position. The exercise is most difficult with the arms straight. Bending the arms decreases the moment arm of resistance.
- In control, the athlete returns to the starting position. Once the required number of repetitions is performed, athlete switches sides and repeats.

> **OTHER VARIATIONS AND SIMILAR EXERCISES** Cable diagonal (low-to-high) rotation, DB/KB/MB low-to-high rotation, halo, MB rotations (standing, seated, kneeling), plate squat rotation press, judo throw, band/tubing rotations, Pallof press, KB high/low windmill, TRX rotation, reach and rotation.

Landmine Bar Rotation (Russian Twist)

Rating: B

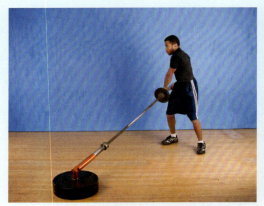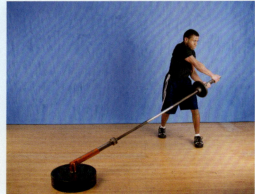

FIGURE 14.60 Landmine bar rotation (Russian twist).

- An Olympic bar is loaded on only one side with the opposite side fixed in a corner acting as a fulcrum for motion. A device that freely allows the bar to rotate (Landmine or Renegade) is recommended (Fig. 14.60).
- Athlete grasps one end of the bar with both arms (one hand over, one under), elbows extended, and at one side.
- While keeping arms straight, the athlete rotates to the opposite side lifting the bar up, extending the bar outward, and across the body to the contralateral side with feet staggered.
- Athlete reverses the action back to the starting position.

OTHER VARIATIONS AND SIMILAR EXERCISES Kneeling, parallel stance, and side rotation.

Skier

Rating: B

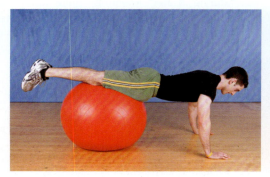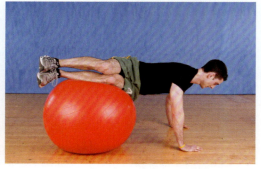

FIGURE 14.61 Skier.

- Athlete begins in a push-up position with shins resting on the SB and knees flexed (Fig. 14.61).
- While maintaining upper-body position, the athlete rotates the trunk quickly to the left (until legs are parallel to the ground) and then back to the right.

OTHER VARIATIONS Exercise can be performed with knees extended.

Turkish Get-Up

Rating: B

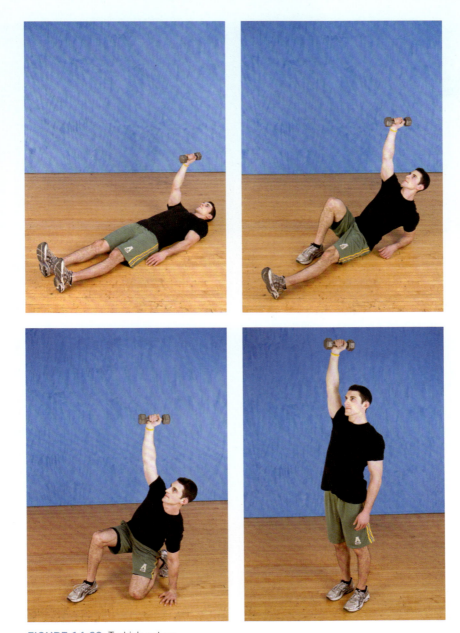

FIGURE 14.62 Turkish get-up.

- Athlete lies supine on the floor with a KB or DB in one hand with arm perpendicular to the floor. Knee on the same side flexes and foot is flat on the floor while athlete flexes the trunk and supports weight on the opposite elbow (Fig. 14.62).
- While weight is supported by back arm, athlete performs a side plank and then tucks the opposite leg under the body (into a lunge position) and begins to rise up to the standing position with KB or DB overhead.
- Athlete reverses the phases and returns to the starting position and performs another repetition.

> **OTHER VARIATIONS** The version shown is a lunge variation. A squat or second lunge variation can be performed. Exercise can be performed with sand bags, barbell (landmine), or core ball.

Good Morning

Rating: A

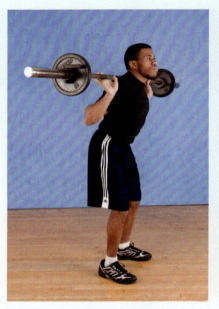
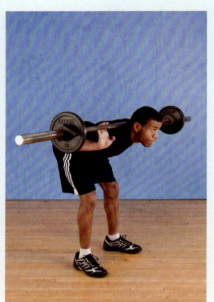

FIGURE 14.63 Good morning.

- Bar is grasped with a closed, pronated grip slightly wider than the shoulder width while it rests on shoulders (similar to back squat). Feet are shoulder width apart with toes pointed slightly outward. Head is straight or slightly upward with eyes focused on a spot on the wall (Fig. 14.63).
- With chest out, shoulders retracted, and lower back flat (hyperextended), torso and hips are flexed at the waist until almost parallel to the floor. Proper hip hinge position is maintained throughout. Lower body remains still.
- Athlete returns to the starting position.

> **OTHER VARIATIONS** Keg/sand bag good morning, DB/KB good morning, good morning on SB/BOSU, or seated.

Back Extension/Hyperextension

Rating: A

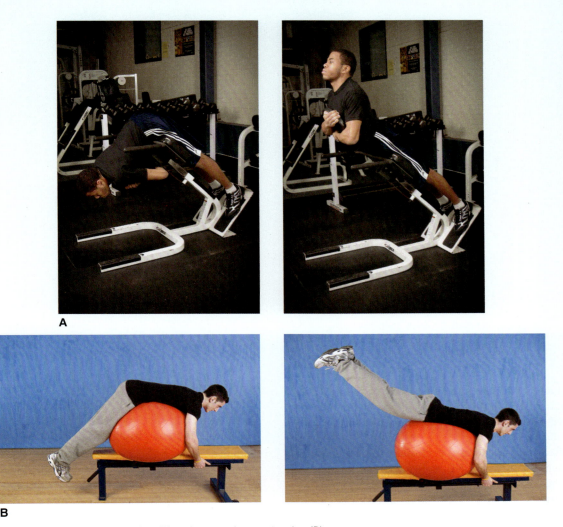

FIGURE 14.64 Hyperextension (**A**) and reverse hyperextension (**B**).

- Upper pad of the Roman chair bench is adjusted so upper thighs lie flat across and there is space for flexion at the waist and knees are not hyperextended. Ankles are positioned under lower pads for support (Fig. 14.64).
- With arms crossed behind head, overhead, or across chest (holding plate, DB, KB, bar, sand bag), the athlete bends forward at the waist in a full ROM while maintaining a flat back and returns to the starting position in control. The exercise is more difficult with arms overhead then across chest.
- Hyperextensions and reverse hyperextensions (panel B) are excellent exercises working the low-back/glute/hamstring muscles. The extended position on a hyperextension bench can be used as a base for combo exercise building (rotations, press-outs, side raises, and rows).

> **OTHER VARIATIONS AND SIMILAR EXERCISES** Machine back extensions, hyperextensions with straight arms (MB, DB, plate, band), twisting hyperextensions, single-arm cross-body rotational back extension, rotations (while maintaining the hyperextended back position), BB back extension, single-leg hyper-extension, reverse hyperextensions, hypers/reverse hypers on SB, glute-ham raise (BW, BB, DB, MB, sand bag), posterior reach, medicine ball overhead repeats, and press-ups.

Kettlebell Swing

Rating: B

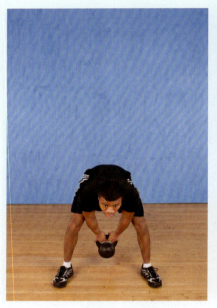 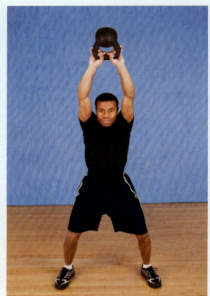

FIGURE 14.65 Kettlebell swing.

- Athlete begins in a semisquat position with chest out and a slight arch in the lower back showing proper hip hinge. KB is grasped between legs with two hands with arms extended (Fig. 14.65).
- KB is lifted (swung) upward explosively via knee, hip, and back extension to where KB rises to or slightly above the level of the head.
- KB is returned to the starting position in control.

> **OTHER VARIATIONS** Exercise can be performed with DB, sand bag, or one arm. A squat can be added at the end (swing squat). Other KB variations include 1- or 2-arm swings with 1 or 2 KBs, alternating swings, rotations, and adding front/back, pirouette, or lateral steps during the up phase of the swing.

Back (Glute) Bridge

Rating: A

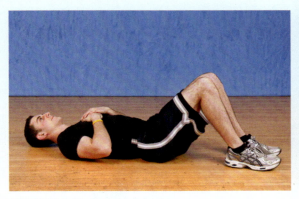 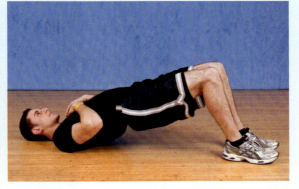

FIGURE 14.66 Back (glute) bridge.

- Athlete lies supine on the floor with arms at side (or across the chest) and knees/hips flexed with feet flat on floor (Fig. 14.66).
- With arms remaining in the starting position, the chest, hips, buttocks, and spine rise (extend) off of the floor to a linear elevated body position (with shoulders supporting upper-body weight) and return back to the starting position. The trainee should focus on pushing through the heels.
- ISOM muscle action can be added at the top of the exercise while the body is in a linear position.
- A progression is to work from 2 legs, to 1 leg, to 1 leg with motion of opposite leg.
- A popular version is the barbell hip thrust and variations.

> **OTHER VARIATIONS AND SIMILAR EXERCISES** Glute bridges on bench, SB/BOSU, bands, single-leg bridge (floor, MB, SB), straight-leg bridge, single-leg bridge with opposite leg motion, TRX bridge, barbell hip thrusts or on Smith machine.

Quadruped (Bird Dog)

Rating: A

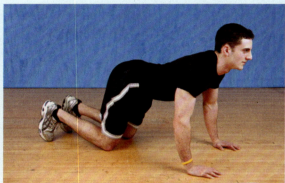
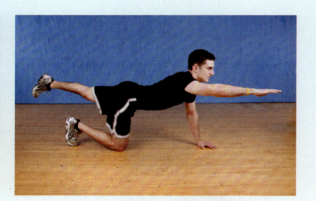

FIGURE 14.67 Quadruped (bird dog).

- The athlete assumes a prone position on all fours with hips and knees flexed, arms vertical to the ground, neutral spine, and torso near parallel to the floor (Fig. 14.67).
- Athlete extends the hip (with knee extended) so that it is aligned with the torso. The contralateral arm (shoulder) is flexed so it too is aligned with the torso. A simpler version entails the athlete either lift the leg only or the arm only. To make the exercise more difficult, an ISOM contraction (5–10 s) can be used at the top position.
- This corrective exercise stresses hip and spinal extensors and is performed most often without additional loading. Athletes should focus on contracting the gluteal muscles tightly.
- The arm and leg are returned to the starting position, and the opposite limbs are trained.

> **OTHER VARIATIONS AND SIMILAR EXERCISES** Quadruped with bent knees, superman (lying prone on the stomach) with both arms and legs extended, superman with ipsilateral arm/leg extension, and SB superman.

Kettlebell Figure 8s

Rating: A

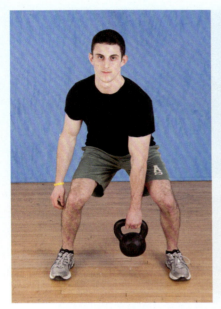
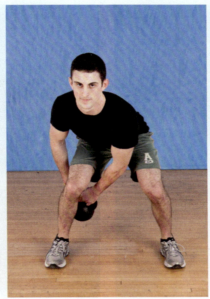
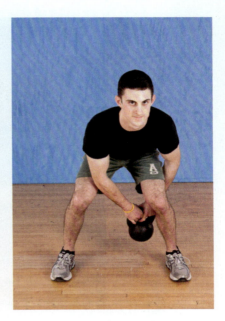

FIGURE 14.68 Kettlebell Figure 8s.

- Athlete bends forward with a flat back in a deadlift position and places KB between the legs with one arm extended (Fig. 14.68).
- KB is passed behind right leg in between the legs to left hand.
- KB is passed behind left leg in between the legs to right hand (forming a figure 8).
- Movements are repeated for the required repetition number.

Manual Resistance Neck (Four-Way)

Rating: A

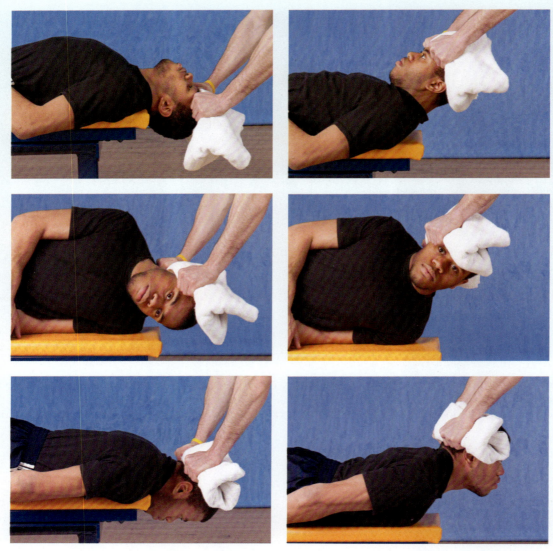

FIGURE 14.69 Manual resistance neck (four-way).

- Athlete begins on all fours or lies on a bench with the neck in the neutral position. A partner applies pressure to the head in four directions (Fig. 14.69).
- Athlete extends the neck against the manual resistance applied by the partner and returns to the starting position. Pressure is applied at multiple points to enable the athlete to laterally flex (right and left) and flex the neck against a resistance.

> **OTHER VARIATIONS AND SIMILAR EXERCISES** Four-way neck machine, neck flexion/extension/lateral flexion with head strap or harness, front/back bridges and rolls and band resistance during various movements.

Tire Flipping

Rating: C

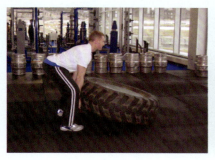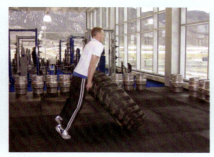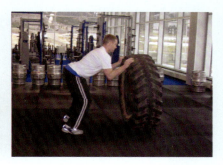

FIGURE 14.70 Tire flipping.

- Athlete begins in a four-point stance with knees and hip flexed using a tire that is at least two times the BW. The height of the tire while it is on the ground should come to approximately knee level (Fig. 14.70).
- Athlete drives the chest into the tire and pushes at ~45°. Hips drive forward using a triple extension (of hips, knees, and ankles) lifting the tire up on its side.
- Athlete jumps under the tire on its way up (rather than curling it!) and places the body in a proper position and extends the arms and continues pushing the tire forward until it flips onto its side. The movement is repeated.
- Other devices besides tires have been developed to be used in a similar manner.
- Tires have uses for other exercises as well.

> **OTHER VARIATIONS AND SIMILAR EXERCISES** Tire drags, *e.g.*, pulling or towing a tire during waling/running, backpedaling, or side shuffling, tire grappling. Drags can be performed with sand bags.

Farmer's Walk

Rating: B

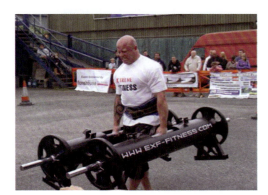

FIGURE 14.71 Farmer's walk.

- Athlete uses heavy DB, KB, plates, hex bar, or a sport-specific farmer's walk device, which enables plate loading of heavy weights (Fig. 14.71).
- Athlete properly bends over, grasps the bar, and lifts the weights into the standing position. Athlete then begins to walk rapidly or run a specified distance while supporting the load in the hands (this exercise is excellent for grip strength training).
- Athlete returns to the staring position and places the weights down on the ground.

> **VARIATIONS AND OTHER TYPES OF CARRIES/WALKS AND LOADING** Hex bar, overhead carries, unilateral carries, stone/sand bag/KB/log carries, team log carries, heavy bag carries, super yoke walks, and loaded treadmill walks.

Sled Push

Rating: B

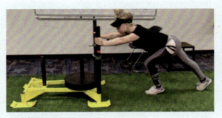

FIGURE 14.72 Sled push.

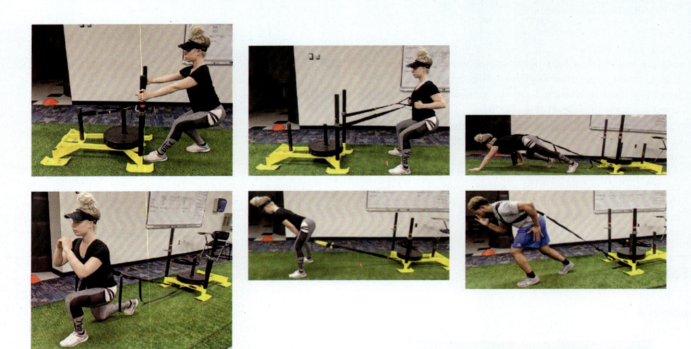

FIGURE 14.73 Sled push variations and similar exercises.

- The athlete assumes a bent-over position with hands placed at a high, moderate, or low position of the sled poles (Fig. 14.72).
- The athlete forcefully pushes the sled as hard or fast as possible until the desired length or time has been reached.
- The heavy sled push is excellent for increasing strength and providing a large metabolic challenge to the athlete.
- Sled drags with light weight are common to enhance speed training.
- Automobiles may also be used in lieu of sleds for heavy training.

OTHER VARIATIONS AND SIMILAR EXERCISES High/low positions, sled drag, sled pull, sled row, bear crawl, squat press, lunge walk, pull through, resisted sprint, duck walk, plank pull, overhead walk, rope pull, and rope drag (Fig. 14.73).

Other Exercises

Sledge Hammer

- The athlete begins by grasping the hammer with one hand above the bottom hand. The exercise becomes increasingly more difficult the farther down the hammer handle is held. The athlete may choose a heavier hammer or grasp the hammer low for strength training or use a lighter hammer or grasp it higher for speed training.
- The athlete assumes a staggered stance with one leg forward. For example, the left leg is forward if the athlete swings from the right side and vice versa.
- The hammer is quickly recoiled and swung as hard and fast as possible while striking the tire. High-rep sets, timed intervals, or time to complete reps may be used to designate an interval.
- **Other Variations and Similar Exercises:** Vertical, horizontal, or diagonal swings may be used. The sledge hammer may also be used as a lever bar for grip, forearm, and upper arm/shoulder training.

Mobility

A number of total body callisthenic or mobility exercises may be performed, some of which have already been described. Often, these are performed using bodyweight but external resistance (*e.g.*, DBs, KBs, weighted vest, bands) may be used for some of the exercises. Some popular mobility exercises include the burpee (which has many variations), jumping jack, duck walk, cartwheel, duck under, hip heist, and front and back shoulder rolls

Gymnastics

Although gymnastics exercises are some of the most difficult exercises to perform, variation or progressions have been increased in popularity given the excellent benefits they provide the athlete in regard to strength, power, balance, coordination, and endurance. Some gymnastic exercises increasing in popularity in strength and conditioning programs include handstands and handstand push-ups, L-hangs or holds, planche progressions, frog stands, front/back levers, and ring exercises such as the iron cross and skin the cat.

Rope/Battling Rope Exercises

Ropes may be used for climbing, pulling, and for oscillation training. Battling ropes are used for wave training to increase strength, endurance, and provide potent metabolic and cardiovascular responses. Waves are generated via multiple movement patterns as the ropes are anchored at a low fixed point. The length and diameter of the ropes and the velocity and amplitude of waves govern the perceived effort and intensity. A large number of exercises can be performed while many can be performed when using different postures (standing, seated, kneeling, lunge, side lunge, plank/side plank, and squatting) and integrated with plyometric and agility drills, *e.g.*, hops, jumps, shuffles. Figure 14.74 and the online appendix depict rope climbing and several popular battling ropes exercises commonly performed in S&C programs including single-arm waves, double-arm waves, double-arm slams, side-to-side waves, grappler hip toss, plank waves, outer and inner circles, snakes (ins and outs), drum solo, Ultimate Warrior shakes, Tsunami, upper cuts, diagonal chops, jumping jacks, and burpees.

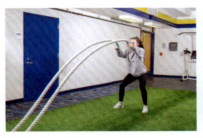
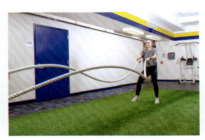
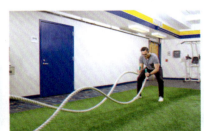
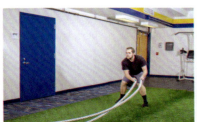
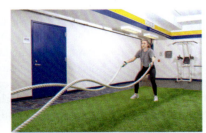
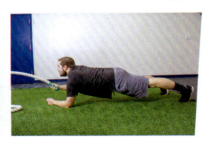

FIGURE 14.74 Battling rope exercises.

> ## Myths & Misconceptions
> ### Several RT Exercises Should Be Totally Avoided in All Circumstances Because They Cause Injury
>
> Some in the sports and fitness industry have painted with a broad brush in labeling some resistance exercises as inappropriate for everyone regardless of training goals or personal situations. Some common exercises criticized are, *e.g.*, the sit-up, BB squat, behind-the-neck press/pull-down, Olympic lifts, and full ROM bench press. These exercises have been touted as injurious to the lower back, knees, and shoulders. All exercises stress joints to induce adaptations. However, distress to joints is to be avoided, but this concern is multifactorial. As Dr. Stuart McGill has stated, "there is no such thing as a safe or dangerous exercise — only an ill-prescribed exercise for an individual." Exercises are not injurious provided the athlete has no preexisting condition and performs the exercises properly. Some exercises will not cause injury but could exacerbate an injury if one has a predisposition. Performing a sit-up for someone with low-back pain is contraindicated. However, a healthy individual can benefit from the sit-up. When exercises do pose a risk of injury, many times it is related to improper technique or loading and not the exercise per se. The choice to include or exclude an exercise in an RT program should be made on an individual basis and not because of misinformation.

Combination Exercises

Combination exercises involve combining two exercises into one. Several exercises can be combined into one. Combination exercises increase the complexity and metabolic responses to resistance exercise. Weight is selected based on the weaker of the two (or three) exercises used. The following table lists some common combination exercises used in RT.

- DB push-up with unilateral row (or T rotation)
- Lunge with torso twist (or shoulder press, lateral raise, curl)
- Clean, front squat, and push press (thruster)
- SB push-up with prone knee-ups
- Step-ups with bicep curl, lateral raise, or shoulder press
- BB pullover and press
- Hyperextension with trunk rotation (or shoulder press, lateral raise)
- DB squat with overhead shoulder press, rotation press, or press out
- Pull-up (or dip) with knee raise or leg scissor
- T-shoulder raises (lateral to front raise)
- Side plank with lateral raise (or hip abduction)

Grip Strength Training

Grip strength has long been recognized as an important component of muscular fitness and performance in sports like strength competitions, weightlifting, powerlifting, wrestling, football, climbing, and gymnastics. Forearm and hand flexor muscles are the primary muscles involved in gripping whereas the wrist extensors provide stability. Grip strength training involves free weight, machine, and cables/bands wrist flexion/extension exercises, various hand gripping devices, radial/ulnar deviation and circumduction with specific devices, finger flexion/extension, abduction and adduction (pinching) exercises, thick bars, and through performance of pulling exercises without the use of ergogenic aids such as lifting straps.

Gripping Exercises: Power gripping (with ball or gripping devices), ISOM BB, KB, sand bag, or DB grip holds, pinch gripping (with weights), power web finger flexion, machine gripping, lever bar wrist rotations, ISOM bar support, thick bar pulling exercises, climbing board hangs, towel exercises, bar grips (thick), and push-ups (on finger tips, fists, or back of hands).

Olympic Lifts and Variations

The Clean, Snatch (Full, Power: From Floor, Above Knee, Below Knee) ("C" Rating)

The Olympic lifts and variations are total-body lifts that recruit most major muscle groups and are the most complex exercises to perform. They are regarded as the most effective exercises for increasing muscle power, as they require fast force production and Olympic weightlifters generate high degrees of power (13). Critical to performance is the quality of effort per repetition (maximal velocity). The clean and jerk (Fig. 14.75 shows the clean) is a two-staged exercise and can result in greater weights being lifted compared to the single-staged snatch (Fig. 14.76). Both lifts require explosive movements of the lower body and trunk, whereas the arms serve as guides and play a secondary role preparing the body to catch the bar. Variations are partial exercises of the full version that can be used to enhance specific performance aspects of the complete lift or for basic strength and power enhancement. For example, full cleans and snatches require the athlete to squat during the catching of the weight. Power cleans and snatches require the athlete to catch the weight in a more vertical position. The bar needs to be pulled a greater distance because of the higher receiving position. These variations are more commonly used among athletes who are not Olympic weightlifters. Other variations (called **transfer exercises**) are described.

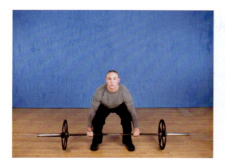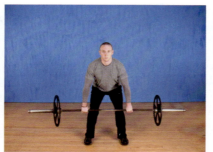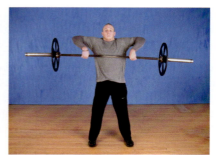
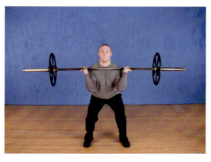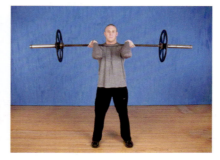

FIGURE 14.75 The clean: beginning, first pull, transition, second pull, and catch positions.

Coaches teach each of these lifts in progressions starting with the clean, the jerk, and later the snatch. Learning the technical aspects of the clean initially assists in the transition to learning the snatch. The following sequences are effective for teaching the Olympic lifts in progression:

Clean: front squat → Romanian deadlift (RDL) → clean pull (mid-thigh, below knee, floor) → high pull → stop or hang cleans (mid-thigh, below knee, floor) → full clean

Front squats help teach the rack position for the catch and squatting technique. The RDL teaches proper hip hinge position during the pull phases. The clean pulls teach proper motion during the pulls and help reinforce the proper sequencing of joint actions of transferring power from the feet to the upper extremities. High pulls assist with developing good pull technique and power. Progressing to the hang or stop clean variations add the ability to learn the turnover and catch to the exercise prior to putting it all together with the full clean.

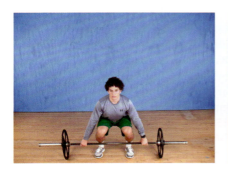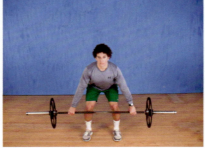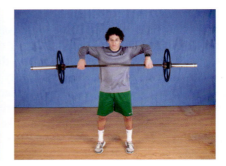
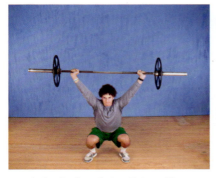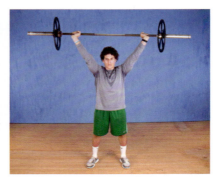

FIGURE 14.76 The snatch: beginning, first pull, transition, second pull, catch, and overhead squat positions.

Jerk: Press behind-the-neck → push press → power jerk → same exercises in the front → the split (footwork) → the jerk

The behind-the-neck position is trained first due to more direct line of bar movement for jerk and better vertical trunk position. The press builds strength. The push press helps teach lower body contribution to pressing. The jerk helps teach the "dive under" and proper overhead bar position. The split helps work on proper footwork ultimately leading to performing the entire jerk exercise.

Snatch: Behind-the-neck press (snatch grip) → overhead squat → drop snatch → heaving drop snatch → snatch RDL → snatch pulls (mid-thigh, below knee, floor) → hang or stop snatch (mid-thigh, below knee, floor) → full snatch

The first exercise teaches proper proprioception of the bar in the overhead position. The second exercise builds upon the first by teaching the athlete to descend/ascend (squat) with the bar in the overhead position. The third exercise builds upon the first two by having the athlete drop into the overhead squat position rather than starting with it and shifting the feet. All three exercises build strength and confidence in the athlete to help prepare for further progressions. The RDL assists with proper hip hinge during pulling. The pulls teach proper motion during pulling and the coordination between joints to transfer power from the feet upward. The hang and stop cleans progress to teaching the athlete to turnover and catch the weight overhead and then putting it all together finally when performing the full snatch.

Ideally, these exercises should be performed on a wooden lifting platform with bumper plates that can easily be dropped without causing damage. Although excessive dropping or throwing of weights is not recommended, the athlete is properly taught to drop the weights when learning the Olympic lifts. This increases safety as there is a greater chance for injury to occur if the bar is not properly dropped on the platform. It is important that the platform remain clear so no ricochet of bar takes place when dropped. If possible, the athlete should attempt to lower his or her center of gravity (COG) as much as possible before releasing the bar. This means the bar will be dropped from a lesser height, which helps preserve equipment as well as ensure safety. The athlete must keep all body segments behind the falling bar and should use hands (on top of bar) to guide bar downward and minimize rebounding.

For the power clean and snatch, similar phases have been identified. These phases include the starting position, the first pull (BB is pulled from the floor), a transition phase prior to the second pull, the second pull, the catch, and the finish typically performed within 1 second. The duration of the lift and muscle power depends upon the loading, size, and skill level of the athletes (14). Critical here is the displacement of the bar and this is highly related to maximum vertical bar velocity (15). Taller athletes need to move the bar a greater distance with higher velocities. One differentiating factor between skilled and lesser-skilled weightlifters is the timing of the phases especially from the transition to the second pull (14).

The Starting Position

The starting position for each lift will vary in some respects but be similar in others. The feet are placed approximately at hip width (similar to a vertical jump position), toes pointed slightly outward, and the bar is located on the floor near (or touching) the shins. The hips and trunk are flexed forming an angle of 25°–50° with the ground, with the hips positioned close to or slightly above the knees (16). The trunk is more upright (larger angle) and hips are higher during the clean because of the narrower grip (using a hook grip) width compared to the snatch. The higher hip position allows heavier loads to be lifted compared to the lower hip position (and less weight) seen with the snatch. Shoulders are positioned directly over or slightly in front of the bar with the body's COG located over the middle of the foot. The low back is kept flat by hyperextending the lumbar spine and retracting the shoulder girdle (sticking the chest out). The head is straight or slightly upward and the arms grasp the bar with elbows extended and out and wrists are flexed. Rotating the elbows outward assists the athlete in maintaining proper bar displacement and keeping the elbow straight throughout pulling. A wide grip width is used for the snatch and a shoulder width grip is used for the clean. For the hang clean or hang snatch, the bar begins either above or below the knee depending on the variation. The stop clean or snatch involves beginning in an upright position, descending to the starting position, and beginning the lift.

First Pull

During the first pull, the bar is pulled toward the body (4–12 cm for the snatch; 3–10 cm for the clean) and is lifted off of the ground to about 31% of the athlete's height for the clean and ~35% for the snatch (16). The first pull is produced mostly by knee extension (~35°–50°) and plantar flexion (to where shins are vertical) with little change in the trunk angle (remains ~30°–32°), and the COG shifts toward the heels. Trunk angle may slightly increase by the end of this phase and elbows remain extended. Shoulders move in front of the bar. This phase typically begins at a knee angle between 80° and 110° but reaches an angle of 145°–155° by conclusion (16). The angle tends to be higher when performing the snatch compared to the clean. In skilled weightlifters observed during competition performing maximal attempts, a rise in force, vertical and horizontal (anterior to posterior) bar velocity, and bar acceleration is seen as the BB is lifted off the floor during this phase (13,15,17). Generally, this phase lasts ~0.50 second and the bar is lifted ~1.5 m·s^{-1} for the snatch and ~1.2 m·s^{-1} for the clean (16).

Transition Phase

The transition (or adjustment) phase is characterized by unweighting, or a reduction in force applied to the ground with a negative bar acceleration and slower vertical bar velocity (despite upward movement of the bar) (13,17,18). Approximately 10° or more of knee flexion is seen (*double knee bend*) with a concomitant increase in trunk extension of 35°–40° (17). Knees may reach an angle range of 125°–135°. The bar reaches the lower third of the thigh for the clean and middle of the thigh for the snatch. Although force applied to the ground and bar acceleration decrease during the transition phase, this phase is critical to optimal lifting technique and performance. Postural realignment occurs, which reduces the back and hip extensor moment arms of resistance; an stretch-shortening cycle (SSC) enhancement is included due to the countermovement; and realignment allows for a second pull with a more vertical torso posture in the strongest area of the ROM, which allows for greater force and power yielding greater bar displacement (17).

Second Pull

The second pull is the most explosive phase and takes ~0.1–0.25 second with the snatch requiring more time than the clean (16). Bar is pulled upward and slightly away from the body by powerful extension of the hip, knee, and ankle joints. A rise in force, bar acceleration, and peak vertical and horizontal bar velocity is seen during the second pull (13,15,17,18). Analyses of Olympic weightlifters show power production is much higher during the second pull than the first pull (19). The second pull poses similar kinetic characteristics to a vertical jump (20). Up to 94% of the work done by a weightlifter is completed by the time the bar reaches peak velocity (19). The bar is pulled slightly away from the athlete and COG shifts toward the toes. Garhammer (13) showed bar velocities during the pull for the snatch compared to the clean tend to be ~10%–20% higher, as the bar is lifted to ~60% of the athlete's stature (18). During competition, bar velocities during the pulling phases are ~1.8–2.1 m·s^{-1} (13,15). Others have reported second pull bar velocities of 1.65–2.05 m·s^{-1} for the snatch and 1.2–1.6 m·s^{-1} for the clean (16). Force applied to the bar decreases at the top of the second pull as the athlete prepares to pull him/her under the bar for the catch. At no time during the pull are the elbows bent.

The Catch

The next phase entails the athletes positioning themselves under the bar for the catch. The bar is still rising in both lifts when the athlete pulls himself or herself underneath during the catch position. The athlete does not pull to max height and then descend underneath. Rather, they occur almost simultaneously (16). The bar reaches ~68%–78% of height for the snatch and 55%–65% of height for the clean. After the second pull, the athlete's feet leave the ground and move laterally into the receiving position. The arms are used to pull the body down under the bar. Optimal bar trajectory entails pulling the bar toward the body during the first pull, moving the bar slightly away from the body during the second pull, and moving the bar closer to the body as the athlete prepares for the catch (resembling an S-shaped pattern of motion) (13,15,18).

The receiving positions for both lifts are critical to optimal performance. For the snatch, after the second pull the feet move out into a squatting position (wider than hip width). The slightly wider stance facilitates stability and brings the hips over the feet. While the feet are moving, the arms pull on the bar, thereby accelerating the athlete's ability to descend under the bar (the athlete facilitates descent and does not merely drop under the bar). Elbows are wide, trunk is upright, wrists turn over, and the bar rotates. Throughout the descent, the athlete applies force to the bar to support the weight in the full squat position. Lastly, the athlete flexes the shoulders, pushes the head forward, and extends hips into an overhead squat finish.

For the clean, similar lower-body movement is seen (feet move out into a squat position). The athlete pulls himself or herself down forcefully and receives the bar at the shoulder position in a lower position than the snatch because the heavier bar is not lifted as high during the second pull. During foot landing, the wrists rotate around the bar, elbows push forward and upward creating a shelf to catch the weight. The bar is caught on the shoulders and chest and the loading forces the athlete down into a deeper front squat position. Upper arms should be parallel to the ground, knees are over feet, and the athlete completes the lift by performing a front squat.

> **⊕ VARIATIONS AND OTHER EXERCISES** DB or KB snatch (above or below knee, from floor), single-leg DB snatch, one-arm snatch (BB, DB, or KB), pressing snatch balance, drop snatch, DB or KB power clean, squat power clean, hang clean (below or above knee), stop clean and stop snatch, DB or KB hang clean, single-leg DB or KB hang clean, KB anchored and alternating clean, KB cross-over clean/snatch, KB bottom's up clean/snatch, squat hang clean, keg cleans/snatch, keg toss, seated SB/bench cleans/snatches, and log cleans.

Interpreting Research
Kinematic Analysis of the Snatch

Gourgoulis V, Aggelousis N, Mavromatis G, Garas A. Three-dimensional kinematic analysis of the snatch of elite Greek weightlifters. *J Sport Sci.* 2000;18:643–52.

Gourgoulis et al. (21) performed a kinematic analysis of the snatch in elite Greek Olympic weightlifters and reported the following:

◆ Knee angles of ~143° (following first pull), ~120° (following transition), and ~156° (following second pull)
◆ Max ankle and hip extension values of 117° and 177°, respectively
◆ Knee extension angular velocity (first pull = ~3.86 rad·s^{-1}; second pull = ~6.32 rad·s^{-1})
◆ Ankle extension angular velocity (first pull = ~1.51 rad·s^{-1}; second pull = ~4.35 rad·s^{-1})

- Hip extension angular velocity (first pull = ~2.81 rad·s^{-1}; second pull = ~8.09 rad·s^{-1})
- Bar displacement (toward lifter = ~6.2 cm; away from lifter = ~3.2 cm)
- Maximal vertical velocity of BB = ~1.67 m·s^{-1}
- Decrease in bar velocity during transition = ~0.05 m·s^{-1}
- Work (first pull = ~612 J; second pull = 413 J)
- Power (first pull = ~1,302 W; second pull = ~2,577 W)
- Phase duration (first pull = ~0.47 s; transition = ~0.15 s; second pull = ~0.16 s; turnover under bar = ~0.23 s)

Hook Grip

To optimally perform the Olympic lifting pulling movements, a strong grip is necessary. Isometric grip strength training is important. Most athletes prefer to use the hook grip. The hook grip (Fig. 14.77) entails wrapping the thumb around the bar and then wrapping the first three fingers around the thumb and bar. This grip configuration allows for greater support during explosive pulling movements. Because the thumb is relatively weak compared to flexion strength of the fingers as a whole, wrapping the thumb around the bar puts the thumb in a better force-producing position as it can then be supported by the flexion strength of most of the fingers. As flexion strength of the fingers and thumb increase, so does the magnitude of friction between the hand and the bar (static friction force = coefficient of static friction × reactive force). Because of the position of the thumb and the greater static friction observed with the hook grip, pain and discomfort are common in athletes accommodating to the hook grip. Bruising can occur, as well as skin irritations from the knurling of the bar when high levels of pressure are applied. Adaptations take place and eventually the discomfort subsides to where the athlete becomes comfortable. Many athletes release the hook grip (in lieu of a normal grip) when the hands rotate to where the palms are facing up (catch in the pull or preparation for the jerk).

Determining Snatch Grip Width

There are two basic ways to estimate proper grip width for the snatch. One method is to have the athlete stand and abduct one arm laterally (parallel to the ground) to the side while making a fist. A tape measure is used to measure the length of the opposite shoulder to the fist. This length is used as the grip width. A second method entails the athlete standing and abducting both arms laterally (parallel to the ground) to the side with elbows flexed. A tape measure is used to determine the length from elbow to elbow as the snatch grip width. Some have recommended using a grip wide enough so that a 49°–63° angle is observed between the arms and the bar or have suggested a position to where the bar comfortably lies in the crease of the hips when trunk/hips are flexed forward with arms fully extended (16). These methods provide a good estimate or at least the starting grip width that can be altered slightly based on technical aspects of the athlete, *e.g.*, shoulder flexibility and strength, elbow joint stability, and pulling mechanics. A good way to assess the grip width is to examine the overhead squat position. The bar should be ~4–6 in. above the head (depending on the comfort level).

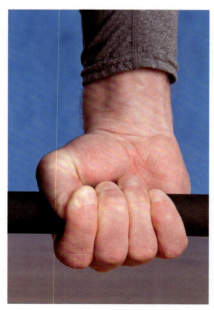

FIGURE 14.77 Hook grip.

Case Study 14.1

Steve is a recent college graduate with a degree in Health and Exercise Science and a concentration in Strength and Conditioning. He was hired by a Division III college and was put in charge of strength and conditioning for the school's football team. As part of his lifting program, Steve required all athletes to perform the power clean because of its utility for power and performance enhancement. However, several incoming freshmen have no experience with Olympic lifting. As a student (and athlete), Steve was properly instructed to teach the power clean in stages (using variations) rather than the complete lift. Thus, Steve grouped these athletes together and began instructional sessions to teach proper technique.

Question for Consideration: If you were Steve, what progressions would you use in order to teach this exercise to this group of athletes?

The Jerk

The jerk is a critical component to Olympic weightlifting (Fig. 14.78). The majority of missed attempts in competition in the clean and jerk result from a missed jerk. The jerk can be described in several phases: the starting position, descent (or half squat or dip), braking, thrust, and split and finish. The athlete starts in the top-front squat position where the hips and shoulders are aligned over the rear segment of the middle of the foot, feet are hip width with toes slightly pointed outward, head slightly back, and arms are relaxed (near parallel to the floor) with elbows in front of the bar as the bar rests in the shelf position. Tensing the arms could result in the athlete pushing the bar forward instead of vertical. The descent or dip provides a countermovement before the explosive thrust of the bar upward. Knee flexion (~114°–132°) and ankle dorsiflexion occur in a vertical manner with COG shifting slightly forward (16). Maximum velocities range within 0.8–1.2 $m \cdot s^{-1}$ with peak velocity occurring halfway through the ROM of the dip with a duration of 0.20–0.25 seconds (22). The end of the dip marks the beginning of the braking phase, which takes ~0.12 seconds, and involves further descent equaling a magnitude of one-third of the overall countermovement depth (16). This phase provides a transition between slowing down the countermovement and subsequent beginning of the thrust. The end of this phase is marked by completely stopped downward movement of the bar. Elite weightlifters squat to ~12%–14% of their standing height to knee angles of ~99°–110°, spend less time braking toward the bottom of the dip than lesser-skilled individuals, and elite weightlifters tend to show horizontal bar displacements of <2 cm compared to lesser-skilled lifters (22).

The thrust encompasses explosive extension of the hips, knees, and ankles driving the bar upward while rising on the toes. Bar velocity ranges between 1.2 and 1.8 $m \cdot s^{-1}$ (16,22). Grabe and Widule (22) showed that the thrust was characterized by peak hip velocities of 4.5–5.0 $rad \cdot s^{-1}$, peak bar velocities of 1.2–1.4 $m \cdot s^{-1}$, max knee angles of 145°–154°, and performed for 0.22–0.28 seconds. Peak vertical bar velocity allows the bar to reach near its maximal height. The remaining bar elevation is brought about by forceful pushing up on the bar from the arms in order to assist in diving under the bar for the split. Most athletes tend to split when performing the jerk; however, some prefer to use the squat position when diving under the bar. For the split, one hip flexes (front leg) and one extends (back leg) to form a stable base support. The back leg lands before the front leg as the feet leave the ground. The split has been characterized by a duration of 0.20–0.28 seconds and max split velocity of 1.6–2.6 $m \cdot s^{-1}$ (front = 1.6–1.8 $m \cdot s^{-1}$; rear = 2.2–2.6 $m \cdot s^{-1}$) (22). The back leg is nearly straight (a little more than 2-ft length posterior from the hip) with a knee angle of ~160° with foot balanced on the toes. The front leg has a knee angle of >90° with shin perpendicular to the floor and is located ~1-ft length in front of the hip. The bar is positioned slightly behind the athlete's head on the same vertical plane as the shoulders and hips. Head is forward, and back is hyperextended. Bar trajectory for the jerk is nearly vertical for the decent and vertical with slight backward movement during the thrust and catch. For the finish, weight is transferred to the rear foot as the front leg pushes backward.

> **OTHER VARIATIONS AND SIMILAR EXERCISES** Power jerk, behind-the neck jerk (clean and snatch grip), and KB/keg/sandbag/DB jerk.

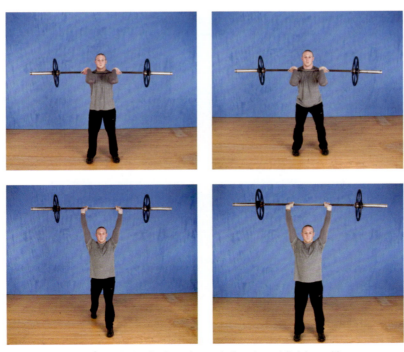

FIGURE 14.78 The jerk: beginning, descent, thrust, and finish positions.

Variations of the Olympic Lifts

Snatch/Clean High Pull

Rating: B

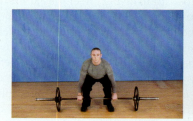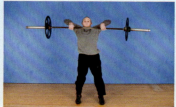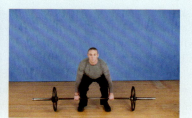

FIGURE 14.79 Snatch/clean high pull.

- Starting position is similar to the snatch (wide grip) or clean (narrow grip). Bar rests on the floor or above/below the knees or on the thigh for high pulls from the hang position (Fig. 14.79).
- With torso erect and elbows fully extended, the bar is explosively lifted upward by extending the hip, knee, and ankle joints. Shoulders remain over the bar for as long as possible while keeping the bar close to the body.
- At maximal plantar flexion, the shoulders are elevated and the bar is pulled high.
- Bar is returned to the starting position or safely released to platform.

- This version is less complex as the athlete does not have to descend under the bar and catch the weight. It is an excellent version to teach athletes new to weightlifting. It can be used to train for power as it is performed explosively with less complexity.

> **OTHER VARIATIONS AND SIMILAR EXERCISES** DB or KB high pull (from floor or hang position), single-leg DB or KB high pull, snatch pull (to knee), and snatch/clean shrugs.

Behind-The-Neck Press (Snatch and Clean Grip)

Rating: B

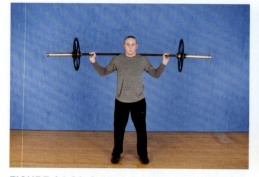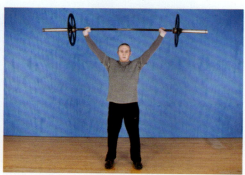

FIGURE 14.80 Behind-the-neck press (snatch and clean grip).

- Athlete assumes a position similar to the back squat with bar resting across the shoulders behind the head. Either a snatch grip or clean grip can be used. Feet are shoulder width or slightly wider apart (Fig. 14.80).

- The bar is pressed upward via shoulder abduction and elbow extension and returned back to the starting position. Wrists should be hyperextended at top of the movement.
- This exercise helps the athlete learn proper overhead position of the bar.

Drop Snatch

Rating: C

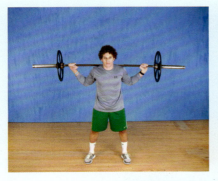
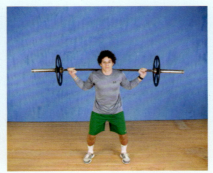
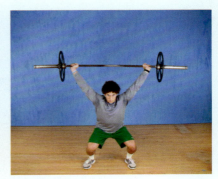
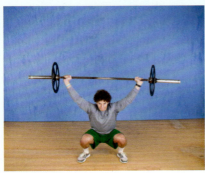
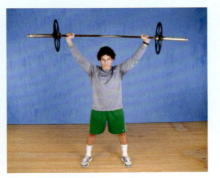

FIGURE 14.81 Drop snatch.

- Athlete begins in a back squat position (bar on shoulders) with a snatch grip and feet hip width apart (Fig. 14.81).
- Athlete dips and drives the bar upward, then jumps feet into the normal squat foot width position and drops as quickly as possible into the low receiving snatch position. Athlete should push up on the bar while dropping; the result is to push the body down into position rather than lifting the bar upward.
- The ascent is synonymous with an overhead squat.
- A common mistake is to press first then drop under. The bar moves very little upward when performed correctly.
- Some variations include the pressing drop snatch and the heaving drop snatch.

Romanian Deadlift

Rating: A

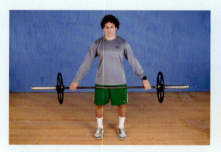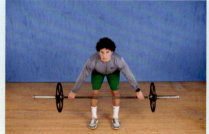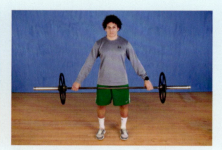

FIGURE 14.82 Romanian deadlift.

- Athlete starts with a snatch grip or clean grip with the bar at hip level. Knees are slightly bent, elbows are extended, chest is out, and back is hyperextended (Fig. 14.82).
- The bar moves downward close to the thigh to a position below the level of the knees. This is brought about by hip/trunk flexion with slight flexion of the knees.
- The bar is lifted back up to the starting position via hip, trunk, knee, and ankle extension.
- This exercise is useful for learning the proper position during pulling movements.

Front Squat

Rating: B

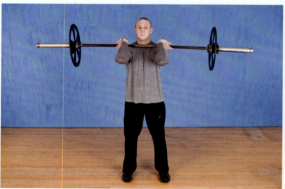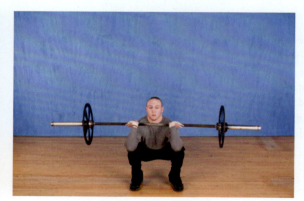

FIGURE 14.83 Front squat.

- Athlete unracks the bar in the shelf or rack position with the bar resting comfortably on upper chest and shoulders, elbows up and in, chest out and lower back hyperextended, wrists relaxed and hyperextended, and feet shoulder width apart (Fig. 14.83).
- Athlete descends to the parallel position (or lower) by flexing the hips, knees, and ankles and maintains an erect torso to keep the bar placed in the proper position.
- Athlete ascends by extending the hips, knees, and ankles while keeping the posture erect.
- Excellent for developing strength and balance and serves as a beneficial transfer exercise for the clean. Common mistakes include shifting weight forward, leaning forward excessively, and tightening wrists/arms to lose rack position.

Overhead Squat

Rating: B

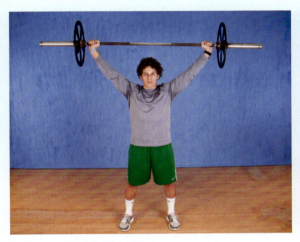 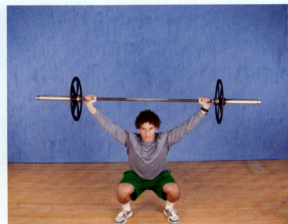

FIGURE 14.84 Overhead squat.

- Athlete grasps BB with a snatch width grip behind the neck and presses it into the overhead snatch position. Shoulders are flexed, elbows are fully extended, the chest is out, low back is hyperextended, and the head is forward. Feet are shoulder width or slightly wider (Fig. 14.84).
- Athlete descends to the parallel position (or lower) by flexing the hips, knees, and ankles and maintains an erect torso with the bar maintained in the overhead position.
- Athlete ascends by extending the hips, knees, and ankles while keeping the posture erect. Some common mistakes are heels coming off of the platform (due to not positioning hips properly during descent possibly due to poor shoulder flexibility), forward movement of the bar, bending the elbows, and excessive forward lean.

> **OTHER VARIATIONS AND SIMILAR EXERCISES** Overhead split squat; can be performed with kegs, DB, KB, and sand bags.

Push Press

Rating: B

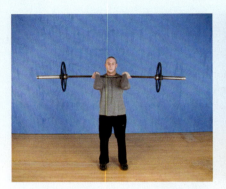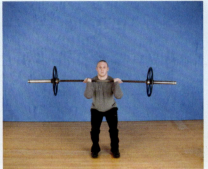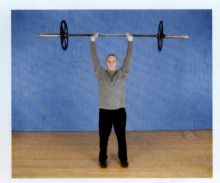

FIGURE 14.85 Push press.

- Bar is grasped with a closed, pronated grip slightly wider than or at shoulder width at the level of shoulders. Elbows are out (arm parallel to the ground) and wrists extended. Feet are slightly wider than shoulder width, and hips and knees are slightly flexed (Fig. 14.85).
- A countermovement (dip) is performed followed by an explosive push of the bar upward by extending the knees, hips, and ankles. BW is shifted to the balls of the feet and the foot is plantar flexed. The bar is pushed from shoulder level until elbows are fully extended overhead.
- Bar is lowered to the starting position, and hips and knees are flexed to absorb the weight of bar.

> **OTHER VARIATIONS AND SIMILAR EXERCISES** DB or KB push press, behind-the-neck push press (clean and snatch grip), keg/sand bag push press, and mastiff bar push press.

 ## Tips for Selecting Exercises

Some general tips for selecting/performing exercises include

1. *Build a base on good technique* — regardless of the exercise; the athlete should have attained good technique prior to progression to heavier weights or more challenging exercises.
2. *Start with basic exercises and progress to more challenging exercises* — the athlete or coach should select some basic exercises to begin and progress to more challenging exercises over time as conditioning improves.
3. *Select exercises that work all major muscle groups* — all major muscle groups should be targeted during RT.
4. *Challenging exercises yield the best results* — in many cases, the exercises that are more difficult and stress several major muscle groups yield better performance results. These core and structural exercises should form the base of the training program. For example, multijoint exercises such as the squat and bench press form the core of many RT programs targeting maximal strength. The Olympic lifts should form the core for power training. The exceptions would be corrective exercises that target susceptible muscle groups for imbalance.
5. *Vary exercises regularly* — exposing the athlete to many exercises can be used as a successful conditioning tool. Over time, coaches can determine which ones work better for certain athletes. Although the coach may have a staple of exercises that form the core of the program, assistance exercises can be varied regularly (every 4–6 wk).

Chapter 14 Resistance Training Exercises   **445**

SUMMARY POINTS

◆ Proper breathing for most exercises entails inhaling during the negative phase and exhaling during the positive phase. There are exceptions where a Valsalva maneuver is beneficial to increasing IAP for exercises that stress the lower back or are explosive.

◆ Joint motion occurs in sagittal, frontal, and transverse planes. Several exercises are multiplanar where motion takes place in two or three planes.

◆ Resistance exercises may be performed using BW, BBs, DBs, SBs, BOSU balls, MBs, thick bars, KBs, bands/tubing, kegs, sand bags, tires, logs, and other implements.

◆ Any alteration of posture, hand/foot width, and hand/foot position changes muscle activation so each exercise variation is treated as a distinct exercise.

◆ A multitude of lower-body, upper-body, and core resistance exercises can be performed so variation in exercise selection can add new dimensions to RT workouts.

◆ The Olympic lifts and variations are the most complex exercises. Because of their reliance on most major muscle groups, the Olympic lifts are performed at explosive velocities and are excellent for increasing total body strength and power.

REVIEW QUESTIONS

1. From the anatomical position, a standing lateral raise (abduction) is performed in
   a. The sagittal plane
   b. The frontal plane
   c. The transverse plane
   d. No plane

2. When performing the squat exercise, the athlete
   a. Should lean forward as far as possible during the descent
   b. Should keep his/her head down facing the ground during each phase
   c. Should drive the hips back so the knees and toes are level during the descent
   d. Should hold his/her breath from start to completion of the set

3. The greatest amount of power produced in the power clean and snatch occurs during the
   a. First pull
   b. Transition phase
   c. Second pull
   d. Catch

4. Which of the following exercises specifically targets the erector spinae muscle group?
   a. Hyperextension
   b. Leg curl
   c. DB fly
   d. Crunch

5. Adding a rotation to a crunch exercise increases the activity of which muscle?
   a. Biceps femoris
   b. Gastrocnemius
   c. Pectoralis major
   d. External oblique

6. The push-up can be made more challenging to shoulder and trunk muscles by performing which exercise?
   a. With one leg abducted and elevated off of the ground
   b. With staggered hands
   c. On an SB
   d. All of the above

7. Using a thick bar during a pulling exercise (deadlift) is a good way to increase grip strength.
   a. T
   b. F

8. The conventional deadlift requires the athlete to keep the arms inside the legs while using a wide stance.
   a. T
   b. F

9. One method used to determine snatch grip width is to have the athlete stand and abduct one arm laterally and measure the length of the opposite shoulder to the fist with a tape measure.
   a. T
   b. F

10. The hyperextension exercise primarily works the quadriceps muscles.
    a. T
    b. F

11. Internal/external rotation shoulder exercises are good for athletes involved in throwing sports.
    a. T
    b. F

12. The bar velocity for the second pull in the snatch is higher than the clean.
    a. T
    b. F

REFERENCES

1. Hackett DA, Chow CM. The Valsalva maneuver: its effect on intra-abdominal pressure and safety issues during resistance exercise. *J Strength Cond Res.* 2013;27:2338–45.

2. Zeller BL, McCrory JL, Kibler WB, Uhl TL. Differences in kinematics and electromyographic activity between men and women during the single-legged squat. *Am J Sports Med.* 2003;31:449–56.

3. Escamilla RF, Fleisig GS, Lowry TM, Barrentine SW, Andrews JR. A three-dimensional biomechanical analysis of the squat during varying stance widths. *Med Sci Sports Exerc.* 2001;33:984–98.

4. Cholewicki J, McGill SM, Norman RW. Lumbar spine loads during the lifting of extremely heavy weights. *Med Sci Sports Exerc.* 1991;23:1179–86.

5. Escamilla RF, Francisco AC, Fleisig GS, et al. A three-dimensional biomechanical analysis of sumo and conventional style deadlifts. *Med Sci Sports Exerc.* 2000;32:1265–75.

6. Escamilla RF, Francisco AC, Kayes AV, Speer KP, Moorman CT. An electromyographic analysis of sumo and conventional style deadlifts. *Med Sci Sports Exerc.* 2002;34:682–8.

7. Gallucci JG, Challis JH. Examining the role of the gastrocnemius during the leg curl exercise. *J Appl Biomech.* 2002;18:15–27.

8. Barnett C, Kippers V, Turner P. Effects of variations of the bench press exercise on the EMG activity of five shoulder muscles. *J Strength Cond Res.* 1995;9:222–7.

9. Signorile JF, Zink AJ, Szwed SP. A comparative electromyographical investigation of muscle utilization patterns using various hand positions during the lat pull-down. *J Strength Cond Res.* 2002;16:539–46.

10. Urquhart DM, Hodges PW, Allen TJ, Story IH. Abdominal muscle recruitment during a range of voluntary exercises. *Man Ther.* 2005;10:144–53.

11. Boyle M. *Functional Training for Sports.* Champaign (IL): Human Kinetics; 2004.

12. Vera-Garcia FJ, Elvira JL, Brown SH, McGill SM. Effects of abdominal stabilization maneuvers on the control of spine motion and stability against sudden trunk perturbations. *J Electromyogr Kinesiol.* 2007;17:556–67.

13. Garhammer J. Biomechanical profiles of Olympic weightlifters. *J Appl Biomech.* 1985;1:122–30.

14. Enoka R. Load-and skill-related changes in segmental contributions to a weightlifting movement. *Med Sci Sports Exerc.* 1988;20:178–87.

15. Isaka T, Okada J, Funato K. Kinematic analysis of the barbell during the snatch movement of elite Asian weight lifters. *J Appl Biomech.* 1996;12:508–16.

16. Drechsler A. The *Weightlifting Encyclopedia: A Guide to World Class Performance.* Whitestone (NY): A is A Communications; 1998.

17. Enoka R. The pull in Olympic weightlifting. *Med Sci Sports.* 1979;11:131–7.

18. Baumann W, Gross V, Quade K, Galbierz P, Schwirtz A. The snatch technique of world class weightlifters at the 1985 world championships. *J Appl Biomech.* 1988;4:68–89.

19. Garhammer J. Power production by Olympic weightlifters. *Med Sci Sports Exerc.* 1980;12:54–60.

20. Garhammer J, Gregor R. Propulsion forces as a function of intensity for weightlifting and vertical jumping. *J Appl Sport Sci Res.* 1992;6:129–34.

21. Gourgoulis V, Aggelousis N, Mavromatis G, Garas A. Three-dimensional kinematic analysis of the snatch of elite Greek weightlifters. *J Sports Sci.* 2000;18:643–52.

22. Grabe SA, Widule CJ. Comparative biomechanics of the jerk in Olympic weightlifting. *Res Q Exerc Sport.* 1988;59:1–8.

CHAPTER 15

Plyometric Training

OBJECTIVES

After completing this chapter, you will be able to:

◆ Define plyometrics and understand the physiology underlying the ergogenic effects

◆ Discuss how plyometric training enhances various components of fitness and athletic performance

◆ Discuss the performance of more than 40 plyometric exercises and variations

◆ Discuss how to properly manipulate acute program variables when designing plyometric training programs

◆ Discuss how to integrate plyometric training with other training modalities

The term *plyometrics* has exhibited a few meanings, spellings, and interpretations over the years depending on whether one is describing pliometrics, classic plyometrics, or modern plyometrics. *Pliometric* exercise translates into "more length" as loaded or explosive eccentric (ECC) muscle actions with no reversible, *e.g.*, concentric (CON), muscle actions are used (1). For example, landing from a jump involves yielding or high ECC loading, where impact forces can exceed the propulsive forces developed during a jump (1). The landing is pliometric where the athlete braces for support (by controlling the degree of hip, knee, and ankle flexion) but does not follow with a CON or propulsion phase, *e.g.*, performing an exercise called a *depth landing*.

Classic plyometrics (note the different spelling) is the term used to describe the origins of plyometric training where it was originally known as "shock training." Shock training consisted mostly of depth jumps and push-ups and variations (*e.g.*, pendulum loadings) where the intensity was very high or ultrahigh and predominately performed by well-trained to elite strength and power athletes. The term *plyometrics* was first coined in the 1970s by track and field coach Fred Wilt (2) but was based on shock training. European athletes were known to use classic plyometric exercises and were achieving superior athletic performances in sports such as track and field, weightlifting, and gymnastics. One such coach/scientist was Dr. Yuri Verkhoshansky, known by many as the modern-day Father of Plyometrics, published his first study in plyometrics in 1964 (known as the *Shock Method* of training) (3,4). Dr. Verkhoshansky preferred the term *shock training* or *shock*

method when describing the classic plyometrics because the high-intensity element distinguished itself from modern plyometrics (4). In fact, Dr. Verkhoshansky has proposed the term *powermetrics* to be used in lieu of plyometrics to limit confusion (4). Classic plyometrics were characterized by this ultra-intense system of depth jumping and loaded pendulum swings where frequency and volume were kept low to avoid overtraining and rest intervals between repetitions and sets were long.

Modern plyometrics, or simply *plyometrics*, is the term commonly used in the United States, which embodies shock training as a segment but also embraces inclusion of exercises that simply consist of *plyometric actions*. Plyometric actions refer to the lengthening or prestretching of skeletal muscles under loading that allows a more forceful CON muscle action (5). Plyometric actions utilize the stretch-shortening cycle (SSC) and are substantially reliant upon loading and the rate of lengthening during the ECC phase (5). Plyometric actions not only include high-intensity movements such as depth jumps and single-leg hops/jumps but also include simple activities such as walking, jogging, hopping, and multidirectional movements where the SSC increases mechanical efficiency. By incorporating the premise of plyometric actions into modern plyometric training, many other exercises have been included in athletic training programs. In fact, modern plyometrics consist of a proposed continuum of exercises from low to high intensity, whereas classic plyometrics consisted entirely of high-intensity exercises. Although some plyometric drills may be considered low or moderate intensity, they are still performed explosively but consist of less ECC loading than classic plyometrics.

447

Myths & Misconceptions
Modern Plyometric Training Consists Entirely of Depth Jumps

Critics of plyometric training have questioned its utility in some populations (*e.g.*, children and adolescents) stating it is too high in intensity. However, the misconception is that plyometrics consist entirely of exercises such as high-intensity depth jumps. That is, they refer to classic plyometrics as the benchmark but fail to recognize the exercise selection differences in modern plyometric training. Although classic plyometric training consisted mostly of depth jumps, it has evolved into a more comprehensive system of training utilizing diverse explosive exercises of low, moderate, and high intensity. If one accepts the terminology/interpretation that modern plyometrics target plyometric actions, then plyometric training consists of jumps, hops, skips, bounding, and upper-body throws, tosses, and passes in addition to power-specific exercises seen in sports, *e.g.*, throws and swings in baseball and kicks, blocks, and strikes in martial arts. These exercises increase force/power and mechanical efficiency of the athlete. Other modes of exercise also include plyometric actions but are considered separate training modalities, *e.g.*, sprint, agility, and resistance training (RT). Plyometric exercises are based on complexity and intensity and can be modified to train many populations. Thus, many individuals benefit from plyometric training independent of the inclusion of depth jumps.

Notwithstanding the terminology differences, plyometrics allow an athlete to reach maximal strength and power in the shortest period of time (5). Interest in plyometric training has increased greatly since the 1970s. Coaches and scientists alike began to attribute the performance enhancement to plyometric training since it was a new training modality. The benefits of plyometric training in enhancing explosive power performance soon were seen by coaches all over the world and became a staple in the training of strength/power athletes into modern day. For example, more than 95% of Major League Baseball (6), 100% of National Basketball Association (7), 100% of National Hockey League strength and conditioning (S&C) coaches (8), and ~94% of National Football League S&C coaches (9) incorporate plyometrics in their athletes' workouts.

Plyometric exercises are classified based on the intensity level. *Maximal plyometrics* involve ultrahigh-intense muscular contractions and typically comprise depth jumps and variations (4). *Submaximal plyometrics* involve low- and moderate-intensity drills that comprise most exercises other than depth jumps (4). In addition, plyometric exercises can be impact-oriented (jumps, hops, skips, plyo push-ups) where the reversible action is stimulated by contact with the ground or object, or non–impact-oriented (strikes, thrusts, throws, passes, and tosses without prior catching of the ball) where the drill is an open chain, *i.e.*, the ECC and CON phases are not augmented by direct contact with the ground or object (4). Both types are included in plyometric training programs. For terminology consistency, it is important to note that plyometric training is described in terms of modern plyometric exercises throughout this chapter.

Physiology of Plyometric Exercise

Plyometric exercise stimulates activation of the SSC. The countermovement initiates the stretch reflex that leads to an ECC muscle action that precedes a brief isometric (ISOM) phase and subsequent CON muscle action. The ECC phase (plus prior delay seen between muscle activation via neural action potentials and muscle contraction [*electromechanical delay*]) is referred to as the *amortization phase*. The length of the ISOM phase between ECC and CON actions is referred to as *coupling time*. The subsequent CON muscle action is augmented by the stretch reflex and the release of elastic energy. The muscle-tendon complex acts like a rubber band when it is stretched. It has elastic potential and the ability to rapidly store and release elastic energy. Elastic energy stored primarily within the series elastic component (tendon, actin, myosin, structural proteins) during an ECC muscle action and elastic force augments muscle force and power during the CON phase when it follows right away (10). Maximal force and power can be expressed when the ISOM coupling time is minimal. It has been recommended that coupling time be <0.15 second, especially in athletes who possess higher percentages of fast-twitch (FT) muscle fibers (4). Thus, minimizing the time of the amortization phase and coupling time is critical for the athlete to develop maximal power. Energy can change forms, and elastic energy is wasted as coupling time increases (elastic energy dissipates into heat energy in proportion to the length of the coupling phase). Elastic energy enhances muscular performance, whereas heat energy has minimal effects. The use of elastic energy is maximized when the CON phase follows the ECC phase immediately. Rapid human movements such as sprinting and plyometrics require high rates of force development since the athlete will have <250 ms to develop force while the feet are in contact with the ground. The second major contributor to the SSC is the stretch reflex. Muscle spindles located within skeletal muscle fibers detect the magnitude and rate of length changes. The response is to send action potentials to the central nervous system where the agonist muscle's force production is enhanced while the antagonist muscles relax. In combination, both mechanisms contribute to SSC function although storage/use of elastic energy contributes to a greater extent (10). With training, more energy can be stored and utilized as muscle force increases (1). Muscle power and rate of force development (RFD) increase. This is critical to athletic performance where force must be maximized in short time periods. Plyometric training is designed to train the SSC via neural adaptations, reflex potentiation, and enhanced elastic potential of skeletal muscles. The selective, or earlier, recruitment of FT motor units is advantageous for acute power performance. Lastly, the FT units stay active or facilitated as activities performed after explosive plyometric exercises are enhanced to a greater extent (11).

Plyometric Training and Athletic Performance

Plyometric training has increased athletic performance in most studies. Lower-body plyometric training can increase jumping height and power (12–19), sprinting ability (13,17,20), agility (17,21,22), peak isokinetic strength (23), and reactive strength index (24). A meta-analysis of 26 plyometric training studies has shown that lower-body plyometric training increases squat jump, countermovement vertical jump, countermovement vertical jump with arm swing, and drop jump performance by 4.7%, 8.7%, 7.5%, and 4.7%, respectively (16). More recent reviews and meta-analyses indicate that lower-body plyometric training of at least 4–12 weeks increases vertical jump performance by 3%–30%, horizontal jump performance by up to 9%, muscle power by 2%–31%, RFD and explosive strength by up to 33%, sprint speed by 1%–14%, agility performance by 2%–23%, and lower-body maximal strength by 3%–45% in athletes and nonathletes (24–26). The increases in jump performance appear dose-related where total impact is related to the magnitude of improvement (25). Vertical lower-body plyometric training augments vertical jump performance but may have less impact on agility and speed performance, whereas horizontal plyometric training may have greater impact on horizontal jump performance and sprint speed (27). Upper-body plyometric training increases power, throwing velocity, and distance (28). In female athletes, plyometric training increases jump performance where large effects are seen beyond 10 weeks of training (29).

Plyometric training increases muscle strength and hypertrophy, as well as induces fiber-type transitions (type IIX to IIA) similar to RT (18,19,24). The combination of plyometrics and RT is most effective for increasing vertical jumping ability (12,30–32), sprinting speed (21,31,32), agility (21), as well as improving motor performance such as kicking velocity (33). Combined RT and plyometric training increases maximal strength (by up to 43%) and power (by up to 37%) (24). However, not all studies show augmentation of RT and plyometric training (34). Wilson et al. (35) showed that 8 weeks of RT consisting of 6 sets of 6–10 reps of squats produced similar increases in vertical jump height to plyometric training consisting of 3–6 sets of 8 reps of depth jumps from 20 to 70 cm heights (21% and 18%, respectively). In addition, 6–9 weeks of plyometric training can increase running economy in moderately trained runners and highly trained endurance athletes (36,37) and can improve 3-km race times in runners (38). Plyometric training enhances swimming block start performance (39), lateral reaction time and sprint ability in tennis players (40), throwing velocity in baseball players (41), and kicking speed in soccer players (42). In addition, plyometric training (alone and in combination with RT, agility, and speed training) is effective for injury prevention by improving landing mechanics (reduced valgus stress), improve ECC muscle control, increasing knee flexion and hamstring muscle activity (prelanding and during landing), and by reducing landing ground reaction force and joint loading especially in female athletes more vulnerable to knee injury (24,25,29).

Sidebar Mechanics of the Vertical Jump

The vertical jump consists of five distinct phases: (a) starting position, (b) countermovement, (c) jump or propulsion, (d) flight, and (e) landing. Athletes begin the vertical jump from a hip-to-shoulder width stance. The countermovement is characterized by rapid hip and knee flexion, ankle dorsiflexion, and shoulder hyperextension. The jump or propulsion phase consists of explosive hip, trunk, and knee extension, plantar flexion, and shoulder flexion. Take-off velocity during the vertical jump is affected by knee extension, 56%; plantar flexion, 22%; trunk extension, 10%; arm swing, 10%; and head swing, 2% (43). In the lower body during propulsion, the hip, knee, and ankle contribute 40%, 24.2%, and 35.8% to the forces applied to the ground, respectively (44). Research has documented the importance of the countermovement and arm-swing in maximizing power and height attained during the vertical jump (45). The arm-swing consists of an explosive forward and upward movement with the thumbs up. The arm-swing helps to keep the torso upright especially as the hips flex. Flight time increases in proportion to the vertical height attained and is dependent upon the power produced by the athlete. The landing style is critical to absorbing shock and minimizing joint stress. Lowering peak ground reaction force and increasing braking (by flexing the knees, hips, and dorsiflexing the ankles for better force distribution and shock absorption) is important (46). Greater stress is seen during a single-leg landing (greater valgus stress on knee, higher muscle activation, less knee flexion to absorb force) than during a double-leg landing (47). Women show greater valgus stress on the knee and greater relative ground reaction force during double-leg landings compared to men (47). Teaching proper landing mechanics is important to reducing the risk of injuries. Proper breathing consists of inhaling during the countermovement, temporary holding of breath during the end of the amortization phase and early max propulsion phase, and exhalation upon elevation off of the ground (48).

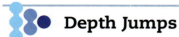 ## Depth Jumps

A staple of plyometric training has been the *depth jump* (or drop jump) since its early introduction in the 1950s into athletic training programs by Dr. Yuri Verkhoshansky (4). The depth jump, one of the most intense types of plyometric exercises, the depth jump has been commonly included in the S&C programs for athletes. The athlete steps off of a box or bench in a relaxed manner, lands (shock), and explosively jumps while spending minimal time on the ground. Biomechanical studies of the depth jump have shown it to be intense, yet effective for maximizing power. It yields a high reactive strength index than other double- and single-leg jumps (49). Bobbert et al. (50–52) have shown that (in comparison to countermovement jumps) depth jumps result in greater peak forces especially in the knees and ankles, whereas the work performed by the hips is lower. The mechanics of the depth jump depend upon individual technique. Peak forces tend to be higher if athletes have minimal flexion of the hips and knees upon landing (a quick rebound) versus athletes who descend lower during the countermovement (50–52). The drop height is another consideration. The higher the drop height, the greater the vertical velocity attained by the athlete during descent, and coupled with the athlete's mass, the higher drop height results in higher levels of force upon ground contact (1). Intensity increases as drop height increases. Most often, drop heights of 20–110 cm are used. Early literature in athletic training recommended 75–115 cm; however, others have recommended more conservative heights of 20–40 cm (52). Peak propulsion force increases in proportion to drop height (50). Bobbert et al. (52) showed that a depth jump from a 60-cm height produced a higher rate of loading and ground reaction force 1.5 times more than a depth jump performed from a 20-cm height. Greater negative work is performed with increasing drop heights (52). The optimal depth jump height is debatable and individualized as the athlete should demonstrate a smooth transition between ECC and CON phases. Some studies show greater vertical jump heights from higher drop heights (40 cm) up to a certain height, whereas some studies show no vertical jump height differences between 20- and 85-cm jump heights (52,53). Similar increases in vertical jump performance following depth jump training at 50- and 100-cm heights were shown (54). Depth jump heights of ~20–40 cm or so may be used initially for athletes beginning depth jump training and gradual progression can take place once the athlete adapts. A vertical jump test from different box heights can be used to find an initial appropriate box height. Vertical jump height is equal or greater with increasing box heights up to a certain point of no additional benefit. That box height corresponding to best vertical jump performance can be used and then progressed upon. Because of the intense nature of the exercise, few sets (39,52,55) of up to 5–8 reps with long (2–10 min) rest intervals for 1–3 days per week have been recommended when maximal depth jumps are performed from large heights and/or with external loading (4).

 ## Plyometric Program Design

Plyometric training, like other modalities, is a composite of several acute program variables that can be manipulated to achieve a target goal. These variables include exercise selection and order, intensity, volume, frequency, and rest intervals (83,84). Designing a plyometric training program for athletes is multifactorial and should include planned progressive overload, specificity, and variation. Many factors need to be considered including the age/training status of the athlete, equipment availability, training surface, and recovery in between workouts, nutrition, and the integration of plyometrics with other training modalities. Although research into plyometric training has increased 25-fold since 2000 (56), most plyometric training studies are not comparative. A wide variety of programs are effective for increasing performance, but few studies directly compared changes when manipulating program variables. Thus, current plyometric guidelines rely mostly on coaches' practical experience with some research support. Some other critical factors to plyometric training include the following:

- The quality of training is most critical. Each rep should be performed with maximal effort, minimal amortization and coupling times, and explosive propulsion.
- Exercise selection should be as specific to the demands of the sport as possible. For lower-body plyometrics, vertical and horizontal movements are recommended. Sport-specific drills can be integrated with plyometric exercises to improve skill development along with power. It is critical for the coach to address limb and rotational dominance in athletes (4,10). Unilateral drills are recommended and important for those athletes that, in part, perform explosively with one leg/arm during propulsion, and bilateral drills are critical for athletes involved in sports where bilateral limb power is needed. Many sports comprise both, so plyometric training programs in these athletes should include uni- and bilateral drills. For example, a right-handed baseball pitcher needs to explosively push off with the right leg against the rubber on the mound and produce high total-body power during counterclockwise rotation during the wind-up, delivery, and follow-through phases of pitching. Thus, single-leg push-offs and lateral hops, as well as counterclockwise MB tosses and throws, can be used to train these actions. Although exercises are included that work the contralateral side or movement to improve muscle balance, emphasis can be given to target these specific movement needs of the athlete's position.
- Gradual progression should be used based on the training level of the athletes. Progression entails increases in intensity via the addition of more complex exercises and perhaps some external loading. Volume can be increased within reasonable limits. Likewise, volume and intensity are inversely related. Low-intensity and moderate-intensity drills should be mastered before progressing to high-intensity drills. It

Interpreting Research
Comparison of the Effects of Bilateral and Unilateral Plyometric Training on Strength and Rates of Force Development

Bogdanis GC, Tsoukos A, Kaloheri O, Terzis G, Veligekas P, Brown LE. Comparison between unilateral and bilateral plyometric training on single- and double-leg jumping performance and strength. *J Strength Cond Res.* 2017;33:633–40.

Bogdanis et al. (57) compared 6 weeks of plyometric training (2 d·wk⁻¹) with either unilateral or bilateral exercises on performance. The program consisted of six plyometric exercises (jumps for distance, countermovement jumps, lateral jumps, box jumps, hurdle jumps, and drop jumps) plus two resistance exercises (leg extension, leg curl) performed for 2–3 sets of 10 reps, while the resistance exercises were performed for 3–4 sets of 3–8 reps with 60%–90% of 1 RM. One group performed the program bilaterally, while the other group performed the workout unilaterally. Both unilateral and bilateral training significantly increased bilateral countermovement jump performance by 12.1% and 11%, respectively. However, unilateral jump performance only increased following unilateral training (by 19%). Drop jump performance increased similar in both groups by 5% and 9%, respectively, for the bilateral and unilateral groups. Reactive strength index (calculated by dividing maximal drop jump height by ground reaction time) only increased following unilateral training. Bilateral maximal ISOM force increased similarly in both groups; however, the sum of unilateral maximal force values increased 2-fold more following unilateral training. Bilateral rates of force development (during the first 100 ms) increased similarly in both groups. However, sums of each leg increased only following unilateral training. These data demonstrated the advantages of incorporating unilateral plyometric exercises into a plyometric training program. Bilateral training produced mostly bilateral improvements, but unilateral training had positive benefits to bilateral and unilateral measurements.

---

has been suggested that athletes have at least a few years of RT and plyometric training experience prior to performing maximal depth jump training (4,10). High-intensity workouts require greater recovery time in between workouts, so frequency must be decreased accordingly.

- Proper technique should always be coached especially when fatigue manifests. Sufficient rest interval lengths should be used to minimize fatigue when peak power is the goal (and not power endurance).
- Plyometric training should take place in an area where there is sufficient space. For horizontal length-specific drills, at least 30–40 yd is recommended. For vertical drills, ceiling height should be higher than the athletes' maximal reach.

Exercise Selection

Plyometric exercises consist mostly of jumps-in-place, standing jumps, multiple hops/jumps, bounding, box drills, depth jumps, and throws (5,48). These exercises can be divided into lower-body and upper-body/trunk/core explosive exercises. *Jumps* involve maximizing the vertical and/or horizontal motion component. *Hops* involve maximizing the repeated motion for a given distance or pattern. *Bounds* are exaggerated horizontal movements where an excessive stride length is used. *Box drills* involve jumping on or off boxes of different sizes for varied intensity. *Depth jumps* involve accentuating the ECC component by stepping off of a box of varied height prior to performing an explosive jump. *Tosses* and *passes* involve the upper torso and arms (in addition to lower body and core power) releasing the ball or object below or in front of the head. *Throws* involve the upper torso and arms (in addition to lower body and core power) releasing the ball or object above, over, or across the head. It is important to note that all of these exercises are performed explosively with minimal amortization and coupling phases. Some drills can be combined to form a more complex drill, *i.e.*, adding a sprint or multidirectional hop/jump to a depth jump. In addition, *ballistic exercises* (discussed in Chapter 12) are plyometric due to the release of the load (minimizing deceleration). Exercises such as the jump squat, bench press throw, ballistic leg press, and ballistic shoulder press target the SSC and increase power. It is advantageous to use equipment designed to safely catch the weight via hydraulic braking when released. Meta-analytic data have shown that best results from plyometric training are seen when multiple lower-body exercises (*e.g.*, countermovement jumps, squat jumps, and depth jumps) are included per workout rather than a fewer number (58).

Exercises

Visit thePoint to view more exercises and variations.

Lower-Body Plyometric Exercises

Two-Foot Ankle Hop ("Pogo")

Intensity: Low

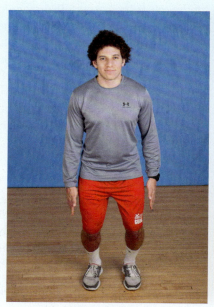 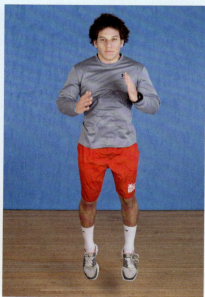

FIGURE 15.1 Two-foot ankle hop.

- The athlete begins with arms at the sides and a shoulder width stance.
- After a countermovement, the athlete jumps straight up (with double-arm action), lands, and explosively jumps upright once again. This exercise stresses the plantar flexor muscles to a high degree (Fig. 15.1).

Side-To-Side Ankle Hop

Intensity: Low

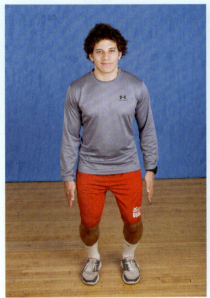 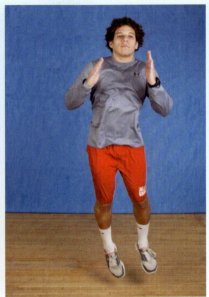

FIGURE 15.2 Side-to-side ankle hop.

- The athlete begins with arms at the sides and a shoulder width stance.
- After a short countermovement, the athlete jumps with both feet side to side spanning ~2–3 ft. Cones may be used as guide markers.
- This exercise may be performed with one leg where the athlete pushes off on the right leg and lands on the left, and vice versa (Fig. 15.2).

Jump-and-Reach

Intensity: Moderate-to-Moderately High (depending on athlete's jump height)

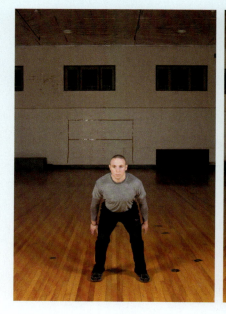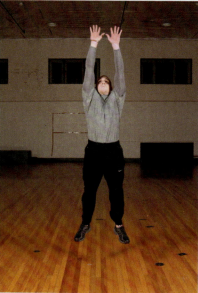

FIGURE 15.3 Jump-and-Reach.

- The athlete begins with arms at the sides and a shoulder width stance.
- After a countermovement (and backswing of arms), the athlete jumps straight up and reaches as high as possible simultaneously, lands, and explosively jumps linearly once again. It helps to have a high target for the athlete to strive for to increase jump height, *e.g.*, rim on a basketball court or Vertec (Fig. 15.3).

> **VARIATIONS** A variation involves turning 90° or 180° prior to the jump and reach to increase sport specificity. The athlete could also place a ball in the hands while jumping.

Squat Jump

Intensity: Low to Moderate

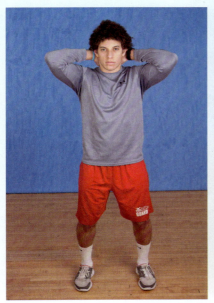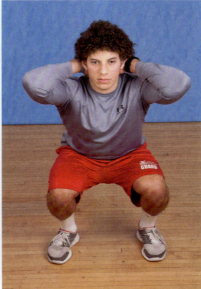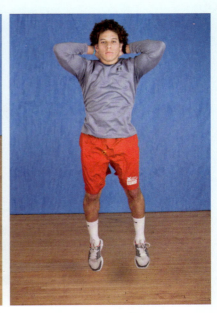

FIGURE 15.4 Squat jump.

- The athlete begins with the fingers interlocked behind the head and a shoulder width stance. This exercise can be performed with a medicine ball (MB), KB, DB, and other forms of resistance as well.
- After a countermovement, the athlete jumps straight up as high as possible, lands, and explosively jumps for another rep (Fig. 15.4).

VARIATIONS Different hand positions can be used. Variations include a dumbbell squat jump and a squat jump with rotation during flight. An advanced variation is to land on just one leg.

CAUTION! Similar to a free weight squat, the athlete should maintain an erect posture during descent and maintain proper knee and toe alignment. The athlete should and softly and the landing directly leads to the countermovement for the next rep.

Knee Jump

Intensity: Low

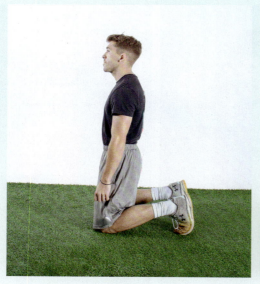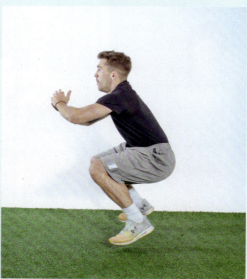

FIGURE 15.5 Knee jump.

- The athlete begins in an erect position while kneeling.
- Following a forceful backward arm swing and countermovement of the hips, the athlete explosively swings the arms forward and extends the hips landing on their feet in a deep squat position (Fig. 15.5).
- The athlete then squats, lowers the body back to the kneeling position, and performs another rep.

> **VARIATIONS** Advanced variations exist where the athlete may eliminate the arm swing (forcing the hips to generate all of the power), external loading can be used, and the athlete could land on a single leg.

Standing Long Jump

Intensity: Low to Moderate

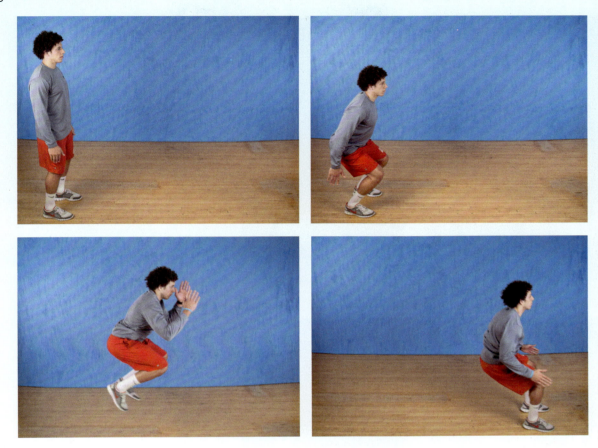

FIGURE 15.6 Standing long jump.

- Athlete begins with arms at the sides and a shoulder width stance with knees slightly bent.
- Following a countermovement (and backswing of arms), the athlete jumps as far forward as possible while using an explosive double-arm action (Fig. 15.6).

CAUTION! Many times the feet will contact the ground in front of the center of gravity (COG) so balance needs to be maintained during landing.

VARIATIONS A variation is to add another jump, multidirectional sprint or agility move, or sport-specific skill to the end.

Barrier Jumps

Intensity: Low to Moderate

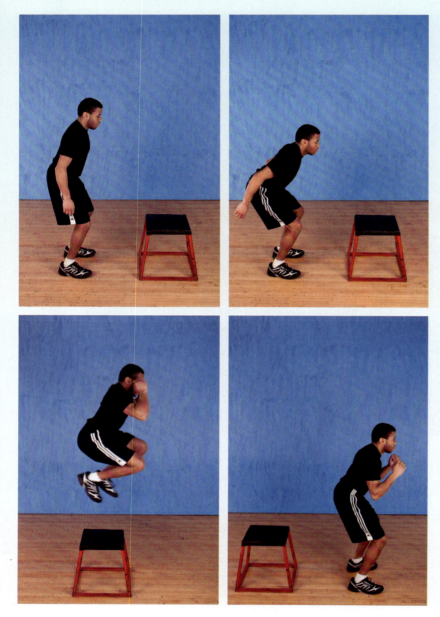

FIGURE 15.7 Barrier jumps.

- The athlete begins with arms at the sides, shoulder width stance, and knees slightly bent.
- After a quick countermovement and arm backswing, the athlete jumps over a barrier using double-arm action. Some common barriers used are cones, hurdles, and boxes. Increasing the height of the barrier increases the intensity (Fig. 15.7).

> **CAUTION!** The athlete must focus to ensure clearing the barrier during jumping to avoid tripping, falling, and risking injury.

> **VARIATIONS** Variations include lateral, backward, and diagonal barrier jumps or hops. Another variation is to add a multidirectional sprint or sport-specific skill to the end.

Cone Hops

Intensity: Low

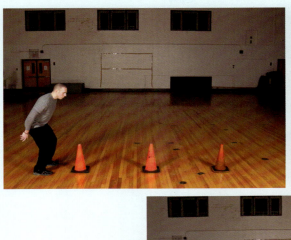
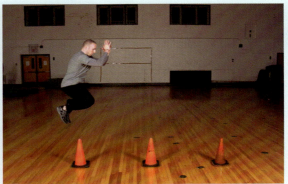
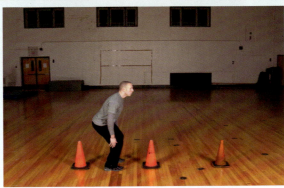

FIGURE 15.8 Cone hops.

- The athlete begins with arms at the sides, shoulder width stance, and knees slightly bent.
- Following a quick countermovement and arm backswing, the athlete jumps forward over a cone using double-arm action. A series of cones can be used for multiple repetitions and the spacing in between cones can alter the intensity (Fig. 15.8).

> **VARIATIONS** Variations include lateral cone hops, backward hops, diagonal hops, or adding 180° rotation to the hop. A multidirectional sprint or sport-specific skill can be added to the end. An advanced variation is to perform hops downhill to accentuate the ECC muscle actions.

Tuck Jumps

Intensity: Moderate to High

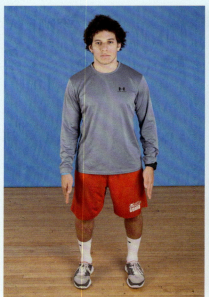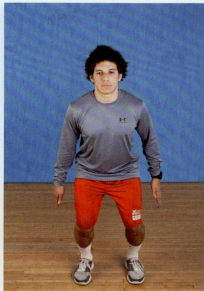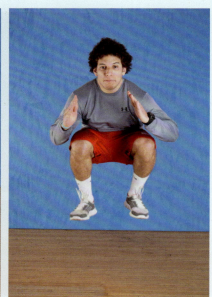

FIGURE 15.9 Tuck jumps.

- The athlete begins with arms at the sides, shoulder width stance, and knees slightly bent.
- After a quick countermovement (and backswing of arms), the athlete explosively jumps vertically as high as possible using a double-arm action. While jumping, the athlete raises the knees to the chest and may temporarily hold that position or grasp the knees with both hands.
- The tuck jump is a good exercise to visualize valgus stress (inward bowing) on the knees during landing. This has been successfully used in the evaluation of female athletes who are more likely to sustain anterior cruciate ligament injuries (Fig. 15.9). Other key coaching points are to ensure the thighs reach parallel at peak of jump and are on the same plane between the right and left limbs, feet should land shoulder width apart, parallel, and at the same time using a soft landing technique.

 VARIATIONS A variation is to use a heel kick (heel to buttocks) instead of a front tuck.

Split Squat Jump

Intensity: Low to Moderate

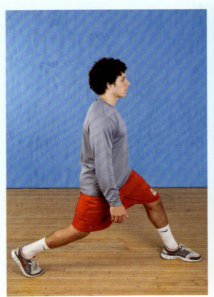 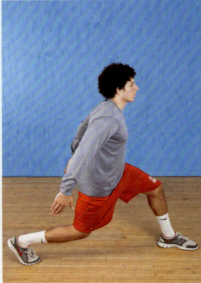 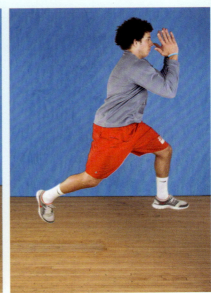

FIGURE 15.10 Split squat jump.

- The athlete begins with arms at the side. One leg is flexed forward while the opposite hip is hyperextended, *e.g.*, resembling a front lunge position. Front knee is flexed ~45°–90°, whereas back knee is slightly flexed.
- After a short countermovement, the athlete explosively jumps vertically while extending the arms upward.
- The athlete lands in the same position held prior to initiating the jump (Fig. 15.10).

> **VARIATIONS** A variation is to cycle the legs during flight, *i.e.*, switch forward/back legs in midair and land in the opposite position (a scissor jump).

Pike Jump

Intensity: Moderate to High

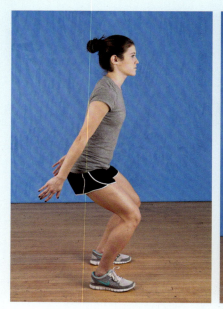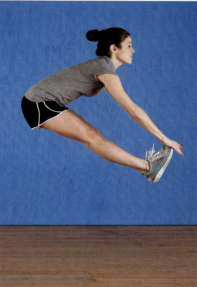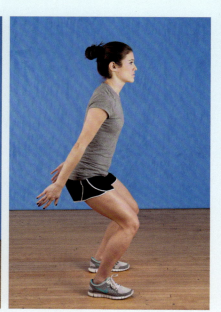

FIGURE 15.11 Pike jump.

- Athlete begins with the arms at the sides, shoulder width stance, and knees slightly bent.
- After a countermovement, the athlete explosively jumps upward. While jumping, the athlete lifts both legs upward while keeping the knees only slightly bent and flexes the shoulders to try to touch the toes during flight. The athlete lands and repeats the jump (Fig. 15.11).

VARIATIONS Variations include widening the legs (abduct the hips) during flight or lifting the legs laterally during flight (Fig. 15.12).

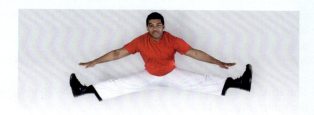

FIGURE 15.12 Pike jump while widening the legs.

Chapter 15 Plyometric Training   463

Single-Leg Vertical Jump

Intensity: High

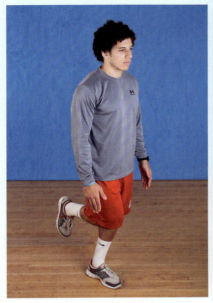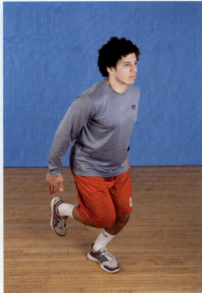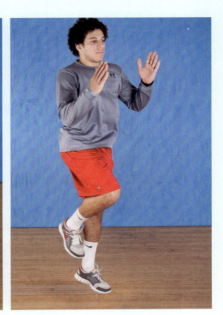

FIGURE 15.13 Single-leg vertical jump.

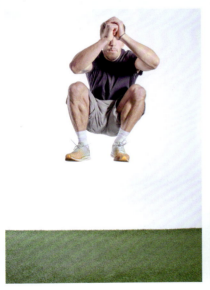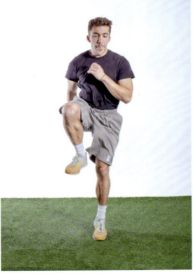

FIGURE 15.14 Single-leg tuck jump.

- The athlete begins with arms at the side. Body weight is placed on one leg, while other nonjumping leg is flexed off of the ground. The front knee is slightly flexed while supporting body weight.
- After a countermovement, the athlete explosively jumps vertically off of the front leg as high as possible using a double-arm action. The athlete lands and explosively performs another jump with the same leg. Some recovery time may be needed in between jumps to maintain balance prior to the next repetition (Fig. 15.13).

VARIATIONS Variations include the single-leg jump and reach and the single-leg tuck jump (Fig. 15.14). The athlete can land and jump off of the opposite leg (cycle legs between reps).

Double-Leg Hops

Intensity: Low to Moderate

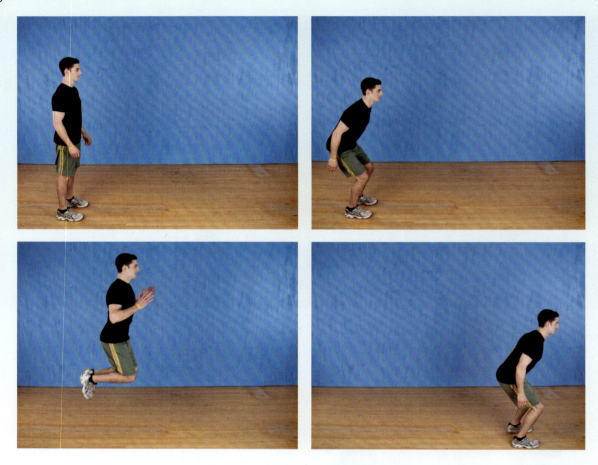

FIGURE 15.15 Double-leg hops.

- Athlete begins with arms at the sides, shoulder width stance, and knees slightly flexed.
- Following a countermovement (and arm backswing), the athlete jumps forward explosively, lands, and repeatedly hops for a specific distance.
- Barriers such as cones, boxes, mini hurdles, and bags can be used as guides (Fig. 15.15).

VARIATIONS Variations include lateral hops, backward hops, and diagonal or zigzag hops. The coach can prescribe specific patterns of hopping to the sport (in shapes of triangle, rectangle, hexagon, a "T, M, W", etc.). Another variation is to perform the hops up stadium steps. A multidirectional sprint or sport-specific skill can be added to the end of the hop sequence.

Single-Leg Hops

Intensity: Moderate to High

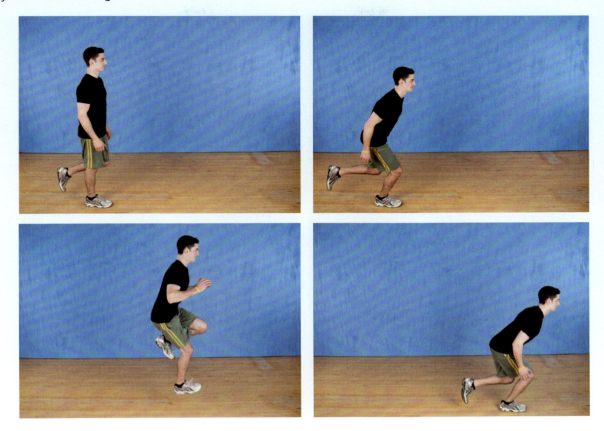

FIGURE 15.16 Single-leg hops.

- Athlete begins with arms at the sides. The jumping leg is slightly flexed while supporting the weight of the body, whereas the nonjumping leg is flexed at the knee ~60°–90°.
- After a countermovement (and arm backswing), the athlete jumps forward explosively, lands, and repeatedly hops for a specific distance (Fig. 15.16).

> **VARIATIONS** Variations include lateral hops, backward hops, and diagonal or zigzag hops. The coach can prescribe specific patterns of hopping to the sport. A multidirectional sprint or sport-specific skill can be added to the end of the hop sequence. Intensity can be increased by performing single-leg hops uphill or up stadium steps.

Standing Triple Jump

Intensity: Moderate to High

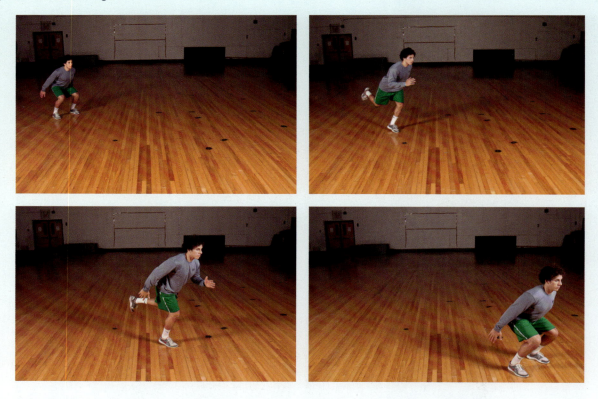

FIGURE 15.17 Standing triple jump.

- The athlete begins with arms at the sides, shoulder width stance, and knees slightly bent.
- Following a countermovement, the athlete jumps forward explosively and lands on one foot. The athlete explosively jumps off of the landing leg and lands on the opposite leg. The athlete explosively jumps off this leg and lands on both feet.
- It helps if the athlete lands on a softer surface such as a landing pit (Fig. 15.17).

> **VARIATIONS** A variation is to begin with a running start instead of standing. Barriers can be used as jump guides.

Single-Leg Box Jump

Intensity: Moderate to High

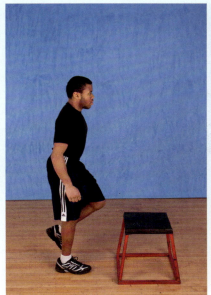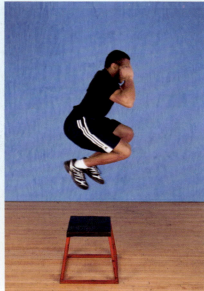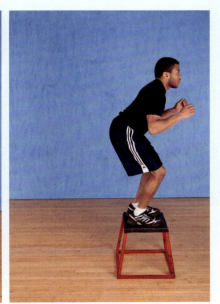

FIGURE 15.18 Single-leg box jump.

- The athlete begins with arms at the sides, support leg on the ground with knee slightly flexed, and nonsupport leg flexed close to or near 90° (Fig. 15.18).
- A box 15–115 cm high is placed in front of the athlete.
- After a countermovement (and arm backswing), the athlete jumps vertically (with double-arm action) and lands on top of the box. The athlete may also land on one (the jumping) leg to increase difficulty.
- Another single-leg box exercise is the *single-leg push-off*. Here, the athlete begins with arms at the sides, front foot on the box, and rear leg in contact with the ground. A box 15–46 cm high should be used (appropriate height should yield jump leg close to parallel to the ground [or hip and knee flexed close to ~90°]). The higher the box the higher the intensity. The athlete explosively jumps vertically (with double-arm action), reaches as high as possible, and lands with the same leg atop the box.

> **CAUTION!** For all box jumps, caution must be used to ensure proper landing on the box. The athlete should land with feet toward the center of the box while maintaining equilibrium.

> **VARIATIONS OF THE SINGLE-LEG PUSH OFF** Variations include alternating legs (landing on the opposite leg while legs cycle in the air), a lateral push-off (where the athlete lands on the same leg), and a lateral push-off where the athlete jumps over the box and lands on the opposite leg (Fig. 15.19).

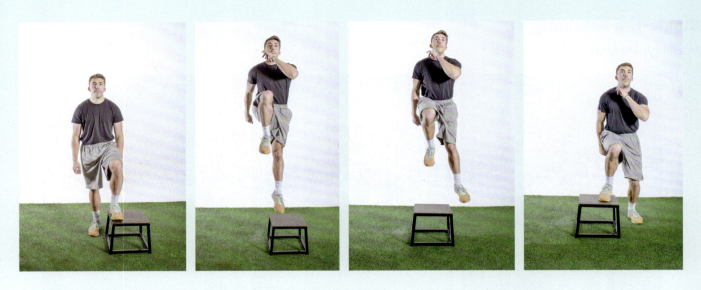

FIGURE 15.19 Lateral push-off and lateral push-off, alternating sides.

Box Jump

Intensity: Low to Moderate

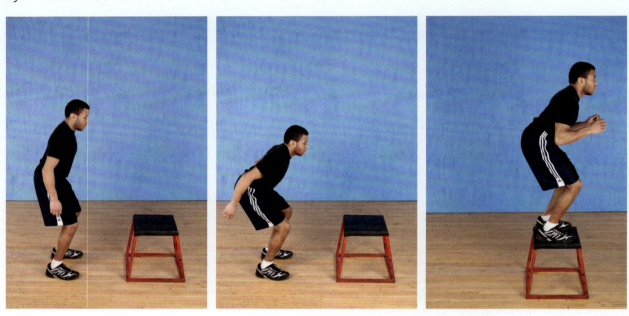

FIGURE 15.20 Box jump.

- Athlete begins with arms at the sides, shoulder width stance, and knees slightly bent.
- A box 15–115 cm high is placed in front of the athlete.
- The athlete jumps explosively up and forward (with double-arm action) on top of the box. The athlete steps off of the box and performs another repetition (Fig. 15.20).
- Box jumps have become a popular exercise choice for many fitness goals.

> **VARIATIONS** Variations of this exercise include a lateral box jump, diagonal box jump, and a squat box jump (with fingers clasped behind the head and no arm action). A multidirectional sprint or sport-specific skill can be added to the end of the drill.

Multiple Box Jumps

Intensity: Moderate to High

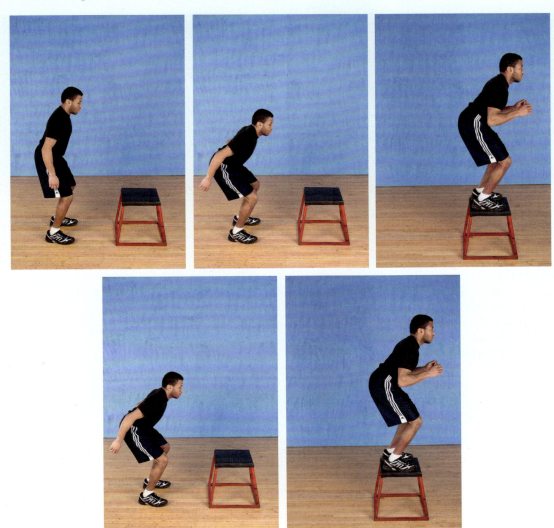

FIGURE 15.21 Multiple box jumps.

- This exercise is similar to the box jump. Multiple boxes are used in succession. Typically, three to five boxes of similar height are used.
- The athlete jumps onto the first box, off onto the floor, and then onto the second box, and repeats until the set is complete (Fig. 15.21).

VARIATIONS Variations to this exercise include lateral box jumps and single-leg landings. Box heights that increase in succession to increase the intensity can be used.

Another variation is to have the athlete jump from a box to stress the element of the landing, *e.g.*, the *depth landing* discussed previously in this chapter. This drill stresses the yielding component, works to develop ECC strength, and is a high-intensity plyometric exercise.

Another variation (*box double leap*) entails the athlete jump on top of the box, then explosively jumps off of the box (with double-arm action) in one motion for height and distance, and sticks the landing. This drill also targets yielding or ECC strength once the athlete jumps off of the box to the floor.

A multidirectional sprint or sport-specific skill can be added to the end of the drill.

Skipping

Intensity: Low

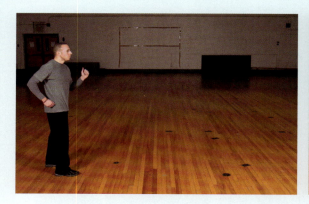 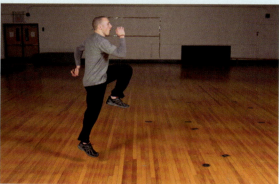

FIGURE 15.22 Skipping.

- Athlete begins with arms at the sides, shoulder width stance, and knees slightly bent.
- After a quick countermovement, the athlete explosively raises one leg (to a 90° knee angle) and the opposite arm (to a 90° elbow angle). Upon return, the opposite limbs are raised, and the cycle is repeated until the targeted number of repetitions has been completed (Fig. 15.22).

> **VARIATIONS** Variations include backward skipping and skipping with double-arm action (as opposed to one).

Alternate Bounding

Intensity: Moderate to High

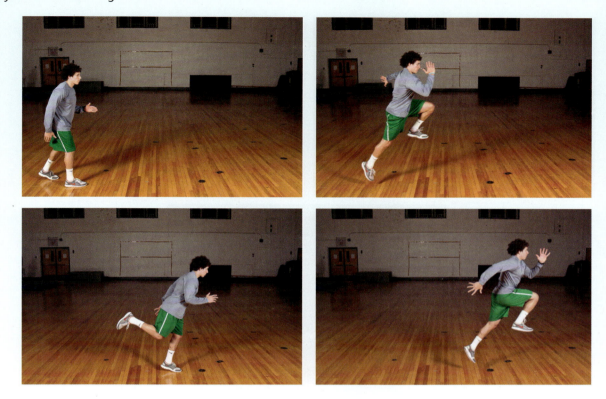

FIGURE 15.23 Alternate bounding.

- The athlete begins with arms at the sides, shoulder width stance, and knees slightly bent.
- After a quick countermovement (preferably from a jog), the athlete pushes off explosively with one leg. The opposite leg will flex forward in an exaggerated manner with the leg parallel to the ground. The athlete reaches forward with the opposite arm. The goal is to cover as much ground as possible during each exaggerated stride.
- Upon landing, the athlete explosively pushes off of the landing foot and repeats (Fig. 15.23).

> **VARIATIONS** Variations to this exercise include double-arm bounding. A multidirectional sprint or sport-specific skill can be added to the end of the drill.

Single-Leg Bounding

Intensity: Moderate to High

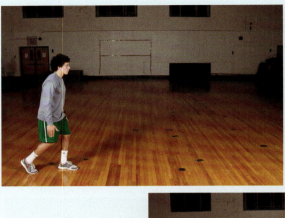
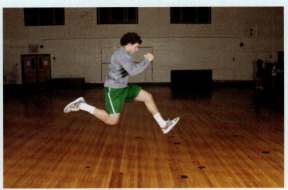
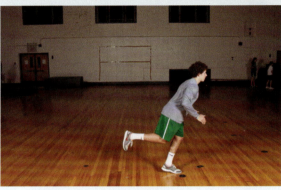

FIGURE 15.24 Single-leg bounding.

- The athlete begins with arms at the sides, shoulder width stance, and knees slightly bent.
- After a quick countermovement (preferably from a jog), the athlete pushes off explosively with one leg. The opposite leg will flex forward in an exaggerated manner with the leg parallel to the ground. The athlete reaches forward with the opposite arm.
- The athlete pushes off and lands on the same foot (different from alternate bounding). The opposite side is drilled following completion of the first side.
- A multidirectional sprint or sport-specific skill can be added to the end of the drill (Fig. 15.24).

Depth Jump (Drop Jump)

Intensity: High to Very High (Depending on Box Height)

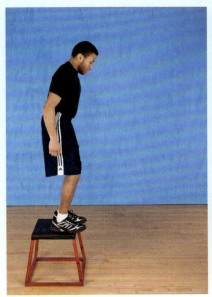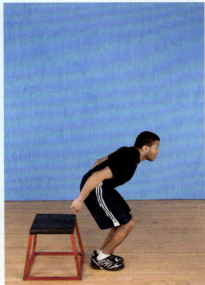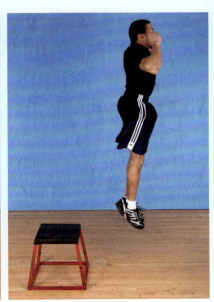

FIGURE 15.25 Depth jump (drop jump).

- The athlete begins with arms at the sides, shoulder width stance, and knees slightly bent on top of a box (with toes near or hanging over the edge of the box). Box heights vary between 20 and 115 cm. Intensity increases as box height increases.
- The athlete steps off of the box, lands on the ground, and explosively jumps vertically (with double-arm action) as high as possible upon landing (Fig. 15.25).

VARIATIONS Many variations can be performed. Several of the jumps discussed in this chapter can be performed once the athlete steps off from the box (jump and reach, squat jump, tuck jump, long jump, pike jump, etc.). A multidirectional sprint or sport-specific skill can be added to the end of the jump. The reverse depth jump is where the athlete steps back off the box and jumps onto the same box.

CAUTION! Athletes must be able to have a smooth transition between ECC and CON phases. If the athlete hesitates to regain stability, then the box height should be reduced. The athlete should not break the exercise into a distinct landing and subsequent jump. Rather, it should be one continuous motion. This is an intense exercise, so volume and frequency should be adapted to allow adequate recovery in between workouts. Because of the intense nature of this exercise, it is recommended that only experienced (at least 1–2 yr) athletes perform this drill.

Depth Jump (Drop Jump) to Another Box or Bench

Intensity: High to Very High

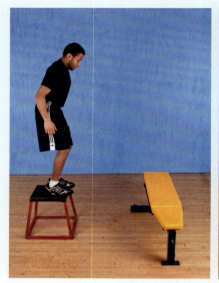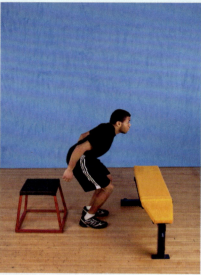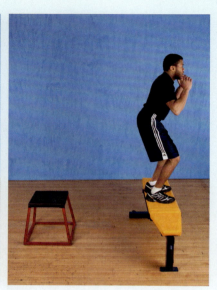

FIGURE 15.26 Depth jump (drop jump) to another box or bench.

- Athlete begins with arms at the sides, shoulder width stance, and knees slightly bent on top of a box (with toes near or hanging over the edge of the box). Box heights vary between 20 and 115 cm. Intensity increases as box height increases.
- The athlete steps off of the box, lands on the ground, and explosively jumps vertically (with double-arm action) as high as possible upon landing.
- The athlete jumps and lands on to a second box or bench. The distance between boxes and height of the boxes can vary based on goals of the exercise. A smaller box with a greater distance from the start box can be used to stress the long jump, whereas a taller box located close to the start box can be used to train the vertical jump. Some have suggested a length of 24 in. in between boxes to start with (5,10) (Fig. 15.26).

VARIATIONS A variation of this exercise (e.g. reverse depth jump) is to use one box. The athlete begins on top of the box facing backward (toward the box as opposed to away from the box). The athlete drops off of the box, lands on the ground, and explosively jumps back on to the top of the box as quickly as possible.

Single-Leg Depth Jump

Intensity: Very High

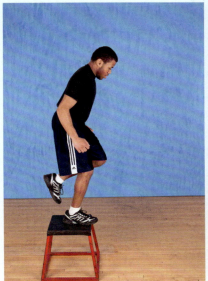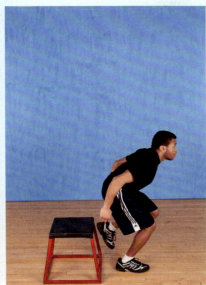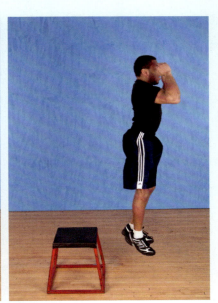

FIGURE 15.27 Single-leg depth jump.

- Similar to the depth jump with the exception, the athlete lands on one foot and explosively jumps off the landing foot (Fig. 15.27).

> **VARIATIONS** This variation is very intense and requires a shorter box in comparison to the double-leg depth jump. It is reserved for trained to highly trained athletes.

Upper-Body and Core Plyometric Exercises

Medicine Ball Chest Pass

Intensity: Low

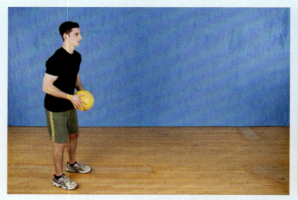
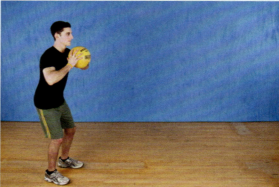
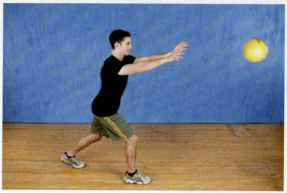

FIGURE 15.28 Medicine ball chest pass.

- Athlete begins with a shoulder width stance with knees slightly bent and grasps an MB or core ball (2–15 lb or more) at chest height with shoulders flexed and abducted with elbows pointing outward.
- After a countermovement, the athlete explosively puts or throws the ball forward. The athlete may maintain his or her stance during the pass or take a step forward to generate momentum.
- The athlete may use a partner, wall, open space, or rebounder when performing this exercise. A partner or rebounder is advantageous because the ball is returned to the athlete after release. This forces the athlete to catch the ball prior to performing the next repetition. Catching the ball and explosively performing another pass stress the SSC to a greater extent (via loaded ECC action). A rebounder is an angled trampoline-like device, which forcefully returns the ball back to the athlete upon contact (Fig. 15.28).

CAUTION! The athlete must focus on catching the MB if a partner or rebounder is used. Failure to properly catch the ball could lead to injury and disrupted technique.

VARIATIONS Variations of this exercise (Fig. 15.29) include performing the chest pass from a running start and seated, squat thrust, or kneeling position. This exercise can also be performed simultaneously with a sit-up where the MB is passed to a partner. A rotation can be added to the chest pass or a side chest throw. Another popular similar exercise is the *wall ball* with usually more than a 10-lb medicine ball. The athlete front squats the medicine ball, throws the ball upward against the wall, catches, and repeats.

This exercise may be preceded by a lower-body plyometric exercise.

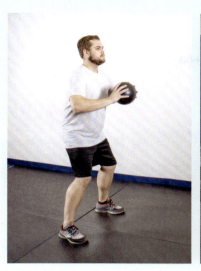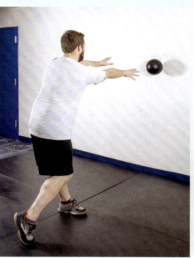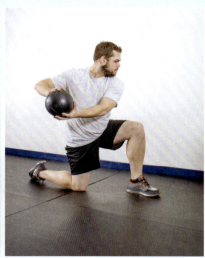

FIGURE 15.29 Standing rotational MB pass and kneeling rotational MB pass.

Overhead Medicine Ball Throw

Intensity: Low

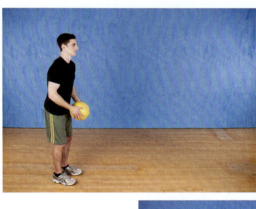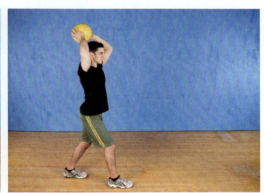
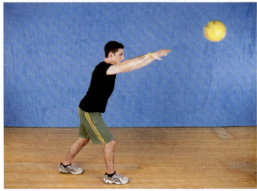

FIGURE 15.30 Overhead medicine ball throw.

- Athlete begins with a shoulder width stance with knees slightly bent and grasps an MB or core ball at chest height.
- The athlete lifts the MB to an overhead position, steps forward with one foot, and explosively throws the ball.
- The athlete may use a partner, wall, open space, or rebounder when performing the exercise (Fig. 15.30).

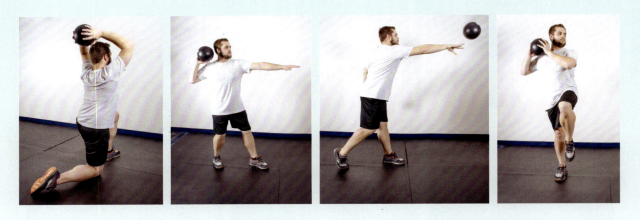

FIGURE 15.31 Kneeling overhead (OH) MB throw, the single-arm OH throw, and the MB baseball throw.

VARIATIONS Variations of this exercise (Fig. 15.31) include performing the overhead MB throw from a staggered stance, running start, and seated or kneeling position. This exercise can be performed with one arm using a lighter MB and a wind-up may be added. This version is used to mimic the demands of throwing a ball and is an excellent exercise for baseball and softball players, quarterbacks, etc. The single-arm overhead throw with a small MB can be performed from a shoulder width stance, staggered stance, running start, or kneeling position. The direction cf the throw can vary (athlete can throw the ball to a partner, off of a wall, for distance, or throw the ball off of the ground).

Medicine Ball Back (Scoop) Throw

Intensity: Low

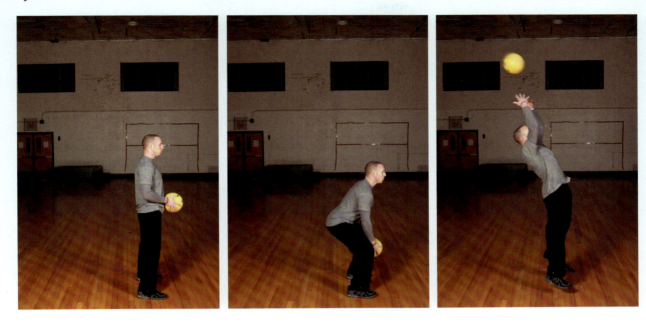

FIGURE 15.32 Medicine ball back throw.

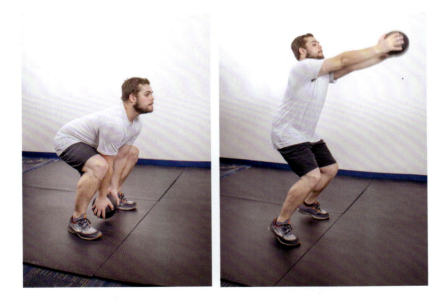

FIGURE 15.33 Medicine ball forward scoop throw.

- The athlete begins with a slightly past shoulder width stance, knees bent, and arms extended in front of the body grasping an MB or core ball.
- A countermovement is performed where the athlete flexes at the hip and knees, and then explosively extends and hyperextends the hips and back, flexes the shoulders, and throws the ball backward as far as possible (Fig. 15.32).

VARIATIONS A variation of this exercise is to perform it seated or throw the ball forward and up instead of back (Fig. 15.33). The exercise may be performed after landing from a broad or depth jump.

Single-Arm Vertical Core Ball Throw

Intensity: Low to Moderate

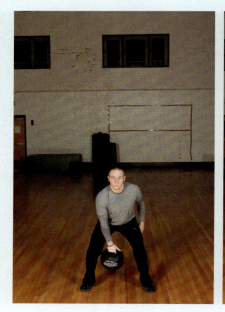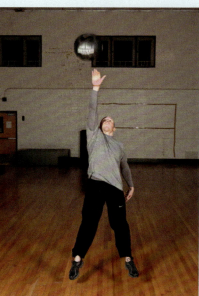

FIGURE 15.34 Single-arm vertical core ball throw.

- The athlete begins with a slightly past shoulder width stance, knees bent, and throwing arm extended in front of the body between the legs grasping a core ball.
- A countermovement is performed where the athlete flexes at the hip and knees and then explosively extends and hyperextends the hips and back, flexes the shoulders, and throws the core ball vertically up as high as possible. This technique is similar to performing a single-arm dumbbell snatch with the exception the core ball is released vertically (Fig. 15.34).

Overhead Medicine Ball Slams

Intensity: Low

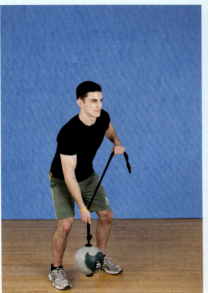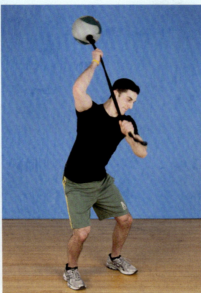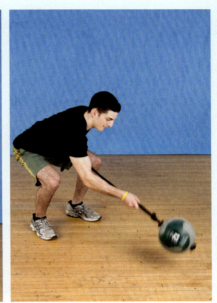

FIGURE 15.35 Overhead medicine ball slams.

- The athlete begins with a slightly wider than shoulder width stance, knees bent, and an MB held at arm's length in front of the body.
- The countermovement entails the athlete extends the hips back and raises the MB to the overhead position.
- Athlete explosively flexes the waist and hips and throws the MB forcefully off of the ground.

- This exercise may be performed with a core ball, slam ball (Fig. 15.35), or keg. If a slam ball is used, the athlete can slam it off of the floor or wall in front of the body. A variation is to use an overhead rotational slam versus a direct overhead vertical slam, or use a single-leg slam. Another variation is to perform side-to-side or diagonal rotational repeat slams off of a wall located directly behind the athlete.

Medicine Ball Underhand Toss

Intensity: Low

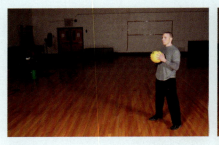 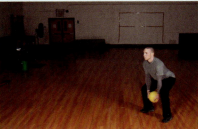 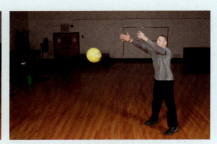

FIGURE 15.36 Medicine ball underhand toss.

- The athlete begins with a slightly wider than shoulder width stance, knees bent, and an MB held at arm's length in front of the body.
- A countermovement is performed where the athlete flexes at the hip and knees, and then explosively extends and hyper-extends the hips and back, flexes the shoulders, and tosses the ball forward.
- The athlete may use a partner, wall, open space, or rebounder when performing the exercise. A partner, wall, or rebounder is advantageous because the ball is returned to the athlete after release (Fig. 15.36).

> **VARIATIONS** A variation is to perform the exercise from the side. Athlete will begin the throw from a side position (where the MB is located lateral to the knee), rotate, and explosively toss the MB understand for distance and/or speed. The exercise may also be performed while doing a back hyperextension in the weight room.

Medicine Ball Side Toss

Intensity: Low

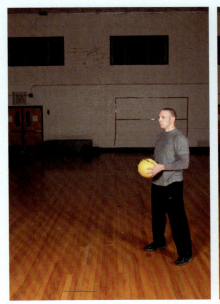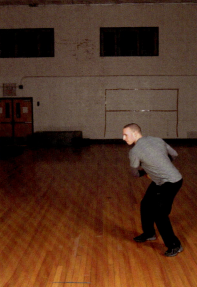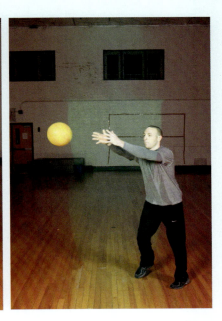

FIGURE 15.37 Medicine ball side toss.

- The athlete begins with a slightly wider than shoulder width stance, knees slightly bent, and arms extended to one side of the body grasping an MB or core ball.
- The countermovement entails the athlete rotate to the side of the MB and explosively tosses the ball in the opposite direction across the body (rotating the opposite side to toss the ball).
- The athlete may use a partner, wall, open space, or rebounder when performing the exercise. This exercise may be performed kneeling, seated, or with a slam ball (against the wall).
- Throws are then performed to the opposite side (Fig. 15.37).

Pullover Pass

Intensity: Low

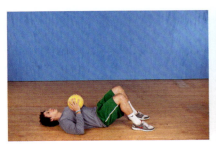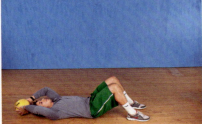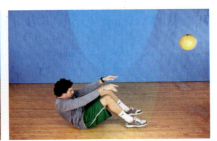

FIGURE 15.38 Pullover pass.

- The athlete lies on the ground or stability ball with knees flexed and feet flat on the floor.
- Athlete lifts the MB or core ball overhead and passes the ball to a partner with straight arms (Fig. 15.38).

> **VARIATIONS** A variation is to incorporate a sit-up or torso rotation while throwing the ball.

Medicine Ball Power Drop

Intensity: *High*

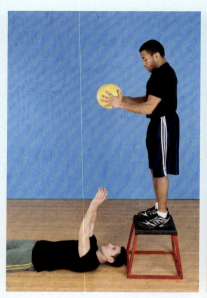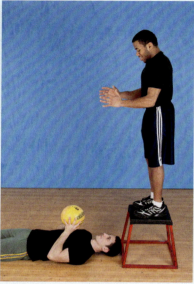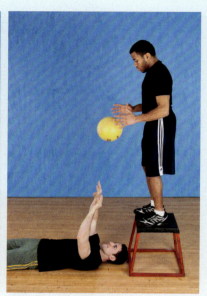

FIGURE 15.39 Medicine ball power drop.

- A partner is needed for this exercise. The partner stands on a plyo box or bench 20–115-cm high holding an MB at arm's length with arms parallel to the ground.
- The athlete begins lying on the ground with arms extended upward and (perpendicular to the floor) with the head near the base of the plyo box or bench. The athlete's arm should be located directly under the MB held by the partner.
- The partner drops the ball and the athlete catches and lowers the ball to chest level (accentuated ECC countermovement).

The athlete then explosively passes (chest presses) the ball back up to the partner (Fig. 15.39).

> **CAUTION!** Caution needs to be used because failure to catch the ball (by either the athlete or partner) could result in injury.

Plyometric Push-Up

Intensity: *Moderate*

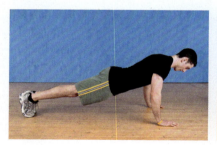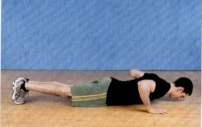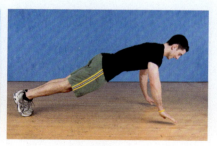

FIGURE 15.40 Plyometric push-up.

- The athlete begins the exercise in a standard push-up position.
- The athlete descends and explosively performs a push-up where the athlete's hands temporarily leave the ground. Some athletes will clap their hands at this point.
- The athlete lands, descends, and continues to perform another repetition (Fig. 15.40).

Depth Push-Up

Intensity: High

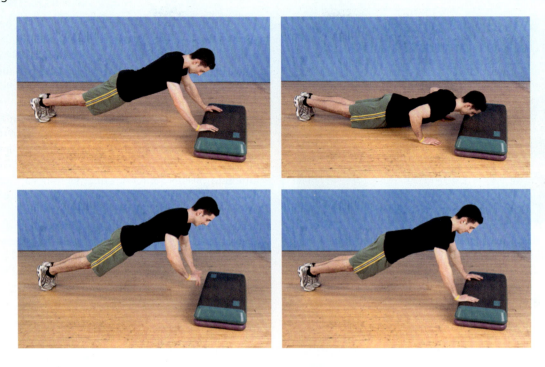

FIGURE 15.41 Depth push-up.

- This exercise is similar to the plyometric push-up except the athlete begins the exercise from an elevated position. MBs, steps, benches, or small boxes can be used for elevation.
- The athlete drops from the elevated height, performs a plyo push-up, and completes the repetition by maintaining the starting position elevated from the ball or box. The athlete needs to explode high enough to ensure he or she can transition to the elevated starting position (Fig. 15.41). Using two boxes or steps laterally placed at the level of each arm is recommended when large elevations are used as it provides a clear path for the head during descent.

Bag Thrusts

Intensity: Low

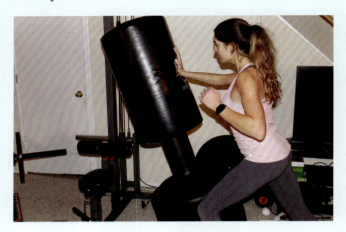

FIGURE 15.42 Bag thrusts.

- A heavy bag or floor bag (Wavemaster) is needed for this exercise.
- The athlete begins with shoulder width stance with feet staggered. The athlete then explosively thrusts hand into the bag (using the limb on the same side of the back leg) (Fig. 15.42).

> **VARIATIONS** Variations of the exercise include a two-handed thrust. The athlete may also use the heavy bag for boxing or martial art strikes. These include various forms of punches, blocks, and kicks.

Pendulum Exercises

Intensity: Low to High

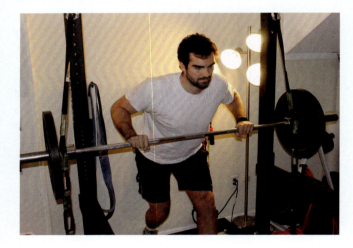

FIGURE 15.43 Pendulum exercises.

- A large MB suspended from a rope hanging from a tall structure is needed for one of these drills. A suspended barbell from a power rack using straps can also be used.
- The athlete can perform multiple throws using an MB or barbell as a pendulum.

- Variations include one- and two-arm overhead throws and chest pass. These can be performed from a standing or kneeling position. Several barbell exercises can also be performed from different postures.
- Catching the ball or barbell is required for these drills, which increases the difficulty (Fig. 15.43).

> **VARIATIONS** A lower-body variation can be performed. The athlete uses a swing-type apparatus suspended from a high support mechanism in close proximity to a wall. Upon swinging, the athlete will contact the wall and explosively push off leading to a subsequent oscillation. The swing can be made heavier to increasing loading during the ECC component to target the yielding phase (1,4). In addition, sturdy uprights can be placed before the swing (in the swings path) to modify the exercise to target the upper body (4). For both variations, the height of the backswing (in addition to loading) affects intensity, *e.g.,* greater backswing yields greater impact force. This variation is a high-intensity drill.

Combination Exercises

Exercises can be combined to form complex drills but ones that also increase sport specificity. Some examples of plyo exercises combined with other modalities or sport-specific movements are the broad jump with lateral or forward sprint, depth jump with MB chest throw, depth jump with lateral sprint, depth jump with football block, and the depth jump with basketball rim touch or dunk.

Intensity

The intensity of plyometric exercises has been defined as the amount of stress placed on involved skeletal muscles, joints, and connective tissues (56) and depends on several factors including the exercise complexity, loading, speed, and the size and length of boxes or barriers used. Historically, plyometric training exercises were generally classified as low, moderate, or high intensity based on body weight, jump height, speed of exercise, and points of contact during landing (59). Recent studies have shown that this classification system does not accurately reflect the true intensity of some exercises (27,60). Researchers have used force plate data (*e.g.*, GRF, during landing and propulsion, RFD, reactive strength index, and joint power absorption) and EMG in an attempt to quantify intensity (27,49,60–62). The Interpreting Research box depicts some results of studies comparing different plyometric exercises.

Plyometric training intensity is related to the magnitude of jump performance improvement (58). The complexity relates to the type of drill used. Double-leg jumps-in-place are low to moderate in intensity, followed by standing jumps, multiple hops and jumps, bounding, box drills, and single-leg exercises (2,5). However, the height attained during a standing jump is critical to where landing forces can exceed that of a depth jump for athletes with high jump capacity (59). Depth jumps are a very intense type of plyometric exercise especially when large boxes are used. Higher loading during landing increases the intensity of the plyometric drill. Loading increases when the mass of the athlete increases (from external loading with weighted vests or weights) and when the velocity of impact increases (from higher jump heights). Single-leg jumps are more intense than comparable double-leg jumps. Single-leg plyometric training may provide more comprehensive increases in jump performance and RFD compared to bilateral-only training (57). In addition, single-leg jumps (hurdle hops) produce higher levels of muscle activation in the gluteus medius, gluteus maximus, and medial and lateral hamstring muscles compared to double-leg hops (63), which could have positive effects on strengthening the lower extremity in reducing risks of knee injuries. Both types of exercises are beneficial, but unilateral training may have greater spillover to activities that involve single-limb movements. Although intensity classification is difficult due to several aforementioned factors, each exercise presented in this chapter is categorized as low, moderate, or high intensity (or hybrid intensity) based on suggested classifications as a guide for exercise selection. The intensity of plyometric training can be increased by adding a low to moderate amount of external loading. For example, using a weighted vest, MB, KB, dumbbells, or other loading device can increase the intensity of plyometric training. Although some studies indicated greater performance improvements with external loading added to plyometric training, the results of a meta-analysis revealed no such performance augmentation (58). The athlete's body weight plays a role as one plyometric drill may be more intense in an athlete of greater size than a smaller athlete. Intensity is increased by using larger barriers or boxes or by setting cones/barriers further apart. This requires the athlete to jump higher or further per repetition. Plyometric training programs begin with low- and moderate-intensity exercises and progresses to higher intensity exercises over time. Table 15.1 illustrates a continuum of plyometric exercises based on intensity. Low-, moderate-, and high-intensity classifications are used although some exercises could be included under multiple headings, and it is important to note that any exercise listed (including low-intensity drills) can be made more intense via methods previously described Case Study 15.1.

> ### Case Study 15.1
>
> Kevin is a heavy school soccer player who wants to begin a plyometric training program. He comes to you for a consultation and wants to know which plyometric exercises would be appropriate for him and specific for the skills needed by a soccer player.
>
> **Question for Consideration:** What plyometric exercises would you recommend for Kevin based on his training level?

Exercise Order

Plyometric exercises can be sequenced in numerous ways. As opposed to RT, there are few sequencing recommendations for plyometric training. Plyometric training studies have used a multitude of sequence combinations and showed positive results. Most sequencing patterns can be beneficial provided adequate recovery is given in between sets and exercises. Low-intensity drills can be included anywhere in sequence. Many coaches prefer to include one or two at the beginning of a workout to help the athlete better warm-up or become more prepared for subsequent high-intensity drills. Low-intensity drills can be performed later in the workout after other key moderate- and high-intensity drills are performed. Moderate- and high-intensity drills are typically performed near the beginning (following appropriate warm-up and low-intensity

Interpreting Research
Kinetic Quantification of Plyometric Exercise Intensity

Ebben WP, Fauth ML, Garceau LR, Petushek EJ. Kinetic quantification of plyometric exercise intensity. *J Strength Cond Res.* 2011;25:3288–98.

Kossow AJ, Ebben WP. Kinetic analysis of horizontal plyometric exercise intensity. *J Strength Cond Res.* 2017;32: 1222–9.

Both studies examined intensity of vertical and horizontal plyometric exercises via force plate data collection. Ebben et al. (60) quantified plyometric intensity by using force plates to measure peak takeoff ground reaction force (with and minus body mass), time to takeoff, flight time, jump height, peak power, landing RFD, and peak vertical landing ground reaction force (with and minus body mass). The exercises studied were line hops, cone hops, squat jumps, tuck jumps, countermovement jumps with and without dumbbells (30% of 1 RM), depth jumps, and single-leg jumps. They found the following:

◆ Line and cone hops produced the lowest time to takeoff while single-leg jumps and loaded jump squats produced the highest.
◆ Highest ground reaction forces during takeoff were seen in cone hops > tuck jumps > line hops and countermovement jumps > loaded jump squat > squat jump > single-leg jump.
◆ Peak power was highest in loaded jump squat > depth jump and countermovement jump > tuck jump > squat jump > single-leg jump > cone hops > line hops
◆ Jump height and flight time were highest for depth jumps, countermovement jumps, and tuck jumps while lowest for line and cone hops

◆ Landing ground reaction forces were highest in depth jump > countermovement jump > loaded jump squat > squat jump > tuck jump > single-leg jump > cone hops > line hops

The authors (59,60) developed a continuum of plyometric intensity (from highest to lowest) where single-leg jumps > depth jumps from high boxes > tuck/pike jumps > jump and reach > loaded jump squats > squat jumps > tall cone hops > short cone hops/pogos/split squat jumps

Kossow and Ebben (27) quantified horizontal plyometric intensity by using force plates to measure peak landing ground reaction force and RFD for the double-leg hop, standing long jump, single-leg long jump, bounding, skipping, power skipping, cone hops, and hurdle hops. They found the following:

◆ Peak vertical GRF was highest in the standing long jump > hops > single-leg long jump > bounding and skipping.
◆ Greatest forces in the sagittal planes were seen in double- and single-leg long jumps; frontal plane = bounding > long jump and single-leg long jump.
◆ Peak RFD was highest in the standing long jump > double leg hop > single-leg long jump > bounding > hurdle hops > skipping.

The results showed that skipping was lower in intensity followed by double leg and hurdle hops and bounding, double-, and single-leg long jumps were more intense.

---

drills), while fatigue is minimal and energy levels are high. Because the intensity level is greater, it is most beneficial to the athlete to perform these drills early to maximize SSC activity. When upper-body plyometric drills are included, the athlete may choose to alternate between lower- and upper-body drills (similar to RT). The rationale is to provide greater recovery in between exercises. Upper-body plyometric exercises can be staggered in between lower-body drills to maximize workout efficiency without compromising SSC performance. Lastly, plyometric exercises may be incorporated into an RT workout (known as complex training) (2,5). A technically similar plyometric exercise can be performed in between sets of a similar resistance exercise. Some sample pairings may include performing squat jumps in between the sets of barbell back squats, tuck jumps in between sets of front squats, box jumps in between sets of hang cleans, a MB chest pass in between sets of the bench press, and bag thrusts (or striking a heavy bag)

in between sets of ISOM wall pushes or the close-grip bench press. Postactivation potentiation occurs during the performance of plyometric drills after resistance exercises. Acute power enhancement may be augmented when using complex training. Although research shows that complex training acutely enhances athletic power (64), short-term training studies have not shown complex training to be more effective for enhancing power or vertical jump performance to a greater degree than performing plyometric and RT separately (65). Thus, integrating plyometric exercises into an RT workout appears equally as effective for enhancing power as separate workouts. Metabolic training, or high-intensity interval training, programs commonly incorporate several plyometric drills (*e.g.*, box jumps, squat jumps) in addition to RT, agility, speed exercises, into the program design. Given the nature of these programs targeting endurance predominately, plyometric exercises can be performed anywhere in sequence.

Table 15.1 Plyometric Exercise Intensity Continuum

Low Intensity	Moderate Intensity	High Intensity
Pogos	Barrier jumps	Pike jump
Side-to-side ankle hop	Tuck jumps	Single-leg vertical jump
Squat jump	Jump and reach	Single-leg hops
Standing long jump	Double leg hops	Depth plyo push-up
Cone hops	Box jumps	MB power drop
Split squat jump	Alternate bounding	Single-leg bounding
Skipping	Multiple box jumps	Depth jump and variations
MB chest pass	Plyo push-up	Pendulum swings
Single-arm vertical CB throw	Triple jump	Single-leg box jump
Overhead MB throw		
MB back throw		
Overhead MB slam		
MB underhand throw		
Pullover pass		
MB side throw		
MB front rotation throw		
Bag thrusts		

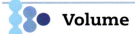

Volume

Volume represents the total number of sets and reps performed during a plyometric workout and depend on training intensity and frequency as well as the impact of other training modalities. For lower-body plyometrics, the number of foot contacts or distance covered denotes training volume. For upper-body or core plyometrics, the number of reps (throws, passes, or tosses) represents training volume.

Similar to other modalities of exercise, plyometric volume and intensity are inversely related. Few guidelines regarding plyometric training volume are available. Meta-analytic data have shown a positive relationship between the number of jumps per session (more than 50 jumps) during lower body plyometric training and performance enhancement (58). However, a minimum volume threshold exists to where further increases will not be advantageous (58). Chu (2) has recommended some guidelines for plyometric training that are listed in Table 15.2.

Table 15.2 Plyometric Training Volumes Based on Experience[a]

Status	Off-Season	Preseason	In-Season
Beginner	60–100	100–250	Depends on sport
Intermediate	100–150	150–300	Depends on sport
Advanced	120–200	150–450	Depends on sport

[a]Numbers represent foot contacts per workout. Warm-up exercises are not included. The wide range of values during preseason indicates variations in intensity. That is, high-intensity drills yield lower volumes, whereas low- and moderate-intensity drills yield higher volumes. In-season volume depends on the sport as volume will be low in sports that are highly plyometric in nature.

Adapted by permission, from Chu DA. *Jumping into Plyometrics*. 2nd ed. Champaign (IL): Human Kinetics; 1998. 29 p.

Frequency

Frequency refers to the number of training sessions per week. Plyometric training typically takes place 1–4 days per week and nearly 80% of plyometric training studies have used frequencies of 2–3 days per week (56). Training frequency will depend on other variables such as intensity and volume, as well as the inclusion of other training modalities. High-intensity training may necessitate a lower frequency especially when depth jumps are performed, and frequency may be lower when other modalities are included. In-season training of athletes necessitates a low training frequency. Sport practices and competitions include plyometric actions so training must be developed around the intensity/volume of plyometric actions seen in the sport. Thus, maintenance plyometric training of 1–2 days per week may suffice which could offset any potential detraining effects. Because of the intense nature of plyometric training, ~48–72 hours of recovery in between training sessions is recommended (2,10). Few frequency comparative studies have been conducted. For example, de Villarreal et al. (13) showed that 1 and 2 days per week (with double the number of drop jumps) frequencies produced greater improvements in vertical jump and sprinting speed than high-frequency (4 d·wk^{-1} with quadruple the number of drop jumps) training. Thus, coaches must use their best judgment in prescribing plyometric training frequencies. Similar to RT, it is the intensity and volume that may be the key variables provided that the frequency selected allows adequate recovery time between workouts.

Rest Intervals

Rest intervals between sets, reps, and plyometric exercises are critical for training adaptations. Adequate rest intervals are needed when maximizing power is the goal. For noncontinuous or single-repetition jumps (depth jump) or throws, intraset rest intervals are useful for maximizing power. For example, 5–10 seconds of rest in between submaximal depth jumps is recommended with 2–3 minutes of rest in between sets (10). However, maximal depth jumps require longer intraset (up to 2–4 min) and interset (>5–10 min) rest intervals (4). Rest interval lengths are exercise-specific and depend on the intensity. More recovery may be needed in between sets for high-intensity drills than low- or moderate-intensity drills. For example, a 30-second rest interval between sets of ankle hops is sufficient but maybe not sufficient when performing sets of box jumps. Work-to-rest ratios of 1:5–1:10 are recommended (2,10). Using a 1:10 ratio, an athlete would rest ~100 seconds if the total set length was 10 seconds. Thus, 1:5 ratio may be applied to low- and moderate-intensity drills and 1:10 ratio to higher-intensity drills. Most plyometric training studies have used rest intervals averaging ~120 seconds (56). Shorter rest interval lengths minimize recovery and train power endurance in the athlete. This could be a goal of the coach during anaerobic conditioning phases, but rest interval prescription for plyometric training targeting maximal power should allow adequate recovery and will be longer in length.

Other Considerations in Plyometric Training Program Design

Designing plyometric training programs depends on additional factors. These include the warm-up, age, training status, surface, and equipment availability.

Warm-Up

All plyometric training programs must begin with a proper warm-up. A general warm-up may be used initially (3–5 min of jogging) followed by a specific warm-up. The specific warm-up exercises selected are used to physiologically prepare the athlete for the workout and facilitate core musculature for the demands of plyometric exercises. They are used to develop fundamental movement skills and coordination transferable to plyometric training. Drills are low in intensity. Some examples of good plyometric training warm-up drills include marching, high-knees, butt kicks, skipping, lunges, back pedaling, side shuffles, cariocas, and progressive form running. These drills are commonly used in preparation for sprint and agility training. In addition, dynamic flexibility and corrective exercises may be used to prepare the body for plyometrics. The warm-up can consist of 10- to 20-m length drills where the athlete performs the set in one direction, rests, and returns back for a second set, or performs a set up and walks back to increase recovery in between sets. If a group of athletes are warming-up together, each athlete can rest a few seconds more while another squad is performing the drill. At least 10 total sets are performed (1–3 sets per drill).

Age

The majority of scientific and practical information regarding plyometric training has focused on young adults and adults typically in their 20s and 30s. However, the use of plyometric training in children, adolescents, and middle-aged to older adults has received attention, and in some cases scrutiny. Part of the issue dealing with plyometric training in these populations has been the diverse terminology in defining plyometrics. Some view plyometrics in classic terms as predominantly depth jumping at high levels of intensity. In contrast, many view plyometrics in modern terms as exercises that stress the SSC which vary greatly in intensity. A proponent of modern plyometrics may propose that plyometrics can be beneficial for most individuals regardless of age. Throughout this chapter, numerous plyometric exercises were illustrated and explained. These exercises vary in intensity and many low-intensity drills are appropriate for many populations. Plyometric training can be safe and effective for individuals regardless of age when properly administered and supervised (66,67).

Plyometric exercises can benefit middle-age and older adults. Muscular power deteriorates at a faster rate than strength loss with aging; therefore, attempts to maintain or improve power can be beneficial to improving fitness. Part of the perception in society is that plyometric exercises are more reserved for young adults. However, plyometric actions are commonly performed in middle-age and older adults who frequently play pick-up games of basketball or racquetball for example. Masters athletes benefit greatly from plyometric training. Precaution must be used regarding potential orthopedic limitations, and plyometrics may be contraindicated for some. Plyometric training guidelines for adults may be used for masters athletes with the exception that volume may be lower and low- to moderate-intensity drills are preferred (10).

Training Status

Plyometric training program design depends on the training status of the athlete. Novice athletes should begin with a basic program composed of low- to moderate-intensity drills and progress to high-intensity drills gradually over time as conditioning and coordination improve. Trained athletes have greater tolerance and can perform higher-intensity drills and a higher volume of exercise. In the past, the strength level of the athlete was considered within the training status domain. Early European coaches recommended that athletes needed to have great strength, *e.g.*, able to squat at least 1.5–2.5 times their body weight and have high levels of ECC and explosive ISOM strength, before beginning plyometric training (4). These guidelines were never intended to apply to submaximal plyometric drills. If this were the case, few athletes would qualify, and this suggestion no longer is relevant for several plyometric exercises. These early suggestions were made due to the fact that depth jumping comprised classic plyometrics, and impact forces could exceed six times the athlete's body weight (4). It would not be logical to force an athlete to have high levels of strength in order to begin a program consisting of basic vertical jumps or pogos. Others have recommended that athletes be able to squat 1.5 times their body weight, bench press their body weight (for heavy athletes) or 1.5 times their body weight (for athletes who weigh <220 lb), perform five plyo push-ups in a row, and be able to perform speed squats and bench presses (five repetitions in <5 s with 60% of body weight) (10). These standards are applied mostly to high-intensity drills. Others have used other prescreening tests such as balance tests (*i.e.*, the Klatt test) or jump tests (*i.e.*, the tuck jump) to assess readiness for plyometric training. A coach may use periodic evaluation of their athletes to determine if that athlete is ready to proceed to more intense training. Although it may be helpful for an athlete to have a solid strength foundation (especially adequate ECC strength), other fitness components are critical including balance, coordination, power, speed, and agility. Because plyometric training improves all of these fitness components, an athlete of lesser conditioning and strength can greatly benefit from plyometric training but mostly via low- to moderate-intensity drills.

Myths & Misconceptions
Plyometric Training Is Harmful for Children and Adolescents

Children and adolescents benefit from plyometric training, and plyometric training can help children and adolescents become physically fit and adequately prepared for various youth sports (85). Many playground activities and games (hop-scotch) children play are plyometric in nature (activate the SSC) so the thought of plyometric training in youth is not novel. Plyometric training in children and adolescents is supported by prominent S&C organizations (68). Some misconceptions concerning plyometric training in youth is that it is unsafe (causes growth plate injuries), and this type of training is inappropriate or unnecessary in youth. However, research does not support the contention that plyometrics are dangerous and a growing body of evidence supports the efficacy of plyometric training in children and adolescents (53,68). Studies investigating youth plyometric training have shown it to be safe and effective for performance improvements (68,69). Youth plyometric training improves jumping ability, running time, push-up performance, and speed (68–70), and these augmentations occur beyond the changes that are associated with typical activity experienced in physical education classes (70). The results from recent meta-analyses concluded that plyometric training of low-to-moderate volume increases lower- and upper-body muscle power, MB throw distance, VJ height and long jump distance, reactive strength index, leg stiffness, sprint speed, agility, balance, and motor performance (*e.g.*, kicking and throwing velocity) in male and female youth ages 6–18 years particularly in children that are in the pre-peak height velocity (10–13 yr of age) and post (16–18 yr of age) maturation stages (71–73). The range of improvements in power measures was ~1%–47% with most studies showing improvements in selected measures ~3%–10% (71). Children and adolescents respond more favorably than adults to plyometric training when it comes to soreness responses after exercise (74). Youth plyometric training programs should begin with low-intensity drills where proper form and technique are stressed. A gradual progression to moderate-intensity drills should be used where the major goals are to increase youth fitness, balance and coordination, and performance. Research has not determined an appropriate minimal age for initiating a plyometric training program but some S&C professionals have had success training children 7–8 years of age provided they have the emotional maturity to listen to instructions and perform the exercises properly (10). The decision to allow a child/adolescent to perform technique-driven plyometrics should be based on individual needs, goals, and interests.

Training Surface

Plyometric training can be performed in a variety of places. The surface selected should be yielding and provide some give to reduce the overall joint stress to the body. However, the surface should not be too yielding. Impellizzeri et al. (75) showed 4 weeks of plyometric training on grass and sand increased jumping and sprint performance. However, grass produced superior results, while less soreness was shown after plyometric training in the sand. Grass and turf fields are popular choices for plyometric training as open fields have the benefit of enabling longer-distance drills to be performed. Matted floors and gymnastics floors are acceptable training surfaces. The mats cannot be too thick as this can excessively increase the amortization phase (10) and not maximize the SSC. Concrete and hardwood floors lack the shock-absorbing ability and may cause undue strain to the athlete. Some studies have examined the potential of aquatic plyometric training. Training in the water has the advantage of increasing resistance during jumping (based on the depth of the water) but the disadvantage of minimizing ECC loading due to the buoyancy of the water. Stemm and Jacobson (76) and Martel (77) showed that aquatic plyometric training increased vertical jump. Other studies showed that aquatic plyometric training increased strength, jump performance, and sprint performance (24). Aquatic plyometric training can be effective especially for single-leg exercises (4). The level of inclination or declination in the surface is important. Often plyometric training will take place on a relatively even surface. However, surface angular alterations can pose a new stimulus for training. Plyometric training uphill increases the metabolic demand and force requirement, whereas plyometric training downhill increases the ECC component, intensity, and results in greater postexercise muscle soreness. One study showed that incline plyometrics augmented jump performance more so than plyometric training on a flat surface (78).

Plyometric Training Equipment

Plyometric training can be performed without any specialized equipment. However, some pieces of equipment may be needed in order to perform some drills. Some common pieces of equipment include cones, boxes, jump ropes, mini hurdles, bands, bags, weighted vests, MBs, slam balls, and core balls. Cones can be used as barriers or guides or can be used as obstacles for various hops and jumps. Cones usually range in size from small (4.5 in.) to large (18 in.). Boxes are used for box jumps, depth jumps, and variations. Plyo boxes come in various sizes but must be sturdy to offset the explosive nature of plyometric exercises. Many boxes will be made of wood or tubular steel capable of withstanding large levels of force. Boxes come in various sizes from small (~6 in.) to large (~42 in. or greater). Smaller boxes are used for hops with larger boxes used for box jumps and depth jumps. Important to box selection is the upper surface. The box top surface should be made of nonskid rubber for greater friction and stability upon landing. The surface dimensions may range from 14 × 14 in. for smaller boxes to 20 × 20 in. for larger boxes. Some smaller boxes have added utilities. There are angled boxes with multiple surfaces that allow for lateral plyometric exercises. Jump ropes come in various forms and sizes with some designed more for speed and some to provide some resistance. Hurdles serve as barriers/obstacles for hops and jumps. Hurdles typically range in size from 6 to 12 in. up to 42 in. or higher. Some hurdles are adjustable which can be used for multiple exercises.

Bands provide resistance to jumping. Several styles are currently on the market. One particular resisted jump training device is the Vertimax (Fig. 15.44). The Vertimax consists of a matted platform with resistance bands attached to a waist harness that gives the athlete resistance during several types of jumps. The loading from the bands creates greater ECC loading upon landing, which serves as a potent stimulus for plyometric training. Several studies have examined jump training with the Vertimax. Rhea et al. (79,80) showed that 12 weeks of training with the Vertimax produced superior increases in vertical jump height and power in athletes than unloaded plyometric training. However, McClenton et al. (81) showed that 6 weeks of depth jump training versus jump training on the Vertimax produced similar increases in performance, and Carlson et al. (82) showed that 6 weeks of jump training on the Vertimax was no more effective than RT or plyometric training for increasing jump performance. Nevertheless, jump training on the Vertimax is effective for enhancing jump performance. Weighted vests can be used for additional resistance during plyometric drills. Various vests are available but typically allow external loading of up to 30 lb or more but caution must be used as external loading may be most appropriate for low- and moderate-intensity drills. Some newer models of weighted vests allow the athlete to add more than 200 lbs but these vests cab be used for more exercises than just plyometric drills. Bags (boxing, football) can be used as obstacles for jumping over. Medicine, core, and slam balls come in various sizes and are used for upper- and lower-body plyometrics.

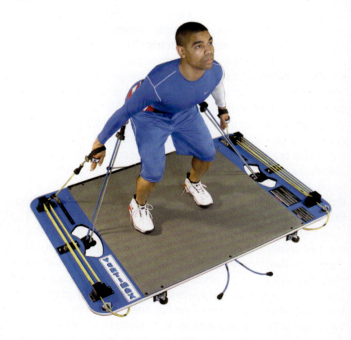

FIGURE 15.44 The vertimax. (Courtesy of Perform Better, Cranston, RI.)

Plyometrics and Safety Considerations

Plyometric training is safe for athletes of all ages provided that common sense is used in the program design, and it is properly supervised. A recent review indicated that participation in plyometric training was not associated with injury incidence (56). The most common reasons for injuries during plyometric training are (a) violation of training guidelines, (b) inadequate warm-up, (c) too high a rate of progression, (d) lack of skill, (e) poor surface selection, (f) improper volume or intensity, and (g) undisclosed predisposition (10). Violations of training guidelines, coupled with high volume with too high intensity (or progressing too much too soon), could result in overreaching and subsequent overtraining of the athlete. Overtrained athletes are more susceptible to injury. For plyometric training, it is the quality of the workout that is important and not quantity per se especially when depth jumps are performed. Volume and frequency need to be carefully prescribed based on the training phase. Inadequate warm-ups force the athlete to embark upon intense, explosive muscular contractions without proper physiologic preparation thereby increasing the risk of injury.

Lack of skill is a particular problem for coaches and athletes. Poor technique among athletes may limit exercise selection. Sufficient coordination, balance, and strength are needed for performance of several plyometric exercises including those moderate to high in intensity. Coaches need to stress proper jumping mechanics with athletes at all phases of training. Critical to proper jump technique is the landing where large levels of force are absorbed by the athlete's body. Peak impact forces during jumping can be greater than the peak propulsion forces. Improper landing can place the athlete at greater risk of injury. Exercise selection can accommodate athletes with subpar skill development. Plyometric drills range in complexity. Beginning exercises may comprise the entire workout for poorly conditioned athletes. The athletes need to demonstrate improvement in technique plus increases in neuromuscular conditioning before progressing to more challenging exercises. Particular caution must be used with larger athletes. Large athletes place greater loading to musculoskeletal system thereby increasing the risk of injury if not careful. The volume of plyometric training should be lower for large athletes and the intensity must closely be monitored (10). It has been suggested that large athletes not perform depth jumps off of boxes >18 in. (10). Plyometric training is safe when athletes are not previously injured. A prior injury or predisposition to injury can place the athlete at greater risk. Careful monitoring of the athletes is necessary. An injury may necessitate altering or temporarily discontinuing plyometric training until medical clearance has been attained. Lastly, proper breathing during plyometrics is important. Similar to high-intensity RT, a Valsalva maneuver is typically used during the ECC and early CON phases of the drill to ensure proper stability, shock absorption, and force and power production during propulsion. Exhalation ensures shortly afterward during the latter stages of the CON action.

Integrating Plyometric with Other Training Modalities

Plyometric training is a modality that is commonly performed with other modalities during a training cycle to optimize athletic performance. A program consisting of plyometric and RT can be employed simultaneously. For example, plyometric training 2 days per week can easily be incorporated into an RT program. Plyometric training can be performed on off-lifting days or on the same day. If performed on the same day, plyometric training may be given priority and performed first. Resistance training can be performed after or later in the day. The muscle groups trained for each workout is important. If only the upper body is resistance trained that day, then lower-body plyometrics can be performed uninhibited and the sequence can vary. It is not recommended that high-intensity lower-body RT and lower-body plyometric training be performed on the same day as the modality-trained second would do so in a semifatigued state. Plyometric drills can also be incorporated into a weight training workout, *e.g.*, complex training.

Plyometric training coincides with sprint and agility training so effective combination programs can be developed. These modalities train similar physiological mechanisms and work in tandem to optimize neuromuscular performance, so integration of these modalities into a workout is common. Plyometric, sprint, and agility drills can be alternated within a workout or trained in sequence. In some sports, athletes need a good aerobic base, and aerobic training may be performed along with plyometric training. It is important to point out that an incompatibility does exist between high-intensity anaerobic and aerobic training modalities. However, low to moderate levels of aerobic training (low frequency) may be performed without compromising performance. If this is the case, it is recommended that plyometric training be performed first followed by aerobic exercise. It is better to perform the two during a workout as aerobic training in between anaerobic training sessions can impede recovery. Flexibility training should be incorporated at the conclusion of a plyometric workout and not before. Table 15.3 depicts some examples of integrating RT and plyometric training. The first two samples are intermediate programs where upper-body/lower-body split or total-body workouts are performed. The third sample is more advanced as it incorporates a higher frequency of plyometric training. Table 15.4 depicts a sample of combined plyometric and sprint training workout using an alternate integration model.

In-season plyometric training necessitates a lower training volume and frequency. The athletes' sport takes presentence so the frequency and volume of plyometric and RT decrease accordingly. Coaches must closely monitor athletic performance in examination of potential overreaching/overtraining, and training volume can be adjusted accordingly. All sports

Table 15.3 Integrating Plyometric and Resistance Training (Upper-Body/Lower-Body Split)

	Day	Resistance Training	Plyometric Training
Upper-body/lower-body split workout	Monday	Upper body	Off
	Tuesday	Lower body	Off
	Wednesday	Off	Total body
	Thursday	Upper body	Off
	Friday	Lower body	Off
	Saturday	Off	Total body
	Sunday	Off	Off
Total-body workout	Monday	Total body	Off
	Tuesday	Off	Upper body
	Wednesday	Total body	Off
	Thursday	Off	Off
	Friday	Total body	Off
	Saturday	Off	Lower body
	Sunday	Off	Off
Advanced upper-body/lower-body split	Monday	Upper body	Lower body
	Tuesday	Lower body	Upper body
	Wednesday	Off	Off
	Thursday	Upper body	Lower body
	Friday	Lower body	Upper body
	Saturday	Off	Total body
	Sunday	Off	Off

Table 15.4 Sample Combined Plyometric and Sprint Training Workout[a]

General Warm-Up	3–5 min of Slow Jogging
Dynamic range of motion drills	1 × 5 drills
High knees	2 × 20 yd
Butt kickers	2 × 20 yd
Lunge walks	2 × 20 yd
Tuck jumps	3 × 10
Gears (10-yd intervals)	3–5 × 40 yd
Double-leg hops with lateral sprints	3 × 30 yd with 20-yd sprints
Box jumps	3 × 8
Sprints	3 × 40 yd
Cooldown	

[a]Specific sprint drills are discussed in Chapter 16.

consist of plyometric actions so practice and competition can be viewed as a training stimulus. Anaerobic sports that require high levels of power and strength necessitate the athlete train intensely during the season to maintain performance. Thus, too much plyometric training can be excessive or counterproductive when the demands of the sport are considered, especially when depth jumps are performed.

Putting It All Together

The program designed should incorporate all of the factors discussed in this chapter. Numerous effective programs can be developed provided that the progressive overload, specificity, and variation are used appropriately and the program is well supervised. Tables 15.5 and 15.6 depict sample plyometric training programs. The key elements are selecting sport-specific exercises and prescribing appropriate levels of intensity and volume. Each repetition should be performed explosively and coaches should constantly monitor technique and stress proper mechanics to their athletes.

Table 15.5	Sample Off-Season Total-Body Plyometric Training Programs[a]

Intermediate Wrestling Program (2×/Week)	**Intermediate Baseball Program (2×/Week)**
Squat jumps — 3 × 10	Tuck jumps — 3 × 10
MB side throw — 3 × 8 (each side)	MB overhead throw — 3 × 8
Single-leg push-off — 3 × 6 (each leg)	Barrier jumps — 5 × 5
Box jumps — 3 × 8	MB kneeling side throw — 3 × 8 (each side)
MB back throw — 3 × 5	Lateral step-ups — 3 × 10
Split squat jump with cycle — 3 × 10	Alternate leg bounding — 3 × 25 yd
Plyo push-up — 3 × 10	
Low- to moderate-intensity drills	
Foot contacts = 120	Foot contacts = 103
Upper-body repetitions = 93	Upper-body repetitions = 72
Alternate exercises	
Single-leg hops	Standing long jump with lateral sprint
Bag/sandbag side throw	Lateral cone hops
Core ball overhead slams	Box jumps
Stadium hops	Slam ball rotations
MB chest pass	MB front rotation throw
Slam ball side rotation slams	

[a]All workouts are to be preceded by a warm-up and finished with a cooldown consisting of stretching. Jump lengths, box heights, barrier heights, etc. are based upon the conditioning of the athlete.

Table 15.6	Sample Off-Season Total-Body Plyometric Training Programs[a]

Advanced Basketball Program (2×/Week)	**Advanced Weightlifting Program (2×/Week)**
Jump and reach — 4 × 10	Tuck jumps — 4 × 10
MB chest pass — 3 × 8	Depth jumps to box — 5 × 3
Depth jumps to box — 5 × 3	Multiple box jumps — 5 × 3
MB overhead throw — 3 × 8	Split squat jump (cycle) — 4 × 10
Single-leg push-off — 4 × 8 (each leg)	MB back throw — 3 × 8
Box jumps — 5 × 5	
Power drop — 3 × 6	
Low- to high-intensity drills	
Foot contacts = 144	Foot contacts = 125
Upper-body repetitions = 66	Upper-body repetitions = 24
Alternate exercises	
Single-leg hops	Squat jumps
Alternate-leg bounding	Double leg hops
Barrier jumps	Single-arm vertical core ball throw
Single-leg depth jumps	Single-leg depth jumps
MB front rotation throw	Depth push-ups

[a]All workouts are to be preceded by a warm-up and finished with a cooldown consisting of stretching. Jump lengths, box heights, barrier heights, etc. are based upon the conditioning of the athlete.

SUMMARY POINTS

- Modern plyometrics are explosive exercises that utilize the SSC and target power, speed, and strength development.
- Plyometric training increases jumping height and power, sprinting speed, agility, muscle strength, hypertrophy, running economy and race times, swimming block start performance, reaction time, throwing velocity, and kicking speed.
- Plyometric exercises consist of hops, jumps, bounding, box jumps, depth jumps, and throws, and the intensity is based on complexity, use of external loading, uphill/downhill, height/distance of jump/throw, height of box, and unilateral versus bilateral exercises.
- Plyometric exercise volume is based upon the number of foot contacts or throws/repetitions. Volume depends on the athlete's training status and whether the athlete is in the off-season, preseason, or in-season training period.
- Plyometric exercises can be performed with just bodyweight and various pieces of equipment including cones, boxes, jump ropes, mini hurdles, bands, bags, weighted vests, MBs, slam balls, and core balls.

REVIEW QUESTIONS

1. The time between the end of the ECC action and beginning of the CON muscle action is known as the
   a. SSC
   b. Coupling time
   c. Isokinetic phase
   d. Relaxation time

2. Which of the following exercises is considered to be the most intense?
   a. Ankle hops
   b. Lateral cone hops
   c. Side to side ankle hops
   d. Depth jumps from a large box

3. An appropriate number of foot contacts of lower-body plyometric drills for a beginner during an off-season program is
   a. 30
   b. 75
   c. 150
   d. 250

4. A plyometric drill involving exaggerated horizontal movements where an excessive stride length is targeted is known as
   a. Bounding
   b. A hop
   c. A box jump
   d. A throw

5. Which of the following would be the most appropriate surface for plyometric training?
   a. Hardwood floor
   b. Concrete
   c. Grass
   d. Sand

6. Greatest CON power output is seen during the _____ phase of the vertical jump.
   a. Starting position
   b. Countermovement
   c. Propulsion
   d. Flight

7. Performing a plyometric exercise in between sets of a similar resistance exercise during a workout is known as complex training.
   a. T
   b. F

8. Plyometric training leads to fiber-type transitions (type IIX to IIA) similar to resistance training.
   a. T
   b. F

9. Double-leg jumps are more intense than single-leg jumps of comparable type.
   a. T
   b. F

10. A low-intensity plyometric exercise simply means that it should not be performed explosively.
    a. T
    b. F

11. A 1:1 work/relief ratio is recommended for most plyometric training programs.
    a. T
    b. F

12. Plyometric training frequency depends on intensity, volume, and the inclusion of other training modalities.
    a. T
    b. F

REFERENCES

1. Zatsiorsky V, Kraemer WJ. *Science and Practice of Strength Training*. 2nd ed. Champaign (IL): Human Kinetics; 2006. p. 1–35.
2. Chu DA. *Explosive Power and Strength*. Champaign (IL): Human Kinetics; 1996. p. 153–65.
3. Verkhoshansky Y. Are depth jumps useful? *Yessis Rev Soviet Phys Ed Sports*. 1968;3:75–8.
4. Verkhoshansky Y, Siff M. *Supertraining*. 6th ed. Ultimate Athlete Concepts. Muskegon, MI; 2009. p. 267–84.
5. Chu DA. *Jumping Into Plyometrics*. 2nd ed. Champaign (IL): Human Kinetics; 1998. p. 1–138.

6. Ebben WP, Hintz MJ, Simenz CJ. Strength and conditioning practices of Major League Baseball strength and conditioning coaches. *J Strength Cond Res.* 2005;19:538–46.

7. Simenz CJ, Dugan CA, Ebben WP. Strength and conditioning practices of National Basketball Association strength and conditioning coaches. *J Strength Cond Res.* 2005;19:495–504.

8. Ebben WP, Carroll RM, Simenz CJ. Strength and conditioning practices of National Hockey League strength and conditioning coaches. *J Strength Cond Res.* 2004;18:889–97.

9. Ebben WP, Blackard DO. Strength and conditioning practices of National Football League strength and conditioning coaches. *J Strength Cond Res.* 2001;15:48–58.

10. Potach DH, Chu DA. Plyometric training. In: Baechle TR, Earle RW, editors. *Essentials of Strength Training and Conditioning.* 3rd ed. Champaign (IL): Human Kinetics; 2008. p. 413–56.

11. Masamoto N, Larson R, Gates T, Faigenbaum A. Acute effects of plyometric exercise on maximum squat performance in male athletes. *J Strength Cond Res.* 2003;17:68–71.

12. Adams K, O'Shea JP, O'Shea KL, Climstein M. The effect of six weeks of squat, plyometric and squat-plyometric training on power production. *J Appl Sport Sci Res.* 1992;6:36–41.

13. De Villarreal ES, Gonzalez-Badillo JJ, Izquierdo M. Low and moderate plyometric training frequency produces greater jumping and sprinting gains compared with high frequency. *J Strength Cond Res.* 2008;22:715–25.

14. Holcomb WR, Lander JE, Rutland RM, Wilson GD. The effectiveness of a modified plyometric program on power and the vertical jump. *J Strength Cond Res.* 1996;10:89–92.

15. Luebbers PE, Potteiger JA, Hulver MW, et al. Effects of plyometric training and recovery on vertical jump performance and anaerobic power. *J Strength Cond Res.* 2003;17:704–9.

16. Marcovic G. Does plyometric training improve vertical jump height? A meta-analytical review. *Br J Sports Med.* 2007;41: 349–55.

17. Marcovic G, Jukic I, Milanovic D, Metikos D. Effects of sprint and plyometric training on muscle function and athletic performance. *J Strength Cond Res.* 2007;21:543–9.

18. Potteiger JA, Lockwood RH, Haub MD, et al. Muscle power and fiber characteristics following 8 weeks of plyometric training. *J Strength Cond Res.* 1999;13:275–9.

19. Vissing K, Brink M, Lonbro S, et al. Muscle adaptations to plyometric vs. resistance training in untrained young men. *J Strength Cond Res.* 2008;22:1799–810.

20. Delecluse C. Influence of strength training on sprint running performance: current findings and implications for training. *Sports Med* 1997;24:147–56.

21. Dodd DJ, Alvar BA. Analysis of acute explosive training modalities to improve lower-body power in baseball players. *J Strength Cond Res.* 2007;21:1177–82.

22. Miller MG, Herniman JJ, Ricard MD, Cheatham CC, Michael TJ. The effects of a 6-week plyometric training program on agility. *J Sports Sci Med.* 2006;5:459–65.

23. Lephart SM, Abt JP, Ferris CM, et al. Neuromuscular and biomechanical characteristic changes in high school athletes: a plyometric versus basic resistance program. *Br J Sports Med.* 2005;39:932–8.

24. Markovic G, Mikulic P. Neuro-musculoskeletal and performance adaptations to lower-extremity plyometric training. *Sports Med.* 2010;40:859–96.

25. Oxfeldt M, Overgaard K, Hvid LG, Dalgas U. Effects of plyometric training on jumping, sprint performance, and lower body

26. muscle strength in healthy adults: a systematic review and meta-analysis. *Scand J Med Sci Sports.* 2019;29:1453–65.

26. Slimani M, Chamari K, Miarka B, Del Vecchio FB, Cheour F. Effects of plyometric training on physical fitness in team sport athletes: a systematic review. *J Hum Kinet.* 2016;53:231–47.

27. Kossow AJ, Ebben WP. Kinetic analysis of horizontal plyometric exercise intensity. *J Strength Cond Res.* 2017;32:1222–9.

28. Singla D, Hussain ME, Moiz JA. Effect of upper body plyometric training on physical performance in healthy individuals: a systematic review. *Phys Ther Sport.* 2018;29:51–60.

29. Stojanovic E, Ristic V, McMaster DT, Milanovic Z. Effect of plyometric training on vertical jump performance in female athletes: a systematic review and meta-analysis. *Sports Med.* 2017;47: 975–86.

30. Kraemer WJ, Newton RU. Training for improved vertical jump. *Gatorade Sport Sci Exchange.* 1994;7:53.

31. Kraemer WJ, Ratamess NA, Volek JS, Mazzetti SA, Gomez AL. The effect of the Meridian shoe on vertical jump and sprint performances following short-term combined plyometric/sprint and resistance training. *J Strength Cond Res.* 2000;14:228–38.

32. Ratamess NA, Kraemer WJ, Volek JS, et al. The effects of ten weeks of resistance and combined plyometric/sprint training with the Meridian Elyte athletic shoe on muscular performance in women. *J Strength Cond Res.* 2007;21:882–7.

33. Perez-Gomez J, Olmedillas H, Delgado-Guerra S, et al. Effects of weight lifting training combined with plyometric exercises on physical fitness, body composition, and knee extension velocity during kicking in football. *Appl Physiol Nutr Metab.* 2008;33: 501–10.

34. Kramer JF, Morrow A, Leger A. Changes in rowing ergometer, weight lifting, vertical jump and isokinetic performance in response to standard and standard plus plyometric training programs. *Int J Sports Med.* 1983;14:449–54.

35. Wilson GJ, Murphy AJ, Giorgi A. Weight and plyometric training: effects on eccentric and concentric force production. *Can J Appl Physiol.* 1996;21:301–15.

36. Saunders PU, Telford RD, Pyne DB, et al. Short-term plyometric training improves running economy in highly trained middle and long distance runners. *J Strength Cond Res.* 2006;20:947–54.

37. Turner AM, Owings M, Schwane JA. Improvement in running economy after 6 weeks of plyometric training. *J Strength Cond Res.* 2003;17:60–7.

38. Spurrs RW, Murphy AJ, Watsford ML. The effect of plyometric training on distance running performance. *Eur J Appl Physiol.* 2003; 89:1–7.

39. Bishop DC, Smith RJ, Smith MF, Rigby HE. Effect of plyometric training on swimming block start performance in adolescents. *J Strength Cond Res.* 2009;23:2137–43.

40. Salonikidis K, Zafeiridis A. The effects of plyometric, tennis-drills, and combined training on reaction, lateral and linear speed, power, and strength in novice tennis players. *J Strength Cond Res.* 2008;22:182–91.

41. Carter AB, Kaminski TW, Douex AT, Knight CA, Richards JG. Effects of high volume upper extremity plyometric training on throwing velocity and functional strength ratios of the shoulder rotators in collegiate baseball players. *J Strength Cond Res.* 2007;21:208–15.

42. Sedano Campo S, Vaeyens R, Phillippaerts RM, et al. Effects of lower-limb plyometric training on body composition, explosive strength, and kicking speed in female soccer players. *J Strength Cond Res.* 2009;23:1714–22.

43. Luhtanen P, Komi RV. Segmental contribution to forces in vertical jump. *Eur J Appl Physiol Occup Physiol.* 1978;38:181–8.

44. Robertson DG, Fleming D. Kinetics of standing broad and vertical jumping. *Can J Sport Sci.* 1987;12:19–23.

45. Harman EA, Rosenstein MT, Frykman PN, Rosenstein RM. The effects of arms and countermovement on vertical jumping. *Med Sci Sports Exerc.* 1990;22:825–33.

46. Hewett TE, Myer GD, Ford KR, et al. Biomechanical measures of neuromuscular control and valgus loading of the knee predict anterior cruciate ligament injury risk in female athletes: a prospective study. *Am J Sports Med.* 2005;33(4):492–501.

47. Pappas E, Hagins M, Sheikhzadeh A, Nordin M, Rose D. Biomechanical differences between unilateral and bilateral landings from a jump: gender differences. *Clin J Sport Med.* 2007;17:263–8.

48. Radcliffe JC, Farentinos RC. *High-Powered Plyometrics.* Champaign (IL): Human Kinetics; 1999. p. 23–115.

49. Ebben WP, Petushek EJ. Using the reactive strength index modified to evaluate plyometric performance. *J Strength Cond Res.* 2010;24:1983–7.

50. Bobbert MF, Mackay M, Schinkelshoek D, Huijing PA, van Ingen Schenau GJ. Biomechanical analysis of drop and countermovement jumps. *Eur J Appl Physiol.* 1986;54:566–73.

51. Bobbert MF, Huijing PA, van Ingen Schenau GJ. Drop jumping I. The influence of jumping technique on the biomechanics of jumping. *Med Sci Sports Exerc.* 1987;19:332–8.

52. Bobbert MF, Huijing PA, van Ingen Schenau GJ. Drop jumping II. The influence of dropping height on the biomechanics of drop jumping. *Med Sci Sports Exerc.* 1987;19:339–46.

53. Asadi A, Arazi H, Ramirez-Campillo R, Moran J, Izquierdo M. Influence of maturation stage on agility performance gains after plyometric training: a systematic review and meta-analysis. *J Strength Cond Res* 2017;31:2609–17.

54. Matavulj D, Kukolj M, Ugarkovic D, Tihanyi J, Jaric S. Effects of plyometric training on jumping performance in junior basketball players. *J Sports Med Phys Fitness.* 2001;41:159–64.

55. Bedi JF, Cresswell AG, Engel TJ, Nicol SM. Increase in jumping height associated with maximal effort vertical depth jumps. *Res Q Exerc Sport.* 1987;58:11–5.

56. Ramirez-Campillo R, Alvarez C, Garcia-Hermoso A, et al. Methodological characteristics and future directions for plyometric jump training research: a scoping review. *Sports Med.* 2018;48:1059–81.

57. Bogdanis GC, Tsoukos A, Kaloheri O, Terzis G, Veligekas P, Brown LE. Comparison between unilateral and bilateral plyometric training on single-and double-leg jumping performance and strength. *J Strength Cond Res.* 2017;33:633–40.

58. Saez de Villarreal ES, Kellis E, Kraemer WJ, Izquierdo M. Determining variables of plyometric training for improving vertical jump height performance: a meta-analysis. *J Strength Cond Res.* 2009;23:495–506.

59. Ebben WP. Practical guidelines for plyometric intensity. *NSCA Perf Train J.* 2006;6:12–6.

60. Ebben WP, Fauth ML, Garceau LR, Petushek EJ. Kinetic quantification of plyometric exercise intensity. *J Strength Cond Res.* 2011;25:3288–98.

61. Ebben WP, Simenz C, Jensen RL. Evaluation of plyometric intensity using electromyography. *J Strength Cond Res.* 2008;22:861–8.

62. Van Lieshout KG, Anderson JG, Shelburne KB, Davidson BS. Intensity rankings of plyometric exercises using joint power absorption. *Clin Biomech (Bristol, Avon).* 2014;29:918–22.

63. Struminger AH, Lewek MD, Goto S, Hibberd E, Blackburn JT. Comparison of gluteal and hamstring activation during five commonly used plyometric exercises. *Clin Biomech (Bristol, Avon).* 2013;28:783–9.

64. Santos EJ, Janeira MA. Effects of complex training on explosive strength in adolescent male basketball players. *J Strength Cond Res.* 2008;22:903–9.

65. Mihalik JP, Libby JJ, Battaglini CL, McMurray RG. Comparing short-term complex and compound training programs on vertical jump height and power output. *J Strength Cond Res.* 2008;22:47–53.

66. Faigenbaum AD, McFarland J, Keiper F, et al. Effects of short-term plyometric and resistance training program on fitness performance in boys age 12 to 15 years. *J Sports Sci Med.* 2007;6:519–25.

67. Faigenbaum AD, Farrell A, Radler T. "Plyo Play": a novel program of short bouts of moderate and high intensity exercise improves physical fitness in elementary school children. *Phys Educ.* 2009;66:37–44.

68. Faigenbaum AD, Kraemer WJ, Blimkie CJ, et al. Youth resistance training: updated position statement paper from the National Strength and Conditioning Association. *J Strength Cond Res.* 2009; 23(Suppl):S60–79.

69. Diallo O, Dore E, Duche P, Van Praagh E. Effects of plyometric training followed by a reduced training programme on physical performance in prepubescent soccer players. *J Sports Med Phys Fitness.* 2001;41:342–8.

70. Kotsamidis C. Effect of plyometric training on running performance and vertical jumping in prepubertal boys. *J Strength Cond Res.* 2006;20:441–5.

71. Behm DG, Young JD, Whitten JHD, et al. Effectiveness of traditional strength vs. power training on muscle strength, power, and speed with youth: a systematic review and meta-analysis. *Front Physiol.* 2017;8:423.

72. Moran JJ, Sandercock GRH, Ramirez-Campillo R, et al. Age-related variation in male youth athletes' countermovement jump after plyometric training: a meta-analysis of controlled trials. *J Strength Cond Res.* 2016;31:552–65.

73. Peitz M, Behringer M, Granacher U. A systematic review on the effects of resistance and plyometric training on physical fitness in youth—what do comparative studies tell us? *PLoS One.* 2018;13:e0205525.

74. Marginson V, Rowlands AV, Gleeson NP, Eston RG. Comparison of the symptoms of exercise-induced muscle damage after an initial and repeated bout of plyometric exercise in men and boys. *J Appl Physiol.* 2005;99:1174–81.

75. Impellizzeri FM, Rampinini E, Castagna C, et al. Effect of plyometric training on sand versus grass on muscle soreness and jumping and sprinting ability in soccer players. *Br J Sports Med.* 2008; 42:42–6.

76. Stemm JD, Jacobson BH. Comparison of land-and aquatic-based plyometric training on vertical jump performance. *J Strength Cond Res.* 2007;21:568–71.

77. Martel GF, Harmer ML, Logan JM, Parker CB. Aquatic plyometric training increases vertical jump in female volleyball players. *Med Sci Sports Exerc.* 2005;37:1814–9.

78. Kannas TM, Kellis E, Amiridis IG. Incline plyometrics-induced improvement of jumping performance. *Eur J Appl Physiol.* 2012;112:2353–61.

79. Rhea MR, Peterson MD, Oliverson JR, Ayllon FN, Potenziano BJ. An examination of training on the VertiMax resisted jumping device for improvements in lower body power in highly trained college athletes. *J Strength Cond Res*. 2008;22:735–40.

80. Rhea MR, Peterson MD, Lunt KT, Ayllon FN. The effectiveness of resisted jump training on the VertiMax in high school athletes. *J Strength Cond Res*. 2008;22:731–4.

81. McClenton LS, Brown LE, Coburn JW, Kersey RD. The effect of short-term VertiMax vs. depth jump training on vertical jump performance. *J Strength Cond Res*. 2008;22:321–5.

82. Carlson K, Magnusen M, Walters P. Effect of various training modalities on vertical jump. *Res Sports Med*. 2009;17:84–94.

83. Fleck SJ, Kraemer WJ. *Designing Resistance Training Programs*. 3rd ed. Champaign (IL): Human Kinetics; 2004. p. 230–6.

84. Gambetta V, Odgers S. *The Complete Guide to Medicine Ball Training*. Sarasota (FL): Optimum Sports Training; 1991. p. 18–52.

85. Mediate P, Faigenbaum A. *Medicine Ball for All Kids: Medicine Ball Training Concepts and Program-Design Considerations for School-Age Youth*. Monterey (CA): Coaches Choice; 2007.

CHAPTER

16 Sprint and Agility Training

OBJECTIVES

After completing this chapter, you will be able to:

◆ Define speed, agility, quickness, reaction ability, and speed endurance

◆ Discuss the roles stride length and stride rate have on speed development

◆ Discuss the mechanics of proper sprint technique relative to the phases of sprinting

◆ Discuss the importance of overspeed and resisted sprint training on speed development

◆ Identify several drills which can improve an athlete's technique, speed, quickness, agility, change of direction, and reactive ability

◆ Discuss relevant elements to change of direction and agility and ways to specifically train each to enhance performance

◆ Discuss the elements of sprint and agility program design

◆ Discuss methods of improving speed endurance

Speed and agility are critical components to several sports. Many have heard coaches say that "speed kills" meaning it is a differentiating factor between teams and athletes in competition. Speed is the change in distance over time, and maximal speed is a critical component to anaerobic sport performance. This is especially important for track and field athletes such as sprinters. However, maximal speed may not be attained until the athlete has run at least 20–40 m in a linear path. In many cases, the athlete may not have the option of running optimally (or unimpeded) for 20–40 m but may have to move rapidly for shorter distances covering multiple directions. Thus, acceleration ability becomes a critical training component. **Acceleration** is the rate of change of velocity over time. In athletic terms, it entails the athlete's ability to reach high velocities in a short period of time following a change of direction (COD), deceleration, or from a static position. Athletes with explosive acceleration ability have a major advantage in sports such as football, basketball, and baseball. Highest rates of acceleration are seen within the first 8–10 strides where the athlete may reach ~75% of his or her max velocity within the first 10 yd (1). Training to increase acceleration is critical to athletic success. Acceleration ability is highly related to reaction time. *Reaction time* refers to the athlete's ability to react to a stimulus. Fast reaction times increase the likelihood of athletic success. For example, the quicker a sprinter reacts to the gun, the better the race time. Goalies in hockey or a baseball player getting

ready to hit a 90-mph fastball may have <0.40 second to react. The quicker the first response, the more likely an athlete will be able to accelerate into a successful position. Sprints of sufficient duration will force the athlete to reach maximal speed and maintain it for as long as possible so speed endurance is critical to many sports. **Speed endurance** also refers to the ability to maintain maximal speed over several repetitions, or repeated sprint ability. Reducing fatigue-induced deceleration is a critical conditioning component. For example, an athlete with the ability to have the same burst of speed in the second half of a game as he or she did in the first half will have good speed endurance. In a linear sprint of sufficient duration (100 m), three distinct phases can be seen (a) acceleration, (b) maximum speed maintenance, and (c) speed endurance or deceleration.

The ability to move rapidly while changing direction in response to a stimulus is **agility**. Agility is quite complex and requires the optimal integration of several physiological systems, components of fitness, anthropometrics, and perceptual-cognitive ability (Fig. 16.1). Although an athlete may have sufficient linear speed, this does not mean he or she will be very agile and coordinated. There is some evidence that linear sprinting ability has only limited transferability to various agility drills especially when there are larger numbers of changes of direction and COD angles (3,4). For example, the ability to backpedal is an independent skill. Maximal backward running velocities range from 60% to 80% of one's sprint speed (4).

500

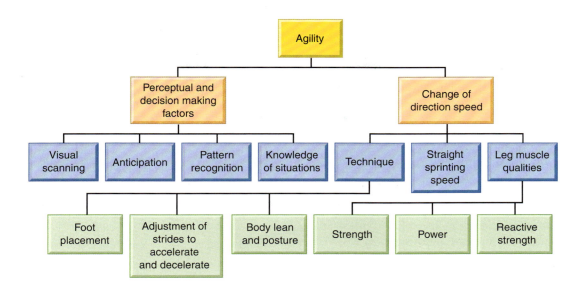

FIGURE 16.1 Components of agility. (Reprinted with permission from Young WB, Farrow D. A review of agility: practical applications for strength and conditioning. *Strength Cond J*. 2006;28:24–9. Ref. 2.)

Backpedalling produces shorter stride lengths, greater stride rates, longer support time, lower peak ground reaction force and time to produce it, and smaller range of motion (ROM) of the hip, knee, and ankle compared to forward sprinting (4). Thus, components of agility must be trained independently in order to maximize athletic performance.

Agility requires the athlete to coordinate several activities including the ability to react and start quickly, accelerate, decelerate, move in the proper direction, and maintain the ability to change direction as rapidly as possible while maintaining balance and postural control. The athlete must adapt to the environment, react quickly, adjust bodily position accordingly, and transition from one skill to another as efficiently as possible. For example, a soccer player may spend ~49% of the time moving linearly, 21% of the time not moving, and ~30% of the time moving in multiple directions accumulating more than 700 changes in direction during a game (5). Agility will allow the athlete to reduce the risk of injury, evade other athletes on the field or court, maintain the proper position to catch, strike, and kick a ball, and maintain the proper position to block or tackle an opponent. Often the athlete may have a small window within which to accelerate or decelerate before a COD takes place. This complexity provides a challenge to the athlete when training for optimal bodily control. The rapid COD may take place from a variety of stable or unstable bodily positions, *e.g.*, standing (unilateral or bilateral), lying (prone or supine), seated on the ground, and/or kneeling positions forcing the athlete to react to a number of situations. The athlete who can change position fluently and rapidly will be more likely to experience success in his or her respective sport. Although the actual practice/competition for the sport increases agility, many strength and conditioning (S&C) coaches see the value of off-season and preseason sport-specific agility training to increase athleticism beyond the improvements seen from just participating in the sport. Training each fitness component throughout the year is important for the athlete just to stay competitive with other athletes.

 ## Increasing Sprint Speed

Sprint speed is the product of stride length and frequency (rate), and faster athletes display higher stride rates and greater stride lengths than slower runners (6). In general, sprint speed is greater in male athletes than female athletes (7). **Stride length** is the length of each stride (from toe-off to heel strike on the same side) during sprinting and is determined by leg length, leg strength and power, and sprinting mechanics. Stride length is improved by increasing the athlete's ability to develop explosive forces applied to the ground (6). This should be a natural occurrence because stride length can be intentionally increased forcibly, a common sprinting error known as overstriding. Overstriding creates equilibrium problems and slows the athlete down. **Stride rate** or *frequency* refers to the number of foot contacts per period of time. Rapid turnover of the feet during the sprint cycle is seen at higher speeds and is a goal of maximal sprint training. Sprint, agility, plyometric, and ballistic training are the most effective ways to increase stride rate. Forcing a greater stride rate can decrease stride length and vice versa. *Maximal sprint speed occurs only when the optimal proportion or combination of stride length and rate are utilized by the athlete.* These are athlete dependent, and it is paramount that the coach closely monitors the technique to prevent flaws, *e.g.*, overstriding, which can slow the athlete down.

Training programs designed to increase maximal speed are multifactorial. Although resistance training (RT), plyometric training, resisted, and nonresisted sprint training increase sprint speed independently (8), an integrated approach is most effective where a combination of plyometric, sprint (nonresisted, overspeed, resisted [chutes, sleds, weighted vests]), and RT (9) is used in the training of athletes. Nonresisted (10), uphill/downhill (11), and resisted sprint training programs (10,12,13) increase acceleration and sprint speed. A review study showed that 6–8 weeks of nonresisted sprint training of 2–3 days per week increased sprint speed (5–100 m) up to 7%, while resisted sprint training increases sprint speed (5–20 m) up to 6% (14). Largest effects in increasing sprint speed from 0 to 10 m and 0 to 20 m are seen with resisted sprint training, while larger effects from 0 to 30 m on beyond are seen with nonresisted sprint training (14). Plyometric training (2–3 d·wk^{-1}, 3–8 wk) may increase sprint speed (5–40 m) by up to 9%, while RT by itself may increase sprint speed by 4%–8% in most studies (14). The combination of sprint and RT is effective for enhancing maximal speed, speed endurance, power, and strength of the lower body (15,16). RT increases muscular strength and power, and in combination with sprint training, enables the athlete to exert greater force with each foot contact leading to an increase in running acceleration and velocity. Maximal strength for sport-specific exercises like the half-squat and hang clean correlate highly to sprint performance (17,18). A number of studies have shown very large relationships of lower body strength (1 RM squat) and sprint speed thereby showing strength increases transfer to enhancing speed (19). Young et al. (20) showed correlations between peak force application and starting ability, acceleration out of the block, and maximum sprinting speed. Thus, a comprehensive sprint enhancement program consists of sprint-specific drills in addition to plyometric, flexibility, and RT (Table 16.1).

Sprint Training

Mechanics of Sprint Running

The phases of sprinting begin with the starting position, acceleration, and maximum speed. The starting position is essential for attaining optimal stability allowing maximal propulsive forces for acceleration. Acceleration is marked by an increase in velocity. Once the athlete begins to accelerate and reaches peak speed or velocity, several phases can be identified that assist the coach in stressing proper technique (Fig. 16.2). Sprinting can be characterized by two major phases: (a) **flight phase** and (b) the **support phase**. The flight phase describes motion of the leg that is not in contact with the ground. It can further be broken into the **early, middle,** and **late flight phases**. The early flight phase describes recovery motion of the back leg from the time it leaves the ground until there is moderate knee flexion and further hip hyperextension. The hip and knee musculature decelerates backward rotation of the thigh and lower leg/foot. The midflight phase describes motion of the back leg as knee flexion increases, and hip flexion positions the thigh in alignment with the torso. The late flight phase describes motion for preparation of ground contact. The hip flexes forward and the knee extends to attain an optimal unilateral landing position and signifies the beginning of the support phase. The support phase describes motion of the leg that is in contact with the ground. It can further be broken into the *early* and *late support phases*. The early support phase describes motion of the leg as it contacts the ground. Braking and shock absorption take place as the hip extends, knee slightly flexes, and the ankle dorsiflexes. The late support phase describes triple extension of the leg to maximize propulsive forces during push-off thereby continuing the motion of the center of gravity (COG) forward. Triple extension involves hip and knee extension and ankle plantar flexion. The final segment of the late support phase concludes with the propulsion leg leaving the ground indicating the beginning of the early flight phase. The cycle repeats for the duration of the sprint. Horizontal and vertical force production is related to sprint performance (*i.e.*, acceleration and maximal speed phases), and elite sprinters are capable of producing greater horizontal forces compared to subelite athletes (21).

Table 16.1	Ways to Increase Components of Sprinting
Sprint Component	**Training Modalities**
Reaction time and start ability	Overspeed training
	Reactive drills
	Power training
Acceleration	Resistance and ballistic training
	Acceleration training
	Resisted and overspeed training
	Basic sprint drills and plyometrics
Stride length	Resistance and ballistic training
	Acceleration training
	Resisted and overspeed training
	Basic sprint, stick/line drills, and plyometrics
	Flexibility training
Stride frequency	Resistance and ballistic training
	Resisted and overspeed training
	Basic sprint drills and plyometrics
	Quick feet drills
Max speed and power	Resistance and ballistic training
	Acceleration training
	Resisted and overspeed training
	Basic sprint drills and plyometrics
	Power training and quickness drills

Adapted with permission from Dintiman G, Ward B, Tellez T. *Sports Speed*. 2nd ed. Champaign (IL): Human Kinetics; 1998. p. 191–220.

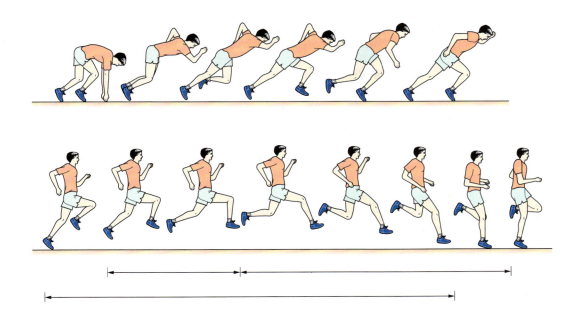

FIGURE 16.2 The flight and support phases of sprinting. (Reprinted with permission from Plisk SS. Speed, agility, and speed-endurance development. In: Baechle TR, Earle RW, editors. *Essentials of Strength Training and Conditioning.* 3rd ed. Champaign (IL): Human Kinetics; 2008. p. 455–85.)

Starting Position

Athletes may begin a sprint from many positions. Often, many positions are encountered during athletic competition. Here, 2-, 3-, and 4-point stances are discussed from a stationary position. From a 2-point stance, the athlete may assume a shoulder width stance with one foot in front of the other with most weight on the front leg. The proper starting position entails the athlete maintains a 3-point (one hand touching the ground) or 4-point (two hands touching the ground) crouch stance with the legs in a staggered stance (with the stronger or dominant leg forward [left leg for a right-handed athlete]) at least 1 foot behind the starting line. Figure 16.3 illustrates the 3-point stance. Bodyweight is evenly distributed with a front knee angle of ~90°, rear knee angle of ~110°–135°, front hip angle of ~40°–50°, a rear hip angle of 80°–90°, and a torso angle of ~42°–45° from the horizontal (4). The height of the COG may range from 0.61 to 0.66 m vertically and is located ~0.16–0.19 m from the starting line horizontally (22). Athletes with stronger arms can maintain a position where the COG is closer to the starting line (22) although weight should be balanced, or the athlete may lose force applied to the ground during propulsion and lose balance forward during initial acceleration. Upon initial motion, both legs explosively push off where the front leg completes its extension as the rear leg swings forward. Knee and hip angles increase while ankle angles decrease. The rear leg produces greater initial force while pushing backward and downward and lifts off first, whereas the front leg plays a vital role in starting velocity and will exert force for a longer period of time (4). In elite sprinters, the front leg applies force for ≤0.37 second and the rear leg produces force for ≤0.18 second (twice as much time for the front leg) (4). Force production is greater in elite sprinters than lesser-trained athletes (22). Simultaneously, the opposite arm swings forward (from a 3-point stance) and up as the rear foot lifts up to increase momentum and reduce inertia. Backward arm countermovement helps forward flexion of the leg. Forward lean of trunk helps overcome inertia while accelerating from the starting position.

Acceleration

Acceleration phase consists of the ability to rapidly increase velocity from the starting position. The back leg drives forward, while the shin is ~45° to the ground. The angle of the shin decreases ~6°–7° with each stride over the first 10 m as the torso gradually reaches an upright position during the first 8–10 strides. Arms are swung back and forth (at a 90° elbow angle)

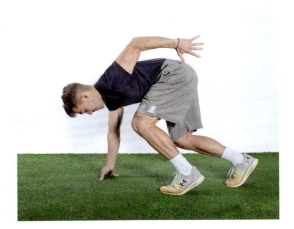

FIGURE 16.3 The 3-point stance starting position for the sprint.

in a sagittal plane, while shoulders remain as relaxed as possible. Wrists remain neutral and fingers are extended. The arms work in opposition to the legs with right arm and left leg moving forward and vice versa. The face, shoulders, hands, and neck muscles remain relaxed. The head begins down in front of the body's COG during acceleration but will eventually extend and form a vertical line with the body when maximal speed is attained. Legs are cycled back and forth in a sagittal plane with high knee action when driving forward and a pawing type of action is used when the ball of the foot strikes the ground. It is important that force be developed through the ball of the foot and not the toes to maximize force applied to the ground (23). The ankles remain dorsiflexed (toes up) for most of the sprint cycle except when the feet come in contact with the ground. Both stride length and frequency increase as speed increases (Fig. 16.4), and the acceleration phase length ranges from 30 to 50 m (22). The athlete's height and/or leg length correlate to stride length, and gender differences in height is a critical factor in viewing differences in max speed, e.g., men typically have longer limbs and faster running speeds (22). At higher speeds, there is a small increase in stride length and a greater increase in stride rate (6). In elite sprinters, support (early and late) phases are ≤0.20 and 0.18 second, respectively, and flight phases (early-to-mid, mid-to-late) are ≤0.70 and 0.90 second, respectively, stride length increases for the first 45 m, stride frequency increases for the first 25 m, forward body lean decreases from ~45° to ~5° within ~20 m, and peak acceleration rate can reach ~11.8 m·s^{-2} (4). Impact forces increase, and ground contact time decreases as speed increases (6). The force applied to the ground increases as speed increases; however, impulse reaches a peak and declines slightly due to shorter foot contact times with the ground (6). Lower-extremity muscle activity increases as velocity increases, and muscle activation during acceleration is ~5% higher than the max speed phase (22). Positive relationships exist between propulsive forces and running velocity during acceleration (22). Athletes with greater acceleration ability typically display higher stride frequencies and reduced ground contact times, as well as superior jump performance, relative strength, and reactive strength index, compared to athletes with less speed and acceleration (24).

Maximum Speed

Stride rate and length are maximized when the athlete reaches peak speed. Stride length at maximal speed is typically around 2.3–2.5 times the athlete's leg length (1). Stride rate plays a more substantial role as the athlete reaches the maximum speed phase (22). Flight phase duration is typically ~0.12–0.14 second, whereas support phase duration is ~0.08–0.10 second in sprinters (4,22). During the support phase, the torso remains erect (<5° forward lean), weight is balanced as only the ball of foot contacts the ground, and horizontal braking forces and vertical displacement are minimized (4). Vertical displacement of the COG decreases as speed increases and elite sprinters with greater speed demonstrate lower vertical displacement values than lesser-skilled athletes (22). The push-off angle of the rear foot during propulsion is ~50°–55°, and peak forces applied to the ground are generated rapidly (<0.04 s in elite sprinters) (4). Weyand et al. (6) have shown that applying greater force to the ground is vital for maximizing sprint speed more so than the movement velocity of the legs during the swing phase. Ground reaction forces during maximal sprints may range from 2.5 to 5 times an individual's body weight (6,25). Leg drive is enhanced by powerful arm action. Elbows are flexed to ~90°, and arms are kept close to body to minimize wind resistance. Flexing the hips (close to 90°) and knees (thigh nearly parallel to the ground during late flight and "heel-to-butt" during midflight) is vital to maximizing hip angular velocity by lowering the hip's moment of inertia during flight. The athlete keeps torso, head/neck, and upper extremity muscles as relaxed as possible. The phase of maximal sprinting affects performance. Athletes transiently slow down during the impact (by ~5%) or braking phase but compensate by increasing velocity during propulsion (22,26). The deceleration during braking is thought to limit maximal speed in addition to the short contact period of propulsion and potential air resistance (27). Muscle activation is greater during impact than in the propulsion phase presumably due to the effects of the stretch-shortening cycle (SSC) (22). Preactivation of lower-body musculature occurs where lower body muscles increase activity up to ~50%–70% of their maximum during preactivation (the period of time directly prior to impact with the ground) to increase stiffness and prepare for shock absorption (28).

Common Errors in Sprinting

Sprinting occurs primarily in the sagittal plane. Thus, movements should be confined to the sagittal plane as much as possible. Proper sprint technique focuses on maintaining correct posture, arm, and leg action. Sprint training entails technique

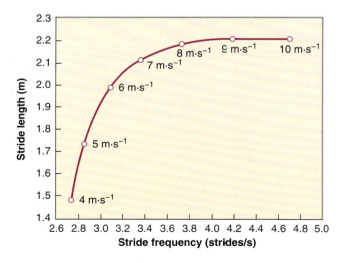

FIGURE 16.4 Stride length and rate relationship to sprint speed. (Reprinted with permission from Plisk SS. Speed, agility, and speed-endurance development. In: Baechle TR, Earle RW, editors. *Essentials of Strength Training and Conditioning*. 3rd ed. Champaign (IL): Human Kinetics; 2008. p. 455–85.)

training in addition to conditioning drills as minor improvements in technique can lead to increases in sprint speed. Deviations lead to unnecessary movements that lower efficiency and reduce speed. Some common errors include the following:

1. Improper stance (hands too far apart, hips too high or low) — can be corrected by narrowing hands and coaching proper hip position
2. Pushing off too high during acceleration — can be corrected by coaching athlete to push downward
3. Rising too quickly during acceleration from the start — can be corrected by coaching athlete to stay low and gradually rise as a *power line* should be formed through the head, spine, and rear leg while maintaining a ~45° torso angle to the ground
4. Excessive head movement — can be corrected by coaching athlete to focus eyes on a target straight ahead
5. Not explosively using the arms to accelerate (movement of the arms counteracts rotational motion initiated by the lower body to help keep the body in proper alignment) — can be corrected by form drills such as arm swings and marches
6. Arm movements occurring out of the sagittal plane (across the body) and not close to the body — can be corrected by coaching front-to-back motion and including form drills such as arm swings, skips, and marches
7. Failing to keep muscles (especially shoulders) as relaxed as possible (fluid, rhythmic motion is important) — can be corrected by coaching athletes to relax and enforcing relaxation during sprints and form drills such as arm swings
8. Excessive bending (flexion/extension) of elbows — can be corrected by coaching the athlete to keep elbow angle close to 90° and including form drills such as arm swings and marches
9. Not fully extending the legs during propulsion (lowers force applied to the ground and could result from weak posterior muscles and tight hip flexors and ankle muscles) — can be corrected by RT, plyometric and sprint drills, and flexibility training
10. Limited hip and knee ROM during lower-body motion — can be corrected by coaching "driving the legs" and through flexibility training, RT, and form drills such as high knees, marching, TRX mountain climbers, and resisted hip flexion
11. Not dorsiflexing the foot during flight — can be corrected by coaching proper foot position (dorsiflexion) and with form drills (skips), flexibility training, and resisted dorsiflexion exercises
12. Failing to maintain upright position during maximal speed — can be corrected by coaching proper body position and core RT and sprint training drills
13. Too much vertical bouncing — can be corrected by coaching the athlete to push off horizontally and minimize vertical motion

Basic Sprint Training Drills

The most specific way to increase sprint speed is by sprinting. However, drills can be used which improve athletic conditioning and technique simultaneously. These drills are used at the beginning of a workout following a general warm-up and dynamic ROM exercises to help prepare the body for more intense sprints and/or plyometric exercises performed later in the workout. Figures 16.5–16.20 depict common basic

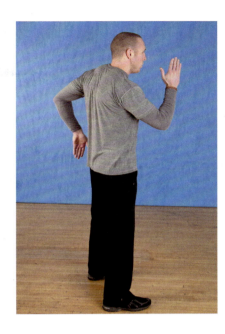

FIGURE 16.5 Standing arm swings. The athlete stands with feet together and swings arms in a sagittal plane with elbows flexed at 90°.

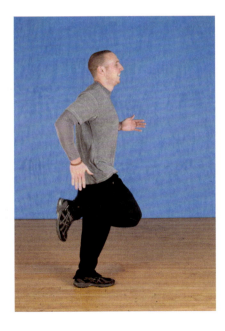

FIGURE 16.6 "Butt kickers." The athlete begins by jogging and pulls the heel of the foot until it bounces off the buttocks. A variation is a drill known as the "wall slide," which is very similar except during recovery the athlete's heel never moves behind the athlete's body.

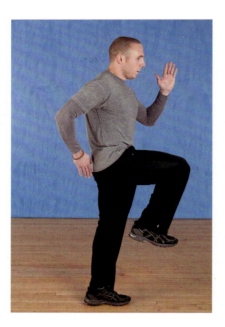

FIGURE 16.7 "High knees." The athlete drives the knees upward with each step trying to maximize ROM with each movement.

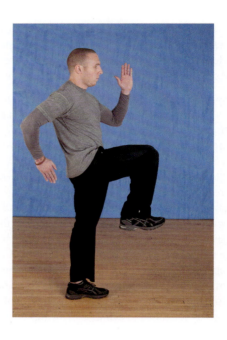

FIGURE 16.9 "A" march. The athlete marches with proper posture and arm action as the knee is fully flexed and the ground foot is plantar flexed when recovery knee is at the highest point. A skip can be used in lieu of marching.

sprint training/technique drills. Drills shown in this chapter were not previously discussed. It is important to note that some linear plyometric drills can be effectively used to enhance sprint speed. For example, drills such as multiple forms of bounding and skipping have high transfer ability to sprinting mechanics. Visit to view more exercises and variations in the online appendix.

Overspeed and Resisted Sprint Training

Overspeed Sprint Training

Overspeed training allows the athlete to attain supramaximal speed, or an assisted speed that is greater than the athlete's maximal effort. The objective is to provide assistance to the

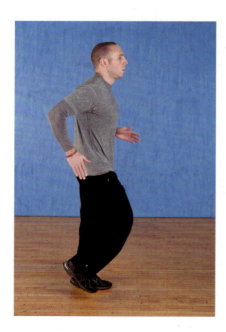

FIGURE 16.8 Ankling. The athlete jogs with very short steps and emphasizes plantar flexion during ground contact.

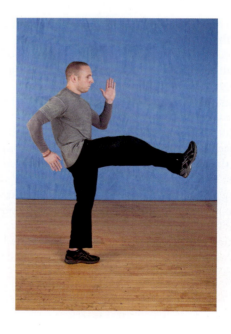

FIGURE 16.10 "B" march. The athlete marches similar to the "A" march (seen in Fig. 16.9) except the recovery leg extends in front of the body.

Chapter 16 Sprint and Agility Training 507

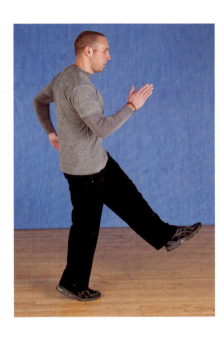

FIGURE 16.11 Straight leg shuffle. The athlete runs with the legs straight and foot dorsiflexed.

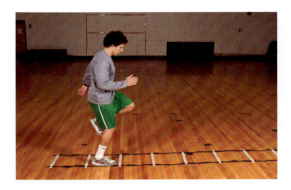

FIGURE 16.13 Ladder runs. To increase foot speed (stride frequency), the athlete runs through an agility ladder as fast as possible while touching one foot down between each rung. Stride length can be emphasized by increasing the slat length or by touching down every second or third run. Sticks can be used in lieu of a ladder.

athlete without altering sprinting mechanics and to improve the quality of effort (4). Overspeed training increases stride length and rate as it poses an intense neuromuscular stimulus and maximizes motor unit recruitment. Supramaximal speed can be achieved with a tail wind, downhill running (~1°–7°), high-speed towing, and high-speed treadmill running (22). The supramaximal velocity attained should not exceed a value >10% or greater than the athlete's own ability, or technical breakdowns could occur such as overstriding and leaning back to augment braking (4). Mero et al. (22) showed that supramaximal sprinting increases stride rate by ~6.9% and stride length by ~1.5%. It is important that the athletes are properly warmed up prior to overspeed training. Overspeed training is most effective when performed early in the workout where the athlete's energy levels are high and fatigue is minimal (23). The intensity is high and can result in greater muscle soreness so adequate recovery in between workouts is essential.

Sprinting with a tailwind is dependent upon environmental conditions. On a gusty day, the athlete could time his or her sprints with the wind and in the same direction. Maximal effort is given and the tailwind propels the athlete forward at a slightly greater speed (increase in speed is related to wind velocity). It is difficult to predict weather patterns so other forms of supramaximal sprinting are more reliable.

Downhill sprinting is a safe form of overspeed training that is practical provided the athlete has access to a training area with a downward slope of at least 50 m. The higher speed attained during downhill sprinting is due mostly to greater force applied to the ground compared to sprinting on a level surface (6). The level of decline need not be high, *e.g.*, at least 1° but up to ~7° (4,23). The steeper the decline, the greater the chance of falling and can produce some technical flaws including overstriding, landing on one's heels, and forcing the athlete to contact the ground beyond the COG (27). Ebben et al. (29) studied downhill sprinting on slopes ranging from 2.1° to 6.9° and showed optimal sprinting kinematics was seen at a decline of 5.8°. At this 5.8° slope, the athletes' maximal speed increased by ~7.1% and acceleration increased by ~6.5% (29). It could be advantageous if a flat or uphill surface is located near the declined surface, which can allow some contrasts in maximal sprinting sets. Paradisis and Cooke (11) showed 6 weeks of downhill sprinting increased sprint speed and stride frequency by 1.1% and 2.4%, respectively. However, a group which combined uphill and downhill sprinting experienced greater improvements in sprint speeds and stride frequency (3.5% and 3.4%, respectively). Downhill sprinting is less metabolically demanding (30) and increases the eccentric (ECC) component. Thus, muscle damage and delayed-onset muscle soreness may ensue, and coaches and athletes must be aware of overuse injuries if the volume and/or frequency of downhill sprinting are too high. Peak impact ground reaction forces may be up to 54% higher (at a 9° decline) during downhill running than running

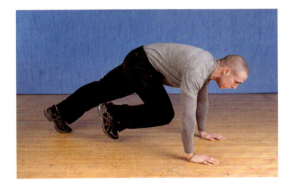

FIGURE 16.12 Mountain climbers. The athlete begins in a push-up position and drives legs forward.

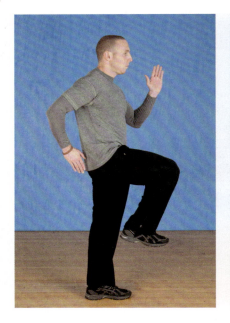 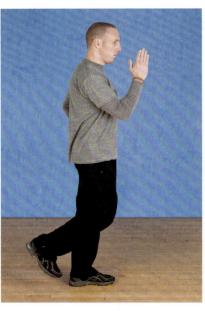

FIGURE 16.14 Pawing. The athlete walks or skips with front leg pulling through and pawing the ground in an exaggerated manner.

uphill (31). Running downhill (as opposed to sprinting) may augment some fitness components. One study showed that 5 weeks (three times per week for up to 20 min per workout) of downhill running (10° slope) at their lactate threshold heart rate (~77% of heart rate max) increased knee extension strength and COD ability (compared to flat running of similar intensity/duration) but did not increase sprint speed, jumping power, or VO_{2max} (32). Flat running did increase VO_{2max} thereby supporting the lower metabolic cost of downhill running (32).

Towing is a popular mode of overspeed training (Fig. 16.18). The athlete is towed or assisted to attain a supramaximal sprint speed. Athletes have used towing to increase their sprint speed since the 1950s (23) although methods used currently are much more efficient, safer, and the popularity of towing has increased. Towing can acutely produce a higher stride length,

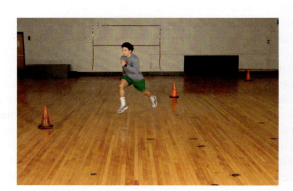

FIGURE 16.16 Gears. Numerous variations of this drill exist of which three are described here. In the first variation, cones (usually five) are placed ~15–20 yd apart. The athlete runs from cone to cone, increasing speed at each cone. This drill is useful for teaching the athlete acceleration and transitioning between speeds. This drill can be varied by altering the pattern of acceleration and decelerations, *e.g.*, accelerate, decelerate, accelerate, decelerate, or accelerate, accelerate, decelerate, accelerate, accelerate. The second variation is known as *ins and outs* (different from the agility ladder drill) where the athlete accelerates, cruises, sprints, cruises, sprints, and decelerates at 10- to 20-yd intervals. The third variation is to use a partner for in-line rolling sprints. The partner stands 10 yd in front of the athlete and begins running. The trailing athlete accelerates and passes the lead athlete and then decelerates. The new trailing athlete accelerates and passes the athlete, and so on. Place exchanges ("changing gears") take place until cessation of the drill. Multiple (>2) athletes can be used.

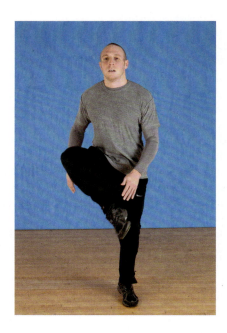

FIGURE 16.15 Drum major. The athlete rotates the forward leg inward and touches the heel to the hand while running forward. The opposite may also be performed to the rear leg (heel to toe) where the athlete touches the foot externally.

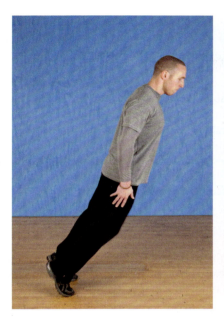 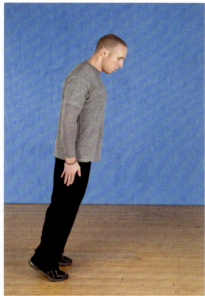 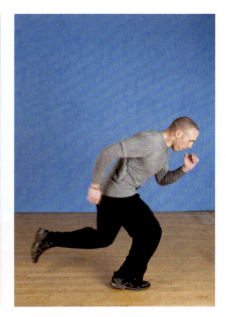

FIGURE 16.17 Falling starts. From a standing position, the athlete either leans/falls forward or is slightly pushed by a partner to initiate the sprint. Upon catching himself or herself (self-imposed reaction), the athlete sprints forward to train his or her acceleration ability.

rate, decreased foot contact times, and sprinting speed and is a potent stimulus to the neuromuscular system (33,34). The magnitude of the towing force is critical to sprint mechanics and the overall training effect. Clark et al. (33) showed that a towing force of >3.8% of the athlete's body weight had negative impacts on sprint training. A small-to-moderate amount of force is all that is needed.

The athlete may be towed in different ways. Elastic tubing can be used and attached around the waist. The opposite end can be attached to another athlete or a stationary object. If a stationary object is used, the athlete will connect the tube in front, back up several yards (at least 20–25 yd depending on the strength and length of tubing used), and begin running while being towed by the elastic tubing. The farther the athlete backs up, the greater the stretching and elastic response of the tubing as more force will be applied to the athlete. Thus, sprinting speed increases during towing. The athlete may connect the other end of the tubing to another athlete. The athlete will attach the tubing to the front, while the athlete doing the towing will have the other end of the tubing attached to his or her rear. The lead athlete begins sprinting thereby increasing the tension applied to the tubing. As a result, the rear athlete is towed forward and stride length and frequency increase. The lead athlete finishes the sprint first and propels the trailing athlete forward for the specified distance. Another way is to ensure that the lead athlete is faster than the trailing athlete. The lead athlete can tow the trailing athlete. At the same time, the lead athlete can use the trailing athlete as resistance (for resisted sprint training).

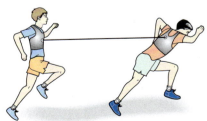

FIGURE 16.18 Overspeed training: towing.

FIGURE 16.19 The "Frankenstein."

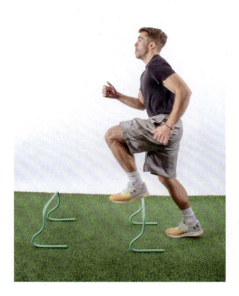

FIGURE 16.20 High knees over hurdles.

Current overspeed trainers sold on the market come in various forms. Bungee cords are used. Latex tubing provides the athlete with a steady force transition during stretching that prevents abrupt motion changes. The tubing may be sheathed in nylon, which helps prevent cuts and backlash that could occur if the tubing rips. Tubing comes with a belt (or harness although a belt is preferred for overspeed towing) for attachment, vary depending on the size of the athlete (above or below 140 lb), may provide various degrees of tension (light, medium, or heavy), and may stretch up to 40 yd or usually three times the original length. Precautions need to be taken with tubing as it can break perhaps leading to an injury for the athlete or it can become loose and disconnected from the belt if not carefully fastened. If any nicks or damage to the tubing is observed, the tubing should be replaced immediately. The athlete should avoid standing too long with the tubing in a stretched position. The athlete should begin sprinting as soon as the desired position is reached. Standing with the tubing stretched for prolonged periods of time can loosen the tubing. In past, it was common for the trailing athlete to be towed by an individual in front riding a bicycle, moped, or other slow-moving vehicle. The use of elastic tubing attached to a stationary object or another athlete is preferred and is safer. Towing is recommended to take place on a grassy surface to lessen the shock on the athlete. The elastic tubing can easily be used on fields and train multiple athletes at a time. Lastly, towing can be used for other drills such as backpedaling and side-to-side movements.

Overspeed training can be performed on an advanced model treadmill. Treadmills that exceed the athlete's max sprint speed can be used to force the athlete to increase stride rate and length. Treadmills that reach high speeds in short periods of time are preferred as a slow increase in belt speed could excessively fatigue the athlete. As with treadmills in general, there are inherent risks and concerns. It is recommended that a spotter be used, and a safety harness (in addition to the support rails) supports the athlete to reduce injury risk. The coach should control the treadmill speed so the athlete can maintain proper form without any additional responsibilities especially during deceleration. The treadmill used should slow belt speed rapidly. It is critical to note that with treadmill sprinting, there is slight deceleration or braking due to belt mechanics with each step. This becomes more pronounced with larger athletes and those sprinting at high speeds (23,35). Some of the braking can be reduced with familiarization.

Resisted Sprint Training

Sprint speed is enhanced through resisted sprint training. The athlete sprints maximally against a resistance. Resistance may come in the form of the following:

- *Wind* — a headwind provides resistance to the athlete. The wind is inconsistent so using a headwind can only occur at sporadic periods of time.
- *Sleds* — a sled or other object that can be dragged posteriorly on the ground (pulling a tire) is a popular means of resisted sprinting (Fig. 16.21). The weight of the sled and plates, plus the coefficient of friction between the sled and surface, determine the resistance encountered by the athlete. The amount of weight on the sled expresses the vertical weight; however, the horizontal force needs to be overcome to provide resistance to the athlete. The frictional force ranges considerably depending on the loading, velocity of the sled, and the surface type so the actual resistance to the athlete may be 30%–50% of the actual weight (36). Sleds are made of steel, have a handle and/or harness attachment, and have a post(s) which hold Olympic plates. Some sleds can be loaded with heavy weights. However, weight selection will depend on goals. Loading prescription is based on a percent of body mass or based on the magnitude of velocity loss during a sprint. For sprint training, low-to-moderate loading (up to 10%–13% of body mass) is used which allows the athlete to maintain proper form, to be explosive, and to

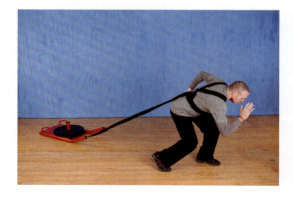

FIGURE 16.21 Sled towing.

reach a speed at least 90% of his or her max (21). To predict the percent of body mass loading to use relative to velocity reduction, Alcaraz et al. (37) developed the following equation:

$$\%Body\ mass = -0.8674 \times \%velocity + 87.99$$

For speed training, <10% of body mass is considered light loading, 10%–20% moderate loading, 20%–30% heavy loading, and >30% very heavy loading (21). The athlete begins in a 3- or 4-point stance, with the sled strap elongated, and maximally accelerates to peak speed as quickly as possible as if he or she were running an unloaded sprint. Sleds can be used for sport-specific power development. Research indicates that peak power is attained at a mean sled resistance of 78%–82% of body mass (with a range of 69%–96% of body mass), which is considerably more weight than is typically used for speed training (38). However, training at this greater loading provides no more advantage to speed development than low-resistance sled training (39). Sleds have attachments on the base, which forces the athlete to bend over farther prior to pushing the sled. Thus, heavier-loaded sleds could be useful for enhancing sport-specific running power and forces the athlete to maintain a low COG. A shoulder harness makes it more difficult to overcome inertia forcing the athlete to lower the COG. This teaches athletes to develop power and stay low. A belt harness is excellent for speed training to maximize sprint speed. Sprints of 10–50 yd with a sled are commonly used. In some cases, an athlete may use a tire in lieu of a sled for resistance. Tires and sleds can also be used for other drills such as backward, side shuffle, and carioca sprints.

- *Parachutes* — *speed chutes* are another popular source of resistance for sprinting. The chute opens as the athlete accelerates and increases resistance as it opens and ascends upward. Chutes come in different sizes and provide different levels of resistance especially at higher speeds of motion. Some newly designed chutes provide variable resistance. For example, they have an adjustable cord-lock on the lines, which can change the shape and diameter of the chute and alter the resistance (more resistance with wide expansion, less resistance with narrow expansion). Some chutes contain a velcro belt, which allows for mid-stride release thereby enabling the athlete to continue sprinting unimpeded. This type of potentiated loaded/unloaded sprint cycling of training has been called *sensation training* (40), or contrast training.
- *Sand* — sand is a highly compliant surface, which increases resistance with each stride. Running in sand increases energy expenditure 1.6 times more than running on a hard surface (41) and can pose a novel stimulus for sprint and speed endurance training. The instability of the sand alters muscular activation of the lower limbs. The greater metabolic demand is due, in part, to decreased mechanical efficiency and SSC activity (41).
- *Weighted Vests* — weighted vests and/or other weighted body wear (pants, suits, shoes, and strength shoes) can

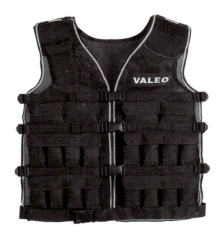

FIGURE 16.22 Weighted vest sprint.

be used for resisted sprint training (Fig. 16.22). Weighted vests are light and durable and have the capacity to add or exchange weights. The vest may come with pockets that can hold small amounts of weights (½–2 lb) totaling perhaps 10–20 lb or more depending on the vest. External loading should not be excessive to impede technique and explosive acceleration. Weighted vests are multipurpose and can be used for plyometric, agility, calisthenics, bodyweight, and sport-specific exercises. A review showed sprint training of 10–50 m with weighted vests of 5%–40% of body mass acutely increased foot contact time and reduced velocity, power, and force; however, the stimulus was shown to increase velocity by ~1.3% and improve sprint times by up to 9% during chronic training with vests of 5%–19% of body mass (42).
- *Harness* — harnesses have multiple purposes. A harness can be used between two athletes (Fig. 16.23). For example, the trailing athlete can provide resistance to the lead athlete. The trailing athlete should supply enough resistance to allow the lead athlete to sprint to at least 85%–90% of their max.

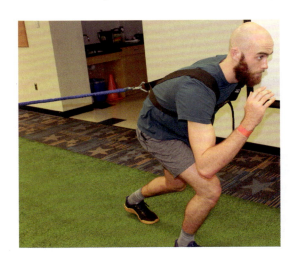

FIGURE 16.23 Towing sprint with resistance.

Some harnesses will have a quick release mechanism that allows the harness cord to disengage, enabling the lead athlete to continue sprinting unimpeded. Some heavy duty harnesses can be attached to heavy objects. For example, athletes have been known to pull cars or trucks. Although this type of training is more oriented toward developing total body power and strength, speed and acceleration are enhanced. Some harnesses have multiple resistance bands that can attach to the ankles, waist, shoulders, and/or arms. These can be used for other modalities besides linear sprinting, *e.g.*, backpedaling, lateral movements, etc.

- *Wearable Resistance* — wearable resistance involves applying an external load to specific segments of the body during sprinting, or any other movement type. Resistance may be applied to the trunk, forearms, upper arms, lateral or medial thigh, medial or distal thigh, and calves. Wearable RT is thought to increase the level of specificity as resistance is applied to specific movements at high velocities. The position of the external loading is important. For example, applying the same resistance load more distally to the thigh (compared to medial thigh) increases the moment of inertia by 4%–14% with loads up to 1 kg thereby providing a greater challenge to the athlete (43). Greater external loading increases the metabolic response to exercise. Studies have examined external loading ranging from 0.5% to 5% of body mass at different segments of the body. Sprint times may not increase (compared to unloaded conditions) unless loading at 5% of body mass is used (44). Lower limb wearable resistance with 3%–5% of body mass increases foot contact time during the first 2 steps and subsequent 10 steps of acceleration by up to 6%, reduces velocity during the acceleration phase by ~2%, and reduces velocity by up to 13% in maximal velocity phase (44). Kinetically, lower limb wearable resistance increases the force-velocity profile of foot contact by up to 11% and has been suggested to assist in increasing horizontal force output during acceleration (44). Chronic (6 weeks) wearable RT increases stride length by 5% but reduces stride frequency by ~5.6% resulting in no change in maximal running velocity (44).
- *Uphill and/or stairs* — sprinting uphill or up stadium stairs provides other sources of resistance. The athlete is forced to contract his or her muscles at a higher magnitude to accelerate his or her COG against the force of gravity. This is particularly true with the hip joint as mechanical advantage of the hip decreases with inclination thereby increasing the torque needed to produce power to move the human body at a specific velocity (45). Sprinting uphill provides a great metabolic challenge to the athlete and is a good way to increase muscle or speed endurance. Because of the added force requirement, uphill sprinting increases acceleration ability. Dintiman et al. (23) have recommended steep inclines (8° or higher) for 10–30 yd for increasing acceleration and start ability, and angles ranging from 1° to 3° for starts and speed endurance for distances >20 yd. Sensation training can be performed if the hill flattens to a plateau. The athlete sprints uphill (to maximize muscle fiber recruitment) and continues to sprint on the flat surface (creating a sense of overspeed training by making the athlete feel like he or she is running faster).

- *Partner* — a partner can physically provide resistance to the athlete to improve acceleration by either holding on to the belt/cord, elastic band, and towel or by placing hands around the athlete's waist. The utility is that the partner supplies resistance for all or only part of the drill. The partner supplies some resistance for 8–10 strides to improve the athlete's starting acceleration. However, the partner may let go and release the athlete (for sensation training) to allow the athlete to sprint maximally for a specified distance without resistance in a variation known as the *partner-assisted release*. This is a version of a *quick release mechanism* thought to enhance speed and power due to neuromuscular potentiation of the high-intensity contraction preceding the release. Quick release techniques have been used in ballistic, resistance, and plyometric training. Because of the need for a high rate of force development (RFD), inadequate time is provided by most explosive exercises <1 second in duration. The resultant force output is lower than what is seen during a slower high-intensity contraction (based on the *force-velocity relationship*). Quick release techniques are used to maximize the force-velocity relationship where a loaded dynamic or maximum isometric (ISOM) contraction (locked against a resistance) is performed for 1–3 seconds (to increase force and motor unit recruitment) and quickly released to allow unresisted motion the rest of the way (46). Upon release, these motor units are still facilitated, force is higher, and the athlete is thought to generate greater speed and power. Thus, it is a technique designed to maximize performance by creating a more favorable force-velocity environment. Sufficient resistance should be applied by the partner before release.

Drills to Increase Acceleration Ability and Speed

Acute sprint speed and technique are altered by the presence of external loading. Most research studies have used resisted sprint loads of 5%–80% of body mass performed for 10–50 m distances for 1–3 sessions per week for study durations of 4–10 weeks (21,47). As loading increases, sprint speed decreases in proportion. Cronin et al. (48) compared sled towing and weighted vest training (with 15% and 20% of body mass) with nonresisted sprints and showed increased sprint times (by 7.5%–19.8%) in both resisted conditions with a concomitant decrease in stride length (−5.2% to −16.5%) and stride frequency (−2.7% to −6.1%). Sled towing and weighted vests increased stance phase duration and decreased swing phase duration, whereas sled towing increased trunk and knee angles and weighted vests decreased trunk angle. Lockie et al. (49) showed that sled towing with 12%–32% of body mass decreased stride length (10%–24% depending on the magnitude of loading) and stride frequency, and increased ground contact time, trunk lean, and hip flexion. Of concern to

Interpreting Research
Resisted Treadmill Sprinting and Ground-Based Sprint Performance

Ross RE, Ratamess NA, Hoffman JR, Faigenbaum AD, Kang J, Chilakos A. The effects of treadmill sprint training and resistance training on maximal running velocity and power. *J Strength Cond Res.* 2009;23:385–94.

Ross et al. (56) investigated the effects of combined resisted/nonresisted sprint training alone or in combination with RT on sprint kinematics. Unique to this investigation was the type of treadmill used for sprint training. A newly designed treadmill (Woodway Force 3.0, Woodway, Inc.) which consisted of a belt that was user-driven (moved in proportion to sprint speed) and contained an electromagnetic braking system, which provided up to 68.2 kg of resistance to the treadmill belt, was studied. The resistance applied occurred within the belt as opposed to the waist, trunk, or limbs, which is characteristic of other resisted sprint training devices. The treadmill training program was performed 2 days per week and consisted of 8–12 sets of maximal sprints for 40–60 m at 0%–25% of each athlete's body mass with rest intervals of 2–3 minutes. The program rotated between loaded and unloaded sprint sets. 30-m sprint times and treadmill sprint velocity improved in both groups. Only the combination sprint/RT group increased treadmill sprint peak power. Interestingly, sprint training also increased 1 RM squat strength. This study showed that treadmill sprint training enhanced land-based sprint performance.

---

resisted sprint training is the loading used. The use of too heavy a load is thought to negatively affect sprinting ability. Sprint start technique and kinematics are not affected by pulling a load of up to 10% of body mass while using a sled (50). However, using loads of 20%–30% of body mass or more, increase time spent in the blocks, decrease stride length during initial steps, increase trunk lean, and produce more horizontal position during propulsion.

Resisted sprinting enhances sprint performance (12,21). A review of the literature showed that loads of 20%–43% of body mass were most specific to increasing acceleration, while loads <10% of body mass were most specific to improving the maximal velocity phase (21). A comparative study showed a load of 20% of body mass produced better improvements in acceleration, whereas loads of 5%–12.5% were better for the max velocity phase (51). Another review found largest acceleration improvements with loads <20% of body mass (47). The larger loads increase horizontal force production thereby targeting acceleration ability (47). Alcaraz et al. (52) showed that resisted sprint training with a sled, chute, or weighted belt was effective for training the maximum speed phase of sprinting. Myer et al. (53) compared inclined treadmill training to partner-resisted sprint training for 6 weeks and showed that both groups increased sprint speed and stride frequency but not stride length with no differences between groups. However, the ability of resisted sprint training to augment sprint performance more than traditional nonresisted sprint and plyometric training is less clear. Clark et al. (54) showed that resisted sprint training with weighted vests or sleds (18% and 10% of body mass) did not augment speed development more than nonresisted sprint training over 7 weeks of training. Spinks et al. (13) showed that resisted and nonresisted sprint training produced similar increases in acceleration over 8 weeks of training. Zafeiridis et al. (10) found nonresisted sprint training more effective for enhancing the maximum speed phase, whereas resisted sprint training was more effective for increasing acceleration.

However, West et al. (55) showed that the combination of resisted (12.6% of body mass) and nonresisted sprint training produced larger improvements in 10- and 30-m sprint times than nonresisted sprint training (of similar volume) alone. A review concluded that resisted sprint training was no more effective than unresisted training when directly compared (47). However, it is recommended that the combination of resisted and unresisted sprint training be used to maximize speed development (21).

Agility Training

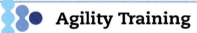

Agility training involves an integrated approach. Agility requires mobility, coordination, balance, power, optimal SSC efficiency, stabilization, proper technique, strength (in the development of forces applied to the ground for impact and propulsion), flexibility, body control, footwork, metabolic conditioning (to reduce fatigue), and a rapid ability to accelerate, decelerate, and change direction (57,58) (Fig. 16.24). There are perceptual and cognitive components to agility such as visual scanning, scanning speed, and anticipation (59). All of these factors work together in improving agility. As a result, some studies have shown low correlations between specific components of fitness and agility. Young et al. (60) found a positive relationship between reactive strength and agility, but leg concentric power (during an isokinetic squat) was poorly correlated to agility. Marcovic (61) and Marcovic et al. (62) have shown that leg extensor strength and power were poor predictors of agility; however, other studies have shown moderate to strong correlations between CON and ECC strength and COD ability especially when the agility test involves large COD angles, *e.g.*, ≥90° (3). Linear sprint speed has shown moderate to high relationships with various

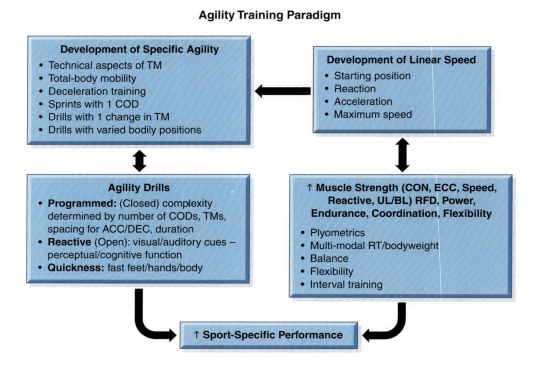

FIGURE 16.24 Agility training paradigm.

agility tests; however, relationships may be stronger if the agility test involves low COD angles (3). Jump power and reactive strength have shown moderate to high correlations with various agility tests (3). In addition, power and speed may not be as strong predictors of agility (compared to balance) in men but may relate higher to agility performance in women (7). These results demonstrate the complex nature of agility especially if the agility or COD test used is not specific to the training methods. Sufficient ECC muscle strength and reactive ability are needed to maximize deceleration and subsequent acceleration. One study showed that the addition of Nordic hamstring curls (2 d·wk⁻¹ for 6 wk) to regular training in team sport athletes improved COD ability by ~2.5% (63). Often, researchers have focused RT programs on bilateral exercises emphasizing vertical force components (64). However, agility movements often occur unilaterally in the vertical-horizontal and/or lateral direction, and require anterior, posterior (breaking and propulsive) and mediolateral force production (64). One study reported similar improvements in pro agility performance following bilateral (back squats) and unilateral (split squats) RT for 5 weeks in rugby players (65) so it appears the unilateral exercises may need to be more specific to cutting maneuvers.

A recent meta-analysis has shown that agility performance may improve by up to ~15% following plyometric training (with a mean increase of 5.3%), up to 12.7% following RT (with a mean increase of 3.3%), up to 6.8% following specific COD training (with a mean increase of 2.4%), and up to 8.2% following combined training methods, *i.e.*, RT, plyometrics, and COD (with a mean of 3.2%) (3). The plyometric training programs consisted largely of countermovement jumps, depth jumps, and other jump variations (bilateral and unilateral). The RT programs were diverse but consisted of exercises such as squats, Olympic lifts and variations, and other lower-body exercises. Programs consisting of squats produced 0.3%–12.7% improvement in COD and program emphasizing Olympic lifts produced 2.5%–9.1% improvements in COD ability (3). Thus, agility training is complex and includes multiple modalities including strength and power, sprint, specific agility, balance and coordination, and flexibility training. In addition to general strength training and conditioning, the application of agility methods should be similar to the loading vectors and movement types seen in athletes.

Technical Aspects of Agility Training

Exercise can improve agility. Some modalities are more effective than others. Plyometric, RT, and flexibility training may positively enhance agility. Although RT by itself may or may not improve agility per se (64,66,67), the increase in strength and power may augment specific components or other modalities of training used to increase agility. Plyometric and sprint training are critical to agility enhancement (3,68). Most often, an integrated workout will take place where plyometrics, sprint, and agility drills will be included to comprehensively train agility.

Although many drills can be used to enhance agility, these drills share some common fundamental movements, which are critical to rapidly changing direction, accelerating, and decelerating. The following list displays some common targets of sport-specific agility drills:

- *Balance* — the ability to maintain equilibrium is critical to agility training. Balance is maintained via input from the visual, vestibular, and proprioceptive systems. The vestibular center lies in the inner ear and responds to head movement and bodily motion by fluid movement. Selected proprioceptive systems (muscle spindles, Golgi tendon organs) and other joint receptors provide feedback to the central nervous system (CNS) to help control equilibrium and kinesthetic awareness. Motion is detected and an appropriate muscular response ensues. Controlling the COG is an underlying component to all agility drills. Balance and stability are greatest when the COG is lowered, the base support is larger, and the line of gravity is centered within the base support. Controlling the COG and base support are critical during agility drills to place the body in a more stable position. Force production is highest in stable positions. A stable athlete can develop greater forces applied to the ground and this, in turn, can increase agility. The ability to maintain equilibrium is vital to agility training. Static balance training includes drills that improve the athlete's ability to stand in place, whereas dynamic balance training drills improve the athlete's ability to maintain equilibrium during motion. Although many exercises may be included, some exercises are designed to target balance improvements more than others. Performing an exercise unilaterally instead of bilaterally, narrowing the base support, performing an exercise in a nonstable environment (stability ball, BOSU ball) or with one's eyes closed, performing a combination exercise, or performing an exercise from an unstable position (performing a shoulder press from a lunge position) are all specific ways to improve balance during RT. Plyometric and sprint drills require the athlete to maintain dynamic balance. Agility drills require high levels of balance and are performed on varying surfaces where rapid movement is crucial. As Verstegen and Marcello (58) have pointed out that a "solid base support creates the foundation on which the athlete can apply positive angles." *Positive angles* refer to the correct position of the hips, knees, and ankles relative to the trunk, which allow the athlete to optimally produce force applied to the ground to accelerate, decelerate, and change directions. During acceleration, a positive shin angle is created as the COG is anterior to the lead foot, whereas a negative shin angle is created during deceleration as the COG is posterior to the lead foot. Proper control of balance allows the athlete to maintain a position where agility can be maximized.
- *Posture* — proper posture is essential to agility training. Preventing excessive amounts of forward lean during acceleration and decreasing forward lean as deceleration increases are critical to properly performing the agility drill. The head should remain in a neutral position and eyes should be focused directly ahead. The athlete should try as best as possible to maintain the power line position during propulsion. Posture is enhanced by strong core

stability so core training is essential. The trunk and hips should be oriented in the direction of the intended movement during COD.
- *Foot contact* — foot contact with the ground is critical to agility. The athlete should maintain a dorsiflexed (toes up) ankle position upon contact with the ground. The dorsiflexed ankle position allows the athlete to quickly explode off of the ground. The athlete lands on the ball of the foot (not the toes) to optimize force applied to the ground. Upon acceleration, the feet rise only slightly off the ground as this reduces time for the next cycles of foot contact. A distinct sound will be heard when the athlete is landing properly and pushing off. The lack of a crisp sound may indicate landing on the toes. Short foot ground contact times and high impact and propulsive forces are critical to maximizing COD performance (69).
- *Arm action* — similar to sprinting, explosive arm action facilitates leg drive and enhances agility performance during acceleration.
- *Reaction* — the ability to react to the stimulus is critical to optimal agility training. Reaction ability comprises vision, hearing, and anticipation, in addition to the appropriate neuromuscular response, which can be enhanced through proper practice over time (58).
- *Quickness* — foot speed and the ability of the athlete to possess a quick first step is critical to agility training. Quickness is dependent upon stance, posture, reactive ability, and knowledge of on which direction movement will initiate.
- *Acceleration/deceleration* — the ability to accelerate and decelerate in many directions forms the core of agility training. Each drill targets the athlete's ability to accelerate and decelerate. During acceleration, there is a forward shift of the COG in response to forward leaning to augment horizontal forces to the ground. Deceleration is needed to slow down or come to a complete stop prior to reaccelerating in a different direction. Deceleration involves large eccentric braking forces applied in short periods of time. The COG is positioned behind the point of the contact foot creating rearward lean thereby resisting momentum of the body. The hips, knees, and ankles flex to lower the COG. In contrast to acceleration, the foot contacts the ground with the heel to increase horizontal braking force and increase ground contact time (70). The torso is more erect relative to the lower body moving the COG posterior to the base of support to enable greater horizontal braking forces (70). The spine remains neutral and head is facing forward. A side-to-side lean and subsequent shift of the COG is needed to produce lateral force in order to change direction and accelerate/decelerate in the frontal plane.
- *Targeted movements* — agility drills involve multiple movements including linear sprints, jumps, backpedaling, side shuffling, side running, cariocas, drop stepping, cross-over stepping, pivoting, and cutting. Cutting is a directional change in as little as a few degrees to 90° (69). Cutting involves *side-step* (lateral foot cutting opposite motion direction), *cross-over* (ipsilateral plant foot cutting same

direction of motion and subsequent crossing of opposite leg over), or *split-step* (jump prior to COD) techniques, each of which involve an initial acceleration, deceleration, COD (with weight acceptance and propulsion in the direction of movement), and final reacceleration (69). Side-stepping involves greater cutting angles, lateral impact and propulsion forces, ground contact time, varied quadriceps and hip abductor muscle activation patterns, and greater knee valgus loading compared to cross-over and split-step cutting techniques, while split-step cutting may enable greater deception and bilateral loading patterns (69).

Change of Direction: The Basics of Agility

The ability to change direction is a critical component to agility performance. COD ability is a composite of several factors shown in Figure 16.1. Each COD requires a braking force for deceleration followed by a subsequent propulsive force for acceleration (and reorientation of the body) in a different direction. Ground reaction forces and foot contact times impact COD ability. COD movements performed at shallow cutting angles (*e.g.*, <75°) are associated with short contact times (<250 ms), whereas movements involving steep cutting angles (*e.g.*, >75°) are associated with longer (>250 ms) foot contact times due to the larger braking component needed (71). Athletes with higher levels of relative strength have higher post COD stride velocity, larger braking and propulsion forces, and greater hip abduction and knee flexion angles during a 45° cut thereby demonstrating the importance of strength during COD movements (72). Increased hip extension force, low COG height, increased knee flexion, low trunk angular displacement during deceleration, and increased lateral trunk tilt during 180° COD can improve COD ability (71).

The complexity of an agility movement is increased with higher numbers of CODs or targeted movements included. Many agility drills will utilize at least one COD with some drills consisting of more than 10 CODs (64). Complex agility drills with several CODs increase the duration of the exercise and requires a higher level of high-intensity muscular endurance to sustain performance (64). Thus, metabolic conditioning is part of the agility training paradigm. Similar to other training modalities, agility training may be performed on a continuum from simple (*i.e.*, emphasizing the basics) to more complex training depending on the training status and abilities of the athlete. Agility training begins with the teaching and proper execution of technique during targeted movement patterns, acceleration, deceleration, and COD. Athletes should be able to demonstrate fundamental technique while performing basic targeted agility movements and be able to properly accelerate, decelerate, and change direction when directed to do so. In some cases, a coach may prescribe more advanced agility drills to athletes who do not have the proper foundation to optimize performance of these drills. This could be problematic if it leads to technical issues. Agility training may progress from simple to more complex movements and from linear sprinting ability to multidirectional movements. Agility training requires an integrated approach of RT, plyometrics, balance, speed, flexibility, metabolic conditioning, and specific agility exercises.

Emphasis on the athlete's ability to decelerate correctly is paramount to agility training and injury prevention and should be targeted early in training. Deceleration training involves a multimodal approach. Deceleration requires balance, mobility, power, and strength, especially ECC strength to control the athlete's COG. RT may target deceleration ability by focusing on the ECC component of the repetition. For example, performing exercises such as barbell squats, front squats, split squats, step-ups, lunges, or deadlifts with an augmented ECC component or lengthened ECC phase can enhance strength that could be beneficial for the strength needed during deceleration. Plyometric exercises (*i.e.*, squat jumps, forward and lateral broad jumps, single-leg hops and jumps) that emphasize proper soft landing technique can augment ECC strength. Foot position during landing can vary to reinforce positions seen during deceleration. For example, athletes may land bilaterally, staggered stance with one foot forward, or unilateral landings with progression. Unilateral exercises increase the intensity during bodyweight movements so jump landing heights should be lower compared to bilateral landings. In addition, holding the landing position is an effective way to increase strength, balance, and coach proper positioning prior to adding additional repetitions or movements to drills. Athletes should be able to consistently demonstrate and land/hold the proper final position of the exercise prior to progressing to subsequent stages of training. Movements initiated off of improper starting positions have little kinesthetic value and may increase the risk of injury. Bodyweight exercises such as lunges, lateral lunges, wall slides, and step-ups can be a valuable part of deceleration training. Emphasizing a slow ECC phase during the descent can be beneficial to increasing ECC strength needed for deceleration. Ultimately, deceleration is emphasized in specific drills involving forward, backward, or side-to-side movements utilizing 2-foot, 1-foot, or lateral braking techniques. In addition, the coach may reinforce deceleration with each drill rather than allowing the athlete to slow down at their own pace at the completion of the drill. One study found forced deceleration at the end of an agility drill augmented some parameters of muscle strength but did not augment agility performance more so than nonreinforced conclusion of agility drills (73). Some examples of specific deceleration and deceleration/COD drills include the following:

- The athlete runs to line or cone (5–10 yd), lowers COG, and decelerates to a complete stop.
- The athlete runs to a cone (5 yd), decelerates, and stops; reaccelerates to the next cone, stops, and repeats to a third cone.
- The athlete runs to cone (5 yd), decelerates, and circles cone; and repeats for three cones.
- The athlete runs forward to a cone or line, decelerates and touches line/cone, back pedals to starting line, decelerates and touches line, and repeats for desired number of repetitions.
- The athlete side shuffles, stops and briefly holds position, and side shuffles back to starting line.

Agility training emphasizes COD in addition to acceleration and deceleration, and the correct technique applied to performing targeted agility movements. Smooth and rapid CODs are crucial to maximizing athletic performance. Performing one basic move and adding one COD or targeted movement to it to stress proper control, technique, and positioning of the COG may be used prior to adding more complex drills later in training. The following gives a few examples of drills that may be used to train the basic components of agility by first stressing one COD or one change from basic movement to a different targeted movement and control of the COG. Cones may be used and placed at various lengths (*e.g.*, 5–10 yd apart) and various cutting angles and targeted movements can be used.

Basic drills with 1 COD

- Linear sprint to a "V" cut: the athlete runs forward linearly for a desired length then sharply cuts at a 45° angle right or left for several steps.
- The athlete sprints 10 yd, decelerates and turns 180° off of L or R leg, and sprints 10 yd to finish.
- The athlete runs 5–10 yd, then performs a lateral (90°) L-cut for 5 yd.
- The athlete side shuffles 5–10 yd, decelerates and touches cone/line, reverses direction, and side shuffles back to starting line.

Basic drills with 1 change in targeted movements

- The athlete sprints 10 yd, decelerates, stops, and then backpedals for 5 yd.
- The athlete sprints 5 yd, switches to backpedaling for 5 yd.
- The athlete performs a broad jump, sticks the landing and rotates COG forward, and subsequently sprints for 10 yd.
- The athlete performs a side jump, sticks the landing and rotates COG forward, and sprints 10 yd.
- The athlete side shuffles for 5 yd, then sprints the final 5 yd.
- The athlete laterally hops and lands on the R leg (holds the position for 2–3 s), laterally hops and lands on the L leg (holds the position for 2–3 s), and sprints for 5–10 yd.
- The athlete backpedals for 5 yd, then performs a side run for the final 5 yd.

Total-body mobility is another factor in agility training. The body must move quickly in multiple planes of motion while maintaining balance. In previous chapters, we discussed bodyweight exercises such as calisthenics (*i.e.*, cartwheels, burpees), tumbling, rolls, duck unders, etc. and multiple-joint/total-body flexibility exercises. These exercises target total body mobility, which ultimately assist in improving agility. In addition, altering the starting position or changing bodily position during a drill can be used to enhance agility. Often, agility drills may begin from basic standing (2-point), 3- and 4-point stances. However, difficulty can be increased if the starting position begins from seated, kneeling, prone, supine, and crawling positions. This is particularly effective for training athletes that encounter many different positions in sport. The following are a few examples of drills utilizing varied bodily positions:

Basic drills from different starting positions

- The athlete begins in a prone position lying on the ground, quickly ascends to their feet, and sprints for 5–10 yd.
- The athlete begins in a 2-point stance, descends to a lying prone position, quickly ascends, and sprints for 5–10 yd.
- The athlete begins in a supine lying position on the ground, rolls to a prone position, quickly ascends to their feet, and backpedals for 5–10 yd.
- The athlete bear crawls for 5 yd, quickly ascends to their feet, and sprints for 5–10 yd.
- The athlete begins in a kneeling position, quickly ascends to their feet, and side shuffles for 5–10 yd.

Agility Equipment

Agility training can be performed with no equipment. A football field with marked lines can be used for many drills. Taped markers can be used on a gym floor for various drills. However, some pieces of equipment expand the types of drills that can be used. *Cones* come in various sizes and are used as markers that guide the movements and COD. Smaller cones force the athletes to reach further when performing drills where the cone needs to be touched upon directional change. *Agility ladders* enable performance of a multitude of quickness drills that are excellent for developing foot speed, balance, and coordination. *Rings* and *agility dots* can be used for a multitude of single- and double-leg movements. *Reaction balls* contain ridges that force the ball to bounce in different directions while the athlete tries to catch it. Use of a reaction ball can help the athlete improve hand-eye coordination, reaction ability, and first-step quickness. *Agility bags* provide obstacles for athletes to perform several multidirectional drills especially front sprints, side shuffling, and backpedaling. *Tires* have been used especially by football players to increase foot speed and agility. *Agility poles* can be set up at various distances and configurations to create an obstacle course for athletes during agility training. *Mini hurdles* and *boxes* may also be used as obstacles in addition to their regular use for hopping and jump drills. *Reaction belts* are excellent for athletes to use during shadow drills. *Jump ropes* are excellent for increasing foot speed. Sport-specific devices and other equipment can be used to train or test agility, reaction ability, and mobility. For example, the Makoto tester (Makoto USA) measures and trains reaction ability, hand-eye coordination, and agility (74) (Fig. 16.25). The athlete stands in the middle of the triangle and reacts to visual and auditory stimuli. Random lighting forces the athlete to strike that area to fine-tune hand-eye coordination, anticipation, and reaction time, and a score is given once the trial time has been completed. Other devices that measure similar abilities are also on the market.

Types of Agility Training Drills

It is essential to minimize the loss of speed during deceleration when training for agility. Drills that require COD of the COG forward, backward, vertically, and laterally train the athlete to

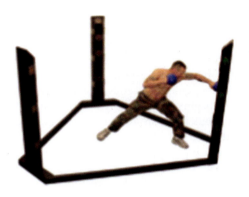

FIGURE 16.25 The Makoto reaction device. (Courtesy of Makoto USA, Centennial, Co.)

optimally move in response to a stimulus. Agility training drills can be classified into three general types: (a) programmed, (b) reactive, and (c) quickness. *Programmed drills* are those that are preplanned (sometimes referred to as *closed skills*). The athlete is aware of the movements prior to beginning the drill. The drills discussed in previous sections are programmed as the athlete knows exactly which targeted movements, drill lengths, and COD angles are used.

Reactive drills are continued based on the visual or auditory information from a coach, other athlete, or object such as a ball. They are not preplanned (sometimes referred to as *open skills*). Athletes from many sports participate in reactive drills as part of their athletic practices and coaches can incorporate numerous sport-specific reactive drills into training or practice sessions. Direct competition forces athletes to react to game situations but reactive drills are used in training as well. For example, from a box jump, the athlete may sprint forward 10 yd. At the yard marker, a coach may be located and will point in a direction for the athlete to continue. If the coach points right then the athlete may cut and sprint to the right or side shuffle to the right. Partner drills may be reactive. *Shadow or mirror drills* involve two athletes attached by a reaction belt (which may have velcro straps to disengage) or not attached. One athlete assumes the lead and the other athlete shadows the athlete's every move. This entire drill is based on reaction. Another example is slap or tag drills. One athlete must tag or touch a partner. A game of *tag* forces one athlete to be evasive and the other to react and apply a tag. Modifications of tag drills can be used from standing positions but sport-specific positions. For example, the *push-up slap* drill involves two athletes facing each other (head-to-head) in a starting push-up position. While maintaining their posture, each athlete tries to slap the hand of the other athlete and the other athlete tries to evade the slap by moving the hand. This not only trains reactive ability but also core strength as the athlete is forced to support his or her prone body weight with one arm for some periods of time. Wrestlers incorporate many reactive drills in their training (as wrestling is a reactive sport) where one athlete may try to slap the partner's foot, while the other tries to evade the slap during takedown simulations. Another drill is to place flags/strings around the wrestlers' waist during shooting drills for takedowns. The athlete who first grabs the other's flag wins the drill. Some reactive drills involve ball tosses and catch which force the athlete to react quickly. For example, the *blind partner toss* involves an athlete standing behind another athlete, throwing a ball against a wall, and the primary athlete reacts by catching the ball wherever it bounces. In baseball or softball, a coach may drop a ball, have the player sprint to the ball, and throw to a base. Medicine balls can be used, thrown against a wall at short distances, and the athlete reacts quickly to catch the ball. Lastly, some drills may consist of closed and open components. That is, part of the drill is predetermined but the rest of the drill is reactive.

Quickness drills are designed to produce fast movements, quick feet and hands. Many agility ladder drills are designed to have rapid movement of the feet. Some quickness drills may involve minimal locomotion but very fast foot movements in a specified area. Some common quickness drills necessitate starting on the ground and quickly popping up to one's feet as fast as possible. Other drills include beginning on the feet, falling to the ground (sprawl in wrestling), and then rapidly getting up. The *resisted let-go* is a useful drill for increasing quickness. One athlete holds or provides resistance to another athlete from the rear (although other angles can be used). The resisted athlete begins to sprint forward or begin a specific agility drill. Resistance is applied at the beginning of the drill. The other athlete then abruptly releases the athlete, eliciting a quick response. In any instance, a drill which forces the athlete to move the body rapidly in any direction can improve quickness.

Programmed drills invoke a more varied response than reactive drills during cutting maneuvers especially in the knee. Besier et al. (75) showed greater stabilization of the knee (via selective activation of medial/lateral, internal/external rotator muscles, and cocontraction of the flexors/extensors) in a programmed cutting maneuver versus generalized cocontraction in reactive cutting. The reactive maneuvers resulted in greater valgus and varus moments on the knee. Programmed drills allow for postural adjustments, while reactive cutting drills increased stress on the knee (76). Stress on the knee is greater during side stepping and crossover steps than linear running (77). These data demonstrate that neuromuscular mechanisms help limit joint distress when the moves are anticipated.

Agility drills come in many forms, and it is beyond the scope of this chapter to depict several hundreds of potential drills (93). Basic agility drills can be used without special equipment or markings. These focus on specific movements and may come in the form of calisthenics such as cartwheels, jumping jacks, forward/backward rolls, shoulder rolls, and other more sport-specific drills such as get-up-and-gos (common in football), sprawl drill (seen in wrestling), pitter-patter (wrestling and football), duck unders (used by boxers), base running drills (baseball and softball), and specific footwork drills (for multiple sports). Several agility drills consist of basic movements such as forward sprints, backpedalling, side shuffling, drop-steps, crossover steps, diagonal steps, and cutting and pivoting. One popular agility drill commonly used in warm-ups and training is the *carioca*. The carioca involves lateral motion where the right leg steps over the left with one step, right leg steps behind the left with the second step, and the cycle repeats with proper hip motion. This drill is performed quickly once proper technique is learned.

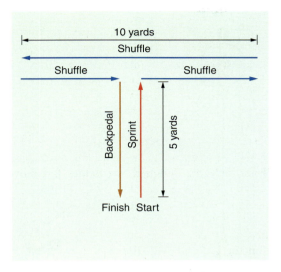

FIGURE 16.26 T-drill.

Many agility drills discussed in this section are composed of the aforementioned movements but utilize multiple CODs and targeted movements. These agility drills are marked by different courses or patterns of movement and are more complex than the single COD/targeted movement change, and deceleration drills discussed in previous sections. The following drills are some examples of agility exercises commonly performed by athletes (Figs. 16.26–16.48). It is important to note that there are numerous drills that can be designed. The coach should choose drills that are similar to motions encountered in the sport and can design patterns that replicate actual movement, *e.g.*, setting cones to replicate a crossing pattern for a football wide receiver. At the end of the drill, a pass may be thrown to the athlete to increase the level of sport specificity. Drills should encompass the basic movements of linear sprints, COD, accelerations/

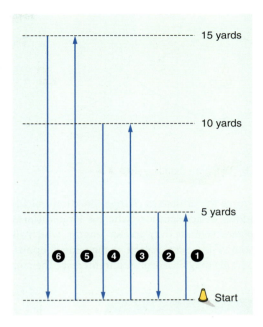

FIGURE 16.28 A 60-yd shuttle run.

decelerations, backpedaling, side and diagonal shuffling, cariocas, cutting, and pivoting. Coaches should constantly monitor technique and be especially instructional to athletes as they touch or run around the cones. Body control is needed to ensure athletes stay close to the cones and do not drift too far away. Correct foot placement, lowering of the COG, deceleration and acceleration, posture, and approach angles are critical when encountering the cones as these can be areas where athletes may lose critical time due to technical flaws. On the field, this may result in a negative play as any additional time taken could mean the difference between making the play and allowing the opponent a major competitive advantage. Cone lengths (and the number of cones) modulate the level of changing direction and pattern of acceleration/deceleration. Close

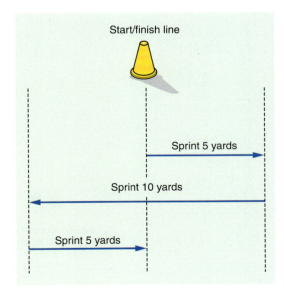

FIGURE 16.27 A 20-yd shuttle (pro agility drill).

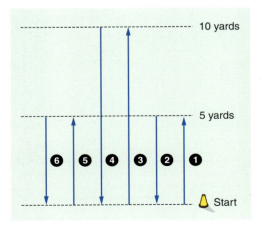

FIGURE 16.29 A 40-yd sprint. Variations: backpedaling or side shuffling. Can change the length of the drill and mix linear sprints with backpedaling and side shuffling.

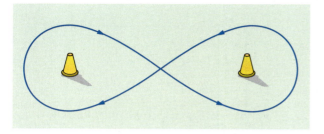

FIGURE 16.30 Figure 8 drill.

distances force the athlete to change direction quickly without large windows of acceleration, whereas large distances enable the athlete to accelerate over greater lengths, which also creates an opportunity for deceleration management upon changing direction. Drills may be integrated to increase the complexity.

Case Study 16.1

Jim is a baseball player who wants to improve his agility over the off-season. He approaches you and wants you to prescribe him some good agility drills he can use to improve his baseball performance. Based on your knowledge of the movement demands of baseball (Jim plays right field), prescribe or design 10 drills which have high baseball specificity. For each one, give an example of how the drill relates to a movement encountered during a baseball game.

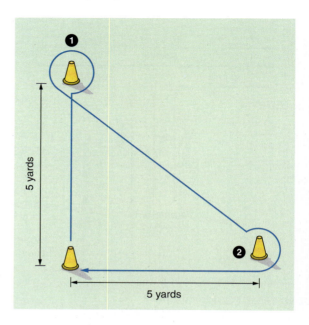

FIGURE 16.32 Right triangle drills. Variations: change the distance between cones, place the second cone on the opposite side, and alter turns at each cone.

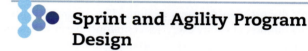

Sprint and Agility Program Design

Although sprint and agility workouts can be performed independently, for most athletes, an integrated approach works very well. Few studies comparing various sprint and

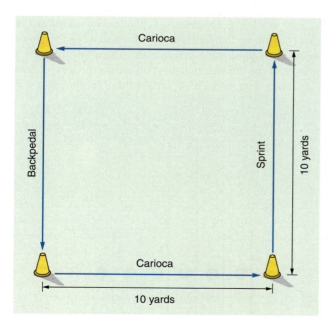

FIGURE 16.31 Square drills. Variations: change cone spacing. A cone can be placed in the middle to add further movements (in the shape of a "*star*").

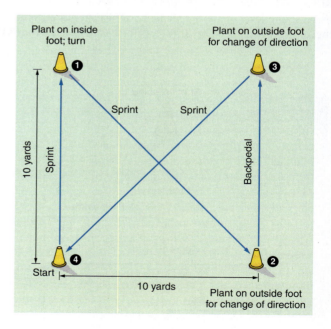

FIGURE 16.33 X-pattern drills. Variations: integrate side shuffling, backpedaling.

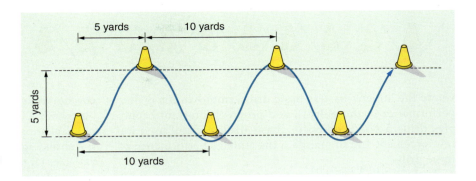

FIGURE 16.34 Z-pattern drills. Variation: change cone spacing.

agility programs for efficacy have been conducted. Most of the available training information is derived from practitioners or from studies where researchers examined the efficacy of one specific agility program so there is wide latitude of design and implementation strategies. Similar to plyometric training, beginning sprint and agility programs should focus on proper technique and footwork using basic drills. Quality is more important than quantity. Basic drills have low levels of footwork complexity, CODs, and number of targeted movements included. Mastery of basic drills leads to progression to more challenging drills. Intensity of drills increases with greater complexity. For sprint training, overspeed and resisted sprint drills are more intense and may be introduced once basic sprint technique is mastered and the athlete has improved sprinting ability (developed a base). When used, these drills are typically performed earlier in the workout when energy is high and fatigue is minimal to facilitate skill acquisition. For agility training, basic drills stressing linear speed and targeted movements should be mastered first. Progressing to mastering single COD (at various angles), deceleration, and the transition from one move to another targeted move can ensue. For footwork drills, basic line drills or ladder exercises (*i.e.*, hopscotch drill, multiple hops) that consist of only one or two major footwork components should be mastered and progress later to more complex drills with larger numbers of foot contacts and motions. Higher intensity agility drills include those with complex movement patterns, include multiple directions, involve high rates of acceleration/deceleration, are reactive, and may incorporate some moderate-to-high plyometric drills in addition to basic agility movements.

Drill progression (upon mastery) is unique. With RT, the athlete can keep increasing load over time. However, with sprint and agility training, there is finite loading (unless external loading is used) so progression entails improving drill times while maintaining optimal technique and mastering more complex drills. Drills can be made more complex by adding other targeted movements, CODs, changing the lengths/position of cones or other agility markers (to affect acceleration and deceleration patterns), or adding a reactive or sport-specific skill to the drill. Agility training progression may be viewed similarly to a martial artist in training. Martial arts progression is based upon a system of belts. Each belt signifies that the athlete has mastered certain skills from a beginning level (white or yellow belt) to advanced levels (black belt and associated ranks). Progression in agility training can be viewed similarly

Myths & Misconceptions
Sprint Speed and Agility Are Entirely Genetically Determined

This statement is partially true in that genetics do play a role in sprint speed and agility. For example, muscular (fiber types, architecture, protein expression, tendon insertion), neural (recruitment, rate, synchronization, coactivation/activation strategies), and skeletal (limb lengths, anthropometrics) factors contribute greatly to maximal sprint speed, and all these have a genetic component to them. Elite athletes may have some performance-enhancing gene polymorphisms that enable higher levels of performance (78). Genetic expression of proteins involved in muscle contraction appear to be up-regulated more in athletes gifted with high sprinting capacity and ability to rapidly accelerate and decelerate. Some of these do not change once the athlete is fully mature, *e.g.*, tendon insertions, limb lengths. However, other factors are trainable and every athlete can improve upon their maximal speed and agility via specific training. Some evidence shows that skill acquisition involved in sprint and agility training may be most trainable during the preadolescent years (4). Proper coaching and/or physical education instruction emphasizing motor development and learning early in life are very beneficial for athleticism later in life. Although genetics may separate the great sprinters from the average sprinters or great athletes from average athletes, every athlete has the ability to improve his or her sprint speed and agility by proper training, diet, and recovery in between workouts.

FIGURE 16.35 Zig-zag drills. Variations: can use agility poles, integrate backpedaling or side shuffling. Cones can be spaced farther apart (with fewer cones, *e.g.*, four) to form the "S" shape.

where the athlete masters basic drills, improves his or her performance in these drills, and progresses to more complex drills. Upon progression, basic drills are still used for reinforcement and to maintain the athlete's performance of these drills.

There is little consensus as to specific guidelines for sprint and agility training. Examination of training programs of some of the world's greatest athletes and practices of elite coaches reflect that there are many ways to train speed, quickness, COD, and agility. However, there are certain recommendations/suggestions that can be used in the design of sprint and agility programs. Manipulation of acute program variables targets specific aspects of speed, quickness, and agility. Similar to other modalities of training, the variation of volume and intensity of sprint and agility is more conducive to progression rather than just increasing each over time as

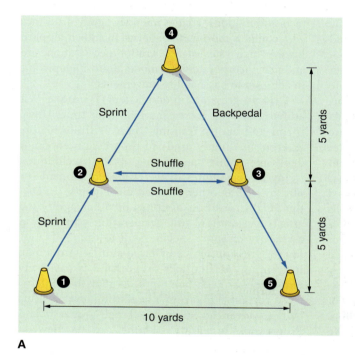

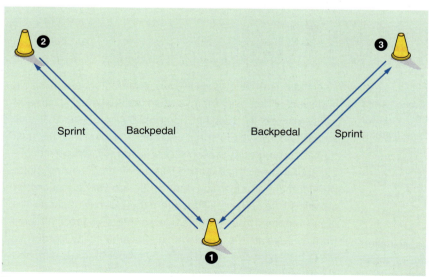

FIGURE 16.36 Letter drills. Cones are placed at strategic locations to form letters of the alphabet, *e.g.*, A (see **A**), V (see **B**), and N. Sprints, backpedaling, and side shuffling are used during each drill.

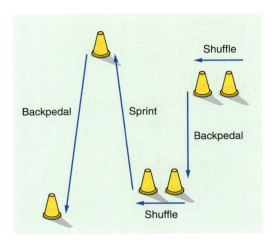

FIGURE 16.37 EKG drill.

overtraining may occur. The following general guidelines can be helpful in program design:

- Structure and Sequencing: the structure of the program needs to be determined right away. That is, whether or not speed and agility workouts will be independent or integrated. The following are structure and sequencing recommendations for both types:
  Sprint training only: general warm-up → dynamic ROM exercises → sprint technique/form drills → overspeed/resisted sprint drills → basic speed → cooldown
  Agility training only: general warm-up → dynamic ROM exercises → targeted agility form drills → basic COD, deceleration, or transition drills → quickness → agility: open, closed (most complex to least complex) → cooldownfacilitate skill acquisition. For agility training

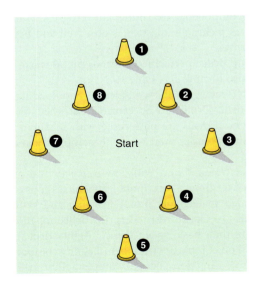

FIGURE 16.38 Diamond reaction drill. A coach is located in the middle to indicate left or right direction to the athlete.

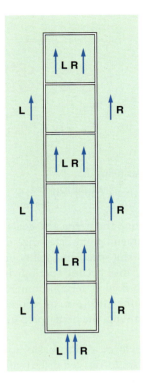

FIGURE 16.39 Hopscotch (ladder drill).

  Integrated sprint/agility training: general warm-up → dynamic ROM exercises → sprint and agility technique → agility (most complex to least complex) → basic speed → cooldown
  Sprint and agility take presentence in sequence if RT is performed the same day.
  Plyometric training can be integrated with sprint and agility training. Plyometric drills may be integrated within sprint and agility workouts or the plyometric exercises may be grouped and performed before or after speed and agility drills.
- Exercise Selection: the types of drills and exercises included are critical to program design. Many drills have been discussed in this chapter and numerous others exist as well. Drill selection should be based on a continuum from basic

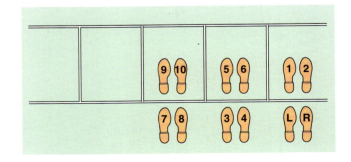

FIGURE 16.40 Ins and outs (ladder drill). Variation: to exit the ladder on the opposite side.

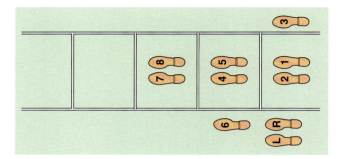

FIGURE 16.41 Icky shuffle (ladder drill).

to complex meeting the needs and goals of the athlete. The following recommendations categorize drills, which should be used in successful speed and agility programs. Similar to other modalities, drill cycling (periodizing many exercises/drills to be performed at certain points in training) can be advantageous to the athlete as the more stimuli the athlete encounters in training, the better prepared he or she are for the competition.

- Sprint training: form drills, basic speed drills (varied lengths), overspeed/resisted drills (with some training experience as a form of progression) — drills target reaction time, acceleration, and maximum speed turnover (stride rate and length).

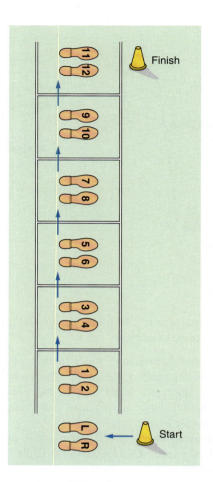

FIGURE 16.43 Left-right shuffle (ladder drill).

- Agility training: sport-specific drills stressing body movement and control, balance exercises, reactive drills, deceleration, COD, basic movement agility drills — patterns and components are simple and progress to more complex as technique mastery is observed and performance improves.
- Warm-up drills: performed after a general warm-up. Some are also form drills (Table 16.2).
- Intensity: refers to the complexity and loading involved in the drill. Drills can be categorized based on intensity. Although all drills are performed with maximal quality of effort, the intensity increases with complexity and external loading.
- Beginner trainees start with low intensity and progress to high over time. Short, more frequent sessions are recommended to facilitate motor learning and skill development. Overspeed/resisted sprint drills are most intense (more than basic speed drills). Agility drill intensity is based on complexity (number of agility components, patterns of direction change). Simple agility drills are performed early and progress to more complex and reactive drills over time. Technique is stressed at all phases of training. Speed is high for each drill so the quality of effort per set/repetition is critical.

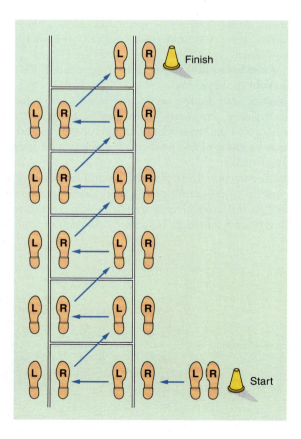

FIGURE 16.42 Side rocker (ladder drill).

Chapter 16 Sprint and Agility Training 525

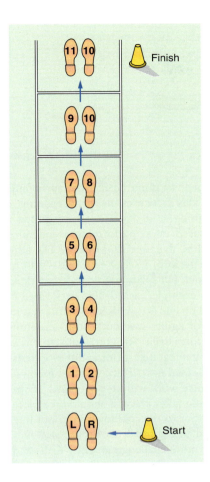

FIGURE 16.44 Two-feet forward (ladder drill).

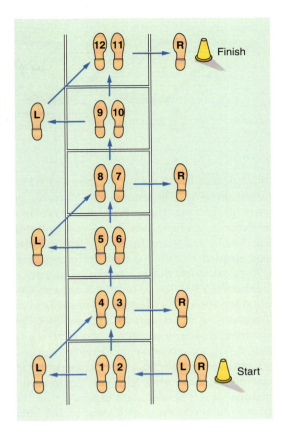

FIGURE 16.45 Two-in lateral shuffle (ladder drill).

- Frequency: the number of sprint/agility workouts per week. Frequency depends on many factors including practice/competition schedule, other modalities of training (resistance, plyometric), diet, and recovery practices.
  1–3 days per week is typically recommended. Higher frequency can be used with caution in advanced athletes. Undulating variations in intensity and volume can accommodate higher training frequencies.
- Volume: the total number of repetitions and work performed. Volume load can be used as the measure which is the product of drill distances and intensity (speed or loading). Volume load is quite variable and depends upon several factors including intensity, frequency, diet, recovery, and training status. Advanced athletes can tolerate higher training volumes but caution still needs to be used. Quality is preferred over quantity.
  1–3 sets for form drills and dynamic exercises; 3–5 sets for sprint and agility workload sets. Volume of overspeed drills should be max 10% of volume. The length/duration of each drill contributes to total volume. For maximal speed and agility training, most drills will be somewhat short in duration to maximize ATP-PC metabolism.

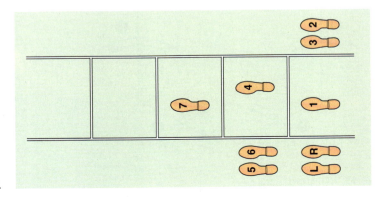

FIGURE 16.46 Zig-zag cross-over shuffle (ladder drill).

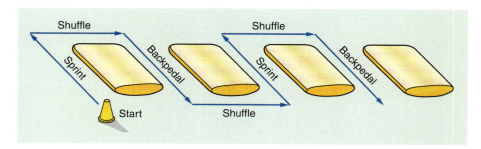

FIGURE 16.47 Bag weaves.

Drills longer in length and/or duration (>10–15 s) begin to stress speed or agility endurance (*anaerobic conditioning*) in proportion. Thus, short, quick, explosive drills are recommended for pure speed and agility development. The United States Track and Field Association has recommended acceleration and maximum speed drills be 20–80 yd in length and that the volume per workout range between 300–500 yd (acceleration) and 300–800 yd (maximum speed) in collegiate athletes (79).

- Rest Intervals: rest in between sets and exercises. Speed and agility training requires adequate recovery in between sets and exercises. A fatigued athlete cannot develop the speed and/or agility needed to optimally train the neuromuscular system. A constant rest interval or work-relief ratio can be used.
  1–3 minutes of rest between sets depending on the intensity and duration of the drill. Work-relief intervals of 1:10–1:20 may be used to target the ATP-PC system and to allow adequate recovery. A shorter ratio (*i.e.*, 1:5) may be used for short-duration sets or when anaerobic conditioning or endurance is a training goal. Less rest is needed between sets of form drills.

Putting It All Together

The program designed can be implemented and periodically assessed. Sprint and agility programs must accommodate other modalities of training such as RT, plyometrics, and depends on whether the athlete is in the off-, pre-, or in-season periods.

Table 16.3 depicts a sample basic 3-day sprint and agility training program. Day 1 focuses on sprint training, day 2 focuses on agility training, and day 3 is an integrated workout. The structure is based upon performing a general warm-up initially followed by dynamic ROM drills. The athlete can select five drills and perform 1 set of each one. Drills may be rotated for each workout. For sprint or integrated workouts, form drills follow. In this example, each drill is performed for 20 yd for 2 sets, *i.e.*, 20 yd up and 20 yd back with little rest in between sets (30 s^{-1}·sec). For agility workouts, basic structural movements replace sprint form drills. Structural movements and form drills are used during integrated sprint/agility workouts. The primary drills are performed next. The cooldown follows if no speed or agility endurance work will be performed. If speed/agility endurance training takes place, it should take place at the end of the workout prior to the cooldown as to not interfere with the maximal speed and agility drills. Progression may take place by incorporating more challenging agility drills and by introducing overspeed and resisted sprint drills.

Table 16.2	Selected Sprint and Agility Training Warm-Up Drills	
Dynamic ROM	**Sprint**	**Agility**
Toe walks	High knees	Ankle hops
Knee circles	Butt kickers	Accelerations
Scorpion	Lunge walks	Side shuffles
Straddled hip circles	Skips	Backpedaling
Lunge with torso rotation	Mountain climbers	Cariocas
BW squat	A and B marches	Side lunges
Press-ups	Ankling	Resisted walks — 4 directions (bands)
Lying hip adduction/abduction	Pawing	45° cuts
Groiner	Resisted knee-ups (bands) Arm swings	

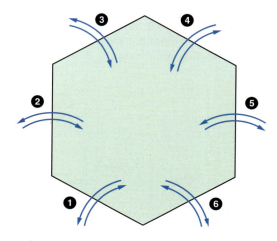

FIGURE 16.48 Hexagon drill.

Table 16.3 Sample 3-Day Sprint and Agility Program

Monday	Wednesday	Friday
General warm-up 3–5-min jog	General warm-up 3–5-min jog	General warm-up 3–5-min jog
Dynamic ROM drills 1 × 5 drills	Dynamic ROM drills 1 × 5 drills	Dynamic ROM drills 1 × 5 drills
High knees 2 × 20 yd	Ankle hops 2 × 10	Mountain climbers 2 × 20 s
Butt kickers 2 × 20 yd	Runs (50% of max) 2 × 20 yd	"B" marches 2 × 20 yd
Lunge walks 2 × 20 yd	Backpedals 2 × 20 yd	Backpedals 2 × 20 yd
"A" march 2 × 20 yd	Side shuffles 2 × 20 yd	Cariocas 2 × 20 yd
Gears (10-yd int) 3–5 × 40 yd	Ladder hopscotch 3×	T-drill 3×
Sprints 5 × 20 yd	Ladder ins and outs 3×	Sprints 6 × 40 yd
Flying sprints 3 × 40 yd	20-yd shuttle 3×	Zig-zag drill 3×
Cooldown	Square drill 3×	60-yd shuttle run 3×
	"V" drill 3×	Cooldown
	Cooldown	

Case Study 16.2

Power training for anaerobic athletes requires an integrated approach consisting of RT, plyometric, sprint, and agility training. Balance between all modalities is imperative to developing effective power training programs.

Questions for Consideration: Consider a training phase where all modalities are included. How might an athlete or coach design a program to include all of these modalities into a weekly workout schedule? Be sure to discuss training frequency, workout structures, general exercise selection, and sequencing.

Speed Endurance Training

Speed endurance reflects the athlete's ability to generate, maintain, and repeat speed performances over time. Athletes with high levels of speed endurance do not experience the same level of fatigue or performance decrement over time as a lesser-conditioned athlete. For example, a basketball player will still have the burst of speed and power late in the second half when the game is on the line or the football player will still have that necessary burst of speed and power in the fourth quarter as they did earlier in the game. Speed endurance training should target the demands of the sport. It is important to break down the sport by analyzing the typical lengths the athlete may sprint, the number of plays or explosive activities seen during a typical game, and the amount of rest seen in between plays. For example, in football, some data show that on offense, a team may have ~12–15 series per game, average ~4.5–5.6 plays per series, with each play lasting ~5.0–5.5 seconds (up to ~13 s for a long play), and have ~25–36 seconds of rest in between plays yielding a work-relief ratio of 1:5 (80). These data provide a valuable framework for S&C coaches to develop a speed endurance training program.

Training targets the ability to *generate speed* by performing drills at 70%–100% of maximal speed for 10–40 seconds bouts with at least a 1:5 work-relief ratio and the ability to *maintain speed* by performing drills at 50%–100% of maximal speed for 5–90 seconds bouts with a 1:1–1:3 work-relief ratio (81). A combination of high-intensity interval training, traditional speed/power/agility/RT, team practice, and aerobic training (to a lesser extent) are used to maximize speed endurance. High-intensity interval training at intensities at or higher than the velocity at VO_{2max} is the primary training modality. Training for **maximal speed** (*i.e.*, 2–10-s bouts with long rest intervals) is critical as increasing sprint speed allows the athlete to move faster. Speed endurance training also encompasses targeting **repeated sprint ability** and **continuous speed performance** (or maintenance) over time. Total volume of speed endurance training depends upon the sport and training status of athletes. Scientific recommendations are sparse and often coaches rely on prior experience and practitioner-based recommendations. Thus, vast number of speed endurance training programs may be successful if the basic tenets of specificity, variation, and progressive overload are adhered to. For example, it has been recommended that speed endurance training involving low-to-moderate intensity drills for moderate distances be performed for 8–20 repetitions for advanced athletes and 5–12 for novice athletes (4). For speed endurance training involving high-intensity drills for short-to-moderate distances, 4–12 repetitions have been recommended for advanced athletes and 4–8 for novice athletes (4).

Speed endurance (and high-intensity interval) training leads to favorable physiological and performance adaptations. In a review of the literature, Iaia and Bangsbo (81) reported that ~4–10 weeks of speed endurance training increased exercise performance lasting 30 seconds (by ~7%), 40–60 seconds (by 13%–25%), 1.5–2.5 minutes (by 4%–36%), 4–6 minutes (by 4%–32%), 8–20 minutes (by 3%–15%), 35–60 minutes (by 2%–4%), time to exhaustion (by 19%–28%), and repeated sprint ability (by ~2%) in trained athletes. Another literature review showed that speed endurance training increased VO_{2max} by ~5%–6%, best sprint time by 0.3%–5.5%, mean sprint time by 0.3%–22%, and improve fatigue index by 13%–54% (82); another meta-analysis showed that 2–12 weeks of repeated sprint training had a large effect on 30 m sprint (5.8%) and moderate effects on repeated sprint ability (2.5%) and running performance (17%) (83). Physiologically, speed endurance training has been shown to lead to muscle fiber-type transitions (e.g., decreased type I, increased type IIa), increase muscle glycogen stores, increase muscle membrane transport proteins (e.g., MCT1, $Na^+/K^+/ATPase$ protein subunits, Na^+/H^+ exchanger isoform 1), increase buffering capacity (mostly in lesser-trained individuals), increase PCr resynthesis, increase VO_{2max}, and increase anaerobic enzyme activity (e.g., PFK, phosphorylase, ATPase, CK, LDH, myokinase) (81,82) all of which enable the athlete to maintain higher speeds for an extended period of time. In addition, relationships between VO_{2max}, lactate threshold, and repeated sprint ability (mean sprint time and sprint performance decrement) have been reported (82). It has been suggested that interval training targeting 80%–90% of VO_{2max} with rest intervals shorter than the work bout may be best to improve buffer capacity (82).

Repeated sprint ability is characterized by the ability to produce high average sprint performances over a series of sprints (82) and is often trained with short series of sprints (3–10 s) with short-to-long rest intervals (83,84). Specifically, *repeated sprint exercise* has been defined as short duration sprints (≤10 s) with brief recovery periods (≤60 s), whereas *intermittent sprint exercise* has been defined as short duration sprints (≤10 s) with long recovery periods (1–5 min) (84). The primary difference is the rest interval length as intermittent sprint exercise demonstrates much smaller performance decrements (Fig. 16.49) (84). Repeated sprint ability is often assessed by examining sprint times (using a number of protocols) per repetition over time, forming a summative composite score of all sprint times, taking the average speed over all reps, or by analyzing fatigue via calculating the **fatigue index** [FI = ((best time − worst time)/best time) × 100] or **percent decrement score** shown below where S is the time of each sprint and S_{best} is the best time.

$$S_{dec}(\%) = \left\{ \frac{(S_1 + S_2 + S_3 + \ldots + S_{final})}{S_{best} \times \text{number of sprints}} - 1 \right\} \times 100$$

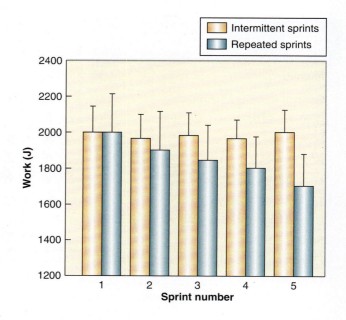

FIGURE 16.49 Repeated vs. Intermittent Sprint Exercise. (From Girard O, Mendez-Villanueva A, Bishop D. Repeated-sprint ability part I—factors contributing to fatigue. *Sports Med.* 2011;41:673–94.)

Repeated sprint ability data can be interpreted in various ways. Figure 16.50 depicts a continuum where RSA data are influenced by maximal speed performance and fatigue rates. For example, an athlete may have a low performance decline slope over time; however, maximal speed or power may not be that high. On the other hand, an athlete may show high speed and power output on the first set or repetition yet also demonstrate dramatic reductions with ensuing repetitions or sets. This is why it is essential to target increasing maximal speed and reducing the slope of decline seen during subsequent sprints with short recovery periods. Although running is often a mode of training, modalities such as cycling, rowing, and swimming may be trained in similar manner to improve repeated speed ability. The ability to maintain other components such as agility and power are critical to athletic success in addition to speed.

Speed endurance training is characterized by longer sprint distances and moderate-to-long rest intervals in between sets and reps for speed maintenance and short distances with short rest intervals to target repeat sprint ability. Drill lengths may range from 30 yd to more than 300 yd and are run at intensities ranging between 75% and 100% of maximal speed (79). Many program design elements are effective for improving speed endurance. For targeting repeated sprint ability, most studies investigated programs using set distances of 5–80 m with work-relief ratios of 1:2–1:10 (82,83). Most studies used training frequencies of 1–3 days per week with one using a 3–6-day-per-week frequency (82,83). Often, 2–6 sets of 3–15 repetitions may be prescribed where a set consists of a desired number of sprints performed with short rest intervals (15–60 s) in between while longer rest intervals (2–5 min) are used in between sets. Each rep is performed at or near maximal speed depending on the level of fatigue. Unlike maximal speed and agility training,

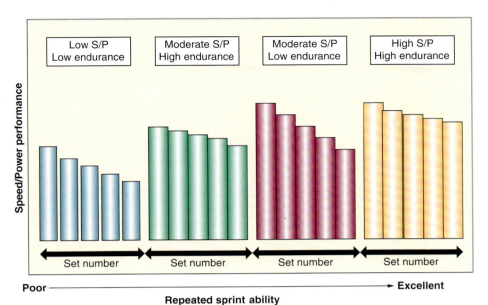

FIGURE 16.50 Repeated sprint ability continuum.

fatigue is not avoided here but becomes important to the conditioning stimulus. Drills consist of repeated sprints (sprints with short rest intervals such as *wind sprints*), interval sprints (where the athlete sprints part of the course and jogs part of the course at regular fixed intervals), repetitive flying sprints, rolling sprints (with groups of athletes where the last athlete sprints to the front upon indication from a coach), or repetitive relays (80). *Pick-up sprints* are effectively used where groups of athletes run on a track as four intervals are used: (a) jog for 25 m, (b) stride for 25 m, (c) sprint for 25 m, and (d) walk for 25 m (23). Partial recovery is seen during the jogging and walking phases. Agility runs such as shuttle runs can be used, so COD ability is challenged by the fatiguing stimulus. Often, training to improve repeat sprint ability may be performed after a practice/training session due to the fatiguing nature of the stimulus. Thus, it is imperative for the coach to balance speed endurance training with other training modalities in order to reduce the likelihood of injuries and overtraining. An example speed endurance workout targeting repeated running sprint ability is shown below:

- General warm-up: 3-minute jog
- Dynamic ROM exercises + core facilitation corrective exercises + form drills
- Practice/training session
- Sprints: 3 sets of 6 repetitions — 40 yd sprints: 20 seconds rest between reps, 2 minutes rest between sets
- Cooldown

Speed endurance training targeting speed maintenance involves longer runs with moderate rest intervals. This may be the case, for example, in training for middle distance events. One critical component is determining the intensity, or speed/time, of the intervals. For example, repeated sprint ability sets involve sprints and maximal or near maximal speed as they are short in distance and duration. However, longer distance sprints may require pacing since an athlete cannot maintain maximal speed throughout and demonstrates an exponential drop in speed with fatigue (85). Although aerobic intervals are used to enhance speed endurance training (as increased aerobic capacity assists in PCr resynthesis and recovery ability), anaerobic intervals play a key role in targeting speed development and maintenance. Historically, running intensities may have been selected for timed interval training via the velocity at VO_{2max} obtained from continuous tests (86). Laboratory testing directly assessing velocity at VO_{2max}, or VO_{2max} prediction continuous field tests such as time/distance trials, the 20 m shuttle run test (Beep test), and the University of Montreal Track test could be used where the average velocity or velocity attained during the final stage could be prescribed for interval training (86,87). However, other intermittent field tests have been developed to better identify a training intensity given the nature of both anaerobic and aerobic system contributions to speed endurance training.

One such method is the *anaerobic speed reserve* (ASR). The ASR is defined as the difference between the speed attained at maximal aerobic capacity (VO_{2max}) and maximal sprint speed (85). Thus, the ASR may be used after determination of both max sprint speed and the speed at VO_{2max} attainment. A negative exponential relationship exists between all-out speed and run duration and is attributed to differences in anaerobic vs. aerobic metabolic power (85). Knowledge of the top-end speed and the maximum aerobic speed can thus aid in predicting performance at any sprint duration up to 4 minutes (85) and be used in the development of intervals an athlete can sustain within their ASR for speed or power endurance training. Bundle et al. (85) developed the following equation to predict running speed at different time intervals (3–240 s) within up to 3.4% of actual speed:

$$\text{Spd}(t) = \text{Spd}_{aer} + (\text{Spd}_{an} - \text{Spd}_{aer}) \cdot e^{(-k \cdot t)}$$

Where Spd(t) is the predicted maximal running speed at time (t), Spd$_{aer}$ is the speed at VO$_{2max}$, Spd$_{an}$ is maximal sprint speed supported by anaerobic power, Spd$_{an}$ − Spd$_{aer}$ is the ASR, e is the base of the natural logarithm, and k is a constant for speed decrement determined by taking the mean of subject individual best fits (0.013). Figure 16.51 depicts this exponential curve over time (panel B). Panel A shows that the curves may differ between sprint-trained athletes (triangles) and endurance-trained athletes (circles). A large ASR may be seen in athletes with high top-end speed coupled with lower speeds at VO$_{2max}$. An athlete can develop an ASR curve to predict speed performance per interval duration for speed endurance training prescription of both interval durations and speed. This can help the athlete maintain a steady performance during an interval rather than falling below the necessary speed. In fact, ASR has been shown to strongly relate to 800 m running performance (88). Cycling anaerobic reserve (known as *anaerobic power reserve*) may be calculated similarly with the exception power output (max vs. power output obtained during VO$_{2max}$) is used (instead of speed) and the decrement constant k = 0.026 (instead of 0.013) given that max power output during cycling is 3.5 times greater than max power output that could be sustained by aerobic power compared to being approximately two times greater during running (89).

Another assessment common to the testing and monitoring of team sport athletes (such as soccer players) is the *Yo-Yo intermittent recovery tests* (90). The YY1R1 is used for individuals with lower fitness levels, whereas the YY1R2 test is used for individuals with higher levels of fitness. The YY1R1 starts at a lower speed with subsequent moderate increases in speed (and typically lasts 10–20 min), while the YY1R2 starts faster (and typically lasts 5–15 min) with more aggressive speed increases (90). These tests have been shown to be reliable and discriminate conditioning levels between elite and lesser team sport athletes (90,91). Both tests were designed to measure repeated interval performance and recovery ability. Studies have shown that 6–8 weeks of speed endurance or high-intensity interval training has improved YY1R1 scores by 15%–35% and YY1R2 scores by 15%–45% (90). Performance of the Yo-Yo tests correlates to VO$_{2max}$ and can be used to predict VO$_{2max}$ (although its accuracy is questionable).

For the test, cones measured 20 and 5 m apart are needed (Fig. 16.52) plus the timing CD and auditory system. The athletes begin aligned with the starting cone, run (upon the start signal) to the finish cone, and immediately return to the start cone thereby arriving before the next beep signal. Once the start cone is reached, athletes then have a 10-second recovery period in which they must jog/walk in between the cones set 5 m apart and then prepare for the next shuttle. The shuttles are repeated while the speed increases as noted by the tempo of the beep signals. Athletes are only allowed two consecutive fail attempts before the test is terminated. Distance is calculated by recording the number of shuttles completed multiplied by 40 (each shuttle is 2 × 20 m). The distance completed is used as an assessment tool for anaerobic conditioning, and the top speed attained during the last successful shuttle (or the equation Yo-Yo speed = speed attained in next to last stage + 0.5 × (n/8) in km·h^{-1} where n = number of runs completed during last stage and 8 represents the number of runs in each stage) may be used for interval exercise prescription (87,92).

One other assessment test used for interval training is the *30–15 intermittent fitness test* (30–15 IFT). Likewise, it could be used as a measure of anaerobic capacity and estimate VO$_{2max}$ and has been to shown to be reliable (86). It consists of 30-second shuttle runs interspersed with 15-second walking intervals. Velocity is set at 8 km·h^{-1} to start for the first 30-second run and then increased 0.5 km·h^{-1} every stage thereafter (86). The athletes are required to run back and forth between 2 lines set 40 m apart and speed is controlled by audio beeps. There are 3-m zones in the middle that allow the athlete to gauge running speeds and serve as start points for subsequent stages after the 15-second recovery intervals. The test is terminated when the athlete can no longer maintain the required running speed or is unable to reach a 3-m zone by the beep three

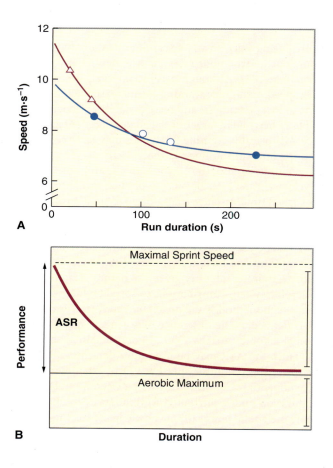

FIGURE 16.51 Anaerobic speed reserve. From Bundle et al. (85) (Panel **A**). ASR is the difference between maximal sprint speed and the speed obtained at VO$_{2max}$ (panel **B**). Different percents of the ASR can be used in the prescription of interval speeds or durations. Within the ASR lies speed values obtained by other means to be used for interval prescription such as incremental tests, the YoYo-1R test, and the 30–15 intermittent fitness test. Panel **A** depicts different ASR curves between an elite sprint athlete and elite endurance athlete.

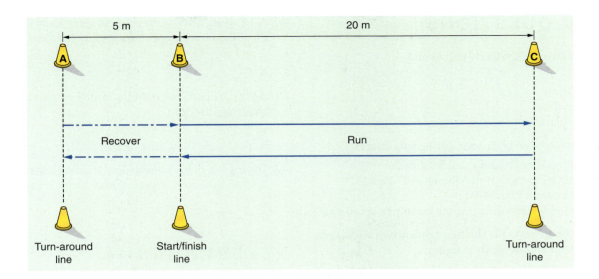

FIGURE 16.52 Yo-Yo intermittent recovery test layout.

consecutive times (86). The final velocity attained is used for intervals and has been shown to significantly correlate to VO_{2max}, jump height, and 10-m sprint speed (86).

Speed endurance training programs are easy to administer. The major components to training progression are the distance sprinted, the number of sprints, and the rest intervals in between sprints. The distance sprinted and the number of sprints can increase, and/or the rest intervals may decrease during speed endurance training progression. When possible, the coach should time each repetition to ensure maximal effort and to use the times to evaluate training especially those last few repetitions at the end of the workout. Comparisons can be made to those repetitions with similar lengths and rest intervals.

SUMMARY POINTS

- Speed, agility, acceleration ability, reaction time, and quickness are essential elements to improving athleticism. An athlete with sufficient linear speed does not mean that he or she will have sufficient agility, reaction time, and quickness. Each component needs to be specifically trained in order to maximize athletic performance.
- Maximal sprint speed is the product of stride rate and length. Increasing stride length and rate through training creates faster athletes.
- Sprinting speed is a skill that can be improved by technical training and conditioning. Coaches need to monitor and institute correct sprinting technique to maximize benefits.
- Sprint training is characterized by the use of form drills, sprints of specific lengths (to mimic athletic demands and target correct metabolic systems), overspeed, and resisted sprint training drills. Technique mastery should be used as a guide before progressing to more intense and complex drills.
- Training for improved agility is multifactorial and requires mobility, coordination, balance, power, optimal SSC efficiency, stabilization, proper technique, strength, flexibility, a rapid ability to accelerate and decelerate, visual scanning, scanning speed, and anticipation.
- Training for speed, agility, and quickness requires an integrated approach consisting of resistance, ballistic, flexibility, balance, and plyometric training in addition to specific sprint and agility training.
- Agility drills may be programmed or reactive. Quickness is best improved by incorporating explosive drills that maximize body movement speed and locomotion.
- Speed endurance is needed by those athletes involved in anaerobic sports where prolonged explosive movements are used with short recovery intervals. Speed endurance training takes place at the end of workouts and can be increased by increasing drill length, increasing drill repetition number, and/or decreasing rest intervals between repetitions.

REVIEW QUESTIONS

1. The rate of change of velocity over time is
   a. Speed
   b. Acceleration
   c. Reaction time
   d. Speed endurance

2. A common technical error seen during sprinting is
   a. Relaxed facial, neck, and shoulder muscles
   b. Explosive arm actions with elbows ~90° angles
   c. Limited knee and hip ROM
   d. Upright torso position during the maximum speed phase

3. Which of the following is the best sequence of drills/exercises for sprint and/or agility training?
   a. General warm-up, dynamic ROM exercises, form drills, overspeed drills, and basic sprinting drills
   b. General warm-up, basic sprint drills, dynamic ROM exercises, overspeed drills, and form drills
   c. Resisted sprint drills, form drills, basic sprint drills, dynamic ROM exercises, and general warm-up
   d. General warm-up, basic agility drills, dynamic ROM exercises, form drills, and overspeed training drills

4. Which of the following drills consists of a backpedaling component?
   a. Sprints with a chute
   b. "Butt kickers"
   c. Cariocas
   d. T-drill

5. Repeated sprints of 200 yd with 2-minute rest intervals in between repetitions are most specific to increasing
   a. Reaction time
   b. Quickness
   c. Acceleration
   d. Speed endurance

6. The Z-pattern drill is an example of a(n) _____ drill.
   a. Agility training
   b. Resistance training
   c. Speed endurance training
   d. Overspeed training

7. Sprint speed is the product of stride length and stride frequency.
   a. T
   b. F

8. The support phase of sprinting describes motion of the leg that is not in contact with the ground.
   a. T
   b. F

9. Overspeed training allows the athlete to attain a speed that is greater than the athlete's maximal effort.
   a. T
   b. F

10. A 1:1 work-relief ratio is used to specifically target the ATP-PC system during sprint and agility training.
    a. T
    b. F

11. Agility, in part, refers to the ability to move rapidly while changing direction.
    a. T
    b. F

12. Towing is a mode of overspeed training where the athlete is assisted to attain a supramaximal sprint speed.
    a. T
    b. F

REFERENCES

1. Lentz D, Hardyk A. Speed training. In: Brown LE, Ferrigno VA, editors. *Training for Speed, Agility, and Quickness*. 2nd ed. Champaign (IL): Human Kinetics; 2005. p. 17–70.

2. Young WB, Farrow D. A review of agility: practical applications for strength and conditioning. *Strength Cond J*. 2006;28:24–9.

3. Falch HN, Raedergard HG, van den Tillaar R. Effect of different physical training forms on change of direction ability: a systematic review and meta-analysis. *Sports Med Open*. 2019;5:53.

4. Plisk SS. Speed, agility, and speed-endurance development. In: Baechle TR, Earle RW, editors. *Essentials of Strength Training and Conditioning*. 3rd ed. Champaign (IL): Human Kinetics; 2008. p. 455–85.

5. Bloomfield J, Polman R, O'Donoghue P. Physical demands of different positions in FA Premier League soccer. *J Sports Sci Med*. 2007;6:63–70.

6. Weyand PG, Sternlight DB, Bellizzi MJ, Wright S. Faster top running speeds are achieved with greater ground forces not more rapid leg movements. *J Appl Physiol*. 2000;89:1991–9.

7. Sekulic D, Spasic M, Mirkov D, Cavar M, Sattler T. Gender-specific influences of balance, speed, and power on agility performance. *J Strength Cond Res*. 2013;27(3):802–11.

8. Lockie RG, Murphy AJ, Schultz AB, Knight TJ, de Jonge XAKJ. The effects of different speed training protocols on sprint acceleration kinematics and muscle strength and power in field sport athletes. *J Strength Cond Res*. 2012;26:1539–50.

9. Delecluse C. Influence of strength training on sprint running performance: current findings and implications for training. *Sports Med*. 1997;24:147–56.

10. Zafeiridis A, Saraslanidis P, Manou V, Ioakimidis P, Dipla K, Kellis S. The effects of resisted sled-pulling sprint training on acceleration and maximum speed performance. *J Sports Med Phys Fitness*. 2005;45:284–90.

11. Paradisis GP, Cooke CB. The effects of sprint running training on sloping surfaces. *J Strength Cond Res*. 2006;20:767–77.

12. Kristensen GO, Van Den Tillaar R, Ettema GJC. Velocity specificity in early-phase sprint training. *J Strength Cond Res*. 2006;20:833–7.

13. Spinks CD, Murphy AJ, Spinks WL, Lockie RG. The effects of resisted sprint training on acceleration performance and kinematics in soccer, rugby union, and Australian football players. *J Strength Cond Res*. 2007;21:77–85.

14. Rumpf MC, Lockie RG, Cronin JB, Jalilvand F. Effect of different sprint training methods on sprint performance over various distances: a brief review. *J Strength Cond Res*. 2016;30:1767–85.

15. Kraemer WJ, Ratamess NA, Volek JS, Mazzetti SA, Gomez AL. The effect of the Meridian shoe on vertical jump and sprint performances following short-term combined plyometric/sprint and resistance training. *J Strength Cond Res*. 2000;14:228–38.

16. Ratamess NA, Kraemer WJ, Volek JS, et al. The effects of ten weeks of resistance and combined plyometric/sprint training with the Meridian Elyte athletic shoe on muscular performance in women. *J Strength Cond Res*. 2007;21:882–7.

17. Davis DS, Barnette BJ, Kiger JT, Mirasola JJ, Young SM. Physical characteristics that predict functional performance in division I college football players. *J Strength Cond Res*. 2004;18:115–20.

18. Wisloff U, Castagna C, Helgerud J, Jones R, Hoff J. Strong correlation of maximal squat strength with sprint performance and vertical jump height in elite soccer players. *Br J Sports Med*. 2004;38:285–8.

19. Seitz LB, Reyes A, Tran TT, de Villarreal ES, Haff GG. Increases in lower-body strength transfer positively to sprint performance: a systematic review with meta-analysis. *Sports Med*. 2014;44:1693–702.

20. Young W, McLean B, Ardagna J. Relationship between strength qualities and sprinting performance. *J Sports Med Phys Fitness*. 1995;35:13–9.

21. Petrakos G, Morin JB, Egan B. Resisted sled sprint training to improve spring performance: a systematic review. *Sports Med*. 2016;46:381–400.

22. Mero A, Komi PV, Gregor RJ. Biomechanics of sprint running. *Sports Med*. 1992;13:376–92.

23. Dintiman G, Ward B, Tellez T. *Sports Speed*. 2nd ed. Champaign (IL): Human Kinetics; 1998. p. 191–220.

24. Lockie RG, Murphy AJ, Knight TJ, de Jonge XAKJ. Factors that differentiate acceleration ability in field sport athletes. *J Strength Cond Res*. 2011;25:2704–14.

25. Weyand PG, Davis JA. Running performance has a structural basis. *J Exp Biol*. 2005;208:2625–31.

26. Mero A. Force-time characteristics and running velocity of male sprinters during the acceleration phase of sprinting. *Res Q Exerc Sport*. 1988;59:94–8.

27. Cavagna GA, Komarek L, Mazzoleni S. The mechanics of sprint running. *J Physiol*. 1971;217:709–21.

28. Mero A, Komi PV. Electromyographic activity in sprinting at speeds ranging from sub-maximal to supra-maximal. *Med Sci Sports Exerc*. 1987;19:266–74.

29. Ebben WP, Davies JA, Clewien RW. Effect of the degree of hill slope on acute downhill running velocity and acceleration. *J Strength Cond Res*. 2008;22:898–902.

30. Baron B, Deruelle F, Moullan F, et al. The eccentric muscle loading influences the pacing strategies during repeated downhill sprint intervals. *Eur J Appl Physiol*. 2009;105:749–57.

31. Gottschall AS, Kram R. Ground reaction forces during downhill and uphill running. *J Biomech*. 2005;38:445–52.

32. Toyomura J, Mori H, Tayashiki K, et al. Efficacy of downhill running training for improving muscular and aerobic performances. *Appl Physiol Nutr Metab*. 2018;43:403–10.

33. Clark DA, Sabick MB, Pfeiffer RP, et al. Influence of towing force magnitude on the kinematics of supramaximal sprinting. *J Strength Cond Res*. 2009;23:1162–8.

34. Corn RJ, Knudson D. Effect of elastic-cord towing on the kinematics of the acceleration phase of sprinting. *J Strength Cond Res*. 2003;17:72–5.

35. Dintiman GB. Acceleration and speed. In: Foran B, editor. *High-Performance Sports Conditioning*. Champaign (IL): Human Kinetics; 2001. p. 167–92.

36. Cross MR, Tinwala F, Lenetsky S, et al. Determining friction and effective loading for sled sprinting. *J Sports Sci*. 2017;35:2198–203.

37. Alcaraz PE, Palao JM, Elvira JL. Determining the optimal load for resisted sprint training with sled towing. *J Strength Cond Res*. 2009;23:480–5.

38. Cross MR, Brughelli M, Samozino P, Brown SR, Morin JB. Optimal loading for maximizing power during sled-resisted sprinting. *Int J Sports Physiol Perform*. 2017;12:1069–77.

39. Cross MR, Lahti J, Brown SR, et al. Training at maximal power in resisted sprinting: optimal load determination methodology and pilot results in team sport athletes. *PLoS One*. 2018;13:e0195477.

40. Smythe R. *Acceleration: An Illustrated Guide*. Portland (OR): Speed City, Inc; 1988. p. 50–108.

41. Lejeune TM, Willems PA, Heglund NC. Mechanics and energetics of human locomotion on sand. *J Exp Biol*. 1998;210:2071–80.

42. Macadam P, Cronin JB, Feser EH. Acute and longitudinal effects of weighted vest training on sprint-running performance: a systematic review. *Sports Biomech*. 2019;1–16.

43. Dolcetti JC, Cronin JB, Macadam P, Feser EH. Wearable resistance training for speed and agility. *Strength Cond J*. 2019;41:105–11.

44. Feser EH, Macadam P, Cronin JB. The effects of lower limb wearable resistance on sprint running performance: a systematic review. *Eur J Sport Sci*. 2020;20(3):394–406. doi: 10.1080/17461391.2019.1629631.

45. Roberts TJ, Belliveau RA. Sources of mechanical power for uphill running in humans. *J Exp Biol*. 2005;208:1963–70.

46. Zatsiorsky VM, Kraemer WJ. *Science and Practice of Strength Training*. 2nd ed. Champaign (IL): Human Kinetics; 2006. p. 30–3.

47. Alcaraz PE, Carlos-Vivas J, Oponjuru BO, Martinez-Rodriguez A. The effectiveness of resisted sled training (RST) for sprint performance: a systematic review and meta-analysis. *Sports Med*. 2018;48:2143–65.

48. Cronin J, Hansen K, Kawamori N, McNair P. Effects of weighted vests and sled towing on sprint kinematics. *Sports Biomech*. 2008;7:160–72.

49. Lockie RG, Murphy AJ, Spinks CD. Effects of resisted sled towing on sprint kinematics in field-sport athletes. *J Strength Cond Res*. 2003;17:760–7.

50. Maulder PS, Bradshaw EJ, Keogh JW. Kinematic alterations due to different loading schemes in early acceleration sprint performance from starting blocks. *J Strength Cond Res*. 2008;22:1992–2002.

51. Bachero-Mena B, Gonzalez-Badillo JJ. Effects of resisted sprint training on acceleration with three different loads accounting for 5, 12.5, and 20% of body mass. *J Strength Cond Res*. 2014;28:2954–60.

52. Alcaraz PE, Palao JM, Elvira JL, Linthorne NP. Effects of three types of resisted sprint training devices on the kinematics of sprinting at maximum velocity. *J Strength Cond Res*. 2008;22:890–7.

53. Myer GD, Ford KR, Brent JL, Divine JG, Hewett TE. Predictors of sprint start speed: the effects of resistive ground-based vs. inclined treadmill training. *J Strength Cond Res*. 2007;21:831–6.

54. Clark KP, Stearne DJ, Walts CT, Miller AD. The longitudinal effects of resisted sprint training using weighted sleds vs. weighted vests. *J Strength Cond Res*. 2010;24(12):3287–95.

55. West DJ, Cunningham DJ, Bracken RM, et al. Effects of resisted sprint training on acceleration in professional rugby union players. *J Strength Cond Res*. 2013;27:1014–8.

56. Ross RE, Ratamess NA, Hoffman JR, Faigenbaum AD, Kang J, Chilakos A. The effects of treadmill sprint training and resistance training on maximal running velocity and power. *J Strength Cond Res*. 2009;23:385–94.

57. Graham J, Ferrigno V. Agility and balance training. In: Brown LE, Ferrigno VA, editors. *Training for Speed, Agility, and Quickness*. 2nd ed. Champaign (IL): Human Kinetics; 2005. p. 71–222.

58. Verstegen M, Marcello B. Agility and coordination. In: Foran B, editor. *High-Performance Sports Conditioning*. Champaign (IL): Human Kinetics; 2001. p. 139–65.

59. Sheppard JM, Young WB. Agility literature review: classifications, training and testing. *J Sports Sci*. 2006;24:919–32.

60. Young WB, James R, Montgomery I. Is muscle power related to running speed with changes of direction? *J Sports Med Phys Fitness*. 2002;42:282–8.

61. Marcovic G. Poor relationship between strength and power qualities and agility performance. *J Sports Med Phys Fitness*. 2007;47:276–83.

62. Marcovic G, Sekulic D, Marcovic M. Is agility related to strength qualities?—Analysis in latent space. *Coll Antropol*. 2007;31:787–93.

63. Siddle J, Greig M, Weaver K, et al. Acute adaptations and subsequent preservation of strength and speed measures following a Nordic hamstring curl intervention: a randomised controlled trial. *J Sports Sci*. 2019;37:911–20.

64. Brughelli M, Cronin J, Levin G, Chaouachi A. Understanding change of direction ability in sport: a review of resistance training studies. *Sports Med*. 2008;38:1045–63.

65. Speirs DE, Bennett MA, Finn CV, Turner AP. Unilateral vs. bilateral squat training for strength, sprints, and agility in academy rugby players. *J Strength Cond Res*. 2016;30:386–92.

66. Fry AC, Kraemer WJ, Weseman CA, et al. The effects of an off-season strength and conditioning program on starters and non-starters in women's intercollegiate volleyball. *J Strength Cond Res*. 1991;5:174–81.

67. Hoffman JR, Maresh CM, Armstrong LE, Kraemer WJ. Effects of off-season and in-season resistance training programs on a collegiate male basketball team. *J Hum Muscle Perform*. 1991;1:48–55.

68. Miller MG, Herniman JJ, Ricard MD, Cheatham CC, Michael TJ. The effects of a 6-week plyometric training program on agility. *J Sports Sci Med*. 2006;5:459–65.

69. Dos'Santos T, McBurnie A, Thomas C, Comfort P, Jones, PA. Biomechanical comparison of cutting techniques: a review and practical applications. *Strength Cond J*. 2019;41:40–54.

70. Hewit J, Cronin J, Button C, Hume P. Understanding deceleration in sport. *Strength Cond J*. 2011;33:47–52.

71. DeWeese BH, Nimphius S. Program design and technique for speed and agility training. In: Haff GG, Triplett NT, editors. *Essential of Strength Training and Conditioning*. 4th ed. Champaign (IL): Human Kinetics; 2016. p. 521–57.

72. Spiteri T, Cochrane JL, Hart NH, Haff GG, Nimphius S. Effect of strength on plant foot kinetics and kinematics during a change of direction task. *Eur J Sport Sci*. 2013;13:646–52.

73. Lockie RG, Schultz AB, Callaghan SJ, Jeffriess MD. The effects of traditional and enforced stopping speed and agility training on multidirectional speed and athletic function. *J Strength Cond Res*. 2014;28:1538–51.

74. Hoffman JR, Kang J, Ratamess NA, Hoffman MW, Tranchina CP, Faigenbaum AD. Examination of a pre-exercise, high energy supplement on exercise performance. *J Int Soc Sports Nutr*. 2009;6:1–8.

75. Besier TF, Lloyd DG, Ackland TR. Muscle activation strategies at the knee during running and cutting maneuvers. *Med Sci Sports Exerc*. 2003;35:119–27.

76. Besier TF, Lloyd DG, Ackland TR, Cochrane JL. Anticipatory effects on knee joint loading during running and cutting maneuvers. *Med Sci Sports Exerc*. 2001;33:1176–81.

77. Besier TF, Lloyd DG, Cochrane JL, Ackland TR. External loading of the knee joint during running and cutting maneuvers. *Med Sci Sports Exerc*. 2001;33:1168–75.

78. Ostrander EA, Huson HJ, Ostrander GK. Genetics of athletic performance. *Annu Rev Genomics Hum Genet*. 2009;10:407–29.

79. Cissik JM, Barnes M. *Sport Speed and Agility*. Monterey (CA): Coaches Choice; 2004. p. 15–85.

80. Hoffman J. *Physiological Aspects of Sport Training and Performance*. Champaign (IL): Human Kinetics; 2002. p. 93–108.

81. Iaia FM, Bangsbo J. Speed endurance training is a powerful stimulus for physiological adaptations and performance improvements of athletes. *Scand J Med Sci Sports*. 2010;20(Suppl 2):11–23.

82. Bishop D, Girard O, Mendez-Villanueva A. Repeated-sprint ability—part II: recommendations for training. *Sports Med*. 2011;41:741–56.

83. Taylor J, Macpherson T, Spears I, Weston M. The effects of repeated-sprint training on field-based fitness measures: a meta-analysis of controlled and non-controlled trials. *Sports Med*. 2015;45:881–91.

84. Girard O, Mendez-Villanueva A, Bishop D. Repeated-sprint ability part I—factors contributing to fatigue. *Sports Med*. 2011;41:673–94.

85. Bundle MW, Hoyt RW, Weyand PG. High-speed running performance: a new approach to assessment and prediction. *J Appl Physiol*. 2003;95:1955–62.

86. Bucheit M. The 30-15 Intermittent Fitness Test: accuracy for individualizing interval training of young intermittent sports players. *J Strength Cond Res*. 2008;22:365–74.

87. Clarke R, Dobson A, Hughes J. Metabolic conditioning: fields tests to determine a training velocity. *Strength Cond J*. 2016;38:38–47.

88. Sandford GN, Kilding AE, Ross A, Laursen PB. Maximal sprint speed and the anaerobic speed reserve domain: the untapped tools that differentiate the world's best male 800 m runners. *Sports Med*. 2019;49:843–52.

89. Weyand PG, Lin JE, Bundle MW. Sprint performance-duration relationships are set by the fractional duration of external force application. *Am J Physiol Regul Integr Comp Physiol*. 2006;290:R758–65.

90. Bangsbo J, Iaia FM, Krustrup P. The Yo-Yo intermittent recovery test: a useful tool for evaluation of physical performance in intermittent sports. *Sports Med*. 2008;38:37–51.

91. Grgic J, Oppici L, Mikulic P, et al. Test-retest reliability of the Yo-Yo test: a systematic review. *Sports Med*. 2019;49:1547–57.

92. Dupont G, Defontaine M, Bosquet L, et al. Yo-Yo intermittent recovery test versus the Universite de Montreal track test: relation with a high intensity intermittent exercise. *J Sci Med Sport*. 2010;13:146–50.

93. McHenry P, Raether J. *101 Agility Drills*. Monterey (CA): Coaches Choice; 2004. p. 51–133.

CHAPTER 17

Aerobic Training

OBJECTIVES

After completing this chapter, you will be able to:

- Discuss factors that affect aerobic endurance performance
- Discuss aerobic endurance training program design and how to manipulate exercise mode, intensity, volume, rest intervals, and frequency to increase $\dot{V}O_{2max}$ and performance
- Discuss how to include different forms of aerobic training into the program
- Discuss aerobic training for endurance and anaerobic athletes
- Discuss the impact altitude has on human performance
- Discuss compatibility issues with concurrent high-intensity aerobic and strength/power training
- Discuss the impact hot and cold environments have on aerobic endurance exercise performance

Aerobic training (AT) constitutes several modes of activities that primarily stress the aerobic energy system and produce a number of cardiovascular (CV), respiratory, and muscular adaptations that increase CV and local muscular endurance. High levels of aerobic fitness are mandatory for endurance athletes such as cyclists, distance runners, triathletes, and swimmers. Increases in aerobic capacity allow the marathon runner to maintain a better pace and reduce event times, allow the cyclist to become more efficient and improve trial times, and allow the swimmer to reduce times during distance events in the pool. However, other groups of athletes benefit from AT for their sports which not only require strength and power but require the athlete to possess sufficient muscular and CV endurance, *i.e.*, boxers, wrestlers, hockey, soccer, and basketball players. The aerobic system assists in acute recovery of anaerobic systems and an increased aerobic capacity allows the athlete to recover faster from workouts and competitions.

Several physiological adaptations (discussed in detail in previous chapters) accompany AT including increases in cardiac output (Q_c), stroke volume (SV), plasma volume, left ventricular size and contractility, blood flow, angiogenesis, red blood cell counts, hemoglobin and 2,3-DPG concentrations, and thermoregulation. In skeletal muscle, AT increases mitochondrial and capillary number and density, oxidative enzyme activity, myoglobin content, fat utilization during exercise and at rest, buffer capacity, and fiber-type transitions (favoring oxidative fibers). Collectively, these changes lead to increases in maximal oxygen uptake ($\dot{V}O_{2max}$) resulting from increased Q_c and arteriovenous (A-$\dot{V}O_2$) difference. The purpose of this chapter is to discuss AT program design, environmental and thermoregulatory considerations, and the effects of high-intensity AT performed concurrently with resistance training (RT).

Factors Related to Aerobic Exercise Performance

Aerobic exercise endurance performance depends on several factors. Figure 17.1 depicts the three most significant factors influencing endurance performance. These are maximal aerobic power or capacity ($\dot{V}O_{2max}$), exercise (*e.g.*, running, swimming, cycling, rowing, etc.), economy, and the lactate threshold (LT). The concept of critical power is another factor to consider (1). Each of these is targeted specifically in training cycles to maximize endurance performance. For example, two athletes with a similar $\dot{V}O_{2max}$ could have profoundly different race times. Although $\dot{V}O_{2max}$ is a stronger predictor of endurance performance in especially in heterogeneous lower-to-moderately fit populations, exercise economy and LT become stronger

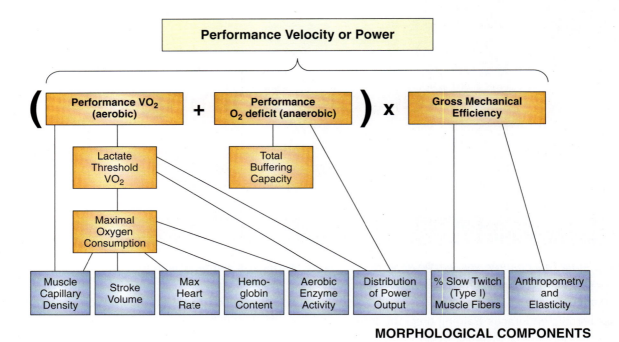

FIGURE 17.1 The major components to endurance performance. (From Joyner MJ, Coyle EF. Endurance exercise performance: the physiology of champions. *J Physiol.* 2008;586(1):35–44.)

correlates at higher fitness levels and may have great impact on determining the results of a race. Hence, periodized endurance training programs typically target these components latter in training.

A higher $\dot{V}O_{2max}$ indicates greater aerobic fitness. Successful professional cyclists possess high $\dot{V}O_2$ maxes, and $\dot{V}O_{2max}$ is a strong predictor of cycling performance in athletes with varied performance capabilities (2,3). Elite male distance runners have $\dot{V}O_{2max}$ values ranging from 70 to 85 mL·kg^{-1}·min^{-1} with values in elite female runners being ~10% lower (4,5). Elite distance runners can maintain an average of 94% of their $\dot{V}O_{2max}$ for a 5-km race and 82% of their $\dot{V}O_{2max}$ for a marathon (5). Studies show high correlations between $\dot{V}O_{2max}$ and performance in endurance events (6). However, athletes with similar $\dot{V}O_{2max}$ values may have largely different endurance performances. As Noakes (5) pointed out, two elite runners (Steve Prefontaine and Frank Shorter), whose best 1-mile run times were <8 seconds different from each other, had a $\dot{V}O_{2max}$ difference of 16%. Thus, aerobic endurance training programs target increased $\dot{V}O_{2max}$ in addition to the other components. $\dot{V}O_{2max}$ can be used to predict race times and vice versa. For example, Mercier et al. (7) developed a nomogram that predicts running times (from 3- to 42-km distances) from $\dot{V}O_{2max}$ values (Fig. 17.2).

The kinetics of $\dot{V}O_2$ during exercise is important. In Chapter 8, the concept of the *slow component of $\dot{V}O_{2max}$* was discussed. $\dot{V}O_2$ may drift or increase at constant work rate that are moderate-to-high in intensity, *i.e.*, above the LT, possibly due to respiratory and muscle fatigue and the recruitment of less efficient type II muscle fibers. This slow component is viewed as metabolic inefficiency, and it is negatively related to $\dot{V}O_{2max}$ (1,8,9).

Individuals with a high $\dot{V}O_{2max}$ display a faster rate of attaining the targeted $\dot{V}O_2$ during the onset of exercise and can reduce the oxygen deficit (9). AT has been shown to reduce the magnitude of $\dot{V}O_2$ slow component during constant-load protocol, which is thought to increase metabolic stability, reduce fatigue development, and limit the need for type II motor unit recruitment (8).

In conjunction with the quantity and kinetics of $\dot{V}O_{2max}$, endurance athletes have greater fuel use efficiency, *e.g.*, preferential metabolism of fat during exercise. An athlete with a high $\dot{V}O_{2max}$ has better oxygen intake, delivery, and utilization. Therefore, the endurance athlete essentially becomes a better "fat-burning machine." When fat is a preferred fuel, glycogen is spared, less lactic acid is formed, and there are fewer pH disturbances. Glycolytic contributions increase during moderate-to-high intensity endurance exercise when the maximum rate of fat oxidation is insufficient to meet the ATP demands of skeletal muscles (4). Athletes predisposed to high endurance performances have a higher proportion of type I muscle fibers. Type I fibers are highly oxidative (resulting in less lactate formation) and are fatigue-resistant. Endurance athletes have higher proportions of type I fibers than anaerobic athletes and sedentary individuals (10). It is thought that endurance athletes have the ability to rotate speed and power production through a larger percent of muscle mass thereby reducing glycolytic stress and lactate production per given muscle fiber (4). The production of less lactate per work rate and improved lactate clearance enable, in part, greater endurance performance.

As a result, the *lactate threshold* (LT) increases in response to AT and enables exercise in a less acidic environment.

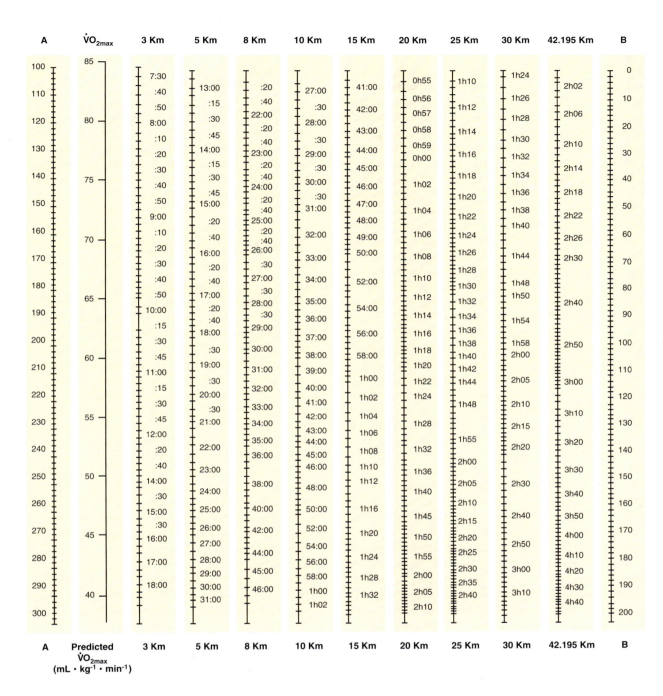

FIGURE 17.2 Prediction of running performance from $\dot{V}O_{2max}$ data. (Reprinted with permission from Mercier D, Leger L, Desjardins M. Nomogram to predict performance equivalence for distance runners. *Track Tech.* 1986;94:3004–3009.)

The LT (LT$_1$) is the first major inflection point where blood lactate increases beyond resting levels. It occurs at a higher percentage of $\dot{V}O_{2max}$ with training and allows the athlete to exercise at a higher intensity. Some coaches use the second major lactate inflection point (onset of blood lactate accumulation or LT$_2$ which occurs at ~4 mmol of lactate) as the threshold intensity. AT shifts the LT curve to the right therefore indicating that absolute (*i.e.*, higher speed or power output per blood lactate level) and relative (*i.e.*, takes place at a higher percent of $\dot{V}O_{2max}$)

improvements may take place. Interestingly, some studies have shown LT to be a better indicator of maximal endurance performance than $\dot{V}O_{2max}$ (11,12). Power output at the LT is a valid predictor of cycling potential (3). *Maximal lactate steady state* is the highest intensity where maximal lactate production equals lactate clearance. It may be used as a predictor of aerobic endurance performance and has been shown to increase during AT (8). Hence, selecting intensities that target these components of LT is critical for AT.

Athletes with high *exercise (i.e., running, cycling, swimming, rowing) economy* have a distinct advantage in endurance sports. Exercise economy refers to the energy cost of exercise at a given velocity. Less energy is expended per exercise velocity or power output thereby increasing the mechanical efficiency of the athlete. Professional road cyclists have high cycling economy compared to amateur cyclists allowing them to achieve high power outputs for extended periods of time (3). In particular, speed at which is produced at the athlete's $\dot{V}O_{2max}$ (often referred to as the *velocity at $\dot{V}O_{2max}$* or v$\dot{V}O_{2max}$) is an important composite of $\dot{V}O_{2max}$, economy, and LT. Some coaches and sport scientists have viewed the v$\dot{V}O_{2max}$ as a better indicator of performance because it demonstrates the speed by which could be attained by aerobic metabolism and, in runners, is often indicative of race times (13). When athletes with similar $\dot{V}O_{2max}$ values are compared, exercise economy becomes a stronger predictor of aerobic endurance performance (3,14), and running economy is higher in elite runners than good runners (15). Oxygen consumption at a given running and cycling speed may vary by up to 40% and 30%, respectively, between different individuals (4). A 5% increase in running economy may improve distance running performance by nearly 4% (16). Several factors affect exercise economy including age, training status, stride length and rate (for running), force production, the stretch-shortening cycle (SSC) and muscular stiffness, flexibility, footwear, and wind resistance (14,15). Wind resistance may account for 2%–8% of the total energy cost in runners (15). Body surface area (*i.e.*, posture), fluid density, relative velocity, and coefficient of drag force contribute greatly to the magnitude of fluid resistance, which can be greatly reduced by drafting (3). Exercise economy increases when RT and AT are performed concurrently. In a review of the literature, Yamamoto et al. (6) showed that concurrent training in highly trained runners improved 3K and 5K times by 2.9% and running economy by 4.6% (range, 3%–8.1%). Another review showed that running economy is related to AT history and can increase via high-intensity interval training (by up to ~8%), RT (by up to 8%), plyometric and/or explosive RT (by up to 6%), and altitude exposure/training (by up to 7%) (17). Figure 17.3 depicts data from Daniels and Daniels (14). In the first graph, male and female runners were compared. At a given velocity, men were able to perform at a lower $\dot{V}O_2$ than women, indicating greater running economy. In the second graph, male distance runners were compared to male runners who competed in 800- to 1,500-m events. At higher velocities, the 800- to 1,500-m runners showed greater running economy than the marathon runners. Other studies have shown that experienced runners have better running economy than untrained individuals (18).

Aerobic Training

Developing an AT program has similar characteristics as other modes. Likewise, the athlete needs to balance the stress of the AT program with other modalities and seasonal demands while optimizing their physiologic environment (*e.g.*, managing stress of school or job, getting proper sleep, proper nutrition, recovery, and minimizing illness and injury). Manipulation of exercise selection, intensity, volume, rest intervals (for interval training), and frequency can target specific goals of AT. There is no single "best method" for AT as many different programs have produced excellent results. As a result, organizations such as the ACSM have provided training guidelines within a general framework to aid the design process but also allow the flexibility to alter each program to meet the needs of the individual. The training of athletes extends beyond general training recommendations. The AT program should be reflective of offering the athlete many stimuli or training approaches and ultimately targeting design elements that the athlete will best respond to. AT programs should be designed to increase $\dot{V}O_{2max}$, LT, and exercise economy, and target elements of speed and power in a cyclical manner. $\dot{V}O_{2max}$ can improve between a range of 5% and 25% (20). No threshold duration exists per workout for optimal increases in aerobic capacity. Rather, the optimal combination of intensity and volume achieves best results.

Interpreting Research
The Importance of Lactate Threshold Differences in Endurance Athletes

Coyle EF, Coggan AR, Hopper MK, Walters TJ. Determinants of endurance in well-trained cyclists. *J Appl Physiol*. 1988;64:2622–2630.

$\dot{V}O_{2max}$ is critical to endurance performance but is one of a few factors, which highly affect performance (exercise economy and LT). Coyle et al. (19) studied 14 cyclists with similar levels of $\dot{V}O_{2max}$. They were subdivided into groups based on LT where one group reached their LT at lower exercise intensity (~65% of $\dot{V}O_{2max}$), and the other group reached their LT at higher exercise intensity (~82% of $\dot{V}O_{2max}$). Subjects were tested at 88% of $\dot{V}O_{2max}$. The high-intensity group's time to fatigue was double the low-intensity group (~61 vs. 29 min). Both groups had similar mitochondrial enzyme activity; however, the high-intensity group had a higher percentage of type I muscle fibers. The vastus lateralis of the low-intensity group showed much higher rates of glycogen utilization and lactate production. More than 92% of the variance in performance was explained by LT and muscle capillary density. The results of this study showed that at similar levels of $\dot{V}O_{2max}$, other factors such as muscle fiber type and LT play critical roles in aerobic endurance performance.

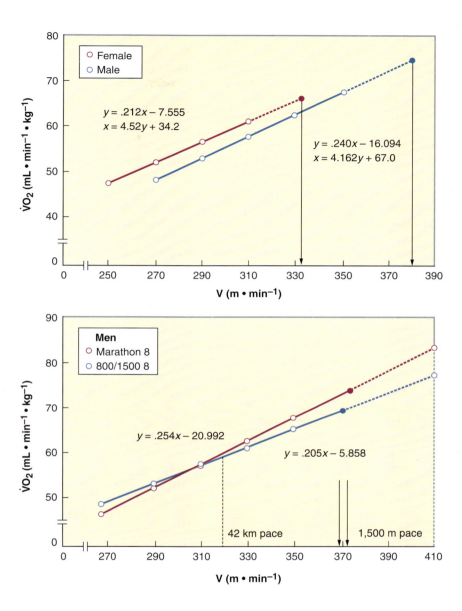

FIGURE 17.3 Running economy. (Reprinted with permission from Daniels J, Daniels N. Running economy of elite male and elite female runners. *Med Sci Sports Exerc*. 1992;24:483–489.)

Modes of Aerobic Exercise

Several modes of aerobic exercise are performed by the athlete (Table 17.1). Each has advantages and brings some unique qualities to AT programs. In general, AT exercises are classified as: (a) those that can be maintained at a constant intensity requiring minimal skill or physical fitness to perform (walking); (b) vigorous intensity endurance activities requiring minimal skill (jogging, cycling); (c) endurance activities requiring skill to perform (swimming, cross-country skiing); and (d) those where skill and intensity are variable during recreational activities (games, sports) (21). The vital elements to aerobic modes of training are its level of continuity and the magnitude of muscle mass involvement. Continuous exercise that stresses large muscle groups produces greater increases in aerobic capacity. *Fitness walking* and *hiking* are aerobic modalities that tend to be lower in intensity and are performed for long durations. Intensity for each can increase by adding an incline (hill) or using hand weights or backpacks (for hiking). *Jogging* and *running* are excellent forms of AT for athletes. Athletes may jog for short distances (at higher speeds), moderate distances (5–10 km), and long distances (half-marathons,

Table 17.1	Modes of Aerobic Training
Walking	Stair climbing, elliptical, and hybrid machines
Hiking	Cycling/spinning
Jogging/running	Aquatics
Aerobic dance/dancing	Swimming
Step aerobics	Rope skipping
Cross-country skiing	Rowing
Skating	Sports

marathons, and ultra-marathons). Running is excellent as it produces a substantial increase in heart rate (HR) and requires a total-body effort. Jogging and running place greater stress on the musculoskeletal system so the chances of overuse injuries increase. Proper volume and frequency are critical to prevent overuse injuries. A good pair of running shoes assists in shock absorption. A firm heel counter, external stabilizer, Achilles pad, midsole, and outsole help protect the body against the rigors of repetitive foot contacts. Athletes who frequently run for distance should change/replace their athletic shoes every 500 miles. Treadmills could be used for indoor running. Treadmills give the athlete the advantage of changing speed and percent grade to a specified level, while forcing the athlete to maintain a certain cadence. Most modern treadmills will monitor HR and allow manual options and preprogrammed protocols to be used. Increasing the percent grade allows the athlete to run hills where the environmental terrain could pose a limitation. Indoor training on treadmills allows the athlete to avoid environmental extremes of very hot, humid, or cold, windy weather, and uncontrollable issues such as traffic. Running on the treadmill belt could be more forgiving on the musculoskeletal system (compared to running on hard surfaces) especially if the athlete is training through periods of overuse or mild injury, and less metabolically challenging per level of running speed than running on the ground.

Stair climbing is an excellent form of AT. Raising the body against gravity (while maintaining an upright posture) requires additional muscle mass involvement. Stair climbing may be performed on cardio machines or steps (although it may be difficult to find an area with enough steps to climb continuously). On machines, the athlete should not rely on the use of hand rails for support as this makes the exercise easier. This could result from weak quadriceps and gluteal muscles or poor endurance. Stair climbing is weight-bearing and can create high levels of fatigue in lower-body musculature. It is effective for increasing muscular endurance but in some lesser aerobically trained athletes, leg fatigue may limit the maximal CV effect initially. Oxygen consumption and leg muscle activation increase as step rate increases (22). *Elliptical trainer machines* have been on the market since the early 1990s, and they combine stair climbing, walking, and running in a low-impact "elliptical-motion like" manner. Like treadmills and stair climbing machines, the intensity (power output, speed) can be controlled throughout. The athlete needs to keep their feet on the pedals during the locomotor movement. An advantage of the elliptical trainers is that they work the upper and lower body simultaneously thereby combining movements not seen during normal stair climbing. Oxygen consumption and ventilation are greater with both arm and leg action (compared to leg action alone) and increase with stride rate and resistance applied (23), and metabolic energy cost is higher during elliptical exercise than cycling at similar percents of max aerobic power (24). Other hybrid machines are available and each company's brand may offer differences in the motion, options, etc. In addition, *vertical climbers* can

increase the physical challenge of AT. Thus, a number of cardio machines are on the market that can provide some unique challenges to athletes.

Cycling is non–weight-bearing and can cause a substantial amount of lower-body fatigue. It is more difficult to attain a higher HR for cycling as it is mostly a lower-body activity (unless arm ergometry is used). Cycling is an effective mode of exercise to increase muscular and aerobic endurance. Proper technique, footwear, and fitting on the bike are important for workout performance, comfort, and reducing incidence of pain or overuse. Hills and faster speeds increase the intensity during outdoor cycling. Outdoor cycling equipment has changed over the years. The tapered helmets and tight clothing help minimize wind resistance, enable greater cycling speeds to be attained, and increase metabolic efficiency. When cycling outdoors, the athlete should wear a protective helmet and adhere to safety/traffic rules. Intensity is easy to control on indoor cycle ergometers. Speed of cycling (in rpms) can increase the power output, and resistance can be added to increase difficulty and cardiometabolic demand. However, the metabolic demand is generally less than that seen during running of a similar intensity. In-door cycling on cycling ergometers can be performed similar to other cardio machines such as a treadmill or stair climber, or in a class setting. Recumbent bikes can also be used, which allows the trainee to sit back (instead of upright or hunched forward like a standard bike) and increase comfort and reduce impact. *Spinning classes* have become popular and is a good way to add variety to cycle training. Spinning classes utilize stationary bikes with weighted flywheels and may focus on different endurance workout types such as continuous or interval templates. Speeds of 60–100 rpms are common depending on whether the trainee is seated flat, standing flat, jumps, or climbing and the level of resistance on the bike. *Arm cycle ergometry* may be used primarily to increase upper body endurance and poses less of a metabolic stimulus compared to maximal lower-body cycling. Maximal arm exercise increases the glycolytic component and lowers the maximal oxygen consumption requirement by 30%, ventilation, and max HR by 10–15 bpm compared to lower-body cycling and running as muscle mass involvement is larger with lower-body cycling (20). At submaximal work rates, arm ergometry produces greater physiologic strain and cardiometabolic demand due to reduced mechanical efficiency and greater recruitment of muscles to stabilize the body (20,25). VO_{2max} during arm ergometry is ~64%–80% of what is seen during leg ergometry (25). In addition, arm cycling can be used for cardio workouts when the legs are recovering from injuries.

Aerobic dance classes have increased in popularity since their inception in the early 1970s by Jacki Sorensen. Aerobics classes integrate many types of movements (walking, stepping, jogging, skipping, kicking, and arm swinging) into a routine to music that varies in length. Aerobics classes may be low-, moderate-, and high-impact. The difference is that in low-impact classes, one foot usually remains on the floor to support body weight, whereas in high-impact classes, exercises are used that require elevation of both feet off the floor leading to greater musculoskeletal loading. Complexity increases with the addition of more challenging movements. *Step aerobics* is popular and increases the intensity by the height of steps used. Steps (usually around 4–12 in.) increase the activity of the SSC. In recent times, other modalities have been added to aerobics classes. RT (dumbbells, bands), core/stability, plyometrics, and balance-type movements have been incorporated into classes to add greater variety and train other components of fitness. For example, some "boot camp" classes have incorporated speed, agility, plyometric, calisthenic and bodyweight, RT, Pilates, yoga, and military-type (army crawls) drills into circuits within each class. The addition of high-intensity interval training to aerobics class setting has added variety and increased the physical challenge. The continuity of each class can be a potent stimulus for increasing aerobic and muscular endurance. Other components of fitness can be trained with different exercises incorporated into the class.

Swimming and *aquatic exercise* provide little orthopedic stress. Swimming is a total-body activity allowing the body to move horizontally through the water. The buoyancy of the water adds resistance to movement but reduces weight-bearing requirements. The buoyancy force allows action-reaction forces during swimming motion to create propulsion. The metabolic response to swimming depends on the stroke used, velocity, gross and propelling efficiency, water temperature (*i.e.*, higher with reduced water temperature), and the level of drag force (20). Energy expenditure during swimming is much higher than running per distance (20). Elite swimmers are more economical than lesser-trained swimmers, *e.g.*, they have lower $\dot{V}O_2$ and energy expenditure per swim velocity (20). More resistance can be added to aquatic exercise by increasing the depth of water or by using aqua dumbbells, fins, and paddles. Swimming is a form of RT and is a total-body exercise, which can increase muscle and aerobic endurance. One limitation is that HRs do not reach as high a level as they do during land-based exercises, *e.g.*, on average 10–13 beats per minute (bpm) less in the water (20). Water cools the body, lessens the effects of gravity on the CV system, and applies compressive force to the body which results in less CV demand and a lower HR. An athlete must know how to swim to reap the CV benefits. Different strokes (breast stroke, side stroke, back stroke, butterfly, and front crawl) can be used to increase variety and muscle activation. The breast stroke is most metabolically demanding, followed by the butterfly, back stroke, and front crawl (26,27). Swim training can increase $\dot{V}O_{2max}$ and LT in trained swimmers (28). Aquatic exercise is similar to aerobics classes (different types including low-impact, toning, deep water running, and kickboxing) or RT workouts with the exception that they take place in the water. Impact is minimal, and there is less thermal stress to the individuals. Swimming skill may not be required for an aquatics class in the shallow end of the pool. Aquatic workouts are also advantageous for therapeutic training modalities where injured athletes are able to condition with minimal joint loading.

Cross-country skiing recruits all major muscles of the body, and the CV demand is very high. As a result, cross-country skiers have high $\dot{V}O_{2max}$ values, similar to or sometimes greater than marathon runners, cyclists, and triathletes (20). A limitation may be the outdoor conditions, but cardio machines that replicate the motions can be used indoors. Coordination is critical when performing cross-country skiing on a machine. The metabolic demand of cross-country skiing on a machine is high and increases with increased limb movement frequency (29).

Rowing and *skating* can increase aerobic capacity. Rowing involves a total-body effort and can lead to high levels of muscle fatigue, which makes it effective for increasing muscle endurance. Competitive rowing over 2,000 m for 6–8 minutes elicits a contribution from the aerobic system at ~70%–87%; and competitive rowers have high $\dot{V}O_{2max}$ values (30). Rowing is performed in the sagittal plane to a large extent and involves bilateral symmetrical actions of the legs and arms. The athlete should maintain a stable trunk position without leaning forward excessively to reduce stress on the lumbar spine. The popularity of indoor rowing ergometry has increased greatly since it is a component of CrossFit training and competition. Skating can provide a CV effect, but it is important to minimize gliding, or the metabolic demands will be lower.

Playing sports (independent of the athlete's main sport) can be viewed as AT to some degree. For example, playing tennis, racquetball, and pick-up games of basketball poses a sufficient aerobic stimulus. However, continuous play is needed to maximize the benefits. The flow of the game and the skill level of the participants are critical. These sports provide a good CV workout when skill level is high, competitive, and continuous play is seen for the majority of the activity. However, an athlete will experience only a small effect if there are constant stoppages due to a lack of skill of the participant, a lack of skill by other players/opponents, or other factors that stop games temporarily (fouls in basketball, retrieving the ball, pauses between points scored and serving in tennis, etc.). The benefit is that sports are competitive and fun to play, which increase motivation and participation. The benefits from sports participation may be augmented when other modes of AT are included in the training program.

The athlete and coach need to decide which modes of training will be included. Each mode has advantages and disadvantages. The pros and cons are compared and modes are selected based on this. Modes that are similar to the demands of the athlete's major sport (*e.g.*, principle of training specificity) should be selected. A running program is specific to many sports that require sufficient aerobic conditioning such as basketball, boxing, and wrestling. Modes that are challenging, yet perhaps not specific, can be integrated in the workout to add variety as they may be used for total conditioning purposes. The ACSM recommends large muscle mass exercise modalities that are continuous and rhythmic in nature (31).

Cross-Training

Cross-training refers to including different modes of exercise into the training program. Cross-training exposes the athlete to many stimuli. As a result, aerobic and anaerobic conditioning improves. Cross-training has the advantage of adding variety and is thought to reduce the likelihood of overuse injuries. It is an effective way to train past plateaus. For example, the advanced runner who has peaked performance with little progression may be best served by including some other modes of training. The increase in fitness from the other modes can have a transfer effect to running and allows the athlete to have mental relief while still training intensely. An athlete can integrate multiple modes of AT in a weekly training program. For example, in a 3-day-per-week program, the athlete can run on Monday, cycle on Wednesday, and stair climb on Friday. Progression can take place on a biweekly basis where either the intensity or volume is increased. If two modalities are used, the athlete can run on Monday, cycle on Wednesday, run on Friday, cycle on Monday, etc. Numerous possibilities exist when cross-training. Most athletes include multiple training modes in their own programs.

Intensity

Intensity selection during AT is critical to changes in aerobic capacity. Intensity prescription must match the goals of the program for that day and may be provided within a range. Intensity and volume/duration are inversely related. A delicate balance is needed to maximize the CV response yet provide enough duration to be a potent stimulus to increase aerobic capacity. Multiple strategies are used, and intensity prescription matches the goals for that workout. LT and exercise economy (in addition to $\dot{V}O_{2max}$) increase endurance performance, and these are often trained at moderately high to high intensities (*i.e.*, at velocities or power outputs at or that surpass the velocity/power at $\dot{V}O_{2max}$). Some researchers have postulated that training at a higher intensity for lower mileage may be more effective for enhancing distance running performance (32). Moderate-intensity, long-duration workouts for 150 and 250 minutes per week are good for weight control and increasing submaximal muscle endurance (33). The ACSM has recommended greater amounts of moderate-intensity exercise (>250 min·wk^{-1}) for clinically significant weight loss (33). Aerobic capacity may increase, but it depends on the athlete's training status. Athletes with high levels of aerobic fitness may not improve their aerobic capacity with low-to-moderate intensity workouts. High-intensity workouts increase aerobic capacity, economy, and LT. *Hill training* (at 85%–90% effort for 30-s to 5-min periods) in runners increases intensity and is associated with faster endurance run times (32). Increasing intensity increases muscle fiber recruitment and CV demands, which have a more profound effect on increasing aerobic and muscle endurance.

There are several ways to monitor or prescribe AT intensity: (a) HR, (b) percentage of $\dot{V}O_{2max}$ or reserve, (c) ratings of perceived exertion (RPE), and (d) use of the aforementioned LT parameters (21). In addition, use of time, speed, or power parameters are commonly used by athletes as intensity guides used with or independent of the previous methods. The most common method used to prescribe intensity is to use HR. There is a very close relationship between HR and oxygen consumption. The first step in intensity prescription is to determine the athlete's maximal HR. Historically, this has been calculated by taking 220 – the athlete's age (HR is in bpm). For example, a 20-year-old athlete's max predicted HR is 200 bpm. However, this formula may underestimate or overestimate measured maximal HR depending on factors such as age and gender. A revised formula: $HR_{max} = 207 - 0.7$ (age) has been recommended as well (20,34). At this point, two methods may be used although more research is needed to better specific the conditions of which each should be used (as other researchers have developed other equations see Ref. (21)). Erroneous determination of HR_{max} could decrease the accuracy of the *heart rate reserve* (*HRR*) values used to determine AT intensity. The next step is to multiply the max HR by the desired training percentage. For example, the 20-year-old athlete desiring to train at 70% intensity would attain an exercise HR of 140 bpm (200 bpm $\times$ 0.70). This is known as the HR_{max} *method*. However, the second method, the HRR method, is preferred. The HRR method, also known as the Karvonen formula (35), takes into account the athlete's resting HR which is a measure of aerobic fitness. The HRR and the percentage of $\dot{V}O_{2max}$ values obtained between 50% and 100% intensities are more closely linear than $\%HR_{max}$ and $\%\dot{V}O_{2max}$ as the $\%HR_{max}$ may yield values of $\%\dot{V}O_{2max}$ that differ by a range of 3%–14% (11). The Karvonen, or HRR, formula is:

$$\text{target HR} = \%\text{INT} (HR_{max} - HR_{rest}) + HR_{rest}.$$

If our athlete has a resting HR of 68 bpm, then his or her target HR (based on the Karvonen formula) would be THR = 0.70 (200 bpm $-$ 68 bpm) + 68 bpm = 174 bpm. Compared to the standard percentage formula, the HRR method does take into consideration one's fitness level (via the resting HR) and provides a better indication of target HR for AT. Figure 17.4 depicts an intensity training zone based on targeted HRs. Many times, a targeted zone is calculated rather than one specific HR. Using the Karvonen formula, a HR zone of 121–180 bpm is shown based on 40%–85% of HRR. Low-, moderate-, and high-intensity AT zones are identified. Age only explains ~75% of the variability of HR so other variables such as training status and exercise mode are critical (11). *The ACSM has recommended 40%–89% of HRR and 64%–95% of HR_{max} for intensity prescription during AT* (21,31). Specifically, moderate and vigorous intensities are recommended for most adults, while light-to-moderate intensities are recommended for deconditioned individuals (31). Athletes benefit from training at the upper end of this range. It is important to point out that HR is a self-correcting variable (changes with improved fitness) for intensity prescription. Submaximal exercise HR is reduced as a CV adaptation. It takes greater effort to reach a target HR as aerobic capacity improves. Thus, maintaining a targeted HR percentage as an intensity guide can still be progressive because the athlete will have to work harder in order to reach the targeted level. The use of HR monitors makes it easy to monitor HR in addition to palpation. Also, many indoor cardio machines enable HR assessment while exercising. For example, an athlete can be given a 12-week AT program with intensity prescription of 60% of HRR for the first 4 weeks, 65% of HRR for the second 4 weeks, and 70% of HRR for the last 4 weeks. Although the athlete maintains the same target HRR

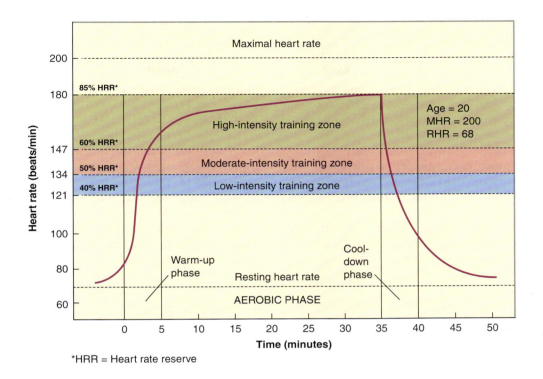

FIGURE 17.4 Intensity zone based on heart rate.

value for 4-week periods, progression takes place within each cycle as it becomes more difficult to reach the desired HR as conditioning improves. Thus, the athlete is forced to continually work harder to maintain the target HRR value.

The second way to prescribe intensity is based on a percentage of $\dot{V}O_{2max}$ or reserve. Selecting a percentage of $\dot{V}O_{2max}$ use the following equation:

$$\text{Target } VO_2 = \%INT(\dot{V}o_{2max}).$$

However, the $\dot{V}O_2$ reserve ($\dot{V}O_2R$) method can be used and is recommended by the ACSM where

$$VO_2R = \%INT(\dot{V}o_{2max} - 3.5) + 3.5.$$

The $\dot{V}O_2R$ method takes into consideration the difference between $\dot{V}O_{2max}$ and resting $\dot{V}O_2$ (3.5 mL·kg^{-1}·min^{-1}) and correlates highly to the HRR method (36). Let us view a 20-year-old athlete with a $\dot{V}O_{2max}$ of 52 mL·kg^{-1}·min^{-1}. Using the first method, if the target intensity is 70% then the target $\dot{V}O_2$ = 36.4 mL·kg^{-1}·min^{-1} (52 × 0.70 = 36.4 mL·kg^{-1}·min^{-1}). Using the $\dot{V}O_2R$ method, the target $\dot{V}O_2$ = 37.5 mL·kg^{-1}·min^{-1} (0.70[52 − 3.5] + 3.5). *The ACSM recommends 40%–89% $\dot{V}O_2R$ for AT (similar to HRR) when the $\dot{V}O_2R$ method is used* (21,31). A limitation of this method is that true $\dot{V}O_2$ data are not readily available (outside of the laboratory setting) so estimation is used.

The ACSM metabolic equations can be used in calculation (21). Variables used in the regression equations include speed, percent grade, work rate, and step height (for those equations used for walking, running, cycling [arm and leg], and stepping). These equations are as follows:

- *Walking*: VO$_2$ (mL·kg^{-1}·min^{-1}) = 0.1 (speed in m·min^{-1}) + 1.8 (speed in m·min^{-1}) (% grade) + 3.5 mL·kg^{-1}·min^{-1}
- *Running*: VO$_2$ (mL·kg^{-1}·min^{-1}) = 0.2 (speed in m·min^{-1}) + 0.9 (speed in m·min^{-1}) (% grade) + 3.5 mL·kg^{-1}·min^{-1}
- *Leg Cycling*: VO$_2$ (mL·kg^{-1}·min^{-1}) = 1.8 (work rate in kg·m^{-1}·min^{-1})/body mass (kg) + 7.0 mL·kg^{-1}·min^{-1}
- *Arm Cycling*: VO$_2$ (mL·kg^{-1}·min^{-1}) = 3.0 (work rate in kg·m^{-1}·min^{-1})/body mass (kg) + 3.5 mL·kg^{-1}·min^{-1}
- *Stepping*: VO$_2$ (mL·kg^{-1}·min^{-1}) = 0.2 (step rate in steps·min^{-1}) + 2.394 (step rate in steps·min^{-1}) (step height in meters) + 3.5 mL·kg^{-1}·min^{-1}

In our previous example, substituting the target VO$_2$ in the equation for running is calculated:

- VO$_2$ (mL·kg^{-1}·min^{-1}) = 0.2 (speed in m·min^{-1}) + 0.9 (speed in m·min^{-1}) (% grade) + 3.5 mL·kg^{-1}·min^{-1}
- 37.5 mL·kg^{-1}·min^{-1} = 3.5 mL·kg^{-1}·min^{-1} + 0.2 (speed) — note: assuming % grade is 0 this latter part is not needed
- 34 mL·kg^{-1}·min^{-1} = 0.2 (speed)
- Speed = 170 m·min^{-1} — speed units are in m·min^{-1}
- Conversion: speed (mph) = speed (m·min^{-1})/26.8
- Speed = 170 m·min^{-1}/26.8
- Speed = 6.3 mph

In our example, the athlete needs to run at 6.3 mph to achieve the target VO$_2$R value. Without performing the calculation, another estimate may be used via metabolic equivalents

(METS). 1 MET = 3.5 mL·kg^{-1}·min^{-1}. Our targeted VO$_2$ of 37.5 mL·kg^{-1}·min^{-1} is equivalent to 10.7 METS (VO$_2$ = 35.7/3.5). A conversion table is used yielding an activity equivalent of 10.7 METS (Table 17.2). Table 17.2 shows running between 6 and 6.7 mph meet the criteria. Thus, METS can be used as an estimate of AT intensity. However, absolute use of METS can result in misclassified AT intensity because they do not consider body weight, sex, and fitness level (21). The ACSM recommends use of relative measures such as HRR and VO$_2$R when prescribing intensity (21). In addition, it is important to note that mode-specific exercise economy affects the intensity prescription where some calculations could underestimate the needed intensity in athletes with high economy.

A third way to prescribe or monitor AT intensity is by using a RPE scale. The most common, the *Borg Scale* (37), is shown in Figure 17.5. It is constructed to increase linearly with work rates in conjunction with HR and oxygen consumption during aerobic exercise. The Borg Scale consists of a continuum of intensity anchors ranging from 6 to 20, *e.g.*, very, very light (*i.e.*, 6–8) to very, very hard (*i.e.*, 19–20). A zero is added to the rating (a rating of 14 = 140 bpm) to estimate HR. A value of 14–17 corresponds to 60%–89% of HRR, 77%–95% of HR$_{max}$, and 64%–90% of $\dot{V}O_{2max}$ (21). The Borg Scale provides accurate estimates in recreational, athletic, and clinical populations provided appropriate calibration methods are used to better gauge the perception zones. Another measure of perceived effort that can be used to regulate AT intensity is the *Talk Test* where an intensity is selected where comfortable speech is possible (21).

There is a minimum intensity, or threshold, needed to improve fitness but varies depending on an individual's current fitness level and other factors such as age, health status, physiologic differences, and genetics (31). Highly trained individuals

Table 17.2	Exercise and Metabolic Equivalents (METS)		
METS	**Exercise**	**METS**	**Exercise**
1.0	Lying/sitting quietly	8.0	Calisthenics — vigorous
2.0	Walking flat — <2 mph	8.0	Circuit training
2.5	Walking flat — 2 mph	8.0	Outdoor cycling — 12–13.9 mph
3.0	Light RT	8.0	Walking flat — 5.0 mph
3.0	Stationary cycling — 50 W	8.5	Step aerobics — 6–8 in. steps
3.0	Walking flat — 2.5 mph	9.0	Running flat — 5.2 mph
3.3	Walking flat — 3 mph	9.0	Stair stepping — 12-in. steps, 30 steps·min^{-1}
3.5	Light calisthenics	10.0	Outdoor cycling — 14–15.9 mph
3.5	Stair stepping — 20 steps·min^{-1}, 4-in. steps	10.0	Running — 6.0 mph
3.8	Walking flat — 3.5 mph	10.0	Step aerobics — 10–12 in. steps
4.0	Water aerobics	10.0	Swimming laps — freestyle, vigorous
4.8	Stair stepping — 30 steps·min^{-1}	10.5	Stationary cycling — 200 W
5.0	Low-impact aerobic dance	11.0	Running — 6.7 mph
5.0	Walking flat — 4.0 mph	11.5	Running — 7.0 mph
5.5	Stationary cycling — 100 W	12.0	Outdoor cycling — 16–19 mph
6.0	Outdoor cycling — 10–11.9 mph	12.5	Running — 7.5 mph
6.0	Vigorous RT	12.5	Stationary cycling — 250 W
6.3	Stair stepping, 12-in. steps, 20 steps·min^{-1}	13.5	Running — 8.0 mph
6.3	Walking flat — 4.0 mph	14.0	Running — 8.5 mph
6.9	Stair stepping, 8-in. steps, 30 steps·min^{-1}	15.0	Running — 9.0 mph
7.0	High-impact aerobic dance	16.0	Outdoor cycling — >20 mph
7.0	Stationary cycling — 150 W	16.0	Running — 10 mph
7.0	Swimming laps — slow, mod effort		

Adapted with permission from Reuter BH, Hagerman PS. Aerobic endurance exercise training. In: Baechle TR, Earle RW, editors. *Essentials of Strength Training and Conditioning*. 3rd ed. Champaign (IL): Human Kinetics; 2008. p. 489–503.

6	
7	Very, very light
8	
9	Very light
10	
11	Fairly light
12	
13	Somewhat hard
14	
15	Hard
16	
17	Very hard
18	
19	Very, very hard
20	

FIGURE 17.5 Borg scale of perceived exertion. The scale with correct instructions can be obtained from Borg Perception, see the home page: www.borgperception.se/index.html. (Reprinted with permission from Borg G. *Borg's Perceived Exertion and Pain Scales.* Champaign (IL): Human Kinetics; 1998.)

need to exercise at near-maximal (*i.e.*, 95%–100% of $\dot{V}O_{2max}$) training intensities to improve $\dot{V}O_{2max}$, whereas 70%–80% of $\dot{V}O_{2max}$ may provide a sufficient stimulus in moderately trained individuals (21,31). For AT, the ACSM (31) uses the following terminology regarding classification of intensity:

- Very light: <30% HRR, VO₂R — <37% $\dot{V}O_{2max}$ — <2 METS — RPE < 9
- Light: 30%–39% HRR, VO₂R — 37%–45% $\dot{V}O_{2max}$ — 2.0–2.9 METS — RPE 9–11
- Moderate: 40%–59% HRR, VO₂R — 46%–63% $\dot{V}O_{2max}$ — 3.0–5.9 METS — RPE 12–13
- Vigorous: 60%–89% HRR, VO₂R — 64%–90% $\dot{V}O_{2max}$ — 6.0–8.7 METS — RPE 14–17
- Near maximal-to-maximal: ≥90% HRR, VO₂R — ≥91% $\dot{V}O_{2max}$ — ≥8.8 METS — RPE ≥ 18

Some athletes aerobically train without direct monitoring of intensity via HRR, VO₂R, or RPE. Rather, intensity is based on *performance parameters*, *e.g.*, speed or power output relative to the distance/duration or work rates prescribed. The goal of the workout or training phase may be the completion of a specified distance or velocity/power output within a time framework as opposed to targeting a specific intensity during the workout. Intensity can be estimated by the pattern of progression used during AT. Many athletes have a designated distance targeted per workout or repetition/set. For example, the athlete may be prescribed a 5-mile run. In week 1, the athlete/coach times the run and establishes a base. In each workout (5 miles is the desired length), the athlete tries to maintain a time frame or improve upon that time. The shorter the time completed, the faster the average running speed. Reduced times indicate better performance but do not quantify the intensity used per se. However, endurance athletes compete against the clock so a performance-parameter training objective is more specific to the competition environment. The use of time trials can be motivational and the athlete (when training on a similar course) may establish mental markers within the event, which provides a guide to where they should be. For example, the athlete may acknowledge that reaching a certain landmark in the course means he or she should be exercising under a certain time. If not, then the athlete needs to increase speed to reach the desired pace. This is seen in many modes such as running, cycling, cross-country skiing, and swimming. In viewing swimming competitions, *e.g.*, the Olympics, on television, often the pace times are shown. These serve as valuable guides to influence coaching strategies. Although not a direct measure of intensity, time trials are commonly used by athletes as a form of overload or progression. In addition, the athlete may be prescribed a fixed workout duration. For example, the athlete may be prescribed a 30-minute run, 2 days per week, for 6 weeks. In each workout, the athlete attempts to cover a larger distance in the same period of time. Greater effort and speed are needed to train farther in the same time period.

Frequency

The frequency of AT is affected by other variables such as intensity, duration, mode, training status, and recovery of the athlete. Frequency will vary depending on whether the athlete is in off-, pre-, or in-season training. High-intensity and/or long-duration workouts may necessitate a reduction in frequency to reduce the risk of overuse injuries and overtraining for non–ultra-endurance athletes. Highly trained athletes have greater tolerance for volume and can handle a higher frequency. Endurance athletes may train 5 days per week in the off-season and incorporate some anaerobic training to improve overall conditioning. However, during the preseason, the athlete may increase volume and frequency greatly for endurance events and may have multiple workouts in a day. Studies have shown that $\dot{V}O_{2max}$ increases similarly between 2- and 5-day frequencies (20,38). However, the intensity may be the critical variable and not the frequency per se. Other physiological adaptations in addition to $\dot{V}O_{2max}$ changes are sought so a higher frequency can be used to target these components (economy, LT, muscle endurance). *The ACSM has recommended 3–5 days of AT per week* (31). For greater specificity, *the ACSM has recommended: ≥5 days per week for moderate-intensity training, ≥3 days per week for vigorous high-intensity training, and 3–5 days per week when combination moderate- and high-intensity workouts are used* (21,31,36). For low- to moderate-intensity AT, frequencies of 5–7 days per week can be used (36). Table 17.3 depicts some different workout strategies relative to AT frequency. These are general recommendations that do not address all of the needs of the athlete. Advanced-to-elite endurance athletes may train with a higher frequency in preparation for a competition, and this may include multiple workouts per day. A high frequency (>250 min·wk⁻¹) is seen by those individuals who are aerobically training for weight loss where moderate intensity, long-duration workouts are often used (33).

Table 17.3 Examples of Intensity Prescription Strategies Based on Aerobic Training Frequencies of 3–6 days per week

FRQ	Monday	Tuesday	Wednesday	Thursday	Friday	Saturday	Sunday
3	H	—	H	—	H	—	—
3	H	—	LM	—	H	—	—
3[a]	LM	—	LM	—	LM	—	—
4	H	LM	—	H	LM	—	—
4	LM	—	H	—	LM	—	H
4[a]	LM	LM	—	LM	LM	—	—
4	H	—	H	—	H	—	LM
5	H	LM	—	H	LM	—	LM
5	H	LM	H	LM	H	—	—
5[a]	LM	LM	LM	LM	LM	—	—
6	H	LM	H	LM	H	LM	—
6[a]	LM	LM	LM	LM	LM	LM	—

[a]LM weeks used for body weight control.

H, high-intensity workout; LM, low-to-moderate-intensity workout.

Myths & Misconceptions
Low-Intensity AT Is the Best Way to Increase $\dot{V}O_{2max}$

It has been suggested that low-to-moderate intensity, long-duration AT is the best way to increase $\dot{V}O_{2max}$. However, a threshold training intensity is needed to increase endurance capacity and, in many cases, the higher the intensity, the larger the $\dot{V}O_{2max}$ improvement. The threshold is based on training status and only surpassing a threshold intensity will lead to improvement. Likewise, a smaller window of adaptation is evident for athletes with a high $\dot{V}O_{2max}$. In a literature review by Swain and Franklin (39), it was shown that individuals with a $\dot{V}O_{2max}$ below 40 mL·kg^{-1}·min^{-1} always increased their aerobic capacity even at intensities as low as 30% of $\dot{V}O_2R$, but individuals with $\dot{V}O_{2max}$ values between 41 and 51 mL·kg^{-1}·min^{-1} showed a threshold (~45% of $\dot{V}O_2R$) where training only above the threshold led to aerobic capacity improvements (39). The majority of studies cited in their review found greater increases in $\dot{V}O_{2max}$ with higher-intensity AT than lower-intensity training (using constant total volume) (39). Figure 17.6 depicts data generated from Swain (36) showing a continuum of adaptations in $\dot{V}O_{2max}$ based on

training intensity and initial training status. Gormley et al. (40) had subjects train at 50%, 75%, and 95% of $\dot{V}O_2R$ (with equal training volumes) and found that a continuum of increases (20.6%, 14.3%, and 10% increases, respectively) were seen for the 95%, 75%, and 50% groups, respectively. Interestingly, Helgerud et al. (41) showed increases in $\dot{V}O_{2max}$ after 8 weeks of interval training at 90%–95% of HR_{max} but failed to observe an increase in $\dot{V}O_{2max}$ with continuous AT at 70% and 85% of HR_{max}. These data demonstrate the utility of interval training in the training of aerobic athletes and show that interval training at high intensities may elicit greater improvements in aerobic capacity than lower-intensity training at a similar volume (36). Based on the available data, the threshold training intensity needed to increase aerobic capacity increases as one's level of aerobic fitness increases and higher-intensity AT leads to greater improvement. Table 17.4 depicts current threshold intensities and subsequent recommendations for AT where progression is the goal (36).

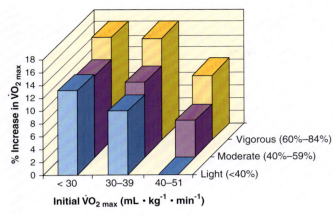

FIGURE 17.6 Increases in $\dot{V}O_{2max}$ at different intensities of training for individuals with various levels of aerobic fitness. Data show greater improvements in $\dot{V}O_{2max}$ with higher intensities of aerobic endurance training. (Reprinted with permission from Swain DP. Cardiorespiratory exercise prescription. In: Ehrman JK, editor. *ACSM's Resource Manual for Guidelines for Exercise Testing and Prescription*. 6th ed. Philadelphia (PA): Lippincott Williams & Wilkins; 2010. p. 448–462.)

Table 17.4 Threshold Intensities of Aerobic Training Needed to Increase Aerobic Capacity

Fitness Level	$\dot{V}O_{2max}$ (mL·kg^{-1}·min^{-1})	Recommended Minimum Intensity
Low to moderate	<40	30% VO_2R or HRR
Average to good	40–51	45% VO_2R or HRR
High	52–59	75% VO_2R or HRR
Very high	≥60	90%–100% VO_2R or HRR

From Swain DP. Cardiorespiratory exercise prescription. In: Ehrman JK, editor. *ACSM's Resource Manual for Guidelines for Exercise Testing and Prescription*. 6th ed. Philadelphia (PA): Lippincott Williams & Wilkins; 2010. p. 448–462.

Volume and Duration

Duration refers to the length of time a workout lasts. *Volume* is the product of training frequency, exercise intensity, and the duration of exercise (21), which is reflective of the total number of cyclical repetitions and distances covered. Both are highly related to each other and depend on the intensity, frequency, and training status of the athlete. AT workouts of moderate intensity are often moderate-to-long in duration. Athletes training for endurance events have been known to exercise at high volumes. High-intensity workouts involve shorter durations and are of low-to-moderate training volumes. For general AT, the *ACSM recommends 20–60 minutes of continuous or intermittent aerobic exercise for healthy adults; 30–60 minutes per day of moderate training, 20–60 minutes per day of vigorous exercise, or a combination* (21,31). In general, the ACSM recommends 300 minutes per week of moderate-intensity AT, or 150 minutes per week of vigorous-intensity AT, or an equivalent combination of both (21). The volume of athletes training for endurance sports exceeds this range frequently. Table 17.5 depicts an example 8-week intermediate AT program based on ACSM guidelines. It is designed to establish an aerobic base for subsequent higher-intensity training. The goals are to increase duration on the lower-intensity workouts and increase intensity on the higher-intensity workout.

There is no optimal volume of training for everyone. Rather, volume (and intensity) relates to the type of training activity. For example, the volume of AT for a marathon runner will be much higher than the volume for a basketball player as the runner must compete for 26 miles, whereas the basketball player must continuously play for two halves but will take frequent breaks due to time-outs, substitutions, and breaks in the action (more anaerobic activity). Volume should be carefully prescribed. Fluctuations in weekly training volumes are common. Many athletes alternate between high-intensity, moderate-volume and moderate-intensity, and high-volume workouts during a training week. Progression in volume may entail the athlete covering a greater distance in a specific or general period of time, adding distance and time, or adding more repetitions or increasing the distance of each repetition (for interval training).

Types of Aerobic Endurance Training Workouts

AT programs can vary greatly in structure, *e.g.*, prolonged low-to-moderate intensity workouts (long slow duration)

Table 17.5	Sample 8-week Base 3-day per week Base Intermediate Aerobic Running Program						
Week	Monday	Tuesday	Wednesday	Thursday	Friday	Saturday	Sunday
1	60% HRR 30 min	—	70% HRR 20 min	—	60% HRR 30 min	—	—
2	60% HRR 30 min	—	70% HRR 20 min	—	60% HRR 30 min	—	—
3	60% HRR 35 min	—	70% HRR 20 min	—	60% HRR 35 min	—	—
4	60% HRR 35 min	—	70% HRR 20 min	—	60% HRR 35 min	—	—
5	60% HRR 40 min	—	75% HRR 20 min	—	60% HRR 40 min	—	—
6	60% HRR 40 min	—	75% HRR 20 min	—	60% HRR 40 min	—	—
7	60% HRR 45 min	—	75% HRR 20 min	—	60% HRR 45 min	—	—
8	60% HRR 45 min	—	75% HRR 20 min	—	60% HRR 45 min	—	—

to higher-intensity workouts intermittent in structure. This section describes some common types of workouts used by endurance athletes.

Continuous Workouts: Long Slow Distance

Long slow distance training (LSD) consists of low-to-moderate-intensity exercise performed for moderate-to-long durations. It may be referred to as *steady-pace training*. It is designed to increase $\dot{V}O_{2max}$ and muscle endurance. Long slow distance training is typically performed between 30 minutes and 2.5 hours at a slower-than-race pace (60%–80% of $\dot{V}O_{2max}$), or a conversational pace. Many endurance athletes perform LSD training 1–2 days per week (11), and some ultra-endurance athletes may include 3–4 LSD workouts per week or more to accumulate additional mileage or to assist in recovery between more intense workouts (13). Because of the lower intensity, LSD workouts may spare muscle glycogen to some degree by a preferential increase in fat utilization. However, the intensity used for LSD training is below the endurance athlete's normal competition pace, so this could be a disadvantage if performed too frequently. The use of LSD training for other athletes with the goal of improving aerobic capacity is common. Often, athletes will start at a comfortable pace for ~30 minutes. For progression, the athlete can increase the time or distance gradually (within a 10% increment) over short-term training periods. It is important to note that this progression strategy applies to LSD workouts, but AT progression also entails the use of other workout types described below.

Pace/Tempo

Pace/tempo training requires the athlete to workout at an intensity similar to or slightly higher than the normal race intensity. Thus, monitoring pace throughout is critical to maintaining the targeted intensity. The intensity corresponds to the LT (~75%–90% of $\dot{V}O_{2max}$). Thus, it is good if the athlete has experience in

racing and has a predetermined pace (for the race length) or if they had had their LT speed measured. Pace/tempo training can increase the LT and improve endurance performance (8). Pace/tempo training can be continuous (20–30 min) or intermittent where short bouts are followed by a recovery period (11). For example, the athlete may run for 20 minutes during a continuous tempo run during a workout or 3×10-minute runs (with 2-min rest intervals between) another workout; both workouts using the same intensity. The purpose is to develop a race type of pace for the athlete. The intensity should not be increased too much; rather, the distance can be increased when appropriate (11). Athletes typically include race/tempo training 1–2 days per week.

Interval Training

Interval training refers to repeated bouts of intense exercise separated by recovery periods that may be generally classified as high-intensity interval training or sprint interval training (21). The key programming variables include the mode, intensity, volume and duration, recovery interval intensity and duration, and the number of interval sets and repetitions (42). The addition of recovery periods enables the athlete to train at a higher intensity during each work bout compared to continuous exercise. Studies show enhanced interval quality (*i.e.*, speed, power) with longer recovery times in between bouts (43). Recovery intervals may either be fixed (*e.g.*, a specific length) or based on work-relief ratios. For example, a work-relief ratio of 1:1 indicates a 30-second rest interval if the work rate interval is 30 seconds.

The prescription of interval training depends on the needs of the athlete. For example, the metabolic demands of soccer will be different from pure aerobic endurance sports such as distance running and triathlon. A number of studies have examined elements of interval training; some in different athletic groups and several in lesser-trained populations. In general, interval training can increase $\dot{V}O_{2max}$, exercise time to exhaustion, LT, economy, and various elements of sports performance (44). Helgerud et al. (45) added 2 days per week of interval training (4 × 4 min of running at 90%–95% of HR_{max} with 3 min of jogging between intervals) to regular soccer practice over 8 weeks and showed $\dot{V}O_{2max}$ increased by 10.8%, LT increased by 16%, running economy increased by 6.7%, and measures of soccer performance (distance covered in a game, number of sprints, and ball involvement) improved only in the interval training group. Acka and Aras (46) compared two interval training programs performed 2 times per week for 4 weeks on rowing ergometry (8 × 2.5 min at 90% of peak power with 3-min rest intervals versus 10 × 30 s at 150% of peak power with 4-min rest intervals) and showed both programs similarly increased VO_2 peak, 2,000 m rowing power, and improved 2,000 m rowing time. Other studies have shown that interval training increases middle distance running and cycling performance by 3%–5% (44). These data, as well as other studies, show why interval training is a fundamental part of the training of athletes. In comparison to continuous AT, interval training was shown to produce similar increases in $\dot{V}O_{2max}$, while some studies have shown interval training more effective for increasing $\dot{V}O_{2max}$ (44). Nevertheless, both form an integral component of the AT of endurance athletes, and interval training may become increasingly important in bringing about further aerobic adaptations in highly trained athletes.

Interval training was discussed in Chapters 12 in relation to speed endurance training (and ways to determine a training intensity including all-out sprints, time trials, progressive $\dot{V}O_{2max}$ testing [to determine $v\dot{V}O_{2max}$], and field testing) and in relation to metabolic training (e.g., high-intensity interval training). To briefly review, anaerobic high-intensity interval training (targeting ATP-PC system) involves 3–10 seconds maximal bursts with at least 60 seconds of rest (or 1:12 to 1:20 work-relief ratios) and anaerobic interval training (targeting glycolysis but still significant aerobic system contributions) involves 10–30 seconds bursts with 1:3 to 1:5 work-relief ratios. These bursts may utilize velocities or power outputs that exceed the $v\dot{V}O_{2max}$ or $p\dot{V}O_{2max}$ (e.g., 115%–170% or more) and contribute to endurance adaptations. Figure 17.7 depicts intensity zones for sprint interval and repeated sprint interval training, as well as intensity zones short and long aerobic interval training in endurance athletes, which is the focus of this chapter.

Interval training for aerobic endurance athletes dates back many years (early 1900s) where athletes such as Paavo Nurmi utilized interval training in the 1920s but became popularized in the 1950s by Olympic champion Emil Zatopek (47). Aerobic endurance athletes use anaerobic and aerobic intervals to increase $\dot{V}O_{2max}$, LT, and economy. Aerobic interval training involves both short and long intervals with recovery periods in between bouts. It is thought that aerobic intervals that elicit

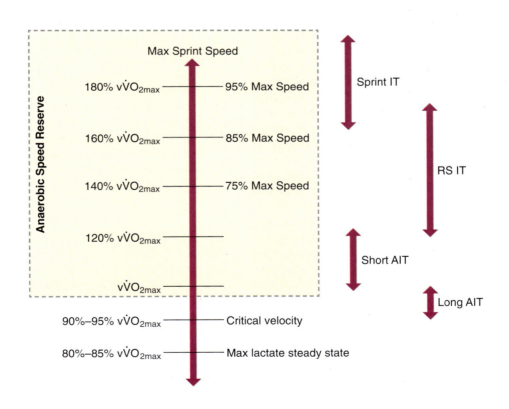

FIGURE 17.7 Intensity zones for interval training. IT, interval training; AIT, aerobic interval training; RS, repeated sprint; $v\dot{V}O_{2max}$, velocity at $\dot{V}O_{2max}$. (Modified from Buchheit M, Laursen PB. High-intensity interval training, solutions to the programming puzzle. Part I: cardiopulmonary emphasis. *Sports Med*. 2013;43:313–38; Billat LV. Interval training and performance: a scientific and empirical practice. Special recommendations for middle- and long-distance running. Part I. Aerobic interval training. *Sports Med*. 2001;31:13–31.)

$\dot{V}O_{2max}$ or close to (*i.e.*, 90%–95%), and the time spent at or near $\dot{V}O_{2max}$, are critical components to aerobic interval training targeting increased aerobic capacity (42). *Short aerobic interval training* involves bursts at 100%–120% of $v\dot{V}O_{2max}$ or $p\dot{V}O_{2max}$ for 15–30 seconds bouts with a 1:1 work-relief ratio (42,47,48). Active recovery (lower-intensity exercise) has been recommended during the rest intervals ≥15 seconds (42,48). The number of sets and reps vary depending on the needs of the athlete. For increasing $\dot{V}O_{2max}$, it has been recommended that 2–3 sets of reps totaling at least 8 minutes are used (48). Compared to continuous AT of similar intensities, short intervals may spare muscle glycogen due to increase lipid oxidation, myoglobin oxygen stores, and potential of some resynthesis of PCr during recovery in addition to enhancing lactate removal (47). Some studies have shown $\dot{V}O_{2max}$ increases of 4%–13% with short aerobic interval training (47), and some studies have shown greater $\dot{V}O_{2max}$ increases than continuous AT provided that the intervals provide sufficient time for the athlete to train at or near their $\dot{V}O_{2max}$ level and large distances are covered at high velocities (47).

Long aerobic interval training involves 1–8 minute bouts at 90%–100% of $v\dot{V}O_{2max}$ or $p\dot{V}O_{2max}$ with work-relief ratios of 1:0.5 to 1:1.5 (47). Figure 17.7 depicts this intensity zone ranging from the $v\dot{V}O_{2max}$ to the critical velocity or critical power intensity. *Critical velocity* (or power) is the intensity between max lactate steady state (MLSS) and $v\dot{V}O_{2max}$, suggested to be the velocity threshold needed to increase $\dot{V}O_{2max}$ and thereby represents the boundary between moderate- and high-intensity aerobic exercise (1,44). It is based on the hyperbolic relationship between speed or power output and time for which it may be sustained (1). The actual relative percent of $v\dot{V}O_{2max}$ is variable based on the training status of the athlete (as endurance athletes display LT, MLSS, and critical velocity values at higher percents of $\dot{V}O_{2max}$) and serves useful in providing a targeted intensity range for long aerobic interval training. Often, 2–5 minute bouts are used for 4–6 intervals for total durations of 12–30 minutes although many variations are effective for increasing endurance performance (42). For increasing $\dot{V}O_{2max}$, Buchheit and Laursen (48) have recommended 6–10 reps × 2-minute intervals, 5–8 reps × 3-minute intervals, and 4–6 reps × 4-minute intervals. The athlete may increase the total time exercising at or near $\dot{V}O_{2max}$ by increasing the length or number of intervals (42). It has been suggested that endurance athletes need ~2 minutes to reach $\dot{V}O_{2max}$ when exercising at $v\dot{V}O_{2max}$ so interval length is at least 2 minutes (13). Of significance is the type of recovery used, *e.g.*, passive (walking) or active exercising at ~50%–70% of $v\dot{V}O_{2max}$. The recovery interval is needed to facilitate recovery, *e.g.*, PCr resynthesis, acid buffering, inorganic phosphate regulation, etc., and to maintain a minimal level of $\dot{V}O_2$ to reduce the time needed to reach $\dot{V}O_{2max}$ in subsequent intervals (42). Buchheit and Laursen (48) have recommended passive recoveries for rest periods of ~2–3 minutes or less and active recoveries for rest periods of 4–5 minutes or more.

Interval training workouts are typically performed 1–2 days per week and may cover up to 8% of the weekly total mileage in 3,000- to 10,000-m runners (49). They are stressful and are commonly placed in between lower-intensity workouts. Many coaches believe interval training to be a critical (and perhaps most beneficial method) for improving distance running performance (32). Over time, the interval segment can be manipulated by manipulating the time or distance covered as well as the recovery intervals. Many variations of intervals are used by the coach and athlete. One model used by coaches and cited in the literature is the Thibault model (48,50) (Fig. 17.8). The number of reps (max of 30) is plotted against the duration (max of 7 min) of each interval. Each of the 6 lines represents the targeted intensity (85%–110% of $v\dot{V}O_{2max}$) for the intervals. For example, if the targeted intensity for a workout is 90% of $v\dot{V}O_{2max}$ and the goal was to perform 3-minute interval bouts, then the model suggests that 8 reps be performed over 2 sets.

Fartlek Training

Fartlek (a Swedish word meaning speed play) training was introduced in the United States in the 1940s and is composed of loosely structured exercise (usually runs but can apply to cycling, rowing, and swimming) performed at various intensities and lengths with mixed periods of hard and easy runs (20,32). They are combinations of other training types. For example, the athlete may run at a moderate pace (~70% of $\dot{V}O_{2max}$) for a period of time and then run at a high intensity for a short time period and repeat the process for the desired length, *i.e.*, the athlete may run at a steady pace for a period of time (6 min) and then run at 30–60 second bursts. Fartlek training is typically performed 1–2 days per week for 20–60 minute workout and can be placed in between lower-intensity workouts (pace/tempo and/or LSD training). Because of the intensity fluctuations, Fartlek training has the potential to increase $\dot{V}O_{2max}$, LT, and running economy (8,11). Because of the fluctuations, it is more difficult to prescribe training HRs. Fartlek training is useful to preparing the athlete to adjusting to competition pace shifts (49).

Repetition Training

Repetition training is a type of high-intensity interval training that constitutes a series of exercise that are faster than current race pace with complete recovery (32). The intensity is greater than the athlete's $\dot{V}O_{2max}$ and last 30–90 seconds (11). Longer recovery periods in between repetitions are used as the intensity is higher, *i.e.*, work-relief ratios of 1:4–1:6 (11,49). There is a potent anaerobic component to repetition training. Thus, speed, economy, anaerobic power, and buffer capacity can increase. Some have recommended that, for middle-distance runners, repetition training constitute a total volume between 2/3 and 1½ times the length of the racing distance (3.3–7.5 km for a 5-km runner) (51). For long-distance runners, repetition training constituting 1/10, 1/5, and 1/3 of the total race distance be used with recovery periods of 5–30 minutes have been recommended (51).

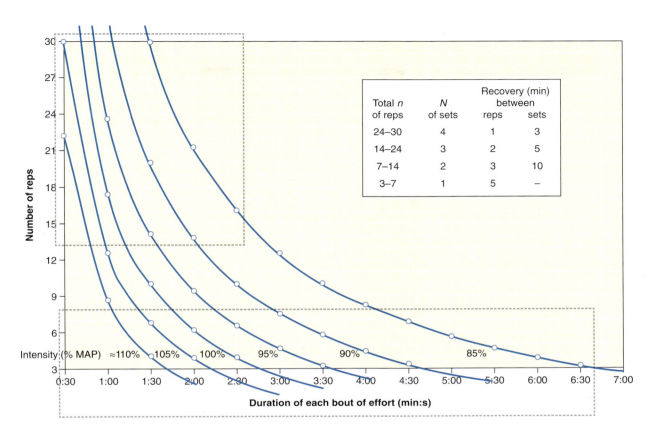

FIGURE 17.8 The Thibault model for interval training programming. (From Thibault G. A graphical model for interval training. *IAAF New Stud Athlet.* 2003;18:49–55). The top box indicates high quantity of training and the lower box indicates quality of training.

Training for Endurance Sports

Training for endurance and ultra-endurance sports entails a multifactorial strategy. It is important for athletes to have already developed an aerobic base. Base AT (off-season training) to increase $\dot{V}O_{2max}$ is critical and consists mostly of moderate-intensity training 5–6 days per week. Specific training can ensue. Periodized training consisting of high-intensity AT coupled or alternated with moderate-intensity, long-duration workouts form the foundation of training for several endurance sports. Supplemental RT and some speed (or perhaps plyometrics) training is included at a lower frequency. For example, a 6-day training routine may comprise one long endurance workout, two to three high-intensity, short-to-moderate-duration workouts (intervals, Fartleks, repetitions, tempos, hills, strides/technique), and two to three low-to-moderate-intensity, moderate-duration workouts used for base training (and facilitate recovery in between high-intensity workouts). Ultra-endurance athletes will utilize a higher frequency of high-volume, long duration workouts per week. Speed work can be incorporated into the high-intensity days, and total-body RT can be performed separately. RT is an important and sometimes overlooked component for the endurance athlete. The goal is not to maximize increases in lean body mass. Mass increase adds weight to the athlete and potentially leads to greater wind resistance encountered both of which can have a negative effect on race speed. Although endurance athletes possess a predominance of ST muscle fibers, strength and power gains do occur, and these can help with race performance. Flexibility training is performed at the end of workouts as part of a cooldown.

Training for the event begins several months in advance. General preparation training consists of increasing $\dot{V}O_{2max}$. Long, continuous training workouts predominate. Special preparation begins a few months before the season or competition. Training volume increases, and greater specificity is added to the training weeks. Higher-intensity workouts are added to improve other facets of race performance, *i.e.*, LT, economy, and speed. Precompetition training is most specialized. Frequency (6–7 d·wk^{-1}) and volume increase. The mileage for long-duration workouts increases and more interval training is added. Brief lower-volume/intensity workouts are included during transitional phases. These equate to unloading weeks in a periodized scheme. For example, a runner preparing for a marathon may use the following pattern for an LSD workout:

Week 1 → 15 miles: Week 2 → 16 miles: Week 3 → 17 miles: Week 4 → 10 miles: Week 5 → 17 miles: Week 6 → 18 miles: Week 7 → 19 miles: Week 8 → 10 miles: Week 9 → 19 miles: Week 10 → 20 miles: Week 11 → 21 miles: Week 12 → 12 miles: Week 13 → 21 miles: Week 14 → 22 miles: Week 15 → 23 miles: Week 16 → 15 miles: followed by a 2-week taper period.

In each week, the volume increases by 1 mile over a 3-week period. The fourth week corresponds to a lower-volume unloading week to allow recovery from the previous weeks of training and transition to another phase of training. Volume progressively increases over time (with the exception of the lower-volume weeks). A tapering period is used 2 weeks before competition as tapering enhances performance. The athlete may overreach (increase volume/frequency in short term) prior to the tapering period, which could result in some plateau. Tapering constitutes a decrease in volume and perhaps frequency to maximize recovery and performance. Final technical points are addressed and race strategies are developed. The taper period corresponds to final nutritional preparations, i.e., carbohydrate loading and increased fluid intake, and final race preparations. By the end of this phase, the athlete is ready for competition.

Endurance athletes from different sports have adopted many training strategies. A triathlon is an ultra-endurance sport, which consists of swimming, cycling, and running. The distances may vary depending on the race. An Ironman triathlon is most rigorous and consists of 3.8-km swim, 180-km cycling, and 42-km run (52). The sequence of events is swimming, cycling, and running. The initial swim reduces optimal cycling power, and subsequent cycling may produce a reduction in running efficiency (52). The triathlete must be proficient in all three modalities. Vleck et al. (53) studied British Olympic and Ironman distance triathletes and showed that Olympic distance triathletes trained 15.6 ± 3.7 hours per week (5.6 ± 2.6-h swimming, 6.3 ± 3.0-h biking, and 3.7 ± 1.4-h running) and Ironman triathletes trained 19.5 ± 7.6 hours per week (6.1 ± 4.5-h swimming, 8.8 ± 4.5-h biking, and 3.9 ± 1.7-h running). Olympic distance triathletes trained 12.0 ± 3.0 times per week (4.0 ± 1.1 workouts swimming, 3.8 ± 1.7 workouts biking, and 4.17 ± 2.0 workouts running) and Ironman triathletes trained 14.3 ± 3.2 times per week (5.1 ± 1.9 workouts swimming, 4.0 ± 2.2 workouts biking, and 4.6 ± 2.0 workouts running) (53). The training consisted mostly of long low-to-moderate-intensity bike rides (>1.5 h) and runs (>1 h), 20- to 60-minute cycling time trials and 20–30 minute continuous or interval runs, and hill work (53). Gulbin and Gaffney (54) showed that Ironman triathletes spent 21.5 ± 10.8 weeks training for the event, and their training distances per week for swimming, cycling, and running were 8.8 ± 4.3, 270 ± 107, and 58.2 ± 21.9 km at paces of 18.1 min·km^{-1}, 31.8 km·h^{-1}, and 4.55 min·km^{-1}, respectively. Triathletes many times have multiworkout days specifically training two of the three competition modalities.

Distance runners use multiple training strategies to enhance performance. A meta-analysis has shown that average weekly running distance, number of weekly runs and runs >20 miles, weekly running hours, running pace, and distance of longest run all were related to marathon finish times in a large group of runners (55). The volume depends on the type of competitive race, e.g., 5 km, 10 km, half-marathon (21.1 km), marathon (42.195 km), and ultra-marathons (50 and 100 km or more). Ultra-marathons are highly stressful on the human body, and ultra-marathoners require a higher volume of training (56). Some elite distance runners train twice a day and run between 100 and 150 miles a week (20). Distance training constitutes base-building,

light, high-quality work, high-intensity intervals, and LT training (32). In fact, elite runners typically alternate between high- and low-to-moderate-intensity workouts and include a substantial amount of speed training to increase LT and running economy (5). Table 17.6 presents data from Kurz et al. (32) who studied several Division I collegiate cross-country runners. The data show shifts in training volume and modes of training over each of the three training phases. They showed the use of speed work, Fartlek training, mileage, and practicing twice per day was associated with slower team times (possibly due to overtraining) during the transition phase. Intervals and tempo training were associated with better running performance. In addition, hill training was related to faster run times during the transition phase. Table 17.7 depicts a sample weekly training program designed for an athlete preparing for a 5-km race. The program is setup so that the longest run of the week takes place on Sunday followed by a day of rest. The rest of training days alternate between high- and moderate-intensity workouts.

Cyclist use multiple training strategies. Professional cyclists may ride 30,000–35,000 km·yr^{-1} and may compete for up to 90 days (2). Typical road races and off-road cross-country cycling events may last between 1 and 5 hours, whereas multistage races consist of several back-to-back days of racing and may total more than 3,800 km as is the case for the Tour de France (2). Similar to other endurance sports, cycling performance is related to $\dot{V}O_{2max}$, peak power output and power output at the LT, LT and blood lactate concentrations, efficiency, and breathing pattern (2). Cyclists have high $\dot{V}O_{2max}$; ranges of 66–85 mL·kg^{-1}·min^{-1} have been reported in male cyclists and 58–68 mL·kg^{-1}·min^{-1} in female cyclists (2). In cyclists with a similar $\dot{V}O_{2max}$, LT and lactate values at peak cycling power are strong predictors of endurance performance (57,58). Some have suggested a power:body mass ratio of >5.5 W·kg^{-1} is a necessary prerequisite for elite cycling (2). Cycling efficiency is related to type I muscle fiber percentages. Cycling programs consist of base training at moderate intensities for long durations (several hours) and progress to higher-intensity interval training as the competitions approach. Interval training is effective to enhance aerobic capacity and muscle endurance when volume increases are no longer augmenting performance. In fact, Tabata et al. (59) have shown that high-intensity interval training produced greater gains in $\dot{V}O_{2max}$ and anaerobic capacity than moderate intensity cycling at 70% of $\dot{V}O_{2max}$.

Case Study 17.1

Angela is a relatively new cross-country runner who is preparing for an upcoming 10-km race. She has some base AT, and her $\dot{V}O_{2max}$ was estimated at 48 mL·kg^{-1}·min^{-1}. She has continued to run recreationally but would now like to try competing. The race is in 15 weeks, and she approaches you to help develop a program to peak her performance at race time.

Question for Consideration: What type of AT program would you prescribe?

Table 17.6 Training Characteristics of Division I Cross-Country Runners

Variable	Transition Phase	Competition Phase	Peaking Phase
Total miles per week	59.5 ± 10.6	72.4 ± 9.1	58.9 ± 10.3
Longest run (miles)	11.5 ± 2.1	13.4 ± 2.2	10.9 ± 1.3
Average number of days per week of:			
Tempo	1.1 ± 0.8	1.6 ± 1.4	2.3 ± 2.0
Short/easy runs	1.9 ± 2.1	2.1 ± 1.8	11.2 ± 7.1
Repetitions	0.1 ± 0.3	0.7 ± 0.6	2.4 ± 2.4
Intervals	0.1 ± 0.3	0.8 ± 0.6	2.7 ± 2.0
Hills	0.6 ± 0.7	0.6 ± 0.7	1.2 ± 4.2
Fartlek	0.5 ± 0.5	0.7 ± 0.5	0.6 ± 0.9
Cross-training	0.5 ± 1.6	0.3 ± 0.6	0.7 ± 1.9
Drills	1.3 ± 2.0	1.6 ± 1.3	5.3 ± 5.9
Weights	1.5 ± 1.4	1.8 ± 0.9	3.6 ± 3.3
Rest	0.5 ± 0.5	0.3 ± 0.5	2.8 ± 1.6
Practice (2× per day)	1.5 ± 1.9	3.5 ± 1.5	7.1 ± 5.4

From Kurz MJ, Berg K, Latin R, DeGraw W. The relationship of training methods in NCAA Division I cross-country runners and 10,000-meter performance. *J Strength Cond Res.* 2000;14:196–201.

Training at Altitude or Hypobaric Conditions

The effects of altitude on human performance became evident at the 1968 Olympic Games held at ~2,340 m in Mexico City where middle distance and long distance running and swimming performances were subpar (60). However, world records in track events were set in all distances up to 800 m where performances were 1%–4% better than the previous-held records (61). The reduced air density creates less drag force and allows augmented short-duration, intense activity. Models have estimated that 100–400 m sprint performance times may be improved by 0.03–0.12 seconds for each 1,000 m increase in altitude (61). However, the effects of altitude have physiological ramifications. In addition to the noted aerodynamic reductions in fluid resistance, it has been well documented that moderate to extreme altitude poses a physiological stress to the athlete via hypoxia (oxygen deprivation). The acute negative effects are less evident during short-duration anaerobic peak strength and power activities, but become more pronounced with greater aerobic contributions to exercise performance. Thus, repeated sprint activity and team sport activity (depending on the length, duration, intensity, and recovery periods in between bouts) may be compromised with earlier onsets of fatigue (61). For example, soccer performance at altitudes of 1,200–1,750 m is reduced as distance covered may be 3%–9% lower and running high-speed acceleration and frequency may be reduced by ~20% (61). However, aerobic performance is compromised but the same factors that acutely reduce performance also serve as a valuable training tool over time. Thus, training at altitude is frequently used to improve performance at sea level or in preparation for competing at moderate to high altitudes. For clarification purposes,

Table 17.7 Sample Precompetition Training Week for Athlete Preparing for 5-km Race

Day	Workout
Monday	Rest
Tuesday	Fartlek runs — 4 miles — fast 30-s, moderate 5 min, repeat …
Wednesday	Easy pace — 3 miles
Thursday	Interval training — 8 × 400 m with 1:1 ratio
Friday	Easy pace — 4 miles
Saturday	Interval training — 6 × 400 m with 1:1 ratio; 3 × 100 m strides — 1:1.5 ratio
Sunday	Long run — 5–7 miles

altitude will be described in the following way using ACSM classifications (21):

- Low altitude = <1,500 m
- High altitude = 1,500–3,500 m
- Very high altitude = 3,500–5,500 m
- Extreme altitude = >5,500 m

In previous chapters, we discussed the aspects of regional hypoxia in relation to blood flow restriction training, and the role of short-term hypoxia (via vascular occlusion) plays in muscle mass development. Here, the focus is on systemic hypoxia brought about via living and/or training in *hypobaric* (low atmospheric oxygen pressure) conditions. The original altitude training began as athletes lived and trained at normal hypobaric altitudes of 1,500–4,000 m known as "live high, train high (LHTH)" dating back to the 1960s (61,62). Although still practiced currently especially by those athletes who live at altitude or routinely train at altitude camps, other methods of altitude, or hypoxic, training have emerged. These systemic approaches include the common method of "live high, train low (LHTL)" under natural hypoxic or simulated conditions (*e.g.*, supplemental oxygen, nitrogen dilution, oxygen filtration), "live high, train low and high (LHTLH)," "live low, train high (LLTH)" or some hybrid types such as "intermitted hypoxic exposure (IHE)," "continuous hypoxic training (CHT)," and "intermittent hypoxia training (IHT)."

The benefits of altitude training derive from acclimatization, physiological adaptations to hypoxic exercise, or a combination of both. The effects may be determined by the duration and magnitude of hypoxia, intensity of training, nutritional status (*e.g.*, hydration levels, iron availability), health, and level of individual responsiveness (63). As altitude increases, barometric pressure and partial pressure of oxygen (PO_2) decrease. The driving force or pressure exerted on oxygen is reduced thereby making it more difficult to extract oxygen from the air and distribute it to the tissue level. Table 17.8 depicts the relationship between altitude, barometric pressure, and PO_2. Although the relative percent of each gas is the same regardless of altitude (*e.g.*, 20.93% for oxygen, 79.04% for nitrogen, and 0.03% for carbon dioxide), the drop in barometric pressure decreases the partial pressure of oxygen. Thus, the result is hypoxia at a level congruent to the altitude level. However, sea level performance ($\dot{V}O_{2max}$) may not change as a result of just living at altitude for a period of time (20). Altitude poses other issues. There is a decrease in temperature with ascending altitude, increase in diuresis, increased likelihood of sleep disorder or poor quality of sleep, and increased exposure to ultraviolet radiation forcing athletes to deal with these stressors in combination with hypoxia (64). There is a greater likelihood of altitude illness especially at higher altitudes. These include *acute mountain sickness* (AMS; or mild altitude sickness), and the more severe *high altitude pulmonary edema (HAPE)*, and *high altitude cerebral edema (HACE)*. Symptoms of AMS are variable but may include headache, nausea, vomiting, fatigue, weakness, and insomnia with hopes they do not lead to more severe symptoms associated with HAPE or HACE. Athletes with *sickle cell trait*

Table 17.8	Relationship between Altitude, Barometric Pressure, and PO_2		
Altitude (m)	Altitude (ft)	Barometric Pressure (mm Hg)	PO_2 (mm Hg)
0	0	760	159
1,000	3,280	674	141
1,500	4,920	634	133
2,000	6,560	596	125
3,000	9,840	526	110
4,000	13,120	462	97
5,000	16,400	405	85
6,000	19,690	354	74
7,000	22,970	308	64
8,000	26,250	267	56
9,000	29,530	230	48

Adapted with permission from McArdle WD, Katch FI, Katch VL. *Exercise Physiology: Energy, Nutrition, and Human Performance.* 6th ed. Philadelphia (PA): Lippincott Williams and Wilkins; 2007. p. 489–502, 615–50.

are at greater risk for sickling (*i.e.*, a medical emergency where RBCs change shape causing decreased blood flow) during exercise and may not be allowed to train or compete at certain altitudes if deemed hazardous by the medical staff. To reduce risks of altitude sickness, it is recommended that athletes acclimatize before or progressively (if possible), ascend to high altitudes at slower rates (*e.g.*, only 600–1,200 m per 24-hour period once above 2,500 m), prehydrate, and initially monitor the intensity of activity during acclimatization (64).

Carotid and aortic chemoreceptors sense reduced PO_2 and reduced arterial saturation elicit cardiorespiratory responses to hypoxia exposure. Acclimatization to chronically reduced inspired PO_2 invokes a series of central and peripheral adaptations that serve to maintain adequate tissue oxygenation. Factors such as elevation, exposure duration, training intensity/volume, and training duration affect the magnitude of adaptation. The most rapid physiological responses to altitude occur during the first few weeks of exposure. It generally takes about 2 weeks (depending on the altitude) to adapt to hypoxia up to 2,300 m and may take an additional week for every additional 610-m increase up to 4,600 m (20). Altitude acclimatization can increase blood hemoglobin concentrations, hematocrit, buffering capacity, and improve structural and biochemical properties of skeletal muscle within several weeks (65,66). Acclimatization to altitude often limits the cardiorespiratory distress from acute or chronic hypoxia (66). However, this positive effect may not improve $\dot{V}O_{2max}$ because the positive effects (increased hematocrit, right shift of the oxyhemoglobin dissociation curve, and increased diffusion capacity within the lungs) may be negated by reduced blood flow to the thorax and periphery, decreased muscle mass, and decreased oxidative enzyme activity (66–68). Other effects that may negate the positive effects of training at altitude are decreased plasma volume, depression of hematopoiesis and increased hemolysis, suppressed immune function (increasing the risk of illness), increased tissue damage via oxidative stress, greater glycogen depletion (via greater sympathetic stimulation), and increased respiratory muscle work upon return to sea level (65). Table 17.9 depicts immediate and chronic responses/adaptations to altitude exposure.

Altitude exposure can reduce body mass and atrophy skeletal muscle, particularly at heights above 6,000 m (68). Weight loss may be the result of reduced lean tissue mass (60%–70%), greater insensible fluid and urine loss, reduced fluid intake and appetite, and increased energy expenditure. Continuous hypoxia can decrease muscle CSA by 10%–22% (69,70). Chronic hypoxia down-regulates mTOR pathway signaling and increases proteolysis via calpain and ubiquitin pathway activity. The changes in mitochondrial and capillary density may reflect a loss of muscle size and not a change in absolute number per

se although new capillary formation may occur (20). Atrophy occurs in FT and ST fibers to a similar magnitude. Hypoxia increases the activity of *hypoxia-inducible factors* (HIFs) which mediate hypoxic effects on skeletal muscle. For example, HIF-1α up-regulates several genes that produce proteins such as glycolytic enzymes, citrate synthase, VEGF, erythropoietin, myoglobin, and other proteins involved in muscular remodeling resulting from hypoxia.

Submaximal and Maximal Aerobic Exercise Performance at Altitude

Submaximal VO_2 for a specific exercise and power output is similar at altitude and at sea level. However, because of the progressive decline in $\dot{V}O_{2max}$ with increasing altitude, the relative difficulty associated with each work rate increases. The impairment is most evident during activities in which a given distance must be traversed in the least amount of time. This decrement increases as the aerobic energy requirements for the activity increase, as high-intensity, anaerobic exercise of short duration may not be affected up to an altitude of 5,200 m (71). At sea level, events lasting 2–5 minutes, 20–30 minutes, and 2–3 hours will be ~2%, 7%, and 17%

Table 17.9	Immediate and Chronic Responses/Adaptations to Altitude Exposure
Immediate	**Chronic**
Plasma volume ↓ (up to 25%)	Acid/base shifts
Acid/base shifts and alkaline body fluids	Hyperventilation
Hyperventilation	Submax HR ↑
Submax HR and cardiac output ↑	Cardiac output and stroke volume ↓
Max cardiac output ↔ or ↓	
Stroke volume ↔ or slight ↓	Catecholamines ↑
Blood pressure ↑	Plasma volume ↓
Catecholamines and SNS activity ↑	Hematocrit, RBC count, 2,3-DPG, EPO, and hemoglobin ↑
Blood lactate ↑ — submax exercise	Capillary and mitochondrial density ↑
↓ arterial saturation (SaO₂) and A-VO₂ difference	Aerobic enzyme content ↑ **or** ↓
↑ glycolysis and CHO use, K⁺, and P_i	Glycolytic enzymes ↑ **or** ↓
$\dot{V}O_{2max}$ ↓	Body weight and lean tissue mass ↓ (5%–15%)
↑ blood lactate — submax exercise	$\dot{V}O_{2max}$ ↓
↓ appetite, sleep	Myoglobin ↑
↓ PCr resynthesis during exercise	Immune function ↓
↓ neural drive and muscle contractility (high altitude) — intense exercise	Glycogen depletion and tissue damage ↑
	↓ blood lactate — max and submax exercise
	↑ energy expenditure, RMR (up to 19%)
	↓ appetite, energy intake

longer, respectively, at 2,300 m (72). The threshold altitude appears to be ~1,600 m for events 2–5 minutes and 600 m for events longer than 20 minutes (20). With continued altitude exposure, acclimatization occurs and the additional difficulty of exercise is reduced.

Acute exposure to altitude increases the blood lactate response to exercise. However, several weeks of exposure to hypoxia unexpectedly reduces the lactate response to exercise, a phenomenon known as the *lactate paradox* (20). The lactate paradox has been controversial and puzzling to physiologists over the years as high-altitude natives, or those individuals acclimated to hypoxic conditions, have shown attenuated blood lactate responses to maximal aerobic exercise in some studies (73) although other research has questioned this concept by failing to show paradoxical lactate levels (74). In those studies supporting the paradox, the attenuation becomes more apparent as altitude increases (73). Although the precise mechanisms are still debatable, the lactate paradox during maximal aerobic exercise may be related to reduced lactate production (rather than clearance from the blood) possibly from up-regulated ATP-coupling pathways decreasing the contribution of fast glycolysis to meet the energy demand (73). Some evidence indicates that the lactate paradox may be transient and dissipate after chronic (>6 wk) exposure to hypoxia (75).

Maximal aerobic capacity is impaired at barometric pressures below 400 mm Hg (above 4,500 m) (66). A loss of 1%–3.2% in $\dot{V}O_{2max}$ for every 305 m of ascent above 1,600 m may be seen (66). Terrados (76) showed that $\dot{V}O_{2max}$ decreased significantly at 1,200 m in sedentary individuals and at 900 m for elite athletes. The $\dot{V}O_{2max}$ decline begins at 600–700 m with a linear reduction of 8% for every additional 1,000 m up to 6,300 m and is more rapid and curvilinear beyond this point (with largest reductions seen in men). Aerobic capacity at 4,000 m may be 75% of sea-level value (20). AT prior to altitude exposure offers little protection against the reductions observed (20). The inability to achieve sea level $\dot{V}O_{2max}$ at altitude makes it difficult for highly trained endurance athletes to perform well. Interestingly, detraining could take place if an athlete trains at altitude at a much lower work rate (62,77). The decrease in $\dot{V}O_{2max}$ occurs because barometric pressure decreases and PO_2 drops such that alveolar oxygen tension and arterial blood saturation are impaired (oxygen availability decreases). The initial response is to increase pulmonary ventilation in order to counteract the low PO_2. Fitness level is critical as highly fit individuals (>63 mL·kg^{-1}·min^{-1}) generally have larger decrements in $\dot{V}O_{2max}$ at altitude than less fit individuals (72). Gore et al. (78) showed a 3.6% decrease in $\dot{V}O_{2max}$ at 580 m in untrained individuals and a 7% decline in endurance athletes. However, at higher altitudes (>7,000 m), this difference due to fitness level diminishes.

Traditional Natural Altitude Training — "Live High-Train High"

Endurance athletes use altitude camps as part of their regular training program. Elite endurance athletes may attend 3–6 altitude training camps per year (63). It has been suggested that repeated exposure to altitude camps facilitates the acclimatization process to subsequent altitude training cycles (63). Frequent use of altitude camps lasting 1–2 weeks (instead of the typical 3- to 4-week duration) interspersed between sea level training may improve performance an average of ~2% in elite endurance athletes (63). Thus, the timing of utilizing altitude camps often coincides with the training phase within a periodized yearly plan. The methods and strategies of using altitude camps have evolved over the years with multiple approaches studied and advances in simulating altitude-related hypoxia (79). Performance at sea level may peak in the short-term (first few days) following altitude training or during a 2nd window (>3 weeks) post altitude training (63).

Traditional altitude camps mostly consisted of living and training at moderate altitudes, *e.g.*, 1,800–2,500 m for 2–4 week durations (79). They consisted of *acclimatization* (where the athlete would accustom themselves to the low PO_2 over a 7–10-d period), *primary training* (2–3 wk of progressive increase in AT intensity and volume), *recovery* (2–5 d of reduced AT volume and intensity), and *return to sea level* (return to regular AT) phases (79). Training at altitude using this LHTH approach may not improve aerobic exercise performance at sea level albeit the scientific literature has been equivocal in studying this phenomenon. Flaws in study design make it difficult to accurately interpret the results of some studies. Bailey and Davies (65) examined 34 studies. Twelve of these studies showed increased endurance performance capacity with altitude training, although only four of these included a control group. Twenty-seven studies did not report a potentiating effect, and fifteen of these included a control group. Overall, $\dot{V}O_{2max}$ increases of up to 17.5% were shown (for altitude exposures of 7–70 d at 1,250–5,700 m) with most not statistically significant. The major problem with training at altitude is that the lower absolute work rates and intensity athletes are forced to adopt. For example, training at 78% of $\dot{V}O_{2max}$ at 300 m would only yield an intensity of 60% at 2,300 m (20). When training high, it is recommended that low-to-moderate intensity, high volume AT is used (63). This could coincide with a general preparation phase where the focus is on hematological changes (63). When training at altitude, it is recommended that at least 7 weeks of sea level training be used in between altitude training cycles to maximize intensity and volume (80). Proper diet, fluid replacement (at least one extra liter of water or carbohydrate-containing beverage), and vitamin/mineral supplementation is important when training at altitude (80), and it is important to note that training at altitude may increase the risk of illness (63).

Live High, Train Low

$\dot{V}O_{2max}$ and performance may be improved the most when athletes live high but train low (LHTL) at higher intensity. This is accomplished by spending several hours per day at high altitude but traveling to a lower altitude for the workouts, or by living and training at sea level but using an altitude simulation device during the nonexercise hours. This move of altitude training began in the early 1990s, and studies have shown the LHTL approach to be more effective than other approaches including LHTH (81). Although $\dot{V}O_{2max}$ increases were shown in elite and subelite athletes, studies have shown performance increases (aerobic endurance power, exercise economy) independent of changes in $\dot{V}O_{2max}$ (65,81). The acute acclimatization can increase RBC production, hemoglobin mass, and erythropoietin, which allow the athlete to train harder at a lower altitude or sea level (20,82). However, the erythropoietin and RBC response is highly variable between athletes and athletes with larger responses tend to produce better performance improvements at sea level versus those who experience limited hematological responses (83). An altitude of 2,000–2,500 m is effective for increasing erythropoiesis during living high, and ~3,100 m may be most effective for increasing nonhematological parameters (79,83). The optimal duration appears to be ~4 weeks for accelerating erythropoiesis but <3 weeks can increase exercise economy and buffer capacity (79). Daily doses of 20–22 hours per day at 2,500 m appear sufficient to increase performance and erythropoiesis, whereas the minimum dose for stimulating erythropoiesis is ~12 hours per day (79). Wilber et al. (77) recommend the following guidelines for living high and training low: *an altitude of 2,000–2,500 m for a minimum of 4 weeks for 22 hours per day*. Stray-Gundersen and Levine (84) have shown living for 4 weeks at 2,500 m increased sea level performance by ~1.5% (with a range of 0%–6%). The benefits lasted for *at least 3 weeks upon return to sea level*. Elite middle distance runners improved their race times by 1.9% following a period of 44 ± 7 days at a simulated altitude of 2,846 m and training at an altitude of 1,700–2,200 m (85). Schmitt et al. (86) studied elite runners, cross-country skiers, and swimmers and showed that 13–18 days of training at 1,200 m coupled with sleeping at 2,500–3,500 m in hypoxic rooms produced greater changes in $\dot{V}O_{2max}$ (7.8% vs. 3.3%) and peak power (4.1% vs. 1.9%) than living and training low while both groups increased

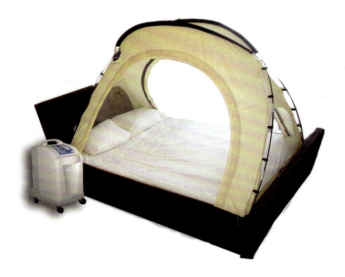

FIGURE 17.9 Altitude tent. (Courtesy of Hypoxico Altitude Training Systems, New York, NY.)

exercise efficiency. Although after 15 days at lower altitude $\dot{V}O_{2max}$ decreased in both groups, peak power was still augmented in the LHTL group. Wehrlin et al. (82) had elite athletes live at 2,500 m for 18 h^{-1} and train at 1,000–1,800 m for 24 days and showed increased serum erythropoietin, hemoglobin, RBC, and hematocrit, and these changes were associated with an increase in $\dot{V}O_{2max}$ and improved 5,000-m running times. Thus, many studies support the concept that LHTL is an effective mode of altitude training. Athletes may simulate altitude via a number of products on the market including hypobaric chambers, hypoxic masks/systems, nitrogen dilution, and altitude tents (see Fig. 17.9). Athletes who live at altitudes can train at sea level (while still at an altitude) by supplemental oxygen to simulate a sea level environment (62).

Myths & Misconceptions
Training at High Altitude Is the Most Effective Mode of Altitude Training

Some have suggested that training high is the best way for the athlete to use altitude to his or her advantage. However, recent studies have shown superior performance enhancement when the athlete lives high but trains low to maintain a sufficient training intensity. Bonetti and Hopkins (81) performed a meta-analysis on altitude/hypoxia endurance training. They classified altitude/hypoxia training studies into six categories and calculated the effects for $\dot{V}O_{2max}$ and other variables. Artificial hypoxia was provided by nitrogen houses, hypobaric chambers, inhalers, and altitude tents.

- LHTH — 14 studies (1,640–2,690 m, 12–30 d)
- LHTL — 6 studies (1,780–2,805 m, 13–28 d)
- Artificial LHTL (8–18 h of long, continuous daily exposure to hypoxia) — 12 studies (2,000–3,500 m, 12–30 d)
- Artificial LHTL (1.5–5 h of brief continuous daily exposure to hypoxia) — 5 studies (3,650–5,500 m, 6–19 d)
- Artificial LHTL (<1.5 h of brief intermittent daily exposure to hypoxia) — 6 studies (3,400–6,000 m, 15–26 d)
- Artificial LLTH — 8 studies (2,500–4,500 m, 9–47 d)

For maximal endurance power output, substantial improvements in subelite athletes were seen with artificial brief intermittent LHTL (1%–4%), LHTL, and artificial, long, and continuous LHTL. In elite athletes, LHTL scored most favorably. For $\dot{V}O_{2max}$, increases were likely with LHTH in subelite athletes but LHTH produced decreases in elite athletes. Other mediators were unclear as to their effects. The authors concluded that naturally LHTL provided the best training strategy for enhancing endurance performance in elite and subelite athletes.

Live High, Train High and Low

A hybrid method of altitude training involves living high but training at high and low altitudes (LHTHL). The differentiating factor is that low-to-moderate intensity AT is performed at the higher altitudes, while high-intensity training is performed at lower altitudes. During precompetitive and competitive training phases, endurance athletes may train with low-to-moderate intensity at altitude but may choose to perform their high-intensity interval sessions at lower altitude. This polarized approach to intensity distribution is widely used by elite endurance athletes and considered by some to be the best practice in elite endurance athletes (63). The LHTLH approach may enhance elite endurance performance by ~1%–2% (63). Chapman et al. (83) examined collegiate cross-country runners over a 4-week altitude camp. They lived at either 1,780, 2,085, 2,454, or 2,800 m and trained at 1,250–3,000 m (higher intensity workouts at 1,250 m and base low-to-moderate intensity training at 1,780–3,000 m). They found only the 2,085 and 2,454 m groups improved sea level 3 km time trial performance by ~2%–3%; $\dot{V}O_{2max}$ increased in all groups except for 1,780 m; and similar increases in erythropoietin and erythrocyte volume were noted thereby demonstrating that the LHTHL approach was very effective especially at the living altitude range of 2,000–2,500 m. The LHTLH approach improves repeated sprint ability and Yo-Yo intermittent recovery test performance (87). Some altitude camps are located within 1 hour driving distance of lower altitude areas where higher intensity AT may be performed.

Simulated Altitude/Hypoxia

The hypoxia associated with different levels of altitude may be simulated (*e.g.*, supplemental oxygen, nitrogen dilution, oxygen filtration) artificially via hypoxic tents, chambers, and altitude masks. Various forms of LHTH, LHTL, LLTH, and LHTLH can be used with simulated hypoxia. The advantage of these devices is they offer the athlete convenience of hypoxia in multiple settings without the other negative consequences of spending significant time at natural moderate-to-high altitudes. The athlete can utilize hypoxia without bearing the cost of having to travel to specific geographic regions. *Intermittent hypoxic exposure* (IHE) refers to exposure to hypoxia from seconds to hours that is repeated for days to weeks with bouts of normoxia in between (79). Early studies were equivocal showing that IHE for 90 minutes to 3 hours per day for 3–5 days per week at 4,000–5,500 m showed either no change in hematological parameters or increased erythropoietin and RBCs with either no or slight performance enhancement (79). Studies using a control group showed no performance enhancement (79). *Intermittent hypoxic training* (IHT) involves living low with intermittent training bouts at altitude (*e.g.*, LLTH). IHT by itself may provide an insufficient stimulus for hematological changes due to the low duration of hypoxic exposure, however, may have a hematological effect when combined with IHE (79). IHT has a positive effect on muscular adaptations with greater up-regulation of HIF-1α and levels of myoglobin, citrate synthase, glycolytic enzyme activity, buffer capacity, and mitochondrial and capillary density compared to sea level training (61,79). Performance changes are equivocal where some studies showed no enhanced aerobic performance, while some studies showed $\dot{V}O_{2max}$ and endurance performance increases (79). If using IHT, Millet et al. (79) have recommended that IHT be used in endurance athletes during precompetition phases 2 days per week for 30–45 minutes of high-intensity exercise per session at simulated altitudes of 2,500–3,000 m, and 3 hours of hypoxia at rest 4–5 times per week when combined with IHE.

Compatibility between High-Intensity Aerobic and Anaerobic Training

One topic of interest in the S&C field is the combined effects of concurrent high-intensity strength/power and AT. Since 1980, several studies have shown an "interference effect" where RT-induced gains in lower-body muscle strength, power, and hypertrophy were attenuated when RT was performed concurrent with high-intensity AT (88–92). Although strength, power, and endurance improve substantially through concurrent training, one or the other may be somewhat attenuated if both are trained rigorously as opposed to focused training on one modality solely. In most cases, power and strength gains may be attenuated although aerobic endurance performance could be limited as well (93). Some studies that have shown an incompatibility examined 3 days per week of RT + 3 days per week of AT on alternating days (training on 6 consecutive days) or 4–6 days per week of combined high-intensity RT and AT (89,92,94). In a meta-analysis, Wilson et al. (95) showed a significant interference effect of simultaneous AT and RT. Large effect sizes were seen for lower-body muscle strength and power reductions with power more susceptible to attenuation than strength. Although power training and AT performed simultaneously in endurance athletes can lead to power and endurance improvements (96), the magnitude of power development may be less than power training alone. Wilson et al. (95) showed that AT mode (*i.e.*, running more than cycling), frequency, and duration were related to the incompatibility. The magnitude of incompatibility depends on the individual's training status, training modes, performance tests used, sequencing of AT and RT, and the volume, frequency, and intensity of AT and RT. In contrast, other studies have shown both modalities can be trained concurrently with no observed interference in strength increases (97–99). Concurrent training may not attenuate aerobic endurance performance as long as the frequency of AT is not sufficiently reduced to accommodate strength and power training.

Key programming issues include whether or not high-intensity AT and RT are performed in the same session, the sequence of each, volume and intensity, and training status of the subjects when examining potential incompatibility. Factors leading to an incompatibility include the following:

- **Inadequate recovery between workouts** — too high a frequency with reference to the volume/intensity of concurrent training could lead to overreaching and possible overtraining. This may be true for lower-body training. If an athlete is RT the lower body 2–3 days per week and performs high-intensity AT on the days in between, it can be argued that a lack of full recovery may occur in between workouts primarily if the athlete is seeking to optimize strength and power gains. Failure to recover completely could negatively impact the athlete's training adaptations and potentially decrease the quality of subsequent workouts. When both AT and RT are performed during the same session (yielding 3 d·wk^{-1} frequency with at least 1 day off in between workouts), the incompatibility is less likely (99–101). These studies show that increasing the recovery period between workouts may minimize the incompatibility. Thus, potential overreaching or overtraining may occur from the culminating effects of insufficient recovery.

- **Residual fatigue** — if high-intensity AT is performed prior to RT during the same workout, then suboptimal effort may be applied during RT due to fatigue and could limit the progression of strength and power development. The same may be applied to RT performed immediately before AT. This "*acute fatigue hypothesis*" entails fatigue may negatively affect the modality performed second in sequence. Performing AT prior to RT limits some measures of strength gains compared to performing RT prior to AT in some but not all studies (88,98). Sale et al. (102) showed that concurrent AT and RT produced greater strength decrements when performed during the same day versus different days, and they suggested that RT performance may have been compromised because half of the workouts consisted of performing AT prior to RT. Bell et al. (88) compared AT before RT and vice versa and found that both increased $\dot{V}O_{2max}$ similarly regardless of the sequence; however, the group that performed RT first attained greater strength gains. A meta-analysis concluded that strength attenuation (but not hypertrophy) takes place when AT is performed prior to RT in sequence (103). Acutely, it is thought that central (reduced neural activation) and peripheral factors (accumulation of metabolites such as inorganic phosphate, H$^+$, and ammonia), depletion of ATP, creatine phosphate and muscle glycogen, and muscle damage may account for the force decrement seen when RT follows AT (104). Some studies showed: (a) a 26.7% reduction in squat performance (3 × 80% of 1 RM) 30 minutes following interval cycling (105); (b) leg press (but not bench press) performance was reduced by 25% (4 h post) and 9% (8 h post) following either interval or LSD cycling protocols (106); (c) squat reps (6 × failure, 80% of 1 RM), but not the bench press, were reduced following 45 minutes of cycling (107); and (d) leg press reps (not bench press) were reduced following an interval running workout (108). Although these studies suggest that lower-body performance may mostly be compromised, upper-body exercise performance could be affected. We examined acute RE performance (5 exercises [high pull, squat, bench press, deadlift, and push press], 3 × 6–10 reps with 70%–80% of 1 RM, 3-min rest intervals) 10 minutes following 4 different AT sessions: (P1) 60% of VO$_2$R for 45 minutes; (P2) 75% of VO$_2$R for 20 minutes; (P3) 90%–100% of VO$_2$R in 3-minutes intervals (1:1 ratio) for 5 sets; and (P4) 75% of VO$_2$R (4.5 mph) uphill (6%–9% grade) for 20 minutes (Fig. 17.10) (109). All aerobic workouts resulted in 9.1%–18.6% fewer reps performed compared to the control protocol (where no AT was performed before RT) with the squat experiencing the greatest reduction. Average power and velocity per set were reduced for the high pull, squat, and bench press following most of the AT protocols. The first three exercises in sequence were most negatively affected in rep, power, and velocity decrements. The interval protocol led to the greatest acute RE performance reductions followed by the 45-minute run.

- **Altered neuromuscular recruitment patterns/adaptations** — a competing adaptation hypothesis based on limitations to neural drive and contrasting skeletal muscle

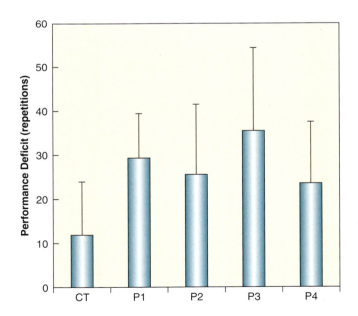

FIGURE 17.10 Repetition deficit following four different aerobic exercise protocols. CT, control protocol; P1–4, each of the aerobic exercise protocols. The performance deficit represents the theoretical maximum number of reps that could have been performed (138) minus the number or reps performed. (From Ratamess NA, Kang J, Porfido TM, et al. Acute resistance exercise performance is negatively impacted by prior aerobic endurance exercise. *J Strength Cond Res.* 2016;30:2667–2681.)

molecular signaling that ultimately could attenuate potential strength/power gains. Intense concurrent training may lead to antagonistic neuromuscular recruitment patterns such as greater fast-to-slow fiber-type (II to I) transitions, elevated cortisol concentrations, attenuated satellite cell density, altered molecular signaling in protein synthesis and mitochondrial biogenesis pathways, growth factor expression (IGF-1, MGF), and attenuated muscle fiber hypertrophy (92,94,110–114).

Strength and endurance training can be performed simultaneously providing adequate recovery is allowed between workouts. Priority can be given to each given the goals of the training phase. It has been suggested that performing RT immediately after low-intensity AT may result in a greater stimulus for endurance adaptation than the low-intensity endurance session alone (115). The critical element for the S&C practitioner is to properly periodize the training program to optimize both components.

Aerobic Endurance Training for Anaerobic Athletes

Several sports rely heavily upon aerobic and anaerobic energy sources (wrestling, boxing, MMA, soccer, hockey, basketball). AT is vital for these athletes as improving CV fitness is important for weight control, enhanced recovery during and between workouts, and stamina. It is important to accurately time aerobic and anaerobic workouts and place them in proper sequence to minimize antagonizing effects. Training periodization is the key. Off-season training should focus on strength and power training with a small amount of AT for base conditioning purposes. The end of the off-season is marked by preseason strength/power testing. Strength and power correlate well with performance of anaerobic sports and need to be emphasized during off-season training. Strength maintenance likely will become the goal during the preseason period as sprint/agility/plyometric workouts increase in frequency to peak power performance. The intensity of AT increases at this time to peak for the beginning of the season. Anaerobic conditioning drills are incorporated to increase buffering capacity and acid-base balance. Maintenance strength training and high-intensity AT can coexist. In-season training is characterized by maintenance programs for most components. Sport participation can maintain and improve conditioning. Specific conditioning may be trained a few days per week depending on the competition schedule. The amount depends on the athlete's playing status. For example, bench players receive less quality practice time and may be less conditioned than starters (38). The S&C coach must increase the amount of non–sport-training to keep their conditioning ready for play. It can be difficult for the coach to balance the rigors of sport practice/competition with training but successful coaches with quality programs will minimize injuries, maximize performance, and prevent end-of-season detraining.

Aerobic Endurance Training in Hot and Cold Environments

The external environment plays a key role in the response to aerobic endurance exercise. Extremes in temperature pose a thermal stress to the athlete. Thermoregulation is critical to environmental adaptations during exercise. The preoptic anterior region of the hypothalamus is the center of thermoregulation and acts like a thermostat to maintain thermal balance, *i.e.*, a normal resting temperature of 37°C or 98.6°F. It responds to sensory information from thermoreceptors in the skin (via unmyelinated C-fibers, myelinated A delta fibers) and changes in the temperature of blood. Thermoregulatory systems work to balance heat gain (exercise, basal metabolic rate [BMR], hormonal control, environment, thermic effect of food) with heat loss (radiation, conduction, convection, and evaporation) with the rates governed by physical properties of the skin (temperature, surface area, moisture) and environment (temperature, air movement, barometric pressure, vapor pressure, clothing) (Fig. 17.11) (20,116). Oxygen consumption and metabolic heat production depends on ambient temperature, body composition, feeding, posture (*e.g.*, higher standing versus seated and sleeping), and increases in proportion to the intensity of exercise by up to 20–25 times resting level in elite athletes (20,116). During exercise ~20%–30% of the energy produced is converted to mechanical work, while 70%–80% is released as heat energy (117).

At rest, radiation, conduction, and convection predominate for maintaining thermal balance. The magnitude of heat transfer depends on the temperature gradient between surfaces, surface area size, and conductivity of materials. Conduction is the heat exchange between two solid surfaces (*e.g.*, body–clothes, body–chair) in direct contact with one another, which accounts for <2% of heat loss during most situations (38). Radiation involves the transfer of energy waves from one body and is absorbed by another. Convection is the heat exchange that occurs between the surface of the body and a fluid medium, *i.e.*, air or water (38), which is why cooling is increased by fans or cold water immersion. Evaporation is most critical for heat dissipation during exercise in the heat. Evaporation of water results from perspiration and quickly cools the body. The human body surface contains ~2–4 million sweat glands to aid in cooling the athlete (20). The cooled skin assists in cooling blood near the body's surface. Water loss from respiratory tracts and sweat collectively prevents excessive increases in core temperature. As temperature outdoors increases, conduction, convection, and radiation lose efficacy in facilitating heat loss, so perspiration becomes critical to cool the body during exercise in the heat. Perspiration evaporation becomes more difficult when the relative humidity is high. *Relative humidity* refers to the ratio of water in the air at a particular temperature to the

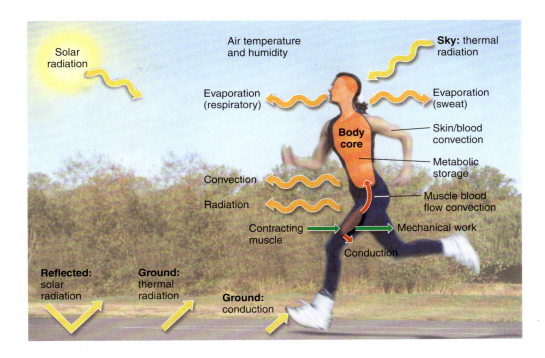

FIGURE 17.11 Regulation of heat exchange. (Reprinted with permission from McArdle WD, Katch FI, Katch VL. *Exercise Physiology: Nutrition, Energy, and Human Performance.* 7th ed. Philadelphia (PA): Lippincott Williams & Wilkins; 2010. p. 615.)

total quantity of moisture that the air could contain (20). A high relative humidity percentage forces the sweat to bead and drip on the athlete rather than evaporate. As a result, cooling mechanisms are reduced, so exercise in hot, humid weather poses a greater risk to fatigue and heat injury than exercise at normal ambient temperature. Blood flow toward the skin increases as a mechanism of body cooling. The hypothalamus sends efferent signaling through the brainstem to induce peripheral active and passive vasodilation to the skin via sympathetic stimulation of vascular endothelium and subsequent smooth muscle relaxation (118). Greater blood flow to the body's surface increases heat loss via radiation and provides some control over increases in core temperature during exercise. At rest, muscle temperature ranges from 33°C to 35°C, and skin blood flow is ~250–300 mL·min^{-1} (118,119). As muscle temperature increases during exercise, heat transfer shifts from muscle to arterial blood which travels to the skin. The rate of transfer of heat from the core to the skin is determined by the temperature gradient and the conductance of skin (119). Blood flow to the skin can be nearly zero during extreme cold temperatures but can increase to 6–7 L·min^{-1} during heat stress (118). Sympathetic (sudomotor) activation of eccrine sweat glands increases the cooling effect (118).

Aerobic Exercise in the Heat

Aerobic exercise performance is impaired by heat stress and the subsequent thermoregulatory response may affect the trainee's willingness to maintain intensity or volume of exercise as core temperature rises (120). $\dot{V}O_{2max}$ may be acutely reduced in excess of 8% in very hot, humid environments and acclimatization may only negate half of this reduction during heat stress (121). Repeated sprint and interval exercise performance may be impaired with large rises in core temperature (122). A paradox exists for the human body during exercise in the heat. Skeletal muscle requires greater blood flow for oxygen and nutrient delivery during exercise. Under normal ambient conditions, up to 80% of Q_c may be diverted to muscle to meet the physical demands of exercise. However, the surface of the skin requires greater blood flow for heat dissipation. Cardiac output must be partitioned, and this can result in a rise in the body's core temperature and can make aerobic exercise more challenging, *e.g.*, the reduced muscle blood flow during the initial stages of exercise makes the workout more anaerobic and can lead to higher elevations of blood lactate, greater muscle glycogen breakdown, lost electrolytes, and fatigue. The reduced blood flow to the skin is seen, in part, to compensate for plasma volume reductions that accompany sweat loss during prolonged exercise in the heat in order to maintain Q_c (20). Circulatory and muscle blood flow supersede thermal regulation in Q_c distribution during exercise in the heat. Thus, core temperature will increase in proportion to intensity. Some studies indicate that aerobic athletes may show no ill effects of exercise in the heat up to ~105.0°F. Athletes with high aerobic capacity have greater thermoregulatory compensation and therefore have better tolerance to exercise in the heat than lesser-trained or untrained individuals. Fatigue coincides with core temperatures of 38°C–40°C (20). Some studies have shown core temperature to rise to 37.3°C when exercising at 50% of $\dot{V}O_{2max}$ and 38.5°C at 75% of $\dot{V}O_{2max}$ (20). Core temperatures above 40°C define *exertional hyperthermia*, where heat production from increased skeletal muscle activity accumulates faster than heat dissipation (123). Heat production in nonelite athletes could increase 15–20 times compared to rest during intense exercise which potentially could raise core body temperature by 1°C every 5 minutes if heat is not removed from the body (123). Brain temperature is higher than core temperature such that at high temperatures, the athlete could experience signs of exhaustion and can potentially collapse. Negative effects of exercising in the heat are exacerbated by obesity, low fitness levels, lack of acclimatization, sleep deprivation, sweat gland dysfunction, some infections, prior history of heat illness, sunburn, and use of certain medications (*i.e.*, stimulants, diuretics, antihistamines) (123). Thermoregulatory recovery following exercise is a complex process. Under normal conditions, muscle and core temperature could take as long as 4–5 times the length of exercise to recover to preexercise levels (124). The addition of heat stress could prolong this time depending on the level of postexercise hypotension and subsequent restoration of mean arterial pressure, as well as hydration status and possible cooling interventions used (124). Prior heat acclimation or high levels of aerobic fitness may not influence the rate of thermoregulatory recovery following exercise (despite marked improvements in thermoregulatory function during exercise) (124).

The intensity, duration, frequency, and number of heat exposures affect the magnitude of acclimatization (125). Although aerobic endurance exercise in normal temperatures can help the athlete acclimatize to a certain extent, exercise in hot, humid conditions is the best way to acclimatize to heat stress. Similar to altitude training camps, athletes have used hot, humid training climates as tools to optimize performance (125). Endurance athletes may benefit from including heat acclimatization camps during preseason and in-season training as part of a periodized training program (125). This suggestion is based on data that show heat acclimation can reduce the negative impact of heat stress (and improves endurance performance) while exercising in hot, humid environments but can also augment performance in cool environmental conditions (126). Lorenzo et al. (126) showed that 10 days of heat acclimation (exercise at 50% of $\dot{V}O_{2max}$ at 40°C) in trained cyclists increased $\dot{V}O_{2max}$ by 5%, time-trial performance by 6%, and LT power output by 5% when exercising in cool conditions in addition to improving performance when exercising during heat stress. Heat acclimatization typically takes around 7–14 days of strenuous exercise where 1.5–2 hours per day of exercise (every third day) >50% of $\dot{V}O_{2max}$ is recommended (119). Each day of exposure to heat strain reduces physiologic strain during acclimation. Table 17.10 presents key physiological changes that improve heat tolerance (121). Heat acclimatization begins on day 1 with 75%–80% of adaptation taking place within the first 4–7 days (121). The ACSM recommends 10–14 days of exercise training in the heat to increase heat acclimatization (123). As acclimatization takes place, athletes may need to adjust training intensity accordingly especially if intensity is low during the first 1–2 weeks of climate adjustment. Heat acclimation is only temporary and will disappear if the individual is no longer exposed to the heat

Table 17.10	Physiological Changes during Acclimatization to Heat
↓ core temperature at rest and exercise	↓ heart rate and SNS activity
↓ skin temperature	↑ stroke volume and myocardial efficiency
↑ sensitivity and rate of sweating (2nd wk)	Spared muscle glycogen
↓ sweating onset threshold	↑ lactate threshold and ↓ lactate response
↑ size and efficiency of eccrine glands	↑ heat shock proteins and thermal tolerance
↑ skin blood flow	↓ RPE during exercise
↑ plasma volume (3%–27%), thirst, total body water (5%–7%), aldosterone, ADH	↓ metabolic rate
↓ electrolyte loss	↑ diluted sweat, ↑ evaporative capacity

stress or exercises. Some studies show that heat acclimation may remain for 1–4 weeks (with rapid losses during the 3rd and 4th weeks) as heart rate improvements are first to subside prior to thermoregulatory changes (121). Critical to longer retainment is exercise even if it occurs in the absence of heat exposure. One day of exercise in heat may be needed for every 5 days spent without heat exposure (121). Heat acclimatization is more pronounced in aerobically fit individuals, and highly trained endurance athletes are less susceptible to heat illness (121). Athletes may acclimatize faster upon repeated exposure to heat stress during subsequent acclimatization training phases (125).

The effects of exercise in the heat are exacerbated by dehydration. Dehydration is most prominent with reductions in body mass of >2% (127) and results in an increased plasma (>290 mOsmol) and urine *osmolality* (>700 mOsmol; *e.g.*, the number of osmoles of solute in fluid) and urine specific gravity (>1.020) (128). Dehydration of >2% reduces maximal race performance in addition to exacerbating thermal stress (129). Fluid loss due to dehydration results in reduced plasma volume, Q_c, heat dissipation, skin blood flow, sweat rates, and increased core temperature and perceived exertion (20,128). As dehydration increases, thermoregulation becomes more difficult. Dehydration of 3%–5% leads to reduced sweat production and skin blood flow thereby reducing heat dissipation (128). One hour of exercise produces ~0.5–1.0 L loss of sweat and rates as high as 3.7 L·h⁻¹ are seen during high-intensity aerobic exercise in athletes, while American football players may lose up to 8.8 L·d⁻¹ (due to large size and equipment) or have sweat rates of 0.6–2.9 L·h⁻¹ with some linemen showing sweat rates of more than 3.0 L·h⁻¹ (20,38,119,128,130). Athletes have sweat rates of

1–2.5 L·h⁻¹ on average and women typically have lower sweat rates and electrolyte losses than men (128). Greater sweat can be lost with higher intensities and/or durations of aerobic exercise. An elite marathon runner may experience up to 5 L of fluid loss (or ~6%–10% of body mass) during competition (20). Sweat rates can be calculated in the following manner (131):

1. Body mass (kg) is recorded before and after 1 hour of exercise in heat.
2. The difference between these two masses is recorded.
3. The mass of wet clothing should be recorded by measuring before and after the exercise session to determine sweat mass trapped in clothing. This value should be added to the difference recorded in step 2. This step may be ignored if nude body mass is used.
4. The mass of fluid consumed during exercise should be recorded and added to the value obtained in step 2. It may be more practical to select a standard amount of fluid to be consumed prior to exercise and only consume that specific amount.
5. The mass of urine lost (if any) should be recorded and subtracted from step 2.
6. The hourly sweat rate (in kg·h⁻¹) equals the value obtained in step 2 once corrected for items in steps 3–5. For example, if 2.0 kg of mass was lost in total during 1 hour of exercise, then the sweat rate = 2.0 kg·h⁻¹ or 2.0 L·h⁻¹.
7. Body mass loss should be replaced during exercise by consuming 1 L of fluid for each kg of body mass lost during exercise to match the sweat rate.

The concentration of sweat contains an average of 35 mEq·L⁻¹ of sodium, 5 mEq·L⁻¹ of potassium, 1 mEq·L⁻¹ of calcium, 0.8 mEq·L⁻¹ of magnesium, and 30 mEq·L⁻¹ of chloride and varies depending on genetics, diet, sweat rate, and level of heat acclimatization (128). Inclusion of electrolytes during fluid replenishment is recommended. The risks of heat illness increase greatly if the athlete begins the workout in a dehydrated state. Dehydration negatively affects CV function, increases heat storage, decreases the time to exhaustion, and reduces endurance exercise performance (128). For each liter of sweat loss, exercise HR increases by ~ 8 bpm with a concomitant decrease in Q_c of 1 L·min⁻¹ (20). Dehydration of 4.3% loss of body mass can reduce walking performance by 48% and decrease $\dot{V}O_{2max}$ by up to 22% (20). Dehydration negatively affects anaerobic exercise performance as well but the response may be lessened in athletes accustomed to dehydration in order to "make weight" such as wrestlers and MMA fighters. Judelson et al. (132) showed that dehydration of 3%–4% results in a ~2% reduction in strength, ~3% reduction in power, and ~10% reduction in high-intensity muscle endurance.

Proper hydration before, during, and after aerobic endurance exercise is critical to optimal CV, thermoregulation, and exercise performance. Thirst often lags behind, so the athlete must drink at intervals to minimize thermal strain. The following recommendations regarding fluid balance may assist athletes during exercise in the heat (20,119,127,128):

- At least 500 mL of water per sports drink should be consumed the night prior to anticipated aerobic exercise in the heat.
- 500 mL of water per sports drink should be consumed upon wakening on the morning of exercise in the heat. Some athletes have prehydrated themselves with a mixture of water (1–2 L) and glycerol (20) although the use of glycerol has not been recommended (128). It is recommended that ~5–7 mL·kg⁻¹ of body mass be consumed at least 4 hours before exercise (128). The fluid (water or sports drink) should taste good and be between 15°C and 21°C.
- 400–600 mL of water should be consumed ~20 minutes before the workout.
- During exercise in the heat (especially prolonged exercise <3 hours), fluid intake (if possible) should match or be close to sweat rate. Sweat rates typically range from 0.4 to 1.8 L·h⁻¹ (128). In general, water/sports drink can be consumed as needed at a rate of 0.4–0.8 L·h⁻¹ (or 0.15–0.3 L every 10–20 min) (128).
- After exercise, ~1.5 L of water per sports drink should be consumed per kg of body mass lost (128).
- In lieu of water, beverages containing a mixture of carbohydrates (5%–8%), amino acids, and vitamins and minerals (sodium, potassium, chloride, magnesium, etc.) can be used to rehydrate, replace lost electrolytes, and provide nutrients for energy during exercise. The ACSM has recommended that a sport beverage contain 20–30 mEq·L⁻¹ of sodium chloride and 2–5 mEq·L⁻¹ of potassium per liter of fluid consumed (128).

Cooling strategies should be used prior to (to remove heat thereby increasing heat storage capacity during exercise), during, and as part of recovery following intense exercise during heat stress. Cooling strategies include cold water immersion, cooling garments or towels, cold fluid ingestion, ice-slurry beverages, cooling packs, fans, cryotherapy, water spray, menthol cooling, and mixed strategies (117,125). Some studies have shown that precooling prior to exercise (especially a mixed strategy followed by cold water immersion) may improve aerobic endurance, interval, and high-intensity exercise performance, while others failed to show any improvements (117,125). The beneficial effects of precooling are attenuated 20–25 minutes into exercise (117). Cold fluid ingestion may enhance performance when ingested before exercise but not during (125). A meta-analysis showed that 15 out of 21 studies showed performance improvements (~9%) when cooling was used during exercise (especially ice vests followed by cold water ingestion) (117). However, some methods of cooling during exercise may be impractical, and the nature of some sports may limit the opportunity to cool. Thus, combining precooling plus attempts to cool during exercise in the heat when possible may be preferred. Cooling strategies used post exercise to restore core, skin, and muscle temperature could help to improve recovery before the next workout and possibly reduce muscle damage (117,125).

Aerobic Exercise in Cold Temperatures

Cold temperatures pose a stress to the athlete during exercise but typically do not limit aerobic performance. Cold environments can increase energy expenditure and may result in some additional fluid loss (133). Higher levels of aerobic fitness have only a small effect on cold tolerance. Precautions need to be taken in order to prevent cold-related injuries such as hypothermia, frostbite, and cold-induced asthma. Cold exposure leads to peripheral vasoconstriction, which decreases peripheral blood flow and convection between the core and outer shell and results in greater insulation and maintenance of core temperature. Heat is lost from the body at a faster rate than it is replaced. Vasoconstriction begins when skin temperature drops to 34°C–35°C and becomes maximal at skin temperatures of 31°C or less in water or 26°C–28°C under local conditions (133). Exposure to cold increases metabolic heat production (*cold-induced thermogenesis*) via shivering. Acclimatizing helps reduce the stress associated with cold temperatures. Chronic exposure to cold temperatures helps the athlete adjust via habituation (less-pronounced cold responses), exaggerated shivering, and greater heat conservation (133). Several factors affect the acute response to cold exposure. Rain and water immersion augment the effects of cold temperatures. Water has a higher thermal capacity for convection than air resulting in greater heat loss. Athletes with higher levels of subcutaneous body fat have greater insulation capacity and a higher level of vasoconstriction to limit heat loss (133). Gender differences exist where women may experience greater heat loss due to lower levels of muscle mass (despite having higher levels of body fat). Cold tolerance decreases with aging due to decreased vasoconstriction and heat conservation and becomes more prominent when the athlete has low blood sugar (which impairs the shivering response) (133).

Precautions need to be taken when exercising in the cold. The temperature, windchill, precipitation, immersion depth (for water), and altitude (colder temperatures with a rise in elevation) need to be monitored and addressed accordingly. Cold temperatures with a high windchill factor require the athlete to prepare accordingly perhaps by adjusting clothing. Proper clothing insulates the athlete, allows for sweat dissipation, and helps maintain core temperature in a cold environment. The ACSM (133) has recommended three layers of clothing: (a) an inner layer in contact with the skin which does not readily absorb moisture but moves it to other layers (lightweight polyester or polypropylene); (b) a middle layer which provides primary insulation (polyester fleece or wool); and (c) an outer layer which maximizes moisture transfer to the environment. The outer layer may not be necessary unless it is raining or very windy (21,133). The level of insulation is modulated based on exercise intensity and duration. Clothing insulation (CLO) should be adjusted to minimize sweating. CLO units can serve as a guide. Table 17.11 depicts various clothing insulation units. Figure 17.12 depicts clothing insulation needs based on aerobic exercise intensity (in MET). The colder the weather, the higher the CLO unit (as evidenced by the down slope of each line). As exercise intensity increases,

Table 17.11	Clothing Insulation Units	
Clothing	**CLO Unit**
Shirt, lightweight pants, socks, shoes, underwear briefs	0.6
Shirt, pants, jacket, socks, shoes, underwear briefs	1.0
Wind/waterproof jogging suit, T-shirt, briefs, running shorts, socks, athletic shoes	1.03
Fleece long-sleeve shirt, fleece pants, athletic socks, and shoes	1.19
Lightweight jacket, thermal long underwear tops and bottoms, briefs, shell pants, athletic shoes, and socks	1.24
Lightweight jacket, long-sleeve fleece shirt, fleece pants, underwear briefs, shell pants, athletic shoes, and socks	1.67
Ski jacket, thermal long underwear bottoms, knit turtleneck, sweater, ski pants, knit hat, goggles, gloves, ski socks, and boots	2.3
Parka with hood, shell pants, fiber fill pant liners, thermal long underwear tops and bottoms, sweat shirt, gloves, thick socks, and boots	3.28
Cold weather expedition suit, thermal long underwear tops and bottoms, sweat shirt, gloves, thick socks, and boots	3.67

Adapted with permission from American College of Sports Medicine. American College of Sports Medicine Position Stand: prevention of cold injuries during exercise. *Med Sci Sports Exerc.* 2006;38:2012–2029.

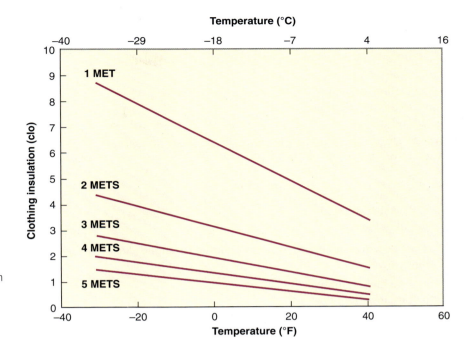

FIGURE 17.12 CLO units for various intensities of exercise. (Reprinted with permission from American College of Sports Medicine. American College of Sports Medicine Position Stand: prevention of cold injuries during exercise. *Med Sci Sports Exerc.* 2006;38:2012–29.)

the CLO unit decreases. Less-insulation clothing is needed as the athlete exercises at progressively higher intensities. Clothing selection must match the potential exercise stimulus. One should not overdress initially to match the cold temperatures at rest but should dress according to the potential clothing insulation needed during exercise. Overdressing can cause too great of heat storage (leading to more sweating) and add weight to the athlete. Wet weather increases the insulation requirement. Up to 50% of heat loss occurs through the head at rest while wearing winter clothing, so knit caps provide needed insulation (31). CLO requirements during exercise are a function of temperature and metabolic rate. Layering is recommended for greater flexibility in balancing insulation needs with heat production (133).

SUMMARY POINTS

- AT elicits a number of beneficial CV, respiratory, metabolic, and neuromuscular adaptations that allow the athlete to improve endurance and performance.
- Aerobic endurance performance is correlated to $\dot{V}O_{2max}$, exercise economy, LT, and muscle fiber types.
- Several modes of aerobic exercise can be used in training. Variation is important to keep motivation high and provide the body with different stimuli.
- Training intensity can be prescribed in three general ways via $\dot{V}O_{2max}$, HR, or RPE. In addition, monitoring of performance (distance covered in a specific amount of time or time to cover a specific distance) can also be used.
- Aerobic endurance training should be performed 2–5 days per week for at least 20–60 minutes based on ACSM guidelines. These guidelines are extended significantly for athletes training for endurance sports.
- Continuous, long duration, pace/tempo, Fartlek, interval, hills, and repetition training are methods used to enhance AT.
- Altitude poses a physiological stress to athletes. Current research suggests that "living high, training low" is more effective than "living high, training high" and "living low, training high" for increasing sea-level $\dot{V}O_{2max}$ and endurance performance.
- High-intensity AT can impede strength and power gains if performed simultaneously with strength training at a high volume and frequency. This incompatibility can be prevented by allowing more recovery in between workouts, performing strength training before AT in sequence when they are performed during the same workout, and through proper periodization phases where emphasis may be placed on one modality while the other modality is maintained.
- Hot and cold environments pose a stress to athletes during AT. Special precautions need to be made to enhance safety and maximize performance.

REVIEW QUESTIONS

1. A mode of AT known for "speed play" is
   a. Interval training
   b. Fartlek training
   c. Repetition training
   d. Hill training

2. Endurance training entails training targeting increases in
   a. $\dot{V}O_{2max}$
   b. Exercise economy
   c. Lactate threshold
   d. All of the above

3. The most recommended means of altitude training currently involves
   a. Live high, train high
   b. Live low, train low
   c. Live high, train low
   d. Live low, train high

4. When using the Borg RPE scale to monitor aerobic exercise intensity, which of the following ranges provides the best stimulus for increasing $\dot{V}O_{2max}$ in a healthy, trained individual?
   a. 6–9
   b. 9–12
   c. 12–14
   d. 14–17

5. The most critical method of heat loss during exercise in the heat is
   a. Evaporation
   b. Convection
   c. Conduction
   d. Radiation

6. Running at 7 mph can elicit an energy expenditure value of _____ MET.
   a. 9
   b. 10
   c. 11.5
   d. 14

7. Aerobic exercise in water generally yields higher HRs compared to land-based activities because the cool water temperature facilitates greater cardiac output.
   a. T
   b. F

8. Hill training can be used to increase the intensity of AT workouts.
   a. T
   b. F

9. The ACSM recommends consumption of a fluid (water or sports drink) with a volume of $\sim$5–7 $mL \cdot kg^{-1}$ of body mass at least 4 hours preexercise hydration.
   a. T
   b. F

10. The heart rate max (HR_{max}) method of aerobic exercise intensity prescription is calculated by multiplying the target intensity (decimal form) by the difference of the max predicted HR and resting HR and then adding the resting HR to the total.
    a. T
    b. F

11. Exercise economy refers to the energy cost of exercise at a given velocity.
    a. T
    b. F

12. The ACSM recommends 20–60 minutes of continuous or intermittent aerobic exercise for increasing aerobic capacity in healthy adults.
    a. T
    b. F

REFERENCES

1. Jones AM, Vanhatalo A. The 'critical power' concept: applications to sports performance with a focus on intermittent high-intensity exercise. *Sports Med.* 2017;47(Suppl):S65–78.
2. Faria EW, Parker DL, Faria IE. The science of cycling: physiology and training—part 1. *Sports Med.* 2005;35:285–312.
3. Faria EW, Parker DL, Faria IE. The science of cycling: factors affecting performance—part 2. *Sports Med.* 2005;35:313–37.
4. Joyner MJ, Coyle EF. Endurance exercise performance: the physiology of champions. *J Physiol.* 2008;586:35–44.
5. Noakes T. *Lore of Running.* 4th ed. Champaign (IL): Human Kinetics; 2003. p. 39–105.
6. Yamamoto LM, Lopez RM, Klau JF, et al. The effects of resistance training on endurance distance running performance among highly trained runners: a systematic review. *J Strength Cond Res.* 2008;22:2036–44.
7. Mercier D, Leger L, Desjardins M. Nomogram to predict performance equivalence for distance runners. *Track Tech.* 1986;94:3004–9.
8. Jones AM, Carter H. The effect of endurance training on parameters of aerobic fitness. *Sports Med.* 2000;29:373–86.
9. Jones AM, Grassi B, Christensen PM, Krustrup P, Bangsbo J, Poole DC. Slow component of VO_2 kinetics: mechanistic bases and practical applications. *Med Sci Sports Exerc.* 2011;43:2046–62.
10. Bergh U, Thorstensson A, Sjodin B, et al. Maximal oxygen uptake and muscle fiber types in trained and untrained humans. *Med Sci Sports.* 1978;10:151–4.
11. Reuter BH, Hagerman PS. Aerobic endurance exercise training. In: Baechle TR, Earle RW, editors. *Essentials of Strength Training*

12. Yoshida T, Udo M, Iwai K, Yamaguchi T. Physiological characteristics related to endurance running performance in female distance runners. *J Sports Sci.* 1993;11:57–62.

13. Daniels J. *Daniel's Running Formula.* 3rd ed. Champaign (IL): Human Kinetics; 2014. p. 33–289.

14. Daniels J, Daniels N. Running economy of elite male and elite female runners. *Med Sci Sports Exerc.* 1992;24:483–9.

15. Saunders PU, Pyne DB, Telford RD, Hawley JA. Factors affecting running economy in trained distance runners. *Sports Med.* 2004;34:465–85.

16. Di Prampero PE, Capelli C, Pagliaro P, et al. Energetics of best performances in middle-distance running. *J Appl Physiol.* 1993;74:2318–24.

17. Barnes KR, Kilding AE. Strategies to improve running economy. *Sports Med* 2015;45:37–56.

18. Morgan DW, Bransford DR, Costill DL, Daniels JT, Howley ET, Krahenbuhl GS. Variation in the aerobic demand of running among trained and untrained subjects. *Med Sci Sports Exerc.* 1995;27:404–9.

19. Coyle EF, Coggan AR, Hopper MK, Walters TJ. Determinants of endurance in well-trained cyclists. *J Appl Physiol.* 1988;64:2622–30.

20. McArdle WD, Katch FI, Katch VL. *Exercise Physiology: Energy, Nutrition, and Human Performance.* 6th ed. Philadelphia (PA): Lippincott Williams & Wilkins; 2007. p. 489–502, 615–50.

21. American College of Sports Medicine. *ACSM's Guidelines for Exercise Testing and Prescription.* 11th ed. Philadelphia (PA): Lippincott Williams & Wilkins; 2020.

22. Halder A, Gao C, Miller M, Kuklane K. Oxygen uptake and muscle activity limitations during stepping on a stair machine at three different climbing speeds. *Ergonomics.* 2018;61:1382–94.

23. Mier CM, Feito Y. Metabolic cost of stride rate, resistance, and combined use of arms and legs on the elliptical trainer. *J Sports Med Phys Fitness.* 2006;77:507–13.

24. Morio C, Haddoum M, Fournet D, Gueguen N. Influence of exercise type on metabolic cost and gross efficiency: elliptical trainer versus cycling trainer. *J Sports Med Phys Fitness.* 2016;56:520–6.

25. Franklin BA. Exercise resting, training and arm ergometry. *Sports Med.* 1985;2:100–19.

26. Barbosa TM, Fernandes R, Keskinen KL, et al. Evaluation of the energy expenditure in competitive swimming strokes. *Int J Sports Med.* 2006;27:894–9.

27. Capelli C, Pendergast DL, Termin B. Energetics of swimming at maximal speeds in humans. *Eur J Appl Physiol.* 1998;78:385–93.

28. Costa MJ, Balasekaran G, Vilas-Boas JP, Barbosa TM. Physiological adaptations to training in competitive swimming: a systematic review. *J Hum Kinet.* 2015;49:179–94.

29. Goss FL, Robertson RJ, Spina RJ, et al. Aerobic metabolic requirements of simulated cross-country skiing. *Ergonomics.* 1989;32:1573–9.

30. Smith TB, Hopkins WG. Measures of rowing performance. *Sports Med.* 2012;42:343–58.

31. American College of Sports Medicine. American College of Sports Medicine Position Stand: the quantity and quality of exercise for developing and maintaining cardiorespiratory, musculoskeletal, and neuromotor fitness in apparently healthy adults: guidance for prescribing exercise. *Med Sci Sports Exerc.* 2011;43:1334–59.

32. Kurz MJ, Berg K, Latin R, DeGraw W. The relationship of training methods in NCAA Division I cross-country runners and 10,000-meter performance. *J Strength Cond Res.* 2000;14:196–201.

33. Donnelly JE, Blair SN, Jakicic JM, et al. American College of Sports Medicine Position Stand. Appropriate physical activity intervention strategies for weight loss and prevention of weight regain for adults [published correction appears in Med Sci Sports Exerc. 2009 Jul;41(7):1532]. *Med Sci Sports Exerc.* 2009;41(2):459–71.

34. Gellish RL, Goslin BR, Olson RE, et al. Longitudinal modeling of the relationship between age and maximal heart rate. *Med Sci Sports Exerc.* 2007;39:822–9.

35. Karvonen M, Kentala K, Musta O. The effects of training on heart rate: a longitudinal study. *Ann Med Exp Biol Fenn.* 1957;35:307–15.

36. Swain DP. Cardiorespiratory exercise prescription. In: Ehrman JK, editor. *ACSM's Resource Manual for Guidelines for Exercise Testing and Prescription.* 6th ed. Philadelphia (PA): Lippincott Williams & Wilkins; 2010. p. 448–62.

37. Borg GA. Psychophysical bases of perceived exertion. *Med Sci Sports Exerc.* 1982;14:377–81.

38. Hoffman J. *Physiological Aspects of Sport Training and Performance.* Champaign (IL): Human Kinetics; 2002. p. 109–19.

39. Swain DP, Franklin BA. VO_2 reserve and the minimal intensity for improving cardiorespiratory fitness. *Med Sci Sports Exerc.* 2002;34:152–7.

40. Gormley SE, Swain DP, High R, et al. Effect of intensity of aerobic training on Vo_{2max}. *Med Sci Sports Exerc.* 2008;40:1336–43.

41. Helgerud J, Hoydal K, Wang E, et al. Aerobic high-intensity intervals improve Vo_{2max} more than moderate training. *Med Sci Sports Exerc.* 2007;39:665–71.

42. Buchheit M, Laursen PB. High-intensity interval training, solutions to the programming puzzle. Part I: cardiopulmonary emphasis. *Sports Med.* 2013;43:313–38.

43. Billat LV. Interval training and performance: a scientific and empirical practice. Special recommendations for middle- and long-distance running. Part II. Anaerobic interval training. *Sports Med.* 2001;31:75–90.

44. Laursen PB, Jenkins DG. The scientific basis for high-intensity interval training. Optimising training programmes and maximizing performance in highly trained endurance athletes. *Sports Med.* 2002;32:53–73.

45. Helgerud J, Engen LC, Wisloff U, Hoff J. Aerobic endurance training improves soccer performance. *Med Sci Sports Exerc.* 2001;33:1925–31.

46. Acka F, Aras D. Comparison of rowing performance improvements following various high-intensity interval trainings. *J Strength Cond Res.* 2015;29:2249–54.

47. Billat LV. Interval training and performance: a scientific and empirical practice. Special recommendations for middle- and long-distance running. Part I. Aerobic interval training. *Sports Med.* 2001;31:13–31.

48. Buchheit M, Laursen PB. High-intensity interval training, solutions to the programming puzzle. Part II: anaerobic energy, neuromuscular load and practical applications. *Sports Med.* 2013;43:927–54.

49. Harter L, Groves H. 3000–10,000 Meters. In: *USA Track & Field, editor. Coaching Manual.* Champaign (IL): Human Kinetics; 1999. p. 109–22.

50. Thibault G. A graphical model for interval training. *IAAF New Stud Athlet.* 2003;18:49–55.

51. Cissik JM. Improving aerobic performance. In: Chandler TJ, Brown LE, editors. *Conditioning for Strength and Human Performance.* Philadelphia (PA): Lippincott Williams & Wilkins; 2008. p. 292–305.

52. Bentley DJ, Millet GP, Vleck VE, McNaughton LR. Specificity aspects of contemporary triathlon: implications for physiological analysis and performance. *Sports Med.* 2002;32:345–59.

53. Vleck VE, Bentley DJ, Millet GP, Cochrane T. Triathlon event distance specialization: training and injury effects. *J Strength Cond Res.* 2010;24:30–6.

54. Gulbin JP, Gaffney PT. Ultraendurance triathlon participation: typical race preparation of lower level triathletes. *J Sports Med Phys Fitness.* 1999;39:12–5.

55. Doherty C, Keogh A, Davenport J, et al. An evaluation of the training determinants of marathon performance: a meta-analysis with meta-regression. *J Sci Med Sport.* 2020;23:182–8.

56. Knechtle B, Nikolaidis PT. Physiology and pathophysiology in ultra-marathon running. *Front Physiol.* 2018;9:634.

57. Bishop D, Jenkins DG, Mackinnon LT. The relationship between plasma lactate parameters, W_{peak} and 1-h cycling performance in women. *Med Sci Sports Exerc* 1998;30:1270–5.

58. Coyle EF, Feltner ME, Kautz SA, et al. Physiological and biomechanical factors associated with elite endurance cycling performance. *Med Sci Sports Exerc.* 1991;23:93–107.

59. Tabata I, Nishimura K, Kouzaki M, et al. Effects of moderate-intensity endurance and high-intensity intermittent training on anaerobic capacity and Vo_{2max}. *Med Sci Sports Exerc.* 1996;28:1327–30.

60. Saunders PU, Pyne DB, Gore CJ. Endurance training at altitude. *High Alt Med Biol.* 2009;10:135–48.

61. Girard O, Brocherie F, Millet GP. Effects of altitude/hypoxia on single- and multiple-sprint performance: a comprehensive review. *Sports Med.* 2017;47:1931–49.

62. Wilber RL. Application of altitude/hypoxic training by elite athletes. *Med Sci Sports Exerc.* 2007;39:1610–24.

63. Mujika I, Sharma AP, Stellingwerff T. Contemporary periodization of altitude training for elite endurance athletes: a narrative review. *Sports Med.* 2019;49:1651–69.

64. Khodaee M, Grothe HL, Seyfert JH, VanBaak K. Athletes at high altitude. *Prim Care.* 2016;8:126–32.

65. Bailey DM, Davies B. Physiological implications of altitude training for endurance performance at sea level: a review. *Br J Sports Med.* 1997;31:183–90.

66. Jackson CG, Sharkey BJ. Altitude, training and human performance. *Sports Med.* 1988;6:279–84.

67. Hochachka PW. Muscle enzymatic composition and metabolic regulation in high altitude adapted natives. *Int J Sports Med.* 1992;13(Suppl):S89–91.

68. Wagenmakers AJM. Amino acid metabolism, muscular fatigue and muscle wasting: speculations on adaptations at high altitude. *Int J Sports Med.* 1992;13(Suppl):S10–113.

69. Hoppeler H, Desplanches D. Muscle structural modifications in hypoxia. *Int J Sports Med.* 1992;13(Suppl):S166–8.

70. MacDougall JD, Green HJ, Sutton JR, et al. Operation Everest II: structural adaptations in skeletal muscle in response to extreme simulated altitude. *Acta Physiol Scand.* 1991;142:421–7.

71. Coudert J. Anaerobic performance at altitude. *Int J Sports Med.* 1992;13(Suppl):S82–5.

72. Fulco CS, Rock PB, Cymerman A. Maximal and submaximal exercise performance at altitude. *Aviat Space Environ Med.* 1998;69:793–801.

73. Hochachka PW, Beatty CL, Burelle Y, Trump ME, McKenzie DC, Matheson GO. The lactate paradox in human high-altitude physiological performance. *News Physiol Sci.* 2002;17:122–6.

74. van Hall G, Lundby C, Araoz M, Calbet JA, Sander M, Saltin B. The lactate paradox revisited in lowlanders during acclimatization to 4100 m and in high-altitude natives. *J Physiol.* 2009;587(Pt 5):1117–29.

75. Lundby C, Saltin B, van Hall G. The "lactate paradox", evidence for a transient change in the course of acclimatization to severe hypoxia in lowlanders. *Acta Physiol Scand.* 2000;170:265–9.

76. Terrados N. Altitude training and muscular metabolism. *Int J Sports Med.* 1992;13(suppl):S206–9.

77. Wilber RL, Stray-Gundersen J, Levine BD. Effect of hypoxic "dose" on physiological responses and sea-level performance. *Med Sci Sports Exerc.* 2007;39:1590–9.

78. Gore CJ, Hahn AG, Scroop GS. Increased arterial desaturation in trained cyclists during maximal exercise at 580 m altitude. *J Appl Physiol.* 1996;80:2204–10.

79. Millet GP, Roels B, Schmitt L, Woorons X, Richalet JP. Combining hypoxic methods for peak performance. *Sports Med.* 2010;40:1–25.

80. Dick FW. Training at altitude in practice. *Int J Sports Med.* 1992;13(Suppl):S203–5.

81. Bonetti DL, Hopkins WG. Sea-level exercise performance following adaptation to hypoxia: a meta-analysis. *Sports Med.* 2009;39:107–27.

82. Wehrlin JP, Zuest P, Hallen J, Marti B. Live high-train low for 24 days increases hemoglobin mass and red cell volume in elite endurance athletes. *J Appl Physiol.* 2006;100:1938–45.

83. Chapman RF, Karlsen T, Resaland GK, et al. Defining the "dose" of altitude training: how high to live for optimal sea level performance enhancement. *J Appl Physiol.* 2014;116:595–603.

84. Stray-Gundersen J, Levine BD. Live high, train low at natural altitude. *Scand J Med Sci Sports.* 2008;18(suppl):21–8.

85. Saunders PU, Telford RD, Pyne DB, Gore CJ, Hahn AG. Improved race performance in elite middle-distance runners after cumulative altitude exposure. *Int J Sports Physiol Perform.* 2009;4:134–8.

86. Schmitt L, Millet G, Robach P, et al. Influence of "living high-training low" on aerobic performance and economy of work in elite athletes. *Eur J Appl Physiol.* 2006;97:627–36.

87. Brocherie F, Millet GP, Hauser A, et al. "Live high-train low and high" hypoxic training improves team-sport performance. *Med Sci Sports Exerc.* 2015;47:2140–9.

88. Bell GJ, Petersen SR, Quinney HA, Wenger HA. Sequencing of endurance and high-velocity strength training. *Can J Sport Sci.* 1988;13:214–9.

89. Dudley GA, Djamil R. Incompatibility of endurance- and strength-training modes of exercise. *J Appl Physiol.* 1985;59:1446–51.

90. Häkkinen K, Alen M, Kraemer WJ, et al. Neuromuscular adaptations during concurrent strength and endurance training versus strength training. *Eur J Appl Physiol.* 2003;89:42–52.

91. Hickson RC. Interference of strength development by simultaneously training for strength and endurance. *Eur J Appl Physiol.* 1980;45:255–63.

92. Kraemer WJ, Patton JF, Gordon SE, et al. Compatibility of high-intensity strength and endurance training on hormonal and skeletal muscle adaptations. *J Appl Physiol.* 1995;78:976–89.

93. Glowacki SP, Martin SE, Maurer A, et al. Effects of resistance, endurance, and concurrent exercise on training outcomes in men. *Med Sci Sports Exerc.* 2004;36:2119–27.

94. Bell GJ, Syrotuik D, Martin TP, Burnham R, Quinney HA. Effect of concurrent strength and endurance training on skeletal muscle properties and hormone concentrations in humans. *Eur J Appl Physiol.* 2000;81:418–27.

95. Wilson JW, Marin PJ, Rhea MR, Wilson SMC, Loenneke JP, Anderson JC. Concurrent training: a meta-analysis examining interference of aerobic and resistance exercise. *J Strength Cond Res*. 2012;26:2293–307.

96. Mikkola JS, Rusko HK, Nummela AT, Paavolainen LM, Häkkinen K. Concurrent endurance and explosive type strength training increases activation and fast force production of leg extensor muscles in endurance athletes. *J Strength Cond Res*. 2007;21:613–20.

97. Balabinis CP, Psarakis CH, Moukas M, Vassiliou MP, Behrakis PK. Early phase changes by concurrent endurance and strength training. *J Strength Cond Res*. 2003;17:393–401.

98. Gravelle BL, Blessing DL. Physiological adaptation in women concurrently training for strength and endurance. *J Strength Cond Res*. 2000;14:5–13.

99. McCarthy JP, Agre JC, Graf BK, Pozniak MA, Vailas AC. Compatibility of adaptive responses with combining strength and endurance training. *Med Sci Sports Exerc*. 1995;27:429–36.

100. Leveritt M, Abernethy PJ, Barry B, Logan PA. Concurrent strength and endurance training: the influence of dependent variable selection. *J Strength Cond Res*. 2003;17:503–8.

101. McCarthy JP, Pozniak MA, Agre JC. Neuromuscular adaptations to concurrent strength and endurance training. *Med Sci Sports Exerc*. 2002;34:511–9.

102. Sale DG, Jacobs I, MacDougall JD, Garner S. Comparison of two regimens of concurrent strength and endurance training. *Med Sci Sports Exerc*. 1990;22:348–56.

103. Eddens L, van Someren K, Howatson G. The role of intra-session exercise sequence in the interference effect: a systematic review with meta-analysis. *Sports Med*. 2018;48:177–88.

104. Leveritt M, Abernethy PJ, Barry BK, Logan PA. Concurrent strength and endurance training: a review. *Sports Med*. 1999;28:413–27.

105. Leveritt M, Abernethy PJ. Acute effects of high-intensity endurance exercise on subsequent resistance activity. *J Strength Cond Res*. 1999;13:47–51.

106. Sporer BC, Wenger HA. Effects of aerobic exercise on strength performance following various periods of recovery. *J Strength Cond Res*. 2003;17:638–44.

107. Reed JP, Schilling BK, Murlasits Z. Acute neuromuscular and metabolic responses to concurrent endurance and resistance exercise. *J Strength Cond Res*. 2013;27:793–801.

108. De Souza EO, Tricoli V, Franchini E, et al. Acute effect of two aerobic exercise modes on maximum strength and strength endurance. *J Strength Cond Res*. 2007;21:1286–90.

109. Ratamess NA, Kang J, Porfido TM, et al. Acute resistance exercise performance is negatively impacted by prior aerobic endurance exercise. *J Strength Cond Res*. 2016;30:2667–81.

110. Babcock L, Escano M, D'Lugos A, Todd K, Murach K, Luden N. Concurrent aerobic exercise interferes with the satellite cell response to acute resistance exercise. *Am J Physiol Regul Integr Comp Physiol* 2012;302:R1458–65.

111. Coffey VG, Pilegaard H, Garnham AP, O'Brien BJ, Hawley JA. Consecutive bouts of diverse contractile activity alter acute responses in human skeletal muscle. *J Appl Physiol*. 2009;106:1187–97.

112. Coffey VG, Zhong Z, Shield A, et al. Early signaling responses to divergent exercise stimuli in skeletal muscle from well-trained humans. *FASEB J*. 2006;20(1):190–2. doi: 10.1096/fj.05-4809fje.

113. Nelson AG, Arnall DA, Loy SF, Silvester LJ, Conlee RK. Consequences of combining strength and endurance training regimens. *Phys Ther*. 1990;70:287–94.

114. Putman CT, Xu X, Gillies E, MacLean IM, Bell GJ. Effects of strength, endurance and combined training on myosin heavy chain content and fibre-type distribution in humans. *Eur J Appl Physiol*. 2004;92:376–84.

115. Baar K. Using molecular biology to maximize concurrent training. *Sports Med*. 2014;44(Suppl 2):S117–25.

116. Cramer MN, Jay O. Biophysical aspects of human thermoregulation during heat stress. *Auton Neurosci*. 2016;196:3–13.

117. Bongers CCWG, Hopman MTE, Eijsvogels TMH. Cooling interventions for athletes: an overview of effectiveness, physiological mechanisms, and practical considerations. *Temperature (Austin)*. 2017;4:60–78.

118. Smith CJ, Johnson JM. Responses to hyperthermia. Optimizing heat dissipation by convection and evaporation: neural control of skin blood flow and sweating in humans. *Auton Neurosci*. 2016;196:25–36.

119. Wendt D, van Loon LJC, van Marken Lichtenbelt WD. Thermoregulation during exercise in the heat: strategies for maintaining health and performance. *Sports Med* 2007;37:669–82.

120. Flouris AD, Schlader ZJ. Human behavioral thermoregulation during exercise in the heat. *Scand J Med Sci Sports*. 2015;25(suppl):52–64.

121. Periard JD, Racinais S, Sawka MN. Adaptations and mechanisms of human heat acclimation: applications for competitive athletes and sports. *Scand J Med Sci Sports*. 2015;25(Suppl):20–38.

122. Girard O, Brocherie F, Bishop DJ. Sprint performance under heat stress: a review. *Scand J Med Sci Sports*. 2015;25(Suppl):79–89.

123. American College of Sports Medicine. American College of Sports Medicine Position Stand: exertional heat illness during training and competition. *Med Sci Sports Exerc*. 2007;39:556–72.

124. Kenny GP, McGinn R. Restoration of thermoregulation after exercise. *J Appl Physiol*. 2017;122:933–44.

125. Racinais S, Alonso JM, Coutts AJ, et al. Consensus recommendations on training and competing in the heat. *Sports Med*. 2015;45:925–38.

126. Lorenzo S, Halliwill JR, Sawka MN, Minson CT. Heat acclimation improves exercise performance. *J Appl Physiol*. 2010;109:1140–7.

127. Ganio MS, Casa DJ, Armstrong LE, Maresh CM. Evidence-based approach to lingering hydration questions. *Clin Sports Med*. 2007;26:1–16.

128. American College of Sports Medicine. American College of Sports Medicine Position Stand: exercise and fluid replacement. *Med Sci Sports Exerc*. 2007;39:377–90.

129. Casa DJ, Stearns RL, Lopez RM, et al. Influence of hydration on physiological function and performance during trail running in the heat. *J Athl Train*. 2010;45:147–56.

130. Davis JK, Baker LB, Barnes K, Ungaro C, Stofan J. Thermoregulation, fluid balance, and sweat losses in American football players. *Sports Med*. 2016;46:1391–405.

131. Armstrong LE. *Performing in extreme environments*. Champaign (IL): Human Kinetics, 2000. p. 15–70.

132. Judelson DA, Maresh CM, Anderson JM, et al. Hydration and muscular performance: does fluid balance affect strength, power and high-intensity endurance? *Sports Med*. 2007;37:907–21.

133. American College of Sports Medicine. American College of Sports Medicine Position Stand: prevention of cold injuries during exercise. *Med Sci Sports Exerc*. 2006;38:2012–29.

CHAPTER 18

Training Periodization and Tapering

OBJECTIVES

After completing this chapter, you will be able to:

◆ Define periodization and understand the benefits of dividing a training year into smaller phases

◆ Define General Adaptation Syndrome and discuss its application to periodized training

◆ Discuss how tapering can be useful for optimizing performance for competition

◆ Discuss different models of periodization and how program variables can be manipulated to achieve a targeted goal

◆ Identify ways in which macrocycles can be developed in athletes during different types of competitive seasons

The physiological responses and adaptations to training were discussed in Part II of this textbook. It is clear that the human body adapts relatively quickly to the stress placed upon it. Thus, variation in the training stimulus is critical to producing continued progress over time. *Periodization* is a systematic method of organizing training into cycles in order to achieve various training goals; and to provide variation, progressive overload, and specificity to the program. It involves the manipulation of acute training program variables within each cycle or phase in order to bring the athlete to maximal performance at the appropriate time while reducing the risk of overtraining (1). It was described as a "purposeful sequencing of different training units" to allow athletes to peak at the right time (2). Athletes and coaches have long been known to vary their training throughout the year; whether it was for 1–2 major competitions per year or within the realm of a team sport or competitive season. The training practices of athletes changed based on whether it was the off-season, pre-season, or in-season periods. Long-term planning was essential for athlete to maximize the benefits of each training period while bringing that improved level of conditioning to the competition or competitive season. Periodization was initially based upon manipulating intensity and volume throughout the training year, although other program variables were altered as well. Flexibility in the periodized program design is a critical component to meet the needs of the athlete or fitness enthusiasts as training periodization has expanded greatly beyond the realm of athletics.

The concept of periodization dates back to the ancient Olympic Games (776 BC–393 AD) where *Philostratus* was thought to have developed a simplified system where Greek Olympians trained during a preparatory phase prior to the Olympics (3). Articles on periodization strategies were seen in the Eastern European sport science literature during the 1920s and 1930s. In Russia, texts were published between 1917 and 1925 by authors such as Kotov, Gorinewsky, and Birsin describing training phases and organization (4). Sport-specific texts describing periodization principles for training in track and field, skiing, boxing, gymnastics, and water sports were published in Russia circa 1938 (4). Programs became more sophisticated as evidenced by the 4-year German training program, which was used in preparation for the 1936 Olympic Games (3). In England circa 1946, Dyson published a text delineating training into noncompetitive, precompetitive, initial competition, main competition, and postcompetitive periods (4). Revisions, adaptations, and application of periodization techniques and methodology continued through the 1950s and 1960s. In 1965, a model of a periodized training program that separated the training year into different phases and cycles was published by Russian sport scientist Leonid Matveyev. He developed the model based on questionnaires concerning the training practices obtained from Russian athletes preparing for the 1952 Olympic Games (3,5). He borrowed the term periodization and based this model on a schedule where there was one major competition per year (3). Variations developed to cater to athletes who had multiple competitions per year or a competitive

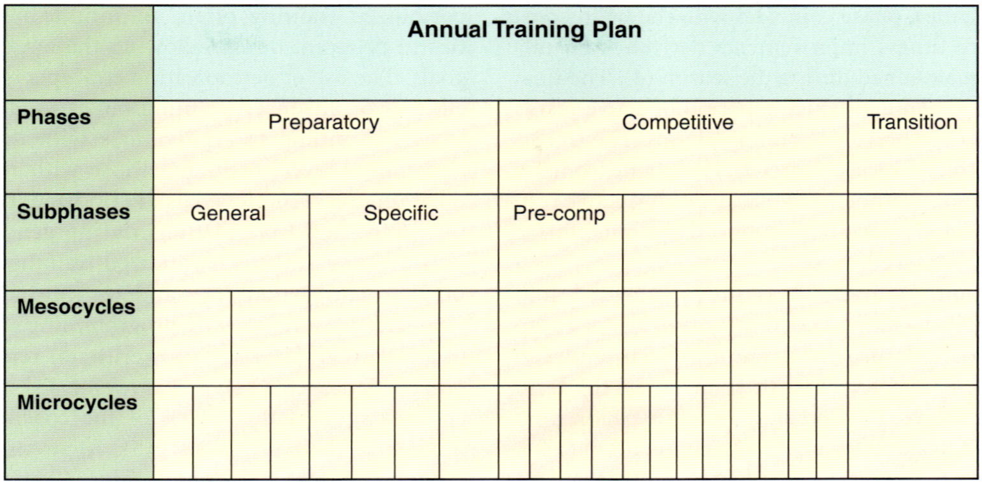

	Annual Training Plan				
Phases	Preparatory		Competitive		Transition
Subphases	General	Specific	Pre-comp		
Mesocycles					
Microcycles					

FIGURE 18.1 Annual training plan proposed by Matveyev. (Reprinted with permission from Bompa TO, Haff GG. *Periodization: Theory and Methodology of Training*. 5th ed. Champaign (IL): Human Kinetics; 2009. p. 125–256.)

season. Periodized training principles were not commonly seen in North America during the first half of the 20th century. European success prompted scientists and coaches from the United States to study Eastern European training methods and develop models based on the work of Matveyev and his predecessors (6). Nevertheless, the underlying goal of periodization was to optimize the training stress and recovery.

Matveyev divided the training year into three distinct phases: *preparatory*, *competitive*, and *transition* (Figs. 18.1 and 18.2). Each training phase is characteristic of a change in volume and intensity. In addition, Matveyev quantified technical training during each phase where allocation to technique increased in proportion to training intensity. The preparatory phase comprises two subphases known as *general* and *specific preparation*. In general preparation training, volume is high and intensity is low. The primary purpose is to prepare the athlete for more intense and sport-specific training in the latter phases.

A physiological base is trained during the preparatory phase to prepare the body adequately for the competition phase. Because intensity is low to moderate, the athlete may experience less stress which helps prepare the athlete for subsequent phases while reducing the risk of overtraining. The second part of the preparatory phase consists of more time devoted to exercises that mimic sport-specific movements in which exercise intensity is increased and volume is reduced. The competitive phase is divided into two phases, precompetition and main competition. The *precompetition* phase consists of the exhibition contests, *e.g.*, preseason games or scrimmages in a sport like American football, while the primary or most important competitions are considered part of the *main competition* phase. The difference is how volume and intensity are manipulated. During the precompetition phase, volume of training is reduced, while intensity of training is increased further. As the main competition phase nears, training intensity reaches its peak while training volume

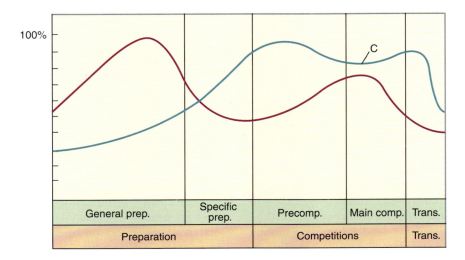

FIGURE 18.2 Matveyev's model of periodization. The *purple line* indicates volume and the *blue line* indicates intensity. (Reprinted with permission from Bompa TO, Haff GG. *Periodization: Theory and Methodology of Training*. 5th ed. Champaign (IL): Human Kinetics; 2009. p. 125–256.)

is reduced. A stabilization phase coincides with the main competition phase where fitness improvements derived from off-season training are maintained during the season (4). The final phase is the *transition phase* in which a period of active rest is used to recover from the previous training phases. The transition phase is restorative and assists in removing fatigue from the athlete from the previous competition phase. During active rest, both training volume and intensity are reduced and other forms of exercise may be introduced.

With periodization, training plans are subdivided into smaller segments called *cycles*. The **macrocycle** refers to an extended training period (usually a training year) and can be broken into different mesocycles. In some cases, the term **monocycle** has been used to describe a yearly periodization macrocycle based on peaking for one major competition (3). A mesocycle refers to several weeks to months of training and consists of smaller microcycles. The duration for each mesocycle is ~1–4 months depending upon the athlete. A **microcycle** consists of smaller units of training, typically around 5–10 days to 4 weeks in length. Microcycles help with the transition between mesocycles and increase specialization within program design.

Although Matveyev's model of periodization was novel, it could not meet the needs of all athletes. In its application to resistance training (RT), it has been criticized for failing to address other program variables such as exercise selection, order, and rest interval length, failing to address which exercises should be included in the volume and intensity calculations (and the level of periodization needed for exercises such as single-joint and core exercises), oversimplifying the volume and intensity relationship between microcycles, failing to address the integration of other modalities of training in addition to RT, and lacking appropriate focus on technical training at all phases, *e.g.*, during low- and moderate-intensity phases in addition to high-intensity phases (4). The model was based on training for one major competition per year excluding athletes with multiple competition seasons or an extended competition season. Often a macrocycle is based on a competition season rather than a single competition. Thus, the structure of Matveyev's periodization model needed to be expanded for athletes with long competitive seasons. The athlete peaks right at the beginning of the competitive season and maintains their performance gains throughout the season. The in-season maintenance phase is characterized by high-intensity training. However, the volume is greatly reduced.

Matveyev's periodization model culminated in peak strength and power. Thus, endurance goals could not be maximized (3). Limitations demonstrated the need for other models and forms of periodization to meet the needs of all athletes. Other models and integrated approaches have since been developed thereby meeting the needs of a larger number of athletes. Thus, periodized training is not one specific template to program design; rather, it is an assortment of methods used to alter and optimize recovery and the training stimulus (7,8). Critics of periodized training often neglect its dynamic nature and focus only on certain components that may limit its applicability. Misinterpretation of this concept creates confusion regarding the efficacy of periodized training. However,

periodized training offers an infinite number of possibilities in program design allowing the targeting of all training goals. The use of periodization concepts is not limited to elite athletes or advanced training but is used successfully as the basis of training for individuals with diverse backgrounds and fitness levels including those with recreational (9) and rehabilitative (10,11) goals. Periodized training is effective for middle-aged populations during general weight training (12). Among athletes, periodized training is most commonly utilized. Ultra-endurance athletes routinely used periodized strategies into their yearly programming (13). More than 95% of strength athletes (*i.e.*, powerlifters) reported using a periodized approach (14). A survey of 137 Division I strength coaches showed that ~93% of the coaches used periodized models in their programs (15). Approximately 95% of high school strength and conditioning (S&C) coaches surveyed reported using periodized training for their athletes (16). Ebben et al. (17–19) and Simenz et al. (20) showed that ~69% of National Football League, 91.3% of National Hockey League, 85.7% of Major League Baseball, and 85% of National Basketball Association S&C coaches use a periodized training model. A survey of elite rugby union coaches showed that 88% used a periodized training strategy (21).

The Importance of Periodized Training

Periodized training enables the athlete or fitness enthusiast to have planned variation in program design to optimize the training stimulus. Periodization helps manage fatigue, provides a basis for the integration of different training modalities, and prepares an athlete for competition. Manipulating the acute training program variables allows the athlete to make the necessary physiological adaptations while reaching their peak condition at the appropriate time. In addition to intensity and volume, it is important to note that other variables are manipulated, *e.g.*, rest intervals, velocity, exercise selection, and order. For example, exercises can be added and removed periodically. This provides the athlete different training stimuli and allows the athlete to train at higher intensities without as great a risk of overtraining. Integrated periodization approaches are common and involve manipulating several variables to meet the needs of the athletes. Altering training volume and intensity in conjunction with appropriately timed short unloading phases (periods of low-intensity, low-volume training) minimizes the risk of **overtraining syndrome**. Several models of periodization are sequential owing to the fact that it is very difficult if not impossible to maintain maximal performance over an extended period of time in trained athletes. Thus, peaking at the right times is essential. Many athletes participate in sports that place importance on an entire season of competition. For these sports, peak condition needs to be achieved by the onset of the competitive year and maintained throughout the competitive season. A *maintenance* (or stabilization) phase ensues, which is designed to maintain the strength, power, and size gains made during the off-season. Exercise intensity is reduced to levels used during the strength mesocycle while training volume is lowered by reducing the number of assistance exercises performed during each workout. Adjustments to training programs are specific to the needs of the particular sport that the athlete plays and the individual's goals. In contrast, athletes who focus on a major competition occurring toward the end of the competitive year will attempt to reach peak condition at that specific point in the season.

General Adaptation Syndrome

Periodized training is rooted in the work of renowned endocrinologist Dr. Hans Selye (22). Selye discussed a **General Adaptation Syndrome**, which has application to the training of athletes. Selye recognized that stress plays a role in disease development and an application has been made to training. General Adaptation Syndrome (Fig. 18.3) comprises three response phases to stressful demands. The initial phase is the *alarm phase* (sometimes referred to as the *shock phase*) and consists of both shock and soreness. Performance during this phase will decrease. This would be synonymous to the initial effects a workout has on the athlete. The second phase is physiological *adaptation* to this new stimulus. The body adapts to the new training stimulus and an improvement in performance ensues. Once the body has adapted, no further adaptations will take place unless the stimulus is altered. The third phase is *exhaustion* (sometimes referred to as *staleness* or *maladaptation*) where constant increases in the exercise stimulus are not accompanied by appropriate rest and/or recovery periods. The body is unable to make any further adaptation, and unless this stimulus is reduced, overtraining could occur. If sufficient recovery is allowed, the body can properly adapt and performance may increase further. Periodization is used to avoid or minimize periods of exhaustion and to maintain an effective exercise stimulus that leads to maximizing athletic potential (23).

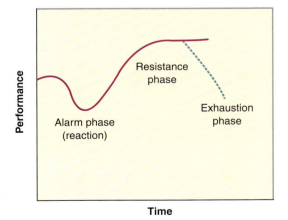

FIGURE 18.3 Selye's general adaptation syndrome. (Reprinted with permission from Selye H. *The Stress of Life*. New York (NY): McGraw-Hill; 1956.)

Tapering and Performance

A **taper** period is one where there is a reduction in workload prior to a major competition to maximize performance (24). Tapering is mostly used when an athlete is peaking for a single competition as opposed to a competitive season. It is common for athletes to overreach near the end of precompetition training and reduce volume and/or frequency (while maintaining or increasing intensity) to induce a rebound in performance (3). Reductions in intensity are counterproductive; thus, it is recommended that tapering be performed at a similar intensity to the peaking phase (3,24). Volume reductions of 50%–90% are effective and correlate positively to performance gains in endurance athletes (24,25). Volume is reduced by shortening workouts and decreasing frequency although volume reductions are preferred while maintaining a similar or slightly reduced frequency (3). Decreasing frequency can enhance short-term performance yet maintain performance over a 2- to 4-week period (3). High-frequency (at least 80% of normal frequency) tapering produces better performance than low-frequency tapering (every third day) and may be necessary for advanced to elite athletes (3,24).

Part of the challenge is to select an appropriate taper type and length. The duration of the taper may depend on the extent of training and overreaching leading up to the tapering period. Figure 18.4 depicts data presented by Bosquet et al. (26) showing that the optimal taper length tends to be ~8–14 days for endurance performance. Figure 18.5 depicts types of tapers used (24). A nonprogressive, or *step taper*, embellishes a standard reduction in training load. For example, a 40% reduction in load would occur immediately and then is maintained for the duration of the taper period. Although it is effective for enhancing performance, it may be inferior to progressive tapers (3,24). A progressive taper involves a systematic reduction in training load (volume). It can be linear or exponential. A *linear taper* involves a gradual reduction in training load throughout the taper period. For example, the athlete could reduce training load by 3%–5% for each workout until the desired load reduction has been attained. A *slow exponential taper* has a slower reduction in training load compared to a *fast exponential taper*. For example, a fast exponential taper may result in a nonlinear load reduction where load may be reduced 45% during the first 1–2 workouts, an additional 10% the next 1–2 workouts, 10% the next 1–2 workouts, and 5% the last 1–2 workouts for a 1.5-week taper. A slow exponential taper may result in a nonlinear load reduction where load may be reduced 25% during the first 1–2 workouts, an additional 15% the next 1–2 workouts, 10% the next 1–2 workouts, and 5% the last 1–2 workouts for a 1.5-week taper. Fast exponential tapers produce greater improvements in performance than linear or slow exponential tapers and have been recommended to peak athletic performance (3,24).

Most studies have shown tapering can augment performance. Aerobic and anaerobic performance improvements of ~0.5%–6% (3% average) can be expected from a proper taper (24). A tapering period of 4–8 days increases muscle glycogen content by 15%–34% (27). Tapering periods of ~2–3 weeks can increase various parameters of judo performance (28),

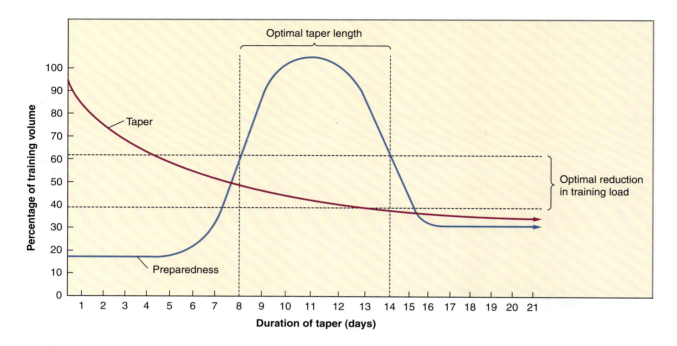

FIGURE 18.4 Tapering and performance. (Reprinted with permission from Bosquet L, Leger L, Legros P. Methods to determine aerobic endurance. *Sports Med*. 2002;32:675–700.)

strength and speed in rugby athletes (29), and track and field throwing performance (30). Vo_{2max} and endurance performance improvements of 1.2%–22% in runners, swimmers, triathletes, and cyclists have been shown during short-term taper periods, *e.g.*, 1–3 weeks (27). Run time to exhaustion (accompanied by increased SERCA1 and Na^+/K^+ pump protein levels) may improve following 10 and 18 days of tapering following intense, high-volume sprint interval training (31). 1,500 m run performance was shown to improve by 3.4% following a 7-day taper (32). Bosquet et al. (33) performed a meta-analysis primarily focused on running, swimming, and cycling endurance performance and showed that optimal tapering involved a 2-week duration where volume was exponentially reduced by 41%–60% without modification of intensity or frequency. Studies failing to show improvements mostly used longer tapering periods of 3–4 weeks (27).

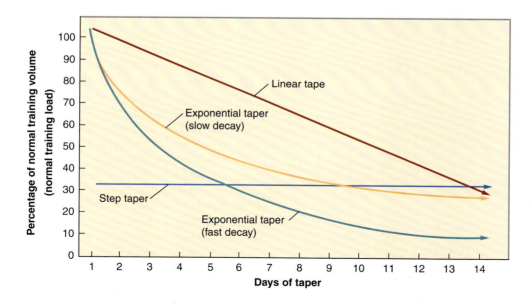

FIGURE 18.5 Common types of tapers used by athletes. (Reprinted with permission from Mujika I, Padilla S. Scientific bases for precompetition tapering strategies. *Med Sci Sports Exerc*. 2003;35:1182–7.)

Strength and power increases of 2%–27% have been shown following tapering periods of 7–35 days (27,34–36). Strength athletes include tapering to enhance recovery, peak performance, rest, psychologically prepare, and reduce risks of injuries (37). Studies show that RT followed by a 3–5 day period of cessation produces superior strength and power performance compared to when testing is performed the day following training (38). Tapering for optimizing strength and power increases involves maintaining or increasing intensity while reducing volume/volume load and frequency by 30%–70% for 1–4 weeks (14,37,39,40). Volume load is high or peaks ~4 weeks before competition (39). Elite powerlifters take ~3–4 days off before a competition and reduce their volume by ~50%–60% during tapering (of ~2.5 wk), while most (70%) remove or reduce assistance exercises from training a few weeks before competition (14,39). Approximately 87% of strongman competitors use a taper in preparation for competition with a mean of ~10 days, reduce volume by ~46%, 50% reduced or removed assistance exercises, and stop training ~4.7 days before a competition (37). Interestingly, lighter athletes had shorter taper lengths than larger athletes and 55% of the strength athletes reported decreasing intensity during the taper period (37). Sixty percent of powerlifters reported using an exponential taper with fast decay and 40% used a step taper (39). Fifty-two percent of strongman competitors use a step taper, 17% use a linear taper, and 16% use an exponential taper (37). Similar tapering patterns were seen in elite weightlifters where very low volume technical work was only performed within 3 days of competition (41). Figure 18.6 depicts changes in volume load and tapering patterns by an elite national level female Olympic weightlifter preparing for three competitions (41). Volume load was highest 4 weeks prior to competition and was decreased by 59%, 47%, and 71%, respectively, during the three 4-week competition phases. Largest reductions were seen during tapering the week before competition.

Basic Models of Periodization

Although there are many ways in which a coach or athlete can vary a training program, some basic models of periodization have been studied mostly in regard to RT although periodization can be applied to aerobic endurance, sprint/agility, and plyometric training programs as well. All are effective for enhancing muscle strength, power, hypertrophy, endurance, and various measures of motor performance. The basic models include the classic (linear), block, undulating (nonlinear), and reverse linear periodization models.

Classical Model of Periodization

The *classical model of periodization* (or *traditional periodization*) was one of the first used and developed from the work of Matveyev (5). Although sometimes referred to as *linear periodization*, a closer examination shows that this model is not linear throughout but intensity and volume can fluctuate at various intervals in more of a wave-like manner. In fact, intensity and/or volume fluctuation can take place within a designated microcycle. For example, over a 4-week period, 1 week may comprise more than 35% of the total monthly volume load, whereas the other 3 weeks may comprise between 15% and 25% of the total volume load per week (4). The term *linear* implies a constant volume and intensity progression,

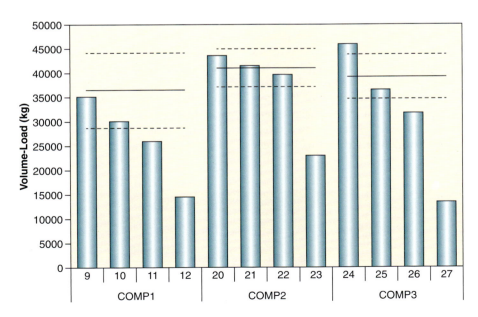

FIGURE 18.6 Tapering patterns used by an elite female weightlifter in preparation for three competitions. COMP = competition number; *black lines* represent normal volume load and *hashed lines* represent the 95% confidence intervals. (From Bazyler CD, Mizuguchi S, Zourdos MC, et al. Characteristics of a national level female weightlifter peaking for competition: a case study. *J Strength Cond Res*. 2018;32:3029–8.)

and this is not the case although the general trend is typically decreased volume and increased intensity. Thus, the term *linear periodization* is somewhat misleading. This model is characterized by high training volume initially and a reduction in volume (with subsequent increase in intensity) with each phase in succession (6) (Table 18.1). The classical model is designed to maximize strength and power, or peak anaerobic performance. This model is commonly used in athletes peaking for strength and power such as powerlifters (14). Each training phase is designed to emphasize a particular fitness component. The initial phase is the *hypertrophy phase* (or strength endurance phase) where muscle growth and muscle endurance improvements are emphasized. A secondary objective is to build a foundation and better prepare the athlete for higher intensities of training later in the cycle. Structural multiple-joint exercises are performed for 3–5 sets per exercise for 8–20 reps for 50%–75% of 1 RM. This phase may last 4–6 weeks but can be longer (9–12 wk) in those athletes with a limited training background. The next phase is a *strength phase* where intensity is increased and volume is decreased (structural multiple-joint exercises performed for 3–5 sets of 4–6 reps [80%–85% of 1 RM] with heavier weights). This phase may last from 1 to 3 months. The subsequent phases include *strength/power* and *peaking phases* that extend upon strength training with high-intensity structural exercise performance and repetitions decrease. The goal is to maximize strength and power by the end of the cycle. More power exercises are included. It has been recommended that power training be emphasized after a strength training phase as strength is the foundation for power development and power may be better developed following appropriate strength training (3). The strength/power phase consists of higher intensity and lower volume (3–5 sets of 2–5 reps). The strength/power phase is critical to translate developed strength into higher power development. The peaking phase occurs prior to the most important competitions of the year. In between phases, unloading weeks are performed where the athlete decreases volume and intensity to facilitate recovery and prepare for the next higher-intensity training phase. Maintenance takes place in-season where lower volume and frequency are seen (1–3 sets of 1–3 reps for structural exercises using a wide range of intensities). Many modifications of this model can be used effectively in athletes in an attempt to reduce some of its inherent limitations. The critical element is that the template be applied to the structural exercises that form the foundation of the program. Every exercise in the training program serves a purpose and other assistance exercises (*e.g.,* complimentary, core, corrective, movement-specific, sport-specific) may follow a different paradigm at various phases.

Block Periodization

Block periodization was developed as an alternative to the traditional model where specific "blocks" were used to target athletic biomotor abilities in a sequential manner and provide better planning for team-sport athletes and for athletes competing several times during the year. Each subsequent training block is augmented by the physiological adaptation taking place from the previous block. For example, Suarez et al. (42) showed in weightlifters that an initial strength-endurance phase increased muscle size, while subsequent strength and power phases (with a taper) increased rate of force development (RFD) in a sequential manner. It involved the implementation of "blocks" designed to target or concentrate on a minimal number of abilities (43). That is, ~60%–80% of the training time may be dedicated to 1–2 targeted abilities per block thereby allowing the athlete to have greater variation in volume and intensity per phase. The most common application described is a triphasic model (one stage) consisting of three mesocycle blocks usually ~2–6 weeks in duration: (a) *accumulation* — a general block where higher volume (reduced intensity) of training is used to develop basic abilities such as endurance, muscle hypertrophy, strength, and movement technique; (b) *transmutation* — focus is on developing specific abilities such as aerobic or anaerobic endurance; and (c) *realization* — precompetition training for maximal speed and power with recovery prior to competition (43). Table 18.2 depicts an example of block periodization applied to RT. The accumulation phase targets muscle hypertrophy via moderate loading for three multiple-joint exercises. The transmutation phase targets strength development with moderately heavy loading and volume reduction. The realization phase targets peaking strength and power development with heavy loading and lower volume.

Comparative studies show that block periodization is effective for targeting strength, power, speed, agility, and

Table 18.1	Classical Model of Periodization in a Strength/Power Athlete			
	Mesocycle			
	Hypertrophy	**Strength**	**Strength/Power**	**Peaking**
Sets	3–5	3–5	3–5	3–5
Repetitions	8–20	4–6	2–5	1–3
Intensity (% 1 RM)	50%–75%	80%–85%	85%–90%	>90%

Table 18.2	Block Periodization Applied to Resistance Training	
Accumulation Phase — Strength/Endurance		
Weeks 1–2		
Back squat	4 × 10–12	60%–65% of 1 RM
Hex-bar dead lift	4 × 10–12	
Bench press	4 × 10–12	
Weeks 3–4		
Back squat	4 × 8–10	65%–70% of 1 RM
Hex-bar dead lift	4 × 8–10	
Bench press	4 × 8–10	
Transmutation Phase — Strength		
Weeks 5–8		
Hang clean	4 × 5–6	75%–80% of 1 RM
Back squat	4 × 5–6	
Hex-bar dead lift	4 × 5–6	
Bench press	4 × 5–6	
Realization Phase — Power		
Weeks 9–10		
Hang clean	4 × 2–3	85%–90% of 1 RM
Back squat	4 × 2–3	
Hex-bar dead lift	4 × 2–3	
Bench press	4 × 2–3	

endurance. Several studies examined block periodization effects on endurance enhancement. As reviewed by Issurin (2), block periodization produced improvements in VO_{2max}, time trial performance, and time to exhaustion in endurance athletes (*e.g.*, skiers, kayakers, and cyclists) with several studies showing superior improvements in various parameters using block compared to traditional periodization. These results were confirmed in a meta-analysis where block periodization provided beneficial effects for increasing VO_{2max} and maximal power output compared to traditional periodization (44). For strength and power training, studies have shown similar and superior maximal strength increases following block periodization compared to traditional (2,45) and that block periodization produced more efficient strength and RFD gains (relative to training volume load) than daily undulating periodization (46). Table 18.3 depicts a multimodality block model for an athlete targeting speed and agility. The main target (speed and agility) is a tertiary focus in phase I where it may command ~10% of the workload, secondary focus in phase II where it may command ~30%–50% of the workload, and primary focus in phase III where it may command ~80% of the workload.

Nonlinear (Undulating) Model of Periodization

Nonlinear (undulating) models enable variation in intensity and volume within each 7–10 days cycle by rotating different protocols (7,47). Nonlinear methods attempt to train the various components of the neuromuscular system within the same cycle. During a single workout, only one characteristic is trained in a given day per structural exercise, *e.g.*, strength, power, muscular endurance, and hypertrophy. The daily variation in programming is known as *daily nonlinear periodization*. For example, in loading schemes for structural exercises in the workout, the use of heavy, moderate, and lighter resistances may be randomly rotated over a week (Monday, Wednesday, Friday), *e.g.*, 3–5 reps, 8–10 reps, and 12–15 reps may be used in the rotation; or a power workout may be used (*e.g.*, 50%–60% of 1 RM, 2–3 reps, high-velocity) (8). This model may be appropriate for athletes who play a varied schedule such as basketball, hockey, baseball, or soccer players that may have several games or competitions in a given week or the schedule of games and travel does not permit a regularly scheduled in-season strength maintenance program. Each exercise needs to be considered independently where structural exercises follow a similar periodization scheme. However, assistance exercises may follow a different periodized scheme depending on program objectives. Thus, each exercise can be periodized within a desired time frame as the goal of each exercise can differ. Another undulating model is *weekly undulated periodization*.

Table 18.3	Basic Block Model for Speed and Agility Training		
Target	**Accumulation**	**Transmutation**	**Realization**
Primary	Max strength	Power	Speed & Agility
Secondary	Power	Speed & Agility	Power
Tertiary	Speed & Agility	Max Strength	Max Strength

Modified from Bompa TO, Haff GG. *Periodization: Theory and Methodology of Training*. 5th ed. Champaign (IL): Human Kinetics; 2009. p. 125–256.

In this model, intensity and volume vary on a weekly basis rather than daily. For example, for structural exercises, an athlete may train at 70% of his or her 1 RM week 1, 80% of his or her 1 RM week 2, and 90% of his or her 1 RM week 3. Volume decreases as intensity increases. The athlete then repeats this cycle for weeks 4–6 and so on. This model has produced similar increases in maximal strength as classical and daily undulated models (48). Lastly, *flexible nonlinear periodization* has increased in popularity where the manipulation of acute program variables could be incorporated into the design of different training days to address physiological needs, recovery, and goals of the athlete. This model increases the flexibility of the programming especially within a competitive season where training disruptions are common, *e.g.*, games, travel, illness, school schedule, etc.

Daily undulating model has compared favorably with the classical model (26). Several studies examining 9–15 weeks of training showed similar strength, lifting velocity, power, and vertical jump increases in athletes and fit individuals using undulating and classical models (48–51). In contrast, the undulating model was more effective for increasing 1 RM bench press, arm curl, and leg press strength following 12 weeks of training than the classic model (52–54). The undulating model was inferior to the classic model for enhancing in-season strength in freshman college football players (55). A meta-analysis of 17 studies comparing traditional and undulating periodization showed that 12 studies found similar strength improvements between the two models, 3 studies favored undulating periodization, and 2 favored traditional (56). The conclusion was both models were similarly effective for increasing muscle strength (56); therefore, both classic and undulating models appear equally effective for maximizing strength (48–51).

> ## Case Study 18.1
>
> Samantha is an Olympic weightlifter preparing for a competition. The competition is 8 months away and will be the only major competition she will be competing in this year. Samantha has been competing for 7 years and was coming off a competition 1 month ago. She is now in transition and seeks your guidance for developing an 8-month periodized macrocycle to get her ready for the competition (Fig. 18.7).
>
> **Question for Consideration:** What training advice would you give Samantha?

Reverse Linear Periodization Model

Models structured in the opposite manner of classic periodization are used to target cardiovascular and a muscular endurance improvement primarily in reference to RT. Reverse linear periodization involves moderate-to-high intensity, low-volume training initially. Intensity decreases and volume increases with each successive phase. Some strength enhancement may be targeted early in training. However, the primary goal is to peak muscle endurance or size at the end of the cycle. By the end of the cycle, the athlete will be training with higher sets and repetitions, with shorter rest intervals, which are effective for enhancing muscular endurance. This model is commonly used by endurance athletes and bodybuilders preparing for competitions and has been shown to be superior for enhancing muscle endurance to other RT periodization models when volume and intensity were equated (57). However, strength improvements following this model are

---

Myths & Misconceptions
Periodized and Nonperiodized Training are Equally Effective for Increasing Long-Term Athletic Performance

Some have suggested that planned training variation is not necessary for progression. Periodized RT increases muscle size, strength, endurance, and power in athletes with a variety of training backgrounds (23,62,63). The effects are most prominent over long-term training periods where the planned variation is effective for reducing plateaus. Several studies compared various periodized models to nonperiodized multiple- and single-set models of training and have shown periodized training is superior for increasing maximal strength, cycling power, motor performance, and jumping ability (1,6,7,52,62,64–72) with the exception of a short-term study, which showed similar performance improvements between periodized and multiple-set nonperiodized models (73). It is thought that longer training periods (at least 4 wk) are

necessary to underscore the benefits of periodized training compared with nonperiodized training (71). Several studies comparing periodized to nonperiodized RT range in duration from 3 to 36 weeks with a mean of ~12 weeks (74). Periodization was shown superior via a meta-analytical review of the literature to nonperiodized RT (75). A recent meta-analysis confirmed greater increases in 1 RM strength with periodized RT regardless of age and sex (74). In addition, periodized endurance training was shown superior to nonperiodized training for improving running performance in runners (59). *Periodized RT (classical, block, reverse linear, undulating, and integrated models) is recommended by the ACSM for progression for strength, power, hypertrophy, and endurance training* (76).

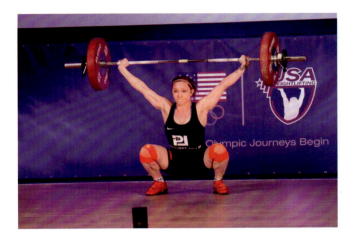

FIGURE 18.7 A competitive Olympic weightlifter. (Photo courtesy of Stephanie Holm.)

inferior compared to linear and undulating models (57,58), and one study reported less muscle hypertrophy compared to traditional periodization (58). For other training modalities, reverse and traditional models may produce similar improvements. For endurance training, reverse and traditional models produced similar performance improvements in swimming and running performance in swimmers, runners, and triathletes (59–61).

 ## Periodization for an Athlete with Multiple Major Competitions

Some sports like track and field require two major competitive seasons, *e.g.*, indoor and outdoor. Thus, periodization involves two major training cycles (sometimes known as *bi-cycles*). Ultimately, the monocycle is divided into two macrocycles similar in structure. Each macrocycle is characterized by classic periodization marked by an increase in intensity and decrease in volume until peaking occurs precompetition. In some programs, the last competition may be most important. Thus, the highest volume may be seen during the first preparatory phase. The preparatory phases of the second macrocycle would be relatively short in duration compared to the first. Changes in intensity are similar during each cycle. The challenge of multicycle training is the reduction in the preparatory phase. It is recommended that bi-cycle periodized programs be limited to more advanced athletes. In other cases, athletes compete in three or more major competitions (tennis, boxing, mixed martial arts) in a single year these training plans are referred to as *tricycles* or *multicycles*.

 ## Periodization for a Strength/Power Athlete in a Team Sport

Power training entails the integration of resistance (heavy RT for strength, ballistic RT to enhance velocity), plyometric, sprint, and agility training. A sample periodized program for an American football player is shown in Figure 18.8. This model follows the classic periodization design (23,62). The preparatory phase's primary objective is to prepare the athlete for more strenuous training and to increase muscle hypertrophy (muscle hypertrophy is desirable in a collision sport like football). This mesocycle may last ~6–8 weeks, and some endurance activities may be performed. The 6- to 8-week strength mesocycle is characterized by an increase in intensity and a reduction in volume. The subsequent strength/power phase incorporates more sport-specific exercises. During this 6- to 8-week mesocycle, training intensity will be further elevated, while training volume is reduced. The use of ballistic and plyometric exercises may be included during this phase. Sport-specific conditioning, agility, and speed training may be included 2–3 days per week. The peaking phase precedes training camp. It is shorter in duration (4–6 wk) and is designed to peak strength and power performance for the start of the season. Training intensity is increased, while training volume is reduced. This is often accomplished by reducing the number of assistance exercises in the program. The onset of training camp initiates the beginning of the preseason period where RT is reduced to 2 days per week maintenance phase (structural exercises with several assistance exercises). Training intensity is similar while repetition number increases. Anaerobic training (sprints or intervals) is continued 2–3 days per week in order to maintain the athletes' sport-specific conditioning level.

 ## Periodization of Sprint, Agility, and Plyometric Training

Periodization of sprint, agility, and plyometric training follows a pattern common to peaking for strength and power (Table 18.4). However, the logistical progression occurs from base training during the off-season to speed-specific training to sport-specific speed and agility training. Plyometric training follows a basic pattern of low-to-moderate-intensity drills to high-intensity drills over time along with a slight increase in volume, *e.g.*, foot contacts. Training during the early preparation phase involves base anaerobic conditioning. The preparatory phase could last 3–6 months for athletes involved in one or two major competitions and 2–3 months for team sports athletes (3). General preparation includes anaerobic conditioning. Volume tends to be somewhat high

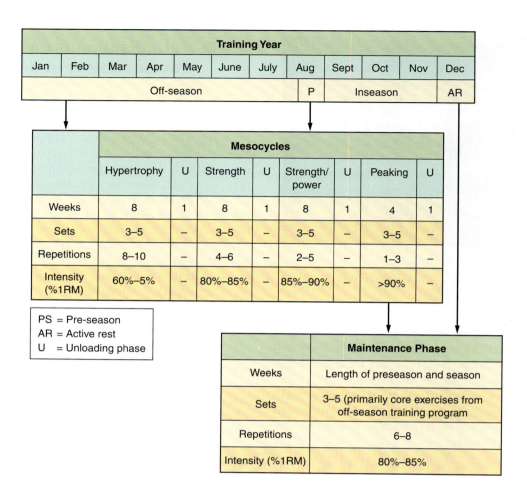

FIGURE 18.8 Periodization for a football player. (Reprinted with permission from Hoffman JR, Ratamess NA. *A Practical Guide to Developing Resistance Training Programs*. 2nd ed. Monterey (CA): Coaches Choice Books; 2008.)

with moderate intensity of drills. Plyometric drills are low to moderate in intensity initially and linear sprint drills stress technique and base building. Interval training is common. Sprinting intensity may range from 70% to 85% of maximal speed for multiple repetitions for 50- to 200-m distances. The purpose is to develop a base for subsequent high-intensity training. Some speed endurance training can be introduced here for those athletes whose sports involve repeated sprints of at least moderate distance. Short interset rest intervals with high-intensity drills (>90%) of maximum for 50–150 m are effective (3). Some low-to-moderate intensity aerobic training (AT) can be performed here as well for those athletes who have a mild-to-moderate aerobic component in their sport. The length of the general preparatory phase may be longer in novice athletes and less for advanced to elite athletes.

Specific preparatory training involves a transition to more specific training. Volume can remain similar but may start to decrease near the end of the phase as intensity increases. Resisted sprint running and overspeed drills can be incorporated here in addition to linear sprints of varying distance. More complex plyometric drills and agility drills are included. The agility drills may be of moderate complexity and work toward increasing complexity and become more reactive as the phase progresses. Precompetition training marks the time where the athlete has peaked strength and power (by the end) and is refining speed and agility by sport-specific training. Speed and agility training is highly sport-specific and in its highest complexity of the precompetition macrocycle. The intensity remains high and volume is gradually reduced. The competitive season is marked mostly by maintenance training. Participation in sport practice and games/competitions assists in maintaining peak performance. However, a 1- to 2-day-per-week (if allowed by the competition schedule) maintenance program (low volume, high intensity) can be valuable for the athlete to maintain performance and reduces the likelihood of mid- to late-season detraining. The transition period marks a time of active rest to allow complete recovery and restoration of body/psyche following a stressful competitive season.

Table 18.4	Sample Annual Training Plan for Strength/Power Athlete										
MO	1	2	3	4	5	6	7	8	9	10	11	12
	Preparatory						Competitive					Transition
	General prep			**Specific prep**			**Precomp**		**Competitions**			**Active rest**
Speed	Anaerobic base			Max speed			Max speed		Maintenance			Other training modalities
	Technique			Overspeed/resisted			Supramax.		High int, low vol			
	Speed endurance			Speed endurance			Sport spec.		Low freq			
				Technique					Sport practice			
Agility				Moderate/high int			Sport spec.		Maintenance			
				Reactive drills			Reactive		High int, low vol			
									Low freq			
									Sport practice			
Plyometrics	Low-to-moderate			Moderate-to-high			High int		Sport practice			
				Sport spec.			Sport spec.					
Strength	Hyper.	Strength		Str/pow		Peak		Maintenance		Maintenance		

Adapted with permission from Bompa TO, Haff GG. *Periodization: Theory and Methodology of Training*. 5th ed. Champaign (IL): Human Kinetics; 2009. p. 125–256.

Periodization of Aerobic Endurance Training

Athletes maximizing aerobic endurance performance benefit from following variations of a reverse linear periodization model where volume is moderate initially and intensity is moderate to high (57) (Table 18.5). The preparatory phase is characterized by AT to increase Vo_{2max}. RT targeting some strength improvements is critical to help increase aerobic exercise economy. By the end of the specific preparatory phase, volume increases and intensity matches the type of aerobic activities performed. During precompetition, combination strategies are employed. The athlete may have 1–3 workouts per week that are longer in duration and of moderate intensity. One workout may be dedicated to longer distance/duration than the other workouts. Throughout the precompetition training phase, the duration of the long run gradually increases with the exception of unloading weeks where volume is reduced. The remaining moderate-to-high distance/duration workouts only increase gradually. The remaining workouts during precompetition are dedicated to higher-intensity AT. Steady-state AT can only take the endurance athlete so far. Interval training (or training targeting lactate threshold and exercise economy improvements) is necessary to provide additional endurance improvements in trained athletes (62). Thus, the athlete during precompetition may train 2–3 days per week at higher intensity and lower volume. Specialized workouts including Fartlek training, hills, intervals, pace/tempo work, and repetition training are performed for greater specialization. Technique work is included and speed drills can be added. While the intensity may remain constant and duration increases with long slow distance workouts, the intensity can increase and volume can remain constant for specialized AT drills. Strength training can continue during precompetition but at a lower frequency and volume, *i.e.*, maintenance training. In some cases, the intensity of strength training can decrease, volume can increase, and rest intervals may decrease to target muscle endurance improvements which may benefit race performance. By the end of the precompetition phase, the athlete is ready for competition and may have partially overreached at this level. A tapering period can be used in the last week where volume is reduced producing a rebound effect to maximize performance during competition.

Periodization of Aerobic and Anaerobic Training Components

Some sports require high muscular strength, power, speed, agility, sufficient levels of muscle endurance, and a sufficient aerobic conditioning level, *e.g.*, wrestling, mixed martial arts, soccer, basketball, and boxing. For these athletes, the general preparatory phase is marked by a classic periodization scheme for RT and a few days per week AT (low intensity, moderate duration) not to impede anaerobic fitness development. During the specific preparatory phase, progressive RT continues (and peaks by the end of the phase) and a 2- to 3-day-per-week sprint, agility, and plyometric program is initiated. During the precompetition phase, RT is reduced to maintenance training (1–3 days per week, high intensity, and low volume), whereas the intensity (complexity) and volume of sprint, plyometric, and agility training increase modestly. Aerobic endurance training increases in intensity and is performed 2–3 days per

Table 18.5	Sample Annual Training Plan for an Endurance Athlete with One Major Competition											
MO	1	2	3	4	5	6	7	8	9	10	11	12
	Preparatory					Competitive						Transition
Endurance	General Base aerobic	Specific Base aerobic intervals, pace		Precompetition Base aerobic — LSD Progressive distance increase Intervals, fartleks, pace, hill. Repetitions Increase intensity, Moderate volume						T	C	Active rest
Speed		Base Technique		Base Technique								
Strength	Strength		Str/End	Endurance		Maintenance						

T, taper; C, competition; LSD, long slow duration.

week. AT can be performed on a separate day or following an anaerobic training workout. By the end of the precompetition phase, the athlete's aerobic endurance increases, anaerobic conditioning is improved and/or maintained, and the athlete is ready for the competition season.

Sample Periodized Strength Training Programs

The coach and athlete can separate the year into basic segments and apply the training principles to each phase of training. Tables 18.6–18.8 provide some examples of periodized strength training programs for athletes. Table 18.6 depicts a sample wrestling strength training program. The program is 15 weeks in length but can be adapted to be longer when unloading weeks are used in between phases. Key qualities include periodized intensity and volume of structural exercises. Loading is increased and volume is decreased (the numbers in parentheses indicate training week numbers). In addition, periodized exercise selection was used where pull-up and push-up progressions were included. Table 18.7 depicts a periodized program for a strength competition athlete. The program initiates from strength/power phases and progresses to sport specific and peak power endurance phases. The program includes several sport-specific exercises the athlete may perform in the competition phase. Table 18.8 depicts a sample program for a boxer. This program consists of periodized intensity and volume for structural exercises as well as inclusion of a variety of sport-specific exercises. All programs depicted are consecutive. That is, unloading weeks are not shown. It is recommended that the coach and athlete include periodic unloading weeks to help the athlete recover from the previous phase and prepare the body for the upcoming training phase.

Table 18.6 Sample Periodized Program for a Wrestler

Monday	Sets × Reps (Week Nos)
Hang clean[a]	3 × 6 (1–4); 5 (5–8); 4 × 5 (9–12); 5 × 3 (13–15)
Bench press	3 × 10–12 (1–4); 8–10 (5–8); 6–8 (9–12); 3–5 (13–15)
Close-grip bench press	3 × 10–12 (1–4); 8–10 (5–8); 6–8 (9–12); 3–5 (13–15)
Shoulder press	3 × 10–12 (1–4); 8–10 (5–12); 6–8 (13–15)
Pull-up progressions	
Wide-grip pull-ups	3 × 10–25 (1–5)
Towel pull-ups	3 × 10–15 (6–10)
Weighted pull-ups or unilateral pull-ups	3 × 8–10 (11–15)
Internal/external rotations	3 × 10
MB Russian twist	3 × 25–50
Stability ball crunches	3 × 25–50
Manual resistance — neck	2 × 10
Wednesday	**Sets × Reps (Week Nos)**
Back squat	3 × 10–12 (1–4); 8–10 (5–8); 4 × 6–8 (9–12); 5 × 3–5 (13–15)
Overhead squat	3 × 6–8 (1–7)
Front squat	3 × 6–8 (8–15)
Unilateral leg press	3 × 8–10 (1–7)
Split squat/lunge	3 × 8–10 (8–15)
Stiff-leg dead lift	3 × 10–12 (1–6); 8–10 (7–12); 6–8 (13–15)
Back extensions	3 × 15–20
Calf raise	3 × 15–20
Thick bar dead lift	3 × 10
Plyometric leg raise	3 × 15–25
Trunk stabilization ("plank")	3 × 1 min

Table 18.6 — Sample Periodized Program for a Wrestler (Continued)

Friday	Sets × Reps (Week Nos)
Power snatch	3 × 6 (1–4); 5 (5–8); 4 × 5 (9–12); 5 × 3 (13–15)
Bent-over barbell row	3 × 10–12 (1–4); 8–10 (5–8); 6–8 (9–12); 3–5 (13–15)
Close-grip lat pull-down	3 × 10–12 (1–5); 8–10 (6–10); 6–8 (11–15)
Weighted dips	3 × 12–15 (1–4); 10–12 (5–8); 8–10 (9–15)
Pullovers	3 × 8–10
Push-up progressions	
Basic	3 × 25–50 (1–5)
Stability ball	3 × 15–30 (6–10)
MB plyo push-ups	3 × 10 (11–15)
Partner plate pass	3 × 25
Weighted curl-ups	3 × 25
Wrist and reverse wrist curls	3 × 10

Intensity — 60%–85% of 1 RM periodized. Rest intervals — 2–3 minutes for core exercises; 1–2 minutes for assistance exercises; 30 seconds to 1 minute for abs.

[a]Progress to power clean.

Reprinted with permission from Hoffman JR, Ratamess NA. *A Practical Guide to Developing Resistance Training Programs*. 2nd ed. Monterey (CA): Coaches Choice Books; 2008.

Table 18.7 — 15-Week Periodized Program for a Strength Competition Athlete

Monday	Tuesday	Thursday	Friday
Weeks 1–4: Strength/Power			
Power clean 5 × 5	Squat 5 × 5–6	Power clean 5 × 5	Dead lift 4 × 5
Bench press 5 × 5–6	Front squat 4 × 5–6	Push press 4 × 5	Box squat 4 × 6
Incline barbell press 4 × 6	Bent-over rows 3 × 6–8	Close-grip bench press 4 × 6	Zercher squat 3 × 5–6
Shoulder press 4 × 6	Power shrugs 3 × 8	Triceps push-downs 3 × 6–8	Reverse hyperext. 3 × 6–8
Sit-ups 3 × 10–15	Good mornings 3 × 8	Barbell curls 3 × 6–8	Glute-ham raise 3 × 10
Weeks 5–8: Strength/Power			
Power clean 5 × 3–5	Squat 5 × 3–5	Power clean 5 × 3–5	Dead lift 5 × 3–5
Bench press 5 × 3–5	Half rack squats 4 × 3–5	Push press 4 × 3–5	DL rack pulls 4 × 3–5
Incline barbell press 4 × 5	Bent-over rows 3 × 5–6	Close-grip bench press 4 × 5	Front squats 4 × 3–5
Shoulder press 4 × 5	Power shrugs 3 × 6	Triceps push-downs 3 × 6–8	Reverse hyperext. 3 × 6–8
Torso rotations 3 × 10–15	Good mornings 3 × 8	Barbell curls 3 × 5–6	Glute-ham raise 3 × 8
Weeks 9–12: Peak Strength/Power — Sport Specific			
Power clean 5 × 1–3	Squat 5 × 1–3	Mastiff log clean & press 4 × 3–5	Dead lift 5 × 1–3
Bench press 5 × 1–3[a]	Quarter rack squats 4 × 3–5	Incline bench press 4 × 3	DL rack pulls 4 × 3–5
Mastiff log clean and press 4 × 3–5	KB swings 3 × 5	Close-grip bench press 4 × 5	Super yoke SQ walks 3 × 20 yd
ISOM lat raise (T-hold) 3 × 20–30 s	Power shrugs 4 × 5	Farmer's walk 2 × 30 yd	Reverse hypers 4 × 5
Torso rotations 3 × 10–12	Thick bar DL 4 × 5	Barbell curls 3 × 5 (+ISOM holds)	One-arm DB rows 3 × 6

Chapter 18 Training Periodization and Tapering **585**

Table 18.7	15-Week Periodized Program for a Strength Competition Athlete (*Continued*)		
Monday	**Tuesday**	**Thursday**	**Friday**
Weeks 13–15: Sport Specific — Peak Power/Endurance[b]			
Power clean 5 × 1–3	Squat 5 × 1–3	Bench press 5 × 1–3[a]	Dead lift 5 × 1–3
Mastiff log clean and press 4 × 3–5[c]	Mastiff stone medley 2–4 × 5 stones	ISOM T-holds 3 × 30–40 s	Super yoke SQ walks 3 × 20 yd
Tire flips 2–4 × 8–10	Truck pulls (with harness) 2–4 × 30 yd	Farmer's walk 2–4 × 40 yd	Loading medley 2–4 times

Periodized core intensity — 70%–100%. Rest intervals — 3–5 minutes for cores; 2–3 minutes for assistance exercises. Off days — 1 day per week for base cardiovascular exercise; 1 day per week for interval training/plyometrics.

[a]Switch to incline bench press if competition includes inclines for max reps — in this case, higher repetitions are performed.

[b]Exercises may change based on specific competitions; sport-specifics are timed so each set is completed as rapidly as possible.

[c]More reps performed if the competition includes this event for max reps; distances for sport-specific events depend upon competition length.

KB, kettle bells.

Reprinted with permission from Hoffman JR, Ratamess NA. *A Practical Guide to Developing Resistance Training Programs*. 2nd ed. Monterey (CA): Coaches Choice Books; 2008.

Table 18.8	12-Week Boxing Strength Training Program[a]	
Monday	**Wednesday**	**Friday**
Weeks 1–4		
Hang clean 4 × 6	Power snatch 4 × 6	Hang clean 4 × 6
Squat 4 × 8–10	Bench press 4 × 8–10	Dead lift 4 × 8–10
DB jump squat 3 × 6	Incline bench press 3 × 8–10	One-arm rows 3 × 8–10
Box step-ups 3 × 10	Dips 3 × 10–15	Weighted pull-ups 3 × 10–15
Good mornings 3 × 8–10	Side lateral raise 3 × 10	Curls 3 × 10
MB side throws 3 × 8–10	Lying triceps ext. 3 × 10	Wrist/reverse curls 3 × 10
Sit-ups 3 × 25–50	Internal/external rotations 3 × 10	Torso rotations 3 × 25
Four-way neck 2 × 10	Scapula stabilizer circuit 2 × 10	Stability ball crunches 3 × 50
Weeks 5–8		
Hang clean 4 × 5	Power snatch 4 × 5	Hang clean 4 × 5
Squat 4 × 6–8	Bench press 4 × 6–8	Dead lift 4 × 6–8
DB jump squat 3 × 6	Alternate DB incline press 3 × 8–10	Bent-over rows 3 × 8–10
Box step-ups 3 × 10	DB jabs, uppercuts, hooks 3 ×15–20	Weighted pull-ups 3 × 10–15
Back extensions 3 × 8–10	SB push-ups 3 × 15–20	Curls 3 × 10
MB side throws 3 × 8–10	Lying triceps ext. 3 × 10	Wrist/reverse curls 3 × 10
Sit-ups 3 × 25–50	Internal/external rotations 3 × 10	Barbell twists 3 × 15
Four-way neck 2 × 10	Scapula stabilizer circuit 2 × 10	KB rotation swings 3 × 15–20

Table 18.8 12-Week Boxing Strength Training Program[a] (Continued)

Monday	Wednesday	Friday
Weeks 9–12		
Hang clean 5 × 3	Power snatch 5 × 3	Hang clean 5 × 3
Squat 4 × 5	Bench press 4 × 5	Dead lift 4 × 5
DB jump squat 3 × 6	Alternate DB incline press 3 × 8–10	Bent-over rows 3 × 6–8
Lunges 3 × 8–10	DB jabs, uppercuts, hooks 3 ×15–20	Weighted pull-ups 3 × 10–15
Back extensions 3 × 8–10	Push-ups (on fists) 3 × 20–25	Curls 3 × 10
Russian twists 3 × 25–50	Triceps push-down 3 × 10	Wrist/reverse curls 3 × 10
Sit-ups 3 × 25–50	Internal/external rotations 3 × 10	Barbell twists 3 × 20
Four-way neck 2 × 10	Scapula stabilizer circuit 2 × 10	KB rotation swings 3 × 15–20

Intensity — 60%–90% of 1 RM periodized. Rest Intervals — 2–3 minutes for core exercises; 1–2 minutes for assistance exercises; 30 seconds to 1 minute for abs. KB, kettle bells; SB, stability ball; MB, medicine ball; DB, dumbbell.

[a]Only includes resistance training workouts; aerobic training, road work, plyometrics/agility, and boxing specific workouts (*i.e.*, heavy bag work, speed bag work, sparring, shadow boxing, etc.) performed separately.

Reprinted with permission from Hoffman JR, Ratamess NA. *A Practical Guide to Developing Resistance Training Programs*. 2nd ed. Monterey (CA): Coaches Choice Books; 2008.

Myths & Misconceptions
Only Athletes Can Benefit from Periodized Training

Some individuals have suggested that periodized training programs are most suitable for athletes with little applicability to other populations. However, studies show that essentially all populations can benefit from periodized training when it has been suitably adapted to meet the needs of those individuals (63). For example, one study showed that a 4-week undulating periodized strength training program produced substantial work-related improvements in patients rehabilitating from lumbar fusion surgery (10). Part of the misconception may develop from the perception among some that all periodized training programs involve some combination of high-intensity resistance, sprint, agility, aerobic endurance, and/or plyometric training. Although that may be the case for athletes, the acute program variables can be manipulated to meet the needs of any population. Periodization simply involves planned variation that can accommodate training at all levels. Several studies have examined periodized programs in untrained populations and showed strength gains and high rates of adherence (63). The key element is that periodized training includes planned variation, and a training program can be varied in numerous ways to meet the needs of a population. There are infinite ways to develop variations of periodization models by manipulating the exercises, order of exercise performance, intensity, volume, rest intervals, and frequency. For example, variations of classic and undulating models can be developed to target intensity and volume ranges that are more appealing to the general population (8–15 reps). A periodized program does not have to culminate in a peaking phase where some exercises are performed for 1–3 reps of heavy weights of more than 95% of 1 RM. Rather, a target zone of low-to-moderate intensities can be used if that meets the goals of the individual. Periodization implies variation and all individuals who exercise need to vary the training stimulus to avoid plateaus and boredom. The keys to improvement are progressive overload, variation, and training specificity (63), and periodized programs include elements of all of these to improve performance and various parameters of health. *The ACSM recommends training periodization for healthy adults and older adults when development of optimal fitness is the goal* (76).

SUMMARY POINTS

- Periodization is the process of manipulating training program variables to bring the athlete to maximal performance at the appropriate time of the year and to reduce the risk of overtraining. It is superior to nonperiodized training for progression in strength and power.
- Several models of periodization are based on the work of Matveyev who divided training into preparatory, competition, and transition phases. The yearly macrocycle can be divided into mesocycles and microcycles to target specific goals.
- Periodized training is rooted in the work of Dr. Hans Selye who characterized adaptation into three segments: alarm, resistance, and exhaustion.
- Tapering for single-competition athletes enhances performance. Although several tapers are used successfully, it is recommended that a 2-week fast exponential taper be used at high intensity with similar frequency and 41%–60% reduction in volume.
- Often-studied models of periodization include the classic, block, undulating, and reverse linear models. All are successful for increasing performance. Some studies show similar improvements between classic and undulating models, whereas some studies show undulating or the classic model superior.
- Periodized programs can be designed for all components of fitness including strength, power, speed, agility, aerobic endurance, muscle endurance, and plyometric training.

REVIEW QUESTIONS

1. A short 1-week cycle that makes up part of a larger cycle is a
   a. Monocycle
   b. Macrocycle
   c. Mesocycle
   d. Microcycle

2. A standard reduction in training volume load after a period of high-intensity training or overreaching (peaking cycle) is known as a
   a. Step taper
   b. Linear taper
   c. Fast exponential taper
   d. Slow exponential taper

3. A progressive rise in intensity with concomitant decrease in volume with each training phase is characteristic of the _____ model of periodization.
   a. Reverse linear
   b. Classic
   c. Daily undulating
   d. Weekly undulating

4. When planning a taper phase, a reduction in training _____ is most recommended.
   a. Intensity
   b. Rest intervals
   c. Volume
   d. None of the above

5. The preparatory phase of training for a soccer player is characterized by
   a. Low volume, low intensity
   b. Low volume, high intensity
   c. High volume, low intensity
   d. High volume, high intensity

6. The first phase of General Adaptation Syndrome characterized by the magnitude of the training stimulus is the
   a. Alarm phase
   b. Adaptation phase
   c. Maladaptation phase
   d. Exhaustion phase

7. Periodization is the process of manipulating acute training program variables to maximize performance and reduce the risk of overtraining.
   a. T
   b. F

8. Periodization of training can only benefit elite athletes and has no application to recreational exercise.
   a. T
   b. F

9. The general preparatory phase consists of high volume, low intensity, and is used to prepare athletes for sport-specific training phases.
   a. T
   b. F

10. Tapering consists a nonlinear reduction in workload prior to a major competition.
    a. T
    b. F

11. Athletes attempting to maximize aerobic endurance performance benefit the most from use of a classical periodization model.
    a. T
    b. F

12. Periodization of sprint, agility, and plyometric training may follow a pattern similar to resistance training when peaking for strength and power.

a. T
b. F

REFERENCES

1. Stone MH, O'Bryant HS, Schilling BK, et al. Periodization: effects of manipulating volume and intensity. Part 1. *Strength Cond J.* 1999;21:56–62.
2. Issurin VB. Benefits and limitations of block periodized training approaches to athletes' preparation: a review. *Sports Med.* 2016;46:329–38.
3. Bompa TO, Haff GG. *Periodization: Theory and Methodology of Training.* 5th ed. Champaign (IL): Human Kinetics; 2009. p. 125–256.
4. Verkhoshansky Y, Siff M. *Supertraining.* 6th ed. Ultimate Athlete Concepts; 2009. p. 313–36.
5. Matveyev L. *Fundamentals of Sports Training.* Moscow: Progress; 1981.
6. Stone MH, O'Bryant H, Garhammer J. A hypothetical model for strength training. *J Sports Med.* 1981;21:342–51.
7. Fleck SJ. Periodized strength training: a critical review. *J Strength Cond Res.* 1999;13:82–9.
8. Kraemer WJ, Beeler MK. Periodization of resistance training: concepts and paradigms. In: Chandler TJ, Brown LE, editors. *Conditioning for Strength and Human Performance.* 3rd ed. New York (NY): Routledge; 2019. p. 371–94.
9. Herrick AB, Stone WJ. The effects of periodization versus progressive resistance exercise on upper and lower body strength in women. *J Strength Cond Res.* 1996;10:72–6.
10. Cole K, Kruger M, Bates D, Steil G, Zbreski M. Physical demand levels in individuals completing a sports performance-based work conditioning/hardening program after lumbar fusion. *Spine J.* 2009;9:39–46.
11. Fees M, Decker T, Snyder-Mackler L, Axe MJ. Upper extremity weight-training modifications for the injured athlete: a clinical perspective. *Am J Sports Med.* 1998;26:732–42.
12. Kerksick CM, Wilborn CD, Campbell BL, et al. Early-phase adaptations to a split-body, linear periodization resistance training program in college-aged and middle-aged men. *J Strength Cond Res.* 2009;23:962–71.
13. Extebarria N, Mujika I, Pyne DB. Training and competition readiness in triathlon. *Sports.* 2019;7:101.
14. Pritchard HJ, Tod DA, Barnes MJ, Keogh JW, McGuigan MR. Tapering practices of New Zealand's elite raw powerlifters. *J Strength Cond Res.* 2016;30:1796–804.
15. Durrell DL, Pujol TJ, Barnes JT. A survey of the scientific data and training methods utilized by collegiate strength and conditioning coaches. *J Strength Cond Res.* 2003;17:368–73.
16. Duehring MD, Feldmann CR, Ebben WP. Strength and conditioning practices of United States high school strength and conditioning coaches. *J Strength Cond Res.* 2009;23:2188–203.
17. Ebben WP, Blackard DO. Strength and conditioning practices of National Football League strength and conditioning coaches. *J Strength Cond Res.* 2001;15:48–58.
18. Ebben WP, Carroll RM, Simenz CJ. Strength and conditioning practices of National Hockey League strength and conditioning coaches. *J Strength Cond Res.* 2004;18:889–97.

19. Ebben WP, Hintz MJ, Simenz CJ. Strength and conditioning practices of Major League Baseball strength and conditioning coaches. *J Strength Cond Res.* 2005;19:538–46.
20. Simenz CJ, Dugan CA, Ebben WP. Strength and conditioning practices of National Basketball Association strength and conditioning coaches. *J Strength Cond Res.* 2005;19:495–504.
21. Jones TW, Smith A, Macnaughton LS, French DN. Strength and conditioning and concurrent training practices in elite rugby union. *J Strength Cond Res.* 2016;30:3354–66.
22. Selye H. *The Stress of Life.* New York (NY): McGraw-Hill; 1956.
23. Hoffman JR, Ratamess NA. *A Practical Guide to Developing Resistance Training Programs.* 2nd ed. Monterey (CA): Coaches Choice Books; 2008.
24. Mujika I, Padilla S. Scientific bases for precompetition tapering strategies. *Med Sci Sports Exerc.* 2003;35:1182–7.
25. Mujika I, Goya A, Padilla S, et al. Physiological responses to a 6-d taper in middle-distance runners: influence of training intensity and volume. *Med Sci Sports Exerc.* 2000;32:511–7.
26. Bosquet L, Leger L, Legros P. Methods to determine aerobic endurance. *Sports Med.* 2002;32:675–700.
27. Mujika I, Padilla S, Pyne D, Busso T. Physiological changes associated with the pre-event taper in athletes. *Sports Med.* 2004;34:891–927.
28. Papacosta E, Gleeson M, Nassis GP. Salivary hormones, IgA, and performance during intense training and tapering in judo athletes. *J Strength Cond Res.* 2013;27:2569–80.
29. Marrier B, Robineau J, Piscione J, et al. Supercompensation kinetics of physical qualities during a taper in team-sport athletes. *Int J Sports Physiol Perform.* 2017;12:1163–9.
30. Bazyler CD, Mizuguchi S, Harrison AP, et al. Changes in muscle architecture, explosive ability, and track and field throwing performance throughout a competitive season and after a taper. *J Strength Cond Res.* 2017;31:2785–93.
31. Skovgaard C, Almquist NWA, Kvorning T, Christensen PM, Bangsbo J. Effect of tapering after a period of high-volume sprint interval training on running performance and muscular adaptations in moderately trained runners. *J Appl Physiol.* 2018;124:259–67.
32. Spilsbury KL, Nimmo MA, Fudge BW, et al. Effects of an increase in intensity during tapering on 1500-m running performance. *Appl Physiol Nutr Metab.* 2019;44:783–90.
33. Bosquet L, Montpetit J, Arvisais D, Mujika I. Effects of tapering on performance: a meta-analysis. *Med Sci Sports Exerc.* 2007;39:1358–65.
34. Izquierdo M, Ibanez J, Gonzalez-Badillo JJ, et al. Detraining and tapering effects on hormonal responses and strength performance. *J Strength Cond Res.* 2007;21:768–75.
35. Ratamess NA, Kraemer WJ, Volek JS, et al. The effects of amino acid supplementation on muscular performance during resistance training overreaching. *J Strength Cond Res.* 2003;17:250–8.
36. Volek JS, Ratamess NA, Rubin MR, et al. The effects of creatine supplementation on muscular performance and body composition responses to short-term resistance training overreaching. *Eur J Appl Physiol.* 2004;91:628–37.
37. Winwood PW, Dudson MK, Wilson D, et al. Tapering practices of strongman athletes. *J Strength Cond Res.* 2018;32:1181–96.
38. Pritchard HJ, Barnes MJ, Stewart RJC, Keogh JWL, McGuigan MR. Short-term training cessation as a method of tapering to improve maximal strength. *J Strength Cond Res.* 2018;32:458–65.
39. Grgic J, Mikulic P. Tapering practices of Croatian open-class powerlifting champions. *J Strength Cond Res.* 2017;31:2371–8.

40. Pritchard HJ, Barnes MJ, Stewart RJ, Keogh JW, McGuigan MR. Higher-versus lower-intensity strength-training taper: effects on neuromuscular performance. *Int J Sports Physiol Perform.* 2019;14:458–63.

41. Bazyler CD, Mizuguchi S, Zourdos MC, et al. Characteristics of a national level female weightlifter peaking for competition: a case study. *J Strength Cond Res.* 2018;32:3029–38.

42. Suarez DG, Mizuguchi S, Hornsby WG, Cunanan AJ, Marsh DJ, Stone MH. Phase-specific changes in rate of force development and muscle morphology throughout a block periodized training cycle in weightlifters. *Sports.* 2019;7:129.

43. Issurin VB. New horizons for the methodology and physiology of training periodization. *Sports Med.* 2010;40:189–206.

44. Molmen KS, Ofsteng SJ, Ronnestad BR. Block periodization of endurance training—a systematic review and meta-analysis. *Open Access J Sports Med.* 2019;10:145–60.

45. Bartolomei S, Hoffman JR, Merni F, Stout JR. A comparison of traditional and block periodization strength training programs in trained athletes. *J Strength Cond Res.* 2014;28:990–7.

46. Painter KB, Haff GG, Ramsey MW, et al. Strength gains: block versus daily undulating periodization weight training among track and field athletes. *Int J Sports Physiol Perform.* 2012;7:161–9.

47. Kraemer WJ, Fleck SJ. *Optimizing Strength Training: Designing Nonlinear Periodization Workouts.* Champaign (IL): Human Kinetics; 2007. p. 1–256.

48. Buford TW, Rossi SJ, Smith DB, Warren AJ. A comparison of periodization models during nine weeks with equated volume and intensity for strength. *J Strength Cond Res.* 2007;21:1245–50.

49. Hartmann H, Bob A, Wirth K, Schmidtbleicher D. Effects of different periodization models on rate of force development and power ability of the upper extremity. *J Strength Cond Res.* 2009;23:1921–32.

50. Hoffman JR, Ratamess NA, Klatt M, et al. Comparison between different off-season resistance training programs in Division III American college football players. *J Strength Cond Res.* 2009;23:11–9.

51. Kok LY, Hamer PW, Bishop DJ. Enhancing muscular qualities in untrained women: linear versus undulating periodization. *Med Sci Sports Exerc.* 2009;41:1797–807.

52. Monteiro AG, Aoki MS, Evangelista AL, et al. Nonlinear periodization maximizes strength gains in split resistance training routines. *J Strength Cond Res.* 2009;23:1321–6.

53. Prestes J, Frollini AB, de Lima C, et al. Comparison between linear and daily undulating periodized resistance training to increase strength. *J Strength Cond Res.* 2009;23:2437–42.

54. Rhea MR, Ball SD, Phillips WT, Burkett LN. A comparison of linear and daily undulating periodized programs with equated volume and intensity for strength. *J Strength Cond Res.* 2002;16:250–5.

55. Hoffman JR, Wendell M, Cooper J, Kang J. Comparison between linear and nonlinear in-season training programs in freshman football players. *J Strength Cond Res.* 2003;17:561–5.

56. Harries SK, Lubans DR, Callister R. Systematic review and meta-analysis of linear and undulating periodized resistance training programs on muscular strength. *J Strength Cond Res.* 2015;29:1113–25.

57. Rhea MR, Phillips WT, Burkett LN, et al. A comparison of linear and daily undulating periodized programs with equated volume and intensity for local muscular endurance. *J Strength Cond Res.* 2003;17:82–7.

58. Prestes J, De Lima C, Frollini AB, Donatto FF, Conte M. Comparison of linear and reverse linear periodization effects on maximal strength and body composition. *J Strength Cond Res.* 2009;23:266–74.

59. Bradbury DG, Landers GJ, Benjanuvatra N, Goods PSR. Comparison of linear and reverse linear periodized programs with equated volume and intensity for endurance running performance. *J Strength Cond Res.* 2020;34:1345–53.

60. Clemente-Suarez VJ, Dalamitros A, Ribeiro J, Sousa A, Fernandes RJ, Vilas-Boas JP. The effects of two different swimming training periodization on physical parameters at various exercise intensities. *Eur J Sport Sci.* 2017;17:425–32.

61. Clemente-Suarez VJ, Ramos-Campo DJ. Effectiveness of reverse vs traditional linear training periodization in triathlon. *Int J Environ Res Publ Health.* 2019;16:2807.

62. Hoffman J. *Physiological Aspects of Sport Training and Performance.* Champaign (IL): Human Kinetics; 2002. p. 109–19.

63. Kraemer WJ, Ratamess NA. Fundamentals of resistance training: progression and exercise prescription. *Med Sci Sports Exerc.* 2004;36:674–88.

64. Kraemer WJ. A series of studies—the physiological basis for strength training in American football: fact over philosophy. *J Strength Cond Res.* 1997;11:131–42.

65. Kraemer WJ, Häkkinen K, Triplett-McBride NT, et al. Physiological changes with periodized resistance training in women tennis players. *Med Sci Sports Exerc.* 2003;35:157–68.

66. Kraemer WJ, Nindl BC, Ratamess NA, et al. Changes in muscle hypertrophy in women with periodized resistance training. *Med Sci Sports Exerc.* 2004;36:697–708.

67. Kraemer WJ, Ratamess N, Fry AC, et al. Influence of resistance training volume and periodization on physiological and performance adaptations in college women tennis players. *Am J Sports Med.* 2000;28:626–33.

68. Marx JO, Ratamess NA, Nindl BC, et al. The effects of single-set vs. periodized multiple-set resistance training on muscular performance and hormonal concentrations in women. *Med Sci Sports Exerc.* 2001;33:635–43.

69. O'Bryant HS, Byrd R, Stone MH. Cycle ergometer performance and maximum leg and hip strength adaptations to two different methods of weight-training. *J Appl Sport Sci Res.* 1988;2:27–30.

70. Stone MH, Potteiger JA, Pierce KC, et al. Comparison of the effects of three different weight-training programs on the one repetition maximum squat. *J Strength Cond Res.* 2000;14:332–7.

71. Willoughby DS. A comparison of three selected weight training programs on the upper and lower body strength of trained males. *Ann J Appl Res Coaching Athletics.* 1992;March:124–46.

72. Willoughby DS. The effects of meso-cycle-length weight training programs involving periodization and partially equated volumes on upper and lower body strength. *J Strength Cond Res.* 1993;7:2–8.

73. Baker D, Wilson G, Carlyon R. Periodization: the effect on strength of manipulating volume and intensity. *J Strength Cond Res.* 1994;8:235–42.

74. Williams TD, Tolusso DV, Fedewa MV, Esco MR. Comparison of periodized and non-periodized resistance training on maximal strength: a meta-analysis. *Sports Med.* 2017;47:2083–100.

75. Rhea MR, Alderman BL. A meta-analysis of periodized versus nonperiodized strength and power training programs. *Res Q Exerc Sport.* 2004;75:413–22.

76. American College of Sports Medicine. American College of Sports Medicine Position Stand. Progression models in resistance training for healthy adults. *Med Sci Sports Exerc.* 2009;41:687–708.

PART IV

Assessment

CHAPTER 19: Assessment and Evaluation

OBJECTIVES

After completing this chapter, you will be able to:

- Discuss the importance of testing and evaluation of athletes
- Discuss the importance of selecting tests that are valid and reliable
- Discuss the importance of selecting assessments, which measure the health-related fitness components of body composition, muscle strength and endurance, cardiovascular endurance, and flexibility
- Discuss the importance of selecting assessments, which measure the skill-related fitness components of power, speed, agility, and balance/coordination
- Discuss the importance of posture and balance testing

Testing and evaluation of athletes are critical components of sports training. Testing serves many functions that benefit the athlete and coach:

- *Testing can identify athletic strengths and weaknesses*: Training programs are designed, in part, to correct weaknesses. "A chain is only as strong as its weakest link" is a common expression used in sports. The results of testing allow the coach and athlete to recognize strengths and weaknesses. For example, if the athlete scores well (top 95%) on various strength measures but is lower on power measures, then it is wise for the coach to prioritize power training. The necessary time needed to increase strength further may impede potential time for the athlete to focus on weaknesses. Power training could take precedence in this athlete. Although strength is a precursor to power development, some athletes have high levels of strength (based on slow-velocity assessments) but do not move at a high enough velocity needed for their sport. Testing results reveal a potential weakness and direct the coach to include more high-velocity exercises to produce balanced athletic development.
- *Evaluation of progress*: Testing is critical to evaluating progress from the athletes' training programs. Although a coach can get a sense of progress from training logs, specific assessments evaluate the efficacy of the training program and serve as a motivational factor for improvement. A regular testing schedule gives the athlete a target date to peak fitness performance.
- *Identifying training loads*: The results of strength assessments serve a basis for intensity prescription for structural exercises during resistance training (RT). For example, one microcycle of the yearly periodized scheme may entail the athlete perform an exercise at 70% of his/her 1 RM. The coach needs to know the 1 RM to accurately prescribe the training load. Strength testing results can be used for load prescription. This applies to aerobic exercise prescription when intensity is prescribed as a percentage of $\dot{V}O_{2max}$ (or $\dot{V}O_2R$).
- *Assessment of athletic talent*: The results of testing can help the coach properly identify athletes participating in certain sports. This may be particularly true for younger athletes. An athlete who scores low on strength and power assessments but high on an aerobic capacity assessment can be directed by a coach to participate in endurance-based sports. Testing can be used as a form of athletic identification for specific sports. The earlier an athlete identifies the qualities needed for success in certain sports, the sooner training can begin to maximize that athlete's potential.

Test Selection and Administration

Tests should be valid, reliable, and used with stringent standards. **Validity** refers to the degree which a test measures what it is supposed to measure (1). Different types of validity can be seen.

Construct validity is the ability of a test to represent the underlying theory or construct. It is of particular interest to the athlete or coach as it is a primary source of validity for the test. For example, the 225-lb bench press test is extensively used at National Football League (NFL) combines. Its ability to assess strength is highly questionable unless the athlete's 1 RM is near 225 lb. An athlete who performs 25 repetitions for the test is truly being assessed on local muscular endurance; therefore, the validity of this test is poor for most athletes. *Face validity* gives the appearance to the athlete and other observers that the test is measuring what it is supposed to. Face validity increases the athlete's motivation and response to the test. *Content validity* refers to the observations of experts regarding a test or a testing battery. A coach can ensure high content validity by performing a needs analysis along with metabolic, kinesiological, and biomechanical breakdowns of the sport to develop a specific test battery. *Criterion-referenced validity* (the extent test scores correlate to sports performance skills) is critical to test selection. For example, 1 RM squat correlates to vertical jump performance. Thus, tests with high criterion-referenced validity relate highly to sport-specific performance and should be included in the testing battery.

Reliability is a measure of the magnitude of repeatability or consistency a test exhibits (1). Tests selected must provide reliable measures of athletic performance. For example, an athlete who scores a peak power output of 4,600 W during a jump squat on 1 day and 5,850 W just 3 days later will not be given reliable results. Clearly some alterations in testing conditions were evident to explain such large variation (it is unlikely for an athlete to increase power this much in 3 days if testing was conducted properly). Reliability depends upon the accuracy of the tester, equipment (use and calibration), and dietary and environmental conditions. Having different coaches perform similar tests (skinfold test, 40-yd dash) can reduce reliability (*intertester reliability*) especially if there is some degree of subjectivity to the test (*i.e.*, postural and mobility screening). Everyone has differences in technique and these differences are reflected by variations in scores. Standardization of testing procedures is mandatory for reliable results. Determination of **test-retest reliability** (correlation between multiple testing days) is mandatory for research purposes but can serve useful to the coach as well. In research, test-retest reliability data of 0.90 or higher is considered excellent, whereas values below 0.70 are considered low, thereby leaving question to the accuracy of the data collected. A test cannot be valid if it is not reliable. Reliability is maximized when standard principles of test selection and administration are strictly adhered to.

The tests selected should be as specific to the sport as possible and should be valid for the fitness component being measured. In fact, sport-specific tests may be developed, validated, and norms generated. A few examples of sport-specific testing may include the Lane agility test for basketball players (2), the sandbag throw conditioning test for wrestlers (3), and specific striking assessments for mixed martial arts fighters (4). Figure 19.1 outlines important testing considerations. Tests should be selected that are metabolically (energy system) and biomechanically (movement pattern) specific to the athlete's sport. The training status of the athlete is important. A well-trained athlete may have very good technique and will be able to apply 100% effort in each trial. A lesser-skilled athlete may have technical difficulties, which could limit his/her level of effort. Test complexity must match the skill set of the athletes. Practice is critical to test selection and administration. A lack of familiarization/practice will result in poor performances that could have been better, provided the athlete had at least 1–2 practice sessions. For example, untrained older women need ~3 times as many familiarization sessions before strength testing than young women (5). Familiarization affects effort and maximal effort can only be applied when the athlete is familiar with the test. In research, a lack of familiarization is evidenced by very large increases in strength over short-term training periods. Experienced athletes require little familiarization but a short practice session could

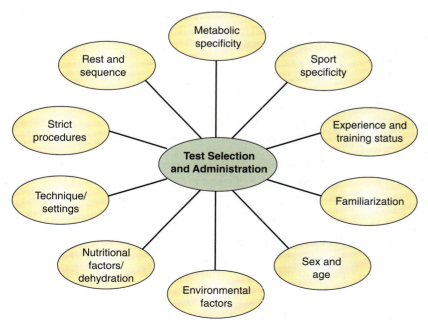

FIGURE 19.1 Factors affecting test selection and administration.

be beneficial. If athletes are not being tested on drills they routinely perform in training, at least 1–2 practice sessions should be given and possibly more depending on individual responses.

The age and gender of the athletes could play a role in test selection and administration. Older individuals need more preparation time for maximal testing. Young (children and adolescents) athletes may require more familiarization as well. Although most tests can be applied similarly for both genders, performance will vary and some caution may be necessary. For example, a pull-up test in men can be used as an assessment of muscle endurance. However, in many women (due to upper-body strength differences), it may be viewed more as a strength test as opposed to an endurance test.

Environmental (temperature, humidity, altitude, precipitation, terrain) factors can affect testing results. Temperature (hot and cold) plays a role indoors and outdoors. For example, testing an athlete's aerobic capacity 1 day in 98°F (with high humidity) weather versus 77°F (with low humidity) has a substantial effect on performance. Greater health risks are prevalent in hot and humid weather. Hot and humid weather negatively affects aerobic more than anaerobic performance (6,7). Temperature plays a role indoors, but it is controllable by the coach. It is important to test the athlete at a similar altitude. Changing altitudes can alter aerobic endurance performance. The level of precipitation is critical. Any moisture or wetness on the surface can affect athletic performance to some degree especially if the athlete is being tested in rainy conditions versus a nonprecipitous day. Lastly, the terrain is important. Maximal athletic performance can vary depending on the surface (grass vs. turf vs. sand vs. hills vs. concrete). The coach should test athletes in the most ideal ways as possible, and attempting to control environmental factors is important. This includes standardizing clothing and footwear, as a new pair of athletic shoes can reduce sprint and agility times compared to an older pair of shoes.

Nutritional factors play considerable roles during testing. An athlete who is nutrient deficient or dehydrated may not perform up to task especially during aerobic endurance assessments. Body composition analyses can be compromised by altered hydration and nutrient status. Adequate fluid, carbohydrate, protein, and micronutrient intake is needed to maximize performance (8). Standardization is important. Standardization includes sports supplements, *e.g.*, creatine monohydrate, which enhances performance (8,9). Testing an athlete on one occasion where nutrient intake is superior to testing on another ccasion can affect the results especially if supplements are not accounted for. Coaches need to be cognizant of athlete's nutritional habits and should encourage a high-quality, nutrient-dense meal the evening before testing as well as adequate food and beverage intake up to ~1–2 hours before testing.

Test administration plays a critical role in measuring athletic performance including the procedures used, settings, equipment, or techniques used during each exercise, range of motion (ROM) used, sequence of testing, and rest intervals between trials. The coach and staff must ensure that strict procedural standardization is employed or results will be affected by errors.

Several administration factors should be addressed prior to testing. The testing staff should be carefully considered and well trained. Everyone needs to function similarly and use standardized procedures. Technique should be synchronized so all testers use similar criteria especially when a large group of athletes are being tested simultaneously. All testers should be highly familiar with the tests and protocols used. If possible, one tester should oversee the testing of a single component. For example, one tester should perform all skinfold tests for body composition and one tester should time all sprint and agility tests for consistency. Multiple testers of the same assessment increases variability. Tests should be well organized and administered efficiently. Athletes should be carefully instructed on test performance and should be encouraged during performance. Fatigue should be minimized so the sequence of tests is critical. Testing can be made more efficient when it occurs on multiple days. However, some tests can be performed in the same day while minimizing fatigue from previous tests. Figure 19.2 depicts a general recommended testing sequence when multiple tests are performed. These tests can be separated into multiple

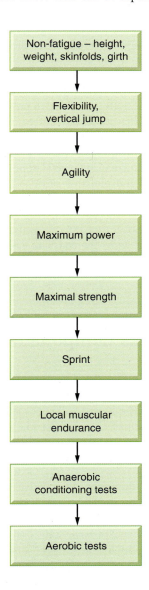

FIGURE 19.2 Recommended sequence of testing.

Myths & Misconceptions
Testing Must Be Performed Frequently to Be Useful

Some have advocated frequent testing of athletes. However, testing can be a useful tool if it is performed at a lower frequency as well. The type of test is important. Some tests (body weight, percent body fat, and flexibility) can be performed frequently (daily) because they are not strenuous on the athlete's body. For example, frequent body weight, percent fat, and hydration status (urine-specific gravity) testing for a wrestler is advantageous based on the needs of the sport for constant monitoring. However, some assessments are more suited for less frequent testing (1 RM strength). Maximal strength testing may occur only a few times in a year. A coach can get a sense of whether the athlete is progressing or not by closely monitoring training logs. A coach can indirectly ascertain if the athlete is improving when his/her training weights/repetitions have increased. The need for testing decreases when the coach can gain valuable information from training logs. The critical component is that testing should not interfere with the athlete's training schedule.

testing days when needed. The sequence involves low-fatigue assessments initially and progresses to more challenging and fatiguing tests.

All steps should be taken by the testing staff to ensure maximal safety of the athletes. This includes the decision to test or not test an athlete with a predisposing injury, illness, or medical condition. Although testing can be beneficial, it is not worth the risk of causing potential damage to an injured athlete. Close monitoring is necessary and constant communication with the athletic training and medical staffs is essential to properly screen athletes at risk for injury. Environmental conditions must be factored. Hot and humid conditions pose a threat to athletes, so caution must be used when planning a testing session on a hot/humid day. Lastly, proper data management is important. All data forms should be designed and prepared prior to testing. Data can be stored in a database for record keeping. Spreadsheets are recommended as they allow the coach not only the ability to monitor testing performance over time but can be used to develop norms and standards. They allow the coach to easily calculate means, standard deviations, or perform some general statistical procedures that are used to compare means over time.

Assessment of Health-Related Fitness Components

Testing of several health-related components of fitness is paramount to a comprehensive testing battery for athletes. These include body composition and anthropometry, muscle strength and endurance, cardiovascular (CV) endurance, and flexibility.

Body Composition and Anthropometry

Body composition describes the relative proportions of fat, bone, and muscle mass in the human body. **Anthropometry** is a term describing measurement of the human body in terms of dimensions such as height, weight (or body mass), circumferences, girths, and skinfolds. In Chapter 2, we discussed various elements of anthropometry including biomechanical elements of size, body types, and limb lengths. Body composition and anthropometric assessments are standard practice for coaches and athletes. Valuable information regarding percent body fat, fat distribution, LBM, limb lengths, and circumferences are gained through body composition assessment. Body composition tests may be useful for evaluating training, diet, or athletic performance, or for reducing the risk factors associated with musculoskeletal injury. Sport performance is highly dependent on the health- and skill-related components of fitness in addition to technique and level of motor skill competency. All fitness components depend on body composition to some extent. For example, an increase in LBM contributes to strength and power development and may contribute to speed, quickness, and agility performance. Reduced nonessential body fat contributes to muscular and cardiorespiratory endurance, speed, and agility development. However, too much additional weight may provide greater resistance to athletic motion and could limit endurance, balance, coordination, and movement capacity. Thus, higher strength-to-mass ratios are needed by some athletes especially endurance athletes and those in sports with weight classes.

There are several ways to measure body composition in athletes including skinfold tests, bioelectrical impedance analysis (BIA), dual X-ray absorptiometry (DXA), underwater weighing, computed tomography (CT) and magnetic resonance imaging (MRI) scans, air displacement plethysmography (ADP; i.e., BOD POD), and near-infrared interactance (NIR) (10,11), although other less practical methods have been used. Each has advantages and disadvantages (Table 19.1). Although DXA use has increased over the several years especially in research settings, underwater weighing is still considered the "gold standard" of body composition assessment and is the preferred method of comparison when validating and developing prediction equations for skinfold analysis. Skinfold assessment, underwater weighing, ADP, and BIA are discussed in more detail in this chapter. Testing consists of analyzing different body composition components. Techniques discussed in this chapter are 2C and 3C models. Body composition models include

- 2 Component (2C): fat mass and lean tissue mass
- 3 Component (3C): fat mass, lean tissue mass, and bone mass; or fat mass, lean tissue mass, and water
- 4 Component (4C): fat mass, bone mass, protein, and water
- 5 Component (5C): fat mass, bone mass, protein, extracellular water, and intracellular water

Chapter 19 Assessment and Evaluation   597

Table 19.1	Advantages and Disadvantages of Popular Body Composition Assessment Techniques	
Assessment	**Advantages**	**Disadvantages**
BMI	Easy to use with minimal equipment	Not valid for athletes
	Noninvasive	Does not account for large muscle mass
Girth	Easy to administer	Girth size not always related to fat content
	Need tape measure	Less accurate than other methods
	Quick with many formulas to select from	
	Good indicator of size changes	
Skinfold	Easy to use once trained	Prone to technician error
	Time efficient and noninvasive	Less accurate for very lean or obese individuals
	Inexpensive	Considers subcutaneous fat
	Many equations to choose from	Potential discomfort via pinching or embarrassment
	Can test many athletes in less time	
Underwater weighing	"Gold standard"	Time consuming
	Very accurate, valid, and reliable when proper procedures used	Requires costly equipment, space
		Requires in-depth examiner knowledge
		Water submersion can be uncomfortable
		Requires measure of lung volume
BIA	Requires little technical expertise	Several confounding variables must be avoided
	Testing is fast	High degree of error if procedures are not strictly followed
	Very easy especially with scale or handheld models	
	Unit is easily transportable	
	Does not require minimal clothing	
ADP	Relaxed atmosphere for individual	Very expensive
	Easy to operate	Equipment not very accessible
	Short measurement time	Must wear minimal, tight clothing
	Good for every population	
	Accurate	
DXA	Very accurate	Very expensive
	Radiation exposure is low	Less accurate when going from one DXA unit to another
	Comprehensive measurements	May require prescription from physician
	Can wear regular clothing	
	Relatively quick measurement time	
	Subject relaxed during test	
	Gives regional measurements	

Modified from Ratamess NA. Body composition. In: T Miller, editor. *NSCA's Guide to Tests and Assessments*. Champaign (IL): Human Kinetics; 2012. p. 15-41.

Height, Body weight, and Body Mass Index

Height and body weight are basic measurements. Height is assessed with a *stadiometer* (a vertical ruler mounted on a wall with a wide horizontal headboard). Height can vary slightly throughout the day where values are higher in the morning. When measuring height, the athlete needs to remove shoes, stand as straight as possible with heels together, take a deep breath, hold it, and stand with head level. Body weight is best measured on a calibrated physician's scale with a beam and moveable weights. Clothing is a major issue and should be standardized (shoes removed, minimal clothing, items removed from pockets). Body weight changes at various times of day due to meal/beverage consumption, urination, defecation, and dehydration/water loss. A standard time (early in the morning) is recommended. Body mass index (BMI) is used to assess body mass relative to height. It is primarily used in untrained or clinical populations (as it may correlate to various disease states) but has little practical value in athletes. It is calculated by

$$\text{BMI}\,(\text{kg}\cdot\text{m}^{-2}) = \text{body mass (kg) / height squared (m}^2)$$

Skinfold Assessment

Skinfold assessments are one of the most popular and practical methods to estimate percent body fat. Skinfold assessment can be relatively accurate provided that a trained coach or technician is performing the measurement with high-quality calipers. Skinfold analysis is based on the principle that the amount of subcutaneous fat (fat immediately below the skin) is directly proportional to the total amount of body fat, and regression analysis is used to estimate total percent body fat. Variability in percent body fat prediction from skinfold analysis is ~±3%–5% assuming that appropriate techniques and equations are used. Body fat varies with gender, age, race or ethnicity, training status, and other factors so numerous regression equations have been developed to predict body density and percent fat from skinfold measurements. Skinfold assessment for athletes is most accurate when prediction equations are used that closely match the population. The number of sites range from 3 to 7. Prediction equations are used to estimate body density, and body density calculation is used to estimate percent body fat. **Body density** is described as the ratio of body mass to body volume.

The procedures for skinfold assessment include:

- The number of sites and equation are first selected (Fig. 19.3).
- A fold of skin is firmly grasped between the thumb and index finger of the left hand (about 8 cm apart) while the subject is relaxed. A larger grasping area (>8 cm) may be needed for large individuals who could max out the measurement capacity of the caliper.
- The jaws of the caliper are placed over the skinfold 1 cm below the fingers of the tester, released, and the measurement is taken within 2–3 seconds.
- All measurements are taken on the right side of the body 2–3 times for consistency to the nearest 0.5 mm. It is important to rotate through all of the sites first as opposed to taking two or three measurements sequentially from the same site.
- For several tests each site is averaged and summed to estimate body density and percent body fat via a regression equation or prediction table.

Table 19.2 depicts several equations used to estimate percent body fat from body density estimates. Those equations most appropriate to use will be selected based on gender, age, ethnicity, and activity level. Those appropriate equations should

have been cross-validated, and general equations have been shown to produce accurate estimates across all segments of the population. Percent body fat can be calculated once body density has been determined. Most often, the Siri (18) or Brozek (19) equations are used although other population-specific equations (Table 19.3) have been developed. Table 19.4 depicts classifications based on percent body fat.

$$\text{Siri Equation:}\,(4.95/B_d - 4.50)\times100$$

$$\text{Brozek Equation:}\,(4.57/B_d - 4.142)\times100$$

Girth Measurements

Girth measurements provide useful information regarding changes in muscle size and body composition. The advantages of taking circumference measurements is that it is easy, inexpensive, does not require specialized equipment (other than a tape measure), and quick to administer. The procedures for girth measurements include (10):

1. The tape measure is applied in a horizontal plane to the site so it is taut and the circumference is read to the nearest half of a centimeter. Minimal clothing should be worn.
2. Duplicate measures should be taken at each site and the average is used. If readings differ by more than 5–10 mm, then an additional measurement is taken.
3. Athletes should remain relaxed while measurements are taken.
4. A large source of error is a lack of standardization of the measurement site. The correct placement of the tape measure per site is as follows:
   a. *Chest* — tape is placed around the chest at level of the fourth ribs after subject abducts arms. Measurement is taken when athlete adducts arms back to starting position and at the end of respiration.
   b. *Shoulder* — tape is placed horizontally at the maximal circumference of the shoulders while athlete is standing relaxed.
   c. *Abdominal* — tape is placed over the abdomen at the level of the greatest circumference (often near the umbilicus) while athlete is standing relaxed.
   d. *Right thigh* — tape is placed horizontally over the thigh below the gluteal level at the largest circumference (upper thigh) while athlete is standing.
   e. *Right calf* — tape is placed horizontally over the largest circumference of the calf midway between the knee and ankle while athlete is standing relaxed.
   f. *Waist* — tape is placed around smallest area of the waist, ~1 in. above the navel.
   g. *Hip* — tape is placed around largest area of the buttocks (with minimal clothing).
   h. *Right upper arm* — tape is placed horizontally over the midpoint of the upper arm between the shoulder and elbow while athlete is standing, relaxed, and elbow is extended.
   i. *Right forearm* — tape is placed horizontally over the proximal area of the forearm where circumference is the largest while athlete is standing relaxed.

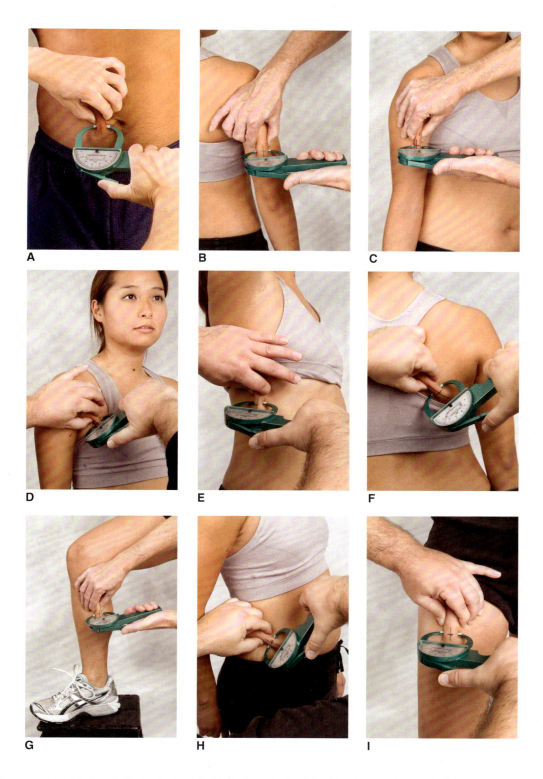

FIGURE 19.3 Common skinfold sites. **A.** Abdominal: vertical fold, 2 cm to the right side of the umbilicus. **B.** Triceps: vertical fold on the posterior midline of the upper arm, halfway between the acromion and olecranon processes, with the arm held freely to the side of the body. **C.** Biceps: vertical fold on the anterior aspect of the arm over the belly of the biceps muscle, 1 cm above the level used to mark the triceps site. **D.** Chest: diagonal fold, one-half the distance between the anterior axillary line and the nipple (men), or one-third of the distance between the anterior axillary line and the nipple (women). **E.** Midaxillary: vertical fold on the midaxillary line at the level of the xiphoid process of the sternum. An alternate method is a horizontal fold taken at the level of the xiphoid/sternal border in the midaxillary line. **F.** Subscapular: diagonal fold (at a 45° angle), 1–2 cm below the inferior angle of the scapula. **G.** Medial calf: vertical fold at the maximum circumference of the calf on the midline of its medial border. **H.** Suprailium: diagonal fold in line with the natural angle of the iliac crest taken in the anterior axillary line immediately superior to the iliac crest. **I.** Thigh: vertical fold; on the anterior midline of the thigh, midway between the proximal border of the patella and the inguinal crease (hip). (From Battista R, et al. *ACSM's Resources for the Personal Trainer*. 5th ed. Baltimore (MD): Lippincott Williams & Wilkins; 2018.)

Table 19.2 — Body Density Prediction Equations from Skinfold Measurements

Sites	Population	Gender	Equation	Reference
2: thigh, subscapular	Athletes	Male	$D_b = 1.1043 = (0.00133 = \text{thigh}) = (0.00131 = \text{subscapular})$	Sloan and Weir (12)
2: suprailiac, triceps	Athletes	Female	$D_b = 1.0764 - (0.00081 \times \text{suprailiac}) - (0.00088 \times \text{triceps})$	Sloan and Weir (12)
3: chest, abdomen, thigh	General	Male	$D_b = 1.10938 - 0.0008267 \,(\text{sum of 3 sites}) + 0.0000016 \,(\text{sum of 3 sites})^2 - 0.000257\,4 \,(\text{age})$	Jackson and Pollock (13)
3: triceps, suprailiac, thigh	General	Female	$D_b = 1.099421 - 0.0009929 \,(\text{sum of 3 sites}) + 0.0000023 \,(\text{sum of 3 sites})^2 - 0.0001392 \,(\text{age})$	Jackson et al. (14)
3: chest, triceps, subscapular	General	Male	$D_b = 1.1125025 - 0.0013125 \,(\text{sum of 3 sites}) + 0.0000055 \,(\text{sum of 3 sites})^2 - 0.000244 \,(\text{age})$	Pollock et al. (15)
3: triceps, suprailiac, abdomen	General	Female	$D_b = 1.089733 - 0.0009245 \,(\text{sum of 3 sites}) + 0.0000025 \,(\text{sum of 3 sites})^2 - 0.0000979 \,(\text{age})$	Jackson and Pollock (16)
4: biceps, triceps, subscapular, suprailiac	General	Male Female 20–29 yr	$D_b = 1.1631 - 0.0632 \,(\text{log sum of 4 sites})$	Durnin and Womersley (17)
4: biceps, triceps, subscapular, suprailiac	General	Male Female 30–39 yr	$D_b = 1.1422 - 0.0544 \,(\text{log sum of 4 sites})$	Durnin and Womersley (17)
7: thigh, subscapular, suprailiac, triceps, chest, abdomen, axillary	General	Female	$D_b = 1.0970 - 0.00046971 \,(\text{sum of 7 sites}) + 0.00000056 \,(\text{sum of 7 sites})^2 - 0.00012828 \,(\text{age})$	Jackson et al. (14)
7: thigh, subscapular, suprailiac, triceps, chest, abdomen, axillary	General	Male	$D_b = 1.112 - 0.00043499 \,(\text{sum of 7 sites}) + 0.00000055 \,(\text{sum of 7 sites})^2 - 0.00028826 \,(\text{age})$	Jackson and Pollock (13)

Table 19.3 — Population-Specific Equations to Calculate Percent Body Fat from Body Density

Population	Age	Sex	Equation
White	7–12	Male	$(5.30/D_b - 4.89) \times 100$
		Female	$(5.35/D_b - 4.95) \times 100$
	13–16	Male	$(5.07/D_b - 4.64) \times 100$
		Female	$(5.10/D_b - 4.66) \times 100$
	17–19	Male	$(4.99/D_b - 4.55) \times 100$
		Female	$(5.05/D_b - 4.62) \times 100$
	20–80	Male	$(4.95/D_b - 4.50) \times 100$
		Female	$(5.01/D_b - 4.57) \times 100$
African-American	18–32	Male	$(4.37/D_b - 3.93) \times 100$
	24–79	Female	$(4.85/D_b - 4.39) \times 100$
American Indian	18–60	Female	$(4.81/D_b - 4.34) \times 100$
Hispanic	20–40	Female	$(4.87/D_b - 4.41) \times 100$
Japanese	18–48	Male	$(4.97/D_b - 4.52) \times 100$
		Female	$(4.76/D_b - 4.28) \times 100$
	61–78	Male	$(4.87/D_b - 4.41) \times 100$
		Female	$(4.95/D_b - 4.50) \times 100$

Adapted with permission from Harman E, Garhammer J. Administration, scoring, and interpretation of selected tests. In: Baechle TR, Earle RW, editors. *Essentials of Strength Training and Conditioning*. 3rd ed. Champaign (IL): Human Kinetics; 2008. p. 249–92; Heyward VH, Stolarczyk LM. *Applied Body Composition Assessment*. Champaign (IL): Human Kinetics; 1996. 82 p. Ref. (20).

Table 19.4	Percent Body Fat Classifications						
%		20–29	30–39	40–49	50–59	60–69	70–79
Age, yr (Men)							
99	Very lean[a]	4.2	7.3	9.5	11.1	12.0	13.6
95		6.4	10.3	13.0	14.9	16.1	15.5
90	Excellent	7.9	12.5	15.0	17.0	18.1	17.5
85		9.1	13.8	16.4	18.3	19.2	19.0
80		10.5	14.9	17.5	19.4	20.2	20.2
75	Good	11.5	15.9	18.5	20.2	21.0	21.1
70		12.6	16.8	19.3	21.0	21.7	21.6
65		13.8	17.7	20.1	21.7	22.4	22.3
60		14.8	18.4	20.8	22.3	23.0	22.9
55	Fair	15.8	19.2	21.4	23.0	23.6	23.6
50		16.7	20.0	22.1	23.6	24.2	24.1
45		17.5	20.7	22.8	24.2	24.9	24.5
40		18.6	21.6	23.5	24.9	25.6	25.2
35	Poor	19.8	22.4	24.2	25.6	26.4	25.7
30		20.7	23.2	24.9	26.3	27.0	26.3
25		22.1	24.1	25.7	27.1	27.9	27.1
20		23.3	25.1	26.6	28.1	28.8	28.0
15	Very poor	25.1	26.4	27.7	29.2	29.8	29.3
10		26.6	27.8	29.1	30.6	31.2	30.6
5		29.3	30.2	31.2	32.7	33.5	32.9
1		33.7	34.4	35.2	36.4	37.2	37.3
$n =$		1,938	10,457	16,032	9,976	3,097	571
Total $n = 42,071.$							
Age, yr (Women)							
99	Very lean[b]	11.4	11.0	11.7	13.8	13.8	13.7
95		14.1	13.8	15.2	16.9	17.7	16.4
90	Excellent	15.2	15.5	16.8	19.1	20.1	18.8
85		16.1	16.5	18.2	20.8	22.0	21.2
80	Good	16.8	17.5	19.5	22.3	23.2	22.6
75		17.7	18.3	20.5	23.5	24.5	23.7
70		18.6	19.2	21.6	24.7	25.5	24.5
65		19.2	20.1	22.6	25.7	26.6	25.4
60		20.0	21.0	23.6	26.6	27.5	26.3
55	Fair	20.7	22.0	24.6	27.4	28.3	27.1
50		21.8	22.9	25.5	28.3	29.2	27.8
45		22.6	23.7	26.4	29.2	30.1	28.6
40		23.5	24.8	27.4	30.0	30.8	30.0
35	Poor	24.4	25.8	28.3	30.7	31.5	30.9
30		25.7	26.9	29.5	31.7	32.5	31.6
25		26.9	28.1	30.7	32.8	33.3	32.6
20		28.6	29.6	31.9	33.8	34.4	33.6
15	Very poor	30.9	31.4	33.4	34.9	35.4	35.0
10		33.8	33.6	35.0	36.0	36.6	36.1
5		36.6	36.2	37.0	37.4	38.1	37.5
1		38.4	39.0	39.0	39.8	40.3	40.0
$n =$		1,342	4,376	6,392	4,496	1,576	325
Total $n = 18,507.$							

[a]Very lean, no <3% body fat is recommended for men.

[b]Very lean, no <10%–13% body fat is recommended for women.

Adapted with permission from *Physical Fitness Assessments and Norms for Adults and Law Enforcement.* Dallas (TX): The Cooper Institute; 2013. For more information: www.cooperinstitute.org

Underwater Weighing (Hydrodensitometry)

Underwater weighing has been the criterion method, or gold standard, for body composition analysis. It is based on Archimedes' principle for determining body density where a body immersed in water encounters a buoyant force that results in weight loss equal to the weight of the water displaced during immersion. Subtracting the athlete's body weight in water from the body weight on land provides the weight of the displaced water. Body fat contributes to buoyancy because the density of fat (0.9007 $g \cdot cm^{-3}$) is less than water (1 $g \cdot cm^{-3}$), whereas lean tissue mass (1.100 $g \cdot cm^{-3}$) exceeds the density of water. Lean tissue density varies based on ethnicity and maturation. Large increases in muscle mass compared to BMD changes can lower body density and result in an overestimate of percent body fat. Body density is calculated and then converted to percent body fat using an equation such as the Siri or Brozek equations. Population-specific equations have been developed to more accurately convert body density data into percent body fat. Test-retest reliability is high when procedures are followed correctly. A tank made of stainless steel, fiberglass, ceramic tile, Plexiglas, or swimming pool (temperature of water should be between $91.4°F$ and $96.8°F$), i.e., at least $4 \times 4 \times 5$ ft is needed and so is a seat suspended from a scale or force transducer for weighing.

The following variables must be known when performing underwater weighing:

- *Residual volume*: The amount of air remaining in the lungs following full expiration. It can be measured or predicted using a combination of age, gender, and height. A substantial amount of air left in the lungs increases buoyancy, which may be mistaken as additional body fat.
- Water density
- Amount of trapped gas in GI system: A predicted constant of 100 mL is used.
- Dry body weight
- Body weight in water

The procedures for underwater weighing include:

- Subjects should wear minimal clothing. A tight-fitting bathing suit that traps little air is recommended. All jewelry should be removed and athlete should have urinated and defecated prior to the procedure.
- Subjects should be 2–12 hours postabsorptive and have avoided foods that increase gas in GI tract. Menstruation may pose a problem for females due to associated water gain; thus, women should not be tested within 7 days of menstruation.
- Subject is weighed on land to determine dry weight.
- Subject enters the tank, removes potential trapped air, and is seated on chair to be weighed (subject fully expires as much air as possible prior to leaning forward to be weighed).
- Subject is weighed 5–10 times while submerged underwater for 5–10 seconds. The highest or average of 3 highest weights are used (weight of chair and belt are considered in calculation).
- Residual lung volume can be measured directly (which increases accuracy) in some systems or estimated based on height and age:

Males : RV (L) = $[0.019 \times$ ht (cm)$] + [0.0155 \times$ age (yr)$] - 2.24$

Females : RV (L) = $[0.032 \times$ ht (cm)$] + [0.009 \times$ age (yr)$] - 3.90$

- Body density is calculated using the following equation:

BD = Mass in air (g)

([Mass in air (g) − mass in water (g)] / density of water) − (RV in mL − GI gas 100 mL)

- Body fat can be calculated using the Siri, Brozek, or population-specific equations

Bioelectrical Impedance Analysis

BIA is a noninvasive and easy-to-administer tool for determining body composition. The underlying principle is that electrical conductivity in the body is proportional to the fat-free tissue of the body. A small electrical current is sent through the body (from ankle to wrist), and the impedance to that current is measured. Lean tissue (mostly water and electrolytes) is a good electrical conductor (i.e., has low impedance), whereas fat is a poor conductor and impedes an electrical current. BIA can measure percent body fat and total body water. A common equation used is $V = pL^2 \cdot R^{-1}$, where V is the volume of the conductor, p is the specific resistance of the tissue, L is the length of the conductor, and R is the observed resistance (11). Accuracy among BIA devices varies greatly. Subjects should not have eaten or consumed a beverage within 4 hours of the test, exercised within 12 hours, or consumed alcohol or diuretics. The subject should have completely voided the bladder within 30 minutes of the test. Most BIA machines use their own equations that account for differences in water content and body density based on people's gender, age, and race or ethnicity, as well as physical activity levels.

The procedures for BIA include:

- BIA device should be calibrated according to the manufacturer's instructions.
- Subject lies supine on a nonconductive surface with arm and legs at the side, not in contact with the rest of the body. The right hand and wrist and right foot and ankle areas are prepared with alcohol and then allowed to dry.
- BIA electrodes are placed on the metacarpal of the right index finger and metatarsal of the right big toe, and the reference (detecting) electrodes are placed on the right wrist and right ankle.
- Current is applied and BIA analyzer computes the results.
- Some BIA devices are simpler to use and require the subject either to stand on the machine like a scale with moistened bare feet or hold the BIA analyzer in both hands.

Air Displacement Plethysmography

Body volume can be measured by air displacement. The BOD POD (a commercial ADP system) uses a dual-chamber (e.g., 450 L subject test chamber, 300 L reference chamber)

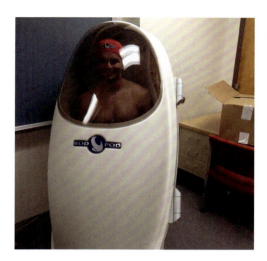

FIGURE 19.4 Photo of ADP testing.

plethysmograph that measures body volume via changes in air pressure within the closed two-compartment chamber. It includes an electronic weighing scale, computer, and software system. The volume of air displaced is equal to body volume and is calculated indirectly by subtracting the volume of air remaining in the chamber when the subject is inside from the volume of air in the chamber when it is empty. Reliability is good but sources of error include variations in testing conditions, the subject not being fasted, air that is not accounted for in the lungs or trapped within clothing and body hair, body moisture, and increased body temperature (Fig. 19.4).

The procedures for ADP include:

- Subject's information is entered in the computer and the unit is calibrated according to the manufacturer's instructions.
- Subject is properly prepared; minimal clothing is worn. Swimsuits, compression shorts, sport bras, and swim caps are recommended. Items such as jewelry and glasses are removed. Percent fat may be underestimated if a swimming cap is not worn.
- Subject's mass is determined via the digital scale.
- Subject enters the chamber and sits quietly during testing while a minimum of two measurements (within 150 mL of each other) are taken to determine body volume.
- Thoracic gas volume is measured during normal breathing (i.e., via the panting method, in which the subject breathes normally into a tube connected within the chamber, followed by three small puffs after the airway tube becomes momentarily occluded at the midpoint of exhalation) or can be predicted via equations.
- Corrected body volume (raw body volume − thoracic gas volume) is calculated, body density is determined, and percent body fat is calculated using prediction equations.

Muscle Strength

The most important reason to assess muscle strength is to evaluate strength training programs. Strength testing comes in various forms depending on the type of strength measured, e.g., dynamic concentric (CON) and eccentric (ECC), isometric (ISOM), or isokinetic (ISOK). The gold standard of dynamic strength testing is the 1 RM, which is performed with free weights and machines. Although other RMs can be used, the 1 RM provides the most accurate strength assessment when performed properly. The 1 RM is the maximal amount of weight that can be lifted once for a specific exercise at a given velocity. High test-retest reliabilities have been shown for 1 RM testing (intraclass correlations ranging from 0.79 to 0.99) (21). One RM testing can be performed with many exercises. However, multiple-joint exercises like the squat, bench press, deadlift, and power clean are most commonly used. The 1 RM power clean may be viewed as a power assessment as well. Although several protocols for strength testing can be effective, the following is a sample of one (21):

1. Following a general warm-up and specific warm-up consisting of selected dynamic flexibility or callisthenic exercises, a light warm-up of 5–10 repetitions at 40%–60% of perceived max is performed.
2. After a 1-minute rest, 3–5 repetitions at 60%–80% of perceived maximum is performed.
3. Step 2 will take the athlete close to the 1 RM. A conservative increase in weight is made, and a 1 RM lift is attempted. If the lift is successful, a rest period of ~3 minutes is allowed. It is important to allow enough rest before the next maximal attempt. A 1 RM should be obtained within 3–5 sets to avoid excessive fatigue. The process of increasing the weight up to a true 1 RM can be enhanced by prior familiarization and expertise of the coaches. This process continues until a failed attempt occurs then weight is adjusted accordingly.
4. The 1 RM value is recorded as the weight of the last successfully completed lift.

It is very important that communication takes place between the athlete and testing staff. A trained staff can recognize an athlete's capacity and determine a proper progression pattern of loading. Feedback from the athlete is critical to determine the loading progressions especially if the lifter has experience and a general idea of the perceived 1 RM. A trial and error approach is seen with athletes with limited experience although an experienced coach may be able to view an athlete and have a certain loading in mind. "How do you feel?" "Are you ready to go?" "How close to your 1 RM do you think you are?" "Can you lift 5 more pounds?" These types of questions and others are vital to the interaction with the athletes as they attempt to exert maximal force. Lastly, rest period length and the number of preliminary repetitions (warm-up) are important. It is essential that the number of repetitions be adequate for proper warm-up but be few enough to not fatigue the athlete. These factors need to be individualized as athletes lifting very heavy weights will require more warm-up sets and longer rest intervals than those lifting lighter weights. Some individuals may require at least 5-minute rest interval between attempts, whereas some individuals need only 1–2 minutes of rest depending on the loading. If a greater number of reps are performed (5–10 RM), it is suggested that fewer warm-up sets be used. Figure 19.5 presents a checklist for strength training (21). This list can provide a guide for coaches

Strength Testing Checklist

- ☐ Has the individual been medically cleared to weight train, and can this individual safety perform strength or endurance testing?

- ☐ Does this individual require any special accommodations?

- ☐ Is the time of day similar between multiple testing sessions?

- ☐ Is muscle strength or endurance to be tested?

- ☐ Is a 1 RM or multiple RM to be used?

- ☐ What is the age and gender of the individual?

- ☐ Was the individual thoroughly familiarized with the testing protocol? How many familiarization sessions were performed?

- ☐ Was proper technique explained and demonstrated (including range of motion, grips, stances, body position, and so on)?

- ☐ Was test-retest reliability of the equipment and protocol performed?

- ☐ What is the individual's training history?

- ☐ Was adequate nutrition intake (and hydration) consumed before testing?

- ☐ Was ambient temperature controlled for?

- ☐ If the individual is experienced, what is his or her perceived or expected RM?

- ☐ What type of muscle action is to be tested?

  - ☐ Concentric?

  - ☐ Eccentric?

  - ☐ Isometric?

- ☐ What type of resistance is to be used?

  - ☐ Dynamic constant external resistance?

  - ☐ Variable resistance?

  - ☐ Isokinetic?

  - ☐ Isometric?

- ☐ For machine-based exercise, what are the appropriate machine settings and starting position of the resistance?

- ☐ Was the individual properly positioned, and does the equipment accurately accommodate the individual?

- ☐ For isometric training, what joint angles will be examined?

- ☐ What is the velocity of movement?

- ☐ Are knowledgeable spotters present?

- ☐ Was the equipment calibrated according to manufacturerrs guidelines?

- ☐ Test specificity:

  - ☐ Were the movement patterns tested similar to those performed during training?

  - ☐ Is there metabolic (energy system) specificity?

- ☐ Were adequate instructions given?

- ☐ Was a proper warm-up performed? Did it include submaximal practice repetitions for testing exercises?

- ☐ Did the individual use proper technique, and did spotters assist in lifting the weight?

- ☐ Was proper breathing patterns used?

- ☐ Was the lifter verbally encouraged throughout the testing protocol, and was a proper lifting environment set for testing?

- ☐ Was visual feedback given for isokinetic testing?

- ☐ Were the proper units of measurement used?

- ☐ What was the individual's 1RM or multiple RM score?

- ☐ Were ergogenics controlled for? What types (if any) were used?

  - ☐ Lifting accessories and apparel?

  - ☐ Nutrition supplements?

  - ☐ Drugs?

- ☐ Did the individual give 100% effort?

- ☐ Were there any other factors that may have affected the test (e.g., illness, injury)?

FIGURE 19.5 Strength testing checklist. (Reprinted with permission from Kraemer WJ, Fry AC, Ratamess NA, French DN. Strength testing: development and evaluation of methodology. In: Maud PJ, Foster C, editors. *Physiological Assessments of Human Performance.* 2nd ed. Champaign (IL): Human Kinetics; 2006. p. 119–50.)

and athletes as it reminds all testers of specific considerations needed prior to and during strength testing. The following protocol is suggested for testing a 6 RM and could be modified to test other RMs (21).

1. Athlete warms up with 5–10 repetitions with 50% of estimated 6 RM.
2. After 1 minute of rest, the athlete performs 6 repetitions at 70% of the estimated 6 RM.

3. Step 2 is repeated at 90% of the estimated 6 RM for 3–6 repetitions.
4. After at least 2–3 minutes of rest, depending on the effort required for the previous set, 6 repetitions are performed with 100%–105% of the estimated 6 RM.
5. After at least 3–5 minutes of rest, if step 4 is successful, increase the resistance by 2.5%–5% for another 6 RM attempt. If six repetitions were not completed in step 4, subtract 2.5%–5% of the resistance used in step 4 and attempt another 6 RM.
6. If weight was removed for step 5 and 6 repetitions were performed, this is the athlete's 6 RM. If the athlete was not successful with this reduced resistance, retesting should occur after 24 hours of rest.

Proper spotting is mandatory for free weight strength testing. Spotters, who are experienced and have a sufficient level of strength and knowledge of correct exercise execution, should be used. The spotter must be able to recognize poor exercise technique and identify hazardous situations. The procedures for proper spotting are exercise specific. Although not all exercises require a spotter, it is recommended that a spotter be present during strength testing for those exercises that involve lifting the weight overhead (shoulder press), lying supine on a bench and lifting the weight over the face or trunk (bench press), or placing the bar on the rear or posterior aspects of the shoulders (back squat). Spotters are not necessary for Olympic lifts or for exercises involving lifting the weight off of the floor. The major difference between spotting for strength training compared to testing is the amount of assistance given to the lifter. It is recommended that a spotter apply minimal force to keep the bar moving during training. However, this is not ideal for strength testing. It is important that fatigue be kept to a minimum. The spotter may provide substantial assistance to spare the lifter unwanted fatigue. The spotter should not touch the bar until failure has occurred. Even the slightest touch gives assistance to the lifter and can overinflate the 1 RM value. Tables 19.5 and 19.6 provide some strength norms and data of various athletic populations.

Table 19.5	Normative Values for Relative Leg Press and Bench Press Strength (1 RM/Body Mass) in a General Population									
	20–29 yr		30–39 yr		40–49 yr		50–59 yr		60+yr	
% Rank	M	F	M	F	M	F	M	F	M	F
Relative Leg Press Strength										
90	2.27	2.05	2.07	1.73	1.92	1.63	1.80	1.51	1.73	1.40
80	2.13	1.66	1.93	1.50	1.82	1.46	1.71	1.30	1.62	1.25
70	2.05	1.42	1.85	1.47	1.74	1.35	1.64	1.24	1.56	1.18
60	1.97	1.36	1.77	1.32	1.68	1.26	1.58	1.18	1.49	1.15
50	1.91	1.32	1.71	1.26	1.62	1.19	1.52	1.09	1.43	1.08
40	1.83	1.25	1.65	1.21	1.57	1.12	1.46	1.03	1.38	1.04
30	1.74	1.23	1.59	1.16	1.51	1.03	1.39	0.95	1.30	0.98
20	1.63	1.13	1.52	1.09	1.44	0.94	1.32	0.86	1.25	0.94
10	1.51	1.02	1.43	0.94	1.35	0.76	1.22	0.75	1.16	0.84
Relative Bench Press Strength										
90	1.48	0.54	1.24	0.49	1.10	0.46	0.97	0.40	0.89	0.41
80	1.32	0.49	1.12	0.45	1.00	0.40	0.90	0.37	0.82	0.38
70	1.22	0.42	1.04	0.42	0.93	0.38	0.84	0.35	0.77	0.36
60	1.14	0.41	0.98	0.41	0.88	0.37	0.79	0.33	0.72	0.32
50	1.06	0.40	0.93	0.38	0.84	0.34	0.75	0.31	0.68	0.30
40	0.99	0.37	0.88	0.37	0.80	0.32	0.71	0.28	0.66	0.29
30	0.93	0.35	0.83	0.34	0.76	0.30	0.68	0.26	0.63	0.28
20	0.88	0.33	0.78	0.32	0.72	0.27	0.63	0.23	0.57	0.26
10	0.80	0.30	0.71	0.27	0.65	0.23	0.57	0.19	0.53	0.25

Reprinted with permission from Hoffman J. *Norms for Fitness, Performance, and Health.* Champaign (IL): Human Kinetics; 2006. p. 1–113.

Table 19.6 — Percentiles for the Bench Press and the Predicted 1 RM for Players in the NFL Combine

% Rank	DB Reps	Pred 1 RM LB	Pred 1 RM KG	DL Reps	Pred 1 RM LB	Pred 1 RM KG	LB Reps	Pred 1 RM LB	Pred 1 RM KG
90	18.0	345	157	28.1	416	189	29.3	423	192
80	17.0	340	155	26.0	400	182	27.0	405	184
70	15.0	325	148	25.0	395	180	26.0	400	182
60	14.0	320	145	24.0	385	175	25.2	396	180
50	13.0	315	143	23.0	380	173	22.5	378	172
40	12.0	305	139	21.6	371	169	21.6	372	169
30	10.0	295	134	20.0	360	164	19.1	356	162
20	10.0	295	134	18.8	353	160	15.4	329	150
10	8.0	280	127	17.0	340	155	13.7	319	145
$\bar{X}$	13.2	315	143	22.8	378	172	22.2	375	170
SD	4.1	28	13	4.4	29	13	5.7	38	17
n		62			68			26	

% Rank	OL Reps	Pred 1 RM LB	Pred 1 RM KG	RB Reps	Pred 1 RM LB	Pred 1 RM KG	TE Reps	Pred 1 RM LB	Pred 1 RM KG
90	30.0	430	195	23.0	380	173	27.4	411	187
80	27.0	405	184	20.0	360	164	24.2	389	177
70	25.6	398	181	19.0	355	161	22.4	377	171
60	24.0	385	175	18.0	345	157	20.4	363	165
50	23.0	380	173	18.0	345	157	19.0	355	161
40	22.0	375	170	17.0	340	155	18.0	345	157
30	21.0	365	166	16.0	335	152	18.0	345	157
20	20.0	360	164	15.0	325	148	17.4	342	155
10	17.0	340	155	14.0	320	145	13.8	320	145
$\bar{X}$	23.3	382	174	17.9	346	157	20.1	361	164
SD	5.1	35	16	3.3	22	10	4.2	28	13
n		97			67			11	

Pred 1 RM, predicted 1 RM; DB, defensive back; DL, defensive line; LB, linebacker; OL, offensive line; RB, running back; TE, tight end.

Reprinted with permission from Hoffman J. *Norms for Fitness, Performance, and Health*. Champaign (IL): Human Kinetics; 2006. p. 1–113.

Isometric Strength Testing

ISOM tests are performed at a static position. The evaluation angle, standardization between athletes, feedback, and motivation all make ISOM testing demanding. Force/torque varies throughout joint ROM; therefore, careful consideration is needed for standardizing joint angles. Some devices used include the hip and back dynamometer, handgrip dynamometer, and ISOK devices (*i.e.*, measuring peak torque at 0°/s). A calibrated force plate can be used with an immovable resistance for several free weight/Smith machine exercises (21). Although peak force/torque assessment is often the primary purpose, rate of ISOM force development can be measured. Fatigue tests (muscle endurance) can be performed with ISOM devices. These tests involve maintaining a certain level of muscular tension over a specified period of time. Many protocols can be used for ISOM testing. All athletes should warm up with low-intensity exercises before testing. Following the warm-up, some practice trials may be performed with submaximal effort (50%–60% of maximal voluntary contraction). The actual test

| | Chapter 19 Assessment and Evaluation | 607 |

Table 19.7 Normative Values of Dominant Grip Strength (kg) in Adults

| | 20–29 yr | | 30–39 yr | | 40–49 yr | | 50–59 yr | | 60–69 yr | |
	M	F	M	F	M	F	M	F	M	F
Excellent	>54	>36	>53	>36	>51	>35	>49	>33	>49	>33
Good	51–54	33–36	50–53	34–36	48–51	33–35	46–49	31–33	46–49	31–33
Average	43–50	26–32	43–49	28–33	41–47	27–32	39–45	25–30	39–45	25–30
Fair	39–42	22–25	39–42	25–27	37–40	24–26	35–38	22–24	35–38	22–24
Poor	<39	<22	<39	<25	<37	<24	<35	<22	<35	<22

Reprinted with permission from Hoffman J. *Norms for Fitness, Performance, and Health.* Champaign (IL): Human Kinetics; 2006. p. 1–113.

requires only 2–3 maximal voluntary efforts. Additional trials may be necessary if, in fact, it appears the athlete is still improving. The peak force for the highest trial is recorded. Table 19.7 provides some norms for maximal grip strength. In addition, some ISOM tests are used to subjectively assess core stability such as the supine bridge, plank, and side plank (22).

Isometric strength testing is used extensively for a number of reasons including the evaluation of training programs and providing normative data for various populations. Although a number of studies measured peak ISOM torque at various positions of the ROM during single-joint exercises, more studies have utilized multiple-joint exercise ISOM strength testing. Multiple-joint ISOM strength testing may have greater applicability to certain athletic movements, and they have shown to be highly related to 1 RM strength of similar movements, e.g., $r = 0.76–0.97$ (23). When converted to system mass (loading plus body weight), peak force produced during ISOM squats and mid-thigh pulls is larger than the force produced during a dynamic 1 RM squat (23). Thus, its assessment provides another useful tool for evaluation. Common exercises tested (in addition to the hip/back dynamometer) include the ISOM squat, leg press, bench press (elbow angles of 90°–135°), and mid-thigh pull at various ROM positions (i.e., knee angles of 90°–140° for the squat and 120°–145° for the mid-thigh pull) and are often assessed during maximal efforts of 3–6 seconds with 2–5 minutes rest intervals between trials (23). Multiple-joint ISOM are reliable ($r = 0.80–0.99$) (24,25). The ISOM mid-thigh pull (shown in thePoint) peak force, impulse, and rate of force development (RFD) have been shown to correlate to change of direction and agility performance time, jump height and reactive strength index, throwing ability, weightlifting (snatch, clean and jerk) performance, sprint speed and power, and maximal strength, e.g., squat, deadlift (25–28). It is performed on top of a force plate (in a power rack or related device) with an immovable barbell placed in a position corresponding to the second pull in Olympic weightlifting. Often the data are expressed and analyzed in time windows, e.g., the first 30, 50, 90, 100, 150, 200, and 250 ms (25,28).

Visit thePoint to view more exercises in the online appendix.

Isokinetic Strength Testing

ISOK testing is performed with a dynamometer that maintains the lever arm at a constant angular velocity. This type of strength evaluation accounts for CON and ECC velocity of movement that is uncontrolled with free weights and machines. The cost of an ISOK dynamometer can be prohibitive, but many laboratories, training rooms, and clinical facilities use them extensively. There have been a large number of studies examining ISOK strength outcomes from training, but many clinical studies examining the potential of ISOK strength measures to predict various types of injuries, e.g., ACL, hamstring strains (29,30). Although many units enable single-joint movements, there are devices on the market that utilize multiple-joint movements that have shown high test-retest reliability (21,31). Due to the complex nature of ISOK testing, there are a number of considerations including the selection of:

1. velocity and order;
2. number of repetitions to be performed;
3. rest intervals;
4. CON and/or ECC muscle action(s);
5. a standardized ROM;
6. standardized test position and proper postural stabilization;
7. equipment calibration and test-retest reliability;
8. feedback, instruction, and familiarization; and
9. gravity compensation.

Studies examining ISOK training have shown velocity-specific strength increases with some spillover above (up to $210°·s^{-1}$) and below (up to $180°·s^{-1}$) the training velocity (21). Training at moderate velocity ($180°–240°·s^{-1}$) produces the greatest strength increases across all testing velocities (21). Testing should match the training velocity, or a spectrum of slow, moderate, and fast velocities can be selected. Three to five repetitions are recommended with rest intervals of 1–3 minutes in between sets to attain peak torque (21). Test-retest reliability for ISOK testing is generally high when position is standardized, equipment is calibrated, and maximal effort is given by the athletes. Optimal ISOK testing allows the athletes to observe their performance via visual feedback as they actually perform the test. In fact, torque may be 3%–19% higher when visual feedback is used (21). Multiple-joint ISOK training (6 weeks of chest press and seated row) has been shown to increase dynamic 1 RM strength by 10.2%–11.2% and muscular endurance (maximal modified push-up performance) by 28.6% in addition to increasing maximal ISOK strength (31). The carryover effects may be attractive to strength training and conditioning professionals seeking to include alternative modalities to RT programs.

Estimating Repetition Maximums

In some cases, estimating a 1 RM or multiple RM may be preferred. Table 19.8 depicts popular prediction equations used by athletes, men and women with little experience, and older adults (21). The load selection ranged from 55% to 95% of 1 RM (for 2–20 reps) with mean ~68%–80% of 1 RM. Prediction is attractive from an administrative standpoint, but its validity is questionable as these equations can underestimate and overestimate 1 RM in certain populations in cross-validation studies (21). Accuracy is greater when <10 reps are performed using nonlinear equations (41,43). Accuracy improves as rep number decreases. Reynolds et al. (41) showed that the highest prediction accuracy for the bench press and leg press was with 5 RM loading compared to 10 and 20 RM loadings in men and women. In a cross-validation study in women, Mayhew et al. (43) compared 14 prediction equations (several shown in Table 19.8) and found most to be fairly accurate in their prediction for the bench press. For total reps to failure, the percent error ranged from −24% to 29%, whereas when total reps were 10 or less, the percent error ranged from −17% to 4%. Accuracy increases with <10 reps, and there is greater accuracy when reps are closer to the 1 RM (2 or 3 reps). Each equation is exercise specific. Many studies

Table 19.8	Formulas Used to Estimate 1 RM Lifting Performance
Reference	**Equation**
Brzycki (32)	1 RM = Wt./1.0278 − 0.0278(# reps)
	%1 RM = 102.78 − 2.78(# reps)
Epley (33)	1 RM = [0.033(Wt.)(# reps) + Wt.]
Lander (34)	1 RM = Wt./1.013 − 0.02671(# reps)
	%1 RM = 101.3 − 2.67123(# reps)
Mayhew et al. (35)	1 RM (lb) = 226.7 + 7.1(#reps w/ 225) (used in college football players)
Cummings and Finn (36)	1 RM = Wt.(1.149) + 0.7119
	1 RM = Wt.(1.175) + # reps (0.839) − 4.2978 (used in untrained women)
Mayhew et al. (37)	1 RM = Wt./{[52.2 + 41.9$e^{-0.055(\text{\# reps})}$]/100}
	%1 RM = 52.2 + 41.9$e^{-0.055(\text{\# reps})}$
O'Connor et al. (38)	1 RM = Wt. (1 + 0.025 × # reps)
Wathen (39)	1 RM = 100 × Wt./[48.8 + 53.8$e^{-0.075(\text{\# reps})}$]
Abadie et al. (40)	1 RM = 8.8147 + 1.1828(7–10 RM)
Reynolds et al. (41)	Bench press 1 RM = 1.1037 × 5 RM (kg) + 0.6999
	Bench press 1 RM = 1.2321 × 10 RM (kg) + 0.1752(LBM) − 5.7443
	Bench press 1 RM = 1.5471 × 20 RM (kg) + 3.834
	% Bench press 1 RM = 55.51 × $e^{-0.0723\,(\text{\# reps})}$ + 48.47
	Leg press 1 RM = 1.0970 × 5 RM (kg) + 14.2546
	Leg press 1 RM = 1.2091 × 10 M (kg) + 38.0908
	Leg press 1 RM = 1.3870 × 20 RM (kg) + 69.2494
	% Leg press 1 RM = 78.17 × $e^{-0.0569\,(\text{\# reps})}$ + 26.41
Macht et al. (42)	In men using the bench press
	1 RM (kg) = 1.11(rep weight in kg) + 6.22
	1 RM (kg) = 1.17(rep weight in kg) + 2.15(reps) − 12.31

Modified from Kraemer WJ, Fry AC, Ratamess NA, French DN. Strength testing: development and evaluation of methodology. In: Maud PJ, Foster C, editors. *Physiological Assessments of Human Performance*. 2nd ed. Champaign (IL): Human Kinetics; 2006. p. 119–50.

used the bench press, thus accuracy appears greater with this exercise. The error rate increases when these equations are applied to other exercises such as the squat and deadlift. For field settings involving large numbers of athletes and limited time or athletes with little RT experience, a case may be made for 1 RM estimation. However, most accurate results are obtained from true RM testing. Lastly, the number of reps performed relative to the 1 RM for different exercises is highly variable. Hoeger et al. (44) showed that at 80% of 1 RM, double the number of reps could be performed for the leg press compared to the leg curl. The amount of muscle mass used and selection of a free weight or machine for the same exercise affect the accuracy.

Muscle Endurance

Local muscle endurance tests involve measuring the ability of selected muscles to perform repeated contractions over time. The contractions can be low to moderate in intensity (*submaximal endurance*) or high in intensity (*high-intensity endurance*). Muscle endurance tests typically come in three categories: (a) performing bodyweight exercises for a maximal number of reps or maximal number of reps in a specified time; (b) reps for a weight training exercise at an absolute percentage of 1 RM; and (c) sustained maximal duration trials.

Bodyweight Exercises

The most common exercises assessed are the partial curl-up, push-up, sit-up, and pull-up. Other exercises such as dips and bodyweight squats have been used. For the partial curl-up test:

- The athlete lies flat on a mat with arms at the side and knees flexed to 90°. An index card can be placed horizontally at the finger tips. The index card is used to standardize ROM.
- With a metronome set to 50 beats · min⁻¹ (to allow 25 curl-ups), the athlete performs curl-ups in a slow manner to the metronome. Shoulder blades are lifted off of the mat (~30°)

and the finger tips must surpass the edge of the index card in order for a repetition to count. The athlete performs as many reps as possible without pausing. Failure to maintain the pace or ROM are criteria to end the test.

- A variation is to perform this test using conventional sit-ups. The athlete can perform as many sit-ups as possible in 1 minute (although some assessments allow 2 min). Here, the athlete gently keeps hands behind his/her head while a partner supports his/her ankles.
- It is important to note that curl-up tests are only moderately related to abdominal endurance and poorly related to abdominal strength; thus, the curl-up test is no longer included in the ACSM Guidelines (45). Sit-up test norms have been published elsewhere (46).

The push-up test is performed in a similar manner:

- For men, a standard push-up position is used for the test. For women, a modified push-up used where knees are placed on the ground and the ankles are crossed.
- Athletes then proceed to perform as many push-ups as possible in good form. Some tests may pose a time limit on the athlete (2 min for the Army standard test). A repetition only counts when full ROM is attained (nearly touching the chest to the ground at the bottom position). An object can be placed low to mark the touching point, *i.e.*, rolled up towel or a tester's fist when assessing male athletes.

Pull-ups can be performed where the athlete must pull his/her body high enough to where the chin surpasses the bar. Bodyweight squats are used where the maximal number attained in 1 minute is recorded (47). Vaara et al. (47) showed the repeated bodyweight squat test may be more indicative of cardiorespiratory endurance and body fat percent rather than the lower-body muscle strength.

Table 19.9 present norms for the push-up test. Table 19.10 depicts norms for pull-ups in college men.

Table 19.9	Fitness Categories for Push-Ups by Age Groups and Sex									
	Age and Sex									
	20–29		**30–39**		**40–49**		**50–59**		**60–69**	
Category	**M**	**F**	**M**	**F**	**M**	**F**	**M**	**F**	**M**	**F**
Excellent	36	30	30	27	25	24	21	21	18	17
Very good	35	29	29	26	24	23	20	20	17	16
	29	21	22	20	17	15	13	11	11	12
Good	28	20	21	19	16	14	12	10	10	11
	22	15	17	13	13	11	10	7	8	5
Fair	21	14	16	12	12	10	9	6	7	4
	17	10	12	8	10	5	7	2	5	2
Poor	16	9	11	7	9	4	6	1	4	1

Reprinted with permission from *ACSM's Guidelines for Exercise Testing and Prescription.* 8th ed. Baltimore (MD): Lippincott Williams & Wilkins; 2010.

Table 19.10	Pull-Up Norms for College Men
Classification	**Number of Pull-Ups**
Excellent	15+
Good	12–14
Average	8–11
Fair	5–7
Poor	0–4

Reprinted with permission from Hoffman J. *Norms for Fitness, Performance, and Health*. Champaign (IL): Human Kinetics; 2006. p. 1–113.

Absolute Repetition Number

Weight training exercises can be performed for a maximal number of reps with a standard load. An important consideration is the resistance to use. Relative loading is based on a percentage of the individual's RM capability, whereas absolute loading has the same resistance for all athletes and all tests (the 225-lb max rep bench press performed at NFL combines for football prospects). For pre- to posttesting, relative muscle endurance performance does not change. Thus, absolute loading is recommended as an increase in the number of reps performed is seen with training. For most individuals, the relationship between strength and absolute muscular endurance is positive, whereas the relationship between strength and relative endurance is negative (21). Any exercise can be used for endurance testing. A specific load needs to be applied among all athletes and test performance is predicated upon the maximal number of repetitions performed with that load. This could be a certain percentage of the athlete's pretesting max or a specific load. Norms can be developed with a large number of athletes performing the test over time. One example is the YMCA Bench Press test (norms have been published elsewhere (46)):

- The loading for the bench press is 80 lb for men and 35 lb for women. A metronome is set at 60 beats · min^{-1} to yield ~30 reps per minute.
- The athlete performs as many repetitions as possible with proper form and ROM (touching the bar to chest). Failing to perform the repetitions in proper ROM, fatigue, and inability to maintain cadence are criteria to terminate the test.

Sustained Maximal Duration Trials

Sustained maximal duration trials usually involve an ISOM muscle action held for maximal time. Many variations can be performed but there are few norms published in athletes. We have used endurance tests including maximal ISOM elbow flexion (90°) against a standard load and grip endurance test where individuals hold or maintain a position against a load for maximal time. The ISOM wall squat test has been used at various depths. One sustained maximal duration test is the *flexed-arm*

hang. The flexed-arm hang (Table 19.11) measures the amount of time an athlete can maintain the final ISOM pull-up position. That is, the athlete maintains his/her position with chin above the bar for as long as possible. Failure to maintain position is criteria for test termination. This test is greatly affected by the athlete's body weight and level of strength.

Measurement of core stability and endurance is a popular bodyweight assessment tool primarily because it is safe, cost-free, and requires little equipment. In fact, trunk muscle endurance contributes to spine stability has been shown to relate to the onset of low-back pain (LBP) more so than muscle strength (48). Some of the more common used bodyweight ISOM trunk endurance tests include the Biering-Sorensen test and modified versions, prone ISOM chest raise, prone double straight-leg raise, trunk flexor test (various positions), plank, and side plank (or bridge). With a few exceptions, these tests have shown good reliability ($r \geq 0.77$) (48,49).

- *Biering-Sorensen test*: The trainee lies prone partially fixed to a table or bench (Fig. 19.6). The upper iliac crest down is supported by multiple straps fixating the lower body to the table. The upper body and trunk is unsupported. To perform the test, the trainee holds the horizontal trunk position (while the arms are folded across the chest) for as long as possible until fatigued, exertion becomes intolerable, or trainee can no longer maintain proper posture (48). A literature review showed mean performance times of 84–195 seconds in men and 142–220 seconds in women (48). McGill et al. (50) reported mean endurance times of 146 ± 51 seconds in men and 189 ± 60 seconds in women. In a group of athletes, mean (± SD) times were 157.4 ± 42.9 seconds in men and 167.4 ± 55.0 seconds in women with a range of 59–320 seconds overall (49). Mean times of 99.6 ± 22.3 seconds were shown in Division I college football players (51). Durations may be lower in trainees with current LBP and the results depend on age, activity level, body size, and percent fat. Mean times have been moderately correlated to vertical jump and power clean performance (51).
- *Prone isometric chest raise test*: The trainee lies in a prone position on a table or the floor (shown in thePoint). This test was adapted from the Biering-Sorensen test. A pillow could be placed under the abdomen to decrease lumbar lordosis. The trainee lifts the trunk off of the table and holds this position for as long as possible. One study reported a mean endurance time of 208 seconds in men and 128 seconds in women (48). Normative data were provided in 548 individuals (age range = 19–77) by Wilson et al. (52). For individuals 19–29, 30–39, and 40–49 in the top 25 percentile, mean endurance times were 187, 190, and 183 seconds in men and 173, 150, and 116 seconds in women, respectively.
- *Prone double straight-leg raise test*: The trainee lies face down in a prone position on the table with arms underneath the forehead. The trainee raises both legs by extending the hips until knee clearance is attained (shown in thePoint). This position is held for as long as possible. The test is terminated when trainee can no longer maintain knee clearance. Normative data were provided in 548 individuals (age range = 19–77) by Wilson

Table 19.11 Flexed-Arm Hang Standards for Youth

Percentile	6	7	8	9	10	11	12	13	14	15	16	17+
Boys												
90	16	23	28	28	38	37	36	37	61	62	61	56
80	12	17	18	20	25	26	25	29	40	49	46	45
70	9	13	15	16	20	19	19	22	31	40	39	39
60	8	10	12	12	15	15	15	18	25	35	33	35
50	6	8	10	10	12	11	12	14	20	30	28	30
40	5	6	8	8	8	9	9	10	15	25	22	26
30	3	4	5	5	6	6	6	8	11	20	18	20
20	2	3	3	3	3	4	4	5	8	14	12	15
10	1	1	1	2	1	1	1	2	3	8	7	8
Girls												
90	15	21	21	23	29	25	27	28	31	34	30	29
80	11	14	15	16	19	16	16	19	21	23	21	20
70	9	11	11	12	14	13	13	14	16	15	16	15
60	6	8	10	10	11	9	10	10	11	10	10	11
50	5	6	8	8	8	7	7	8	9	7	7	7
40	4	5	6	6	6	5	5	5	6	5	5	5
30	3	4	4	4	4	4	3	4	4	4	3	4
20	1	2	3	2	2	2	1	1	2	2	2	2
10	0	0	0	0	0	0	0	0	0	1	0	1

Note: Time listed in seconds.

Adapted by permission from Presidents Council for Physical Fitness, Presidents Challenge Normative Data Spreadsheet (online). Available at www.presidentschallenge.org.

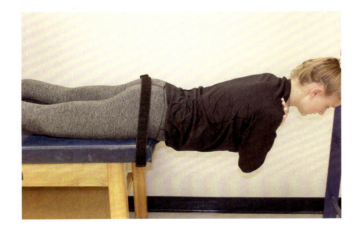

FIGURE 19.6 The Biering-Sorensen test.

et al. (52). For individuals 19–29, 30–39, and 40–49 in the top 25 percentile, mean endurance times were 130, 123, and 95 seconds in men and 126, 111, and 87 seconds in women, respectively.

- *Isometric trunk flexor test*: Also known as the sit-up hold or V-sit test, the trainee sits upright on a table at a 60° angle relative to the table (variations exist where different angles are used). The knees and hips are flexed 90°, and the feet are stabilized (Fig. 19.7). A triangular reference block may be used to standardize the angle. A variety of data have been reported in different studies. For example, Durall et al. (53) reported mean endurance times of 140.8 ± 116 seconds in women and 143.8 ± 67.5 seconds in men. McGill et al. (50) reported mean endurance times of 144 ± 76 seconds in men and 149 ± 99 seconds in women. Evans et al. (49) reported mean endurance times of ~223.0 ± 134 seconds in

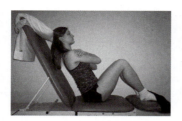

FIGURE 19.7 The isometric trunk flexor (60°) endurance test. (From Durall CJ, Greene PF, Kernozek TW. A comparison of two isometric tests of trunk flexor endurance. *J Strength Cond Res.* 2012;26:1939–44.)

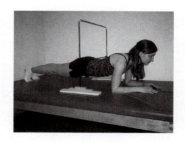

FIGURE 19.8 The plank test. (From Durall CJ, Greene PF, Kernozek TW. A comparison of two isometric tests of trunk flexor endurance. *J Strength Cond Res.* 2012;26:1939–44.)

male and female athletes. However, they also reported mean endurance times of ~360 seconds in a small group of nonathletes. Mean times of 113.8 ± 51.9 seconds have been reported in Division I college football players (51). McGill et al. (50) has recommended that the ratio of endurance times between this test and the Biering-Sorensen test be <1.0.

- *Side plank (bridge) test:* The trainee lies on his/her side with the legs extended with the top foot placed in front of the lower foot. The trainee lifts the hips off of the ground and maintains a straight body position supporting themselves on the feet and elbow (shown in thePoint). Upper arm may be placed at side or across the chest. This position is held for as long as possible. The test is terminated when trainee can no longer maintain the planked position. The test should be performed on the right and left sides. McGill et al. (50) reported mean endurance times of 94 ± 34 (right) and 97 ± 35 (left) seconds in men and 72 ± 31 (right) and 77 ± 35 (left) seconds in women, 39%–65% of their Biering-Sorensen time. Evans et al. (49) reported mean endurance times 79.6–92 (±32-46) seconds for the right and left sides in men and women. Mean times of 95.9–100.8 ± 24.4–31.9 seconds have been reported in Division I college football players, and these times were related to sprint performance (51). Mean times of 87.0–92.6 ± 23.0–25.8 seconds have been reported in male high school soccer players (54).
- *Plank (prone bridge) test:* The trainee assumes a prone position with hips elevated off of the ground (without sagging or excessively piking the hips) and maintains a straight "planked" position while supported on the feet and forearms (Fig. 19.8). This position is held for as long as possible. The test is terminated when trainee can no longer maintain the planked position. Durall et al. (53) reported mean endurance times of 79.7 ± 34.8 seconds in women and 126.1 ± 51.9 seconds in men. Mean times of 124.0 ± 48.8 seconds were shown in male high school soccer players (54).

Flexibility and Muscle Length

Flexibility depends on several factors including tendon and ligament stiffness, muscle viscosity and bulk, distensibility of the joint capsule, and muscle temperature. Flexibility is joint specific so no single test can measure total-body flexibility (45). Joint flexibility can be measured for a multitude of joints in multiple planes (depending on the joint assessed). Under normal (noninjury) conditions, the shoulder, spine, and hip regions may typically be targeted with routine flexibility assessment in athletes although some sports may require other areas of emphasis. Flexibility can be assessed by goniometers, electrogoniometers, a Leighton flexometer, inclinometer, and a tape measure. For some tests, visualization of anatomical landmarks may be sufficient to determine a certain level of flexibility on a "pass or fail" basis. Goniometers (Fig. 19.9) are most practical as a plastic goniometer is inexpensive and easy to use to quantitatively assess static flexibility. It acts similar to a protractor. The center of the goniometer is placed at the joint axis of rotation and the arms are aligned with the bony segments. The Leighton flexometer is a type of gravity-based goniometer used to measure flexibility. Inclinometers measure the angles of slope and therefore can be used to assess joint ROM. Both inclinometers and flexometers can be strapped to the athlete or held by hand and the ROM is recorded. Electrogoniometers are attached to body segments and can measure static and dynamic ROM. These are used in laboratory settings. Joint ROM can be assessed in angular motion terms (degrees or radians) and linear terms (inches, centimeters) with use of a tape measure (Fig. 19.9). Table 19.12 presents normal joint ROM for eight major joints in the human body.

Sit-and-Reach Test

Perhaps the most common indirect assessment of flexibility is the *sit-and-reach test*. It is used to assess lower back, gluteal, and hamstring muscle flexibility (45). Several variations of this test exist. This test is not only affected by flexibility but may also rely upon abdominal girth and limb/torso lengths. Thus, a *modified sit-and-reach test* is used, which establishes a zero point based on limb/torso lengths (Fig. 19.10). It is important to note that the ACSM recommends other methods of assessing flexibility as the sit-and-reach test shows poor relationships to low back pain and may be considered questionable as a measure of hamstring flexibility (45). The sit-and-reach test is a linear

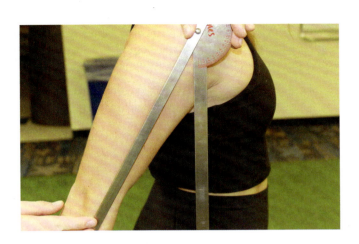
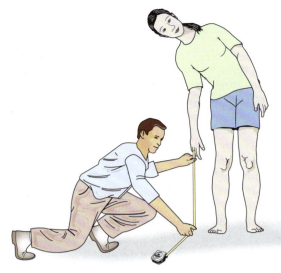

FIGURE 19.9 Plastic goniometer and tape measure ROM measurement.

Table 19.12 Average Ranges of Joint Motion

Joint	Joint Motion	ROM (degrees)
Hip	Flexion	90–125
	Hyperextension	10–30
	Abduction	40–45
	Adduction	10–30
	Internal rotation	35–45
	External rotation	45–50
Knee	Flexion	120–150
	Rotation (when flexed)	40–50
Ankle	Plantar flexion	20–45
	Dorsiflexion	15–30
Shoulder	Flexion	130–180
	Hyperextension	30–80
	Abduction	170–180
	Adduction	50
	Internal rotation	60–90
	External rotation	70–90
	Horizontal flexion	135
	Horizontal extension	45
Elbow	Flexion	140–160
Radioulnar	Forearm pronation (from midposition)	80–90
	Forearm supination (from midposition)	80–90
Cervical spine	Flexion	40–60
	Hyperextension	40–75
	Lateral flexion	40–45
	Rotation	50–80
Thoracolumbar spine	Flexion	45–75
	Hyperextension	20–35
	Lateral flexion	25–35
	Rotation	30–45

Reprinted with permission from Hoffman J. *Norms for Fitness, Performance, and Health*. Champaign (IL): Human Kinetics; 2006. p. 1–113.

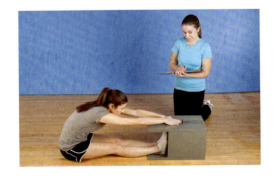

FIGURE 19.10 The sit-and-reach test.

assessment of ROM. Notwithstanding these limitations, the procedures for the modified sit-and-reach are as follows:

- A sit-and-reach box or tape measure/stick is needed. Following a proper warm-up, the athlete sits shoeless with feet against the sit-and-reach box. The athlete's starting position is determined by having the athlete place arms together with right hand over left hand, feet flat against the box with knees fully extended, and back against the wall. The athlete reaches forward by protracting only the shoulder girdle to determine the starting position. This calibrates the starting point and limits limb/torso length bias.
- While keeping the knees extended, the athlete slowly bends at the waist forward as far as possible (without bouncing) and pushes the sliding device maximally to achieve the greatest ROM possible. This final position is held momentarily. It is important to make sure the athlete keeps feet flat against box, does not bend knees, and does not ballistically reach when performing the test. The score is recorded.
- The best of three trials is recorded. If the best trial is the third trial, then additional 1–2 trials can be given. This may occur if the warm-up is insufficient. Norms for modified sit-and-reach performance data for men and women have been published elsewhere (55).

Trunk Rotation Test

Another test is the *trunk rotation test*. This can be performed with essentially no equipment or a specialized device (an Acuflex rotation tester). The procedures are as follows:

- A vertical line is marked on a wall. The athlete stands with his/her back to the wall (with a shoulder width stance) at approximately arm's length away.
- The athlete rotates to the right as far as possible (with arms straight in front and parallel to floor), touches the wall, and this position is marked. The athlete then rotates to the left, touches the wall, and the position is marked. Feet must remain stationary while trunk, shoulders, and knees are free to move.
- The distance from the line is measured. A positive score is one where the mark exceeds the vertical line and a mark before the vertical line indicates a negative score.
- *Scoring*: >20 cm = excellent; 15–20 cm = very good; 10–15 cm = good; 5–10 cm = fair; 0–5 cm (or a negative score) = poor.

Shoulder Elevation Test

The shoulder elevation test measures flexibility of the shoulder and pectoral areas but also requires a certain level of muscle strength to elevate the arms against gravity. To perform, the trainee first grasps a stick in front of the body using a pronated grip. Arm length is determined by measuring the distance from the acromion process to the top of the stick. The subject then assumes a lying prone position on a mat where the chin touches the floor. The trainee extends the arms straight overhead while holding the stick (shown in thePoint). The trainee slowly raises the stick upward as high as possible while maintaining chin contact with the mat and keeping the elbows fully extended. The highest position is held for 1–2

seconds while a measurement is taken. The tester measures the length from the floor to the top position of the stick held by the trainee. Multiple trials should be used, typically at least three. Scoring may be accomplished by either recording the highest length attained from the floor (*i.e.*, using that as the score) or by using the following formula:

$$\text{Shoulder elevation score} = \text{Arm length (inches)} - \text{Best height attained (inches)}$$

A value of <6 or <5.5 in men and women is considered excellent; 6–8.24 and 5.5–7.49 is good; 8.25–11.49 and 7.5–10.74 is average; 11.5–12.5 and 10.75 to 11.75 is fair; and more than 12.5 and 11.75 is considered poor (56).

Pass/Fail Tests

Visualization for a number of ROM tests can be done without special equipment. These subjective tests provide the trainer or coach with basic information that could be used in training to target weak areas or muscle imbalances. Although goniometers and ROM-assessing equipment can be used, therapists and medical professionals have identified acceptable levels of ROM that can be easily assessed with minimal equipment. Very few normative data exist for some of these tests. Some of these potentially nonquantitative tests include assessments for prone/supine transversus abdominis muscle activation, pectoralis major and minor length, shoulder flexion, internal and external rotation, supine straight leg raise, FABER, Thomas test, Ober test, supine hip abduction/adduction, wall angel, supine lat stretch, and seated and prone hip external/internal rotation (57–59).

- *Prone/supine transversus abdominis muscle activation test*: The trainee lies supine on a table (but may be tested in a prone position as well) with knees bent to ~90° and arm at the side of the body. The tester may place their hand under the trainee's lordotic curve of the spine (or could use a pressure cuff or stabilizer to provide biofeedback). The trainee performs abdominal hollowing and contracts the transversus abdominis muscle by squeezing the naval in and up toward the spine without moving the spine, pelvis, rib cage, and without breath-holding (59). Although not a flexibility test, maintaining a proper neutral spine is important for all modalities of exercise.
- *Pectoralis minor length*: The pectoralis minor muscle is prone to shortening after prolonged exposure to scapular protraction resulting from postural issues or muscle imbalances. Shorter pectoralis minor length limits scapular ROM and external rotation during arm elevation, thereby increasing the risk of impingement (60). For this test, the trainee lies supine on a firm surface with arms at the sides (shown in thePoint). The posterior aspect of the acromion is palpated and its distance to the surface is measured. Values >1 in. may be indicative of shortened length (57,60); however, the mass of the trainee is important as large individuals may result in higher values and this technique has not strongly correlated to actual pectoralis minor length (60). However, it is simple to implement and may have some practical benefit. Other ways including palpating origin/insertion points such as the coracoid process and the 4th rib

and measuring the distance with a tape measure may be more accurate (60).

- *Shoulder internal/external rotation test*: The trainee lies supine on a table with the arm abducted to 90° and the elbow flexed 90°. The shoulder is externally rotated as far as possible or until the forearm is lying on table (shown in thePoint). The trainee passes if they can attain this final position. For internal rotation, the trainee begins in the same position but this time internally rotates the arm forward as far as possible. A "pass" is scored if they can attain ~70° of internal rotation from this position (57).
- *Supine straight leg test*: The trainee lies supine on the ground with hands under the lordotic curve of the spine. The right leg is lifted as high and far as possible without flexing the knee or arching the back (shown in thePoint). The final position is held for 1–2 seconds. The same procedures are followed for the left leg. The trainee targets 90° of hip flexion.
- *The FABER (flexion, abduction, and external rotation) test*: This test is used to assess hip ROM and identify hip pathology such as hip, lumbar spine, or sacroiliac joint dysfunction. The trainee lies supine on the table with the leg placed in a figure-4 position (hip flexed, externally rotated, and abducted with the lateral ankle placed on the contralateral thigh proximal to the knee) while supporting the contralateral pelvis (Fig. 19.11). A "pass" is scored if the bent leg attains a parallel position to the table without pelvic movement (57). Therapists and medical professionals have used this as a provocation test to assess pathology by applying force to the bent leg around the knee to check for the presence of pain. The perpendicular length from the lateral femoral epicondyle to the table may be measured to quantitatively assess hip ROM and symmetry between limbs.

Bagwell et al. (61) reported mean FABER lengths of 12.4 ± 2.8 cm (with no differences between men and women) with a noted difference of 3.7 cm between different testers. Values of ~7–9 cm were shown in professional golfers and greater lengths are associated with a history of LBP (62).

- *Thomas test*: The Thomas test is used to assess flexibility of the hip flexor and abductor/adductor muscles. The modified Thomas test requires the trainee to sit near the end of a table, lean back, and lie supine while bringing both knees to the chest. One leg is held tightly at knee level while the other leg drops and is relaxed (shown in thePoint). The lumbar spine must remain flat and in contact with the table during the test. The hanging leg is examined. Goniometers can be used to measure joint angles. Through visualization, a "passing" test is indicative of the hip to rest on the table while the knee is flexed and in line with the hip. If the thigh is elevated off of the table, then the hip flexors (psoas group) may be tight. Athletes were shown to have their legs to hang ~11°–12° below the horizontal (58,63) or have ~6°–10° of hip extension (64). If the knee does not flex beyond ~80°, then the quadriceps (mostly rectus femoris) may be tight. If the hip abducts, then the tensor fascia latae may be tight. Athletes have been shown to have leg abduction of up to 15° so some slight abduction may be seen in some athletes (63).
- *Supine hip abduction/adduction test*: The trainee lies supine on a table or the floor with legs straight. One leg is abducted to at least 45° without movement of the pelvis or hip rotation (shown in thePoint). The other leg is adducted without rotating the hip or lifting the leg. Movement of at least 10°–30° of adduction is recommended (57).
- *Prone hip external/internal rotation test*: The trainee lies prone on a table or floor with arms at the sides. One knee is flexed to 90°. The hip externally rotates to the side as far as possible without flexing or lifting the hip or rotating spine and pelvis (shown in thePoint). Attaining an angle of 35° is desired (57). From the same position, internal hip rotation is performed. Attaining an angle of 45° is desired (57).
- *Ober test*: Since 1935, the Ober test has been used to evaluate tightness in the tensor fascia latae muscle and the iliotibial (IT) band although recent evidence suggests it may be more indicative of tightness in the gluteus medius and minimus muscles and the hip joint capsule (65). Nevertheless, it provides an indication of tightness in the hip region. The trainee lies on their side on a table with the knees and hips (especially the bottom knee and hip) slightly to moderately flexed. The tester stands behind the trainee and firmly stabilizes the pelvis of the upper leg while grasping the leg, flexing the knee, and moving it into hip extension and abduction to where it is aligned with the trunk. The leg is slowly lowered toward the table in adduction allowing gravity to induce the motion (Fig. 19.12A). Supporting the hip throughout is critical to endure the leg does not internally rotate or flex to facilitate lowering, which would lead to a false result. To judge, a negative test results when the leg drops naturally below the horizontal without pain indicating a normal IT band. A positive test results when the leg remains elevated or abducted above the neutral position over the bottom leg indicating IT band tightness. A *modified Ober test* was described in 1952

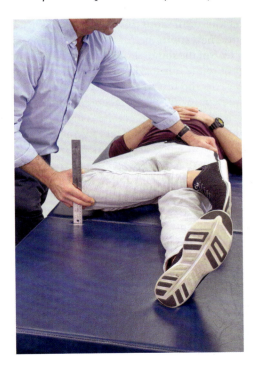

FIGURE 19.11 The FABER test.

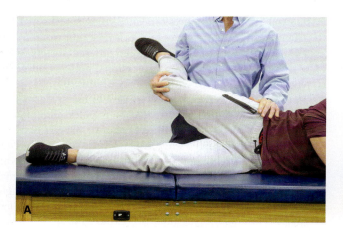 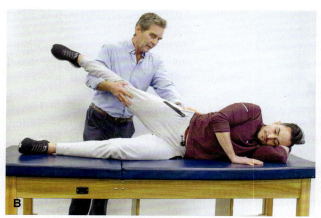

FIGURE 19.12 **A, B.** The Ober test.

and is often preferred (65). The difference is that the upper tested leg remains straight as opposed to a 90° flexed knee position in the original test (Fig. 19.12B). This is believed to reduce the potential influence of the rectus femoris on influencing the results. Ferber et al. (58) showed that in 300 recreational athletes the average ROM seen during the modified Ober test was −24.6° ± 7.3° from the horizontal and suggested that −23° be used as a criterion value for the test.

- *Wall angel test:* The trainee stands back (flat back position without arching) to a wall with feet ~5 in. away from the wall. The shoulders are abducted and elbow flexed to 90° to form an "L" shape (shown in thePoint). To correctly perform the test, the head, back, and arms should be flat against the wall. Failure to attain the correct "L" position could be indicative of thoracic spine immobility, tight latissimus dorsi, and pectoral muscles.
- *Supine shoulder flexion (lat stretch) test:* The trainee lies supine on a table or the floor with the arms at the side, back flat, and legs extended. The arms (shoulders) are flexed overhead as far as possible with palms facing ceiling (shown in thePoint). If the arms can reach the table or floor, then mobility is sufficient. The extended leg position provides a small degree of slack to the latissimus dorsi muscle allowing a deeper overhead position to be reached. If this final position is not attained, having the trainee forcefully flex the shoulders further could induce lumbar extension. This is indicative of lat restriction. In step 2 from the final position, the trainee flexes the hips and knees bringing the knees closer to the chest. If the arms extend upward when the leg position is changed, this is indicative of lat tightness. Further flexion of the hips leading to posterior tilt of the pelvis extends the arms further, thereby augmenting the effect of lat restriction. Greater shoulder ROM is seen with the legs extended when a lat restriction is present.

Posture and Functional Performance

Posture relates to the alignment and function of all segments of the human body at rest and during motion. Proper posture is important for optimal alignment, proper length-tension relationships of skeletal muscle during contraction, and optimal force transmission and absorption throughout the kinetic chain (66). The control of posture during exercise is critical to optimal performance and relates highly to having good core stability and strength. Postural assessment allows the coach to determine potential muscle imbalances (length and strength), weakness, and can be applied to target specific areas with the training program. Although posture can be critiqued during any type of exercise or motor skill, some postural assessments can be performed early, which can be used to detect issues that can manifest later during more complex exercise performance. Posture may be assessed statically and dynamically.

Functional performance relates to the ability to perform basic athletic skills with stability, mobility, bodily control, and balance (67,68). Basic movements form the base necessary to build upon to perform more complex athletic skills. Functional qualities critical to sports performance include good mobility (especially in the hips and shoulders), ability to shift weight from one foot to the other to maintain balance, transfer power from the core to the limbs, and learn to control posture and bodily movement (67,68). Poor technique and mobility lead to poor posture and subsequent compensation that can place the athlete at greater risk for injury. Thus, testing of basic functional skills may be seen as a precursor to more advanced training.

Postural and performance screening can be done by viewing the athlete's performance in training or during sport practice. However, some screening protocols have been developed. One protocol is known as the *Functional Movement Screen* (67–70). It consists of applying a 0–3 score (0 = pain during movement, 1 = unable to perform prescribed movement, 2 = can perform movement but needs to compensate and has difficulty, and 3 = good performance of skill) to selected movements such as squatting, stepping, lunging, reaching, striding, kicking, pushing, and rotation (please see https://www.acsm.org/get-stay-certified/fms for ACSM FMS video). The coach or trainer may use the measuring device, hurdle, and measuring stick or dowel that comes with the kit. The maximum score is 21 as there are 7 tests with a 3-point optimal score. For tests of asymmetry involving separate performance and scoring of right and left sides, the lower score of the two (if there is a difference between right and left sides) is used for calculating total points. It is recommended that each movement be viewed independently based on the objectives of each screening test as opposed to only viewing the total point score as the main assessment outcome (69). The movements assessed include

- *The overhead (deep) squat* — this test assesses total body mobility and core stability. A broomstick or dowel is held in an overhead position with a moderate grip width while the athlete squats as deep as possible. To start, the trainee may place the dowel on the head with an elbow angle of 90°. The dowel is then pressed directly overhead to attain the starting position. The feet are shoulder width apart and pointed straight ahead. The ideal technique involves heels flat on the ground, knees aligned over toes (with no valgus collapse), the stick or dowel aligned over the feet, and torso upright at a position parallel to the tibias (minimal forward lean). Deviations result in a lower score and can indicate limited mobility of the shoulders, thoracic spine, hips, and ankles. Up to three repetitions may be performed.
- *Hurdle step* — this test assesses mobility of the lower body, core stability, single-leg stability and control, and asymmetries in stepping. A mini hurdle is used and is set to a height of the top of the athlete's tibial tuberosity. The athlete takes a hip width stance with toes aligned directly beneath the hurdle and feet together. The dowel is placed on the rear shoulders with both hands supporting it in place. The athlete steps over the hurdle and touches the heel to the floor while keeping the opposite (support) leg extended and supporting body weight and then returns to the starting position. Optimal performance involves the hips, knees, and ankles remaining aligned within the sagittal plane, minimal to no movement of the lumbar spine (no leaning or lateral flexion), head focusing straight ahead, balance control, dowel remains parallel to the hurdle, and no contact between the foot and hurdle. The hip should be flexed directly upward with no external rotation to clear the hurdle. The athlete performs the test on the opposite side next. Deviations result in a lower score and could indicate poor stability of the support leg or poor mobility of the stepping leg.
- *In-line lunge* — a 2 × 6 board or the FMS measuring device is needed. The tester measures the length of the athlete's tibia with a yardstick and marks this length on the board (from the athlete's toes) as the athlete steps on the board with one foot. A dowel is held behind the back with right arm up and left arm down so that it touches the head, spine, and sacrum. The athlete lunges and places the heel of the lead leg (left in this example) on the mark and lowers the back knee until it touches the board. The athlete performs the test on the opposite side next. Optimal performance involves no torso movement, feet remain in a sagittal plane, knee touches the board behind the lead heel, and balance is maintained throughout. Deviations result in a lower score and could indicate poor hip mobility, balance, low stability in the knee and ankle, and an imbalance between adductor weakness and abductor tightness.

- *Shoulder mobility* — first, hand length is measured from the distal wrist crease to the tip of the middle finger. The trainee stands with feet together, makes a fist with each hand, placing the thumb inside the fist, and assumes a maximally adducted/internally rotated position with one arm and an abducted and externally rotated position with the other arm. The tester measures the distance between both of the athlete's fist along the back with a tape measure. Optimal performance involves attaining a ROM with both arms, *i.e.*, within one hand's length when measured. The athlete performs the test using the opposite limb arrangement. Deviations result in a lower score and could indicate poor shoulder ROM, poor scapular and thoracic spine mobility, and excessive development and shortening of the pectoralis minor and latissimus dorsi (leading to rounded shoulders). A clearing exam is performed after the test where the trainee places the palm of the hand on the opposite shoulder and lifts the elbow as high as possible while maintain hand-shoulder contact. The goal is to examine the potential for shoulder impingement-related pain during this movement. Pain is considered a "positive" test. This test is not part of the total point scoring. However, the presence of pain during the clearing test would lead to a score of "0" for the shoulder mobility test.
- *Active straight-leg raise* — this is a measure of hip flexibility and core stability. The athlete lies supine with head on the floor, feet straight, and palms up with a 2 × 6 board positioned under the athlete's knees. The athlete lifts the leg with a dorsiflexed ankle position and an extended knee while the opposite leg remains straight (while the lower back remains on the floor). Once the athlete reaches the final position (as far back as the leg will reach before the knee begins to bend), the tester aligns a dowel through the medial malleolus of the ankle perpendicular to the floor. The athlete performs the test using the opposite leg. Optimal performance involves the dowel located between the mid-thigh and hip area of the opposite leg. Deviations result in a lower score and could indicate poor hamstring flexibility and tightness of the hip flexors associated with anterior pelvic tilt. Up to three repetitions may be performed.
- *Trunk stability push-up* — this test assesses core stability more so than upper body strength. The athlete assumes a prone position with hands shoulder width apart and thumbs aligned with top of the head (men) or chin (women). From that position, the athlete performs a push-up with no lag in the lumbar spine. Optimal performance involves being able to do a push-up with proper posture. Poor performance may indicate a lack of strength and/or poor trunk stabilization. Up to three repetitions may be performed. A clearing exam is performed after the test. A spinal extension test, the press-up, is performed to see if any pain is present. This test is not part of the total point scoring.
- *Rotary stability* — this test assesses core and shoulder stability. A 2 × 6 board or the FMS board is used for alignment while the athlete assumes a quadruped position on the floor. The athlete lifts the arm (flexes the shoulder) and leg (hip extension) on the same side of the body by ~6 in. The athlete

then flexes both limbs to where the elbow touches the knee. The athlete performs the same skill with the opposite side. Optimal performance involves the athlete maintaining posture, moving both limbs in the desired ROM, and not having the limbs cross over the board. Poor performance may indicate poor trunk stabilization and rotational strength. A clearing exam is performed after the test. A spinal flexion test is used to see if pain is produced. This test is not part of the total point scoring. A variation used in functional screening is the *seated rotation test*. The athlete sits upright on the floor with back straight and legs crossed in a doorway. The athlete holds a dowel on the front shoulders with arms crossed on top. The athlete rotates as far as possible to the right and then to the left. A good score is seen when the athlete is able to touch the dowel to the wall (68).

The FMS was shown to have poor to high interrater reliability (*i.e.*, 0.37–0.98) (69,71,72) and good test-retest reliability (73). Values are higher when coaches or trainers are trained in using this assessment. The results are more consistent when the same tester conducts the tests over time as greater variability ensues among different testers. Studies in various groups of athletes have shown mean composite scores of 12.0–17.5 (73–77) with similar mean scores found between high school, collegiate, and professional athletes (76). Early studies suggested a composite score of 14 to be a threshold value for injury prevention. Higher risks of injury were shown in male and female athletes who have scored 14 or less (69,71,78); however; other studies have shown no such relationships (76). Composite scores alone may not be the best predictor but individual results (plus results from other assessments) may provide coaches and trainers with more meaningful information on weakness to address. FMS asymmetry scores between right and left sides or the presence of pain during a FMS test are associated with injury risk (78,79). Chronic training involving specific corrective or movement-specific exercises has been shown to increase FMS scores within 4–8 weeks (74,80,81).

Aerobic Capacity

Aerobic capacity assessments estimate $\dot{V}O_{2max}$. Because most athletes and coaches will not have access to metabolic carts to directly assess maximal aerobic capacity, prediction from field tests is most practical. These tests have been validated and typically require variables such as heart rate (HR) or test time to predict $\dot{V}O_{2max}$. Estimates of $\dot{V}O_{2max}$ from the HR response to exercise are based on the assumptions that a steady-state HR is obtained for each work rate, a linear relationship exists between HR and work rate, the max work load achieved is indicative of the $\dot{V}O_{2max}$, max HR for a given age is uniform, and mechanical efficiency is similar between athletes (45). In some cases (1.5-mile run), several athletes can be tested simultaneously. Critical to the accuracy of these estimates is the effort level put forth by the athlete. Aerobic capacity can be underestimated if the athlete does not perform with maximal effort. The most common modes include field tests, cycle ergometer/treadmill, and step tests.

Field Tests

Field tests include running and walking assessments of fixed length or a specified time. Three common running field tests are the 1.5-mile run, 12-minute run, and the multistage 20-m shuttle run tests. The procedures are as follows:

- *1.5-Mile run* — this test is commonly performed on a quarter-mile track. Following a proper warm-up, the athlete(s) begin at the starting line and runs as rapidly as possible (at a steady pace) for 6 laps (1.5 miles) until crossing the finish line. The coach (with a stopwatch) begins timing on "go" and stops timing when the athlete crosses the finish line. The time is recorded. $\dot{V}O_{2max}$ can be estimated by the following equation:

$$\dot{V}O_{2max} \text{ of } (mL \cdot kg^{-1} \cdot min^{-1}) = 3.5 + (483 / run \text{ time in minutes})$$

Or can be estimated with gender-specific equations (82):

$$Men : \dot{V}O_{2max}(mL \cdot kg^{-1} \cdot min^{-1}) = 91.736 \\ - (0.1656 \times body \text{ mass in kilograms}) - (2.767 \\ \times run \text{ time in minutes})$$

$$Women : \dot{V}O_{2max}(mL \cdot kg^{-1} \cdot min^{-1}) = 88.020 \\ - (0.1656 \times body \text{ mass in kilograms}) - (2.767 \\ \times run \text{ time in minutes})$$

- *Cooper 12-minute run* — this test is performed on a track with markings at each 100-m interval. The athletes begin at the starting line and upon the signal "go," run as rapidly as possible (at a steady pace) for 12 minutes. Upon the signal to "stop," the distance the athlete successfully completed is measured. For example, 6.5 laps = 2,600 m. The distance is recorded. $\dot{V}O_{2max}$ can be estimated by the following equation:

$$\dot{V}O_{2max} (mL \cdot kg^{-1} \cdot min^{-1}) = 0.0268 \text{ (distance covered)} - 11.3$$

- *Multistage 20-m shuttle run* — has variations and is known as the *beep test* or *Progressive Aerobic CV Endurance Run (PACER)* test as it has been adapted to other segments of the population (children and adolescents) since its development in the early 1980s (83). A flat, nonslippery area marked with parallel lines or cones separated by exactly 20 m and the beep test CD/multimedia package are needed for this field test. A shorter 15-m variation can be used if athletes are tested in a small facility (which requires a conversion chart). A scorekeeper is used to record completed laps/shuttles. The CD provides audio cues (beeps) that allow the athlete to set a pace during running. The athlete continuously runs between the two lines or cones (touching the line each time) at a pace based on the stage or level of the test. For example, a beep starts the test, the athlete runs 20 m, and returns 20 m upon the next beep. Sufficient pacing is important to ensure that athletes do not overwork during initial stages. The test is progressive where the beeps are closer together with each successive stage, thereby forcing the athlete to run at a faster pace until the athlete can no longer maintain the pace. There are ~21 levels each lasting a minute with most athletes completing between 6 and 15. An additional sound or triple beep may be used to indicate completion of a level. The test ends when athletes can no longer keep pace with the beeps on two successive trials. Athletes should be allowed multiple practice sessions before testing to familiarize themselves to the beep cadence. The final score is the level (indicated by the number or corresponding velocity) or number of laps attained before athlete cannot maintain pace for successive shuttles. There are different variations of the test. The original version developed by Leger and Lambert (83) begins with a starting velocity of 8.0 km·h⁻¹ and progresses 0.5 km·h⁻¹ with each stage (every 2 min) of the test. Another variation using adults and children begins with a starting velocity of 8.5 km·h⁻¹ and progresses 0.5 km·h⁻¹ with each minute (stage) of the test (84). Other studies were conducted that allowed prediction of $\dot{V}O_{2max}$ from the number of levels completed (85) and number of laps/shuttles completed (86). Validity and test-retest reliability of the test are good (83,85,86) with reliability being greater in adults than children (84). Research shows that men ($\dot{V}O_{2max}$ of ~58–59 mL·kg⁻¹·min⁻¹) complete an average of 11.4–12.6 levels with 105–121 total shuttles (laps) and women ($\dot{V}O_{2max}$ of ~47.4 mL·kg⁻¹·min⁻¹) complete an average of 9.6 levels with 85 total shuttles (85,86). $\dot{V}O_{2max}$ can be estimated using the following equations:

Adults (mean age of 26 yr): $\dot{V}O_{2max}$ (mL · kg⁻¹ · min⁻¹)
= 5.857 (speed in km · h⁻¹) − 19.458 (83)

Adults and children (8−19 yr): $\dot{V}O_{2max}$ (mL · kg⁻¹ · min⁻¹)
= 31.025 + 3.238 (speed in km · h⁻¹) − 3.248 (age in years)
+ 0.1536 (age in years × speed in km · h⁻¹)
where speed begins at 8.0 + 0.5 (stage number) (84)

Adults (19 − 36 yr): $\dot{V}O_{2max}$ (mL · kg⁻¹ · min⁻¹)
= 14.4 + 3.48 (level completed) where level completed
(number) is the last fully completed stage of the test (85)

Men (26 − 47 yr): $\dot{V}O_{2max}$ (mL · kg⁻¹ · min⁻¹)
= 18 + 0.39 (laps or shuttles completed)(86)
— Note: this equation is based on a
small number (i.e., 9) of subjects.

Norms for the 1.5-mile run and 12-minute run tests are presented in Table 19.13, and $\dot{V}O_{2max}$ norms are presented in Table 19.14.

Cycle Ergometer Tests

Cycle ergometer tests are single- or multistage submaximal tests where $\dot{V}O_{2max}$ is predicted from exercise HR. Accurate assessment of HR is mandatory. A HR monitor is preferred. Palpation can be used but introduces a large magnitude of error. Factors that affect HR (hot/humid temperature, caffeine, stress)

must be controlled for greater accuracy. Two common cycle ergometer tests are the Åstrand-Rhyming and YMCA tests.

- *Åstrand-Rhyming test* — is a single-stage submaximal test lasting 6 minutes in duration. The pedal rate is standardized at 50 rpm. HR is measured after the first 2 minutes. If HR ≥120 bpm, the athlete continues at the initial work rate. If HR ≤120 bpm, the athlete increases work rate to the next increment level. HR is measured during the 5th and 6th minutes of the exercise and averaged to be used in the nomogram (Fig. 19.13). $\dot{V}O_{2max}$ data must then be corrected for age using the nomogram in Table 19.15 (45). The workload varies in the following manner:
  - Untrained men: 300 or 600 kg·m·min⁻¹ (50 or 100 W)
  - Trained men: 600 or 900 kg·m·min⁻¹ (100 or 150 W)
  - Untrained women: 300 or 450 kg·m·min⁻¹ (50 or 75 W)
  - Trained women: 450 or 600 kg·m·min⁻¹ (75 or 100 W)
- *YMCA submaximal cycle ergometer test* — this test consists of 2–4 stages that last 3 minutes each. The initial workload is set at 150 kg·m·min⁻¹. The workload for the second stage depends on the HR measured in the last minute of the first stage. The HR measured during the last minute of each stage is plotted against work rate. The line is then extrapolated to the athlete's age-predicted maximal HR and a perpendicular line (b) is dropped to the axis to determine work rate (45,89) (Fig. 19.14). The work rate in kg·m·min⁻¹ is converted to watts using the following formula:

$$\text{Work rate (W)} = \text{work rate (kg} \cdot \text{m} \cdot \text{min}^{-1}) / 6.12$$

Using the athlete's body mass (kg), $\dot{V}O_{2max}$ is calculated via the following equation:

$$\dot{V}O_{2max} − ([10.8 \times \text{work rate}] / \text{body mass}) + 7$$

Normative data for the YMCA protocol are published elsewhere (90).

Step Tests

Several step tests have been developed over the years. These involve different step heights, rates, and stage durations. Heart rate is typically used in the prediction of $\dot{V}O_{2max}$. One example is the Queens College step test developed by McArdle et al. (91):

- *Queens college step test* — males and females use step height of 16.25 in. However, the step rate in men is 24 steps·min⁻¹ and women is 22 steps·min⁻¹ set to a metronome. The duration of the test is 3 minutes and HR is taken at the conclusion of the test. $\dot{V}O_{2max}$ is calculated via the following equations:

$$\dot{V}O_{2max} (\text{men}) = 111.33 − (0.42 \times \text{HR})$$

$$\dot{V}O_{2max} (\text{women}) = 65.81 − (0.1847 \times \text{HR})$$

Table 19.13 — Percentile Ranks for Distance Run during 12-Minute Run (Top) and for 1.5-Mile (2.41-km) Run Time (min:s) (Bottom)

Distance Run during 12-Min Run

Percentile	Age (yr)									
	20–29		30–39		40–49		50–59		60+	
MEN	N = 1,675		N = 7,095		N = 6,837		N = 3,808		N = 1,005	
	ML	KM	ML	KM	ML	KM	ML	KM	ML	KM
90	1.74	2.78	1.71	2.74	1.65	2.64	1.57	2.51	1.49	2.38
80	1.65	2.64	1.61	2.58	1.54	2.46	1.45	2.32	1.37	2.19
70	1.61	2.58	1.55	2.48	1.47	2.35	1.38	2.21	1.29	2.06
60	1.54	2.46	1.49	2.38	1.42	2.27	1.33	2.13	1.24	1.98
50	1.50	2.40	1.45	2.32	1.37	2.19	1.29	2.06	1.19	1.90
40	1.45	2.32	1.39	2.22	1.33	2.13	1.25	2.00	1.15	1.84
30	1.41	2.26	1.35	2.16	1.29	2.06	1.21	1.94	1.11	1.78
20	1.34	2.14	1.29	2.06	1.23	1.97	1.15	1.84	1.05	1.68
10	1.27	2.03	1.21	1.94	1.17	1.87	1.09	1.74	0.95	1.52
Women	N = 764		N = 2,049		N = 1,630		N = 878		N = 202	
90	1.54	2.46	1.45	2.32	1.41	2.26	1.29	2.06	1.29	2.06
80	1.45	2.32	1.38	2.21	1.32	2.11	1.21	1.94	1.18	1.89
70	1.37	2.19	1.33	2.13	1.25	2.00	1.17	1.87	1.13	1.81
60	1.33	2.13	1.27	2.03	1.21	1.94	1.13	1.81	1.07	1.71
50	1.29	2.06	1.25	2.00	1.17	1.87	1.10	1.76	1.03	1.65
40	1.25	2.00	1.21	1.94	1.13	1.81	1.06	1.70	0.99	1.58
30	1.21	1.94	1.16	1.86	1.10	1.76	1.02	1.63	0.97	1.55
20	1.16	1.86	1.11	1.78	1.05	1.68	0.98	1.57	0.94	1.50
10	1.10	1.76	1.05	1.68	1.01	1.62	0.93	1.49	0.89	1.42

1.5 Mi (2.41 km) Run Time (min:s)

Percentile	Age (Yr)				
	20–29	30–39	40–49	50–59	60+
Men	N = 1,675	N = 7,095	N = 6,837	N = 3,808	N = 1,005
90	9:09	9:30	10:16	11:18	12:20
80	10:16	10:47	11:44	12:51	13:53
70	10:47	11:34	12:34	13:45	14:53
60	11:41	12:20	13:14	14:24	15:29
50	12:18	12:51	13:53	14:55	16:07
40	12:51	13:36	14:29	15:26	16:43
30	13:22	14:08	14:56	15:57	17:14
20	14:13	14:52	15:41	16:43	18:00
10	15:10	15:52	16:28	17:29	19:15
Women	N = 764	N = 2,049	N = 1,630	N = 878	N = 202
90	11:43	12:51	13:22	14:55	14:55
80	12:51	13:43	14:31	15:57	16:20
70	13:53	14:24	15:16	16:27	16:58
60	14:24	15:08	15:57	16:58	17:46
50	14:55	15:26	16:27	17:24	18:16
40	15:26	15:57	16:58	17:55	18:44
30	15:57	16:35	17:24	18:23	18:59
20	16:33	17:14	18:00	18:49	19:21
10	17:21	18:00	18:31	19:30	20:04

Reprinted with permission from Hoffman J. *Norms for Fitness, Performance, and Health*. Champaign (IL): Human Kinetics; 2006. p. 1–113.

Table 19.14 Percentile Values for Maximal Aerobic Power (mL·kg·min^{-1})

Percentile	20–29	30–39	40–49	50–59	60+
Men					
90	51.4	50.4	48.2	45.3	42.5
80	48.2	46.8	44.1	41.0	38.1
70	46.8	44.6	41.8	38.5	35.3
60	44.2	42.4	39.9	36.7	33.6
50	42.5	41.0	38.1	35.2	31.8
40	41.0	38.9	36.7	33.8	30.2
30	39.5	37.4	35.1	32.3	28.7
20	37.1	35.4	33.0	30.2	26.5
10	34.5	32.5	30.9	28.0	23.1
Women					
90	44.2	41.0	39.5	35.2	35.2
80	41.0	38.6	36.3	32.3	31.2
70	38.1	36.7	33.8	30.9	29.4
60	36.7	34.6	32.3	29.4	27.2
50	35.2	33.8	30.9	28.2	25.8
40	33.8	32.3	29.5	26.9	24.5
30	32.3	30.5	28.3	25.5	23.8
20	30.6	28.7	26.5	24.3	22.8
10	28.4	26.5	25.1	22.3	20.8

Reprinted with permission from Hoffman J. *Norms for Fitness, Performance, and Health*. Champaign (IL): Human Kinetics; 2006. p. 1–113.

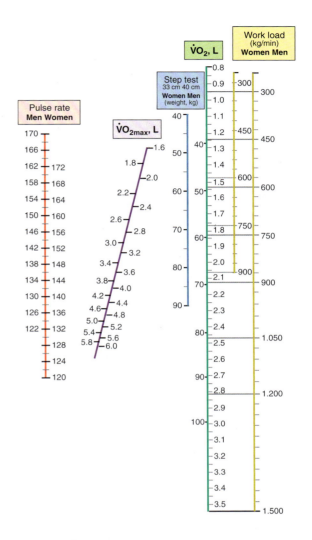

FIGURE 19.13 Åstrand-Rhyming test nomogram. (Reprinted with permission from Åstrand PO, Rhyming I. A nomogram for calculation of aerobic capacity [physical fitness] from pulse rate during submaximal work. *J Appl Physiol*. 1954;7:218–21.)

Table 19.15 Age Correction Factor for the Åstrand-Rhyming Cycle Ergometer Test

Age	Correction Factor
15	1.10
25	1.00
35	0.87
40	0.83
45	0.78
50	0.75
55	0.71
60	0.68
65	0.65

Lactate Threshold

In Chapter 8, we discussed the concept of the lactate threshold (LT), and in Chapter 17, we discussed the importance of LT in maximizing endurance competition performance. Measurement of LT provides the athlete with a specific intensity or workload that can be trained at specific intervals. The simplest way to assess LT is to use a portable calibrated lactate analyzer with strips, lancets, and alcohol wipes. A fingertip is prepped with alcohol, lancets that are used to pierce the skin and produce a blood droplet, and the analyzer with strip is used to draw blood into the reservoir and measure blood lactate concentrations. Gloves should be worn (especially if a partner is taking the sample) and blood waste disposed of properly. Different protocols can be used once the trainee has warmed-up but usually involve running or cycling. Testing should be as specific to training program as possible. Progressive ramp protocols (similar to those used for $\dot{V}O_{2max}$ testing) in 2–3 minutes stages are recommended (with intensity increases of 5%–15%

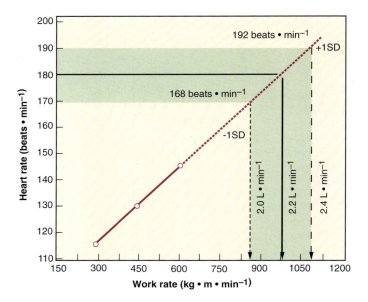

FIGURE 19.14 Relationship between HR and work rate in relation to max aerobic capacity; b = extrapolated work rate. (Reprinted with permission from Thompson W, editor. *ACSM's Guidelines for Exercise Testing and Prescription*. 8th ed. Baltimore (MD): Lippincott Williams & Wilkins; 2010.)

and velocity (Fig. 19.15). The optimal expression of power consists of many physiological and biomechanical factors discussed in previous chapters including muscle fiber types, energy metabolism, muscle size and architecture, neural activation, inter- and intramuscular coordination, torque/leverage, and the stretch-shortening cycle (93). Tests of peak power are explosive and short in duration (a few seconds) and predominantly stress the ATP-PC system. Some of these peak power tests include 1 RM Olympic lifts, jump tests, jump squats on force plate or transducer, medicine ball throws, Margaria-Kalamen test, and RFD tests. Other tests measure power endurance, *i.e., anaerobic capacity* tests. These track power over time (Wingate test) or measure the amount of time it takes to complete a pattern of movement (300-yd shuttle and line drill). Because these tests are longer in duration (15–90 s), they stress the glycolytic energy system so the maintenance of power is most critical.

per stage) so that a sample can be taken near the end of a stage or at regular time intervals. The test should begin at a low intensity so blood lactate can remain at resting levels early in the test. For example, one treadmill running protocol we have used consists of 2-minute stages at a speed of 6.0 mph with increments in percent grade of 2.5% per stage until exhaustion. For flat running, we have used a protocol consisting of 2-minute stages (starting at 5.0 mph) with increments in velocity of 0.5 mph each stage until exhaustion (92). Blood samples can be taken from different sites at the end of each stage. When the test is complete, blood lactate data can be plotted versus speed (or workload). The deflection point where blood lactate increases beyond resting level is the LT. This corresponding workload can be used as a guide for interval training targeting improvements in LT. Recall from Chapters 8 and 17 that LT can increase as a function of training. Thus, periodic assessment may be beneficial to accurately update training programs.

Assessment of Skill-Related Fitness Components

Testing of several skill-related components of fitness is paramount to a comprehensive testing battery for athletes. These include peak power, anaerobic capacity, speed, agility, and balance.

Power

Power testing is critical to assessing anaerobic athletes. **Power** is the rate of performing work and is the product of force and velocity. Peak power occurs at the optimal combination of force

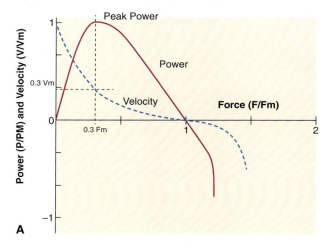

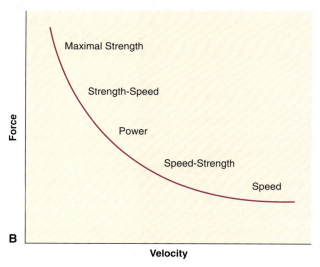

FIGURE 19.15 The relationships between force, velocity, power, and speed. Panel **A** shows the relationship of peak power to force and velocity. Panel **B** shows the force-velocity relationship with the curve labeled from maximal strength (high force, low velocity) to speed (low force, high velocity). (First graph from Peterson MD. Power. In: *NSCA's Guide to Tests and Assessments*. Champaign (IL): Human Kinetics; 2012. p. 217–52.)

Power tests may be adapted to reflect greater sport specificity. A few examples are also listed in this section.

Vertical and Broad Jumps

Jump tests are predicated upon the correlation between power and jump height or distance. They are easy to administer and provide valuable information relating to athletic success. This section discusses two jump tests, the vertical and broad jumps although other types of jumps can be assessed.

Vertical Jump

- A tape measure, chalk, or special device like the *Vertec* is needed.
- When using a wall (*Sargent jump test*), the athlete stands against a wall with dominant arm flexed vertically as high as possible. The athlete has chalk on his/her fingers. The initial step is to determine the starting height as the athlete reaches high, touches the wall, and sets the starting height. Using a countermovement, the athlete jumps as high as possible and touches the highest possible point on the wall (marking it with chalk on the fingertips) with the use of arm swing. The distance between marks is measured. The best of three trials is recorded.
- When using a Vertec, the athlete sets the starting position. The Vertec is adjustable and has color-coded vanes (Fig. 19.16). The very first vane marks the reading on the Vertec. A red vane is placed every 6 in., and blue and white vanes are 1 in. apart, marking whole and half inch measures, respectively. The athlete stands erect with the dominant arm flexed vertically as high as possible and touches (and moves) the corresponding vanes. This demarcates the starting height. For testers, it is important to make sure the athlete extends the body as far as possible (without rising on the toes) or the vertical jump height can be overexaggerated. The height of the Vertec is adjusted (raised) so that the athlete will touch and move a vane (and not the top one) when jumping maximally. Using a countermovement, the athlete jumps as high as possible touching the highest possible vanes. The highest vane touched demarcates the finish height. For subsequent jump trials, it is advantageous for the coach to leave 1–2 vanes (0.5–1.0 in.) under the highest one attained in place. This gives the athlete a target height to shoot for when jumping maximally. Starting height is subtracted from the finish height and the difference is the vertical jump height. The best of three trials is recorded. If the third trial is the best, then a fourth (or fifth) trial should be used.
- Power can be calculated from vertical jump height. This can be useful for differentiating between two athletes with similar vertical jump heights. Larger athletes must produce more absolute power to jump a certain height than smaller athletes. Thus, assessment of power (peak and mean) may be advantageous in addition to just using vertical jump height. Originally, the *Lewis formula* was used to estimate peak power from vertical jump height using the following equation:

$$\text{Power (W)} = [\sqrt{4.9} \times \text{body mass (kg)} \times 9.807] \times [\sqrt{\text{jump height (m)}}]$$

However, cross-validation against jumps from a force plate showed that the Lewis formula underestimated mean and peak power by up to 70% (46). Since, other equations have been developed. It is critical to selecting equations based on technique standardization (*i.e.*, arm swing vs. no arm swing, countermovement vs. squat, etc.) and in populations that match as closely as possible the testing population. Estimation error is expected when using any equation, depending on age, gender, and activity level of the population tested. Thus, selecting the most specific equation and consistently using it throughout athletic assessment can provide the coach or practitioner with acceptable estimates and can provide an indication of the efficacy of the training program used.

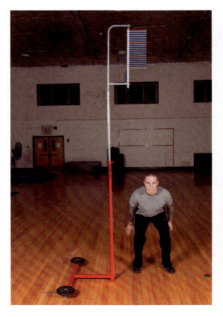
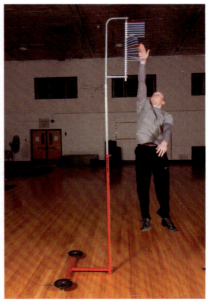

FIGURE 19.16 Vertical jump with a Vertec.

Harman et al. (94) developed the following accurate regression equations for estimating peak and mean power during the vertical jump:

$$\text{Peak power (W)} = 61.9 \text{ (jump height in cm)} + 36 \text{ (body mass in kg)} + 1,822$$

$$\text{Mean power (W)} = 21.1 \text{ (jump height in cm)} + 23 \text{ (body mass in kg)} + 1,393$$

Johnson and Bahamonde (95) developed the following equations:

$$\text{Peak power (W)} = 78.6 \text{ (jump height in cm)} + 60.3 \text{ (mass in kg)} + 15.3 \text{ (ht in cm)} - 15.3 \text{ (ht in cm)} - 1,308$$

$$\text{Mean power (W)} = 43.8 \text{ (jump height in cm)} + 32.7 \text{ (mass in kg)} - 16.8 \text{ (ht in cm)} + 431$$

Sayers et al. (96) developed the following equation in 108 male and female athletes and nonathletes:

$$\text{Peak power (W)} = 60.7 \text{ (jump height in cm)} + 45.3 \text{ (mass in kg)} - 2,055$$

Canavan and Vescovi (97) developed the following equation in 20 college women:

$$\text{Peak power (W)} = (65.1 \cdot \text{VJ height (cm)}) + (25.8 \cdot \text{BM (kg)}) - 1.413.1$$

Amonette et al. (98) developed the following equations in 415 youth/adult men (mostly athletes) of different ages:

$$\text{Peak power (W)} = 12 - 15 \text{ years} : (61.9 \cdot \text{VJ height (cm)}) + (40.8 \cdot \text{BM (kg)}) - 1,680.7$$

$$\text{Peak power (W)} = 16 - 18 \text{ years} : (63.6 \cdot \text{VJ height (cm)}) + (46.2 \cdot \text{BM (kg)}) - 2,108.2$$

$$\text{Peak power (W)} = 19 - 24 \text{ years} : (83.0 \cdot \text{VJ height (cm)}) + (54.5 \cdot \text{BM (kg)}) - 3,436.8$$

$$\text{Peak power (W)} = \text{Overall} : (63.6 \cdot \text{VJ height (cm)}) + (42.7 \cdot \text{BM (kg)}) - 1,846.5$$

Norms for vertical jump performance in athletes are presented in Table 19.16. Variations of the basic vertical jump test can be used. For example, the *one-step vertical jump test* is commonly used especially in a sport such as basketball where jumping off of a single-leg is common to the sport (2). The test is similar to the vertical jump test except the athlete first places one foot back, steps, and then jumps vertically off of both feet as high as possible. In addition, jump height can be determined from

Table 19.16	Vertical Jump Norms for Athletes	
% Rank	**Men (cm)**	**Women (cm)**
91–100	86.35–91.45	76.20–81.30
81–90	81.30–86.34	71.11–76.19
71–80	76.20–81.29	66.05–71.10
61–70	71.10–76.19	60.95–66.04
51–60	66.05–71.09	55.90–60.94
41–50	60.95–66.04	50.80–55.89
31–40	55.90–60.94	45.70–50.79
21–30	50.80–55.89	40.65–45.70
11–20	45.70–50.79	35.55–40.64
1–10	40.65–45.69	30.50–35.54

Reprinted with permission from Chu DA. *Explosive Power and Strength*. Champaign (IL): Human Kinetics; 1996. p. 167–80. Ref. (99).

other types of jumps in addition to squat, counter-movement, and one-step jumps. The depth jump may be used (described in Chapter 15). This is especially useful when determining the appropriate height of the box used during plyometric training or as a measurement of the reactive strength index (see Chapter 2).

Broad Jump (Standing Long Jump)

The broad jump assesses horizontal power development. Other variations including the 2-hop or 3-hop tests involve performance of consecutive repetitions of broad jumps emphasizing the landing and subsequent SSC activation prior to the next subsequent jump. Here, the total length covered by 2 or 3 jumps is recorded. For a single-repetition broad jump

- A flat area (at least 15 ft in length) (grass field, gym floor, etc.), a tape measure, and a masking tape are needed. Tape serves as a start marker and can be used to secure the tape measure lengthwise. The athlete starts with his/her toes just behind the starting line.
- Using a countermovement with arm swing, the athlete jumps forward as far as possible. The athlete should land on both feet for the trial to count. The athlete should land with feet straddled over the tape measure. A point at the athlete's rearmost heel is marked and the distance is measured. The best of three trials is recorded.
- Table 19.17 presents norms for the broad jump in athletes.

Force Plate and Transducer Assessments

Many types of technologies can be used to assess power including force plates, linear position transducers, accelerometers, video analysis, and timing mats. Force plates and linear position transducers can be used for a number of different

Table 19.17	Broad Jump Norms for Athletes	
% Rank	Men (m)	Women (m)
91–100	3.40–3.75	2.94–3.15
81–90	3.10–3.39	2.80–2.94
71–80	2.95–09	2.65–2.79
61–70	2.80–2.95	2.50–2.64
51–60	2.65–2.79	2.35–2.49
41–50	2.50–2.64	2.20–2.34
31–40	2.35–2.49	2.05–2.19
21–30	2.20–2.34	1.90–2.04
11–20	2.05–2.19	1.75–1.89
1–10	1.90–2.04	1.60–1.74

Reprinted with permission from Chu DA. *Explosive Power and Strength*. Champaign (IL): Human Kinetics; 1996. p. 167–80.

exercises and movements. Jump squats performed on a force plate (Fig. 19.17) or with a position transducer attached to the bar or athlete's belt can provide power data for the coach. Force plates contain strain gauges or load cells that directly measure ground reaction force from the athlete. Force output (and moments) can be measured in three planes of motion. Force-time data are generated such that impulse, momentum, and flight time can be determined, as well as velocity-time data. RFD data can be generated directly from the force-time curves or from software calculation. Considering that power is the product of force and velocity, power curves can be generated yielding peak and mean power output data. Many jumps can be tested in addition to depth, squat, and countermovement jumps and testing can occur in multiple planes (*i.e.*, lateral jumps). Repeated jump tests and tests of power endurance can be used. We have used a 20-repetition squat jump test (with 30% of pretraining squat 1 RM) to generate power-time curves

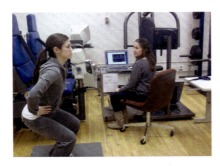

FIGURE 19.17 Force plate testing of a vertical jump. Here, an athlete is preparing to perform a vertical jump test consisting of three successive jumps on the force plate. Power-time curves from the previous set-off jumps can be seen on the monitor screen. (Photo courtesy of The College of New Jersey Human Performance Lab.)

and to calculate fatigue rates (highest power output − lowest power output/highest power output × 100) in athletes and have seen fatigue index rates of 13%–21% (100). Bosco et al. (101) described a test where repeated maximal countermovement vertical jumps are performed consecutively for 15 to 60 seconds. Flight time, foot contact time, and number of jumps completed per interval are recorded. Average power and fatigue rate may be calculated. Modified protocols (with fewer reps) have been used where foot contact time is used as the key measure of assessing *reactive strength* (2). One test, the 10-to-5 repeated jump test, involves performing 11 maximal jumps where foot contact times of <250 ms are desired for reps to count (2). The five highest jumps are totaled to produce a reactive strength score (2).

Some types of force plates can be set in the floor, whereas some are portable. Several unilateral and bilateral exercises can be performed on force plates from running to jumps to various ground-based weight training, plyometric, and sport-specific exercises. Unilateral tests can be used to assess potential imbalances. For example, right-to-left differences of more than 15% may indicate some type of injury or may be seen as increasing the risk of injury (102). Thus, comparison of single-leg movements via force, power, velocity, and flight time data can be used to assess the athlete's unilateral kinetic performance (102). Athletes can be assessed on force plates under sport-specific conditions, *e.g.*, jumping to spike a volleyball or rebound in basketball, and pushing off during pitching in baseball. Depth jumps have been used where the athlete steps off of boxes of various heights, lands on the plate, and jumps as explosively as possible. Flight time can be divided by contact time with the plate during landing to calculate the *reactive strength index* (102). Power data can be expressed in absolute or relative terms. Normalized power data (to body weight) can provide the coach additional data especially for those athletes who require a high strength/power-to-mass ratio like a high jumper who is competing against gravity versus a football player where absolute total-body power is essential (102). Relative power measures allow for comparisons among athletes of different body weights.

The technology used in designing a force plate can be incorporated into sport-specific equipment. Force transducers can be systematically placed in sport-specific training equipment to measure force and power. Placing force transducers into a blocking sled can measure sport-specific force and power in a football player. Force/pressure transducers can be placed into footwear to measure forces produced during various tasks. They have been placed within treadmills to measure force and velocity during sprinting (103). Special boxing dynamometers were developed to measure force during straight punches in boxers (104). Critical is the placement of transducers, the planes of detection, and the potential for damage and movement as a result of striking. Thus, reliability is of concern. However, these pieces of equipment appear to provide meaningful data to researchers and coaches when used over time as a tool in the athletic assessment box. The most critical element is that sport-specific tests can be used to truly measure athletic performance during direct motor skill applications.

Although force plates are typically found in biomechanics or exercise physiology laboratories, position and velocity transducers and accelerometers are more practical and affordable for coaches to use. Accelerometers (such as the Myotest) can be attached to the belt or mounted to a barbell to measure power and velocity (105). Transducers are applied to bars or the body and measure displacement during movement. Studies have shown them to be valid and reliable during kinetic testing (106). The Tendo unit is used to measure power in athletes (Fig. 19.18). It consists of a position transducer that is applied to one (or both) end of the bar and is interfaced with a microcomputer for data collection. It measures bar displacement and time, thereby allowing bar velocity to be calculated for each repetition. The weight on the bar or body weight is input (to compute force) and power (peak and average) is calculated for each repetition. Instant feedback is provided so athletes can be made aware of their subsequent effort for each repetition. Transducers enable power assessment for any resistance exercise, traditional or ballistic, although ballistic exercises are preferred, e.g., jump squats, bench press throw, and Olympic lifts. The Ultimate Fighting Championship Institute uses linear position transducers in conjunction with the loaded landmine punch throw test as a measure of power specificity for striking (4). We reported peak and average power data for several exercises including the high pull, back squat, bench press, incline bench press, bent-over barbell row, deadlift, seated shoulder press, and push press (92,107). The best systems combine transducer data with force plate data in calculation of power. Tendo transducers are reliable ($R = 0.87$–0.94) measures of power during standardized performance of bench press and barbell back squat (108,109).

Although several exercises can be used for assessment, the jump squat and bench press throw are used most primarily because they are ballistic exercise that yields high-power outputs. Ballistic exercises minimize the deceleration phase and increase power development throughout the exercise ROM. Loaded and unloaded jump squats are used for power assessment.

When used as an assessment, jump squats that yield the highest power outputs are recommended. Earlier studies showed loaded jump squats (30%–60% of 1 RM) yielded highest values, whereas some recent studies have indicated jump squats with body weight only yield highest values (102,110,111). A meta-analysis showed 0%–30% of 1 RM to be optimal loading for producing peak power during jump squats (112). The bench press throw with 30%–60% of 1 RM was shown to produce peak power output (23), although a recent meta-analysis showed 0%–30% of 1 RM may be optimal for producing peak power (113). Safety is increased when these exercises are performed on a device that has a braking system in place. The coach should select an absolute loading scheme and use that with successive power assessments. Power improvements are greater when the same preloading is used for power testing. Because power-loading curves are bell shaped, changing the loading assesses power on a different segment of the curve, which can skew power measurements erroneously. A change in power can reflect a different segment of the curve rather than an adaptation to training.

Power output generated from ballistic assessments is variable when comparing data from one study to another. It is very difficult to compare power outputs from athletes in one study to athletes from another study as there has been little consistency in power data obtained. It is difficult to establish norms for jump squat power as each plate or transducer yields values different from other laboratory's measurements. It is necessary for the coach or staff to generate their own norms based on power data generated from one device.

RFD assessments can be used. There are several ways to measure RFD as force plates generate RFD data during tests such as jump squats or any exercise performed on the plate. A common RFD assessment involves ISOM testing. An ISOM squat (performed on top of a force plate), mid-thigh pull, or leg press (when a force plate or strain gauge is built into the sled) can be used. The bar or sled is fixed at a specific joint angle where it cannot move, e.g., with stoppers, pins in a rack, or ultra-heavy weights added to the bar or sled. The athlete is instructed to produce as much force as possible in the shortest amount of time. From the data generated, several variables of interest can be used. For example, if the athlete's peak force was 4,000 N pretesting, variables such as time to produce 4,000 N (100% of peak force) or time to a specific force output, e.g., 60%, 70%, 80%, and 90% of peak force, can be determined. This test can be applied after several weeks or months of training. A reduction in the time to produce these various levels of force indicates an increase in RFD. Thus, RFD tests measure how fast an athlete can produce submaximal or maximal force and can be a valuable tool in athletic assessments. However, because force plates, strain gauges, load cells, and transducers are needed, the cost may be high and prohibitive for some athletic settings.

Margaria-Kalamen Test

The Margaria-Kalamen test measures power by assessing the athlete's ability to ascend stairs as rapidly as possible. It has been used, albeit sparingly, to assess an athlete since its inception in the 1960s (55). The procedures are:

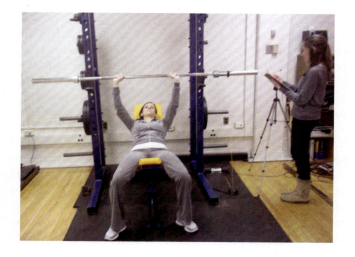

FIGURE 19.18 Use of a transducer during an incline bench press. (Photo courtesy of The College of New Jersey Human Performance Lab.)

Table 19.18	Normative Values (in W) for the Margaria-Kalamen Stair Sprint Test									
	Age and Gender									
	15–20 yr		20–30 yr		30–40 yr		40–50 yr		50 + yr	
Category	M	F	M	F	M	F	M	F	M	F
Excellent	2,197	1,789	2,059	1,648	1,648	1,226	1,226	961	961	736
Good	1,840	1,487	1,722	1,379	1,379	1,036	1,036	810	809	604
Average	1,839	1,486	1,721	1,378	1,378	1,035	1,035	809	808	603
Fair	1,466	1,182	1,368	1,094	1,094	829	829	642	641	476
Poor	1,108	902	1,040	834	834	637	637	490	490	373

Adapted from Fox E, Bowers R, Foss M. *The Physiological Basis for Exercise and Sport*. 5th ed. Dubuque (IA): Wm C. Brown. 1993:676. With permission of The McGraw-Hill Companies: based on data from Kalamen J. *Measurement of Maximum Muscular Power in Man*. Doctoral Dissertation. The Ohio State University; 1968, and Margaria R, Aghemo I, Rovelli E. Measurement of muscular power (anaerobic) in man. *J Appl Physiol*. 1966;21:1662–4.

- A staircase with nine or more steps (at least 7-in. high and a lead-up area of ~20 ft) and an electronic timing device are needed. The height of each step needs to be measured and the elevation from the third to the ninth step needs to be calculated (6 × step height) *a priori*. The electronic timer start switch is placed on step 3 and the stop switch is placed on step 9.
- The athlete sprints 20 ft toward the stairs and then rapidly ascends the stairs three steps at a time. Timing begins when the athlete touches the third step and ends upon touching the ninth step. This time is used for calculation.
- Power is calculated via the following formula:

$$\text{Power (W)} = [\text{Body mass (kg)} \times \text{vertical height from steps 3 to 9 (m)}] / \text{time(s)} \times 9.81$$

- Norms for the Margaria-Kalamen test are shown in Table 19.18.

Upper-Body Power Assessments

Several tests can be used to assess upper-body power. The bench press throw is common. This test involves explosively throwing the bar upward. A linear position transducer is used to measure power. Transducers can be used for other upper-body exercises as well. The plyo push-up on a force plate can be used (data shown in Fig. 19.19). High reliability for the plyo push-up on a force plate for determining peak power has been shown (114). Wang et al. (114) reported peak power values of ~939 W in recreationally resistance-trained men. They also developed prediction equations for upper-body power (when flight time is known) using the plyo push-up:

Upper Body Peak Power $= (11.0 * \text{body mass (kg)})$
$+ (2012.3 * \text{flight time (sec)}) - 338$

Upper Body Mean Power $= (6.7 * \text{body mass (kg)})$
$+ (1004.4 * \text{flight time (sec)}) - 224.6$

Several different MB throws (side throws, overhead throws, and underhand throws) can be used. The distance the ball is thrown relates highly to upper-body (or total-body) power. Studies have shown MB tests to be valid and reliable indicators of power. Stockbrugger and Haennel (115) showed that the backward MB toss was a reliable test of power and correlated highly to vertical jump performance. Values of 12–15.4 m have been shown using 3-kg MBs in athletes (82). Cowley and Swensen (116) showed front and side MB throws to provide reliable power data. Ikeda et al. (117) found the side MB throw reliable in men but less reliable in women for predicting trunk rotation power. Overhead throws have greater specificity to athletes such as basketball players or soccer players who use this motion regularly in the sport. Thus, several throws can be useful to the coach when developing an upper-body power protocol. Backward throws have a greater lower-body component, whereas side throws test rotational power. Direct upper-body power has been assessed using the MB chest pass.

Medicine Ball Chest Pass

- This test can be performed from a standing or seated position. A seated position isolates the upper body to a greater extent. Medicine balls vary, but one standard size can be used ~2%–5% of the athlete's body weight. When standing, a shoulder width stance is used. When seated, a back support is helpful as the athlete needs to keep contact with the support during the throw (a belt can be used). The athlete could sit against a wall as well. The toes should be aligned with a tape marker to set the starting line.
- The athlete passes or puts the MB as far as possible at an angle <45°. Upon landing, the center of the ball is marked

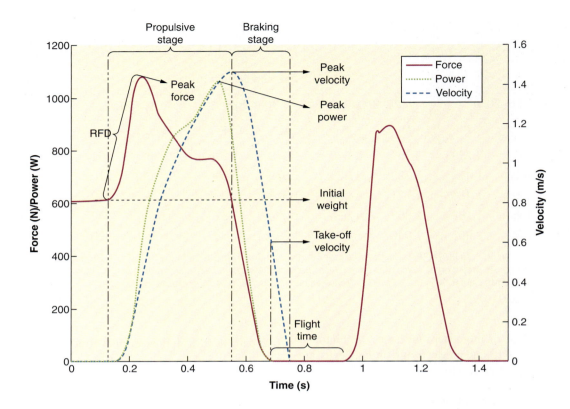

FIGURE 19.19 Force, velocity, and power curves during a plyo push-up on a force plate. (From Wang R, Hoffman JR, Sadres E, et al. Evaluating upper-body strength and power from a single test: the ballistic push-up. *J Strength Cond Res.* 2017;31:1338–45.)

and the distance from the starting line is measured. Some coaches prefer to chalk the ball for accuracy. Thus, the chalk will mark the landing spot and will make it easier to identify the correct location.

- The best of three throws is recorded. Norms are difficult for this test because coaches use different size MBs, and standing versus seated will produce different results. Adolescent athletes using the seated pass were shown to pass a 3-kg MB ~3.8–4.3 m (118), whereas Division III college football players have shown 3-kg MB pass values of 5.3–5.8 m (119). It is recommended that each coach store data and produce his/her own norms when standardized procedures are used.

Anaerobic Capacity Tests

Anaerobic capacity tests measure power endurance. They typically last 15–90 seconds in duration. Three common tests of anaerobic capacity are the Wingate anaerobic power, 300-yd shuttle, and line drill tests.

Wingate Anaerobic Power Tests

The Wingate anaerobic power test is an all-out maximal cycle ergometry test lasting 30 seconds (although shorter and longer variations have been used). Cycling is performed against a resistance relative to the athlete's body mass, e.g., 0.075 kg per kilogram of body mass on a Monark cycle ergometer. Although it is mostly used in laboratory settings, the Wingate test has been used to a lesser extent in the testing of athletes since its development in the early 1970s at the Wingate Institute in Israel (120). It is a reliable measure of anaerobic power (120). Several useful variables can be determined including absolute and relative peak power, average power, minimum power, time to peak power, total work, and the fatigue index. A mechanically braked cycle ergometer is needed with a sensor attached to the frame, which can measure flywheel revolutions per minute. Most units are interfaced with a computer and software program that performs all of the calculations for the athletes and coaches. The Wingate test can be applied to measure upper-body anaerobic power as an arm cycle ergometer can be used (45,89). The procedures for the Wingate test are as follows:

- Athlete sits comfortably on the cycle and warms up for ~5 minutes at a comfortable pace (60–70 rpm) against a light resistance or ~20% of the test resistance. A couple of short sprints are performed as part of the warm-up.
- Upon the signal "go," the athlete pedals as fast as possible (against zero resistance to overcome inertia) and the resistance is applied to the flywheel at the onset (0.075 kg per kilogram of body mass). The athlete pedals as fast as possible throughout the 30-second test duration. It is important to monitor technique and prevent standing during pedaling.
- Duration of the test may be modified depending on the athletes. For example, we used Wingate tests of 1 minute in wrestlers to further assess power endurance (121).
- Norms for men and women are presented in Table 19.19.

Table 19.19 — Norms for the Wingate Anaerobic Power Test

% Rank	Peak Power Men (W)	(W·kg⁻¹)	Mean Power Men (W)	(W·kg⁻¹)	Peak Power Women (W)	(W·kg⁻¹)	Mean Power Women (W)	(W·kg⁻¹)
90	822	10.89	662	8.2	560	9.02	470	7.3
80	777	10.39	618	8.0	527	8.83	419	7.0
70	757	10.20	600	7.9	505	8.53	410	6.8
60	721	9.80	577	7.6	480	8.14	391	6.6
50	689	9.22	565	7.4	449	7.65	381	6.4
40	671	8.92	548	7.1	432	6.96	367	6.1
30	656	8.53	530	7.0	399	6.86	353	6.0
20	618	8.24	496	6.6	376	6.57	337	5.7
10	570	7.06	471	6.0	353	5.98	306	5.3

Reprinted with permission from Maud PJ, Schultz BB. Norms for the Wingate anaerobic test with comparison to another similar test. *Res Q Exerc Sport*. 1989;60:144–51. Ref. (122).

- For the upper body Wingate test, the athlete grasps the handles of the arm cycle ergometer while seated in contact with bench positioned so that the athlete has slight bend of the elbows at the farthest distance. The arm cycle ergometer wheel axle is aligned with subject's shoulder joint. Following a 5-minute warm-up (60 RPMs at ~25–35 W) with all-out sprints at the end of each minute, the tester counts down from 5 to 0 while subject pedals at fastest speed with no load, says "go", applies the resistance (~4%–5% of body weight), and subject continues to pedal with maximum effort for 30 seconds. Repeated upper body Wingate tests (*i.e.*, 3–5 max 30-s bouts) are used to assess power endurance. Norms are shown in Table 19.20.

300-Yard Shuttle

- For this test, two parallel lines 25 yd apart (on a flat surface) and a stopwatch are needed. When possible, multiple athletes can be tested at once with additional testing personnel.
- The athlete assumes a starting position at one line (after a proper warm-up). Upon the signal "go," the athlete sprints as fast as possible to other line (25 yd away) making foot contact with it. The athlete immediately sprints back to the starting line, and this process is repeated for six continuous round trips. Each roundtrip is 50 yd; therefore, six roundtrips total 300 yd (123) (Fig. 19.20).
- Time is kept from the "go" signal until the athlete touches the final line at the 300-yd mark. After the first trial, 5 minutes of rest is given and a second trial is performed. The average of both trials is calculated and recorded. Norms for the 300-yd shuttle run are presented in Table 19.21.

Line Drill

- Often referred to as a *suicide drill*, the line drill is performed on a basketball court although it can be modified for other areas. It involves four back-and-forth sprints to all lines on a basketball court.
- The athlete begins from a starting position at the baseline and sprints to the foul line and back. The athlete then sprints from the baseline to the half-court line and back. The athlete then sprints from the baseline to the far foul line and back. Lastly, the athlete sprints from the baseline to the far baseline and back. The athlete must touch each line upon arrival, or the test is terminated and repeated.
- The stopwatch begins upon "go" and stops when the athlete touches the final baseline. The total run is ~470 ft for college and 420 ft for high school athletes (124).
- Two minutes of rest is given in between trials and the athlete may run four in total and may take the average for his/her final score (124).
- There are limitations in the literature regarding norms for the line drill test. Times of 26–31 seconds (mean of 28.5) have been shown in male basketball players (88) and means of 30–32 seconds have been shown in female basketball players (125).

Speed

Assessments of speed involve maximal linear locomotion. Short sprint tests assess maximal speed and acceleration ability, whereas long sprint tests assess speed endurance. Sprint assessments discussed in this chapter are the 10-yd dash, 40-yd dash, and 120-yd sprint.

Table 19.20 Norms for the Upper-Body Wingate Anaerobic Power Test

Category	<10	10–12	12–14	14–16	16–18	18–25	25–35	>35
Peak power in males								
Excellent	206	192	473	473	575	658	565	589
Very good	164	171	389	411	484	556	501	510
Good	143	159	343	379	438	507	469	471
Average	122	148	296	348	393	458	437	433
Below overage	101	137	253	316	347	409	405	394
Poor	80	126	207	284	301	360	373	356
Very poor	60	115	162	252	256	311	341	317
$\bar{X}$	112	143	275	332	370	433	421	413
SD	42	22	91	63	91	98	64	77
Peak power in females								
Excellent	201	176	214					
Very good	152	159	199					
Good	135	141	184					
Average	119	124	170					
Below average	102	106	156					
Poor	86	89	140					
Very poor	53	55	110					
$\bar{X}$	127	133	177					
SD	33	35	30					

From Hoffman J. *Norms for Fitness, Performance, and Health.* Champaign (IL): Human Kinetics; 2006. p. 1–113.

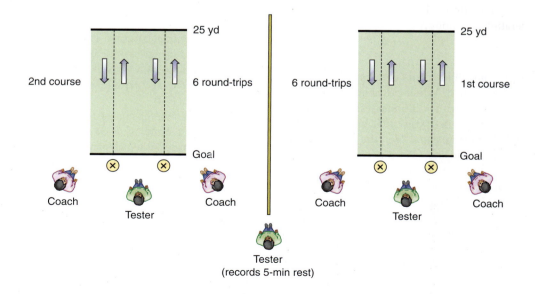

FIGURE 19.20 The 300-yd shuttle run.

Table 19.21	Norms for the 300-yd Shuttle Run			
% Rank	Baseball	Men's Basketball	Women's Basketball	Softball
90	56.7	54.1	58.4	63.3
80	58.9	55.1	61.8	65.1
70	59.9	55.6	63.6	66.5
60	61.3	56.3	64.7	67.9
50	62.0	56.7	65.2	69.2
40	63.2	57.2	65.9	71.3
30	63.9	58.1	66.8	72.4
20	65.3	58.9	68.1	74.6
10	67.7	60.2	68.9	78.0

Reprinted with permission from Hoffman J. *Norms for Fitness, Performance, and Health.* Champaign (IL): Human Kinetics; 2006. p. 1–113.

10-Yard Dash

- The 10-yd dash is a measure of acceleration. A 10-yd marked area (with room for deceleration) and a stopwatch or electronic timing device are needed.
- Following a proper warm-up, the athlete assumes a starting position using either a 3- or 4-point stance at the starting line. Upon the "go" signal, the athlete sprints as fast as possible through the 10-yd marker. A coach begins the stopwatch on "go" and stops timing once the first segment of the athlete's body crosses the finish line. It is important that the same coach time each athlete for better accuracy and consistency. If an electronic timer is used, infrared sensors are placed at the finish line to stop timing. A start switch is used at the starting line where timing begins once the athlete lifts off during acceleration and stops once the athlete crosses the infrared beam.
- Multiple (3 to 4) trials can be used with 3–5 minutes of rest in between. Studies have shown times of 1.63 to 1.80 and 1.90 to 2.00 seconds in male and female athletes, respectively (126). Division I college football players (all positions) were shown to run times on an average of 1.81 seconds (127). Professional baseball players were shown to have times of 1.52–1.59 seconds (128).

40-Yard Dash

- A 40-yd marked area (with room for deceleration) and a stopwatch or electronic timing device are needed for this assessment. Other distances have been used to assess athletes, *e.g.,* 60 and 100 m; however, the 40-yd dash is most commonly used.
- Following a proper warm-up, the athlete assumes a starting position using either a 3- or 4-point stance at the starting line. Upon the "go" signal, the athlete sprints as fast as possible through the 40-yd marker. A coach begins the stopwatch on "go" and stops timing once the first segment of the athlete's body crosses the finish line. It is important that the same coach time each athlete for better accuracy and consistency. If an electronic timer is used, infrared sensors are placed at the finish line to stop timing. A start switch is used at the starting line where timing begins once the athlete lifts off during acceleration and stops once the athlete crosses the infrared beam.
- Following a rest period of at least 3 minutes, a 2nd and 3rd trial is run. Norms are presented in Table 19.22. Analysis of NFL Combine data from 2002 to 2016 has shown a range of times of 4.24–6.06 seconds with a mean of 4.81 ± 0.31 seconds (129).
- Power may be calculated by the following: Power $(N \cdot m \cdot s^{-1})$ = body weight (N) × velocity $(m \cdot s^{-1})$
- Deceleration may be assessed as it has been suggested that athletes decelerate within 7–8 steps following a maximal sprint (130).
- Repeated 40-yd dashes assess speed endurance. One test used by the National Association of Speed and Explosion (NASE) is the NASE Repeated 40-s test (130). It involves running ten 40-yd sprints. The rest interval in between varies from sport to sport but may range from 15 to 30 seconds. The best and worst sprint should not deviate by more than 0.2–0.3 second (130). If so, the athlete may need to focus on specific speed endurance training to improve.

120-Yard Dash

- This assessment is conducted similarly to the 40-yd dash with the exception it is three times the distance. However, more relevant information can be determined by the coach. Each 40-yd interval is measured separately. This gives coaches information on all three phases of sprinting (130).
- Three timers are needed: one to start the test and conclude at the 40-yd mark, one to begin timing at the 40-yd mark and conclude at the 80-yd mark, and one to begin at the 80-yd mark and conclude at the 120-yd mark. A variation is to have all three timers begin timing on "go" and stop upon completion of the 40-, 80-, and 120-yd mark, respectively. The interval times are determined via subtraction of the 40-yd time from the 80-yd time and 80-yd time from the 120-yd time. An electronic timing device can be used and is preferred but three sets of infrared sensors would be needed for each 40-yd interval.
- The athlete begins in a 3- or 4-point stance and sprints as fast as possible throughout the 120-yd distance.
- The initial 40 yd is the *stationary 40-yd dash* and times recorded relate similarly to the performance of a normal 40-yd dash. Norms for 40-yd dash times can apply for this segment.
- The second segment is known as the *flying 40-yd dash* because it begins with the athlete already at full speed. Acceleration can be assessed by subtracting the flying

Table 19.22

Percentile Ranks for 40-yd (36.6 M) Sprint Times (Sec) among American Football Players (Top) and College Football Players Participating in the NFL Combine (Bottom)

American Football Players

% Rank	High school (14–15 yr)	High school (16–18 yr)	High school (14–15 yr) E	High school (16–18 yr) E	NCAA DIII	NCAA DI	NCAA DI E
90	4.86	4.70	5.08	4.98	4.59	4.58	4.75
80	5.00	4.80	5.17	5.10	4.70	4.67	4.84
70	5.10	4.89	5.28	5.21	4.77	4.73	4.92
60	5.20	4.96	5.31	5.30	4.85	4.80	5.01
50	5.28	5.08	5.43	5.40	4.95	4.87	5.10
40	5.38	5.17	5.52	5.46	5.02	4.93	5.18
30	5.50	5.30	5.63	5.63	5.12	5.02	5.32
20	5.84	5.45	5.84	5.73	5.26	5.18	5.48
10	6.16	5.73	6.22	5.84	5.47	5.33	5.70
$\bar{X}$	5.40	5.15	5.54	5.41	4.99	4.92	5.17
SD	0.53	0.45	0.52	0.35	0.35	0.32	0.37
n	113	205	94	151	538	757	608

College Football Players Participating in the NFL Combine

% Rank	DB	DL	LB	OL	QB	RB	TE	WR
90	4.41	4.72	4.57	5.07	4.60	4.44	4.66	4.42
80	4.45	4.80	4.62	5.15	4.70	4.50	4.78	4.46
70	4.48	4.87	4.66	5.21	4.75	4.55	4.80	4.50
60	4.51	4.90	4.72	5.25	4.79	4.58	4.83	4.52
50	4.54	4.90	4.76	5.30	4.81	4.62	4.90	4.55
40	4.57	4.96	4.78	5.33	4.86	4.65	4.96	4.57
30	4.59	5.03	4.81	5.40	4.91	4.69	4.99	4.61
20	4.62	5.09	4.86	5.47	4.99	4.74	5.02	4.65
10	4.67	5.15	4.92	5.56	5.10	4.82	5.07	4.68
$\bar{X}$	4.54	4.97	4.75	5.31	4.84	4.62	4.89	4.55
SD	0.11	0.19	0.13	0.20	0.17	0.16	0.15	0.10
n	111	100	62	155	41	67	42	98

E, electronic timing device; other measurements were from handheld stopwatches; DB, defensive backs; DL, defensive linemen; LB, linebackers; OL, offensive linemen; QB, quarterbacks; RB, running backs; TE, tight ends; WR, wide receivers.

Data collected from 1999 NFL combine.

Reprinted with permission from Hoffman J. *Norms for Fitness, Performance, and Health.* Champaign (IL): Human Kinetics; 2006. p. 1–113.

40 time from the static 40 time. Acceleration is good if the athlete's difference is <0.7 second (130).

- The third segment is known as the *speed endurance 40 segment* because it measures the athlete's ability to maintain maximal speed. It is determined by subtracting the speed endurance 40 time from the flying 40 time. Speed endurance is good if the difference is <0.2 second (130).

Agility

Agility tests assess the athlete's ability to rapidly accelerate, decelerate, and change direction in a controlled manner using forward, backward, and/or side shuffling types of movements. Cones and stopwatches (or more accurate timing devices) are used for agility testing. Tape and tape measures are needed to measure and mark off appropriate distances. Similar to sprint testing, it is important that the same coach or tester measure all tests for each athlete to increase consistency and reduce human-related errors in timing. Nimphius et al. (131) described more than 30 drills used in agility testing, each ranging from 1 to 20 changes of direction, 8–60 m in total distance, and completion times ranging from 1.5 to 22 seconds. Coaches should select drills with high movement specificity seen in the sport. Although a multitude of drills can be used for assessment, the 505 change of direction test (and change of direction deficit), T-test, hexagon test, pro agility, three-cone drill, Edgren side step, and Davies tests are discussed.

505 Change of Direction (COD) Test

The 505 COD test involves a 15-m sprint, COD 180° turn, and subsequent 5-m sprint (Fig. 19.21). The 505 COD test may help distinguish between dominant and nondominant limb performance differences because it uses one single 180° turn. Several studies have shown asymmetries between limbs when comparing scores (132–134).

- A marked area, tape measure, and timing devices are needed for this test.
- After a warm-up, the athlete stands on the starting line with a 2-point split stance.
- Upon "go," the athlete accelerates maximally for 15 m to the 3rd line marker, touches the line with their foot, turns 180° quickly on the right or left leg, and sprints maximally for 5 m to the 2nd line marker (or finish).
- Timing begins at the 10-m marker and stops after the athlete crosses the finish line marker.
- The test should be repeated for the opposite limb. At least 2–3 minutes of rest should be used in between trials. Multiple trials should be performed for each leg and the times recorded.

The time of the test (as well as other agility drills) has been suggested to be a measure of COD ability. Some studies have shown time ranges of 2.39–2.67 seconds in various groups of male and female athletes (132–134). However, this notion has been challenged because much of the drill consists of linear sprints (*i.e.*, acceleration) and only 31% of the time is spent changing direction (134). Nimphius et al. (134) recommend calculating the *change of direction (COD) deficit* from the 505 test. The COD deficit is calculated by subtracting the 10-m sprint time from the 505 test time. The difference is thought to represent COD time. Nimphius et al. (134) reported times of 0.617 and 0.670 seconds for dominant and nondominant limbs, respectively, in cricket athletes. Other studies have shown COD deficits of 0.469–0.638 in a wide group of male and female athletes using both dominant and nondominant limbs (132,133).

T-Test

- Four cones and a stopwatch are needed. Three cones are aligned in a straight line 5 yd apart and a fourth cone is aligned with the second cone 10 yd apart forming a "T" shape.
- Following a warm-up, the athlete sprints forward 10 yd, shuffles to the left 5 yd to the cone, shuffles back right 10 yd to other cone, shuffles left to the middle cone, and back pedals back to the starting cone. The athlete faces forward at all times and does not cross his/her feet. Cones are touched at each marker.
- The athlete begins on "go" and timing stops when the athlete backpedals past the starting cone at the completion of the drill. T-test times <9.5 and 10.5 seconds in men and women athletes, respectively, are excellent; 9.5–10.5 seconds (men) and 10.5–11.5 seconds (women) are good; and 10.5–11.5 seconds (men) and 11.5–12.5 seconds (women) are average.

Hexagon Test

- This test requires adhesive tape, a tape measure, and a stopwatch. A hexagon is formed with each side measuring 24 in. to form angles of 120° (55).

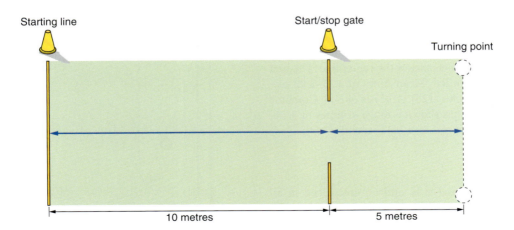

FIGURE 19.21 The 505 agility test.

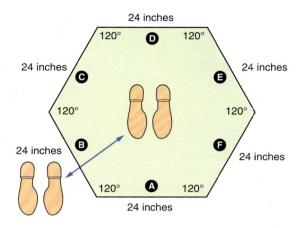

FIGURE 19.22 The hexagon test.

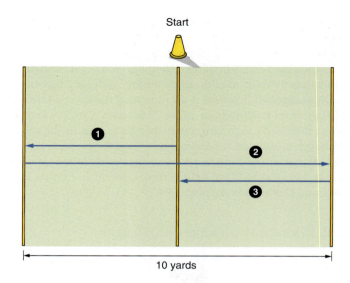

FIGURE 19.23 Pro-agility test.

- Following a proper warm-up, the athlete begins by standing in the middle of the hexagon. Upon the signal "go," the athlete begins double-leg hopping from the center of the hexagon to each side and back to the center. The athlete starts with the side directly in front and continues clockwise until the drill is complete (which requires three revolutions). Thus, the athlete will jump 18 times and back to the center in a clockwise direction (Fig. 19.22).
- The trial is stopped for violations including landing on the line (rather than over it), loss of balance, or taking extra steps. The best of three trials is recorded.
- Norms for this drill are limited. Studies have shown values of ~12.3 seconds in male athletes, ~14.2 seconds in college men, 12.9–13.2 seconds in female athletes, and 14.3 seconds in college women (45,55).

Pro-Agility Test (20-Yard Shuttle Run)

- This drill can be performed on a football field with parallel lines 5 yd apart or another marked area. A stopwatch is needed.
- The athlete begins straddling the center line in a 3-point stance. Upon the signal "go," the athlete sprints 5 yd to the line on the left (touching the line with hand and foot), then sprints right for 10 yd to the furthest line (touching the line), and then sprints left for 5 yd through the center line (Fig. 19.23). Timing ends when the athlete passes the center line. The best time of 2–3 trials is recorded. Mean times of 4.35–4.92 seconds were shown in athletes (126). Analysis of NFL Combine data from 2002 to 2016 has shown a range of times of 3.75–5.56 seconds with a mean of 4.39 ± 0.27 seconds (129).

3-Cone Drill

- For this drill, three cones (A, B, and C) are placed in an upside-down "L" configuration with each cone separated by 5 yd (Fig. 19.24). A stopwatch is needed for timing.
- The athlete begins behind the starting line at cone A, sprints to cone B and back to cone A, then sprints to the outside of cone B, rounds cone B and sprints to cone C, rounds cone C, sprints back to cone B, and then sprints back to cone A at the finish point.
- Timing begins on "go" and finishes when the athlete crosses the finish point. The best of three trials is recorded. Few norms are available for this test. Table 19.23 presents some data obtained from the 1999 NFL combine (46). Analysis of NFL Combine data from 2002 to 2016 showed a range of times of 6.42–9.12 seconds with a mean of 7.28 ± 0.42 seconds (129).

Edgren Side-Step Test

- A 12-ft area is needed where lines (tape) are placed 3 ft apart. Five taped lines are needed altogether. A gymnasium floor is recommended.

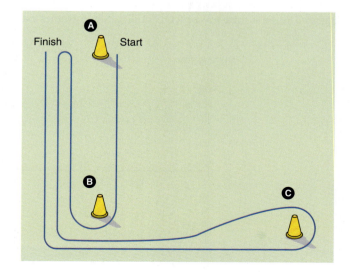

FIGURE 19.24 Three-cone drill.

Table 19.23 Three-Cone Drill Scores (S) from the 1999 NFL Combine

% Rank	DL	LB	DB	OL	QB	RB	TE	WR
90	7.22	7.05	6.87	7.66	7.06	7.17	7.12	6.85
80	7.45	7.16	6.97	7.82	7.13	7.29	7.16	7.01
70	7.52	7.30	7.07	7.98	7.19	7.32	7.27	7.10
60	7.64	7.38	7.09	8.07	7.31	7.36	7.38	7.19
50	7.71	7.49	7.14	8.15	7.36	7.47	7.42	7.28
40	7.78	7.54	7.22	8.28	7.40	7.53	7.48	7.35
30	7.89	7.61	7.29	8.38	7.54	7.60	7.57	7.41
20	8.07	7.70	7.39	8.51	7.59	7.71	7.71	7.49
10	8.47	7.84	7.47	8.66	7.70	7.82	8.04	7.58
Avg	7.75	7.46	7.17	8.18	7.29	7.48	7.47	7.26
SD	0.43	0.30	0.22	0.43	0.57	0.27	0.34	0.30

Reprinted with permission from Hoffman J. *Norms for Fitness, Performance, and Health.* Champaign (IL): Human Kinetics; 2006. p. 1–113.

- Following a proper warm-up, the athlete begins the test by straddling the center line. On "go," the athlete side steps to the right to the outside line, side steps left to the furthest line, and repeats side shuffling back and forth for 10 seconds (Fig. 19.25). A tester counts the number of lines crossed during the 10-second period.

Davies Test

- This is an upper-body agility/strength test (66). Two pieces of tape are placed 36 in. apart. Athlete assumes a push-up position with each hand placed over one piece of tape.

- The athlete moves the right hand to touch the left (while maintaining correct posture) and returns to the starting position. The athlete then moves the left hand to touch the right hand and returns to the starting position while maintaining proper core position throughout. The athlete repeats these alternating movements as rapidly as possible for 15 seconds. The test can be adapted to be performed for a longer duration, *e.g.*, 60 seconds.
- The number of touches is recorded. The athlete is given three trials and the highest number is recorded. Better performance is seen with higher numbers of touches.

Balance

Balance is the ability to maintain static and dynamic equilibrium and controlling the center of gravity relative to the base support. The assessment of balance can be of great value to the athlete. Athletes with poor balance or inferior performance on balance tests are at greater risk of ankle and knee injuries (135,136). For unilateral testing, differences in balance ability between dominant and nondominant leg can be assessed and compared. Balance training reduces incidence of recurrent ankle sprains and ACL injuries in soccer and volleyball players (135). Athletes have superior balance compared to nonathletes with gymnasts and soccer players scoring very high among groups of athletes tested (137–140). It is thought that balance training promotes greater joint stability and stiffness resulting from higher agonist and antagonist muscle activation, thereby reducing the risk of injury (135). Thus, balance testing can be used to monitor stability increases during training. Balance training (also known as neuromuscular, proprioceptive, or sensorimotor training) embodies a combination of all training modalities in addition to specific balance exercises.

Balance can be tested in different ways. The basic modes to test balance include timed static standing tests (eyes closed or on

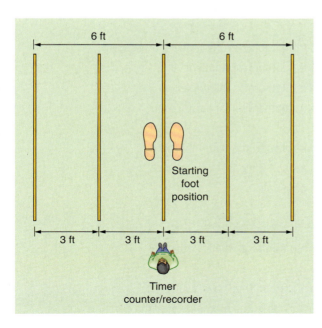

FIGURE 19.25 Edgren side step test.

one leg), dynamic unilateral standing tests that involve a measureable movement with opposite limb or upper extremities, balance tests using unstable surfaces (stabilometers, wobble board, BOSU, pads, foam rollers, stability balls), standing tests on force plates (to measure *postural sway* or total shifts of the center of pressure during a prescribed time), and using specialized balance testing equipment (NeuroCom System, Biodex Stability Systems, Tetrax System). The following are some balance tests used:

- *Single-leg squat* — a measure of balance, neuromuscular control, and strength that places the athlete in a position seen in many sports. This test has been shown to be reliable in athletes especially when the testing staff has assessment experience (141). The athlete stands with hands on hips, a shoulder width stance, and eyes focused straight ahead. Feet should be positioned straight ahead. The athlete squats on one leg while the opposite leg is elevated (knee and hip flexed). The exercise ROM depends on strength level as well as body size so ROM can be adjusted based on the individual athlete. The coach looks at posture (erect torso), hip position, and knee movement. Too great of an inward movement of the knee (valgus stress) is contraindicated. This test is particularly effective in testing female athletes who are much more likely to sustain an ACL injury than their male athlete counterparts. Excessive valgus stress places the knee at greater risk for injury so close monitoring of hip and knee position during this test can identify problems that could adversely affect athletes on the field or court. Excessive valgus motion could be indicative of weak hip abductors and external rotators, reduced ankle dorsiflexion ROM, and increased hip adductor activity. In addition to the presence of valgus motion, the coach should look to make sure the shoulders and pelvic girdle remain level, and the tested knee aligns with the foot. The trainee should avoid rotating the pelvis inward or outward, knee valgus motion, and elevating or dropping the opposite hip as compensation for weakness or balance issues (142). Excellent single-leg squat assessment would be indicative of hip flexion >65°, <10° of hip abduction or adduction, and <10° of knee valgus motion (143). A number of scoring systems are used to grade the single-leg squat assessment including 3 and 4 point scales and quantitative scoring (141,144), and techniques have varied between studies (*i.e.*, hands on hips vs. crossed on chest vs. flexed parallel to ground, standing on box vs. floor). Crossley et al. (144) developed criteria for "good," "fair," and "poor" performances of the single-leg squat (Table 19.24). They found that subjects scoring "good"

Table 19.24 Single-Leg Squat Criteria

	Criterion	To Be Rated "Good"
A	Overall impression across the 5 trials:	
	Ability to maintain balance	Participant does not lose balance
	Perturbations of the person	Movement is performed smoothly
	Depth of the squat	The squat is performed to at least 60° of knee flexion
	Speed of the squat	Squat is performed at ~1 per 2 seconds
B	Trunk posture	
	Trunk/thoracic lateral deviation or shift	No trunk/thoracic lateral deviation or shift
	Trunk/thoracic rotation	No trunk/thoracic rotation
	Trunk/thoracic lateral flexion	No trunk/thoracic lateral flexion
	Trunk/thoracic forward flexion	No trunk/thoracic forward flexion
C	The pelvis "in space"	
	Pelvic shunt or lateral deviation	No pelvic shunt or lateral deviation
	Pelvic rotation	No pelvic rotation
	Pelvic tilt (take note of depth of squat)	No pelvic tilt
D	Hip joint	
	Hip adduction	No hip adduction
	Hip (femoral) internal rotation	No hip (femoral) internal rotation
E	Knee joint	
	Apparent knee valgus	No apparent knee valgus
	Knee position relative to foot position	Center of the knee remains over the center of the foot

From Crossley KM, Zhang WJ, Schache AG, Bryant A, Cowan SM. Performance on the single-leg squat task indicates hip abductor muscle function. *Am J Sports Med*. 2011;39:866–73.

had greater earlier onset of gluteus medius activation, greater hip abduction strength (but not hip external rotation strength), and greater side plank strength than those ranked as "poor."

- *Anterior reach* — the athlete begins with feet oriented with a marker located perpendicular to a tape measure. With hands positioned on the hips, the athlete extends a leg out as far as possible (while balancing on the opposite leg) keeping the front foot close to the floor without touching. The induced flexion of the support knee requires some degree of muscle strength and balance to perform. The distance reached with the front leg is measured. The best score of 3–4 trials is recorded for each leg. Balance must be maintained and the reaching leg cannot touch the floor for the trial to count.

- *Single-leg balance test* — the athlete stands on one leg (without shoes) with the opposite leg bent and off of the ground. Hips remain level and head focused straight ahead. The eyes begin open but then are closed for 10 seconds. A negative test indicates good balance, whereas a positive test indicates equilibrium issues or a sense of imbalance.

- *Standing stork test* — the athlete stands on one leg with the contralateral hip and knee flexed such that the toes are touching the opposite knee. Hands remain on the hips. Upon "go," the athlete plantar flexes onto his/her toes and the coach begins timing with a stopwatch. The athlete remains in this position for as long as possible. Multiple trials can be used and the longest time is recorded. For men, holding this position for >50 seconds is excellent, 40–50 seconds is above average, and <20 seconds is poor. For women, holding this position for >30 seconds is excellent, 20–30 seconds is above average, and <10 seconds is poor. Familiarization is very important for this test as great variability can be seen. Thus, the athlete should be given a few practice sessions prior to testing.

Landing tests — examining postural control and balance during landing is critical to optimizing technique during power movements especially in prescreening of athletes for potential injuries. Landing tests involve either stepping off of an elevation or jumping and landing bilaterally or unilaterally. Single-leg tests involving drop landings, drop vertical jump, hops, and sidestep cutting have been used to assess risk factors for injury. Single-leg hops (*i.e.*, triple hop, 6 m timed hop) may be evaluated by distance covered or the time needed to cover a specified distance. Trainers and coaches may look for knee valgus motion, internal rotation, and degree of flexion, in addition to balance, stability, and posture. Assessment is important in the coaching of "soft" landing. Some coaches and trainers have used the Klatt test where balance and stability are monitored during single-leg landing after the trainee jumps off of a small box (with the contralateral leg flexed in front of body and arms parallel to ground with hands clasped). Soft landing is indicative of greater hip and knee ROM, and less ground reaction force and an 11% reduced time of peak ACL force (145). One bilateral landing test is the *Landing Error Scoring System* (LESS). The LESS test involves standing on a 30-cm box, jumping forward and landing bilaterally on a marked line on the floor, and maximally jumping vertically as high as possible (Fig. 19.26). Two video cameras are placed ~10 feet away in front and to the right of the landing area. At least 3 trials are performed after a warm-up and practice repetitions. Scoring is based on errors that occur through a 17-point subjective technical grading sheet for at least 2 of the 3 trials recorded (Table 19.25). Padua et al. (146) developed the following classifications: <4 = very good; 4 = good; 5–6 = moderate; >6 = poor. In their study, they reported that 14% of women were in the very good group, compared with 29% of men, and 36% of women were in the poor group compared with 23% of men. Inclusion of specific plyometric, balance, and functional exercises has the capacity to improve LESS scores (147).

- *Stabilometer balance test* — stabilometers consist of platforms that are adjusted to move in all planes of motion relative to horizontal position (5°) (Fig. 19.27). The test involves the athlete's ability to maintain balance for a period of time. Some tests use a maximal time limit of 30 seconds and test the athlete's balance within that time frame. The degree of

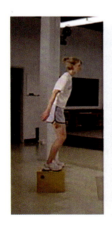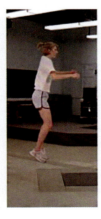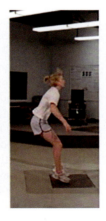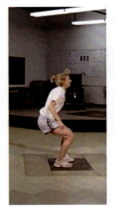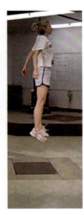

FIGURE 19.26 The Landing Error Scoring System (LESS) test. (From Padua DA, Marshall SW, Boling MC, et al. The Landing Error Scoring System (LESS) is a valid and reliable clinical assessment tool of jump-landing mechanics. *Am J Sports Med*. 2009;37:1996–2002.)

Table 19.25 Assessment Criteria for the Landing Error Scoring System (LESS)

#	Criterion		
1.	Knee flexion angle at initial contact flexed >30°	Yes = 0	No = 1
2.	Hip flexion angle at initial contact; hip flexion?	Yes = 0	No = 1
3.	Trunk flexion angle at initial contact	Flexed = 0	Not flexed = 1
4.	Ankle plantar flexion at initial contact	Toe-to-heel = 0	Heel-to-toe = 1
5.	Knee valgus angle at initial contact; knee over midfoot?	Yes = 0	No = 1
6.	Lateral trunk flexion angle at initial contact	No flexion = 0	Lateral flexion = 1
7.	Stance width at contact – > shoulder width?	Yes = 1	No = 0
8.	Stance width at contact – < shoulder width?	Yes = 1	No = 0
9.	Foot position at contact – internally rotated >30°	Yes = 1	No = 0
10.	Foot position at contact – externally rotated >30°	Yes = 1	No = 0
11.	Symmetrical foot contact	Yes = 0	No = 1
12.	Knee flexion displacement during contact >45°	Yes = 0	No = 1
13.	Hip flexion at max knee flexion	Yes = 0	No = 1
14.	Trunk flexion at max knee flexion	Yes = 0	No = 1
15.	Knee valgus displacement	Lateral to big toe = 0	Medial to big toe = 1
16.	Joint displacement in sagittal plane	Soft = 0	Average = 1
			Stiff = 2
17.	Overall impression	Excellent = 0	Average = 1
			Poor = 2

deviation depends on the athlete's ability so an appropriate angular deviation needs to be selected to accurately assess the athlete within the required time period. The time the athlete remains in balance is recorded. Multiple trials can be used and the best time is recorded. Like force plates, stabilometers can be quite costly.

- *Force plate tests* — several postural sway tests (which measure the deviation of the COP) can be performed on a force plate. Many tests are unilateral and vary in duration (*i.e.*, 20 s) (148), *i.e.*, a single-leg balance test. Some tests involve the athletes closing their eyes as well. Variables such as the total length of path, sway velocity, front-to-back sway, and medial-to-lateral sway can be assessed. Single- and double-leg landings can be assessed via a force plate. Studies show improvements (less postural sway) following balance training (149).
- *Balance Error Scoring System (BESS)* — the BESS requires a foam pad (~2.5 in. thick), stop watch, and score card. Testing consists of 6 separate 20-second balance tests performed under different conditions with no shoes. The 6 conditions involve (a) single-leg stance, (b) double-leg stance, and (c) tandem stance performed both on a hard surface like the floor and on the foam pad (Fig. 19.28). The trainee stands with hands on hips and eyes closed for all tests. For double-leg stance, feet are kept side-by-side and touching (150). For single-leg stance, the trainee stands on the nondominant foot and the opposite hip is flexed 30° and knee is flexed ~45°. For tandem stance, the trainee stands heel-to-toe with the nondominant foot in the back (heel of the dominant foot should be touching the toe of the nondominant foot). Each trial lasts

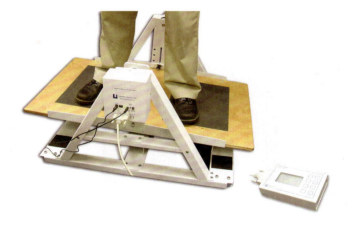

FIGURE 19.27 A stabilometer (Lafayette Instruments Inc., model 16030) used for balance testing. It has fully integrated timing functions, electronic angle measurement for increased accuracy, and allows a wide range of testable parameters including variable test times, selectable angle limits, and digital tilt angle readout.

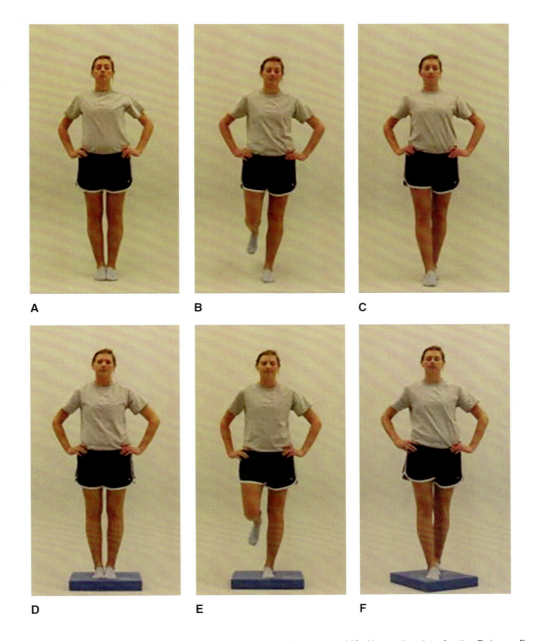

FIGURE 19.28 The Balance Error Scoring System (BESS) test. (From Iverson GL, Koehle MS. Normative data for the Balance Error Scoring System in adults. *Rehabil Res Pract.* 2013;2013:846418.). Panels **A** through **F** demonstrate the 6 conditions of the test.

20 seconds and a spotter can be present to assist in case the trainee loses balance. Errors are recorded for each trial when the trainee (a) moves hands off of the hips; (b) opens eyes; (c) loses balance or falls; (d) abducts or flexes hip >30°; (e) lifts forefoot or heel off of surface; and (f) remains out of proper testing position for more than 5 seconds. The maximum number of errors per trial is 10; therefore, the worst possible score attained would be 60. The lower the score, the better the balance. Norms are presented in Table 19.26.

- *Star Excursion Balance Test (SEBT)* and the *Y Balance Test* — the SEBT incorporates a single-leg stance on a support leg with maximum reach of the opposite leg. It is a screening tool to measure dynamic balance and identify potential injury risks. The athlete stands in the center of a grid with 8 lines (120 cm) extending out at 45° increments (Fig. 19.29). The 8 lines represent the anterolateral, anterior, anteromedial, medial, posteromedial, posterior, posterolateral, and lateral directions. However, the anterior, medial, and posterior directions may suffice in the testing of athletes (140). The athlete maintains a single-leg stance while reaching with the contralateral leg as far as possible for each taped line lightly touches the furthest point possible (151). The athlete then returns to a bilateral stance and the coach measures the distance from the center of the grid to the touch point with a tape measure. The best (or average) of three trials is recorded and the same is performed for the opposite side.

Table 19.26 Normative Data for the Balance Error Scoring System

Age	N	Mean	Median	SD	Superior	Above Average	Broadly Normal	Below Average	Poor	Very Poor
20–29	65	11.3	11.0	4.8	0–5	6–7	8–14	15–17	18–23	24+
30–39	173	11.5	11.0	5.5	0–4	5–7	8–15	16–18	19–26	27+
40–49	352	12.5	11.5	6.2	0–5	6–8	9–16	17–20	21–28	29+
50–54	224	14.2	12.0	7.5	0–6	7–8	9–18	19–24	25–33	34+
55–59	197	16.5	15.0	7.6	0–7	8–10	11–20	21–28	29–35	36+
60–64	148	18.0	16.5	7.8	0–8	9–12	13–22	23–28	29–40	41+
65–69	77	19.9	18.0	7.1	0–12	13–15	16–24	25–32	33–38	39+

From Iverson GL, Koehle MS. Normative data for the Balance Error Scoring System in adults. *Rehabil Res Pract*. 2013;2013:846418.

Reach distances are normalized to leg length. Fifteen seconds of rest is given between reaches. Trials are discarded if the athlete does not touch the line, lifts the stance foot from the center grid, loses balance, or does not maintain start and return positions for one full second. Studies have shown moderate-to-good intratester reliability (0.67–0.96) (87) and improvements following balance training (149).

The Y Balance Test (YBT) is the instrumented SEBT version and was developed to reduce the length of the SEBT to include only the 3 aforementioned directional movements (shown in thePoint). The YBT requires the trainee to balance on one leg while reaching as far as possible with the other leg in only the anterior, posterolateral, and posteromedial directions. The score is calculated by summing the 3 directions and normalizing the quantity to leg length. A Y Balance kit is helpful but other measuring devices can be used. After a warm-up and practice trials, the trainee performs at least 3 trials for each leg in each direction. The test is performed while the subject stands on the center foot plate (with hands on hips) and slides each piece as far as possible in each direction. Loss of balance results in a failed attempt and trainee must slide the box at the side and not place weight on top. Also, the trainee cannot kick the box to extend the length. Some studies have shown the YBT to be predictive of injury, whereas others did not (152). Some studies have shown mean composite scores of 97%–102% where athletes score higher than nonathletes (152). However, scores for the anterior direction (~60%–76%) are considerable lower than posteromedial (95%–117%) and posterolateral (88%–115%) (87,152,153). Studies have shown that 8 weeks of specific strength and balance training can improve scores on the test by 6%–8% (87).

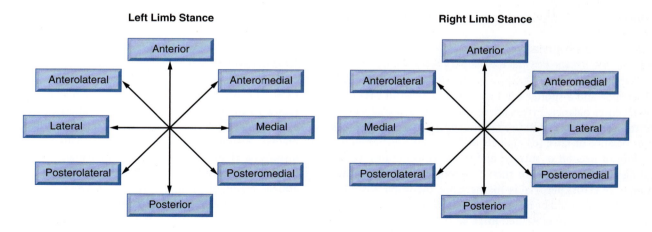

FIGURE 19.29 The star excursion balance test configuration. (Reprinted with permission from Olmsted LC, Carcia CR, Hertel J, Schultz SJ. Efficacy of the star excursion balance tests in detecting reach deficits in subjects with chronic ankle instability. *J Athl Train*. 2002;37:501–6.)

Case Study 19.1

Darryl is a recent college graduate who is now the official strength and conditioning coach of a collegiate Division II basketball team. In addition to developing the team's yearly strength and conditioning program, Darryl must also design the team's testing battery.

Question for Consideration: Based on your knowledge of the sport of basketball and the needs of a basketball player, what type of testing battery can Darryl develop for his team to assess the critical health- and skill-related components of fitness paramount to basketball?

SUMMARY POINTS

◆ Tests selected should be valid, reliable, and sport specific. The testing battery should include at least one test each for the major health- and skill-related components of fitness specific to the athlete's sport.

◆ The testing staff should be well trained, familiarized to testing procedures and equipment used, aware of each athlete's situation, and should be assigned to specific athletes when multiple testing sessions are planned per year.

◆ Results of tests are compared to norms for the athlete's age-matched means for that sport, or the coach can develop his/her own norms and use that data for comparison.

◆ Testing the health-related fitness components includes assessments for body composition, muscle strength and endurance, cardiovascular endurance, and flexibility, in addition to postural screening.

◆ Testing the skill-related fitness components includes assessments for power, speed, agility and mobility, and balance/coordination.

REVIEW QUESTIONS

1. In assessing the effectiveness of the program you recently designed, you want to test the athlete's agility. Which one of the following assessments would be most appropriate?

   a. 120-yd dash
   b. 1.5-mile run
   c. Medicine ball chest pass
   d. T-test

2. Which of the following strength tests can also be used as a measure of total-body power?

   a. 1 RM bench press
   b. 1 RM power clean
   c. 1 RM squat
   d. 1 RM deadlift

3. A 21-year-old male athlete performs a grip strength test and records a max value of 68 kg. His grip strength is classified as

   a. Excellent
   b. Good
   c. Average
   d. Poor

4. The Wingate test is a measure of

   a. Maximal strength
   b. Flexibility
   c. Anaerobic capacity
   d. Aerobic endurance

5. Which of the following is an assessment of maximal sprinting speed?

   a. T-test
   b. 40-yd dash
   c. Stork test
   d. Margaria-Kalamen test

6. The multistage 20-m shuttle run is an assessment of maximal aerobic capacity.

   a. T
   b. F

7. Reliability is a measure of repeatability or consistency a test exhibits.

   a. T
   b. F

8. Skinfold analysis is considered the "gold standard" of body composition assessment.

   a. T
   b. F

9. The hexagon test is an assessment of agility.

   a. T
   b. F

10. When selecting a test sequence when multiple assessments are performed during the same session, a lower-body muscle endurance test should be performed before a maximal agility test.

    a. T
    b. F

11. Posture relates to the alignment and function of all segments of the human body at rest and during motion.

    a. T
    b. F

REFERENCES

1. Harman E. Principles of test selection and administration. In: Baechle TR, Earle RW, editors. *Essentials of Strength Training and Conditioning*. 3rd ed. Champaign (IL): Human Kinetics; 2008. p. 237–47.

2. Wen N, Dalbo VJ, Burgos B, Pyne DB, Scanlan AT. Power testing in basketball: current practice and future recommendations. *J Strength Cond Res*. 2018;32:2677–91.

3. Wright GA, Isaacson MI, Malecek DJ, Steffen JP. Development and assessment of reliability for a sandbag throw conditioning test for wrestlers. *J Strength Cond Res*. 2015;29:451–7.

4. UFC Institute. *A Cross-Sectional Performance Analysis and Projection of the UFC Athlete*. Las Vegas, NV. Volume 1. 2018.

5. Ploutz-Snyder LL, Giamis EL. Orientation and familiarization to 1RM strength testing in old and young women. *J Strength Cond Res*. 2001;15:519–23.

6. American College of Sports Medicine. American College of Sports Medicine Position Stand: exercise and fluid replacement. *Med Sci Sports Exerc*. 2007;39:377–90.

7. American College of Sports Medicine. American College of Sports Medicine Position Stand: exertional heat illness during training and competition. *Med Sci Sports Exerc*. 2007;39: 556–72.

8. Ratamess NA. *Coaches Guide to Performance-Enhancing Supplements*. Monterey (CA): Coaches Choice Books; 2006.

9. Volek JS, Ratamess NA, Rubin MR, et al. The effects of creatine supplementation on muscular performance and body composition responses to short-term resistance training overreaching. *Eur J Appl Physiol*. 2004;91:628–37.

10. Ratamess NA, Ehrman JK. Body composition status and assessment. In: *ACSM's Resource Manual for Guidelines for Exercise Testing and Prescription*. 6th ed. Philadelphia (PA): Lippincott Williams & Wilkins; 2009. p. 264–81.

11. Ratamess NA. Body composition. In: Miller T, editor. *NSCA's Guide to Tests and Assessments*. Champaign (IL): Human Kinetics; 2012. p. 15–41.

12. Sloan AW, Weir JB. Nomograms for prediction of body density and total body fat from skinfold measurements. *J Appl Physiol*. 1970;28:221–2.

13. Jackson AS, Pollock ML. Generalized equations for predicting body density of men. *Br J Nutr*. 1978;40:497–504.

14. Jackson AS, Pollock ML, Ward A. Generalized equations for predicting body density of women. *Med Sci Sports Exerc*. 1980;12:175–81.

15. Pollock ML, Schmidt DH, Jackson AS. Measurement of cardiorespiratory fitness and body composition in the clinical setting. *Compr Ther*. 1980;6:12–27.

16. Jackson AS, Pollock ML. Practical assessment of body composition. *Phys Sports Med*. 1985;13:76–90.

17. Durnin JVGA, Womersley J. Body fat assessed from total body density and its estimation from skinfold thickness: measurements on 481 men and women aged from 16 to 72 years. *Br J Nutr*. 1974;32:77–97.

18. Siri WE. The gross composition of the body. *Adv Biol Med Physiol*. 1956;4:239–80.

19. Brozek J, Grande F, Anderson J, et al. Densitometric analysis of body composition: revision of some quantitative assumptions. *Am N Y Acad Sci*. 1963;110:113–40.

20. Heyward VH, Stolarczyk LM. *Applied Body Composition Assessment*. Champaign (IL): Human Kinetics; 1996. 82 p.

21. Kraemer WJ, Fry AC, Ratamess NA, French DN. Strength testing: development and evaluation of methodology. In: Maud PJ, Foster C, editors. *Physiological Assessments of Human Performance*. 2nd ed. Champaign (IL): Human Kinetics; 2006. p. 119–50.

22. Friedrich J, Brakke R, Akuthota V, Sullivan W. Reliability and practicality of the core score: four dynamic core stability tests performed in a physician office setting. *Clin J Sport Med*. 2017;27:409–14.

23. McMaster DT, Gill N, Cronin J, McGuigan M. A brief review of strength and ballistic assessment methodologies in sport. *Sports Med*. 2014;44:603–23.

24. Drake D, Kennedy R, Wallace E. The validity and responsiveness of isometric lower body multi-joint tests of muscular strength: a systematic review. *Sports Med Open*. 2017;3:23.

25. James LP, Roberts LA, Haff GG, Kelly VG, Beckman EM. Validity and reliability of a portable isometric mid-thigh clean pull. *J Strength Cond Res*. 2015;31:1378–86.

26. Beckham G, Mizuguchi S, Carter C, et al. Relationships of isometric mid-thigh pull variables to weightlifting performance. *J Sports Med Phys Fitness*. 2013;53:573–81.

27. Townsend JR, Bender D, Vantrease W, et al. Isometric mid-thigh pull performance is associated with athletic performance and sprinting kinetics in Division I men and women's basketball players. *J Strength Cond Res*. 2019;33:2665–73.

28. Wang R, Hoffman JR, Tanigawa S, et al. Isometric mid-thigh pull correlates with strength, sprint, and agility performance in collegiate rugby union players. *J Strength Cond Res*. 2016;30: 3051–6.

29. Green B, Bourne MN, Pizzari T. Isokinetic strength assessment offers limited predictive validity for detecting risk of future hamstring strain in sport: a systematic review and meta-analysis. *Br J Sports Med*. 2018;52:329–36.

30. Undheim MB, Cosgrave C, King E, et al. Isokinetic muscle strength and readiness to return to sport following anterior cruciate ligament reconstruction: is there an association? A systematic review and a protocol recommendation. *Br J Sports Med*. 2015;49:1305–10.

31. Ratamess NA, Beller NA, Gonzalez AM, et al. The effects of multiple-joint isokinetic resistance training on maximal isokinetic and dynamic muscle strength and local muscular endurance. *J Sports Sci Med*. 2016;15:34–40.

32. Brzycki M. Strength testing: predicting a one-rep max from reps-to-fatigue. *J Phys Edu Recreat Dance*. 1993;64:88–90.

33. Epley B. Poundage chart. In: *Boyd Epley Workout*. Body Enterprises; Lincoln (NE); 1985.

34. Lander J. Maximum based on reps. *NSCA J*. 1985;6:60–1.

35. Mayhew JL, Ware JS, Bemben MG, et al. The NFL-225 test as a measure of bench press strength in college football players. *J Strength Cond Res*. 1999;13:130–4.

36. Cummings B, Finn KJ. Estimation of a one repetition maximum bench press for untrained women. *J Strength Cond Res*. 1998;12:262–5.

37. Mayhew JL, Ball TE, Arnold MD, Bowen JC. Relative muscular endurance performance as a predictor of bench press strength in college men and women. *J Appl Sport Sci Res*. 1992;6:200–6.

38. O'Conner B, Simmons J, O'Shea P. *Weight Training Today*. St. Paul (MN): West Publishers; 1989.

39. Wathen D. Load assignment. In: Baechle T, editor. *Essentials of Strength Training and Conditioning*. Champaign (IL): Human Kinetics; 1994. p. 435–46.

40. Abadie BR, Altorfer GL, Schuler PB. Does a regression equation to predict maximal strength in untrained lifters remain valid

when the subjects are technique trained? *J Strength Cond Res.* 1999;13:259–63.

41. Reynolds JM, Gordon TJ, Robergs RA. Prediction of one repetition maximum strength from multiple repetition maximum testing and anthropometry. *J Strength Cond Res.* 2006;20:584–92.

42. Macht JW, Abel MG, Mullineaux DR, Yates JW. Development of 1RM prediction equations for bench press in moderately trained men. *J Strength Cond Res.* 2016;30:2901–6.

43. Mayhew JL, Johnson BD, LaMonte MJ, Lauber D, Kemmler W. Accuracy of prediction equations for determining one repetition maximum bench press in women before and after resistance training. *J Strength Cond Res.* 2008;22:1570–7.

44. Hoeger WK, Barette SL, Hale DF, Hopkins DR. Relationship between repetitions and selected percentages of one repetition maximum. *J Appl Sport Sci Res.* 1990;1:11–3.

45. American College of Sports Medicine. *ACSM's Guidelines for Exercise Testing and Prescription.* 11th ed. Philadelphia (PA): Lippincott Williams & Wilkins; 2020.

46. Hoffman J. *Norms for Fitness, Performance, and Health.* Champaign (IL): Human Kinetics; 2006. p. 1–113.

47. Vaara JP, Kyrolainen H, Niemi J, et al. Associations of maximal strength and muscular endurance test scores with cardiorespiratory fitness and body composition. *J Strength Cond Res.* 2012;26:2078–86.

48. Moreau CE, Green BN, Johnson CD, Moreau SR. Isometric back extension endurance tests: a review of the literature. *J Manipulative Physiol Ther.* 2001;24:110–22.

49. Evans K, Refshauge KM, Adams R. Trunk muscle endurance tests: reliability, and gender differences in athletes. *J Sci Med Sport.* 2007;10:447–55.

50. McGill SM, Childs A, Liebenson C. Endurance times for low back stabilization exercises: clinical targets for testing and training from a normal database. *Arch Phys Med Rehabil.* 1999;80:941–4.

51. Nesser TW, Huxel KC, Tincher JL, Okada T. The relationship between core stability and performance in Division I football players. *J Strength Cond Res.* 2008;22:1750–4.

52. Wilson G, Wilson L, Affleck M, Hall H. Trunk and lower extremity muscle endurance: normative data for adults. *J Rehabil Outcome Meas.* 1998;2:20–39.

53. Durall CJ, Greene PF, Kernozek TW. A comparison of two isometric tests of trunk flexor endurance. *J Strength Cond Res.* 2012;26:1939–44.

54. Imai A, Kaneoka K. The relationship between trunk endurance plank tests and athletic performance tests in adolescent soccer players. *Int J Sports Phys Ther.* 2016;11:718–24.

55. Harman E, Garhammer J. Administration, scoring, and interpretation of selected tests. In: Baechle TR, Earle RW, editors. *Essentials of Strength Training and Conditioning.* 3rd ed. Champaign (IL): Human Kinetics; 2008. p. 249–92.

56. Johnson BL, Nelson JK. *Practical Measurements for Evaluation in Physical Education.* 4th ed. Minneapolis (MN): MacMillan Publishing; 1986.

57. Cressey E, Hartman B, Robertson M. *Assess and Correct: Breaking Barriers to Unlock Performance.* Indianapolis (IN): self-published; 2009.

58. Ferber R, Kendall KD, McElroy L. Normative and critical criteria for iliotibial band and iliopsoas muscle flexibility. *J Athl Train.* 2010;45:344–8.

59. Lee AY, Kim EH, Cho YW, Kwon SO, Son SM, Ahn SH. Effects of abdominal hollowing during stair climbing on the activations of local trunk stabilizing muscles: a cross-sectional study. *Ann Rehabil Med.* 2013;37:804–13.

60. Borstad JD. Measurement of pectoralis minor muscle length: validation and clinical application. *J Orthop Sports Phys Ther.* 2008;38:169–74.

61. Bagwell JJ, Bauer L, Gradoz M, Grindstaff TL. The reliability of FABER test hip range of motion measurements. *Int J Sports Phys Ther.* 2016;11:1101–5.

62. Vad VB, Bhat AL, Basrai D, et al. Low back pain in professional golfers: the role of associated hip and low back range-of-motion deficits. *Am J Sports Med.* 2004;32:494–7.

63. Harvey D. Assessment of the flexibility of elite athletes using the modified Thomas test. *Br J Sports Med.* 1998;32:68–70.

64. San Juan JG, Suprak DN, Roach SM, Lyda M. Lower extremity strength and range of motion in high school cross-country runners. *Appl Bionics Biomech.* 2018;2018:6797642.

65. Willett GM, Keim SA, Shostrom VK, Lomneth CS. An anatomic investigation of the Ober test. *Am J Sports Med.* 2016;44:696–701.

66. Clark MA, Lucett SC, Corn RJ. *NASM Essentials of Personal Fitness Training.* Philadelphia (PA): Lippincott Williams & Wilkins; 2008. p. 99–138.

67. Cook G. Baseline sports-fitness testing. In: Foran B, editor. *High-Performance Sports Conditioning.* Champaign (IL): Human Kinetics; 2001. p. 19–48.

68. Cook G. *Athletic Body in Balance.* Champaign (IL): Human Kinetics; 2003. p. 31–8.

69. Cook G, Burton L, Hoogenboom BJ, Voight M. Functional movement screening: the use of fundamental movements as an assessment of function—part 1. *Int J Sports Phys Ther.* 2014;9:396–409.

70. Cook G, Burton L, Hoogenboom BJ, Voight M. Functional movement screening: the use of fundamental movements as an assessment of function—part 2. *Int J Sports Phys Ther.* 2014;9:549–63.

71. Bonazza NA, Smuin D, Onks CA, Silvis ML, Dhawan A. Reliability, validity, and injury predictive value of the functional movement screen. *Am J Sports Med.* 2016;45:725–32.

72. Teyhen DS, Shaffer SW, Lorenson CL, et al. The functional movement screen: a reliability study. *J Orthop Sports Phys Ther.* 2012;42:530–40.

73. Schultz R, Anderson SC, Matheson GO, Marcello B, Besier T. Test-retest and interrater reliability of the functional movement screen. *J Athl Train.* 2013;48:331–6.

74. Bodden JG, Needham RA, Chockalingam N. The effect of an intervention program on functional movement screen test scores in mixed martial arts athletes. *J Strength Cond Res.* 2015;29:219–25.

75. Miller JM, Susa KJ. Functional movement screen scores in a group of Division IA athletes. *J Sports Med Phys Fitness.* 2019;59:779–83.

76. Pollen TR, Keitt F, Trojian TH. Do normative composite scores on the functional movement screen differ across high school, collegiate, and professional athletes? A critical review. *Clin J Sport Med.* 2021 Jan;31(1):91–102.

77. Rowan CP, Kuropkat C, Gumieniak RJ, Gledhill N, Jamnik VK. Integration of the functional movement screen into the National Hockey League combine. *J Strength Cond Res.* 2015;29:1163–71.

78. Moore E, Chalmers S, Milanese S, Fuller JT. Factors influencing the relationship between the functional movement screen and injury risk in sporting populations: a systematic review and meta-analysis. *Sports Med.* 2019;49:1449–63.

79. Chalmers S, Fuller JT, Debenedictis TA, et al. Asymmetry during preseason Functional Movements Screen testing is associated with injury during a junior Australian football season. *J Sci Med Sport.* 2017;20:653–7.

80. Bagherian S, Ghasempoor K, Rahnama N, Wikstrom EA. The effect of core stability training on functional movement patterns in college athletes. *J Sport Rehabil.* 2019;28:444–9.

81. Yildiz S, Pinar S, Gelen E. Effects of 8-week functional vs. traditional training on athletic performance and functional movement on prepubertal tennis players. *J Strength Cond Res.* 2018;33:651–61.

82. Housh TJ, Cramer JT, Weir JP, Beck TW, Johnson GO. *Physical Fitness Laboratories on a Budget.* Scottsdale (AZ): Holcomb Hathaway Publishers, Inc.; 2009. p. 50–162.

83. Leger LA, Lambert J. A maximal multistage 20-m shuttle run test to predict Vo$_{2max}$. *Eur J Appl Physiol Occup Physiol.* 1982;49:1–12.

84. Leger LA, Mercier D, Gadoury C, Lambert J. The multistage 20 metre shuttle run test for aerobic fitness. *J Sports Sci.* 1988; 6:93–101.

85. Ramsbottom R, Brewer J, Williams C. A progressive shuttle run test to estimate maximal oxygen uptake. *Br J Sports Med.* 1988;22:141–4.

86. Paliczka VJ, Nichols AK, Boreham CAG. A multi-stage shuttle run as a predictor of running performance and maximal oxygen uptake in adults. *Br J Sports Med.* 1987;21:163–5.

87. Filipa A, Byrnes R, Paterno MV, Myer GD, Hewett TE. Neuromuscular training improves performance on the star excursion balance test in young female athletes. *J Orthop Sports Phys Ther.* 2010;40:551–8.

88. Hoffman JR, Epstein S, Einbinder M, Weinstein Y. A comparison between the Wingate anaerobic power test to both vertical jump and line drill tests in basketball players. *J Strength Cond Res.* 2000;14:261–4.

89. Hoffman J. *Physiological Aspects of Sport Training and Performance.* Champaign (IL): Human Kinetics; 2002. p. 109–19.

90. YMCA of the USA. In: Golding LA, editor. *YMCA Fitness Testing and Assessment Manual.* Champaign (IL): Human Kinetics; 2000. 247 p.

91. McArdle WD, Katch FI, Katch VL. *Exercise Physiology: Energy, Nutrition, and Human Performance.* 6th ed. Philadelphia (PA): Lippincott Williams & Wilkins; 2007. p. 250–1.

92. Ratamess NA, Kang J, Porfido TM, et al. Acute resistance exercise performance is negatively impacted by prior aerobic endurance exercise. *J Strength Cond Res.* 2016;30:2667–81.

93. Peterson MD, Miller T. Power. In: *NSCA's Guide to Tests and Assessments.* Champaign (IL): Human Kinetics; 2012. p. 217–52.

94. Harman EA, Rosenstein MT, Frykman RM, Rosenstein RM, Kraemer WJ. Estimation of human power output from vertical jump. *J Appl Sport Sci Res.* 1991;5:116–20.

95. Johnson DL, Bahamonde R. Power output estimate in university athletes. *J Strength Cond Res.* 1996;10:161–6.

96. Sayers SP, Harackiewicz DV, Harman EA, Frykman PN, Rosenstein MT. Cross-validation of three jump power equations. *Med Sci Sports Exerc.* 1999;31:572–7.

97. Canavan PK, Vescovi JD. Evaluation of power prediction equations: peak vertical jumping power in women. *Med Sci Sports Exerc.* 2004;36:1589–93.

98. Amonette WE, Brown LE, De Witt JK, et al. Peak vertical jump power estimations in youth and young adults. *J Strength Cond Res.* 2012;26:1749–55.

99. Chu DA. *Explosive Power and Strength.* Champaign (IL): Human Kinetics; 1996. p. 167–80.

100. Ratamess NA, Kraemer WJ, Volek JS, et al. The effects of amino acid supplementation on muscular performance during resistance training overreaching. *J Strength Cond Res.* 2003;17:250–8.

101. Bosco C, Luhtanen P, Komi PV. A simple method for measurement of mechanical power in jumping. *Eur J Appl Physiol.* 1983;50:273–82.

102. Newton RU, Kraemer WJ. Power. In: Ackland TR, Elliott BC, Bloomfield J, editors. *Applied Anatomy and Biomechanics in Sport.* 2nd ed. Champaign (IL): Human Kinetics; 2009. p. 155–75.

103. Ross RE, Ratamess NA, Hoffman JR, Faigenbaum AD, Kang J, Chilakos A. The effects of treadmill sprint training and resistance training on maximal running velocity and power. *J Strength Cond Res.* 2009;23:385–94.

104. Smith MS, Dyson RJ, Hale T, Janaway L. Development of a boxing dynamometer and its punch force discrimination efficacy. *J Sport Sci.* 2000;18:445–50.

105. Comstock BA, Solomon-Hill G, Flanagan SD, et al. Validity of the Myotest® in measuring force and power production in the squat and bench press. *J Strength Cond Res.* 2011;25:2293–7.

106. Cronin JB, Hing RD, McNair PJ. Reliability and validity of a linear position transducer for measuring jump performance. *J Strength Cond Res.* 2004;18:590–3.

107. Ratamess NA, Chiarello CM, Sacco AJ, et al. The effects of rest interval length manipulation of the first upper-body resistance exercise in sequence on acute performance of subsequent exercises in men and women. *J Strength Cond Res.* 2012;26:2929–38.

108. Faigenbaum AD, Ratamess NA, McFarland J, et al. Effect of rest interval length on bench press performance in boys, teens, and men. *Pediatr Exerc Sci.* 2008;20:457–69.

109. Hoffman JR, Ratamess NA, Kang J, Rashti SL, Faigenbaum AD. Effect of betaine supplementation on power performance and fatigue. *J Int Soc Sports Nutr.* 2009;6:1–10.

110. Cormie P, McCaulley GO, McBride JM. Power versus strength-power jump squat training: influence on the load-power relationship. *Med Sci Sports Exerc.* 2007;39:996–1003.

111. Kawamori N, Haff GG. The optimal training load for the development of muscular power. *J Strength Cond Res.* 2004;18: 675–84.

112. Soriano MA, Jimenez-Reyes P, Rhea MR, Marin PJ. The optimal load for maximal power production during lower-body resistance exercises: a meta-analysis. *Sports Med.* 2015;45:1191–205.

113. Soriano MA, Suchomel TJ, Marin PJ. The optimal load for maximal power production during upper-body resistance exercises: a meta-analysis. *Sports Med.* 2017;47:757–68.

114. Wang R, Hoffman JR, Sadres E, et al. Evaluating upper-body strength and power from a single test: the ballistic push-up. *J Strength Cond Res.* 2017;31:1338–45.

115. Stockbrugger BA, Haennel RG. Validity and reliability of a medicine ball explosive power test. *J Strength Cond Res.* 2001;15:431–8.

116. Cowley PM, Swensen TC. Development and reliability of two core stability field tests. *J Strength Cond Res.* 2008;22:619–24.

117. Ikeda Y, Kijima K, Kawabata K, Fuchimoto T, Ito A. Relationship between side medicine-ball throw performance and physical ability for male and female athletes. *Eur J Appl Physiol.* 2007;99:47–55.

118. Santos EJAM, Janeira MAAS. Effects of reduced training and detraining on upper and lower body explosive strength in adolescent male basketball players. *J Strength Cond Res.* 2009;23:1737–44.

119. Hoffman JR, Ratamess NA, Klatt M, et al. Comparison between different off-season resistance training programs in Division III American College football players. *J Strength Cond Res.* 2009;23: 11–9.

120. Bar-Or O. The Wingate anaerobic test. An update on methodology, reliability and validity. *Sports Med.* 1987;4:381–94.

121. Ratamess NA, Hoffman JR, Kraemer WJ, et al. Effects of a competitive wrestling season on body composition, endocrine markers, and anaerobic exercise performance in NCAA collegiate wrestlers. *Eur J Appl Physiol.* 2013;113:1157–68.

122. Maud PJ, Schultz BB. Norms for the Wingate anaerobic test with comparison to another similar test. *Res Q Exerc Sport*. 1989;60:144–51.

123. Gillam GM. 300 yard shuttle run. *NSCA J*. 1983;5:46.

124. Semenick D. The line drill test. *NSCA J*. 1990;12:47–9.

125. Delextrat A, Cohen D. Strength, power, speed, and agility of women basketball players according to playing position. *J Strength Cond Res*. 2009;23:1974–81.

126. Triplett NT, Miller T. Speed and agility. In: *NSCA's Guide to Tests and Assessments*. Champaign (IL): Human Kinetics; 2012. p. 253–74.

127. Mann JB, Ivey PA, Mayhew JL, et al. Relationship between agility tests and short sprints: reliability and smallest worthwhile difference in National Collegiate Athletic Association Division-I football players. *J Strength Cond Res*. 2016;30:893–900.

128. Hoffman JR, Vasquez J, Pichardo N, Tenebaum G. Anthropometric and performance comparisons in professional baseball players. *J Strength Cond Res*. 2009;23:2173–8.

129. Hedlund DP. Performance of future elite players at the National Football League scouting combine. *J Strength Cond Res*. 2018;32:3112–8.

130. Dintiman G, Ward B, Tellez T. *Sports Speed*. 2nd ed. Champaign (IL): Human Kinetics; 1998. p. 1–44.

131. Nimphius S, Callaghan SJ, Bezodis NE, Lockie RG. Change of direction and agility tests: challenging our current measures of performance. *Strength Cond J*. 2018;40:26–38.

132. Dos Santos T, Thomas C, Comfort P, Jones PA. Comparison of change of direction speed performance and asymmetries between team-sport athletes: application of change of direction deficit. *Sports*. 2018;6:174.

133. Lockie RG, Farzad J, Orjalo AJ, et al. A methodological report: adapting the 505 change-of-direction speed test specific to American football. *J Strength Cond Res*. 2017;31:539–47.

134. Nimphius S, Callaghan SJ, Spiteri T, Lockie RG. Change of direction deficit: a more isolated measure of change of direction performance than total 505 time. *J Strength Cond Res*. 2016;30:3024–32.

135. Hrysomallis C. Relationship between balance ability, training and sports injury risk. *Sports Med*. 2007;37:547–56.

136. Trojian TH, McKeag DB. Single leg balance test to identify risk of ankle sprains. *Br J Sports Med*. 2006;40:610–3.

137. Bressel E, Yonker JC, Kras J, Heath EM. Comparison of static and dynamic balance in female collegiate soccer, basketball, and gymnastics athletes. *J Athl Train*. 2007;42:42–6.

138. Davlin CD. Dynamic balance in high level athletes. *Percept Mot Skills*. 2004;98:1171–6.

139. Matsuda S, Demura S, Uchiyama M. Centre of pressure sway characteristics during static one-legged stance of athletes from different sports. *J Sports Sci*. 2008;26:775–9.

140. Thorpe JL, Ebersole KT. Unilateral balance performance in female collegiate soccer athletes. *J Strength Cond Res*. 2008;22:1429–33.

141. Raisanen A, Pasanen K, Krosshaug T, et al. Single-leg squat as a tool to evaluate young athletes' frontal plane knee control. *Clin J Sports Med*. 2016;26:478–82.

142. National Academy of Sports Medicine. In: McGill EM, Montel I, editors. *Essentials of Sports Performance Training*. 2nd ed. Burlington (MA): Jones and Bartlett Learning; 2019. p. 81–151.

143. Bailey R, Selfe J, Richards J. The single leg squat test in the assessment of musculoskeletal function: a review. *Physiother Ireland*. 2010;31:18–23.

144. Crossley KM, Zhang WJ, Schache AG, Bryant A, Cowan SM. Performance on the single-leg squat task indicates hip abductor muscle function. *Am J Sports Med*. 2011;39:866–73.

145. Laughlin WA, Weinhandl JT, Kernozek TW, et al. The effects of single-leg landing technique on ACL loading. *J Biomech*. 2011;44:1845–51.

146. Padua DA, Marshall SW, Boling MC, et al. The Landing Error Scoring System (LESS) is a valid and reliable clinical assessment tool of jump-landing mechanics. *Am J Sports Med*. 2009;37:1996–2002.

147. Root H, Trojian T, Martinez J, Kraemer WJ, Distefano LJ. Landing technique and performance in youth athletes after a single injury-prevention program session. *J Athl Train*. 2015;50:1149–57.

148. Hrysomallis C. Preseason and midseason balance ability of professional Australian footballers. *J Strength Cond Res*. 2008;22:210–1.

149. Zech A, Hubscher M, Vogt L, et al. Balance training for neuromuscular control and performance enhancement: a systematic review. *J Athl Train*. 2010;45:392–403.

150. Iverson GL, Koehle MS. Normative data for the Balance Error Scoring System in adults. *Rehabil Res Pract*. 2013;2013:846418.

151. Olmsted LC, Carcia CR, Hertel J, Schultz SJ. Efficacy of the star excursion balance tests in detecting reach deficits in subjects with chronic ankle instability. *J Athl Train*. 2002;37:501–6.

152. Engquist KD, Smith CA, Chimera NJ, Warren M. Performance comparison of student-athletes and general college students on the functional movement screen and the Y balance test. *J Strength Cond Res*. 2015;29:2296–303.

153. Plisky PJ, Gorman PP, Butler RJ, et al. The reliability of an instrumented device for measuring components of the star excursion balance test. *N Am J Sports Phys Ther*. 2009;4:92–9.

INDEX

Note: Page numbers followed by '*f*' indicate figures; page numbers followed by '*t*' indicate tables and page numbers followed by '*b*' indicate boxes.

A

Accelerometers, 36
Acceptable macronutrient distribution range
    (AMDR), 49
Acclimatization to heat, 562*t*
Accommodation, 237
Acetylcholine, 84
Acetyl-CoA carboxylase (ACC), 189–190
Aconitase, 187
Actin filaments, 98–99
Action force, 35
Action potential, neural communication
    integration, 76–77
    neurotransmitters, 77–78
    propagation, 77–78
Active insufficiency, 24–25
Active stretch, 256–257
Active warm-up, 251–255
Actomyosin complex, 100
Acute mountain sickness (AMS), 554
Acute program variables, 287, 288*f*
Adenosine phosphate (ADP), 178–179
Adenosine triphosphate (ATP), 179*f*
    aerobic metabolism, 187–193, 188*f*–187*f*
    energy system contribution and athletics, 193,
        193*t*–194*t*
    glycolysis, 181–187, 182*f*
    hydrolysis of, 179, 183
    lactate, 184, 185*f*
    metabolic acidosis and buffer capacity, 186–187
    phosphocreatine systems, 179–181
Adenylate kinase, 179
Adequate intake (AI), 49
Adipocytes, 189–190
Adipose triglyceride lipase (ATGL), 188–189
Adrenaline, 166
Aerobic capacity assessment
    cycle ergometer tests, 619, 628
    fields tests, 618–619, 620*t*–621*t*
    lactate threshold, 621–622
    step tests, 619
Aerobic dance class, 540–541
Aerobic endurance, 239
Aerobic endurance training, 546*b*, 547*f*, 557*b*
    altitude training
        acclimatization, 554–555
        barometric pressure, 554, 554*t*
        benefits, 554
        human performance, 553–554
        immediate and chronic adaptations, 554–555,
            555*t*
        LHTL approach, 556–557, 557*f*
        maximal aerobic capacity, 555–556
        partial pressure of oxygen, 554
        physiological responses, 554–555
        sea level performance, 554

        submaximal $\dot{V}O_2$, 555–556
    anaerobic athletes, 560
    cold temperatures, 564–565
    endurance sports training, 551–552
    Fartlek training, 550
    frequency, 545, 546*t*
    heat, 561–563
    vs. high-intensity strength/power, 558–560
    hot and cold environments, 560–565, 561*f*
    intensity selection
        aerobic capacity, 542
        heart rate, 542, 543*f*
        hill training, 542
        RPE scale, 544, 545*f*
        $\dot{V}O_{2\,max}$, 544–545, 544*t*, 547*f*
    interval training, 548–550
    long slow distance training, 548
    modes, 539*t*
        aerobic dance class, 540–541
        cross-country skiing, 541
        cross-training, 541–542
        cycling, 540
        jogging and running, 539–540
        rowing and skating, 541
        stair climbing, 540
        swimming and aquatic exercise, 541
    pace/tempo training, 548
    repetition training, 550
    types of, 547–550
    volume and duration, 547, 548*t*
Aerobic endurance training for anaerobic athletes,
    560
Aerobic exercise
    catecholamines, 166–167
    β-endorphin, 167
    endurance performance
        exercise economy, 538, 539*f*
        lactate threshold, 536–537
        $\dot{V}O_{2\,max}$, 535–536, 537*f*
    estradiol, 169–170
    growth hormone, 160
    insulin, 163
    thyroxine and triiodothyronine, 167
Aerobic metabolism
    aerobic training adaptations, 191–192
    anaerobic training adaptations, 192–193
    beta oxidation, 187
    CHO metabolism, 187
    electron transport chain, 187, 189*f*
    energy yield
        carbohydrates, 187–188
        fats, 191, 192*f*
    Krebs cycle, 187, 188*f*–187*f*
    lipid metabolism, 188–191, 190*f*
    mitochondria, 187
Aerobic training, 3
    cardiovascular responses, 217–221

    glycogen, 184
    metabolism, 191–192
Afterload, 218
Agility, 500–501, 501*f*
    bags, 517
    ladders, 517
    poles, 517
    tests assessment
        505 change of direction (COD) test, 633, 633*f*
        3-cone drill, 634, 634*f*, 635*t*
        Davies test, 635
        Edgren side-step test, 634–635, 635*f*
        hexagon test, 633–634, 634*f*
        pro-agility test, 634, 634*f*
        T-test, 633
Agility training, 13
    3-day Agility program, 526, 527*t*
    change direction, 516–517
    components, 500–501, 501*f*
    equipment, 517, 518*f*
    Makoto reaction device, 517, 518*f*
    paradigm, 513–514, 514*f*
    program design
        drill progression, 521–522
        exercise selection, 523–524, 527
        frequency, 525
        intensity, 524
        plyometric training, 523
        rest interval, 526
        structure and sequencing, 523
        volume, 525–526
    technical aspects
        acceleration/deceleration, 515
        arm action, 515
        balance, 515
        exercise, 514
        foot contact, 515
        posture, 515
        quickness, 515
        reaction, 515
        targeted movements, 515–516
    total-body mobility, 517
    training drills
        bag weaves, 519–520, 526*f*
        carioca, 518
        diamond reaction, 519–520, 523*f*
        EKG, 519–520, 523*f*
        hexagon drill, 519–520, 526*f*
        hopscotch, 519–520, 523*f*
        Icky shuffle, 519–520, 524*f*
        Ins and outs, 519–520, 523*f*
        left-right shuffle, 519–520, 524*f*
        letter drills, 519–520, 522*f*
        programmed, 518
        quickness, 518
        reactive, 518
        right triangle drills, 519–520, 520*f*

648 Index

20-yd shuttle, 519–520, 519f
60-yd shuttle run, 519–520, 519f
side rocker, 519–520, 524f
40-yd sprint, 519–520, 519f
square drills, 519–520, 520f
T-drill, 519–520, 519f–526f
two-feet forward, 519–520, 525f
two-in lateral shuffle, 519–520, 525f
X-pattern drills, 519–520, 520f
zig-zag, 519–520, 522f, 525f
zig-zag cross-over shuffle, 519–520, 525f
Z-pattern, 519–520, 521f
warm-up drills, 526t
Agonist muscles, 96–97
Air displacement plethysmography, 602–603
Albumin, 154
Aldolase, 181
Alleles, 104
Alternate bounding, 471, 471f
Altitude tent, 557f
American College of Sports Medicine (ACSM), 287
Amine hormone, 147
Amino acids, 51–52
functions of, 53t
Amortization phase, 448–449
5′ AMP-activated protein kinase (AMPK), 188
Anabolic steroids, 146
Anaerobic exercise training
ATP-PC, 179
cardiovascular responses, 217–221
β-endorphin, 167
insulin, 163
lactate concentration, 185
metabolism, 192–193
Anaerobic speed reserve (ASR), 529, 530f
Anatomical position, 367–368
Androgen receptor, 158–159
Anemia, 63
Angle of pennation, 27–29
Angular (rotary) motion, 23
Ankling, 505–506, 506f
Annual training plan, 571–572, 571f, 581t–582t
Antagonist muscle activation, motor units, 84
Anterior cross-arm stretch, 265, 265f
Anterior cruciate ligament (ACL) tear, 288
Anthropometry, 596–603
Antidiuretic hormone (ADH), 146
Antioxidants, 64–65
Apolipoprotein, 227
Appetite regulating hormones, 169
Appositional growth, 132
Arterial compliance, 217
Arterial stiffness, 217
Arterial vasodilation, 216f
Arteries, 211
Arterio-venous oxygen difference, 213–214
Articular/hyaline cartilage, 140–141
Ascending pyramids, 309–310
Åstrand-Rhyming test, 619, 621t, 621f–622f
Athletes
basal metabolic rate estimation, 195–197
blood doping, 215b
breath control, lifting, 368b
energy system contribution, 193, 193t–194t
Atrioventricular node (AV node), 212–213
Autocrine action, 145
Autogenic inhibition, 257
Autonomic nervous system, 89–91, 90f

B

Back (Glute) Bridge, 427, 427f
Backpedalling, 500–501
Bag thrusts, 486, 486f
Balance assessment
anterior reach, 637
fitness components, 17
force plate tests, 638
one-leg DB standing shoulder press, 397f
single-leg balance test, 637
single-leg squat, 636–637
stabilometer balance test, 637–638, 638f–640f
standing stork test, 637
star excursion balance test, 639–640, 640f
Balance discs, 346, 347f
Balance error scoring system (BESS), 638–639, 639f
Ballistic stretching, 257
Barbell lunge, 379, 379f
Barbells, 340–341, 341f
Baroreceptors, 219
Barrier jumps, 458, 458f
Bar rotation, 422, 422f
Basal ganglia, 78
Basal metabolic rate (BMR)
ACSM'S metabolic equations, 197t–198t
energy expenditure during exercise, 196–197, 197t
resting energy expenditure, 195–196
resting metabolic rate, 195–197, 196t
Basic strength exercises, 292
Battling rope exercises, 433, 433f
Beep test, 618–619
Behind-the-neck press, 440, 440f
Behind-the-neck triceps stretch, 267, 267f
Bench press, 385, 385f
Bent-knee sit-up, 415, 415f
Bent-knee twists, 416, 416f
Bent-over barbell row, 391, 391f
Bent-over shoulder/pectoral stretch, 264, 264f
Beta oxidation, 187
Biceps stretch, 268, 268f
Biering-Sorensen test, 610, 611f–612f
Bilateral-access hypothesis, 88
Bilateral deficit, 88
Bilateral facilitation, 88
Bilateral training, 241–242
Bioelectrical impedance analysis, 602
Bioenergetics, 178
Biological value (BV), 52
Biomechanics (see Force production)
Biotin (vitamin H), 59t–60t
Bipennate muscles, 27
Blood
blood vessels, 211, 212f
components, 213–217, 213f–214f
doping, 215b
flow, 215–217
lipids and lipoproteins, 226–227
pressure, 217, 219–220, 220f, 225–226
volume, 226
Bodybuilding, 7–8, 14, 14f, 160
Body composition, 12
advantages and disadvantages of, 597t
girth measurements, 598
height, bodyweight, and body mass index, 597–598
skinfold assessment, 598, 599f, 600t

Body density, 598, 600t, 602
Body fat, 201–204
classifications, 601t
Body mass, 195
Bohr effect, 214
Bone(s)
adaptations to exercise, 132–133
anatomy, 128–130
growth, 132–134
human voluntary movement, 128
matrix, 129–130
remodeling, 130–133, 131f, 132f
size and strength, training to increase, 135
Bone alkaline phosphatase (BAP), 131–132, 134
Bone mineral density (BMD)
bone markers, 134
and muscle mass and strength, 133
training guidelines, 133
Borg scale, 544, 545f
BOSU balls (Balance Trainer), 346, 346f, 347f
Box jump, 468, 468f
Brainstem, 78
Branched-chain amino acids (BCAAs), 53–54
Breakdown sets, 322
Breath holding, intraabdominal pressure, 40–41
Buffer capacity, 186–187
Bundle of His, 212–213
Buoyancy of water, 354–355
Butterfly stretch, 274, 274f
Butt kickers, 505–506, 505f

C

Cable rotations, 421, 421f
Calcium, 61t–62t
Calf (Toe) raise, 383, 383f
Caloric balance, 48
Canaliculi, 129–130
Capillary density, 191–192
Carbaminohemoglobin, 215
Carbohydrates, 49–51, 49t, 49f
functions of, 49t
structure of, 52t
Carbonic anhydrase, 186, 214–215
Cardiac dimensions, 222–223
Cardiac muscle, 96
hypertrophy, 222
Cardiac musculature, 210–211
Cardiac output (Qc), 217, 219, 219f, 223–224, 223f
Cardioacceleration training, 218
Cardiocytes, 210–211
Cardiorespiratory system
heart (see Heart)
respiratory system (see Respiratory system)
Cardiovascular drift, 218
Cardiovascular endurance, 12
Cardiovascular function, 217
Carioca, 518
Cartilage adaptations, 140–141
Catalase, 64–65
Catch, 437
Catch-up growth, 137
Catecholamines, 166–167
Cell body, 76–77
Central command, 229
Central nervous system (CNS), 75–76
Cerebrum, 78, 79f

Index **649**

Chains, 346–349, 348*f*
Chain size information, 321, 321*f*
505 change of direction (COD) test, 633, 633*f*
Chemical buffer, 186
Chemiosmotic hypothesis, 187
Chemoreceptors, 229–230
Chloride, 61*t*–62*t*
Cholesterol, 55, 146
CHO loading, 184
Chromatids, 104
Chromium, 61*t*–62*t*
Chromosomes, 104, 104*f*
Chylomicrons, 55
Citrate synthase, 187, 191–192
Classical model, 575–576, 576*t*
Classic plyometrics, 447
Clean, 434–437
    grip, 440, 440*f*
    high pull, 440, 440*f*
    and jerk, 434–437, 435*f*
Closed-chain kinetic exercise, 241
Clothing insulation (CLO), 564–565, 564*t*, 565*f*
Cluster training method, 324–325
Cobalamin (B$_{12}$), 59*t*–60*t*
Coefficient of friction, 36–37
Coefficient of restitution, 39–40
Cold-induced thermogenesis, 564
Collagen, 129–130, 139
Combination exercises, 434, 487
Combining exercises, 322–323
COMMOV (Contraction of Other Muscle groups and other MOVements), 316*b*
Compact bone, 128–129
Compensatory acceleration technique, 313–314
Competitive lifting sports
    bodybuilding, 7–8
    modes, 16–17
    performance, 16–17
    powerlifting, 8
    strength competitions, 8
    weightlifting, 7
Complete proteins, 52
Complex training, 487–488
Concentric hypertrophy, 222
Concentric (CON) muscle action, 13, 23–24
    cardiac output, 219
    corrective exercise programming, 315–316
    exercise selection, 291
    force production, velocity, 26–27
    functional isometrics, 320
    GH response, 155
    heart rate response, 218
    hydraulic resistance machines, 343
    musculotendinous stiffness, 254
    partial repetitions, 320
    pneumatic resistance machines, 343
    PNF stretching, 257
    repetition velocity, 313
    specificity, 239–240
    stretch-shortening cycle, 26
    stroke volume response, 218–219
Concurrent activation potentiation, 41
Conduction, 560–561
3-Cone drill, 634, 634*f*, 635*t*
Cone hops, 459, 459*f*
Cones, 517
Connective tissue adaptations
    components of, 135–141

skeletal system, 128–135
    stimuli for, 126–127
Construct validity, 593–594
Content validity, 593–594
Contract-relax PNF stretching, 258
Contract-relax with agonist contraction, 258
Contract-relax with antagonist contraction, 258
Contrast loading combinations, 325
Convection, 560–561
Cooldown, 282–283
Cooper 12-minute run test, 618
Copper, 61*t*–62*t*
Core balls, 344–346, 346*f*
Core exercises
    Back (Glute) Bridge, 427, 427*f*
    bar rotation, 422, 422*f*
    bent-knee sit-up, 415, 415*f*
    bent-knee twists, 416, 416*f*
    cable rotations, 421, 421*f*
    Crunch (Curl-Up), 414, 414*f*
    dead bug, 414*f*
    difficult, 413
    farmer's walk, 431, 431*f*
    good morning, 424, 424*f*
    hyperextension, 425, 425*f*
    kettlebell figure 8s, 429, 429*f*
    kettlebell swing, 426, 426*f*
    kinesiology of, 413*t*
    lying leg raise, 419, 419*f*
    manual resistance neck (four-way), 430, 430*f*
    medicine ball woodchop, 420, 420*f*
    plank, 418, 418*f*
    proper position for, 413
    quadruped, 428, 428*f*
    side bends, 417, 417*f*
    skier, 422, 422*f*
    sled push, 432, 432*f*
    stability ball exchange, 419, 419*f*
    stability ball roll-out, 418, 418*f*
    tire flipping, 431, 431*f*
    Turkish get-up, 423, 423*f*
Cori cycle, 185
Corrective exercise programming, 315–316
Corticomuscular coherence, 80
Corticotrophin-releasing hormone (CRH), 146
Cortisol, 164–166
Costameres, 102–103
Countermovement vertical jump (CMJ), 26
Creatine kinase (CK), 179
Criterion-referenced validity, 593–594
Critical velocity, 550
Cross-bridge cycling, 100–102, 101*f*
Cross-country skiing, 541
Cross education, 88, 241
Cross-links, 135–136
Cross-training, 541–542
Crunch (Curl-Up), 414, 414*f*
Curvilinear motion, 22
Cycle ergometer tests, 619, 628
Cycling, 540
Cytochrome C oxidase, 191–192

D

Davies test, 635
Dead bug, 413, 414*f*

Deadlift, 378, 378*f*
Decline bench press, 386*f*
Dendrites, 76–77
Depth jump, 473, 473*f*, 474*f*
Depth landing, 447
Depth push-up, 485, 485*f*
Descending pyramid, 310
Descending sets, 322
Detraining, 244
Diamond reaction, 519–520, 523*f*
Diaphysis, 128–129
Diencephalon, 78
Dietary reference intakes (DRI), 48–68
    antioxidants, 54–57, 54*f*–55*f*, 57*t*, 64–65
    carbohydrates, 49–51, 49*t*, 49*f*
        glycemic index and glycemic load, 50–51, 51*t*, 51*b*
    lipids, 54–57, 54*f*–55*f*, 57*t*
    microbiome, microbiota and probiotics, 67–68
    protein, 51–54, 52*t*–53*t*, 52*f*
    vitamins and minerals, 57–67, 58*f*, 59*t*–60*t*, 64*f*
    water, 57
Diet-induced thermogenesis, 195
Digestible indispensable amino acid score (DIAAS), 52
2,3-Diphosphoglycerate (2,3-DPG), 214
Disaccharides, 49
Double-leg hops, 464, 464*f*
Downhill sprinting, 507–508
Drop jump, 473, 473*f*
Drop sets, 322
Drop snatch, 441, 441*f*
Drum major, 505–506, 508*f*
Dumbbell fly, 388, 388*f*
Dumbbell lateral raise, 400, 400*f*
Dumbbells, 341–342
Dynamic constant external resistance, 13
Dynamic flexibility exercises, 251–253, 252*b*
Dynamic (sliding) friction, 36–37
Dynamic method, 324
Dynamic stretching, 257
Dynamic warm-up, 254–255

E

Eccentric hypertrophy, 222
Eccentric (ECC) muscle action, 13, 23–24
    BP response, 220
    cardiac output, 219
    corrective exercise programming, 315–316
    exercise selection, 291
    force production, velocity, 26–27
    functional isometrics, 320
    GH response, 155
    glucocorticoid receptor, 165
    heart rate response, 218
    hydraulic resistance machines, 343
    muscle IGF-1 adaptations, 162
    pliometric exercise, 447
    pneumatic resistance machines, 343
    PNF stretching, 257
    repetition velocity, 313
    specificity, 239–240
    stretch-shortening cycle, 26
    stroke volume response, 218–219
    variable resistance training, 321–322
    water and environment, 354–355

650 **Index**

Edgren side-step test, 634–635, 635f
Elastic bands and tubing, 346–349
Elastic cartilage, 140–141
Elastic energy, 448–449
Elasticity, 127
Elastin, 135
Electrolytes, 63
Electromechanical delay, 448–449
Elliptical trainer machines, 540
Empty calories, 48
Endergonic reactions, 178
Endochondral ossification, 132
Endocrine action, 145
Endocrine hormones (*see* Hormones)
Endomysium, 97–98
β-Endorphin, 167
Endosteum, 128–129
Endurance sports training, 551–552, 553t
Endurance training
    aerobic (*see* Aerobic endurance training)
    oxygen consumption, 224–225
Energy, 178, 195–196
Energy availability (EA), 65
Energy metabolism, specificity, 240
Enolase, 181
Epimysium, 97–98
Epiphyses, 128–129
Ergogenic, 180
Essential amino acids, 51–52, 52t
Estimated average requirement (EAR), 48
Estrogens, 169–170
Evaporation, 560–561
Excess postexercise oxygen consumption (EPOC),
    197–198
Excitation-contraction coupling, 100
Exercise
    acute testosterone response to, 155–156
    androgen receptor, 158–159
    appetite regulating hormones, 169
    ATP-PC, 179
    balance, 397b, 397f
    basal metabolic rate, 195–197
    blood
        lipids and lipoproteins, 227
        pressure, 219–220, 220f, 225–226
        volume, 226
    body fat reduction, 201–204
    carbohydrate intake and muscle glycogen, 184b
    cardiac dimensions, 222–223
    cardiac output, 219, 219f, 223–224, 223f
    catecholamines, 166–167
    cortisol, 165
    creatine, 180
    economy, 538, 539f
    β-endorphin, 167
    energy expenditure, 197t, 201
    estrogens, 169–170
    exercise order, 14
    fluid-regulatory hormones, 168–169
    glucagon, 164
    glycogen, 183
    growth hormone, 160
    heart rate response, 218
    indirect calorimetry, 193–195
    insulin, 163–164
    insulin-like growth factors, 161–162
    leptin, 169

luteinizing hormone, 158
    oxygen consumption, 197–201, 221, 224–225
    plasma volume, 220–221
    pulmonary adaptations to, 230–231, 230f
    respiratory muscle-specific training, 231–232
    SHBG, 158
    stroke volume response, 218–219
    thyroid hormones, 167–168
Exercise balls, 344–346, 346f
Exercise kinesiology, 367–368
Exercise selection, 14
    agility training, 523–524, 527
    resistance training program design, 291–293
    sprint training, 523–524, 527
Exergonic reactions, 178
Exertional hyperthermia, 561–562
Expiratory reserve volume, 228

F

FABER (flexion, abduction, and external rotation)
    test, 615, 615f–616f
Face validity, 593–594
F actin, 99
Falling, 505–506, 509f
Farmer's walk, 431, 431f
    bars, 353
Fartlek training, 550
Fascia, 138–139
Fascicles, 29–30, 97–98
Fast exponential taper, 573
Fast glycolysis, 181
Fatigue tests, 606–607
Fat-soluble vitamins, 57–58
Fatty acid transport protein (FATP), 189–190
Female athlete triad, 65b
Ferritin, 63
Fiber-type transitions, 109–110, 109f
Fibroblasts, 135
Fibrocytes, 135
Fibrous, 99
Fick equation, 221
Filamin (Filamin-C), 98–99
Firing rate, motor units, 83
First pull, 436
Flat bones, 128
Flexed-arm hang, 610, 611t
Flexed arms above head stretch, 266, 266f
Flexibility assessment, 238
    exercises, 3
    factors affecting, 256
    fitness components, 12
    goniometer and ROM measurement, 612, 613t,
        613f
    injury prevention, 255–256
    and injury prevention, 255–256
    modified sit-and-reach test, 612–614
    pass/fail tests, 614–616
    performance effects, 255
    progressive overload, 238
    resistance training, 259b
    shoulder elevation test, 614
    sit-and-reach test, 612–614, 613f
    stretching (*see* Stretching)
    training, 254–255
    training guidelines, 281–282, 282t

    trunk rotation test, 614
    types, 256–260
Flexible nonlinear periodization, 577–578
Flexion, abduction, and external rotation (FABER)
    test, 615, 615f–616f
Fluoride, 61t–62t
Foam rolling, 258–260
Folic acid, 59t–60t
Force couples, 23
Forced expiratory volume, 228
Forced negatives, 319–320
Forced repetitions, 322
Forced vital capacity, 228
Force plate tests, 638
Force production
    action/reaction forces and friction, 35, 35f–36f
    body size, 40
    mass and inertia, 38–39
    momentum and impulse, 39–40
    muscle architecture (*see* Skeletal muscle)
    muscle actions, 23–24
    muscle length, 24–26
    stability, 38
    strength and conditioning, 40–42
    torque and leverage, 30–35
    velocity role, 26–27, 27f
Force–velocity relationship, 27f, 28b
Forward lunge stretch, 270, 270f
Forward triceps stretch, 268, 268f
Frankenstein, 505–506, 509f
Frank–Starling mechanism, 218
Free inorganic phosphate, 178–179
Free radical, 64–65
Free weights
    vs. machines, 292–293
        movement-specific training, 242–243
        unilateral *vs.* bilateral training, 241–242
    open- *vs.* closed-chain kinetic exercises, 241
    resistance training modalities
        advantages, 343–344
        barbells, 340–341, 341f
        disadvantages, 343–344
        dumbbells, 341–342
        free-weight equipment, 342
        vs. machines, 343–344, 345b
        RT machines, 342–343, 342f
Frequency, 14
Friction, 36–37
Frontal plane, 367–368, 370f
Front squat, 442, 442f
Fulcrum, 31–32
Fumarase, 187
Functional isometrics, 320
Functional movement screen, 616–617
Functional residual capacity, 228
Functional syncytium, 210–211
Fusiform muscles, 27

G

G actin, 99
Gate control theory, 257
Gears, 505–506, 508f
Gene expression, 107–108
General adaptation syndrome, 573, 573f
General preparation training, 571–572

General-to-specific model of progression, 244, 244f, 290–291, 291f
General warm-up, 251, 252f
Giant sets, 323
Girth measurements, 598
Global positioning system (GPS), 36
Globular, 99
Glucagon, 164
Gluconeogenesis, 181
Glutathione peroxidase, 64–65
Glycemic index (GI), 50–51, 51t, 51b
Glycemic load (GL), 50–51, 51t, 51b
Glycerides, 54
Glycogenolysis, 181
Glycogen synthase, 183
Glycolysis, 181
    control of, 183
    fast, 181
    glycogen metabolism, 183–184
    lactate, 184, 185f
    metabolic acidosis and buffer capacity, 186–187
    reactions of, 181, 182f, 183
    slow, 181
    training adaptations, 184
Golgi tendon organs (GTO), 84
Gonadotropin-releasing hormone (GnRH), 146
Good morning, 424, 424f
Grip strength, 434
Gross motor coordination, 13
Ground reaction force, 35, 36f
Growth hormone, 146, 160–161
Growth plate, 132
Gymnastics exercises, 433

H

Haldane effect, 215
Half-life, 150
Hammer curl, 409, 409f
Health-related fitness component assessment
    aerobic capacity assessment
        cycle ergometer tests, 619, 628
        fields tests, 618–619, 620t–621t
        lactate threshold, 621–622
        step tests, 619
    body composition and anthropometry
        girth measurements, 598
        height, body weight, and body mass index, 597–598
        skinfold assessment, 598, 599f, 600t
    flexibility assessment
        goniometer and ROM measurement, 612, 613t, 613f
        modified sit-and-reach test, 612–614
        pass/fail tests, 614–616
        shoulder elevation test, 614
        sit-and-reach test, 612–614, 613f
        trunk rotation test, 614
    muscle endurance test
        absolute repetition number, 610
        bodyweight exercises, 609, 610t
        sustained maximal duration trials, 610–612, 611t
    muscle strength
        isokinetic strength testing, 607–608
        isometric strength testing, 606–607

leg press and bench press strength, 605t
    proper spotting, 605
    repetition maximums estimation, 608–609, 608t
    strength testing checklist, 604f
Heart
    anatomy, 210–211, 211f
    blood components, 213–217, 213f–214f
    blood flow, 215–217
    blood vessels, 211, 212f
    cardiac musculature, 210–211
    cardiovascular function, 217
    cardiovascular responses to exercise, 217–221
    chronic adaptations at rest and during exercise, 221–227
    extrinsic regulation of, 213
    intrinsic regulation of, 212–213, 212f
    regulation of, 212–213
Heart rate, 217
    variability, 217–218
Heat exchange, regulation of, 561f
Heat shock proteins, 105
Heavy bags, 354
Heavy negatives, 319–320
Hematocrit, 213
Hemoconcentration, 150–151
Hemoglobin, 213
Hexagon drill, 519–520, 526f
Hexagon test, 633–634, 634f
Hexokinase, 181
High altitude cerebral edema (HACE), 554
High altitude pulmonary edema (HAPE), 554
High-density lipoproteins, 55
High-fat diets, 57
High-intensity endurance, 12
High knees, 505–506, 506f, 510f
Hiking, 539–540
Hold-relax PNF stretching, 258
Hold-Relax with antagonist contraction, 258
Hook grip, 438, 438f
Hopscotch, 519–520, 523f
Hormones
    action, 145
    activity, 148–152, 149f
    appetite regulating hormones, 169
    catecholamines, 166–167
    concentrations in the blood, 150–151
    cortisol, 164–166
    definition, 145
    β-endorphin, 167
    estrogens, 169–170
    fluid-regulatory hormones, 168–169
    functions and emdocrine glands, 146f, 147, 147t–148t
    glucagon, 164
    growth hormone, 160
    insulin, 163–164
    insulin-like growth factors, 161–163
    leptin, 169
    negative feedback control, 152
    receptor interaction, 152–153, 153f, 154f
    releasing hormones, 146
    testosterone, 154–159
    thyroid hormones, 167–168
    types of, 146–147
Hormone-sensitive lipase, 188–189
Human strength curves
    ascending strength curve, 34–35, 35f

descending strength curve, 35, 35f
    moment arm
        ascending-descending torque curve, 34
        during elbow flexion, 34
    physiological and biomechanical factors, 34
    sticking region, 33–34
Hydrodensitometry, 602
Hydrolysis, 178–179
Hydroxyapatites, 129–130
Hyperextension, 425, 425f
Hyperplasia, 118
Hypertonic solution, 51b
Hypertrophy, 12
    phase, 575–576
Hypervolemia, 226
Hypobaric conditions, 553–558
Hyponatremia, 63
Hypothalamus, 78
Hypotonic solution, 51b
Hypoxia-inducible factors (HIFs), 555

I

Icky shuffle, 519–520, 524f
Incline bench press, 386, 387f–388f
Incomplete proteins, 52
Individualization, 244
Inflatable ball, 344–346, 346f
Ins and outs drill, 519–520, 523f
Inspiration, 228
Inspiratory capacity, 228
Inspiratory muscle training (IMT), 231
Inspiratory reserve volume, 228
Insulin-like growth factors, 161–163
Insulin resistance, 163–164
Insulin sensitivity, 163–164
Integrated models, 310
Integrative training, 10
Intensity, 14
30–15 Intermittent fitness test, 530–531
Intermittent hypoxic exposure (IHE), 558
Intermittent hypoxic training (IHT), 558
Internal/external shoulder rotations, 401–402
Intertester reliability, 594
Interval training, 193
Intra-abdominal pressure (IAP), 40–41, 40f, 218–219
    abdominal contraction, 40–41
    breath holding, 40–41
    lifting belts, 40–41
    trunk muscle training, 40–41
Intramembranous ossification, 132
Intramuscular triglycerides, 188–189
Intrapulmonary pressure, 227–228
Intrathoracic pressure (ITP), 40–41, 218–219
Iodine, 61t–62t
Iron, 61t–62t
Irregular bones, 128
Isocitrate dehydrogenase, 187
Isoinertia, 13
Isokinetic strength (ISOK) testing, 607–608
Isometric (ISOM) muscle action, 13, 23–24
    blood flow, 215–216
    corrective exercise programming, 315–316
    exercise selection, 291
    forced repetition, 322

652 **Index**

Isometric (ISOM) muscle action (*Continued*)
force production, velocity, 26–27
functional isometrics, 320
gripping exercises, 434
manual or partner resistance, 340, 340*f*
pliometric exercise, 447
PNF stretching, 257
repetition velocity, 320
specificity, 239–240
stretch-shortening cycle, 26
Isometric strength (ISOM) testing, 606–607
Isometric trunk flexor test, 611–612, 612*f*

J

Jerk, 439, 439*f*
Jogging and running, 539–540
Joint hypermobility syndrome, 256
Jump-and-reach, 454, 454*f*
Jump ropes, 517

K

Kegs, 351–352, 352*f*
Ketogenic diet, 56–57
α–Ketoglutarate dehydrogenase, 187
Kettlebell, 352–353, 352*f*, 426, 426*f*, 429, 429*f*
Kettlebell figure 8s, 429, 429*f*
Kettlebell swing, 426, 426*f*
Kilocalories, 48
Kinematics, 22
Kinesiology
core exercises, 413*t*
lower body exercises, 372, 372*t*
upper-body exercises, 384, 384*t*
Kinetics, 22
Knee jump, 456, 456*f*
Kneeling hip adductor stretch, 274, 274*f*
Kneeling overhead medicine ball throw, 477, 478*f*
Krebs cycle, 187, 188*f*–187*f*

L

Lactate, 184, 185*f*
Lactate dehydrogenase (LDH), 181
Lactate paradox, 556
Lactate threshold (LT), 185, 536–537, 538*b*, 621–622
Lacunae, 129–130
Ladder runs, 505–506, 507*f*
Landing Error Scoring System (LESS) test, 637*f*, 638*t*
L-arginine, 217
Lateral push-off, 467, 468*f*
Lat pull-down, 392, 392*f*
Lat stretch, 266, 266*f*
Law of Laplace, 222
Law of mass action, 180
Lean body mass, 11
Left-right shuffle, 519–520, 524*f*
Leg curl, 381, 381*f*
Leg extension, 382, 382*f*
Leg press, 377, 377*f*
Length-tension relationship, 24, 25*f*

Leptin resistance, 169
Letter drills, 519–520, 522*f*
Lever
effort arm, 31–32
first-class, 31–32, 31*f*
mechanical advantage, 32
resistance arm, 30
second-class, 31–32, 31*f*
third-class, 31–32, 31*f*
Lifting accessories
belts, 41
bench press shirts, 42
lifting suits, 41–42
slingshot, 42
weightlifting shoes, 42
wraps, 41
Linear periodization, 575–576
Linear taper, 573
Line drill, 629
Line of gravity, 38
Linoleic acid, 55
Linolenic acid, 55
Lipids, 54–57, 54*f*–55*f*, 57*t*
metabolism, 188–191, 190*f*
Lipolysis, 188–189
Lipoprotein lipase, 188–189
Live high-train high (LHTH), 556
Live high, train high and low (LHTHL), 558
Live high, train low (LHTL) approach, 556–557, 557*f*
Local muscular endurance, 12
Logs, 353
Long aerobic interval training, 550
Long bones, 128–129
Long-chain fatty acids, 54–55
Longitudinal (strap) muscles, 27
Long slow distance training, 548
Low-density lipoproteins, 55
Lower body exercises
barbell lunge, 379, 379*f*
Calf (Toe) Raise, 383, 383*f*
deadlift, 378, 378*f*
kinesiology, 372*t*
leg curl, 381, 381*f*
leg extension, 382, 382*f*
leg press, 377, 377*f*
major muscles, motion, 373*f*
plyometric exercise
alternate bounding, 471, 471*f*
barrier jumps, 458, 458*f*
box jump, 468, 468*f*
cone hops, 459, 459*f*
depth jump, 473, 473*f*, 474*f*
double-leg hops, 464, 464*f*
drop jump, 473, 473*f*
jump-and-reach, 454, 454*f*
knee jump, 456, 456*f*
lateral push-off, 467, 468*f*
multiple box jumps, 469, 469*f*
pike jump, 462, 462*f*
side-to-side ankle hop, 453, 453*f*
single-leg bounding, 472, 472*f*
single-leg box jump, 467, 467*f*
single-leg depth jump, 475, 475*f*
single-leg hops, 465, 465*f*
single-leg tuck jump, 463, 463*f*

single-leg vertical jump, 463, 463*f*
skipping, 470, 470*f*
split squat jump, 461, 461*f*
squat jump, 455, 455*f*
standing long jump, 457, 457*f*
standing triple jump, 466, 466*f*
tuck jumps, 460, 460*f*
two-foot ankle hop, 452, 452*f*
squat, 375, 375*f*
step-ups, 380, 380*f*
Low-pulley row, 395, 395*f*
Lung volumes and capacities, 228–229
Luteinizing hormone (LH), 158
Lying hip external rotation stretch, 277, 277*f*
Lying leg raise, 419, 419*f*
Lying torso stretch, 270, 270*f*
Lying Triceps Extension (Skull Crushers), 406, 406*f*

M

Macrocycle, 579
Macronutrients, 47–48
Magnesium, 61*t*–62*t*
Main competition phase, 571–572
Maintenance training, 10
Makoto tester, 517
Maladaptation, 573
Malnutrition, 47
Malonyl CoA decarboxylase, 189–190
Maltodextrins, 51*b*
Mammalian target of rapamycin (mTOR), 113–114
Manganese, 61*t*–62*t*
Manual/partner resistance, 340, 340*f*
Manual resistance neck (four-way), 430, 430*f*
Mass, force production, 38–39
Matveyev's model, 571*f*, 572
Maximal inspiratory mouth pressure, 231
Maximal lactate steady state, 536–537
Maximal plyometrics, 448
Maximum voluntary ventilation (MVV), 228
Mechanotransduction, 102–103, 132–133
Medicine balls, 344, 344*f*
back throw, 479, 479*f*
chest pass, 476, 476*f*, 477*f*, 627–628
front rotation throw, 489*t*, 495*t*
power drop, 484, 484*f*
side toss, 483, 483*f*
underhand toss, 482, 482*f*
woodchop, 420, 420*f*
Medicine ball chest pass test, 476, 476*f*, 477*f*, 627–628
Medicine ball woodchop, 420, 420*f*
Medium-chain fatty acids, 54–55
Mesocycle, 571*f*, 572
Metabolic acidosis, 186–187
Metabolic equivalents (METS), 543–544, 544*t*
Metabolic responses and adaptations
ATP (*see* Adenosine triphosphate (ATP))
metabolic demands and exercise, 193–204
Metabolic training programming, 316–318, 318*b*
Metabolism, 178
Metaboreflex, 231
Metarterioles, 211
Microbiome, 67–68
Microbiota, 67–68

Index 653

Microcycle, 572
MicroRNAs, 107–108
1.5-Mile run test, 618
Minerals, 57–67, 58*f*, 59*t*–60*t*, 64*f*
  functions, intake, deficiency, and food sources, 61*t*–62*t*
Mini hurdles and boxes, 517
Minimal essential strain, 133
Minute ventilation (V_E), 228–229
Mitochondrial density, 191–192
Mitogen-activated protein kinase (MAPK) molecules, 114, 114*f*
Mobility exercises, 433
Modern plyometrics, 447–448
Modified Ober test, 615–616
Modified sit-and-reach test, 612–614, 613*f*
Molybdenum, 61*t*–62*t*
Moment arm of force, 30
Moment arm of resistance, 30
Moment of inertia, 39
Monocarboxylate transporter (MCT), 185
Monocycle, 572
Monosaccharides, 49
Monounsaturated fatty acids (MUFAs), 54–55
Motor nervous system, 75–76
Motor units
  activation potentiation, 82–83
  alpha motor nerve, 81, 81*f*
  antagonist muscle activation, 84
  firing rate, 83
  recruitment
    muscle mass activation, 82
    selective, 82
  synchronization, 83–84
Mountain climbers, 505–506, 507*f*
Movement patterns, specificity, 240–243
Movements assessment
  active straight-leg raise, 617
  hurdle step, 617
  in-line lunge, 617
  overhead squat, 617
  rotary stability, 617–618
  shoulder mobility, 617
  trunk stability push-up, 617
Movement-specific resistance device, 349
Multipennate muscles, 27
Multiple box jumps, 469, 469*f*
Multiple-joint exercises, 292
Multiple-set program, training volume
  heavy to light system, 310
  integrated/undulating model, 310
  light to heavy system, 308–309
  load/repetition system, 308–309
  set structure systems, 308–309, 309*f*
Multipoundage system, 322
Multistage 20-m shuttle run test, 618–619
Muscle actions, 13
  concentric (*see* Concentric (CON) muscle action)
  eccentric (*see* Eccentric (ECC) muscle action)
  isomeric (*see* Isometric (ISOM) muscle action)
  specificity, 239–240
Muscle activation
  bench and shoulder press, 387, 387*b*, 387*f*–388*f*
  lat pull-down, 393*b*, 394*f*
Muscle architecture, 27–30

Muscle endurance test
  absolute repetition number, 610
  bodyweight exercises, 609, 610*t*
  sustained maximal duration trials, 610–612, 611*t*
Muscle fibers, 97–98
Muscle group split routines, 293–295
Muscle groups training, specificity, 240
Muscle hypertrophy
  factor influenzing
    circulatory, 115–116
    mechanical, 115–116
    metabolic stress, 116–117
    muscle action, 116
    nutritional, 115–116
    nutritional factors, 117
    training program, 116
  fiber types, 115
  protein synthesis, 110–111
  signaling pathway, 113–115
  training modalities, 118
Muscle memory, 107
Muscles
  adaptations, 96–97
  agonist, 96–97
  anatomy, 97–98, 97*f*
  antagonist, 96–97
  characteristics and adaptations, 103–119
    aerobic training, 119
    fast-twitch, 108
    fiber types in athletes, 108–109
    gene expression and MicroRNAs, 107–108
    hyperplasia, 118
    muscle fiber formation and repair, 105–107
    muscle hypertrophy, 110–112
    slow-twitch, 108
    structural changes, 119
  insertion, 96–97
  length
    active and passive length-tension, 24, 25*f*
    cross-bridge formation, 24
    length-tension relationship, 24, 25*f*
    stretch-shortening cycle, 26
  muscle fiber organization
    myofilaments, 99, 99*f*
    sarcomere, 98–99
    skeletal muscle's graded responses, 102
    sliding filament theory, 99–102
  neutralizer, 96–97
  origin, 96–97
  spindles, 26, 86–87
  stabilizer/fixator, 96–97
  strength assessment
    absolute, 11
    allometric scaling, 11
    isokinetic strength testing, 607–608
    isometric strength testing, 606–607
    leg press and bench press strength, 605*t*
    proper spotting, 605
    relative, 11
    repetition maximums estimation, 608–609, 608*t*
    Sinclair formula, 11
    strength testing checklist, 604*f*
    strength-to-mass ratio, 11
    Wilks formula, 11
Muscular endurance, 12
Myelin sheath, 76–77

Myocardium, 210–211
Myofascia, 258–259
Myofascial release, 258–260
Myofibril, 97–98
Myofilaments, 99, 99*f*
Myogenesis, 105–106
Myokinase, 181
Myonuclear domain, 98
Myonuclei domain theory, 107
Myosin, 97–98
Myosin heads, 99
Myostatin, 105–106
MyPlate, 48*f*

N

National Strength and Conditioning Association (NSCA), 8–9, 19–20
Needs analysis, 287
Negative feedback systems, 152
Negative nitrogen balance, 51–52
Nerve cells
  axon hillock, 76–77
  axons, 76–77
  cell body, 76–77
  dendrites, 76–77
  myelin sheath, 76–77
  neural communication, 77–78
  neurons, 76–77
  presynaptic terminal, 76–77
  supporting cells, 76–77
Nervous system
  autonomic, 89–91, 90*f*
  brain centers, 78–80
  descending corticospinal tracts, 80
  functional organization, 75–76
  motor units, 81–84
  nerve cells, 76–78, 77*f*
  neuromuscular junction, 84, 85*f*
  sensory, 84–87
  unilateral *versus* bilateral training, 88
Neural adaptations, 75–76
  electromyography, 87
  muscle hypertrophy, 87
  training program, 87
Neuromuscular junction (NMJ), 84, 85*f*
Neurons, 76–77
Neurotransmitter, 84
Niacin (B₃), 59*t*–60*t*
Nitric oxide synthase, 217
Noncontinuous set, 323–325
Nonessential amino acids, 51–52, 52*t*
Nonlinear (undulating) model, 577–578
Nonperiodized training, 578*b*
Nuclear factor of activated T cells (NFAT), 109–110
Nutrients, 47–48
  balance, 48
Nutrition, 47
  dietary reference intakes, 48–68
    antioxidants, 54–57, 54*f*–55*f*, 57*t*, 64–65
    carbohydrates, 49–51, 49*t*, 49*f*
    lipids, 54–57, 54*f*–55*f*, 57*t*
    microbiome, microbiota and probiotics, 67–68
    protein, 51–54, 52*t*–53*t*, 52*f*
    vitamins and minerals, 57–67, 58*f*, 59*t*–60*t*, 64*f*
    water, 57

654   Index

Nutrition (*Continued*)
nutrients, 47–48
practical considerations, 68–69
during exercise or competition, 69
post exercise or competition, 69
precompetition strategies, 68–69

O

Ober test, 615–616, 616f
Oligosaccharides, 49
Olympic lifts
behind-the-neck press, 440, 440f
catch, 437
clean and jerk, 434–437, 435f
drop snatch, 441, 441f
first pull, 436
front squat, 442, 442f
hook grip, 438, 438f
jerk, 439, 439f
overhead squat, 443, 443f
push press, 444, 444f
Romanian deadlift, 442, 442f
second pull, 437
snatch, 434–437, 435f, 440, 440f
snatch/clean high pull, 440
starting position, 436
transition phase, 436–437
Onset of blood lactate accumulation (OBLA), 185
Open-chain kinetic exercise, 241
Oscillation bench press, 347, 348f
Osmolality, 51b, 562–563
Osmosis, 180
Osteoarthritis, 141
Osteoblasts, 131–132
Osteocalcin, 131–132, 134
Osteoclasts, 130–131
Osteocytes, 129–130
Osteon, 129–130
Overhead medicine ball
slams, 481, 481f
throw, 477, 477f
Overhead squat, 443, 443f
Overloads, 322
Overspeed training
downhill sprinting, 507–508
supramaximal speed, 506–507
tailwind, 507
towing, 508–509, 510f–511f
treadmills, 510
tubing, 509–510
warm up, 506–507
Overtraining syndrome, 572–573
Overweight implements, 242–243
Oxford technique, 310
Oxidative stress, 64–65
Oxygen consumption, 221, 221f, 224–225, 224f
EPOC, 197–198
fast component of, 197
oxygen deficit, 197
resistance exercise and, 198–201
rest interval manipulation, 201b
slow component of, 197
Oxygen deficit, 197
Oxygen-hemoglobin dissociation curve, 213–214, 213f–214f
Oxytocin, 146

P

Pace/tempo training, 548
Pantothenic acid (B_5), 59t–60t
Paracrine action, 145
Parallel bar dips, 389, 389f
Parallel elastic component, 24
Partial pressure of oxygen and carbon dioxide, 214f
Partial repetition, 320–321, 320f
Partner hip flexor stretch, 272, 272f
Partner quadriceps stretch, 276, 276f
Pass/fail tests, 614–616
Passive insufficiency, 24–25
Passive stretching, 256–257
Passive warm-up, 251
Pawing action/drill, 505–506, 508f
Pectoralis minor length, 614–615
Pectoral wall stretch, 263, 263f
Pendulum exercises, 486, 486f
Peptide hormones, 146–147
Performance parameters, 545
Perimysium, 97–98
Periodized training, 586b
aerobic and anaerobic training components, 582–583
aerobic endurance performance, 582, 582t
athlete with multiple major competitions, 579
boxing strength training program, 585t–586t
classical model, 575–576, 576t
general adaptation syndrome, 573, 573f
Matveyev's model, 571f, 572
nonlinear (undulating) model, 577–578
reverse linear periodization model, 578–579
sprint, agility, and plyometric training, 579–580, 581t
strength athlete, team sport, 579, 580f
strength competition athlete, 584t–585t
tapering and performance, 573–575, 574f
wrestler, 583t–584t
Periosteum, 128–129
Peripheral nervous system, 75–76
Personal experience, 18
Phosphagen repletion, 180
Phosphocreatine (PC), 179
energy, 179
equation, 179
phosphagen repletion, 180
training adaptations, 180–181
Phospholipids, 55–56
Phosphorous, 61t–62t
Physio balls, 344–346, 346f
Physiologic cross-sectional area (PCSA), 29, 29f
Pike jump, 462, 462f
Piriformis stretch, 277, 277f
Plank, 418, 418f
Plank (prone bridge) test, 612, 612f
Plasma volume, 220–221
Plasticity, 127
Platelets, 213
Plyometric push-up, 484, 484f
Plyometric training, 3
anaerobic sports, 493–494
athletic performance, 449
classic, 447
depth jumps, 450, 455b
frequency, 490

maximal, 448
modern, 447–448
off-season total-body training program, 494, 495t
physiology of, 448–449
program design
age, 490–491
equipment, 492, 492f
exercise selection, 451–452 (*see also* Plyometric exercises)
training status, 491
training surface, 492
warm-up, 490
resistance training, 493, 494t
safety considerations, 493
sample off-season total-body programs, 494, 495t
shock training, 447
sprint training workout, 493, 494t
submaximal, 448
volume, 489, 489t
Poisson's ratio, 127
Polypeptides, 146–147
Polysaccharides, 49
Polyunsaturated fatty acids (PUFAs), 54–55
Positive nitrogen balance, 51–52
Post-activation performance enhancement (PAPE), 253–254
Post-activation potentiation (PAP), 253–254
Posterior parietal cortex, 78
Posterior shoulder hyperextension, 264, 264f
Post exercise hypotension, 220
Posture and functional performance, 616–622
Potassium, 61t–62t
Power fitness components, 12–13
Powerlifting, 8, 15, 15f
Power Plate vibration training system, 356–357, 356f
Power testing
anaerobic capacity tests, 628–629
broad jump, 624
force plate and transducer assessments, 624–626
Margaria–Kalamen test, 626–627, 627t
upper-body power assessments, 627–628
vertical jump, 623–624
Power-to-mass ratio, 38–39
Preacher curl (Olympic/EZ curl bar), 410, 410f
Prebiotics, 68
Precompetition phase, 571–572
Preexhaustion, 297
Prehabilitation, 10
Preinitiation complex, 152–153
Press-up stretch, 271, 271f
Pre-stretch augmentation percent (PSA), 26
Presynaptic terminal, 84
Pretzel, 268, 268f
Principle of reversibility, 244
Pro-agility test, 634, 634f
Probiotics, 67–68
Procollagen, 135–136
Professional practice, 17–18
Proficiency, 18
Programmed drills, 518
Progressive aerobic CV endurance run (PACER) test, 618–619
Progressive overload
aerobic endurance, 239
flexibility, 238
power, speed, and agility, 238–239

resistance training, 237–238
Prolactin inhibiting hormone (PIH), 146
Prone double straight-leg raise test, 610–611
Prone hip abductor stretch, 280, 280f
Prone hip external/internal rotation test, 615
Prone isometric chest raise test, 610
Prone/supine transversus abdominis muscle
    activation test, 614
Proopiomelanocortin, 167
Proper nutrition, 47
Proprioceptive neuromuscular facilitation (PNF)
    stretching
    benefits, 259
    muscle relaxation, 257
    variations, 258
Protein, 51–54, 52t, 52f
    functions of, 53t
    quality, 52
Protein digestibility–corrected amino acid score
    (PDCAAS), 52
Protein-efficiency ratio (PER), 52
Pullover, 395, 395f
Pullover pass, 483, 483f
Pull-up, 392, 392f
Pulsatility, 150
Push press, 444, 444f
Push-pull exercise pairing, 297b
Push-up, 390, 390f
Plyometric exercises
    exercise order, 487–488
    intensity of, 487, 488b, 489t
    lower-body
        alternate bounding, 471, 471f
        barrier jumps, 458, 458f
        box jump, 468, 468f
        cone hops, 459, 459f
        depth jump, 473, 473f, 474f
        double-leg hops, 464, 464f
        drop jump, 473, 473f
        jump-and-reach, 454, 454f
        knee jump, 456, 456f
        lateral push-off, 467, 468f
        multiple box jumps, 469, 469f
        pike jump, 462, 462f
        side-to-side ankle hop, 453, 453f
        single-leg bounding, 472, 472f
        single-leg box jump, 467, 467f
        single-leg depth jump, 475, 475f
        single-leg hops, 465, 465f
        single-leg tuck jump, 463, 463f
        single-leg vertical jump, 463, 463f
        skipping, 470, 470f
        split squat jump, 461, 461f
        squat jump, 455, 455f
        standing long jump, 457, 457f
        standing triple jump, 466, 466f
        tuck jumps, 460, 460f
        two-foot ankle hop, 452, 452f
    rest intervals, 490
    upper-body
        bag thrusts, 486, 486f
        depth push-up, 485, 485f
        kneeling overhead medicine ball throw, 477, 478f
        medicine ball back throw, 479, 479f
        medicine ball chest pass, 476, 476f, 477f
        medicine ball power drop, 484, 484f
        medicine ball side toss, 483, 483f

medicine ball underhand toss, 482, 482f
        overhead medicine ball slams, 481, 481f
        overhead medicine ball throw, 477, 477f
        pendulum exercises, 486, 486f
        plyometric push-up, 484, 484f
        pullover pass, 483, 483f
        single-arm vertical core ball throw, 480, 480f
Pyridoxine (B_6), 59t–60t
Pyruvate dehydrogenase, 187
Pyruvate kinase, 181

Q

Quadrate (quadrilateral) muscles, 27
Quadruped, 428, 428f
Quality training technique, 325
Quaternary structure, 51–52
Queens College Step Test, 619
Quickness drills, 518

R

Radius of gyration, 39
Range of motion, specificity, 240
Rate of force development, 12–13
Rate pressure product, 226
Reaction balls, 517
Reaction belts, 517
Reaction force, 35
Reaction time, 13, 500
Reactive drills, 518
Reactive hyperemia, 215–216
Reactive oxygen species (ROS), 64–65
Reactive strength (RS), 26
Reactive strength index modified (RSImod), 26
Reciprocal inhibition, 257
Recommended dietary allowance (RDA), 48
Recruitment, motor units
    muscle mass activation, 82
    postactivation potentiation, 82–83
    selective, 82
Rectilinear motion, 22
Reflex potentiation, 86–87
Rehabilitation, 10
Relative energy deficiency in sport (RED-S), 65b
Relative humidity, 560–561
Relaxation, 102
Releasing hormones, 146
Reliability, 594
Repetition, 13
    frequency, 314–315
    training, 550
    velocity
        hypertrophy training, 313–314
        isokinetic resistance exercise, 320
        muscle endurance training, 314
        strength training, 313–314
Residual fatigue, 559, 559f
Residual volume, 228
Resistance exercises, 371
Resistance training (RT)
    androgen receptor response, 158–159
    ATP-PC, 179
    β-endorphin, 167
    benefits of, 10, 10t

blood pressure, 226
bone growth, 137b
cardiovascular responses, 217–221
catecholamines, 166
combination exercises, 434
competitive forms, 14–17
core exercises, 413, 413t
cortisol, 164–166
exercise order and selection, 14
fitness components
    health-related, 10–12
    skill-related, 12–13
frequency, 14
frontal plane, 370f
glucocorticoid receptor, 165–166
glycogen, 183
grip strength training, 434
growth hormone-binding protein, 161
IGF-1, 162
individuals, 10, 10t
intensity, 14
intramuscular signaling, 165–166
lower body exercises, 372, 372t
metabolic response, 202f–203f
muscle action, 13
Olympic lifts and variations, 434–439
oxygen consumption, 197–201
progressive overload, 237–238
repetition, 13
repetition velocity, 14
respiratory muscle-specific training, 231–232
resting growth hormone, 160–161
resting TE concentration, 156–157
rest periods/intervals, 14
sagittal plane, 369f
tendon growth, 140b
testosterone, 156–157
tips for selecting exercises, 444
training modalities (see Resistance training
    modalities)
transverse plane, 371f
upper-body exercises, 384
Resistance training equipment and safety
    injury prevention, 357
    safety and effectiveness, 358
    safety checklist, 359b
    spotter, 362b
Resistance training modalities
    automobiles, 350
    balance discs, 346, 347f
    body weight
        partner's weight, 339–340
        push-up, 336–337, 337f
        TRX, 337–339, 339f
        weight and strengthening exercises, 336–340
    BOSU balls, 344–346, 346f
    chains, 346–349, 348f
    elastic bands and tubing, 346–349
    exercise balls, 344–346, 346f
    free weights
        advantages, 343–344
        barbells, 340–341, 341f
        disadvantages, 343–344
        dumbbells, 341–342
        free-weight equipment, 342
        vs. machines, 343–344, 345b
        RT machines, 342–343, 342f

656 Index

Resistance training modalities (*Continued*)
  machines
    advantages, 343–344
    cable pulley machine, 342, 342*f*
    disadvantages, 343–344
    hydraulic resistance machines, 343
    isokinetic machine, 343
    plate-loaded machines, 342–343, 343*f*
    pneumatic resistance machines, 343
    Smith machine, 342
  manual/partner resistance, 340, 340*f*
  medicine balls, 344, 344*f*
  movement-specific resistance device, 349
  Olympic lifts and variations, 344
  ropes and battling ropes, 349–350, 350*f*–351*f*
  sleds, 350, 351*f*
  springs, 346–349
  stability balls, 344–346, 346*f*, 347*b*
  strength implements
    Farmer's walk bars, 353
    kegs, 351–352, 352*f*
    kettlebell, 352–353, 352*f*
    logs, 353
    sandbags and heavy bags, 354
    stone lifting, 354, 355*f*
    Super Yoke, 354
    tires and sledgehammers, 353, 353*f*
  vibration devices and training, 356–357
  water and environment, 354–355
Resistance training program design
  advanced techniques
    breakdown sets, 322
    combination exercises, 322–323
    combining exercises, 322–323
    forced repetitions, 322
    functional isometrics, 320
    heavy and forced negatives, 319–320
    noncontinuous set, 323–325
    overloads, 322
    partial repetition, 320–321
    quality training, 325
    spectrum repetition, 325
    variable resistance training, 321–322
  ballistic training and maximal strength, 304*b*
  corrective exercise programming, 315–316
  exercise order and workout structure,
    293–297
  exercise selection, 291–293, 293*t*
  individualization, 287–291
  intensity
    ACSM recommendation, 299–300
    dose-response, 297–298, 298*f*
    intensity classification, 297, 298*t*
    intensity increasing methods, 304–305, 304*f*
    power training, 300–302
    repetition number, 300*t*–301*t*, 310
  repetition velocity, 313–314
  rest interval, 310–312, 311*f*
  training status, 290–291
  training volume
    hormonal system, 306
    metabolic systsm, 306
    multiple-set program, 308–310
    muscular system, 306
    nervous system, 297–298
    set number per workout, 306
    volume load, 305

Resisted sprint training
  external loading, 511
  ground-based performance, 513*b*
  harness, 511–512, 511*f*
  headwind, 510
  parachutes, 511
  partner, 512
  sand, 511
  sled towing, 510–511, 510*f*–511*f*
  speed chutes, 511
  treadmill performance, 513*b*
  uphill and/or stairs, 512
  wearable resistance, 512
  weighted vests, 511, 511*f*
Respiration, 210
Respiratory exchange ratio (RER), 193–195
Respiratory muscle-specific training, 231–232
Respiratory quotient (RQ), 193–195
Respiratory system
  breathing control, 229–230, 230*f*
  function, 227–228, 228*f*
  lung volumes and capacities, 228–229
  pulmonary adaptations to training, 230–231, 230*f*
  respiratory muscle-specific training, 231–232
Resting metabolic rate (RMR), 193–195, 196*t*
Reverse curl, 412, 412*f*
Reverse linear periodization model, 578–579
Reverse wrist curl, 411, 411*f*
Riboflavin (B$_2$), 59*t*–60*t*
Ribosome biogenesis, 112–118
Right triangle drills, 519–520, 520*f*
Rings and agility dots, 517
Rolling friction, 36–37
Romanian deadlift, 442, 442*f*
Rope exercises, 433
Rowing, 541
Running economy, 538, 539*f*
Ryanodine receptors, 100

S

Sagittal plane, 367–368, 369*f*
Saltatory conduction, 77–78
Sandbags, 354
Sarcolemma, 98
Sarcomere, 97–98
Sarcoplasm, 98
Sargent jump test, 623
Satellite cells, 105–106
Saturated fats, 54–55
Scapula retraction/protraction, 402, 402*f*
Seated dumbbell biceps curl, 408, 408*f*
Seated posterior lean, 265, 265*f*
Seated shoulder press, 396–397, 396*f*
Seated toe touch stretch, 272, 272*f*
Seated triceps extension, 405, 405*f*
Second messenger systems, 152, 153*f*
Second pull, 437
Selective androgen receptor modulators (SARMs),
  159
Selenium, 61*t*–62*t*
Self-myofascial release, 259, 260*f*
Semi-leg straddle, 269, 269*f*
Semistraddle stretch, 272, 272*f*
Sensory nervous system
  Golgi tendon organs, 84

muscle spindles, 86–87
Series elastic component, 24
Sesamoid bones, 128
Sex hormone-binding globulin (SHBG), 158
Shock training, 447
Short aerobic interval training, 549–550
Short bones, 128
Short-chain fatty acids, 54–55
Shoulder internal/external rotation test, 615
Shoulder rotation stretch, internal/external, 267,
  267*f*
Shrug, 398, 398*f*
Sickle cell trait, 554
Side bends, 417, 417*f*
  stretch, 271, 271*f*
Side plank (bridge) test, 612
Side rocker, 519–520, 524*f*
Side-to-side ankle hop, 453, 453*f*
Simulated altitude/hypoxia, 558
Sinclair formula, 11
Single-arm lat stretch, 266, 266*f*
Single-arm vertical core ball throw, 480, 480*f*
Single-joint exercises, 292
Single-leg balance test, 637
Single-leg bounding, 472, 472*f*
Single-leg box jump, 467, 467*f*
Single-leg depth jump, 475, 475*f*
Single-leg hops, 465, 465*f*
Single-leg squat, 636–637
Single-leg tuck jump, 463, 463*f*
Single-leg vertical jump, 463, 463*f*
Sinoatrial node (SA node), 212–213
Sit-and-reach flexibility test, 256, 612–614, 613*f*
Sit-up hold test, 611–612
Skating, 541
Skeletal muscle, 96
  bones (*see* Bone(s))
  muscle (*see* Muscles)
  muscle fiber arrangement, 27–30, 28*f*
    angle of pennation, 27–29
    muscle fascicle length, 29–30
    nonpennate muscles, 27–29
    pennate muscle fibers, 27–29
Skeletal system
  appendicular skeleton, 128
  axial skeleton, 128, 128*f*
Skewed pyramid, 310
Skier exercise, 422, 422*f*
Skill-related fitness component assessment
  agility tests
    505 change of direction (COD) test,
      633, 633*f*
    3-cone drill, 634, 634*f*, 635*t*
    Davies test, 635
    Edgren side-step test, 634–635, 635*f*
    hexagon test, 633–634, 634*f*
    pro-agility test, 634, 634*f*
    T-test, 633
  balance
    anterior reach, 637
    force plate tests, 638
    single-leg balance test, 637
    single-leg squat, 636–637
    stabilometer balance test, 637–638, 638*f*–640*f*
    standing stork test, 637
    star excursion balance test, 639–640, 640*f*
  posture and functional performance, 616–622

power testing
anaerobic capacity tests, 628–629
broad jump, 624
force plate and transducer assessments, 624–626
Margaria–Kalamen test, 626–627, 627*t*
upper-body power assessments, 627–628
vertical jump, 623–624
speed
10-yard dash, 631
40-yard dash, 631, 632*t*
120-yard dash, 631–632
Skinfold assessment, 598, 599*f*, 600*t*
Skipping, 470, 470*f*
Slam balls, 344–346, 346*f*
Sledge hammer, 433
Sledgehammers, 353, 353*f*
Sled push, 432, 432*f*
Sliding filament theory
cross-bridge cycling, 100–102, 101*f*
excitation-contraction coupling, 100
relaxation, 102
Slow exponential taper, 573
Slow glycolysis, 181
Smooth muscle, 96
Snatch, 434–437, 435*f*, 440, 440*f*
drop, 441, 441*f*
grip, 440, 440*f*
grip width, 438
high pull, 440, 440*f*
kinematic analysis, 437
Snatch/clean high pull, 440
Sodium, 61*t*–62*t*
Spatial summation, 102
Specific gravity, 354–355
Specificity
energy metabolism, 240
movement patterns, 240–243
muscle action, 239–240
muscle groups training, 240
range of motion, 240
velocity, 240
Specific warm-up, 251
Spectrum repetition/contrast loading combinations, 324–325
Spectrum repetitions, 325
Speed, 13
assessment
10-yard dash, 631
40-yard dash, 631, 632*t*
120-yard dash, 631–632
endurance, 500
Speed endurance, 500
Speed endurance training
continuous speed performance, 527–528
fatigue index, 528
intermittent sprint exercise, 528, 528*f*
maximal speed, 527–528
repeated sprint ability, 527–528, 528*f*, 529*f*
speed maintenance, 529
wind sprints, 528–529
Spinning classes, 540
Split squat jump, 461, 461*f*
Spongy/trabecular bone, 128–129
Sports adrenal medulla, 166
Sports anemia, 215
Sport-specific devices, 517

Springs, 346–349
Sprint training
acceleration, 500
3-day Agility program, 526, 527*t*
basic drills
"A" march, 505–506, 506*f*
ankling, 505–506, 506*f*
"B" march, 505–506, 506*f*
butt kickers, 505–506, 505*f*
drum major, 505–506, 508*f*
falling, 505–506, 509*f*
Frankenstein, 505–506, 509*f*
gears, 505–506, 508*f*
high knees, 505–506, 506*f*, 510*f*
ladder runs, 505–506, 507*f*
mountain climbers, 505–506, 507*f*
pawing, 505–506, 508*f*
standing arm swings, 505–506, 505*f*–510*f*
straight leg shuffle, 505–506, 507*f*
components of, 501–502, 502*t*
errors in, 504–505
mechanics of running
acceleration phase, 503–504, 504*f*
early flight phase, 502
flight phase, 502, 503*f*
late flight phase, 502
maximum speed, 504
middle flight phase, 502
midflight phase, 502
starting position, 503, 503*f*
support phase, 502, 503*f*
overspeed training
downhill sprinting, 507–508
supramaximal speed, 506–507
tailwind, 507
towing, 508–509, 510*f*–511*f*
treadmills, 510
tubing, 509–510
warm up, 506–507
program design
drill progression, 521–522
exercise selection, 523–524, 527
frequency, 525
intensity, 524
plyometric training, 523
rest interval, 526
structure and sequencing, 523
volume, 525–526
resisted
external loading, 511
ground-based performance, 513*b*
harness, 511–512, 511*f*
headwind, 510
parachutes, 511
partner, 512
sand, 511
sled towing, 510–511, 510*f*–511*f*
speed chutes, 511
treadmill performance, 513*b*
uphill and/or stairs, 512
wearable resistance, 512
weighted vests, 511, 511*f*
speed and technique, 512–513
speed endurance, 500
speed endurance training, 527–531
stride length, 501
stride rate, 501

Square drills, 519–520, 520*f*
Squat, 375, 375*f*
front, 442, 442*f*
jump, 455, 455*f*
overhead, 443, 443*f*
Squat stretch, 276, 276*f*
Stability ball (SB), 346–349, 347*b*
exchange, 419, 419*f*
roll-out, 418, 418*f*
slaps, 403, 403*f*
Stability, force production, 38
Stabilometer balance test, 637–638, 638*f*–640*f*
Stadiometer, 597–598
Stair climbing, 540
Staleness, 573
Standing adductor stretch, 278, 278*f*
Standing arm swings, 505–506, 505*f*–510*f*
Standing biceps curl (olympic/EZ curl bar), 407, 407*f*
Standing hamstring stretch, 278, 278*f*
Standing long jump, 457, 457*f*
Standing quadriceps stretch, 275, 275*f*
Standing Shoulder Press (Military Press), 396–397, 396*f*
Standing stork test, 637
Standing triple jump, 466, 466*f*
Star excursion balance test, 639–640, 640*f*
Starting position, 436
Static friction, 36–37
Static stretching, 257, 261
anterior cross-arm stretch, 265, 265*f*
behind-the-neck triceps stretch, 267, 267*f*
bent-over shoulder/pectoral stretch, 264, 264*f*
biceps stretch, 268, 268*f*
butterfly stretch, 274, 274*f*
flexed arms above head stretch, 266, 266*f*
forward lunge stretch, 270, 270*f*
forward triceps stretch, 268, 268*f*
internal/external shoulder rotation stretch, 267, 267*f*
involving several muscle groups, 281–282, 281*f*
kneeling hip adductor stretch, 274, 274*f*
lying hip external rotation stretch, 277, 277*f*
lying torso stretch, 270, 270*f*
neck extensors, flexors, and lateral flexors, 262, 262*f*
neck rotation, 261*f*
partner hip flexor stretch, 272, 272*f*
partner quadriceps stretch, 276, 276*f*
pectoral wall stretch, 263, 263*f*
piriformis stretch, 277, 277*f*
posterior shoulder hyperextension, 264, 264*f*
press-up stretch, 271, 271*f*
pretzel, 268, 268*f*
prone hip abductor stretch, 280, 280*f*
seated posterior lean, 265, 265*f*
seated toe touch stretch, 272, 272*f*
semi-leg straddle, 269, 269*f*
semistraddle stretch, 272, 272*f*
side bend stretch, 271, 271*f*
single-arm lat stretch, 266, 266*f*
squat stretch, 276, 276*f*
standing adductor stretch, 278, 278*f*
standing hamstring stretch, 278, 278*f*
standing quadriceps stretch, 275, 275*f*
step stretch, 280, 280*f*
straddle stretch, 273, 273*f*

658 Index

Static stretching (*Continued*)
supine hamstrings stretch, 279, 279*f*
supine hip flexion, 269, 269*f*
wall calf stretch, 279, 279*f*
Static warm-ups, 254–255
Steady-pace training, 548
Step aerobics, 540–541
Step stretch, 280, 280*f*
Step-ups, 380, 380*f*
Steroid hormones, 146, 152–153, 154*f*
Stone lifting, 354, 355*f*
Straddle stretch, 273, 273*f*
Straight leg shuffle, 505–506, 507*f*
Strength competition, 15–16, 584*t*–585*t*
Strength-to-mass ratio, 11, 38–39
Strength training and conditioning (S&C)
aerobic endurance, 239
competitive lifting sports, 7–9
critical components, 237, 238*f*
definition, 3
detraining, 244
early origins, 4
force production, 40–42
individualization, 244, 245*f*
nineteenth-century advances, 4–5, 5*f*–6*f*
professional
duties, 19*b*, 20
education and proficiencies, 17–19
memberships and certifications, 19–20
responsibilities, 20
responsibility of, 17
roles, 20
progression and program design, 243–244, 244*f*
progressive overload, 237–239
science and medicine, 4
specificity, 239–243
supervision, 244–246, 246*f*
tactical strength training and conditioning, 9
training variation, 243
Stress
compression, 126
definition, 126
deformation, 126
shear, 126
stress-strain relationship, 127, 127*f*
tension, 126
torsion, 126
Stress relaxation, 257
Stress–strain relationship
elasticity, 139
linear strain, 127
plasticity, 127
Poisson's ratio, 127
shear strain, 127
for tendon, 127
Stretching
active stretch, 256–257
dynamic stretching, 257
passive stretching, 256–257
PNF stretching, 257–258
Stretching-induced force deficit, 254
Stretch reflex, 86
Stretch–shortening cycle (SSC)
bench press performance, 26

fast-twitch (FT) muscle fibers, 26
stretch reflex, 26
Stroke volume, 217–219
Submaximal muscular endurance, 12
Submaximal plyometrics, 448
Succinate dehydrogenase (SDH), 187
Succinyl-CoA-synthetase, 187
Sulfur, 61*t*–62*t*
Superoxide dismutase (SOD), 64–65
Supersets, 322
Supervision, 244–246, 246*f*
Super Yoke, 354
Supine hamstrings stretch, 279, 279*f*
Supine hip abduction/adduction test, 615
Supine hip flexion, 269, 269*f*
Supine shoulder flexion (lat stretch) test, 616
Supine straight leg test, 615
Supplementary motor area (SMA), 78
Supporting cells, 76–77
Supramaximal speed, 506–507
Surfactant, 227–228
Suspension training, 337–339
Swimming and aquatic exercise, 541
Swiss balls, 344–346, 346*f*
Synchronization, motor units, 83–84
Synovial fluid, 140–141

T

Tailwind, 507
Targeted energy system, 288
T-drill, 519–520, 519*f*–526*f*
Tendon
ligament and fascial adaptations, 138–140
stiffness, 139
Terminal cisternae, 98
Tertiary structure, 51–52
Testosterone (TE), 154–159
acute systemic responses, 155–156
androgen receptor and signaling, 158–159
ergogenic effects of, 154
luteinizing hormone, 158
reponse and muscle strength, 155–156
resting TE concentrations, 156–157
sex hormone-binding globulin, 158
skeletal muscle steroidogenesis, 157
Test–retest reliability, 618
Test selection and administration
age and gender, 595
close monitoring, 596
data management, 596
environmental factors, 595
familiarization affects, 594–595
nutritional factors, 595
recommended testing sequence, 595–596, 595*f*
reliability, 594
testing frequency, 596*b*
validity, 593–594
Tetanus, 102
Thiamin (B_1), 59*t*–60*t*
Thomas test, 615
Thyroid hormones, 152–153, 167–168
Thyrotropin-releasing hormone (TRH), 146

Tidal volume, 228
Tire flipping, 431, 431*f*
Tires, 353, 353*f*
Tolerable upper intake level (UL), 49
Torque
angular motion, 30
centric and eccentric forces, 30
human strength curves, 33–35, 34*f*
linear motion, 30
moment arm, 30*f*, 33
bodily proportions, 33
tendon insertion, 33
system of lever, 31–32, 31*f*
Total-body lifts, 315
Total-body workout, 293–296, 295*t*
Total lung capacity, 228
Towing, 508–509, 510*f*–511*f*
Training variation, 243
Transcranial magnetic stimulation (TMS), 80
Trans fatty acid, 54–55
Transfer exercises, 434
Transition phase, 436–437
Transmural pressure, 223
Transport (binding) proteins, 150
Transverse planes, 367–368, 371*f*
Treadmills, 510
Triad, 98
Triceps pushdown, 404, 404*f*
Tri-sets, 323
Tropomyosin, 99
Troponin, 99
T-rotation, 390*f*
Trunk contraction, 40–41
Trunk rotation test, 614
T-test, 633
Tubing, 509–510
Tuck jumps, 460, 460*f*
Tumor suppressor tuberous sclerosis complex (TSC1/TSC2), 113–114
Turkish get-up, 423, 423*f*
Twitch, 102
Two-feet forward drills, 519–520, 525*f*
Two-foot ankle hop, 452, 452*f*
Two-in lateral shuffle drills, 519–520, 525*f*
Tyrosine, 166

U

Underwater weighing, 602
Underweight implements, 242–243
Undulating models, 310
Unilateral training, 241–242
Unipennate muscles, 27
University of Montreal Track test, 529
Unsaturated fats, 54–55
Upper-body exercises
bench press, 385, 385*f*
bent-over barbell row, 391, 391*f*
decline bench press, 386*f*
dumbbell fly, 388, 388*f*
dumbbell lateral raise, 400, 400*f*
hammer curl, 409, 409*f*
incline bench press, 386, 387*f*–388*f*
internal/external shoulder rotations, 401–402
inverted row, 391*f*

Index 659

kinesiology of, 384, 384*t*
lat pull-down, 392, 392*f*
low-pulley row, 395, 395*f*
Lying triceps extension (Skull Crushers), 406, 406*f*
parallel bar dips, 389, 389*f*
preacher curl (olympic/EZ curl bar), 410, 410*f*
plyometric exercise
    bag thrusts, 486, 486*f*
    depth push-up, 485, 485*f*
    kneeling overhead medicine ball throw, 477, 478*f*
    medicine ball back throw, 479, 479*f*
    medicine ball chest pass, 476, 476*f*, 477*f*
    medicine ball power drop, 484, 484*f*
    medicine ball side toss, 483, 483*f*
    medicine ball underhand toss, 482, 482*f*
    overhead medicine ball slams, 481, 481*f*
    overhead medicine ball throw, 477, 477*f*
    pendulum exercises, 486, 486*f*
    plyometric push-up, 484, 484*f*
    pullover pass, 483, 483*f*
    single-arm vertical core ball throw, 480, 480*f*
pullover, 395, 395*f*
pull-up, 392, 392*f*
push-up, 390, 390*f*
reverse curl, 412, 412*f*
reverse wrist curl, 411, 411*f*
scapula retraction/protraction, 402, 402*f*
seated dumbbell biceps curl, 408, 408*f*
seated shoulder press, 396–397, 396*f*
seated triceps extension, 405, 405*f*
shrug, 398, 398*f*
stability ball slaps, 403, 403*f*
standing biceps curl (Olympic/EZ curl bar), 407, 407*f*
Standing shoulder press (Military Press), 396–397, 396*f*
triceps pushdown, 404, 404*f*
T-rotation, 390*f*
upright row, 399, 399*f*
wrist curl, 411, 411*f*

Upper/lower-body split, 293–295, 297, 315
Upright row, 399, 399*f*

V

Valgus stress, women athletes, 289*b*
Validity, 593–594
Valsalva maneuver, 41, 218–219
Variable resistance training, 321–322
Ventilatory muscle-specific training, 231–232
Ventilatory threshold, 228–229
Venules, 211
Vertical climbers, 540
Vertical jump mechanics, 449*b*
Very low-density lipoproteins (VLDL), 55
Vibration devices and training, 356–357
Vitamin A (retinoids, beta carotene), 59*t*–60*t*
Vitamin C (ascorbic acid), 59*t*–60*t*
Vitamin D, 59*t*–60*t*
Vitamin E (α-tocopherol), 59*t*–60*t*
Vitamin K, 59*t*–60*t*
Vitamins, 57–67, 58*f*, 59*t*–60*t*, 64*f*
    functions of, 58*f*, 59*t*–60*t*
    intake, deficiency and food sources, 59*t*–60*t*
Volume load, 305
Volume overload, 221–222
V-sit test, 611–612

W

Walking, 540–541
Wall angel test, 616
Wall calf stretch, 279, 279*f*
Warm-up
    aerobic training, 251–253
    design, 251–253
    dynamic *vs.* static warm-up, 252*b*, 254–255
    general warm-up, 251, 252*f*
    high-intensity, 253–254, 253*f*
    high-intensity exercises, 251–253
    passive warm-up, 251
    performance effects, 253
    physiology, 253
    postactivation performance enhancement, 253–254
    vs. postactivation potentiation, 253–254, 253*f*
    resistance exercise, 251–253
    specific warm-up, 251
    sport-specific warmups, 254
Water, 57
Water-soluble vitamins, 57–58
Weekly undulated periodization, 577–578
    tennis program, 327*t*
    wrestling program, 326*t*
Weight lifting, 7, 15, 15*f*
    belts, intraabdominal pressure, 41
    oxygen consumption, 225
Weight training, 5
Whole-body vibration devices, 356–357, 356*f*
Wilks formula, 11
Wingate anaerobic power test, 628–629, 629*t*
Wrestler, periodized training, 583*t*–584*t*
Wrist curl, 411, 411*f*

X

X-pattern drills, 519–520, 520*f*

Y

300-Yard shuttle, 629, 630*f*, 631*t*
Y balance test (YBT), 639–640
YMCA Submaximal Cycle Ergometer Test, 619
Yo-Yo intermittent recovery tests, 530, 531*f*

Z

Zig-zag cross-over shuffle, 519–520, 525*f*
Zig-zag drills, 519–520, 522*f*, 525*f*
Zinc, 61*t*–62*t*, 64
Z-pattern drills, 519–520, 521*f*

CCS0321